P9-BHW-499

GEORGE W. HUNTER, III, Ph.D.,
Col. U.S.A. (Ret.)

Clinical Professor of Parasitology, Department of Community Medicine, University of California, San Diego, School of Medicine, La Jolla, California. Professor Emeritus, University of Florida, College of Medicine, Gainesville, Florida. Formerly, Resident Coordinator of LSU-ICMRT and Research Professor of Medical Parasitology, Department of Tropical Medicine and Medical Parasitology, Louisiana State University, School of Medicine, New Orleans, Louisiana. Chief, Section of Parasitology–Entomology, Fourth Army Area Medical Laboratory, Fort Sam Houston, Texas. Professor of Parasitology, Affiliated Units of the Graduate School, Baylor University Medical School, Houston, Texas.

J. CLYDE SWARTZWELDER, Ph.D.

Professor Emeritus. Formerly Professor of Medical Parasitology and Head of Department of Tropical Medicine and Medical Parasitology; Director, LSU International Research and Training Programs in Tropical Medicine, Louisiana State University, School of Medicine, New Orleans. Consultant in Parasitology, Veterans Administration Hospital; Visiting Scientist, Charity Hospital of Louisiana, New Orleans. Formerly, Chief (Major, AUS), Field Survey Branch, Tropical Disease Control Division, Office of the Surgeon General, U.S. Army

DAVID F. CLYDE, M.D., Ph.D., D.T.M.&H.

Professor of Tropical Medicine and Head of Department of Tropical Medicine and Medical Parasitology, Louisiana State University, School of Medicine, New Orleans. Member, Expert Advisory Panel on Malaria, World Health Organization. Formerly Professor of International Medicine; Director, International Health Program, University of Maryland School of Medicine, Baltimore. Deputy Chief Medical Officer and Senior Consultant (Epidemiology), Ministry of Health, United Republic of Tanzania.

TROPICAL MEDICINE

Fifth Edition

W. B. SAUNDERS COMPANY Philadelphia • London • Toronto

W. B. Saunders Company: West Washington Square
Philadelphia, PA 19105

1 St. Anne's Road
Eastbourne, East Sussex BN21 3UN, England

1 Goldthorne Avenue
Toronto, Ontario M8Z 5T9, Canada

Library of Congress Cataloging in Publication Data

Hunter, III, George William, 1902–

Tropical medicine.

First-2d ed. by T. T. Mackie, G. W. Hunter, and C. B. Worth; 3d-4th ed., by G. W. Hunter, W. W. Frye, and J. C. Swartzwelder, published under title: A manual of tropical medicine.

Includes index.

1. Tropics—Diseases and hygiene. I. Swartzwelder, John Clyde, joint author. II. Clyde, David F., joint author. III. Mackie, Thomas Turlay, 1895–1955 A manual of tropical medicine. IV. Title. [DNLM: 1. Tropical medicine. WC680 H944m]

RC961.H8 1975 616.9'88'3 74–17757

ISBN 0–7216–4847–9

Listed here is the latest translated edition of this book together with the language of the translation and the publisher.

Polish (*3rd Edition*)—Lekarskich, Warsaw, Poland

Spanish (*4th Edition*)—La Prensa Medica Mexicana, Mexico D.F., Mexico

Tropical Medicine ISBN 0–7216–4847–9

Last digit is the print number: 9 8 7 6 5

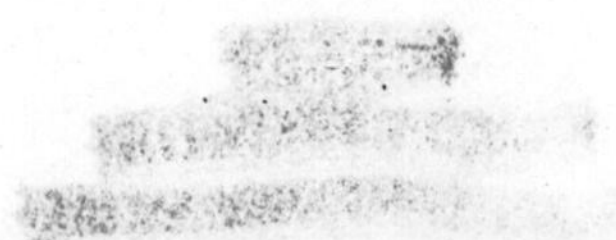

The Authors and Collaborators
of the Fifth Edition of *Tropical Medicine*
Wish to Dedicate This Book to

ALL THOSE PERSONS WHO ARE CONCERNED WITH THE HEALTH, WELFARE AND CONTROL OF DISEASE AMONG THE CITIZENRY OF COUNTRIES IN THE TROPICS, SUBTROPICS AND TEMPERATE ZONES

The reader should consult the manufacturer's labeling for full prescription information on drugs referred to in this book.

Contributors

STANLEY H. ABADIE, Ph.D.
Professor of Medical Parasitology and Microbiology and Dean, School of Allied Health Professions, Louisiana State University Medical Center. Visiting Scientist, Charity Hospital of Louisiana; Consultant, Veterans Administration Hospital, New Orleans, Louisiana.

Methods and Procedures

ROBERT ABEL, Jr., M.D.
Assistant Professor of Ophthalmology, Jefferson Medical College of Thomas Jefferson University, Philadelphia. Assistant, Corneal Service, Wills Eye Hospital, Philadelphia, Pennsylvania; Assistant, Department of Ophthalmology, Wilmington Medical Center, Wilmington, Delaware.

Toxoplasmosis (with Herbert E. Kaufman and Joseph H. Miller)

MICHAEL PHILIP ALPERS, M.B.
Senior Research Fellow, Department of Microbiology, Perth Medical Centre, Western Australia.

Kuru

VICTOR M. AREÁN, M.D.
Clinical Professor of Pathology, University of South Florida College of Medicine, Tampa, and University of Florida College of Medicine, Gainesville. Pathologist, Saint Anthony's Hospital, St. Petersburg; Consultant, Veterans Administration Hospital, Tampa, Florida.

American Trypanosomiasis

FRANCISCO BIAGI, M.D.
Professor of Medical Parasitology, Universidad Nacional Autónoma de México. Consultant to the American British Cowdray Hospital and Hospital Infantil Privado, Mexico City, Mexico.

Leishmaniasis—Introduction, Kala-Azar, Cutaneous and Mucocutaneous Leishmaniasis

ROBERT E. BLOUNT, Jr., M.D., LTC., M.C., U.S.A.
Chief of Medicine, U.S. DeWitt Army Hospital, Fort Belvoir, Virginia.

Plague

MERLIN L. BRUBAKER, M.D.
Clinical Associate Professor of Tropical Medicine, Louisiana State University Medical Center, New Orleans. Regional Advisor: Leprosy, Venereal Diseases and Treponematoses, World Health Organization/Pan American Health Organization. Formerly Director, U.S.P.H.S. Hospital, Carville, Louisiana.

Syphilis, Yaws and Endemic Syphilis, Pinta, Leprosy, Gonococcal Infections, Granuloma Inguinale

WILLY BURGDORFER, Ph.D.
Head, Rickettsial Diseases Section, Rocky Mountain Laboratory, National Institute of Allergy and Infectious Diseases, Public Health Service, U.S. Department of Health, Education, and Welfare, Hamilton, Montana.

Rickettsial Diseases—Introduction, Epidemic (Louse-borne) Typhus, Murine (Flea-borne) Typhus, Queensland Tick Typhus, Rickettsialpox, Trench Fever, The Relapsing Fevers

CHARLES C. J. CARPENTER, M.D.
Professor and Chairman, Department of Medicine, Case Western Reserve University School of Medicine. Physician-in-Chief, University Hospitals of Cleveland, Cleveland, Ohio.

Cholera

CLYDE G. CULBERTSON, M.D.
Professor of Pathology, Indiana University School of Medicine. Consultant, Lilly Research Laboratories, Indianapolis, Indiana.

Naegleria and Hartmannella (or Acanthamoeba) Infections

VINCENT J. DERBES, M.D.
Professor of Medicine and Chief, Section of Allergy-Dermatology, Tulane University School of Medicine. Consultant, Charity Hospital of Louisiana, Baptist Hospital, Ochsner Foundation Hospital, and U.S. Public Health Hospital, New Orleans, Louisiana.

The Fire Ant (with Rodney C. Jung)

DAVID P. EARLE, M.D., M.A.C.P.
Professor of Medicine, Northwestern University Medical School. Attending Physician, Northwestern Memorial Hospital, Chicago, Illinois.

Epidemic Hemorrhagic Fever

ANNA C. GELMAN, M.P.H.
Assistant Professor of Epidemiology, Columbia University School of Public Health, New York, New York.

Tropical Disease Gazetteer

ROGER H. GROTHAUS, Ph.D., LTC., M.S.C., U.S.N.
Chief, Entomology Division, Naval Medical Field Research Laboratory, Camp Lejeune, North Carolina.

Class Insecta (Hexapoda), Control of Arthropods of Medical Importance (with Donald E. Weidhaas)

JEAN-JACQUES GUNNING, M.D., Capt., M.C., U.S.N.
Director of Clinical Services and Chief of Medicine, Naval Regional Medical Center, Camp Pendleton, California. Clinical Associate Professor, Department of Tropical Medicine and Medical Parasitology, Louisiana State University Medical Center, New Orleans, Louisiana.

Leptospirosis and Rat-bite Fevers

FRANK HAWKING, D.M., F.R.C.P., D.T.M.
Formerly Head, Parasitology Division, National Institute for Medical Research, London. Research Associate, Brunel University, Uxbridge, England.

The Trypanosomidae, African Trypanosomiasis

ARISTIDES HERRER, Sc.D.
Head, Leishmaniasis Department, Gorgas Memorial Laboratory, Republic of Panama. Clinical Associate Professor of Medical Parasitology, Louisiana State University Medical Center, New Orleans, Louisiana.

Bartonellosis

HARRY HOOGSTRAAL, Ph.D., D.Sc.
Head, Medical Zoology Department, U.S. Naval Medical Research Unit No. 3, American Embassy, Cairo, Egypt.

Class Arachnida

RODNEY CLIFTON JUNG, M.D., Ph.D., F.A.C.P.
Clinical Professor of Medicine, Tulane University School of Medicine. Senior in Internal Medicine, Touro Infirmary; Senior Physician in Medicine, Charity Hospital of Louisiana; Consultant, St. Charles Hospital, New Orleans, Louisiana.

The Fire Ant (with Vincent J. Derbes)

HERBERT E. KAUFMAN, M.D.
Professor and Chairman, Department of Ophthalmology, Shands Teaching Hospital, University of Florida College of Medicine, Gainesville, Florida.

Toxoplasmosis (with Robert Abel and Joseph H. Miller)

HUGH L. KEEGAN, Ph.D.
Professor (Medical Entomology), Department of Preventive Medicine, University of Mississippi School of Medicine, Jackson, Mississippi.

Selected Animals Hazardous to Man

RONALD KENNETH MACPHERSON, M.Sc., M.D., F.R.A.C.P.
Professor of Environmental Health and Principal, School of Public Health and Tropical Medicine, University of Sydney, New South Wales, Australia.

Effect of Heat (with John P. O'Brien)

EMILE A. MALEK, Ph.D.
Professor of Parasitology, Department of Tropical Medicine, Tulane University Medical Center, New Orleans, Louisiana.

Medically Important Mollusks

JEAN MAYER, Ph.D., D.Sc., A.M.(Hon.), M.D.(Hon.), S.D.(Hon.)
Professor of Nutrition, Lecturer in the History of Public Health, and Master of Dudley House, Harvard University. Consultant in Nutrition, Children's Hospital Medical Center, Boston, Massachusetts.

Nutritional Diseases (with Frederick J. Stare)

JOSEPH HENRY MILLER, Ph.D.
Professor, Department of Tropical Medicine and Medical Parasitology, Louisiana State University Medical Center. Scientist, Visiting Staff, Charity Hospital of Louisiana, New Orleans, Louisiana.

Toxoplasmosis (with Herbert E. Kaufman and Robert Abel), *Pneumocystis Pneumonia*

HAROLD D. NEWSON, Ph.D.
Associate Professor, Departments of Entomology and of Microbiology and Public Health, Michigan State University, East Lansing, Michigan.

Medically Important Arthropods—Introduction, Order Diptera

JOHN P. O'BRIEN, M.D., F.R.C.P.A.
Post-Graduate Lecturer in Pathology, University of Sydney. Consultant Pathologist, St. Vincent's Hospital and Lewisham Hospital, Sydney, New South Wales, Australia.

Cutaneous Diphtheria, Effect of Heat (with Ronald K. Macpherson), *Tropical Ulcer*

RICHARD A. ORMSBEE, Ph.D.
Staff Member, Rocky Mountain Laboratory, National Institute of Allergy and Infectious Diseases, Public Health Service, U.S. Department of Health, Education, and Welfare. Lecturer in Microbiology, University of Montana, Hamilton, Montana.

American Spotted Fevers, Related Spotted Fevers and Rickettsioses, Q Fever

JOHN WILLARD RIPPON, Ph.D.
Associate Professor of Medicine, The University of Chicago. Consultant, Veterans Administration Hospital, Hines, Illinois.

Mycotic and Actinomycotic Diseases

WESLEY W. SPINK, M.D.
Regents' Professor of Medicine and Comparative Medicine, Professor Emeritus, University of Minnesota Medical School, Minneapolis, Minnesota.

Brucellosis

FREDERICK J. STARE, M.D., Ph.D., S.D.(Hon.), D.Sc.(Hon.), A.M.(Hon.)
Professor of Nutrition, Harvard University; Head, Department of Nutrition, Harvard School of Public Health. Associate in Medicine, Peter Bent Brigham Hospital, Boston, Massachusetts.

Nutritional Diseases (with Jean Mayer)

PHILLIPS THYGESON, M.D.
Professor Emeritus of Ophthalmology, University of California, San Francisco, School of Medicine, San Francisco, California.

Trachoma

ROBERT TRAUB, Ph.D., Col., U.S.A.(Ret.)
Professor of Microbiology, University of Maryland School of Medicine, Baltimore, Maryland. Member, Commission on Hemorrhagic Fever and Associate Member, Commission on Rickettsial Diseases, Armed Forces Epidemiological Board. Consultant, World Health Organization and the National Institutes of Health.

Scrub Typhus (Chigger-borne Rickettsiosis) (with Charles L. Wisseman, Jr.)

DAVID MERRILL WEBER, M.D., F.A.C.P., Capt., M.C., U.S.N.
Officer-in-Charge, U.S. Navy Unit for Medical Research and Training, Gorgas Memorial Laboratory, Republic of Panama. Tropical Disease Consultant, Gorgas Hospital, Canal Zone. Clinical Associate Professor, Department of Tropical Medicine and Medical Parasitology, Louisiana State University Medical Center, New Orleans, Louisiana.

The Diarrheal Diseases and Food-borne Illnesses

DONALD E. WEIDHAAS, Ph.D.
Laboratory Director, Insects Affecting Man Research Laboratory, Agricultural Research Service, U.S. Department of Agriculture, Gainesville, Florida.

Class Insecta (Hexapoda), Control of Arthropods of Medical Importance (with Roger H. Grothaus)

CHARLES L. WISSEMAN, Jr., M.D.
Professor and Chairman, Department of Microbiology, and Assistant Professor of Medicine, University of Maryland School of Medicine, Baltimore, Maryland. Medical Staff, University of Maryland Hospital. Director, Commission on Rickettsial Diseases, Armed Forces Epidemiological Board. Consultant to Surgeon General of the Army, National Institutes of Health, World Health Organization and Pan American Health Organization.

Scrub Typhus (Chigger-borne Rickettsiosis) (with Robert Traub)

TELFORD H. WORK, M.D., D.T.M.&H., M.P.H.
Professor of Infectious and Tropical Diseases, Departments of Public Health and of Microbiology and Immunology, University of California, Los Angeles, Center for the Health Sciences, Los Angeles, California.

Exotic Virus Diseases, Enteric Virus Diseases, Respiratory Virus Diseases

GUY PARRY YOUMANS, M.D., Ph.D.
Professor and Chairman, Department of Microbiology, Northwestern University Medical School. Attending Staff, Northwestern Memorial Hospital, Chicago, Illinois.

Tuberculosis

MARTIN DUNAWAY YOUNG, Sc.D., D.Sc.(Hon.)
Visiting Professor of Parasitology, College of Veterinary Medicine and Department of Immunology and Microbiology, University of Florida College of Medicine, Gainesville, Florida.

Malaria

Foreword

During World War II, the then dean of tropical medicine in the United States, Colonel Richard P. Strong, in response to the urgent needs of the period, organized a superb course on tropical medicine at the Army Medical School in Washington. This course in tropical medicine, incorporating the contributions of a distinguished group of visiting lecturers, provided the format and substance of the first edition of the *Manual.* Subsequent editions, ever more multi-authored to insure authoritative coverage of a diverse subject material, have successfully preserved the original concise, yet comprehensive, format. The needs of the physicians and of other professionals dealing with tropical disease and the health problems of the developing areas of the world have been well served.

Today there is insufficient appreciation of the broad societal significance of tropical diseases and their impact on the United States. Since World War II the health gap has widened, as has the economic gap, between the developed and developing areas of the world. To be sure, yaws has been suppressed, and smallpox is being confined to an ever smaller geographic area. At the same time, however, pandemic cholera has appeared in Sub-Sahara Africa, malaria is resurgent in many areas, Shiga dysentery has produced high mortality in Central America, and schistosomiasis spreads as man increasingly relies on impounded water. For more than half of mankind, the burdens of endemic preventable infections and parasitic disease have not been lightened, but indeed worsen in synergistic lockstep with malnutrition as global production of food lags behind an expanding human population. Belatedly, economic planners and those concerned with population control are beginning to appreciate that mass misery due to ill health negates efforts directed at improving economic productivity and at stabilizing growth of human populations. The effective utilization of the huge sums of money now being contributed by the more affluent countries for the benefit of those less privileged will require a massive expansion of health-related activities. The supply of professional health workers skilled in the containment of tropical diseases, and of those capable of developing new knowledge of infectious and of parasitic diseases to meet the continuum of new problems posed by an ever-changing human ecology, likewise should be rapidly expanded. This societal need must be faced by those responsible for graduate education in the health professions.

There are few physicians in the United States who do not encounter problems in the area of tropical medicine with surprising regularity. Each day tens of thousands of citizens from the United States travel through or reside in the poorly sanitated areas of the world. There, the traveler, often poorly indoctrinated in approaches to personal preventive measures, like an innocent "sentinel monkey," ingests, inhales, or contacts potential pathogens or is exposed to vectors harboring such agents. With rapid jet air travel, return to the United States via plane may be a matter of hours after exposure. The immediate diagnosis and treatment of the patient with incipient cerebral malaria, or the recognition of acute African trypanosomiasis, are essential and may be lifesaving.

There is, however, a disturbing misconcept inherent in the term "tropical medicine," for many tropical diseases are not exotic on the domestic scene. In some areas of the United States, diseases such as ascariasis, trichuriasis, and amebiasis are commonly seen. Symptomatic giardiasis is now encountered with increasing frequency in individuals who have not left the United States. The prevalence of some ectoparasites of man is directly proportional to hair length and to the degree of communal living. The training of the physician to provide primary medical care—a popular concept in contemporary medical education—logically should incorporate knowledge of indigenous "tropical diseases," as well as of those truly exotic.

This new edition arrives at an opportune time. It should assist in the preparation of the greatly expanded cadre of physicians and scientists needed to integrate health into the economic developmental process in the poorly sanitated areas of the world. It will provide the physician practicing in the United States with an authoritative reference source in an area of continuing medical importance.

THOMAS H. WELLER, M.D.
Richard Pearson Strong
Professor of Tropical Public
Health and Chairman of the
Department, School of Public
Health, Harvard University

Preface to the Fifth Edition

The First Edition of *A Manual of Tropical Medicine* was prepared during World War II to meet the needs of the Armed Forces in the tropical and subtropical areas of the world. A concise presentation of the practical aspects of the important tropical diseases, stressing both the epidemiological and clinical aspects, resulted in wide acceptance of the *Manual* as a textbook and reference—for medical and graduate students, clinicians, and other military and nonmilitary personnel in medicine, public health, microbiology and allied fields. Because of the expansion of health and medical education programs on a worldwide basis and changing needs, the book has been revised four times. With this, the Fifth Edition, it adopts the shortened title *Tropical Medicine*.

Political, social and economic trends during the past four decades have involved nations of the world in activities which dispersed their citizens to all areas of the world. This migration back and forth has increased the need for trained personnel in all disciplines encompassed by medicine and public health in the tropics and subtropics. The activities and responsibilities of the United States in the field of international health, which are being carried on in cooperation with many countries, are consonant with this nation's desire to contribute to the improvement of the standards of world health. The contribution of the United States to international health and medical education by means of professional cooperation and technical assistance in the attack on diseases of the tropics and subtropics is one of our finest exports and is symbolic of our country's humanitarian principles.

In the preparation of this edition, we continued to be challenged by the need to present to medical workers a concise yet explicit statement of the etiology, epidemiology, pathology, clinical characteristics, diagnosis, treatment, control and prophylaxis of the important infectious diseases, nutritional and physical disorders and other conditions constituting the health problems of the tropics. Although many of these diseases are also endemic or have their counterparts in the subtropical and temperate zones, the main attack on them must continue to be in developing countries in the tropics. There a multiplicity of adverse social and economic factors makes the task seem increasingly difficult. Principal among these factors are (1) an explosive population increase related to a high birth rate, (2) predominantly rural economies inadequate to provide the revenues from which national social and health services and improved communications must be financed, and (3) uncontrolled slum urbanization overwhelming local sanitation resources.

It is increasingly apparent that the fundamental remedies for the present proliferation of tropical diseases and malnutrition must come through enlightened political and economic practices in the areas of advancement of agricultural and industrial techniques, acceptance of an appropriate policy of family planning, and establishment of a network of health care centers throughout each developing nation. Advice on these matters from international agencies and developed countries, however well-intentioned, will be fruitless unless a genuine national commitment exists on the part of the recipient.

A number of principal revisions and changes have been made in the Fifth Edition. The section on mycotic and actinomycotic diseases has been completely rewritten. Also, the section on viral diseases has undergone substantial rewriting and revision. New chapters include those on simple goiter and venereal diseases in the tropics. Additional subjects that have been included are infections by *Capillaria philippinesis*, *Schistosoma intercalatum* and *Angiostrongylus costaricensis*. Coverage of primary amebic meningitis due to *Naegleria* and *Hartmannella* spp. has been rewritten and expanded. Also, the material on amebiasis has been revised substantially in cognizance of modern concepts of the infection and disease. A more practical and clinical approach has been taken in the presentation on diarrheal diseases, making the content on this group of entities more useful for the clinician and student. Extensive changes also have been made, with new contributors, in the coverage of rickettsial diseases, toxoplasmosis, leishmaniasis, tuberculosis, leptospirosis, rat-bite fevers, *Pneumocystis* pneumonia and effects of heat. The addition of practical information on diagnosis and treatment of infestations by arthropods and on envenomization by insects should assist the physician in the management of such conditions. Treatment has been updated throughout. The numerous figures in the previous edition have been augmented with many new illustrations of value for clinical understanding and teaching of tropical diseases.

We have continued to include some of the more important references, both old and new, at the end of each chapter. It should be realized, however, that there has been no attempt to make such a listing complete, since this obviously would not be feasible.

The broad expanse of tropical medicine includes so many diseases and specialties that authoritative presentation is best obtained by the contributions of collaborators. Individuals recognized for special knowledge and for basic research in specific fields were invited to contribute to this revision. The contribution of each collaborator is indicated in the byline of each chapter or section heading. Chapters with no indicated authorship were written or revised by the authors.

THE AUTHORS

Acknowledgments for the Fifth Edition

As in the other editions, materials have been drawn from numerous medical, scientific and technical journals, recent monographs and abstracting journals, such as the *Tropical Diseases Bulletin,* without which such a revision would have proved an impossible undertaking.

We wish to express once again our deep appreciation to those individuals cited in the first four editions of *A Manual of Tropical Medicine* and especially to Dr. T. T. Mackie and Dr. C. Brooke Worth, two of the original coauthors who contributed so much to the writing of the earlier editions. The coauthors also express their appreciation to Dr. William W. Frye for his significant contributions as coauthor of the third and fourth editions.

We wish to thank our former collaborators who furnished the basic manuscripts covering subjects in their special spheres of interest. In many instances they provided or added original material. We gratefully acknowledge the help of the following persons who so generously collaborated in earlier editions: Drs. R. Tucker Abbott, George R. Callender, Gordon E. Davis, Paul D. Ellner, John P. Fox, Irving Gordon, Arthur P. Long, Harry Most, Albert B. Sabin, Arvey C. Sanders, Emanuel Suter and H. W. Wade.

Others including Drs. Bettie M. Catchings, Antonio Peña Chavarria, Dorothy Clemmer, John H. Cross, Jane E. Deas, Dieu-Donne J. Guidry, Chamlong Harinasuta, Graham E. Kemp, Max C. Miller, Adele H. Spence, George A. Thurber, Ernestine H. Thurman, Harold Trapido, Kenneth Walls, Lionel G. Warren and Rodrigo Zeledon advised and assisted the authors in correlating material in their specialized fields for the current edition.

Grateful appreciation is also due the Armed Forces Institute of Pathology for many of the illustrations of pathology. Many cuts *not* bearing a special acknowledgment were furnished through the courtesy of this group.

Appreciation is also expressed to Dr. Robert L. Simmons and Mr. Kenneth W. Brown for photographic assistance and to Mr. Donald M. Alvarado and Mr. Robert O. Beach for the art work for the previous edition, which made possible many excellent figures still used in this edition. Many new illustrations for the fifth edition were prepared with the assistance of Donald M. Alvarado, Joseph A. Burkhardt, Elizabeth M. Candelario, Dr. Mark R. Feldman, Eugene R. Miscenich, Felix P. Schillesci, Jr. and Eugene Wolfe.

Special appreciation is due to Mrs. Helen Outen and Mrs. Arah Russell for their aid in the preparation of the typescript; also to Fern E. Hunter for her editorial and secretarial assistance.

Finally, the authors wish once again to express their sincere gratitude to the publisher, W. B. Saunders Company, for their deep interest, constructive criticisms and invaluable assistance, which made this fifth edition possible.

THE AUTHORS

References

Listed below are a number of general references on tropical medicine. Interested students will find additional information or even different viewpoints in this material. Other references, including appropriate books, deal with more limited topics and are listed at the end of each chapter. It should be emphasized that these references are not intended to be complete. Many contain bibliographies that will permit the student to delve into the literature of a given subject more thoroughly.

Adam, Paul and Zaman: Medical and Veterinary Protozoology. An Illustrated Guide. Churchill Livingstone, Edinburgh, 1971.

Ansari (ed.): Epidemiology and Control of Schistosomiasis (Bilharziasis). S. Karger AG, Basel, 1973.

Arthur: Ticks and Disease. Row, Peterson & Co., Evanston, Illinois, 1962.

Barua and Burrows (eds.): Cholera. W. B. Saunders Co., Philadelphia, 1974.

Batten: The Surgery of Trauma in the Tropics. The Williams & Wilkins Co., Baltimore, 1961.

Beeson and McDermott (eds.): Cecil-Loeb Textbook of Medicine. 14th ed. W. B. Saunders Co., Philadelphia, 1975.

Brown: Basic Clinical Parasitology. 3rd ed. Meredith Corporation, New York, 1969.

Brumpt: Précis de Parasitologie. Vols. I and II. Masson et Cie., Paris, 1949.

Cançado (ed.): Doença de Chagas. Hospital das Clinicas. Belo Horizonte, Brasil, 1968.

Cavier and Hawking (eds.): Chemotherapy of Helminthiasis. International Encyclopedia of Pharmacology and Therapeutics. Vol. I, Section 64. Pergamon Press, New York, 1973.

Chatterjee: Parasitology (Protozoology and Helminthology) in Relation to Clinical Medicine. 9th ed. K. D. Chatterjee, Calcutta, 1973.

Ciba Foundation: Symposium 20 (new series), Trypanosomiasis and Leishmaniasis with Special Reference to Chagas Disease. Elsevier, Excerpta Medica, North-Holland, Amsterdam, 1974.

Coatney, Collins, Warren and Contacos. The Primate Malarias. U.S. Government Printing Office, Washington, D.C., 1971.

Cochrane and Davey: Leprosy in Theory and Practice. The Williams & Wilkins Co., Baltimore, 1964.

Cruickshank et al.: Medical Microbiology. A Guide to the Laboratory Diagnosis and Control of Infection. 12th ed. Vol. 1. Microbial Infections. Churchill Livingstone, Edinburgh, 1973.

Davey and Wilson: Davey and Lightbody's The Control of Diseases in the Tropics. A Handbook for Medical Practitioners. H. K. Lewis, London, 1971.

Davis: Drug Treatment in Intestinal Helminthiases. W.H.O., Geneva, 1973.

Dawes (ed.): Advances in Parasitology. Vols. 1–11. Academic Press, New York, 1963–1973.

De Carneri: Parassitologia Generale e Umana. 5th ed. Casa Editrice Ambrosiana, Milano, 1974.

Faust, Russell and Jung: Craig and Faust's Clinical Parasitology. 8th ed. Lea & Febiger, Philadelphia, 1970.

Ford: The Role of the Trypanosomiases in African Ecology. A Study of the Tsetse Fly Problem. Clarendon Press, Oxford University Press, London, 1971.

Gentilini et al.: Médecine Tropicale. Flammarion Médecine-Sciences, Paris, 1972.

Greenberg: Flies and Disease. Vol. I (1971): Ecology, Classification and Biotic Associations. Vol. II (1973): Biology and Disease Transmission. Princeton University Press, Princeton, New Jersey.

Gsell and Mohr (eds.): Infektionskrankheiten. Band IV. Rickettsiosen und Protozoenkrankheiten. Springer-Verlag, Berlin-West, 1972.

Horsfall: Medical Entomology. Arthropods and Human Disease. The Ronald Press Co., New York, 1962.

Hughes (ed.): Health Care for Remote Areas. Kaiser Foundation International, Oakland, California, 1972.

Ingram and Mount: Man and Animals in Hot Environments. Springer-Verlag, Berlin-West, 1975.

Jelliffe (ed.): Diseases of Children in the Subtropics and Tropics. 2nd ed. Edward Arnold (Publishers) Ltd., London, 1970.

Kenney: Scope Monograph on Pathoparasitology. Upjohn Co., Kalamazoo, Michigan, 1973.

King: A Medical Laboratory for Developing Countries. Oxford University Press, London, 1973.

Maegraith: Adams and Maegraith Clinical Tropical Diseases. 5th ed. Blackwell Scientific Publications, Oxford, 1971.

Maegraith and Gilles: Management and Treatment of Tropical Diseases. Blackwell Scientific Publications, Oxford, 1971.
Marcial-Rojas (ed.): Pathology of Protozoal and Helminthic Diseases. The Williams & Wilkins Co., Baltimore, 1971.
Marshall (ed.): Essays on Tropical Dermatology. Vol. 2. Excerpta Medica, Amsterdam, 1972.
Middlemiss: Tropical Radiology. Pitman Press, Bath, 1961.
Minton: Venom Diseases. Charles C Thomas, Publisher, Springfield, Illinois, 1974.
Mulligan and Potts: The African Trypanosomiases. Geo. Allen & Unwin, London, 1970.
Nnochiri: Medical Microbiology in the Tropics. Oxford University Press, London, 1974.
Owen: Man's Environmental Predicament. An Introduction to Human Ecology in Tropical Africa. Oxford University Press, London, 1973.
Pal and Whitten (eds.): The Use of Genetics in Insect Control. Elsevier North-Holland Publishing Co., Amsterdam, 1974.
Pampana: A Textbook of Malaria Eradication. 2nd ed. Oxford University Press, London, 1969.
Piekarski: Medizinische Parasitologie in Tafeln. 2nd ed. Springer-Verlag, Berlin-West, 1973.
Preventive Medicine in World War II. Vols. IV and VII. Communicable Diseases. Medical Department, United States Army. Edited by J. B. Coates, Jr., Col. MC, E. C. Hoff, and P. M. Hoff. U.S. Government Printing Office, Washington, D.C., 1958, 1964.
Rippon: Medical Mycology. The Pathogenic Fungi and the Pathogenic Actinomycetes. W. B. Saunders Co., Philadelphia, 1974.
Russell, West, Manwell and Macdonald: Practical Malariology. 2nd ed. Oxford University Press, London, 1963.
Shaper, Hutt and Fejfar (eds.): Cardiovascular Disease in the Tropics. British Medical Association, London, 1974.
Shuvalova (ed.): Tropicheskiye Bolezni. Meditsina, Leningrad, 1973.
Somerset: Ophthalmology in the Tropics. The Williams & Wilkins Co., Baltimore, 1962.
Spencer et al.: Tropical Pathology. Springer-Verlag, Berlin-West, 1973.
Spillane: Tropical Neurology. Oxford University Press, London, 1973.
Wilcocks and Manson-Bahr: Manson's Tropical Diseases. 17th ed. Baillière Tindall, London, 1972.
Wilkie: Jordan's Tropical Hygiene and Sanitation. 4th ed. The Williams & Wilkins Co., Baltimore, 1965.
Williams and Jelliffe: Mother and Child Health: Delivering the Services. Oxford University Press, London, 1972.
Woodruff: Medicine in the Tropics. Churchill Livingstone, Edinburgh, 1972.

In addition, the interested student should consult such compendia as the *Current List of Medical Literature, Tropical Diseases Bulletin* and *Biological Abstracts.*

Contents

Section III

SPIROCHETAL DISEASES

Section IV

BACTERIAL DISEASES

Section IX

MISCELLANEOUS CONDITIONS

Section X

MEDICALLY IMPORTANT ANIMALS

Section XI

MEDICALLY IMPORTANT ARTHROPODS

SECTION I
Virus Diseases

CHAPTER 1
Exotic Virus Diseases

TELFORD H. WORK

Introduction

Tropical diseases have long been conveniently ascribed to regions in the torrid zone. However, the burgeoning population of the earth and accelerating movement of human hosts harboring short incubation pathogens cause diverse disease syndromes that transcend a strictly geographic distribution. Currently, consideration should also be given to what is considered exotic to conventional medical problems of temperate urban localities. This would include epidemiologic situations characteristic of arctic and subarctic areas that might simulate disease occurrence at high altitudes in equatorial latitudes.

No constellation of pathogens manifests this ubiquitous distribution more than the causative agents of virus diseases. Viruses that caused pandemic pox diseases, and others that were mosquito transmitted, were long considered the tropical virus diseases. It is now necessary to grasp concepts of tick-borne virus disease transmission as a temperate as well as a tropical zone phenomenon. Viruses cause severe disease in the immunologically unprotected transient through a maintenance cycle wherever substandard sanitation occurs. Person-to-person or fecal-oral routes of virus transmission are now recognized as basic disease mechanisms throughout the tropics. This has been recognized in the past decade in the etiologic association of viruses with human diseases surpassing in numbers, varieties, syndromes, attack rates, prevalence and general impact other recognized causative agents of human disease. This requires the practitioner, researcher and student alike to appreciate the variety of epidemiologic and pathogenic mechanisms utilized by the many agents. The integration of variable classifications will prove most useful in suspecting a viral etiology, selecting appropriate diagnostic procedures, and defining epidemiologic mechanisms of transmission so that measures of control and prevention can be introduced. In this era there are few effective measures for treatment of virus diseases. Prevention and control are the primary medical weapons of a diverse team of health specialists.

To influence a virus disease situation favorably, it is necessary to have a knowledge of (1) possible etiologic agents, (2) diverse epidemiologic patterns that might be elucidated, (3) methodology of epidemiologic investigation that may be applied and (4) demonstrated means of control and prevention. These factors set the specialist in virus diseases apart from others who use antibiotics and chemotherapy to treat afflicted patients.

Viruses are the most successful parasites in the causation of enzootic, epizootic and epidemic disease because they carry with them in their minuscule particulate form little more than programming genetic material by which they selectively exploit the protein and lipid cellular constituents of host cells, tissues and organs of a susceptible host in which they must necessarily replicate intracellularly. The tropisms directed by their enzymatic and nucleic acid constitution infiltrate susceptible cells in diverse ways, but often more precisely than the parasitism of protozoal and metazoal organisms that classically have dominated the field of tropical medicine for the past half century.

For these reasons no consistent classification by morphology, physicochemical characteristics, tropisms, pathogenesis, clinical signs, epidemiology, prognosis or sequelae can be reliably applied. Usually application of two or more of these considerations is required to formulate a hypothesis that will lead to correct investigation and diagnosis.

Having outlined these difficulties it may be more understandable, in reviewing the diseases caused by some three or four hundred recognized viral pathogens, why the structure and organization of these chapters have been formulated in such an imperfect way.

Considered first are arbovirus infections and diseases. These are essentially all zoonotic in origin and primarily, although not exclusively, vector-borne. It therefore follows that most of the other identifiable zoonotic diseases—those transmissible from other animals to man—are logical extensions of an examination of diseases frequently occurring in, although not confined to, tropical regions.

The second grouping is related to the problem of substandard or nonexistent sanitation in which there is no safe separation of excretions from intake of fluids and food required for life. This has been the accepted sphere of enteric disease in the tropics, although certain of the viral pathogens included in the second chapter do not cause enteric disease but are encompassed by the epidemiology of enteric transmission involving the infectious process by the fecal-oral route.

A third categorization deals with agents transmitted by oral contact, aerosols and airborne mechanisms and those affecting the respiratory tree. Again, even though their clinical manifestations may range from systemic disease to skin manifestations, portal of entry and pathogenesis have been the theme for their inclusion.

The fourth component focuses on exanthematous diseases not only because visible signs stimulate consideration of viral causation of such lesions, but also because of the importance of differentially recognizing what might masquerade as smallpox at a time when the World Health Organization Global Smallpox Eradication Campaign has presently driven the disease back to foci in eastern India, Bangladesh and Ethiopia.

Based upon the above, a compilation of information has been attempted in a form thought to be most helpful to a variety of professionals and students who will use this book as an introduction to virus diseases in the tropics.

It appears that the only truisms that remain are: (1) etiologic diagnosis of a virus disease depends upon isolation of the virus from the patient during an early stage of infection, with demonstration of a rise in titer of antibodies to that agent in at least two sera taken sequentially several days apart during the acute and convalescent stages; and (2), with very few exceptions, there is no specific treatment for most virus diseases, only symptomatic relief and physiologic support to minimize effects from the process of infection in the patient. On the other hand, a number of prophylactic measures such as specific vaccines, water purification and mosquito screens can prevent infections. Well defined control measures effectively applied following early diagnosis of a specific infection can save inestimable numbers from disease and entire communities from epidemic extension of virus infections, which usually appear so insidiously that they are recognizable only to the alert, well informed and thinking health professional.

Arbovirus Infection and Diseases

Definition. *Ar*thropod-*bo*rne *viruses (arboviruses)* are those that infect susceptible vertebrates by the bite of an arthropod in which replication has occurred during an extrinsic incubation period following ingestion of the virus from another viremic vertebrate. Arthropods other than insects, such as ticks, may be effective vectors.[1] The arthropod is generally infected and infectious for life. It therefore often becomes as effective a reservoir as a vector.

Arbovirus infection of vertebrates is usually asymptomatic, as is characteristic of most successful parasites. Following an incubation period during which the arbovirus replicates in specific cells and tissues, humoral dispersion of the virus stimulates a specific immune response. Viremia is of limited duration. The immunity that follows is usually prolonged, probably for the life of the vertebrate host.

Strictly speaking, the term arboviruses is properly confined to those viruses that are hematophagously ingested and that replicate within an arthropod vector. A quarter century of epidemiologic search for the medical importance and public health significance of these agents[2] has discovered many that are notably not arthropod-borne. These include the arenaviruses[3] and such viruses as Modoc and Rio Bravo of Group B of mammalian tissue origin, which do not replicate in mosquito or tick tissues and therefore are probably not arthropod-borne.

Early in these investigations, resistance to inactivation by deoxycholic acid (DCA) and diethyl ether was a chemical characteristic excluding filterable agents from inclusion among the arboviruses. Nodamura and Colorado tick fever viruses are exceptions that tend to prove the rule; such DCA- and ether-sensitivity led to their characterization as lipid-enveloped, cuboid, ribonucleic acid core (RNA) viruses, now classified as togaviruses in the most recent International Nomenclature and Classification.[4] But further molecular chemical characterization and electron microscopy have turned up arthropod-transmitted deoxyribonucleic acid (DNA) and bullet-shaped helical rhabdoviruses, e.g. vesicular stomatitis virus, which are natural arboviruses, but not togaviruses[5] (Fig. 1–1).

Arbovirus must therefore be considered an ecologic definition in terms of epidemiologically and antigenically associated zoonotic viruses. They are described in the "International Catalogue of Arboviruses Including Certain Other Viruses of Vertebrates."[6]

Arboviruses are commonly among the

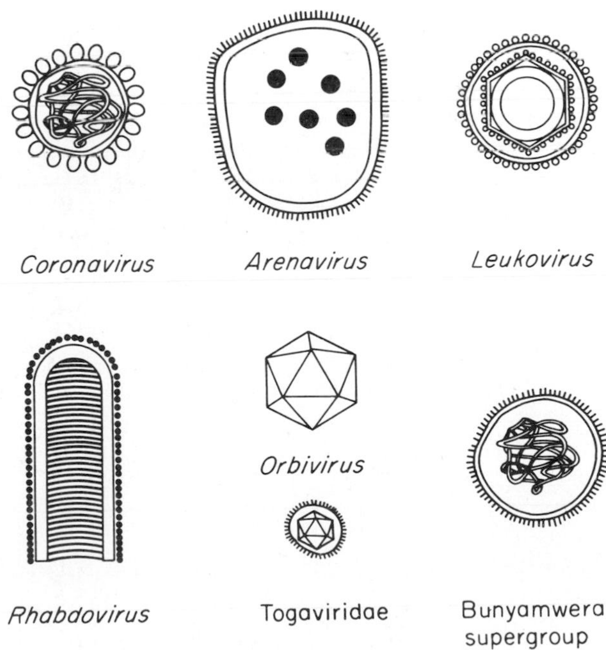

Figure 1–1. Diagram illustrating the shapes of some arboviruses. (From Fenner, F. J. 1974. Biology of Animal Viruses. Academic Press, New York. Used with permission.)

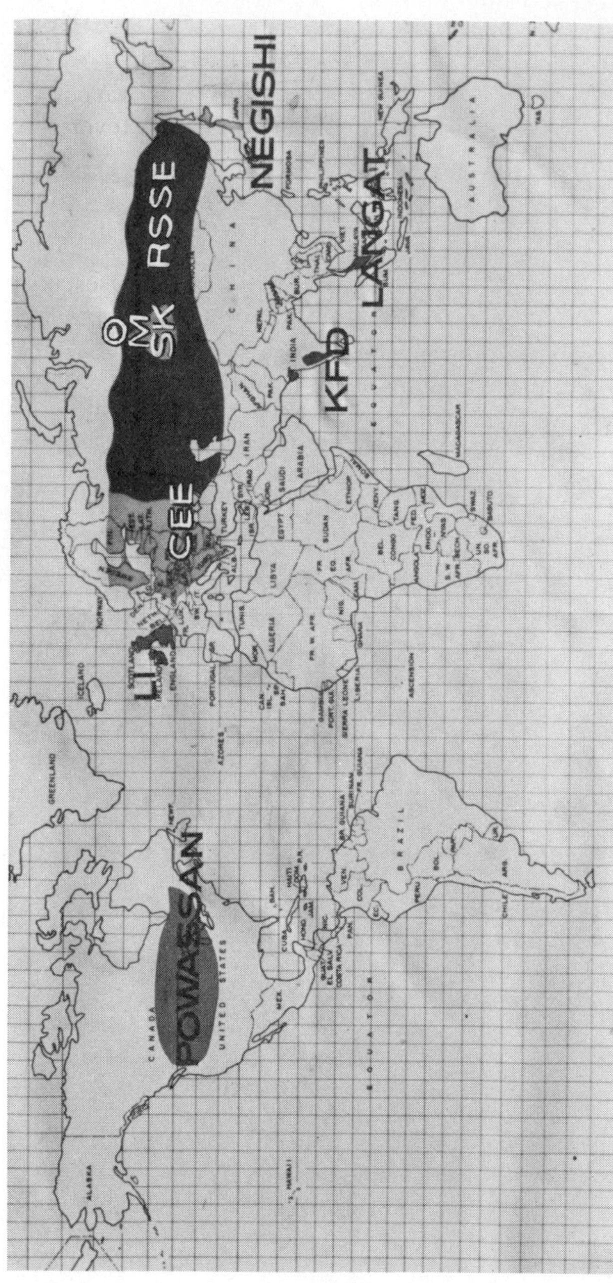

Figure 1–2. Schematic distribution of the tick-borne Russian spring-summer complex of arbovirus Group B.

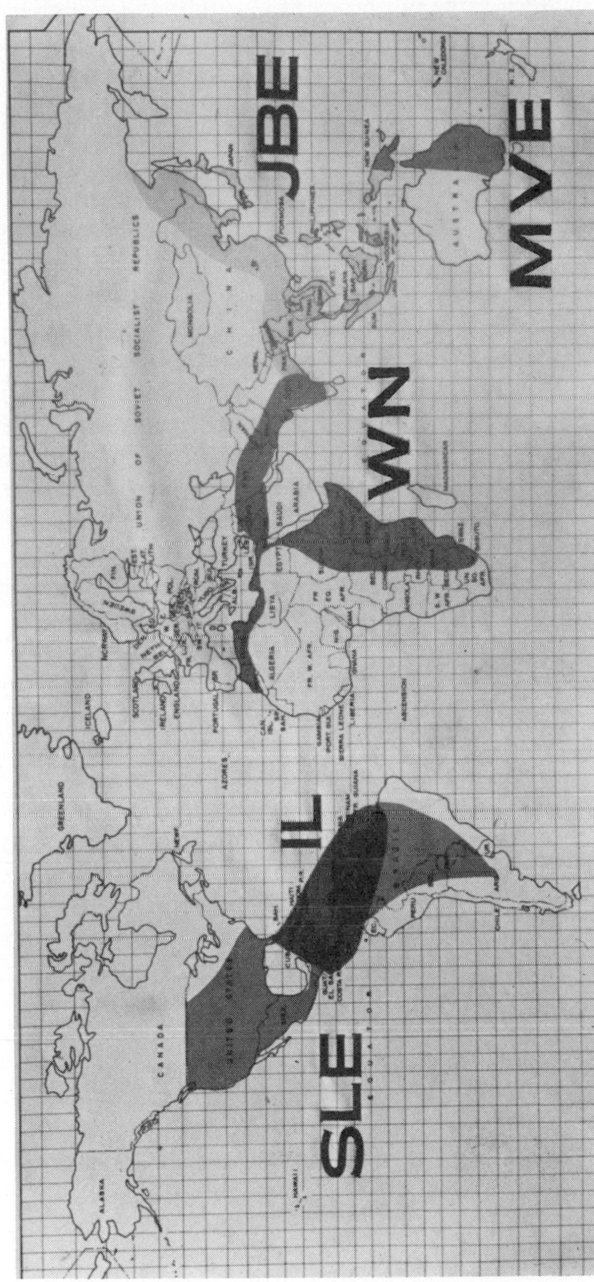

Figure 1–3. Schematic distribution of the Japanese B encephalitis and West Nile complex of arbovirus Group B.

smallest in size (25 to 50 nm), but others such as the Bunyaviridae may approach or exceed 100 nm. Their discovery, characterization and compilation into more than 40 antigenic groups, representing almost 400 agents, derives as much from the conceptual zoonotic approach of isolation from arthropods and nonhuman vertebrates as from the occurrence of human disease. While more than 100 of these agents have now been associated with human infection and disease, it is important to remember that many if not most have been isolated from arthropod vectors or vertebrate hosts or both. These were often the initial source of diagnostic strains that eventually were used in the laboratory to establish serologically the etiologic diagnosis of human disease. The corollary is that etiologic association with human disease may await isolation of an arbovirus from its silent cycle vertebrate host or arthropod vector.

Those viruses that are mechanically transmitted on the mouthparts of insects by the "flying needle" mechanism, such as rabbit myxomatosis and fowlpox, are clearly excluded, as are togaviruses, such as rubella, which have no ecologically associated mechanism of maintenance and transmission.

Casals' antigenic group concept has provided some order in an otherwise chaotic plethora of infectious agents by serologically demonstrating that many arboviruses are antigenically related.[2] Alphabetical and other designations, presented in subsequent tables, were given to groups of antigenically related agents, those with particularly close affinities being subordinated into a complex such as the mosquito-borne Japanese B–West Nile[7] and tick-borne Russian spring-summer complexes[8] of arbovirus Group B (Figs. 1–2 and 1–3).

Etiology. Overt arbovirus disease in man usually occurs as an infection tangential to a silent arthropod-vertebrate cycle of maintenance in nature. While most arbovirus infections, even in man, may be asymptomatic or very mild, the numerous causative agents can and do produce disease that ranges from self-limiting but incapacitating fever and headache, to hemorrhagic disease, which may be fatal, or central nervous system disease dissociating the patient from his environment, frequently resulting in severe permanent sequelae or death.

It can also be generalized that many of the recognized arbovirus pathogens can cause any one or a combination of these clinical manifestations on occasion. This emphasizes the importance of the virus laboratory in establishing a correct diagnosis.

Epidemiology. Human disease resulting from arbovirus infection is often an insidious event that challenges the clinical acumen of the physician and requires precise interpretation of significant information in taking the history. Such information can best be obtained by comprehensive consideration of how the patient invaded or became tangentially associated with the natural cycle of arbovirus maintenance and dissemination.[9] Figure 1–4 displays the four basic cycles by which arboviruses exist and shows the mechanisms and loci in the cycles where man may be exposed to infection.

Once an arbovirus infection is suspected, determination of the possible occupational or environmental exposure may provide the clue that directs the clinician to selection of the best laboratory approach to establishing a diagnosis.[9] Sometimes of even greater importance is the direction of effort to isolation of the causative virus from the arthropod vector or vertebrate host where, because arboviruses are parasites of animals other than man, such agents can most successfully be sought.

Seasonal occurrence may reflect factors in the ecologic situation. There may be rain, which has resulted in an abundance of mosquitoes, or a multiplication of susceptible vertebrate hosts during the bird spring breeding season, or the more frequent exposure of human hosts because of out-of-door summer work or recreation in biotopes occupied by infected man-biting vectors.

Detection of sporadic cases, which may herald onset of an epidemic during a favorable season with appropriate combinations of virus, reservoir and vector, justifies considerable thoughtful attention of physicians

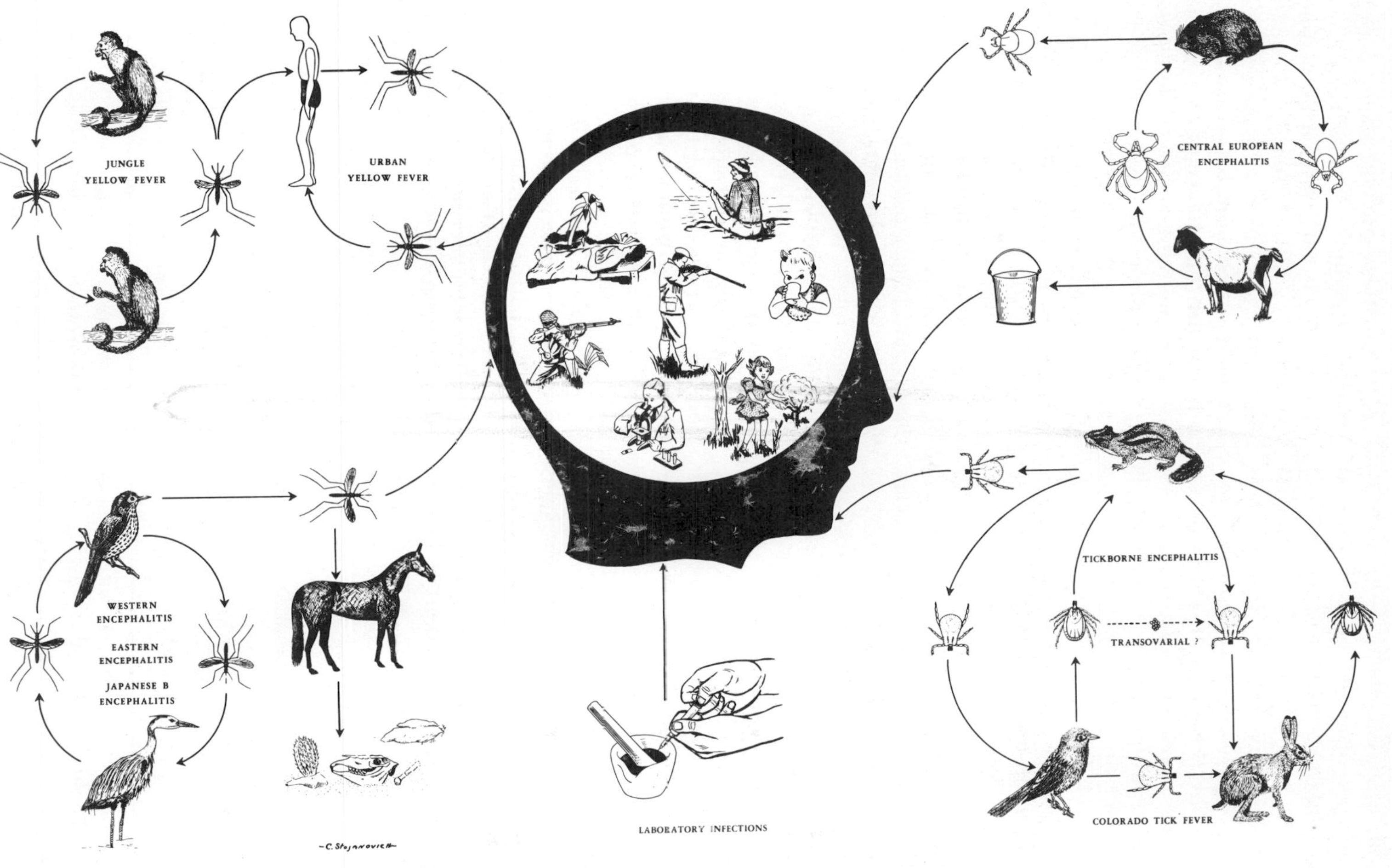

Figure 1–4. The four basic arbovirus cycles showing their relationship to man.

and public health authorities. If it can be afforded and supported by an adequate laboratory, a surveillance system, including routine examination of mosquitoes for virus and vertebrate hosts for virus and antibody conversion, is an even more timely mechanism for detection of any virus activity that poses a threat.

Because of the many mechanisms involved in dissemination of virus outside a man-to-man transmitted cycle, epidemiologic patterns of season, duration, age and sex vary widely. However, because infection usually produces prolonged immunity, significant attack rates in all age groups indicate invasion of a new arbovirus; disease confined to children indicates reintroduction or intermittent overflow from a wild cycle to the humans who are susceptible. Particular selection of age or sex groups usually focuses on locality and mechanism of exposure, although incontrovertible confirmation of such assumptions is often tedious, and even frustrating to the point of failure.

Distribution. With such a plethora of different mechanisms for successful biologic survival, the adaptation of arboviruses must be considered a continuous process not only in time but in relation to geographic distribution, dissemination, focalization, confinement, displacement and elimination. Such biologic processes are doubtless the explanation of such a great number and variety of arboviruses, many of them antigenically related derivatives from an original "genetic stem," but accommodated to a geographic diversity of situations that fosters maintenance and transmission of arboviruses in all inhabited continents of the world.

It is this global dissemination of arboviruses that makes it impossible to separate the strictly tropical from other arbovirus diseases. Reference has been made to the ecologic, geographic and antigenic diffusion of related arboviruses. These are noted in the subsequent sections dealing with clinical syndromes (Tables 1–1 to 1–6).

Schematic examples are presented in Figures 1–2 and 1–3, showing the distribution of two antigenic complexes of arbovirus Group B.

The mosquito-borne Japanese B–West Nile complex, which includes Japanese B encephalitis (JBE), Murray Valley encephalitis (MVE), St. Louis encephalitis (SLE), Ilheus (IL) and West Nile (WN) viruses, appears to occur largely in the tropical and subtropical latitudes, with epidemic summer-fall occurrence in more temperate regions. On the other hand, the tick-borne Russian spring-summer complex, which includes Russian spring-summer encephalitis (RSSE), Omsk hemorrhagic fever (OHF), Central European meningoencephalitis (CEE), louping ill (LI), Powassan encephalitis (POW), Negishi (NEG), Langat (LAN), and Kyasanur Forest disease (KFD), seems to occur predominantly in temperate regions, except for Langat and Kyasanur Forest disease, which are localized deep within the tropics. To unravel the evolutionary history of these close antigenic relations provides one of the most intriguing biologic challenges encompassed in arbovirology.

The issue is raised here only to emphasize the global distribution of arboviruses and the diseases they cause and to demonstrate how misleading it would be to focus only on their distribution within tropical zones.

Pathology. Although man is usually infected with arboviruses by bites from infected hematophagous arthropods, infection can occur by ingestion, as with milk-borne diphasic meningoencephalitis, or by inhalation and mucous membrane contamination, which are the frequent cause of accidental laboratory infections. The actual sequence of events leading to establishment of infection, replication of the virus and causation of overt disease is not accepted in detail for many arboviruses. It is generally understood that the virus is carried by the blood to the cells or tissues for which the virus has tropism. After invading such cells, the virus disappears into an eclipse phase during which it cannot be detected.

Fluorescent antibody visualization of antigen distribution and tissue titration from vital organs over time following infection indicate that there are several mechanisms for establishment of infection and pathogenesis of viral dissemination.[10] The virus replicates at the site where biting mouthparts of the vector arthropod were inserted. There shortly follows concentration and replication of the virus in the lymph drainage adjacent to the site of the bite. Almost simultaneously virus is also detectable at widely separated sites, reflecting humoral dissemination of the original virus replicates.

Virus is found in spleen, lymph nodes and bone marrow, but contrary to previous belief, experimental infections with some arboviruses indicate that the reticuloendothelial system is no more susceptible to or productive of virus than many other tissues to which virus was initially disseminated. These other sites include: striated and smooth muscle fibers, osteo-, chondro- and odontoblasts of mesodermal origin; epithelium and salivary glands of the oral cavity, convoluted tubules of the kidney, adenohypophysis, and islets of Langerhans of entodermal origin; and adrenal medulla, olfactory mucosa, retina, peripheral ganglia and sites in the sympathetic nervous system, as well as neurons and glial cells of the central nervous system (CNS), which are of ectodermal origin.

Replication at these sites pours virus into the circulating blood. As a viremia the virus is carried to susceptible tissues where its concentration in excess of that removed by the immune response determines its invasiveness. Hence, with neurotropic viruses there must be sufficient quantity of virus escaping from capillary circulation in the brain to move through intracellular spaces to invade and replicate in enough neurons to produce damage resulting in neurologic dysfunction encompassed by disease manifestations of encephalitis.

This process occupies the incubation period. Many highly neurotropic viruses have low neuroinvasiveness, and therefore low encephalitis attack rates because the neurotropic virus does not replicate rapidly enough nor in sufficient quantity (titer) to surpass humoral antibody defense or cell-mediated inflammatory defense—as manifest by perivascular cuffing—to allow sufficient virus to invade and damage enough neurons to result in clinical disease. This explains why highly infectious pathogenic viruses of severe encephalitis, such as St. Louis and Japanese B, produce CNS disease in very few of the persons who sustain infection as a result of mosquito transmission of virus. On the other hand there are highly infectious, pathogenic, neurotropic viruses, such as West Nile and Venezuelan equine encephalitis, which produce high attack rates of febrile illness but low attack rates of neuroinvasive encephalitis.

The mechanism for extravasation of red cells by increased capillary permeability seems to be an immunologic phenomenon because there is no increase in virus titer associated with sites of hemorrhagic sequelae. Often no virus at all is recoverable from these sites when humoral immunity is demonstrable. Such gross or microscopic changes are characteristic of some of the hemorrhagic fevers, but may be manifest to a limited extent in arbovirus infections with other more prominent clinical signs.

Cell-mediated immune reactions are suspected of being responsible for delayed CNS signs associated with arboviral encephalitis. The hypothesis, supported by some experimental data, is that slower pathogenesis induces a cell-mediated response as observed in perivascular cuffing by thymus-derived and other cellular elements. Consequent increased intracranial pressure produces indirect damage to the CNS.[11]

Such pathophysiologic mechanisms have led to controversy about how severe manifestations of arbovirus encephalitis should be handled. Those favoring immune mechanisms of resistance to an excessive viremic dissemination of virus in the brain recommend conservative supportive treatment to encourage a humoral immune response and cell-mediated resistance at the capillary level. Others suggest that immunosuppression will inhibit intracerebral perivascular inflammation and decrease consequent edema and intracranial pressure. Animal experiments have shown delayed manifestation of severe CNS signs but there has been evidence of ultimate massive neuron destruction by increased viral invasion. Since neuron destruction is irreversible and controlled clinical trials with immunosuppressives cannot presently be justified, the conservative supportive approach remains the treatment of choice.

The rapidity of subsequent invasion of other cells and the tissue destruction that results in manifest host response in overt disease depend on the nature and type of arbovirus. The incubation period, which is relatively limited, ranges from as short as 24 hours, as with Venezuelan equine encephalitis, to 10 days, which is not unusual for St. Louis encephalitis. It may be observed that the shorter the incubation period, the more explosive the clinical onset and course, the longer incubation being more insidious and very often more damaging.

There is histologic evidence of tropic selection for specific tissues, such as the liver in yellow fever, which is characterized by midzonal necrosis and Councilman bodies, or perivascular cuffing and neuronophagia of the cerebrum in acute arbovirus encephalitis. These lesions are demonstrable to the point of being diagnostic when they are observed in appropriate specimens. However, much else occurs that is not well understood. Leukopenia and thrombocytopenia are common in many arbovirus infections. There is still no explanation for the mechanism leading to late development of capillary permeability with focal necrosis in many organs and extravasation of red cells into different widely separated tissues, as is commonly observed in the hemorrhagic fevers. There is usually too high a titer of antibody circulating by the time this occurs to attribute these changes directly to virus invasion, replication and cell destruction.

The pathologic manifestations are therefore quite varied, reflecting not only the nature of the arbovirus but the tissue susceptibility and the physiologic and organic condition of the individual host as well.

Clinical Characteristics. Although infection with any of these viruses may involve any organ system, as manifest by a variable complex of symptoms and signs, certain antigenically differentiated types display selective proclivity for particular tissues. Such tropism and sequential manifestations of various types and phases of pathogenesis allow classification into different clinical categories. The more detailed discussion of arbovirus diseases that is presented later will follow this general classification of clinical characteristics:

1. Fever with malaise, headache, and pains of general and localized distribution
2. Fever with malaise, headache, arthralgia and rash
3. Fever with malaise, headache, general and localized pains, rash and lymphadenopathy
4. Hemorrhagic fevers
   a. Fever associated with prostration, hepatitis, nephritis, toxemia and hemorrhagic manifestations (mosquito-borne)
   b. Fever with headache, general and localized pain, prostration and hemorrhagic signs (mosquito-borne)
   c. Rodent-associated viral hemorrhagic fevers
   d. Tick-borne viral hemorrhagic fevers
   e. Primate-associated hemorrhagic fevers
5. Fever associated with central nervous system involvement ranging from meningoencephalitis to severe encephalitis with sequelae (mosquito- and tick-borne)

It is again emphasized that infection of man by any arbovirus may be subclinical or may consist of only a mild febrile episode. However, regardless of the severity, the incubation period is usually relatively short, ranging from 2 to 10 days. Onset of fever is sudden, frequently associated with headache and malaise. Symptoms of coryza and complaints of an influenza-like syndrome in its early stages do not exclude suspicion of an arbovirus infection.

Although dengue fever has long been characterized by a saddleback fever curve, this is an exception. Sustained fever is reportedly characteristic and is an important clinical differentiation from malaria, the fever usually falling by lysis in association with diminution of other clinical signs and symptoms.

The febrile phase is the period in which most recognizable associated signs appear, such as conjunctivitis, leukopenia, pleocytosis in spinal fluid and hemorrhagic complications.

Certain signs detectable by laboratory examination are reliably associated with pathogenic processes characteristic of different arboviruses. For example, those infections that depress the hematopoietic system, such as dengue and other agents producing hemorrhagic phenomena, manifest a marked leukopenia and thrombocytopenia. Meningoencephalitis and encephalitis are accompanied by a pleocytosis in the spinal fluid, initially polymorphonuclear but shifting to lymphocytic if the acute process is prolonged.

Convalescence is often noticeably slower and complete recovery longer delayed than with other types of acute infectious diseases, reflecting the systemic involvement that is characteristic of arbovirus infections. In syndromes marked by leukopenia and thrombocytopenia, there may be a mild compensatory leukocytosis following the febrile phase.

Diagnosis. While no specific treatment is available for any arbovirus disease, it is of considerable importance not only to the physician and the patient but also to the community public health to establish a definitive diagnosis. This can be done only with adequate laboratory facilities and can be established with certainty only by isolation of the causative virus and demonstration of a rise in titer of antibodies against the virus in paired acute and convalescent sera of the patient.

In the absence of such definitive results, circumstantial evidence of considerable significance can be obtained by application of a multiplicity of laboratory serologic procedures – in vitro hemagglutination-inhibition (HI), complement-fixation (CF), and neutralization (NT) tests being the most important. Because of the diversity and complexity of these test procedures, reference should be made to detailed laboratory methods and laboratory tests.[12]

Subsequent sections of this presentation deal with particular types of disease syndromes, but the approach to establishing a diagnosis is the same for all. First, attempt to isolate the virus. Second, with the isolate or other suspected etiologic agent, demonstrate the occurrence of infection by showing the development of specific antibodies in the patient's sera.

Isolation of Virus. As soon as an arbovirus etiology is suspected, a specimen of blood should be collected to inoculate for virus isolation. Because other secretions and fluids may also contain virus (possibly of a different type etiology), a throat swab, cerebrospinal fluid and stool should also be collected for examination.

If the patient dies, *substantial* portions of all organs and tissues should be collected at autopsy. These should include not only portions of all major areas of the brain – a virus may be selective for the cerebral region it invades – but also lung, spleen, liver, kidney, adrenal, myocardium, skeletal muscle and lymphatic tissue; heart blood or clot for postmortem serum should also be collected. Portions should be preserved in 10 per cent formalin for later histologic examination.

For expeditious transmission to a nearby laboratory, refrigeration on wet ice is adequate. Otherwise, the blood should be allowed to clot, cooled at 4° C (39.2° F) for clot retraction and the serum separated. Clot and serum should be frozen in separate containers to avoid hemolysis on dry ice. Some arboviruses such as that causing Colorado tick fever are adherent to the red cells, so if such a virus is suspected, the clot should be preserved and inoculated too. The postmortem tissue specimens, each in a separate sterile container, and the cerebrospinal fluid (CSF) and throat washings should also be frozen for dispatch to the laboratory.

At the laboratory the specimens should be prepared for inoculation under refrigerated conditions to minimize deterioration of any virus. The serum, CSF, throat washings and centrifugates of the tissue suspensions should each be inoculated intracerebrally into a litter of suckling mice. Even though certain tissue culture systems have been found sensitive to infection with many arboviruses, the suckling mouse remains the most comprehensively susceptible to the largest number of known arboviruses, particularly at the unknown (usually low) titer characteristic of clinical specimens.

Isolation of an arbovirus from clinical material is the exception rather than the rule for many reasons: viremia has passed, neutralizing antibody or interferon may be present, there may be loss of virus during collection and transportation to the laboratory. But the reward of such an isolation is always worth the effort, and the sooner the specimen is collected and the mouse inoculated, the better.

It should be re-emphasized here that there may be a better chance of capturing the causative virus from suspected arthropod vectors and reservoir vertebrates collected in the same area.

Illness or death of an inoculated mouse indicates the time for harvest and passage. Subsequent filtration and chemical sensitivity tests establish its nature as a filterable agent, chemically compatible with the arboviruses. Further characterization and identification involves serologic procedures similar to those used to establish development of antibody in the patient, except for the use of antigenic group and specific hyperimmune antisera for agents suspected from the history, clinical course and regional location of the case. Previous serologic surveys of human arbovirus infections in the area may be invaluable in providing such clues.

SEROLOGY. Technical details of serologic test procedures do not belong here. But consideration of the principles underlying their use and interpretation serves to direct attention of the clinician toward collecting the right specimens at the right time.

Inherent in the response to an arbovirus infection are three types of antibody: (1) Neutralizing (NT) antibody is the first to appear, early in the acute phase of the disease, rapidly rising to high titer, then declining to some extent to level off for prolonged duration, usually for life. It is the most type-specific, reacting with little cross-reaction and highest titer to the homologous infecting arbovirus. (2) Hemagglutination-inhibiting (HI) antibody appears shortly after the NT antibody and parallels its rise and early fall; it is broadly reactive with viruses antigenically related to the infecting agent and therefore can give a clue as to the type of infection in the absence of the homologous agent. Although its decline may be more precipitous and to a lower level than NT antibody, and possibly of more limited duration, it usually is detectable long after disappearance of (3) complement-fixing (CF) antibody, which appears 10 to 14 or more days after onset of the disease and increases in titer to a maximum in 1 to 2 months, following which it begins a decline that usually reaches a low or undetectable level in 1 or 2 years. Heterologous reactivity is usually much more restricted than in HI but is greater than with NT antibodies. The CF test, therefore, is useful in demonstrating an antibody titer rise later in the course of arbovirus infection. Should the homologous infecting agent not be in the test, there is often a positive reaction due to some heterologous crossing; its presence in substantial titer indicates a recent infection.

The earlier the blood is drawn in the acute illness, the better the chance of sampling a viremia leading to isolation of virus. Even if the blood has been taken too late to recover the virus, the antibody titer will be at its lowest in relation to the titer in a specimen collected 8 or more days later for demonstration of the all-important 4-fold or greater rise in titer of the specific homologous or heterologous antibody; this will establish a serologic diagnosis.

Sequential bleedings a week apart may provide serum specimens that will demonstrate a 4-fold or greater fall in titer, which is also diagnostic. If the diagnosis is suspected or if the patient is seen late in the course of illness, careful attention should be given to the spacing and collection of more than one serum specimen. (See Fig. 1–5.)

Single serum specimens collected from

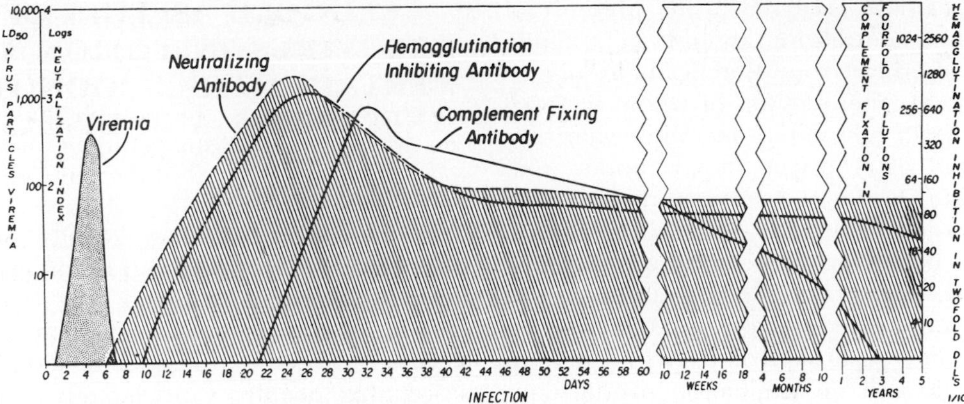

Figure 1–5. Hypothetical diagnostic features of three arbovirus infections of man.

convalescent or apparently normal household, occupational or neighborhood associates of the patient may be tested against a variety of arbovirus antigens. Such a serologic survey not only provides evidence of which agents have been active or may be indigenous to the area, but the complement-fixation titers indicate how recently the virus may have been disseminated. This is particularly important in trying to detect arboviruses that may be causing febrile illness in children living in a tropical environment.

Once having determined a specific diagnosis in one or more patients, the serologic survey will provide information on the percentage of susceptibles, the geographic distribution of those already infected and what the incidence of inapparent infection may be—all important facts for intelligent handling of public health control and prevention.

Prophylaxis. Identification of the primary vector to man or that which serves the natural maintenance cycle, and detailed definition of its bionomics, provide information essential for effective vector control measures. This is by far the most important long-term and emergency effort toward prevention of arbovirus transmission.

Vector control measures vary according to the type and behavior of the arthropod transmitter. They may include well engineered environmental sanitation to eliminate such vectors as the *Culex pipiens* complex, use of an interior adulticide to control *Aedes aegypti,* mosquito nets to protect against sylvan vectors or use of protective clothing and repellents to prevent tick infestation.

Although vaccination for yellow fever with attenuated 17D has proved successful in the prevention of sylvan and urban yellow fever, it is obvious that arboviruses are too numerous to rely on vaccine prophylaxis among those most exposed environmentally or occupationally. Nevertheless, formalin-inactivated virus vaccines for Russian spring-summer encephalitis and Japanese B encephalitis have been prepared and administered to large numbers of people, and beneficial results have been reported. However, the time required for development of adequate immunity precludes their effective use in an epidemic.

Experimental attenuated arbovirus vaccines for special situations are under development. That for Venezuelan equine encephalitis has too high a reaction rate for general use. That for western equine encephalitis has been tried only in horses. Those for dengue require still further evaluation in regard to heterologous protection in the light of recent characterization of a multiplicity of dengue types. The utility of a broad spectrum immunization scheme for antigenic group protection remains to be proved in man. Its general utility is doubtful and not only because it is a complex procedure. Multiple infections with Group B arboviruses have occurred in the presence of high titer neutralizing antibody to a multiplicity of other Group B antigens.

Finally, the question of whom to vaccinate, when, how often and with what type and kind of arbovirus vaccine under what conditions brings the realization that vaccination for a multiplicity of arbovirus infections is not likely to become a prophylactic panacea. Primary efforts continue to be directed toward vector control. Only continuation and expansion of the virologic, entomologic and epidemiologic investigations will enlarge the useful knowledge necessary to evaluate and control a rapidly increasing number of arbovirus and associated zoonotic diseases.

CLINICAL ASPECTS OF ARBOVIRUS INFECTION AND CERTAIN OTHER ZOONOTIC INFECTIONS AND DISEASES OF MAN

Ecologic rather than zonally defined geographic factors are the predominant influence governing occurrence of arbovirus disease. Endemic foci shift. Epidemic excursions periodically project into societies of susceptible people. Consequently, an adequate clinical consideration of disease caused by what have often been called the tropical viruses entails a comprehensive presentation of all those known to produce human dis-

Table 1–1. Fever with Malaise, Headache and Pains of General and Localized Distribution

Virus	*Serologic Group*	*Vector*	*Known Geographic Range of Infection*
Mucambo	A	Mosquito	Brazil (Pará) São Paulo, Surinam, French Guiana, Trinidad
Kunjin	B	Mosquito	Northern (tropical) Australia, Sarawak, Borneo
Sepik	B	Mosquito	New Guinea
Banzi	B	Mosquito	South Africa, Rhodesia, Mozambique
Spondweni	B	Mosquito	South Africa, Mozambique, Nigeria, United Republic of Cameroon
Wesselsbron	B	Mosquito	South Africa, Bechuanaland, Rhodesia, United Republic of Cameroon, Nigeria
Zika	B	Mosquito	Uganda, Nigeria, C. African Republic, Malaya
Bussuquara	B	Mosquito	Brazil (Pará), Colombia, Panama
Rio Bravo	B	Probably none but vertebrate (bat)	California, New Mexico, Texas, Southwestern North America
Apeu	C	Mosquito	Brazil (Pará)
Caraparu	C	Mosquito	Brazil, Panama, Surinam, French Guiana, Trinidad
Itaqui	C	Mosquito	Brazil (Pará)
Madrid	C	Mosquito	Panama
Marituba	C	Mosquito	Brazil (Pará)
Murutucu	C	Mosquito	Brazil (Pará), French Guiana
Oriboca	C	Mosquito	Brazil (Pará), Surinam, French Guiana, Trinidad
Ossa	C	Mosquito	Panama
Restan	C	Mosquito	Surinam, Trinidad
Calovo (Batai)	Bunyamwera	Mosquito	Czechoslovakia, Austria, Yugoslavia
Germiston	Bunyamwera	Mosquito	South Africa, Angola, Rhodesia, Mozambique, Uganda
Ilesha	Bunyamwera	Mosquito	Nigeria, United Republic of Cameroon, C. African Republic, Uganda, Ghana

ease. Under sections titled according to the previous outline of clinical characteristics, the arboviruses associated with different predominant syndromes have been organized into tables that also list the type of vector, the serologic group (which may assist in laboratory diagnosis) and the known geographic range of infection (Table 1–1).

The arthropod vectors have been listed in the tables not only to assist in eliciting an appropriate history of exposure to arthropod bite but to emphasize that the etiologic virus which will most frequently establish a serologic diagnosis is most often isolated from arthropod vectors collected in the locality.

Significant or pathognomonic etiologic, epidemiologic, clinical, pathologic, diagnostic and prophylactic features are mentioned under these headings in each section as a guide to the differentials in a categorical clinical syndrome that may help the physician and public health worker in recognizing and dealing effectively with a specific etiologic entity.

FEVER WITH MALAISE, HEADACHE AND PAINS OF GENERAL AND LOCALIZED DISTRIBUTION

Etiology and Epidemiology. Although it has long been generally accepted that

Table 1–1. FEVER WITH MALAISE, HEADACHE AND PAINS OF GENERAL AND LOCALIZED DISTRIBUTION

Virus	*Serologic Group*	*Vector*	*Known Geographic Range of Infection*
Guaroa	Bunyamwera	Mosquito	Colombia, Brazil, Panama
Inkoo	California	Mosquito	Finland
Tahyna	California	Mosquito	France, Czechoslovakia, Yugoslavia, Italy, Germany, Austria, U.S.S.R., Kenya, Mozambique
Guama	Guama	Mosquito	Brazil (Pará), Trinidad, Surinam, French Guiana
Catu	Guama	Mosquito	Brazil (Pará), Trinidad, French Guiana
Oropouche	Simbu	Mosquito	Brazil, Trinidad
Bwamba	Bwamba	Mosquito	Uganda, Nigeria, C. African Republic
Zinga	Ungrouped	Mosquito	Republic of Congo
Phlebotomus, Naples	Phlebotomus	*Phlebotomus* (sandfly)	Italy, Egypt, Iran, Pakistan
Phlebotomus, Sicilian	Phlebotomus	*Phlebotomus* (sandfly)	Italy, Egypt, Iran, Pakistan
Chagres	Phlebotomus	Mosquito	Panama
Candiru	Phlebotomus	?	Brazil (Pará)
Punta Toro	Phlebotomus	*Lutzomyia*	Panama
Vesicular stomatitis (Indiana)	VSV	*Lutzomyia* (sandfly) Mosquito	United States, Mexico, Costa Rica, Panama, Venezuela, Colombia, Ecuador, Peru
Chandipura	VSV	*Phlebotomus*	India, Nigeria
Piry	VSV	?	Brazil (Pará)
Ganjam*	Ganjam	Hard tick	India
Dugbe	Ganjam	Hard tick	Nigeria, C. African Republic
Kemerovo	Kemerovo	Hard tick	Western Siberia, Egypt
Quaranfil	Quaranfil	Soft tick	Egypt, South Africa
Colorado tick fever	Ungrouped	Hard tick	Western United States
Nairobi sheep disease	Ungrouped	Hard tick	Kenya, Uganda

*Recent serologic results suggest that Ganjam virus may be a strain of Nairobi sheep disease virus.

culicine genera are the mosquito vectors of arboviruses—in contrast to anophelines for malaria—accumulating experimental and field data show that there is a definable diversity of selective replication plasm in a variety of not only mosquito genera but other arthropods as well. Bwamba virus and many of the Bunyamwera group viruses were either originally isolated from anopheline mosquitoes or shown to be primarily transmitted by them.

The sandfly fever complex, occurring in at least three continents, involves as different a dipteran vector as the hard and soft tick vectors of other febrile disease viruses. These vector variations are the key to the epidemiology and distribution of the variety of arboviruses that cause disease of such obscure clinical differences that no specific etiologic agent can confidently be assumed on clinical grounds alone. That is why the clinician must consider aspects of geographic range, ecologic association and observable vectors in seeking a diagnosis. (See Table 1–1.)

Clinical Characteristics. A number of these infections are known only by one or a few cases, often etiologically established too late to permit definitive clinical laboratory studies. But a third of those listed, which is a substantial number of those studied in sufficient clinical detail, are associated with significant, sometimes marked, leukopenia. Conjunctival inflammation and unduly severe and prolonged prostration, with slow convalescence, are clinical clues that point toward an arbovirus infection. This type of infection often contrasts strikingly to the rapid response and recovery from bacterial and parasitic infections for which there is specific chemotherapy.

Because of the relatively mild and self-limited nature of this group of arbovirus infections, some experimental exposure of human volunteers and laboratory infections have been studied in detail. One of these, sandfly fever, is characteristic. It has an incubation period averaging 3 to 4 days, but that may be as long as 9 days. There is a sudden onset of headache and fever followed by burning and pain in the eyes associated with conjunctival inflammation. This is followed by malaise, generalized pain and anorexia, nausea and vomiting associated with severe prostration for the febrile period, which may last as long as 9 days. There may also be a relative bradycardia following the acute onset.

Other infections may occur as the result of laboratory exposure.[13] More than 350 such arbovirus infections have been documented, many of them with viruses listed here. A history of laboratory exposure is important to elicit. One disease, vesicular stomatitis, Indiana type, has resulted from laboratory exposure but also from handling or contact with diseased animals which have vesicular lesions or crusts. Isolations of this virus have been reported from arthropods and there is growing evidence of natural transmission by phlebotomine sandflies in some situations.

Treatment. Treatment is symptomatic: analgesics for headache and pain, antipyretics for the fever. Bed rest and supportive treatment such as maintenance of proper hydration and nutrition may shorten the course of convalescence. Protection of the patient from arthropod bite early in the acute stage, when a viremia may be present, may abort further dissemination of the virus.

Prophylaxis. There are no vaccines for these arboviruses. Detection of the arthropod vector and expeditious introduction of vector control measures are the only really effective protection.

FEVER WITH MALAISE, HEADACHE, ARTHRALGIA AND RASH

Etiology and Epidemiology. The divergent virus vector identities producing a similar clinical disease are noted here by the phlebotomine-borne Changuinola virus appearing as the cause of a syndrome belonging predominantly to mosquito-borne Group A arboviruses. Uruma virus from the Bolivian Amazonia is so closely related antigenically to Mayaro that it is now considered a strain of the latter (Table 1–2).

The extensive but scattered recognition

Table 1–2. Fever with Malaise, Headache, Arthralgia and Rash

Virus	*Serologic Group*	*Vector*	*Known Geographic Range of Infection*
Ross River	A	Mosquito	Queensland, New South Wales, Victoria, Australia
Mayaro	A	Mosquito	Brazil, Trinidad
Sindbis	A	Mosquito	South and East Africa, Egypt, Israel, India, Malaya, Philippines, Australia
Chikungunya	A	Mosquito	South, East, Central and West Africa, India, Thailand, Malaya
O'nyong-nyong	A	Mosquito	East Africa and Senegal
Bunyamwera	Bunyamwera	Mosquito	South, East and West Africa
Changuinola	Changuinola	*Lutzomyia*	Panama

of chikungunya and Sindbis fevers from Africa through South Asia to Australasia indicates the probability that these viruses and the diseases they cause will be described from many more localities in that vast range if considered frequently enough by physicians and diagnostic laboratories (Table 1–2). Ross River virus, which is the cause of epidemic polyarthritis in Australia, appears to be an antigenically related complex of viruses with local enzootic foci from which they seasonally emerge in epidemic excursions transmitted by a variety of culicine mosquitoes.

It is notable that o'nyong-nyong virus is another that in its extensive epidemic manifestations in East Africa was transmitted by man-biting *Anopheles funestus* and *A. gambiae.* The bionomics of these anophelines was doubtless responsible for distribution of the disease and the remarkable dynamics of its epidemic movement. Antigenically very similar to culicine-transmitted chikungunya virus, this difference in vectors is probably the most significant factor in the epidemiologic variations in the two diseases.

Clinical Characteristics. Leukopenia associated with an acute onset, followed by arthralgia or rash or both, is as clear a clinical orientation toward an etiology by one of these arboviruses as a clinician can have, particularly if the geographic and ecologic association is correct. The predominant role of Group A arboviruses in the causation of this febrile arthralgia/rash syndrome might ultimately require reclassification of Kunjin virus from Table 1–1 to these other Group A agents.

A disease called epidemic polyarthritis, associated with marked pain in the joints, occurred in the Murray Valley of Australia in 1956. It was subsequently serologically shown to be caused by infection with Ross River virus, which has been responsible for epidemic polyarthritis in widely separated localities in Australia.

Treatment. Treatment should be symptomatic, with the use of analgesics and antipyretics and maintenance of hydration and nutrition. Management should include measurement of fluid intake and output and careful correction of fluctuations in hydration and electrolyte balance, which will be discussed later.

Prophylaxis. No vaccine exists for any of these agents. Selective vector control and protection from mosquito bite are most important.

FEVER WITH MALAISE, HEADACHE, GENERAL AND LOCALIZED PAINS, RASH AND LYMPHADENOPATHY

Etiology and Epidemiology. West Nile virus is the Afro-Asian member of the Japanese B–West Nile complex of arbovirus Group B. Millions of human infections have been experienced from the western Mediterranean and North Africa, South and East Africa, and through the Middle East to the Bay of Bengal Coast of India, and possibly as far as Borneo (Table 1–3, Fig. 1–3). The distribution is environmentally dependent on cyclic association of West Nile virus with a wild avian host cycle maintained by transmission by various *Culex* mosquitoes, i.e. *Culex theileri* in South Africa, *C. univittatus* and *C. antennatus* in Egypt, *C. molestus* in Israel. Epidemiologic behavior of the disease ranges from high attack rates in infant residents of the Nile Delta, where it occurs as an endemo-epidemic disease in June or July through September of each year, to significant attack rates in all ages in north European immigrants into Israel in almost annual summer epidemics. Elsewhere it appears to infect early in life, producing a preponderantly immune adult population.

Dengue viruses are believed to be transmitted exclusively by *Aedes* mosquitoes, which are found scattered in different ecologic and urban habitats throughout and beyond the West Nile virus–infected regions. Although a number of *Aedes* species have been demonstrated experimentally to be potential dengue vectors, only urban *Aedes aegypti,* sylvan *A. albopictus* and urbosylvan *A. polynesiensis* in Oceania have been strongly implicated as vectors of dengue.

Although there is evidence that dengue antibodies occur in wild primates in Malaya and in bats in tropical Australia, there is no proof of a vertebrate reservoir other than that manifest by the man-*Aedes*-man cycle which has been repeatedly or continually observed in sporadic, endemic and epidemic appearance of dengue virus activity throughout the tropical world, wherever *Aedes aegypti* or closely related species become prevalent (Tables 1–3, 1–4). For almost 3 years (1963 to 1966) epidemic dengue moved from Jamaica eastward through Puerto Rico and southward along the Lesser Antilles Islands to the Paria Peninsula of eastern Venezuela, and thence westward along the South American coast. The singular absence of dengue from Trinidad, where *Aedes aegypti* mosquitoes have been eradicated, is a clear example of protection against human dengue by the elimination of the historic vector.

Dengue now appears to be endemic in many urban *Aedes aegypti*–infested localities in the Caribbean area as a manifestation of failure in eradication of or reinfestation by *Aedes aegypti.* The disease has erupted frequently in South American and Caribbean countries in the past few years. An estimated several hundred thousand cases clinically and epidemiologically compatible with dengue were experienced on the Caribbean coastal plain of Colombia in late 1971 and early 1972, and sporadic outbreaks documented as dengue-2 have been occurring in Puerto Rico from 1969 to the present (1975). Dengue has been considered such a continuous problem by the Pan American Health Organization that a special committee has

Table 1–3. Fever with Malaise, Headache, General and Localized Pains, Rash and Lymphadenopathy

Virus	*Serologic Group*	*Vector*	*Known Geographic Range of Infection*
West Nile	B	Mosquito	In Africa: From South and West Africa to Suez; In Europe: Rhone River Delta and other parts of the Mediterranean littoral to the near East; In Asia: Israel, India, Malaysia, Borneo
Dengue-1	B	Mosquito	Hawaii, Oceania, New Guinea, Japan, Malaysia, Thailand, India
Dengue-2	B	Mosquito	Circumglobal in *Aedes aegypti*–infested areas of tropics
Dengue-3	B	Mosquito	Caribbean, Oceania, Philippines, Thailand
Dengue-4	B	Mosquito	Philippines, Thailand, India

been established to monitor the extent, intensity and type of dengue virus infection.[14] There is apprehension that increasingly frequent outbreaks of different types of dengue will result in dengue hemorrhagic fever similar to the disease that has spread through Southeast Asia in the past 20 years.

Because of the antigenic variety in the dengue complex, the epidemiologic behavior of dengue disease is often perplexing. For instance, dengue-4 produces disease annually in South India, while dengue-2 occurs only occasionally.

Sporadic cases occur in persons who take up residence in an *Aedes*-infected area. Infant or childhood dengue occurs when natives are environmentally exposed to endemic *Aedes*-transmitted dengue. All ages may be attacked in areas in which epidemiologic factors favor periodic introduction of new antigenic types of dengue. Such a phenomenon was observed in the 1963–1964 Caribbean dengue epidemic in which an antigenically new type of dengue (3) swept through all age groups in Jamaica, Puerto Rico, the Virgin Islands and on to northern South America, an area in which there was substantial prior immunity to dengue-2.

This explains why dengue is an ever-present threat wherever human-feeding *Aedes* mosquitoes are present. Explosive epidemics occur when large numbers of nonimmune persons are moved into localities endemic for dengue, as in military operations in the Pacific or, more recently, the sending of Peace Corps and other civilian officials into many tropical countries in support of various assistance programs. Vacationers who suffer a febrile illness after return to their temperate zone homes from a sojourn in tropical America should be thoroughly checked for the diagnosis of dengue.

Clinical Characteristics. West Nile virus infection, occasionally referred to as Mediterranean dengue during World War II and more recently epidemic among north European immigrants in Israel, in almost all cases falls within the clinical range of classic dengue. More than one-third of West Nile fever patients manifest a denguelike rash. West Nile virus infection of the aged may result in severe or fatal encephalitis, indistinguishable from St. Louis or Japanese B encephalitis. If geographic location of such a case leads to suspicion of West Nile virus as the etiology of an arbovirus encephalitis, the description and discussion of the diseases listed in Table 1–6 will prove more pertinent and useful.

The dengue syndrome is perhaps the most widespread tropical arbovirus disease, having been the subject of some of the most intensive clinical studies of natural and experimental infection in man. According to Sabin's detailed description, the usual incubation period is from 5 to 8 days, with a range of from 2½ to 15 days, depending upon the amount of virus introduced. Headache, backache, fatigue, stiffness, anorexia, chilliness, malaise and occasionally rash may appear 6 to 12 hours before the first rise in temperature. In about half the patients the onset is sudden, with a sharp rise in temperature, severe headache, pain behind the eyes, backache, pain in the muscles and joints, and chilliness, but only rarely a shaking chill. Fever persists for 5 to 6 days in typical cases and usually terminates by crisis. A saddleback or diphasic type of temperature curve is seen in some patients with dengue but is not observed in the majority and cannot be regarded as pathognomonic. Anorexia and constipation are common, and epigastric discomfort with colicky pain and abnormal tenderness of the abdomen may be seen. Altered taste sensation also constitutes a common symptom early in the disease. Marked weakness and dizziness, photophobia, drenching sweats, sore throat, cough, epistaxis, dysuria, hyperesthesia of the skin, pain in the groin and testicles, and delirium are occasionally encountered. The lymph nodes are frequently enlarged, the spleen only rarely. Nuchal rigidity is absent even when the patient complains of a stiff neck.

A rash usually appears on the third to the fifth day and rarely lasts for more than 3 or 4 days. It is usually maculopapular, fading on pressure; occasionally it may be scarlatiniform. Although it is usually first seen on the chest, trunk and abdomen, as shown in Figure 1–6, it eventually spreads to the

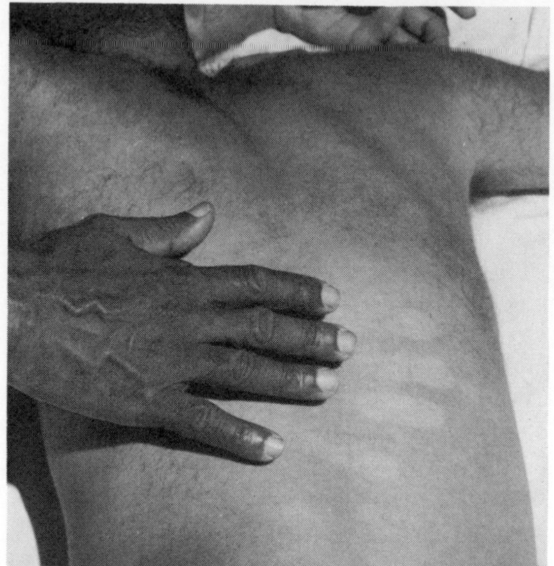

Figure 1–6. Pressure blanching of erythematous, macular rash of dengue. (Courtesy of Dr. Telford H. Work.)

extremities and frequently to the face. On the last day of fever, or shortly after defervescence, another type of eruption occurs in many patients. This consists of small petechiae over the dorsum of the feet and legs and occasionally also in the axillae, over the dorsum of the wrists, hands and fingers, and on the buccal mucosa and hard and soft palates.

An example of the characteristic changes in the leukocytes is shown in Figure 1–7. The most marked leukopenia occurs several days after onset of fever and is the result of a diminution in the neutrophils. The blood picture, as a rule, returns to normal within a week after defervescence.

Classic dengue is not fatal but may be temporarily incapacitating because of fever and pain, hence its importance as a tropical disease among military forces. Otherwise, sporadic cases occur as a painful annoyance sufficient to focus attention on the feasibility and advisability of eliminating the *Aedes aegypti* vector by well established means.

Diagnosis. Because of difficulties encountered in adapting most strains and types of dengue virus to a laboratory detection system, such as illness and death in suckling mice inoculated intracerebrally with acute blood serum, diagnosis is seldom established by virus isolation. It sometimes requires a number of passages in suckling mice to obtain a repeatable mortality. A new technique developed by Rosen amplifies dengue virus titer by inoculation of mosquitoes and subsequent identification by fluorescent antibody or tissue culture techniques.[15]

A more specific serologic diagnosis may be accomplished by demonstration of a rise in titer in two or more serial acute and convalescent sera by HI, CF and NT tests against all four types of dengue virus. Because of close antigenic relationships, the specific dengue type can only be suggested, particularly in patients possessing antibodies resulting from prior infection with a group B arbovirus, including 17D vaccination for yellow fever.

Although diagnosis of most cases will be on clinical grounds, it is important to establish a virologic diagnosis when suspected cases occur where *Aedes aegypti* mosquitoes are prevalent or when representatives of a nonimmune population assigned to work or live in such an area report clinical illness suggestive of classic dengue.

Treatment. There is no antiviral treatment. Maintenance of hydration, relief of pain by analgesics and diminution of fever by antipyretics are the basic measures for lessening the misery of a patient suffering from the dengue syndrome. Careful observation and management of such infections in an area where hemorrhagic dengue has been known to occur may prevent progression of patients into hemorrhagic complications or shock. This entails monitoring hemorrhagic phenomena such as tourniquet test and hematocrit level as described on pages 28 to 31. Good nursing may be critically important when classic dengue is first recognized in such an area.

Prophylaxis and Control. Experimental attenuated live virus vaccines for dengue types 1 and 2 have been tried, resulting in some success. However, the usual unpredictable distribution and occurrence by age and

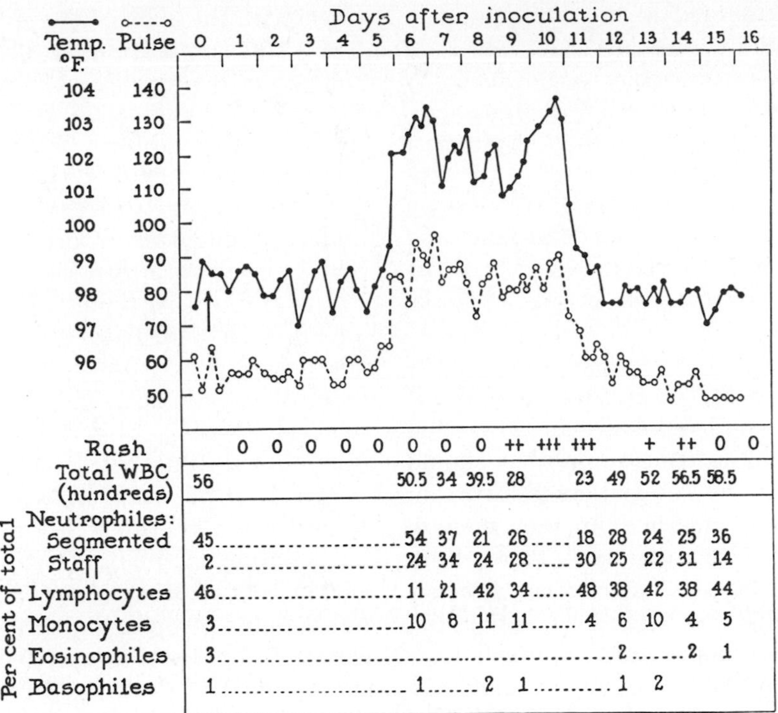

Figure 1–7. Graphic representation of temperature and pulse rate of a human volunteer inoculated experimentally with the Hawaiian strain of dengue virus by means of the bites of eight infected *Aedes aegypti* mosquitoes; arrow indicates day on which the patient was bitten. Time of appearance of rash is also indicated, as well as total and differential blood counts. (Sabin, A. B. 1959. *In* Rivers, T. M., and Horsfall, F. L., Jr.: Viral and Rickettsial Infections of Man. 3rd ed. J. B. Lippincott Co., Philadelphia. Used by permission of the National Foundation.)

locality make routine use questionable, except in such personnel as the military when operations are anticipated in an area of high risk. Some persons suffer a mild febrile reaction following vaccination. The vaccine is not commercially available.

Practical measures of protection from *Aedes aegypti* bite in urban areas by repellents and proper clothing, screened windows or mosquito nets over beds must be provided when effective efforts cannot be made to eliminate the species from the household, the community or even the nation by well documented mosquitocidal and sanitary methods. An insecticide, Abate, has been demonstrated effective in inhibiting stored water container breeding of *A. aegypti.* Technology has been developed for aerial spraying of ultra low volume malathion for extensive urban mosquito control. While this is expensive, those are situations where such application may be worth the cost.

THE HEMORRHAGIC FEVERS

Except for military authorities of eastern Europe and eastern Asia, the hemorrhagic fevers were largely unknown until 2 decades ago. The United Nations troop encounter with hemorrhagic nephrosonephritis in Korea late in 1951 stimulated a search for knowledge of the Russian and Japanese encounters with this disease in eastern Siberia and Manchuria in preliminary episodes of World War II.[16] This exposed two other diseases in the Soviet Union, tick-borne Crimean and Omsk hemorrhagic fevers, which are interesting associated subjects in geographic pathology that had been elucidated in 1942 and 1948 by Soviet investigators.[17]

Discovery of tick-borne Kyasanur Forest disease in India in 1957 brought into perspective a global complex of diseases that included dengue hemorrhagic fever, first clinically documented in the Philippines in 1954, Argentinian hemorrhagic fever in 1955 and Bolivian hemorrhagic fever in 1962. Then *Aedes aegypti*–borne dengue hemorrhagic fever spread through Southeast Asia, Marburg disease associated with African green monkeys exploded in German pharmaceutical facilities in Marburg and Frankfurt in 1967,[18] and Lassa fever began its West African devastation at Jos, Nigeria, early in 1969.

This array of hemorrhagic diseases displays a variety of geographic, pathologic, epidemiologic and etiologic features that convey some basic conclusions that should alert physicians and researchers to a current transience of confidence in our medical knowledge of virus diseases (Table 1–4). Some of these entities have been characterized as virus diseases because of application of modern virologic and epidemiologic methodology. Others are new human diseases due to new ecologic associations incurred either by changing human habitat and agricultural practices, or by the shifting nature of viral pathogens. Still others are the result of human-caused acceleration of vector-borne virus infections. The resulting implications are 2-fold: (1) viral hemorrhagic diseases will erupt in new geographic situations, and (2) it is likely that new viral hemorrhagic fevers are yet to be described. For these reasons it is as important to understand the varied etiology and epidemiology of all as it is to direct a course of inquiry and examination that will establish the etiology of one already described.

FEVER ASSOCIATED WITH PROSTRATION, HEPATITIS, NEPHRITIS, TOXEMIA AND HEMORRHAGIC MANIFESTATIONS (MOSQUITO-BORNE)

Etiology and Epidemiology. Yellow fever was the first recognized and elucidated arbovirus disease of the tropics.[19] It is the classic hemorrhagic fever. Yellow fever remains the most dramatic, serious arbovirus disease of the tropics. In spite of development and application of prophylactic vaccines in tens of millions of people, and the control and eradication of *Aedes aegypti* in many countries of the New World, sylvan and epidemic yellow fever have continued to occur within, and adjacent to, the recognized endemic yellow fever areas of Africa and South and Central America.

A progressive epidemic began in Panama in late 1948. During the following decade it progressed through Central America to southern Mexico. There have been epidemics in eastern Nigeria, a Sudanese outbreak in the Blue Nile region, and a severe outbreak in adjacent areas of southwestern Ethiopia in 1960 to 1962.

Routine vaccination was stopped in Senegal in 1960, resulting in an accumulation of nonimmune people, primarily children. An explosive epidemic erupted in 1965 in the center of that country, threatening extension to adjacent West African territory where yellow fever vaccination has also been less rigorously applied in recent years.

Simultaneously, in the vast areas of continental South America where the mosquito–nonhuman primate cycle continues natural maintenance of yellow fever transmission, hundreds of cases of human sylvan yellow fever have been reported. Cases and deaths were reported from the Paraná River regions of Paraguay, Brazil and Argentina in 1966. Almost annually fatal cases of yellow fever have been reported from Peru, Colombia and Venezuela. There has been a resurgence of sylvan yellow fever in Ecuador in 1975 due to opening of eastern regions of the country to oil exploitation. The disease has periodically recurred in Bolivia and Venezuela, and sylvan yellow fever reappeared in eastern Panama in 1974. Sporadic human deaths from yellow fever, such as occurred in Uganda, and scattered epidemics reported from the Congo are further testimony that yellow fever is still not under very comprehensive control. Although yellow fever can be controlled by quarantine, the changing political and social conditions in the tropics of Africa and the New World permit it to remain a major medical problem. It will continue to appear, often unexpectedly, in a number of places.

Being the prototype of all arboviruses, the antigenic group to which yellow fever virus belongs has been given the generic name *flavivirus.* Its nucleocapsid is formed on the endocytoplasmic reticulum. It is a togavirus about 40 nm in diameter with a lipid coat sensitive to inactivation by diethyl ether and deoxycholic acid.

The spherical virus particles are found free in the cytoplasm of the salivary glands of infectious *Aedes aegypti* mosquitoes after an extrinsic incubation period of 10 or more days, depending upon the ambient temperature. The mosquito infects the primate host during ingestion of blood. After an eclipse phase a viremia develops. The virus is present in blood of a sick primate or man for at least 3 days after onset of disease signs.

An increasing variety of etiologic entities are being characterized as hemorrhagic fever. Because they are clinically indistinguishable in many respects from classic forms of yellow fever, this disease warrants special consideration here. In fact, a proper evaluation of the clinical, pathologic and diagnostic criteria characterizes yellow fever as one of the hemorrhagic fevers.

Human infection results from two basically different cycles of virus transmission, *urban* and *sylvan.* The urban cycle is the simple man-mosquito-man, *Aedes aegypti*–transmitted yellow fever described for more than 3 centuries in tropical and summer temperate port city epidemics in West Africa and the New World. Because of recent extensive control and eradication of *Aedes aegypti*, the urban mosquito vector has limited and scattered distribution, particularly in countries of the Western Hemisphere. However, in areas such as the southeastern United States where *A. aegypti* continues to breed, introduction of a viremic case in a human or other primate is a potential source of infection to the classic vector. After a 1- to 2-week extrinsic incubation period, such mosquitoes can initiate infection of secondary and subsequent cases, leading to epidemic urban yellow fever. To eliminate this threat and that of reinfestation of areas in the Caribbean from which it has been eradicated, a major effort to eradicate *Aedes aegypti* from United States territory was initiated in 1964, but budget cuts in 1968 terminated the effort within the United States in 1969.

Sylvan yellow fever differs according to the ecologic situation. In the rain forests of South America, species of tree top *Haemagogus* mosquitoes maintain transmission in wild primate epizootics. The incidence of overt disease and death depends on species susceptibility of the monkeys involved. Howler (*Alouatta* sp.) and spider (*Ateles* sp.) monkeys have a high case fatality rate producing extensive epizootic deaths in sylvan areas when yellow fever strikes through canopy mosquito transmission. *Cebus* monkeys, on the other hand, rarely succumb to sylvan yellow fever.

Once infected, the mosquito vector remains infectious for life. It therefore may serve as an effective reservoir as well as a vector. In the intermittently dry forest areas in parts of Central America, survival of durable *Sabethes* mosquitoes is proposed as an explanation of the progressive but pulsating extension of sylvan yellow fever through the jungle primate population of that geographic area. It is when human invasion of the forest or human-directed change in the terrain brings man in juxtaposition with the otherwise remote tree top *Haemagogus* and *Sabethes* mosquitoes that the sporadic or clustered cases of sylvan yellow fever occur in Latin America.

In East Africa the mosquito-primate cycle is maintained by a forest canopy mosquito, *Aedes africanus,* that is not known to feed upon man with sufficient frequency to transmit yellow fever to human populations. However, some of the infected primates, as viremic raiders of semisylvan African village gardens, are fed upon by *Aedes simpsoni.* After an appropriate extrinsic incubation period, this peridomestic village mosquito transmits the virus to garden cultivators or village hut dwellers, and thence from person to person.

The apparent low occurrence of overt disease in East African village populations that possess serologic evidence of high in-

Table 1–4. AN EPIDEMIOLOGIC CLASSIFICATION OF THE HEMORRHAGIC FEVERS

Category	*Disease*	*Virus*	*Abbreviation*	*Antigenic Group*	*Vector*	*Reservoir*	*Geographic Distribution*
Mosquito-borne	Yellow Fever	Yellow Fever	YF	Flavivirus YF-Den Complex of Group B	Urban *Aedes aegypti* Sylvan Neotropical *Haemagogus* spp. *Sabethes chloropterus* Ethiopian *Aedes africanus* *Aedes simpsoni*	Urban *Homo sapiens* Sylvan Neotropical *Cebus* spp. *Ateles* spp. *Alouatta* spp. Ethiopian *Cercopithecus* spp. *Colobus* spp.	Tropical Central and South America, Tropical Africa
	Dengue HF Dengue shock syndrome	Dengue-1 Dengue-2 Dengue-3 Dengue-4	DEN-1 DEN-2 DEN-3 DEN-4	Flavivirus YF–DEN Complex of Group B	Urban *Aedes aegypti* Rural *Aedes albopictus*	Urban *Homo sapiens* Sylvan Other primates not proved	Philippines, Vietnam, Thailand, Malaysia, Indonesia, Burma, India, South Pacific Islands
Tick-borne	OMSK HF	OMSK HF	OMSK	Flavivirus RSS Complex of Group B	*Dermacentor pictus* *D. marginatus* *D. silvarum* *Ixodes persulcatus* *Haemaphysalis concinna*	*Ondatra zibetica*	Western Siberia
	Kyasanur Forest disease	Kyasanur Forest disease	KFD	Flavivirus RSS Complex of Group B	*Haemaphysalis spinigera* *H. turturis* *H.* spp. *Ixodes petaurista* *I.* spp.	*Presbytis entellus* *Macaca radiata* *Rattus r. wroughtoni* *R. blanfordi* *Suncus murinus*	Mysore, India

	Crimean HF	Crimean HF	CHF	CONGO	*Hyalomma marginatum* *H. anatolicum* *Boophilus microplus*	Small mammals Cattle	Bulgaria, U.S.S.R. Pakistan
			CON	CONGO	*Hyalomma anatolicum* *H. marginatum* *H. rufipes* *H. truncatum* *Amblyomma variegatum* *Boophilus decoloratus*	Cattle	Nigeria, Zaire, Uganda
Rodent-associated	Argentinian HF	Junin	JUN	Tacaribe of Arenaviruses	*Calomys laucha* *C. musculinus* Contact/Excreta	*Calomys laucha* *C. musculinus*	Buenos Aires, Córdoba, Santa Fe Provinces of Argentina
	Bolivian HF	Machupo	MAC	Tacaribe of Arenaviruses	*Calomys callosus* Contact/Excreta	*Calomys callosus*	El Beni, Santa Cruz Departments of Bolivia
	Lassa fever		LAS	Tacaribe of Arenaviruses	*Mastomys natalensis* *Homo sapiens* Contact/Excreta	*Mastomys natalensis*	Jos Plain, Nigeria, Sierra Leone, Liberia, West Africa
	Korean HF	KHF (?) Unknown	KHF	Unknown	Unknown	Epidemiologically associated with *Clethrionomys* sp. *Apodemus* sp.	European U.S.S.R. Primorye, U.S.S.R. (See Chapter 4)
Monkey-associated	Marburg fever		MAR	Ungrouped	*Cercopithecus aethiops* Secretions, blood, tissues	*Cercopithecus aethiops*	Uganda, Rhodesia, East Africa

cidence of inapparent infection may reflect a racial factor of resistance to yellow fever. However, the devastating epidemics in the Sudan and in Ethiopia do not bear out the refractory susceptibility of all Africans. There may be as yet undefined variations in virulence between strains of yellow fever virus that do not have detectable antigenic differences.

Why yellow fever has never invaded Asia where there is widespread distribution of man-biting *Aedes aegypti* mosquitoes, which transmit other arboviruses such as dengue and chikungunya to millions of people, has not been satisfactorily explained. The development of related antibody by endemic and epidemic occurrence of other Group B arbovirus infections does not seem to be an adequate explanation. Several dengue and even West Nile and Japanese B encephalitis virus infections sometimes occur in the same individual. There are also large, exposed, apparently susceptible populations that are devoid of immunity to any Group B arbovirus.

In spite of quarantine practices and immunization requirements of various Asian nations, the country boat traffic across the Arabian Sea and accelerating air travel must periodically introduce infected *Aedes aegypti* and viremic persons into *Aedes aegypti*–infected environments. The occurrence of a clinically similar hemorrhagic fever, tick-borne Group B arbovirus Kyasanur Forest disease, has emphasized the catastrophic potential for, but continued absence of, yellow fever in India. A sixth of the world's human population, essentially nonimmune to yellow fever, seems oblivious to the disease that threatens millions living in similar tropical situations in Africa and Latin America.

While severity may vary according to age, in an unimmunized population all age groups are afflicted. Epidemic yellow fever is being recognized more frequently in children, particularly in West Africa, as a result of the decline in active yellow fever immunization programs. Therefore, yellow fever should be suspected in cases of hepatitis, hemorrhagic disease or fever of undetermined etiology in these geographic regions of Africa. There are a number of clinicopathologic similarities of Rift Valley fever of East Africa that favor its differential consideration when yellow fever is suspected in that geographic area. This is because Rift Valley fever is a sylvan infection in an endemic area where observations of yellow fever as a human disease are sporadic and often obscure.

What is known about the clinical manifestations of Rift Valley fever stems from cases occurring as a result of field examination of infected animals or laboratory exposure to the virus. Evidence of liver involvement and necrosis in Rift Valley fever, and its widespread occurrence in an *Aedes*–wild animal cycle in East Africa, requires its consideration here. In spite of clinical and epidemiologic similarities, the liver lesions of yellow fever and Rift Valley fever are histologically distinguishable.

Clinical Characteristics. As with so many other arbovirus infections, inapparent, subclinical and mild febrile yellow fever virus infections occur, eliciting an immune response that protects these individuals against further infection for life. In such diverse areas as East African and South American rain forests, obscure infections may occur in a majority of exposed persons, particularly children. Although mortality rates have exceeded 50 per cent in some epidemics, the range is usually 5 to 10 per cent. These severe cases characterize yellow fever as the most fulminating of all arbovirus hemorrhagic fevers.

After a relatively short incubation period of 3 to 6 days, there is sudden onset of fever, often exceeding 40° C (104° F), headache and generalized pain, especially in the low back and extremities. Other early striking signs are markedly injected and inflamed conjunctivae, photophobia, leukopenia and thrombocytopenia.

During this initial onslaught, systemic dispersion of the viscerotropic virus produces extensive midzonal and periportal parenchyma cell necrosis in the liver. Increased blood bilirubin, prolonged prothrombin time and jaundice result; however, even in severe cases, the jaundice may not be apparent. Detection of jaundice in darker skinned patients is further complicated by the obscurative conjunctival inflammation.

The systemic invasion is also selective for the kidney and heart. Nephron damage, with sloughing of the tubular epithelium and accumulation of detritus in the lumina, is reflected by leakage of protein, manifested by early diagnostic appearance of albuminuria. Renal shutdown often follows, producing oliguria and abnormal increase in blood urea.

The initial febrile tachycardia slows relative to continued high temperature (classic Faget's sign), possibly reflecting dilatation of a damaged myocardium. This may cause a fall in blood and pulse pressure, which can result in shock. During the shift from the several day invasive phase to systemic toxemia there may be a period in which the fever subsides and the patient appears to be recovering. Such a hopeful condition may only precede the more severe stage, which terminates fatally, usually during the second week after onset. Prognosis, therefore, should be made with conservative reservations. Unusually early appearance of increased bilirubin, urea, albuminuria, oliguria and hemorrhagic signs is ominous, regardless of the current clinical appearance of the patient.

Hemorrhagic signs vary from the simple bleeding of gums through the variety of hemorrhagic manifestations of the other hemorrhagic fevers, to the dreaded "black vomit," the hematemesis that sometimes precedes or accompanies delirium, coma and impending death.

Diagnosis. Severe onset of high fever, headache, myalgia and prostration followed by hepatomegaly, jaundice, vomiting, hemorrhagic signs, oliguria and albuminuria in a patient exposed in a recognized area of yellow fever virus activity should focus suspicion on this etiology. It is again emphasized that many infections may be subclinical and many overt cases mild. To prevent both local and international spread, laboratory confirmation of the suspected diagnosis should be expeditiously sought.

There may be a polymorphonuclear leukocytosis followed by a leukopenia with predominance of mononuclear cells after one week. Diminution of chloride excretion in the urine may be detected and hypoglycemia may occur accompanied by increase in guanadine-like substances in the blood.

In differential diagnosis, dengue and hemorrhagic dengue must be considered, since they occur in similar tropical situations. Hepatitis A or B may be the most difficult differential diagnoses to make in a yellow fever endemic area. Lassa fever, caused by a hepatotropic arenavirus, must also be considered. Appearance of acute febrile jaundice in children, originally diagnosed as hepatitis A or B, may be the first sign of an impending epidemic of yellow fever. Since jaundice and hemorrhagic vomiting also occur in severe malaria and leptospirosis, these must be ruled out.

Viruses can readily be isolated from blood serum collected in the first few days of acute illness by inoculation into suckling mice. Serial acute and convalescent sera will show the appearance and the rise in titer of neutralizing and hemagglutination-inhibiting antibodies during the first week to 10 days of disease and will be followed by development of specific complement-fixing antibodies in the second week. Because yellow fever virus belongs antigenically in arbovirus Group B, most closely related to the dengue viruses, detection of Group B antibody rise by hemagglutination-inhibition or complement-fixation is not sufficient to establish a diagnosis. Either a virus must be isolated and identified as yellow fever, or in vitro serologic titers and neutralization indices must be greater for yellow fever than other Group B arboviruses.

Yellow fever virus may also be isolated from *Aedes aegypti* mosquitoes collected in the area or from monkeys in an associated epizootic.

Viruses have been isolated from liver obtained at postmortem examination 10 days after onset of the disease. In sylvan or rural situations, where refrigeration and virologic facilities are not available, postmortem diagnosis is established by use of the viscerotome, which is inserted into the liver through a slit in the skin to obtain a segment of liver that is preserved in 10 per cent formalin. Later, histologic examination reveals characteristic liver diseases, including eosinophilic inclusions called Councilman bodies that are considered pathognomonic of yellow fever by some. However, these appear in postmortem liver tissues of other viral hemorrhagic fevers that occur outside the recognized yellow fever zones.

Treatment. Because the clinical manifestations of yellow fever are a result of viscerotropic invasion of the virus, there is no treatment for the virus infection. Whether any regimen alters the already established course of the disease is questionable. Supportive measures may relieve suffering of the patient somewhat; antipyretics and sponge baths to diminish high fever and analgesics for headache and myalgia may be given. It is important to counter the dehydration caused by vomiting through carefully controlled fluid replacement, which can usually be accomplished by provision of fruit juice and milk. Serious kidney dysfunction and electrolyte imbalance may require parenteral administration of appropriate fluids, but the frequent occurrence of myocardial damage requires that caution be exercised in the use of any measure that might put further strain on the heart. If hemorrhagic complications are severe, blood transfusion may be necessary but should be guided by careful and frequent measurement of hematocrit and blood pressure. Intravenous glucose may be administered to combat hypoglycemia, 10 to 20 ml of 7.5 per cent solution of gluconate for guanidine intoxication; large doses of vitamin K have also been given early in the disease. There are no valid statistics that favor an active therapeutic regimen over cautious supportive care of the severely ill.

Early abnormal or excessive rise in blood bilirubin and the appearance of oliguria and albuminuria indicate a poor prognosis, even though the patient may not appear to be so seriously ill. These indicate the extent of organic damage. It is at this stage that comfortable rest and good nursing care may make a critical difference in the outcome.

Prophylaxis. Epidemic urban yellow fever was eliminated from the Western Hemisphere by control of *Aedes aegypti* mosquitoes. Where the *Aedes aegypti* is prevalent in an area susceptible to introduction of yellow fever, a possibility exists that transmission to nonimmune natives can occur, as has been demonstrated by recent African epidemics. *Aedes aegypti* control is, therefore, an important specific preventive measure against yellow fever.

However, the elimination of sylvan yellow fever in the jungles of South America and Africa is presently inconceivable because of the multiplicity of arboreal mosquito vectors and the vast areas involved.

Sporadic cases among nonimmune persons living or working in these forest areas will continue to occur, particularly in South America, where yellow fever moves through in 10- to 15-year cycles as the primate populations, decimated in the previous epizootic of yellow fever, are replenished. While protective clothing, screens, mosquito nets and repellents are temporary aids in the prevention of any mosquito-borne infection, continuous protection against yellow fever in such situations is provided by use of chick embryo and tissue culture attenuated live 17D yellow fever virus vaccine.[20] The attenuation of the virus eliminated viscerotropism for man. Its neurotropic nature has been manifest by the rare occurrence of postvaccinal encephalitis in infants. However, no more than 15 patients, all under 1 year of age, have been reported in a 25-year period. All recovered without sequelae. One case of 17D postvaccinal encephalitis in a 3-year-old child who died 12 days after vaccination has been documented.

Considering that possibly two hundred million persons have been vaccinated with 17D, with only an occasional mild febrile reaction observed 1 to 7 days following subcutaneous injection of 0.5 ml of vaccine, this is probably the safest prophylactic live virus vaccine in use in public health practice. Its limitation is that lyophilized ampules of the chick embryo tissue containing the vaccine virus must be maintained frozen until rehydration. It must then be used within 1 hour, but can be injected by jet gun as well as by syringe and needle. Because it is a live virus, an infection with viremia is induced that produces an immune reaction with development of detectable neutralizing antibodies in 90 per cent of those vaccinated. No case of yellow fever has ever been reported in a person properly vaccinated with 17D.

Another vaccine that is used in Africa is known as the Dakar or French neurotropic vaccine. Its advantage is its durability in gum arabic at warm ambient temperatures for as long as 24 hours[20] compared to the viability of rehydrated 17D for only 1 hour. The French attenuated mouse brain vaccine in gum arabic can also be applied by the scratch technique, along with smallpox. Detrimental effects from such scratch application are secondary infections, sometimes with tetanus. Postvaccinal encephalitis after use of the Dakar vaccine has occurred frequently enough in children to limit its use in persons over 10 years of age.

FEVER WITH HEADACHE, GENERAL AND LOCALIZED PAIN, PROSTRATION AND HEMORRHAGIC SIGNS (MOSQUITO-BORNE)

Etiology and Epidemiology. When hemorrhagic manifestations appear as an epidemic component or clinical result of infection with mosquito-borne dengue viruses, ominous epidemiologic and clinical implications necessitate their consideration as separate diseases (Table 1–5). These have variously been called Philippine, Thai and Southeast Asian hemorrhagic fevers in descriptions in the literature since their occurrence was first noted, beginning in 1954.

In epidemics of febrile illness, encompassing classic dengue and dengue hemorrhagic fever, virologic or serologic diagnosis of chikungunya virus infection was established. While mild hematologic changes could be detected, none of these cases presented severe hemorrhagic complications or shock. Chikungunya virus as a cause of hemorrhagic fever is therefore rare or in doubt, although it has been considered a contributory cause of hemorrhagic disease in India. Because continued geographic extension lessens the significance of such geographic terms, it is medically more rational to refer to these syndromes as hemorrhagic dengue.

Aedes aegypti is the established vector. This explains the urban, peridomestic occurrence of cases, seasonally associated with conditions such as heavy rainfall, which favors an increase in the numbers of *A. aegypti*. However, cases can occur at any time of year, reflecting the year-round presence of infected *A. aegypti* mosquitoes associated with domestic containers of water that provide for peridomestic breeding of this anthropophilic mosquito vector. *Aedes albopictus*, which has a more sylvan habitat, has also been implicated as a vector.

Attack rates are highest in young children, maximum hospitalization occurring in the 3- to 5-year age group. It is also noteworthy that epidemics of dengue infection in large urban Southeast Asian areas, such as Bangkok, produce hemorrhagic disease almost always in children of Oriental races,

Table 1–5. FEVER WITH HEADACHE, GENERAL AND LOCALIZED PAIN, PROSTRATION AND HEMORRHAGIC SIGNS

Virus	*Serologic Group*	*Vector*	*Known Geographic Range of Infection*
Dengue-1	B	Mosquito	Philippines, Vietnam,
Dengue-2	B	Mosquito	Thailand, Malaysia,
Dengue-3	B	Mosquito	India, Indonesia,
Dengue-4	B	Mosquito	South Pacific Islands

classic dengue being the clinical picture in Caucasians afflicted in the same epidemic. While this may reflect greater protection from bites by infected *A. aegypti*, it is also a possible supporting evidence of the hypothetical double dengue infection in the pathogenesis of hemorrhagic fever.

Pathogenesis and Pathology. Highest attack rates of DSS are in children, most of whom are suffering a second infection with dengue that produces quick anamnestic response of IgG immunoglobulin, which is thought to form immune complex aggregations at the endothelial sites of virus multiplication, thereby setting off vascular permeability that loses formed constituents of blood-plasma protein and erythrocytes into the interstitial tissues of organs and skin.[22] The extent of this hemorrhagic diathesis may be immunologically determined and marks the clinical extent and prognosis of the disease.

Double dengue hemorrhagic disease has not been observed in Caucasian children. The disease in Oriental infants is rare in the first few months owing to maternal antibody. Its peak at 6 to 8 months is thought to be due to sensitization of the primary infection immunologic reaction to declining maternal antibody titer, producing typical double dengue immune complex DSS.[22]

Experimental studies in monkeys as well as serologic study of human cases has shown that when the second infection is with dengue-2 virus, following any of 1, 3, or 4, the severity is greater and the prognosis more serious. However, any combination of two different dengue virus infections occurring within 3-month to 5-year intervals can precipitate DHF. Also demonstrated experimentally and by serologic study of multiple type dengue infections, persons subsequently exposed to infections by a third or fourth constituent of the dengue spectrum are refractory to DHF because of solid immunity.

While actual antibody complexing at the sites of dengue virus replication has not yet been definitely proved, there are data that show extreme difficulty in isolating dengue virus from hemorrhagic tissues collected from fatal cases of DHF and DSS. This would indicate a tight antibody-virus combination. What is not explained is the rapidity of recovery once hemodynamics are restored to normal, which is in distinct contrast to the pathogenic evolution of the other viral hemorrhagic fevers.

Postmortem studies of patients who died at this stage, usually 5 to 7 days after onset of fever, show interstitial pneumonitis, focal necrosis in liver and myocardium, depletion and abnormal cellular constitution of lymph nodes and spleen, sloughing of tubular epithelium in the kidney, hemorrhages in the adrenals, effusion in the perirenal and other anatomical spaces, and extravasation of blood into interstitial spaces and lumina of various organs. Most of these abnormalities are nonspecific manifestations of toxic phenomena that could result in death or could be the result of uncompensated shock.

The postmortem findings range from mild to severe changes. Until larger series are studied, it can only be surmised that death results from nonspecific systemic decompensation rather than directly from viral destruction of tissues and organs. Perhaps the most striking feature of this disease is the rapid recovery of the young once physiologic integrity is restored, versus the more prolonged course in older patients who appear to have greater immunologic integrity but slower physiologic response.

Diagnosis. Early description of dengue infections with demonstrated alteration in hematologic findings led to a broad diagnosis of dengue hemorrhagic fever. It became obvious that a series of cases in young children who rapidly went into shock with frequent fatal outcome was clinically different from others showing hemorrhagic signs but no shock. Rapidity of recovery in survivors of shock compared to prolonged convalescence in the others led to distinction between the two syndromes.

Dengue hemorrhagic fever (DHF) has been characterized as serious illness 2 or more days after onset of fever with a hypoproteinemia (protein level of 5.5 gm per 100 ml or less) with thrombocytopenia, prolonged bleeding time (greater than 5 minutes) and/or elevated prothrombin time. *Dengue shock syndrome* (DSS) includes, in addition to these signs, shock as manifest by hypotension or pulse pressure less than 20 mg Hg and a hematocrit greater than 20 per cent with increase in serum transaminases.[21]

Onset in children is classic dengue with fever and maculopapular rash that blanches with pressure. In older patients the fever is more severe, with headache, myalgia and the rash.

Dengue hemorrhagic fever appears on the third and fourth day of fever with hemorrhagic phenomena ranging from positive tourniquet test (Grade I) to other hemorrhagic signs such as skin petechiae, bleeding gums, epistaxis, hematemesis and melena (Grade II). In such cases there is almost always marked pharyngeal inflammation. Dengue shock syndrome is detected by early signs of circulatory failure with tachycardia, hypotension, pulse pressure less than 20 mg Hg, cold clammy skin and restlessness due to anxiety of impending shock (Grade III). Undetected or untreated this serious condition can progress to profound shock with imperceptible pulse and blood pressure (Grade IV).

Palpation of an enlarged liver is a common physical sign and may cause the patient pain.

The marked leukopenia of early classic dengue may be missed if the patient is not seen until hemorrhagic signs or shock appear. Persistent leukopenia is not uncommon, but a normal or relatively increased leukocyte count with continued thrombocytopenia appears to reflect circulatory congestion, hemoconcentration and generalized tissue damage during the hemorrhagic phase of the disease.

Treatment. The aim of treatment is to control the leakage of plasma that results from increased vascular permeability, the primary pathophysiologic problem. This leads to tissue anoxia and metabolic acidosis, which if inadequately compensated results in death. The key indicator is a sudden increase in hematocrit level, which indicates plasma loss.

Early leukopenia and the ever-present thrombocytopenia may reflect disseminated intravascular clotting. This loss of thrombocytes plus anoxic vascular permeability allow for hemorrhagic diathesis, which is marked by gastrointestinal and other hemorrhages.

Using the hematocrit as a guide to early treatment, administration of plasma, plasma expanders, electrolytes (as guided by blood chemistry and urinalysis), and other fluids should prevent shock. It often brings about dramatic improvement that in a few hours may become lasting recovery.

If detected early, the preshock state may be treated satisfactorily in outpatient clinics. Attendants and relatives of such dengue patients are to be instructed that any sign of restlessness, abdominal pain, cold extremities or skin lesions should bring immediate transport to hospital for antishock monitoring and treatment.

Dengue hemorrhagic fever patients without shock can be supportively treated by oral fluids to combat the dehydration that results from fever, anorexia and vomiting. Fruit juice or electrolyte- and dextrose-containing beverages are better than plain water.

In the very young, febrile convulsions are a possibility but antipyretic salicylates are to be avoided because they may precipitate acidosis and hemorrhage. Acetaminophen is the antipyretic of choice.

Parenteral fluid therapy should be guided by hematocrit determination if early measures for fluid and electrolyte balance are unsuccessful. The volume and concentrations should be those presented for diarrheal dehydration. DSS requires immediate administration of intravenous fluid to expand plasma volume. This can be accomplished by intravenous lactated Ringer's or isotonic saline at 20 ml per kg. If shock continues start plasma or a plasma expander such as dextran at a rate exceeding 10 ml per kg per hr. Intravenous fluids should be continued after there is clinical improvement and hematocrit begins to fall; they can be terminated 48 hours after recovery from shock or when hematocrit drops below 40 per cent and urine volume and restored blood pressure indicate that circulatory blood volume has been restored.

Oxygen therapy may be necessary in severe shock. This may require sedatives because of restlessness and apprehension. Chloral hydrate or paraldehyde are the drugs of choice. In rare cases of massive blood loss, transfusion may be necessary, so a precautionary measure early in shock might be to group and cross-match the patient's blood.

Control and Prevention. Since there is no means for attacking dengue virus infection, efforts must be directed toward breaking the cycle of transmission. This means mosquito vector control. Since dengue is highly vector-dependent, vector control measures can be targetted against peridomestic breeding in water containers by use of larvicides, such as the application of granules of Abate to water containers. In emergencies such as epidemics, adulticide spraying or fogging of *Aedes aegypti*–infested premises or aerial spraying with low volume malathion can be recommended. Because DHF is hypothetically a result of sequential dengue virus infections, use of live attenuated virus vaccines is contraindicated.

Eradication of *Aedes aegypti* from urban areas is the surest means for preventing dengue virus transmissions.

RODENT-ASSOCIATED VIRAL HEMORRHAGIC FEVERS

The arenaviruses are not arthropod-borne. Because they are zoonotic, because they were isolated and virologically and epidemiologically characterized as suspect arboviruses, and because the syndromes they cause require differential diagnosis from a number of arbovirus diseases, it is useful to consider them along with the arbovirus hemorrhagic fevers.

Etiology. As enveloped viruses they are inactivated by exposure to sodium deoxycholate. Morphologically they are distinguished by "sandlike" particles in the nucleocapsid, which are actually ribosomes incorporated from the cells in which they replicate. It is these distinctive particles that led to the name arenavirus (Fig. 1–1).

Although the prototype of the family is neurotropic lymphocytic choriomeningitis virus, those viruses involved in the causation of hemorrhagic fevers—Lassa, Junin and Machupo—are hepatotropic and produce extensive damage to liver cells. This produces widely disseminated hemorrhagic phenomena that probably are secondary to hepatic dysfunction, rather than the primary viral replication and destruction or immune complex pathologic changes seen in other hemorrhagic diseases.

Argentinian and Bolivian Hemorrhagic Fevers

Although the causative arenaviruses of Argentinian and Bolivian hemorrhagic fevers are distinct members of the Tacaribe Group, and the areas of their endemic occurrence are geographically separate, they are considered together here because of the epidemiologic and clinical similarities of the disease they produce. As represented in Table 1–4, Junin virus, the cause of Argentinian hemorrhagic fever, and Machupo virus, which was isolated from Bolivian hemorrhagic fever, are viruses of rodents, particularly of the genus *Calomys,* which inhabits cultivated fields, grasslands and forest edges adjacent to rural communities of the lowlands east of the Andes in the southern portion of South America. The indigenous rodents serve as reservoirs in which the virus is maintained in an immunotolerant state and transmitted horizontally to others by contact with infected excreta and tissues, and vertically from mother to offspring through milk and other effluvia.[23] If infection occurs within 9 days of birth, a viremia is initiated that can result in chronic viremia with failure of antibody response sufficient to terminate virus circulation. This leads to chronic infection of salivary tissues and kidneys with resulting infectious secretions and urine.

In weanling rodents a similar immunotolerant chronic viremia condition may be produced or a prolonged viremia ultimately leads to a neutralizing antibody response that clears virus from the blood but is insufficient to eliminate viremia from infected kidneys. *Calomys* therefore serves not only as a reservoir of the virus within the rodent population but as a vector as well. There is no evidence that the rodents suffer hemorrhagic disease. However, there is a significant fall in fertility with consequent drop in population as a consequence of neonatal infection.

It is when man transgresses the enzootic habitat of the infectious rodents, as occurs in the corn harvest on the pampas of Argentina, or when infectious *Calomys callosus* enter human habitations, as occurred in San Joaquin of El Beni in eastern Bolivia, that human hemorrhagic fever with case fatality rates ranging from 10 to 30 per cent occurs.

Clinical Characteristics. After an incubation period of 1 to 2 weeks, there is insidious onset of fever and muscle pains. This is accompanied or soon followed by headache and inflammation of the conjunctivae. Blood count shows mild to marked leukopenia, which often continues for the duration of the fever. Such a febrile course may last unremittently for 10 to 14 days or suddenly end after a few days. So far, there is no objective basis for prognosticating a self-limited febrile illness or one that will progress to hemorrhagic complication.

Hemorrhagic signs may appear by the fifth day of fever. These can consist only of bleeding gums, and petechiae of the soft palate and skin of the torso. More severe hemorrhage is marked by epistaxis, hemoptysis, hematemesis and melena, which reflects extensive internal bleeding.

A fall in blood and pulse pressure may occur with a rise in hematocrit indicating onset of shock before the usual signs of classic shock appear. This is the time for implementing supportive treatment.

Neurologic signs frequently appear. These range from tremor of the tongue to intensive tremor of the extremities. Pathogenesis of these signs is unexplained because when the patients recover there is no neurologic deficit and no other sequelae.

Diagnosis. Suspicion of a hemorrhagic fever depends upon careful physical examination with recognition of hemorrhagic signs such as initial bleeding, leukopenia and the all-important abnormal increase in hematocrit associated with high fever, generalized myalgia or low back pain and prostration. Geographic pathology and epidemiologic cues such as habitat type, seasonal occurrence and occupational exposure are important leads to diagnosis before an epidemic becomes obvious by the recognition of a number of diseased people.

Inoculation of acute serum specimens and throat washings into suckling hamsters may establish a virologic diagnosis. Appearance of detectable antibodies is delayed sometimes until 3 weeks after onset, so negative serologic reactions in paired sera from first suspected cases do not rule out an etiology of Junin or Machupo virus infection. Additional sequential and convalescent sera must be collected and tested to serologically identify the causative agent by complement-fixation or neutralization tests. Such diagnostic tests should be referred to an appropriately secure laboratory. Fatal laboratory infections, especially with Junin virus, have been reported.

Treatment. In Argentina it has been customary to give convalescent plasma. If given early enough in the illness—up to 5 days after onset—as passive immunotherapy, there is an impression that it effectively slows or halts further pathogenesis of the disease. No controlled evaluation of the treatment has been accomplished. As has been observed in Lassa fever, this clinical improvement following convalescent serum treatment may be peculiar to arenavirus infection, which characteristically shows a long viremia with slow immune response.

When hemorrhagic signs first appear and hematocrit begins to rise, maintenance of fluid balance becomes imperative. If this can be accomplished with obligatory fluid intake, while monitoring blood hematocrit levels and frequent urinalyses, intravenous fluid administration can be avoided. If not, because of inability of the patient to swallow or inadequacy of oral ingestion due to vomiting, intravenous fluids and blood expanders are indicated, recognizing the possibility of pulmonary edema and circulatory collapse due to overload of the failing cardiovascular system.

Prevention. Because particular species of rodents are recognized reservoirs and vectors of Machupo and Junin viruses, it would appear that rodent control is the method of choice in eliminating exposure of people, as was demonstrated in the dramatic fall in attack rate in San Joaquin, Bolivia, following household trapping of *Calomys.*[24] However, an infected rodent population scattered through vast agricultural areas, as is the case with mal de Rostrojos among the grain harvesters of Argentina, poses practical problems of feasibility of technique in terms of safety and cost.

Biologic control by replacing arenavirus infection of rodents with the antigenically related Pichinde virus, which is nonpathogenic for man, has been suggested. But such an approach also poses problems of safety and practicability.

An attenuated strain of Junin virus has been tried as a vaccine for Argentinian hemorrhagic fever. As yet, the trials have not been extensive enough to measure feasibility in significantly lowering attack rates among those rurally exposed. Therefore, early diagnosis of suspect cases followed by whatever environmental controls are indicated and feasible is the best that can be recommended at present.

Simpler, more expeditious and continual ecologic surveillance for rodent infection and transmission may be the most effective long-term approach to the control and eventual prevention of the South American hemorrhagic fevers which do have a distinctive geographic pathology that can be continually defined.

Lassa Fever

Etiology and Epidemiology. Lassa fever results from infection with an hepatotropic arenavirus. It is highly infectious, highly pathogenic and highly virulent. While its presently recognized area of endemicity is in several countries of West Africa, the epidemic potential is undefined because of the notorious patient-to-contact and laboratory infectivity of Lassa virus.[25] It causes hemorrhagic disease of high attack and case fatality rates.

It is named Lassa for the locality from which the index case was brought to a mission hospital on the Jos Plateau of Nigeria. From there the first human cases of the disease were described and the first patient-to-medical attendant transmission was observed in 1969.[26] Outbreaks have subsequently been characterized in Liberia and Sierra Leone where similar ecologic habitats support populations of *Mastomys natalensis,* a rodent of the family CRICETIDAE which also includes *Calomys,* the reservoir genus of the South American hemorrhagic fevers.

Epidemiologic features of Lassa fever were initially derived from perception of a series of catastrophic and fatal events that demonstrated the dangers of exposure to the virus and to patients suffering with the disease.[27] More recent work by immune survivors of the infection and the handling of clinical and field-collected specimens in high security facilities have begun to formulate a picture of extensive geographic distribution in West Africa with some foci of endemic infection of human populations in which inapparent or subclinical infections have occurred.

Pathogenesis. Although the liver has been demonstrated to be a target organ by electron microscopic visualization of Lassa virus in postmortem tissue, the clinical signs and progression of disease and postmortem histopathologic examination show involvement and dysfunction of many organs and tissues. Whether this is due to general dispersion and replication of the virus with tissue destruction, or liver dysfunction with consequences of liver failure or toxemia, is not known.

Clinical Characteristics. As with the other hemorrhagic diseases, onset is usually that of an insidious febrile illness. Only after appearance of hemorrhagic signs, or the occurrence of a number of typhoidlike illnesses in a geographically suspect population group, will the possibility of Lassa fever be suggested as a differential from anicteric liver disease, yellow fever or typhoid.

The clinical course, only a few days to 2 weeks after exposure, is one of fever, headache, myalgia, abdominal and/or thoracic pain, nausea, vomiting, diarrhea, and bradycardia relative to the temperature. By the second week there have developed inflammation of conjunctivae, papulovesicular or ulcerative pharyngitis, maculopapular rash on face or body, lymphadenopathy and a leukopenia that was probably an early manifestation if a complete blood count was done at the beginning of the illness.

In the second week following onset, hemorrhagic signs appear that range from petechial skin hemorrhages to hemoptysis, hematemesis, melena and vaginal hemorrhage. At this stage the blood pressure falls, pulse pressure diminishes, and there is albuminuria followed by oliguria (as kidney function shuts down), delirium and shock. The patient may become afebrile just prior to death. In those who survive, some may show a vacillating sequence of febrile episodes with one or several associated signs but ultimate convalescence in which febrile relapses may occur in the third or fourth week.

Diagnosis. Because Lassa fever occurs in tropical localities of West Africa where malaria, yellow fever, typhoid fever, leptospirosis and relapsing fever occur, the differential diagnosis presents a challenging array of possibilities. The laboratory may establish the validity of the differential. But, as with other arenavirus infections, the immune response, as reflected in antibodies that are specific and can be detected serologically, is delayed, sometimes for weeks.

Facilities for safe virologic diagnosis are not available in Africa, although convalescent sera from recovered suspect cases can be sent to the W.H.O. Regional Reference Laboratories for the CF test against inactivated Lassa antigen.

When suspicion of Lassa fever as a sporadic case or cluster occurs to the physician, it is important to take precautions by (1) isolating the patient from all except essential medical personnel, (2) avoiding contact with potentially infectious oral secretions, blood and urine, and (3) handling all blood specimens obtained for routine diagnostic purposes aseptically with thermal inactivation of sera to be used in diagnostic serologic tests.

Treatment. Perhaps because of the unique delay in antibody response characteristic of arenavirus infections, the use of convalescent plasma or serum may produce effective passive immunity that could inhibit further spread and replication of Lassa virus. Improvement in seriously ill patients has been observed following such convalescent serum therapy.[28] The long viremia of arenavirus infections must be remembered in selecting donors of convalescent plasma because too early a bleeding may still contain virus.

Otherwise, early detection of plasma loss internally should guide replacement therapy as described for the South American hemorrhagic fevers. Neglect in responding to early pre-shock signs will delay measures of responding to hypovolemia until shock occurs, when it may be too late to reverse the pathophysiologic changes that usually result in death.

TICK-BORNE VIRAL HEMORRHAGIC FEVERS

Kyasanur Forest Disease (KFD) and Omsk Hemorrhagic Fever (OHF)

Etiology and Epidemiology. The KFD and OHF viruses are small togaviruses of the Russian spring-summer antigenic complex of Flavivirus Group B. They are tick transmitted, by species listed in Table 1–4 (Fig. 1–8).

In their recognized disease region these agents produce overt fatal hemorrhagic disease in aberrant vertebrate hosts: KFD in langur, *Presbytis entellus* and *Macaca radiata* monkeys in Mysore State in India; and OHF in *Ondatra zibetica* in Omsk and Novosibirsk Oblasts of western Siberia. This indicates that while these vertebrate hosts may be involved terminally or tangentially as providers of virus by viremia to tick vectors, or by contact with infectious blood and tissues, they are not basically involved in the silent sylvan cycle of virus maintenance and transmission. Epizootic disease and deaths that

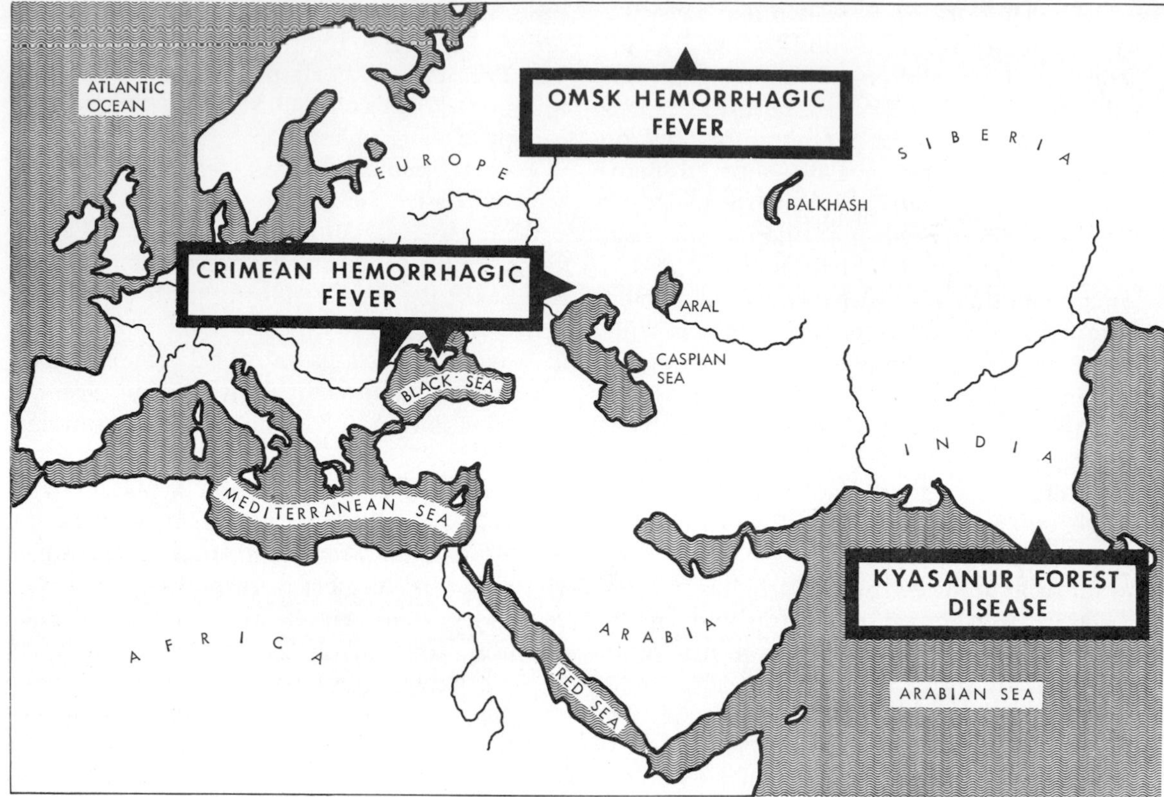

Figure 1–8. Geographic distribution of Crimean and Omsk hemorrhagic fevers and Kyasanur Forest disease. (Work, T. H. 1963. Tick-borne viral hemorrhagic fevers. *In* Hull, T. G. (ed.): Diseases Transmitted from Animals to Man. 5th ed. Charles C Thomas, Springfield, Illinois. Used by permission.)

periodically decimate monkeys[29] and muskrats mark these animals as sentinels of tick-transmitted virus infections originating in other small mammals—the vole *Suncus murinus* and forest species of *Rattus* for KFD, and the water vole *Arvicola terrestris* and the suslik *Spermophilus erythrogenus* for OHF.[30]

Since its initial discovery and virologic and epidemiologic elucidation in India in 1957, KFD has annually recurred in epidemics of varying intensity as its endemic area has slowly expanded and new susceptibles and occupationally exposed villagers have encountered *Haemaphysalis spinigera* and other infected ticks.

Omsk hemorrhagic fever was initially characterized in Omsk and Novosibirsk Oblasts of Siberia in 1945 to 1948, at which time it was attributed to *Dermacentor pictus* tick transmission. Subsequently, cases and outbreaks are more commonly associated with direct contact with blood and tissues of infected muskrats by the occupationally exposed fur trappers and skinners. The infection results in a high disease attack rate with a case fatality of 5 to 10 per cent in treated patients.

Clinical Characteristics. Although KFD and OHF viruses are antigenically distinct, and their geographic pathology widely separated, their clinical manifestations in man are sufficiently similar to be related simultaneously.

Three to 8 days following a sylvan infestation by infected ticks, or occupational exposure to infectious blood or tissues, or to laboratory fomites, there is a sudden onset of fever, headache, and conjunctival inflammation. Myalgia rapidly develops involving the extremities and lumbar region and is often marked by meningismus. A papulovesicular eruption often appears on the soft palate. By the third day diarrhea may occur. Hemorrhagic signs begin to appear in the form of bleeding gums and nasal hemorrhage. Hemoptysis, hematemesis, bloody stool, and melena indicate internal bleeding not attributable to any specific lesion.

These clinical developments are associated with a marked leukopenia (leukocyte count of 2000 or less) and thrombocytopenia (blood platelet count of 100,000 or less), which parallel the febrile phase that lasts 5 to 14 days. There may be a mild leukocytosis during defervescence. Convalescence may encompass a second febrile episode in the third or fourth week after onset.

In fatal cases, death occurs in the second week owing to various complications: hypovolemic shock, hemorrhagic diathesis filling the lung with blood, and secondary bacterial pneumonia.

Skin rash and petechiae characteristic of other hemorrhagic diseases do not occur and neurologic signs are rare. Convalescence is slow, with apparent fine tremors of the tongue, fingers and extremities reflecting more muscular weakness than neurologic deficit. Complete recovery, without sequelae, may take 6 weeks to 2 months.

Treatment. Being a viral infection, there is no specific therapy and the viremia with immune response is so rapid that passive immunotherapy is not likely to be of assistance. Attention is therefore directed toward supportive measures, the most important of which are maintenance of hydration, detecting hypovolemia and providing fluids by mouth or intravenously—physiologic saline, plasma expanders, plasma or whole blood as indicated by periodic blood determination and urinary output.

Prevention and Control. It is difficult in a hot climate to prescribe antitick infestation measures such as acaricide-saturated clothing covering the extremities. In certain occupational pursuits such as tick-collecting, dimethyl phthalate has been used effectively. Avoidance of tick infestation and tick bites by frequent mutual search for ticks on the body is recommended. Protective gloves and clothing while handling potentially infectious blood and carcass tissues are important.

Initial efforts at vaccination of those at high risk of exposure to KFD virus in India, by a formalin-inactivated Russian spring-summer encephalitis virus mouse brain immunogen, failed to give significant protection against closely related KFD virus. Inactivated tissue culture virus and attenuated KFD virus vaccines have been developed and experimentally tested with protective effect in primates. No field trials in persons occupationally exposed have been undertaken.

For OHF no vaccine prophylaxis has been reported.

Crimean Hemorrhagic Fever and Congo Virus Infections

Etiology and Epidemiology. Crimean hemorrhagic fever (CHF) and Central Asian hemorrhagic fever (CAHF) were initially considered separate entities because of different geographic range, different vectors, higher case fatality rates of CAHF, and high risk of infection of attending medical personnel by exposure to hemorrhagic cases of CAHF.[31] Since isolation of CHF virus in 1967, an antigen has been available for neutralization (NT) testing against convalescent CAHF sera. CAHF has been considered the same as CHF because of identical cross NT results. CHF therefore has a more extensive and scattered range from Bulgaria to Central Asia and southward into Pakistan, and possibly into Central Africa[32] (Fig. 1–8).

Dispersion of the nymphal tick vectors, *Hyalomma marginatum*, by rooks, *Corvus frugilegus*, accounts for scattered rural distribution in cattle-raising enterprises. Highest attack rates are among milk maids who encounter infected ticks on cow teats, and among field hands who are infected by ticks in pastures where cattle serve as hosts to adult ticks. CHF is therefore a rural disease with highest attack rates in important occupational groups.

Clinical Characteristics. With an incubation period as short as 3 days and as long as 9 days, there is onset of fever, headache, conjunctival inflammation, myalgia and hemorrhagic complications characteristic of the other tick-borne viral hemorrhagic fevers. There is marked leukopenia and thrombocytopenia. By contrast to KFD and OHF, there is often capillary extravasation into the skin, producing petechiae and extensive ecchymoses in pressured areas of the extremities and trunk. This reflects capillary fragility that can be used as a diagnostic test.

While demonstrated to be antigenically identical with CHF virus, Congo virus has been isolated from blood of severe febrile human illnesses in Zaire and Uganda. The same virus has been isolated from ticks in Pakistan and Nigeria, as presented in Table 1–4. Characteristic hemorrhagic disease has not yet been described from these areas except for those detailed elsewhere as other African hemorrhagic fevers. It is therefore important to consider this virus in differential diagnosis of hemorrhagic disease in Africa, South Asia and the Middle East, and to request its consideration in laboratory virologic and serologic diagnostic tests.

Treatment. This is supportive as with the other hemorrhagic fevers, and is aimed at preventing progression into shock and maintenance of erythropoietic elements in the circulating blood.

Prevention and Control. No vaccine is available. Because of the recognized rural and bovine-associated occupational attack rates, prevention of tick infestation, tick bite and tick crushing is basic to breaking the chain of tick-man transmission. The role that cattle play as hosts to virus-infected ticks has been investigated. Experimental methods of acaricidal dips and sprays have been successfully tried, ridding cattle of tick infestation for as long as 11 days. However, because of the widespread avian distribution by rooks, and the long-distance movement of cattle as is customary from northern to southern Nigeria, there seems little chance of controlling potential carriers of reservoir ticks. Education of those at risk in methods of avoiding or quickly counteracting tick infestation is presently the only effective approach to prevention.

PRIMATE–ASSOCIATED HEMORRHAGIC FEVERS

Marburg Virus Disease

Etiology and Epidemiology. Marburg virus disease is caused by an exceptionally large bullet- or bent sausage–shaped virus 700 to 1000 nm or larger.[33] The virus was initially observed and the disease characterized in persons exposed to infected organs or tissue cultures of vervet *Cercopithecus aethiops* monkeys collected and air-shipped from Uganda in East Africa between June and August of 1967. The virus is hepatotropic, and infection occurred by contact with monkey organs and tissue cultures rather than by association with infected animals. However, secondary human cases occurred, apparently because of intimate human contact with patients or their effluvia, particularly acute blood specimens.

Of the 31 cases of the initial outbreak in laboratories in Marburg and Frankfurt in West Germany and Belgrade, Yugoslavia, seven patients died, thus manifesting high attack and case fatality rates. Because of associated monkey deaths in animals exposed under different circumstances en route and after arrival of the monkeys in their European animal quarters, the infection was considered to have originated in Uganda but to have been transmitted to other primates en route. These fatalities suggested that the maintenance reservoir in East Africa was in vertebrates other than green monkeys.

A series of three cases, of which one died, occurred in South Africa in February-March 1975. The index case was exposed in Rhodesia, which extends southward almost 2000 miles along the suspected range of Marburg virus reservoirs. It is important to note that these cases were initially thought to be Lassa fever on clinical grounds, but firm diagnosis was established by electron microscopic visualization and subsequent immunofluorescent identification of Marburg virus[34] (Fig. 1–9).

Clinical Characteristics. A week to 10 days following intimate exposure to infec-

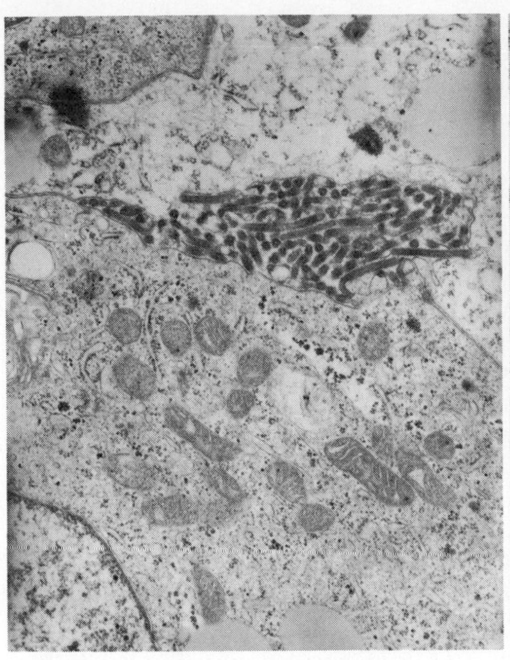
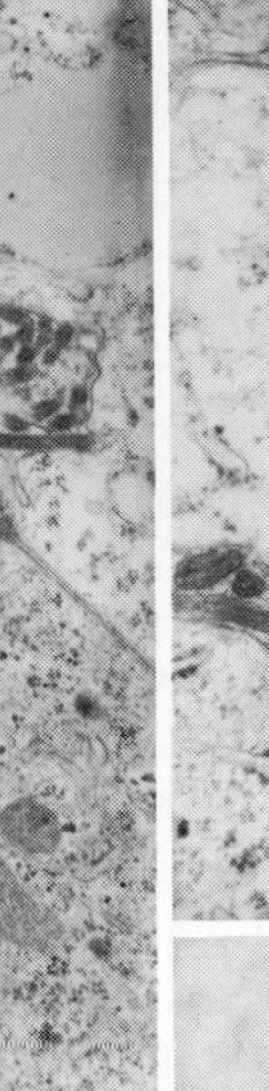
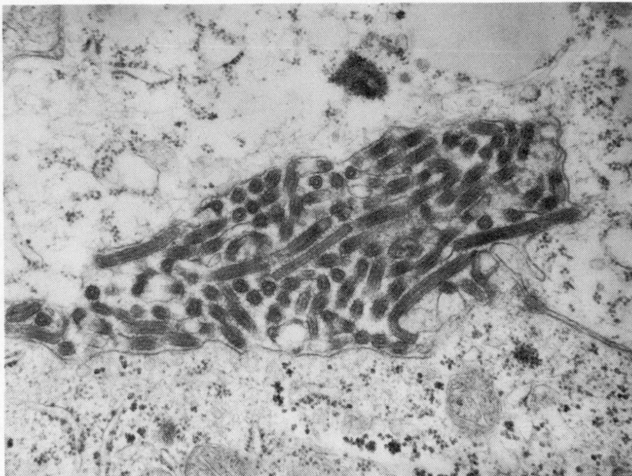
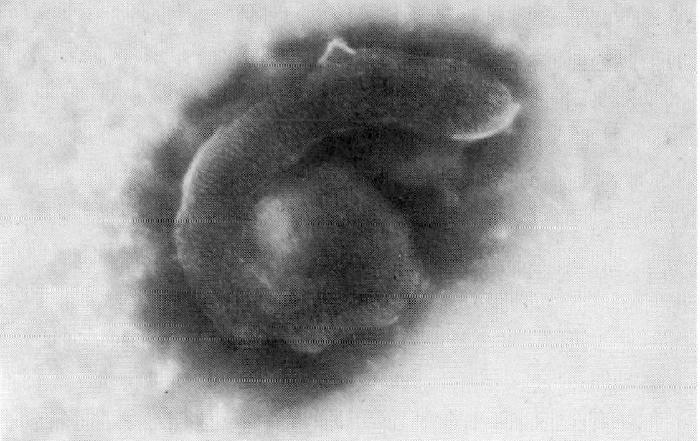

Figure 1–9. Marburg virus isolated from blood of fatal human case infected in Rhodesia in February 1975, extending the known range of the pathogen southward in East Africa by almost two thousand miles. Initially associated with laboratory exposure to primate tissues, the enzootic reservoir or vector is still unknown. These electron photomicrographs established a specific diagnosis of hemorrhagic fever, initially clinically suspected to be Lassa fever. (By permission of Dr. Frederick A. Murphy, Virology Division, Center for Disease Control, Atlanta, Georgia.)

tious organs or tissue culture of primates or intimate contact with effluvia of acute onset or blood of a patient, the illness begins and follows a course similar to many other viral hemorrhagic diseases. Invariably, there is headache and fever, soon followed by inflammation of the conjunctivae. There then may ensue a macular rash, petechiae, a maculopapular eruption on the pharynx, bradycardia, signs of internal hemorrhage, leukopenia, thrombocytopenia, prostration, myalgia, myocarditis, meningismus, albuminuria, delirium, shock and death, or lytic fall in temperature with long convalescence without sequelae. The involvement of the liver is anicteric but manifest by abnormal serum glutamic oxaloacetic transaminase and serum glutamic pyruvic transaminase levels.

Diagnosis. Suspicion of the infection can be established by history of geographic, primate or case exposure. Careful closed system collection of blood for inoculation into guinea pigs or postmortem tissues for electron microscopic examination or fluorescent antibody screening is presently the only route to establishing a definitive diagnosis. With these basic procedures in mind, differential laboratory diagnosis of typhoid, yellow fever, other arenavirus infections and tick-borne hemorrhagic fever viruses must be undertaken.[35] This will require of the physician reference to the nearest W.H.O. Reference Virus Laboratory or, through appropriate channels, communication with the Center for Disease Control in Atlanta, Georgia, where all reagents and high security facilities are available for definitive virologic and serologic diagnosis.

Treatment. This involves early detection of preshock indications and appropriate prevention of hypovolemia. There is no evidence that passive immune measures are effective in this fulminating infection.

Prevention and Control. Since the original outbreak was etiologically associated with African green monkeys recently received from East Africa, a 3-week quarantine of such animals has been recommended to allow appearance of the disease in infected monkeys. Obviously, the high risk of infection from blood and secretions of patients calls for extreme care in handling the patient and his effluvia in a condition of total isolation.

Other Monkey-Related Virus Infections

Information on monkeypox (p. 85), Tanapox (p. 85), and infections with simian herpes viruses (p. 85) is presented in Chapter 4.

FEVER ASSOCIATED WITH CENTRAL NERVOUS SYSTEM INVOLVEMENT RANGING FROM MENINGOENCEPHALITIS TO SEVERE ENCEPHALITIS WITH SEQUELAE (MOSQUITO- AND TICK-BORNE)

Etiology and Epidemiology. The viruses listed in Table 1-6 were formerly designated the arthropod-borne neurotropic viruses. Three decades ago they constituted the largest recognized problem of diseases caused by arboviruses—that of epidemic encephalitis.

The foregoing presentation of other arbovirus diseases puts the encephalitides into better perspective. They still constitute an arbovirus disease component of great importance. Their multiple antigenic nature, the diverse epidemiologic situations in which sporadic and epidemic cases occur, and the largely helpless position of the physician or community when the first cases of epidemic encephalitis are recognized establish that there is no complex of infectious disease problems that requires more sophisticated understanding than the arbovirus encephalitides.

The clinical manifestations vary according to the localization and dispersion of the virus in the central nervous system. Since the primary differences are the antigenic character of the different viruses and the epidemiologic situations in which infection occurs, it is useful to consider them in accordance with these features.

Western equine encephalitis (WEE), eastern equine encephalitis (EEE) and Venezuelan equine encephalitis (VEE) are designated the equine encephalitides. All are caused by culicine mosquito-transmitted Group A togaviruses. The appellation "equine" results from their causation of equine encephalitis. Such disease in horses, mules and donkeys can mark the beginning of encephalitis virus transmission and serve as a warning that human cases may soon occur. Vectors of WEE and EEE are infected from a wild bird cycle, and transmission to man is dependent on species-selective feeding of the mosquito vector.

Western equine encephalitis virus transmission occurs throughout the Western Hemisphere from Canada to Argentina. Occurrence of epidemic human disease is manifest in the Great Plains and western United States where *Culex tarsalis* is the primary vector. Central nervous system (CNS) attack rates relative to numbers of persons infected are relatively low.

Eastern equine encephalitis virus in the United States has a widespread wild bird–*Culiseta melanura* silent enzootic cycle from Louisiana and Florida to New Jersey and Massachusetts that breaks out in explosive epidemics only when a human-biting mosquito enters the cycle. In addition to equine disease, pheasant flock epizootics, particularly in game farms along the east coast, signal entry of virus transmission into areas of increased risk. When human infection occurs there is a high CNS attack rate with high case fatality and irreversible sequelae rates.

The titer and duration of viremia in

equines with WEE and EEE infections is insufficient to infect mosquitoes, so such animals are considered dead end infections tangential to the avian maintenance and amplification cycles.

Venezuelan equine encephalitis,[36] on the other hand, usually produces a high titer viremia in equines, which in an epizootic-epidemic situation may be the primary source of virus to a large variety of mosquito vectors. In contrast to geographically widespread WEE and EEE enzootic dispersion,

Table 1–6. Fever Associated with Central Nervous System Involvement Ranging from Meningoencephalitis to Severe Encephalitis with Sequelae

Virus	*Serologic Group/Complex*	*Vector*	*Known Geographic Range of Infection*
Western equine encephalitis	A	Mosquito	Canada, Western and Eastern U.S.A., Mexico, Guyana, Brazil, Argentina
Eastern equine encephalitis	A	Mosquito	Eastern Canada and U.S.A., Mexico, Dominican Republic, Jamaica, Panama, Trinidad, Guyana, Colombia, Brazil, Argentina, Thailand (?)
Venezuelan equine encephalitis	A	Mosquito	Florida, Mexico, Panama, Colombia, Venezuela, Trinidad, Guyana, Brazil, Ecuador, South Texas
Japanese B encephalitis	B	Mosquito	Japan, China, Taiwan, Thailand, Malaya, Burma, India, Guam, Philippines, Indonesia, Korea
Murray Valley encephalitis	B	Mosquito	Australia, New Guinea
St. Louis encephalitis	B	Mosquito	Atlantic to Pacific Coastal Regions of U.S.A., Caribbean Islands including Jamaica, Haiti and Trinidad, Panama, Brazil, Argentina
Ilheus	B	Mosquito	Guatemala, Honduras, Panama, Colombia, Venezuela, Trinidad, Guyana, Surinam, Brazil
California encephalitis	California Complex	Mosquito	California, Great Basin, Rocky Mountain states, North and South Central states, Ohio Valley, Southeastern states, Florida and Louisiana
Inkoo	California Complex	Mosquito	Finland
Powassan	B	Tick	Ontario, Canada, upper New York, South Dakota, Colorado, California
Russian spring-summer encephalitis	B	Tick	Far Eastern and Western Siberia, Manchuria, China
Diphasic meningoencephalitis and Central European encephalitis	B	Tick (aberrant by milk)	Central and Eastern Europe from the Baltic to the Balkans
Louping ill	B	Tick	British Isles, Eire
Negishi	B	Tick (?)	Japan

antigenically distinguishable strains of VEE virus are maintained in multiple isolated foci of *Culex (Melanoconion)* species that feed on rodents which have a limited home range but reproduce rapidly, resulting in a frequent population turnover that provides new susceptibles.[37] While epizootic pulsations and epidemic excursions occur from these foci, pandemics such as that which swept from Central America through Mexico and into Texas in the period 1969 to 1972[38] are due to VEE virus strains recognized to have caused extensive epizootic epidemics in Ecuador, Colombia and Venezuela in the past. That these explosive epizootics and epidemics pass through focal enzootic and endemic areas indicates that a separate vertebrate-vector cycle occurs, probably primarily utilizing the equine host and vectored by almost any mosquito that feeds on such equines and man. In this respect, epidemic VEE is distinctly different from the species-specific mosquito vector–wild bird cycle of WEE and EEE and focally enzootic VEE. Because of this, and because disease attack rates with epidemic VEE are very high, the appearance of equine VEE epizootics wherever they occur is a forewarning of potential human epidemics of major dimensions.

The second group belongs in the Japanese B–West Nile complex of arbovirus Group B.[7] All are *Culex* mosquito–transmitted: Japanese B encephalitis (JBE) virus by *Culex tritaeniorhynchus* in Japan and Southeast Asia, *C. gelidus* in Malaysia and *C. vishnui* complex in India; Murray Valley encephalitis (MVE) virus by *C. annulirostris* in Australia; St. Louis encephalitis (SLE) virus by *C. tarsalis* in rural localities of western North America and *C. pipiens quinquefasciatus* in urban and suburban situations from Texas, the Mississippi Valley, and the Ohio Valley east to New Jersey, and *C. nigripalpus* in subtropical Florida and true tropical localities such as Jamaica.

All the JBE–WN complex encephalitis viruses appear to have an enzootic reservoir in wild birds. This may be a key factor in their wide dispersal and extensive annual summer-fall distribution in the temperate and subtropical latitudes. They appear to be maintained more or less continuously in tropical habitats. Seasonal occurrence of the mosquito-borne encephalitides in the temperate zone also reflects the availability of a new brood of nonimmune avian hosts that serve in the buildup of a circulating virus reservoir for infection of mosquitoes during peak periods of vector breeding and transmission. This produces epidemic peaks in late summer and early fall in the temperate zone, even though in equatorial areas cases may appear in every month of the year.

Equine cases of JBE have been reported in Singapore and Burma but are not of epidemiologic importance because JBE in human populations occurs where equines are rare or nonexistent. On the other hand, swine, which do not suffer overt disease, provide an important reservoir infectious to vector mosquitoes because of prolonged high titer viremia and prolific reproduction of new nonimmune offspring in communities where pork is a major source of meat protein. This includes most areas in Asia where JBE is increasingly reported not only as a seasonal epidemic disease of cooler climates but as a continual sporadic and epidemic occurrence in true tropical climates that support continued breeding of mosquito vectors.

While initially discovered to be a disease in India only in 1955,[7] recent epidemics in West Bengal mark JBE as a disease problem of major importance in that area.[39] Endemic JBE was shown to be widespread in lowland Thailand in 1956, but recent epidemics in upland Chiengmai[40] reflect an extension to new habitats of susceptible human populations.

Japanese B encephalitis and SLE have low CNS attack rates ranging from 1 in 200 to 1 in 500 infections.[41] In an immunologically virgin population JBE attacks all age groups, whereas SLE produces highest attack and case fatality rates in the elderly. Murray Valley encephalitis probably affects all age groups.

The California encephalitis complex includes several antigenic types of virus that are definitively characterized as belonging to a distinctly different group of mosquito-borne arboviruses of the Bunyamwera supergroup. It appears that most are transmitted by *Aedes* and *Culiseta* mosquitoes, many of which have a sylvan habitat. Accumulating evidence indicates that California complex viruses have mammalian rather than avian reservoir hosts, which, by genetic isolation, helps to explain their different regional antigenic and epidemiologic characteristics.

Human pathogenicity for each of the California complex viruses has not been established beyond recognition that the prototype BFS–283 was associated in the early 1940s with acute febrile CNS disease in the San Joaquin Valley of California and La Crosse with annual epidemics of encephalitis in the Ohio Valley, Wisconsin and elsewhere in the Middle West.[42] Less severe human disease is attributed to Tahyna and related viruses in Europe, the encephalitogenic potential not yet having been established.

Although present in the tropics, primary activity of California complex viruses has so far been defined primarily in temperate and subarctic regions. Even in warmer climates such as the Imperial Valley of California, transmission has been detected in *Culiseta inornata* mosquitoes, which are active in winter at temperatures close to freezing. The puzzle of early seasonal transmission in late spring, soon after thaw of frigid conditions, was solved by demonstration that the virus is transovarially transmitted through the egg, which is the mechanism by which certain *Aedes* mosquito vector species, such as *Aedes triseriatus*, survive through the winter.[43] That the occurrence of many undiagnosed acute febrile CNS disease cases is due to California encephalitis virus is certain, for when this cause has been considered and appropriately tested in the virus laboratory, such an etiology was established in many geographically separated localities.

The tick-borne Group B encephalitis viruses (Table 1–6) occur across the Palearctic region of Eurasia with one representative (Powassan) present in Canada and the northern United States. Those of the Eurasian continent have been called Russian spring-summer encephalitis (RSSE) or Far Eastern tick-borne encephalitis in Siberia and diphasic meningoencephalitis or Central European encephalitis (CEE) in Europe, including European Russia. These names generally correspond to the geographic distribution of their principal vectors, *Ixodes persulcatus* for RSSE and *Ixodes ricinus* for CEE, although their ranges overlap in European Russia. A wide variety of small mammals and birds upon which these ticks feed has been implicated in the zoonotic cycle of these viruses, and a secondary route of infection for man through virus secreted in goat's milk has been demonstrated for CEE. *Ixodes ricinus* is also the vector of the related louping ill virus of the British Isles and Eire. In North America, Powassan virus is transmitted by species of *Ixodes* and has, in addition, been isolated from *Dermacentor andersoni*. There is no information on the vectors or zoonotic hosts of Negishi virus, isolated from a fatal case of encephalitis in Japan, although, on the basis of its close antigenic relationship to the tick-borne encephalitis viruses, ticks may be suspect. The several year life span of ticks in northern climates provides a ready explanation for the persistence of the tick-borne encephalitis viruses in regions where they occur. Human infections result from man's intrusion into favorable tick habitats or on occasion, among urban dwellers, from the consumption of virus-contaminated milk. These agents are also highly infectious in the laboratory and numerous laboratory-contracted cases have occurred.

Pathogenesis. Details of arbovirus pathogenesis are given in the introductory information in this chapter (p. 8). The diverse manifestations of viral encephalitis reflect the quantity and dispersion of neuronal invasion and destruction.[44] A viremia follows initial replication of neurotropic virus elsewhere. A high titer is necessary for sufficient virus to escape from the capillaries into the interfaces of glial and neuronal cells. If sufficient neurons are affected, clinical signs appear.

The transient signs observed in many of the arbovirus encephalitides manifest the wide distribution of affected centers in the brain. Stiff neck indicates involvement of the meninges. The cerebellum and basal nuclei can be involved, as are various physiologic control centers. Hyperthermia results from destruction of the heat-regulating center, so the temperature should be carefully observed. Symptoms simulating poliomyelitis can occur by involvement of the spinal cord with anterior horn cells affected at different levels.

Later humoral immune response may produce a hypersensitivity reaction with perivascular inflammation. The frequency of this late complication, which may lead to secondary neurologic signs owing to increased intracranial pressure, is unknown. Therefore, at the present time, the use of corticosteroids to inhibit such inflammation and pressure is contraindicated because they delay the humoral immune response, thus prolonging and accelerating viremia which increases risk of viral invasion of the CNS.

Clinical Characteristics. Clinical manifestations range from inapparent infection or mild febrile episodes of a nondescript nature to fulminating febrile CNS disease resulting in coma, paralysis and death. The incidence of inapparent infection or mild disease varies according to the age of the infected person and the antigenic type of infecting arbovirus. Eastern equine and California encephalitis are most severe in children, while serious consequences of SLE virus infection occur most frequently in those at or past middle age.

The mosquito-borne Group A equine encephalitides have relatively shorter incubation periods of 3 to 7 days; however, longer periods have sometimes been observed. Onset of VEE as soon as 24 hours after infection has been known to occur.

The Group B mosquito-borne viruses, and those of the tick-borne complex, generally require a longer incubation period during which the pathogenesis may be more insidious, producing the severe paralyses and mental deterioration seen commonly in Japanese B encephalitis and Russian spring-summer encephalitis.

Central nervous system involvement is the principal clinical characteristic of the encephalitides as a group. The systemic consequences of infection, which occur later than the neuronal destruction, attributable directly to virus invasion, are often the precipitating cause of death.

The course of pathogenesis in most arbovirus encephalitides is remarkably similar, the rate and extent of CNS involvement reflecting the antigenic nature of the virus and the age and other constitutional factors of the patient.

A short incubation period and a fulminating infection that is characteristic of VEE (and sometimes WEE) and of the first phase of the diphasic form of Russian spring-summer encephalitis often cause a leukopenia, which is a manifestation of first stage viral multiplication in the lymphatics and the hematopoietic system. The clinical picture is a variable combination of fever, headache, malaise, stiff neck, occasional vomiting, sore throat, coryza and back pain lasting from 1 to 7 days. The syndrome often is not unlike influenza and may be diagnosed as such if an arbovirus etiology is not suspected on the basis of a history of exposure to mosquito or tick bite within an appropriate incubation period. It is from serum or spinal fluid of early acute cases characterized by this first phase syndrome that the causative virus can often be isolated.

Many patients suffer only a short illness with fairly prompt and complete recovery. However, this may be only a prodrome followed by temporary clinical improvement or apparent recovery before signs of central nervous system involvement appear.

A variation of this course is characteristic of some cases of WEE and California encephalitis that begin with a mild fever and headache. The temperature climbs gradually day after day and the headache increases and localizes in the frontal region. The patient becomes lethargic. Spontaneous vomiting and convulsions occur and may be the prelude to delirium and coma. Recovery is slow, with fall in temperature occurring by lysis. Appetite gradually returns, but convalescence is prolonged.

Severe cases of the equine encephalitides and SLE, most recognized cases of Japanese B encephalitis and the second stage of tick-borne diphasic meningoencephalitis, or the more severe Far Eastern form of Russian spring-summer encephalitis, correspond to the second phase of pathogenesis in which there is extensive viral invasion of the central nervous system. This gives rise to the symptoms and signs that direct clinical attention to the diagnosis of an encephalitis.[45]

There is sudden rise in or onset of high temperature, severe headache, stiff neck, prostration, conjunctivitis, photophobia, irritability and vomiting, with somnolence progressing to delirium, convulsions, coma, shifting sensory and motor neurologic changes, paralysis and death from hyperthermia or respiratory failure. In this phase there is often a relative leukocytosis and a shift from monocytic to polymorphonuclear pleocytosis in the cerebral spinal fluid accompanied by increase in protein.

Of considerable clinical significance at this time is the rapid shift in neurologic signs, entailing appearance and disappearance of normal and abnormal reflexes unilaterally, cranial nerve changes, alteration in muscle tone from flaccidity to spasticity, and the possibility of eliciting response from comatose patients by strong pressure on muscles or by other painful stimuli.

If death does not occur during the acute phase of the illness, there is slow recovery during which permanent neurologic damage may be assessed. The most severe is decerebrate rigidity or athetosis, focal upper and lower motor neuron paralyses, and prolonged coma which has been characterized as "sleeping sickness" by the layman, loss of intelligence, irreversible emotional instability as manifest by stupor, laughing and crying, and incoordination of movements.

Some patients show continued improvement over a long period of time while others have such irreversible neurologic damage that they may be permanently bedridden or require full-time institutional care. Some who display an apparent complete recovery may later show emotional instability under stress or inability to concentrate, or may just no longer do well in school or at other demanding mental tasks.

Differential Considerations. Acute febrile CNS disease has a multitude of causes including endocrine disturbances, toxins, protozoal and metazoal parasites, mycoses, bacteria and viruses. Leads to the causation of the disease are often established by a careful history. Epidemiologic association with sources, contacts or environmental exposures may be the key. Cerebrospinal fluid examination and culture may provide the clues. Reference should be made to general medicine texts for details characterizing each category of CNS disease. Attention is directed here to consideration of viral etiology once other classes of agents are ruled out.

Rabies is considered in detail subsequently. Very often suspect arbovirus encephalitis turns out to be due to *Herpesvirus hominis, Herpesvirus simiae,* lymphocytic choriomeningitis or postvaccinial virus infections, or a rare case of so-called postinfectious exanthemic virus disease such as measles or other exanthemic virus.

Over a long period of study, in 5 to 10 per cent of acute fulminating cases, encephalitis is due to *Herpesvirus hominis,* which, under conditions presently unknown, crosses the blood-brain barrier to invade the CNS. Epidemiologic association is an early clue. If the acute encephalitis occurs outside the usual mosquito or tick transmission season, herpes encephalitis should be considered. Serologic study of paired sera may show a rise in titer of specific antibody. Brain biopsy for other suspicions can show inclusion bodies characteristic of herpes virus invasion of the neurons.

Monkey B virus infection simulates herpes encephalitis but occurs almost invariably following association with animal colony primates. History of monkey bite should provide the lead, although such a direct inoculation need not be the mechanism as cases have occurred in the suspect presence of airborne fomites. An interim period of several years from primate exposure to onset reflects latency characteristic of herpes virus. When any herpes virus encephalitis occurs the prognosis is not good, for if the patient survives, the CNS destruction is so extensive that the victim becomes a physical and/or mental invalid.

Lymphocytic choriomeningitis virus, which was periodically recovered and labeled an arbovirus from mosquito virus studies, is now known to be latent in mice, especially some laboratory colonies used for the isolation of arbovirus. It is an arenavirus that is maintained asymptomatically in a wild rodent reservoir, most commonly the house mouse.[3] It is also maintained in other small mammals, and a recent nationally extensive epidemic associated with pet hamsters shipped from a large wholesaler in the United States caused almost 200 cases of acute febrile CNS disease that were suspected of being aseptic meningitis or encephalitis. While the acute illness may be severe, there is usually full recovery and low mortality.

Enterovirus infections are considered in Chapter 2 but may masquerade as arbovirus CNS disease until a virus is isolated or serologic rise in titer is established.

Epidemic influenza may encompass cases of encephalitis due to influenza virus infection of the CNS. The neurotropic proclivities vary from strain type to strain type.

Diagnosis. Suspicion of a viral source may be missed during the first acute phase, when there is a possibility of isolating an etiologic agent from blood, cerebrospinal fluid (CSF) or throat washings. But there is little question of the diagnosis when the neurologic signs appear. Pleocytosis in the spinal fluid strengthens the suspicion. Venezuelan equine encephalitis virus is recoverable from the pharynx up to 2 weeks after onset of illness, even after full recovery. This can be utilized for diagnosis by virus isolation even after the viremia has subsided. On the other hand, SLE and JBE viruses have been isolated from the blood only a few times because the long incubation period allows a humoral antibody response that controls and eliminates the viremia. Such antibodies can be detected by hemagglutination inhibition test (HI) within 3 days after onset of fever. This means that a presumptive diagnosis of SLE and JBE can be made serologically in a few hours and returned to the physician while the patient is still acutely ill.[7]

Specific etiologic diagnosis can be established only by laboratory examination. Isolation of the causative agent should be attempted from serum and CSF specimens collected as early as possible in the acute febrile stage. If the patient dies early in the course of disease, tissues of the brain, lung, liver, spleen or kidney may yield the viral pathogen. The diagnosis is established serologically by a rise in titer of antibody in two or more sequentially collected sera tested against viruses suspected on the basis of seasonal, environmental or geographic clues.

Treatment. There is no specific treatment for any of the neurotropic arbovirus infections. Once clinical disease is recognized, the best supportive treatment available may modify the more severe complications. The importance of good and constant nursing care cannot be overemphasized. This will provide for maintenance of a patent airway should respiratory difficulty develop, avoid tissue damage during convulsions, prevent bedsores, maintain hydration, and promptly dispose of vomitus and excreta from the incontinent patient.

Perhaps the most important lifesaving measure during the acute stage is the control of hyperthermia when the heat-regulating centers of the brain are affected. The means range from ice and sponge baths to artificial hibernation. A respirator should be available for patients who go into respiratory failure.

The *contraindications* to use of corticosteroids have been discussed previously. The problems of managing the convalescent patient are of a different order, ranging from prevention of bedsores and pneumonia to physical therapy and psychiatric assistance.

Prophylaxis. Formalin-inactivated mouse brain and tissue culture virus vaccines have been developed for those occupationally and recreationally exposed to the tick-borne RSS complex viruses. They appear to be effective. An attenuated live Langat virus vaccine is currently under study in Russia and the United Kingdom for infections caused by this group of agents.[45]

Of less evident effectiveness are the killed virus vaccines for Japanese B encephalitis. Such a vaccine used in American military personnel in the Far East during and after World War II was not effective. The Japanese, however, report success with their most recent killed virus vaccine.[39]

Laboratory workers have received apparent protection from a three-dose plus annual booster of diluted inactivated chick embryo–grown EEE and WEE virus vaccines. An attenuated live WEE virus vaccine is currently under study.

A VEE virus strain (TC–83), partially attenuated by passage in guinea pig heart tissue culture, has been developed. But the severity and rate of overt reactions make it useful only for those with a high risk of environmental or laboratory exposure. Being a live virus vaccine, it should give long protection, but overt VEE virus disease has occurred following accidental infection of those possessing neutralizing antibody as a result of vaccination. However, the use of this vaccine for the immunization of equines, the amplifying hosts of this virus, reduces the source of infection for vector mosquitoes and may be expected to prevent or abort spillover of infection to man.

Transfusion from donors of fresh whole blood containing high titer specific antibody has been used prophylactically following laboratory exposure to specific agents. Specific immune globulin preparation is currently being developed, but this material is not yet available in quantity sufficient for general use, even for laboratory workers.

Therefore, vector control aimed at the specific mosquito or tick vector is the mainstay of prevention and control where potential exposure or transmission is significant in endemic or epidemic situations. Persons entering a potentially infected area should be protected by appropriate clothing, repellents and acaricides as outlined in Chapter 72. Screening of dwellings and use of mosquito nets in sleeping quarters have proved effective in areas where mosquito vectors invade domestic premises searching for a human blood meal.

Rabies

Etiology and Epidemiology. Rabies is the classic neurotropic virus infection that is clinically manifested as a viral encephalitis. It is an example of low infectivity, but high pathogenicity, and the epitome of high virulence for the canine and human central nervous system (CNS). The virus is a zoonotic bullet-shaped rhabdovirus, which, if the infectious process is successful in establishing an infection at the tissue site of inoculation, replicates and proceeds via the peripheral neurons toward the central nervous system.

The essentially irreversible CNS neuron invasion and destruction produces a fulminating encephalitis that is rarely therapeutically inhibited. Rabies is therefore the model for conceptualization of zoonotic disease. Zoonoses are those infectious conditions of nonhuman animals transmissible with disease consequences in man.

The usual infectious process transmitting the virus to man involves wild or domestic canine bites that inject infectious virus from the infected salivary gland into the subcutaneous or mucous membrane tissues of a susceptible human being. Reliance of the virus on neuronal progression to the CNS provides the one means by which invasion of the CNS can be inhibited.

A knowledge of the etiology of rabies encephalitis is basic to an understanding of current concepts of early treatment and prophylaxis that can prevent CNS invasion. Also, an understanding of the epidemiology of rabies is essential for rational measures for preventing implementation of the process that results in infection, which virtually always leads to fatal acute febrile encephalitis or paralytic respiratory failure.

As a zoonotic infection rabies virus is maintained in vertebrate wildlife, particularly bats, skunks, foxes and, in certain parts of the world, other canines such as wolves. When rabid, the secretions from virus-infected salivary glands of these reservoir animals are inoculated into others as the infection is maintained in their wild kingdom. Threat to an associated human population is therefore monitored by an active surveillance of wildlife, looking for overt disease and laboratory detection of infection by isolation of virus from salivary gland or brain, visualization of Negri bodies (stainable eosinophilic intracellular conglomerates of rabies virus material) (Fig. 1–10) or immunofluorescent demonstration of antibody combined with tissue containing rabies virus.[46]

Rabies virus has long been considered a unique agent, but recent work in Africa has revealed several previously unknown viruses to be serologically related. Two of these appear to be insect transmitted. It is possible that further research on these newly discovered viruses may ultimately lead to a greater understanding of the natural history of rabies and perhaps also to better means of control and prevention.

Although human rabies is rare in the United States owing to such continued surveillance and extermination of wildlife reservoirs, and because of such measures as basic public health canine control by licensing, animal immunization and canine collection, most other areas of the world, particularly in the tropics, annually report almost a thousand human cases, which is only a small percentage of those that actually occur. In addition, domestic animal rabies due to wild reservoir exposure, such as vampire bats in tropical America, takes such a toll of cattle that there is a significant depletion of protein supply and huge economic loss. Therefore, while medical attention must be primarily focused on human exposure and human disease, it is equally important to grasp the basic concepts of wildlife rabies, which is the ultimate source of rabies as it affects human society.

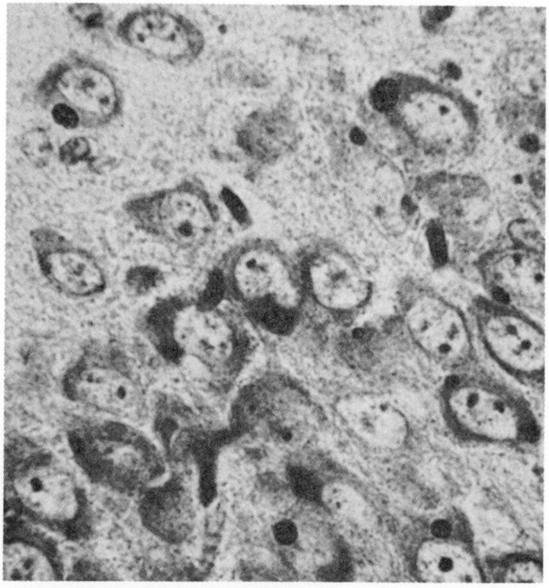

Figure 1–10. Intracytoplasmic inclusion bodies: Negri bodies of rabies.

Aggressive canines, whether they are rabid wolves of the mountains in Iran or street dogs in Cairo, are the most frequent infectors of man. Such feral and urban reservoirs stem from a canine cycle that is quite simple. Bat rabies, on the other hand, was originally recognized as a problem in the American tropics where the vampire bat transmitted the disease derriengue to cattle while taking their usual blood meal. What was not understood was the long duration of survival and infectivity of reservoir bats.

In the 1950s the unusual behavior of insectivorous or frugivorous bats exposed another zoonotic cycle. It was recognized that colonial bat populations served as vector reservoirs when human disease occurred in human cave visitors who were exposed only to excrement and atmospheric fomites. From these events emerged recognition that bats were another important zoonotic source that must be considered in pursuing an exposure history, because children often pick up apparently "tame" bats and other infected animals such as skunks and are subsequently bitten.

Certain insular territories in the world such as Great Britain, Australia and Hawaii have managed to eradicate rabies or remain rabies-free through stringent quarantine of canines. Other countries such as Sweden and the Netherlands have eradicated rabies through animal control efforts.

An animal need not appear rabid to transmit the virus because the salivary glands can be infected for several days, perhaps a week, prior to onset of CNS symptoms. The low infectivity of rabies virus is mainly manifest by the rarity of laboratory infections and the absence of reports of man-to-man transmission, particularly in health care delivery situations where medical personnel are in close contact with a rabid patient during terminal stages of the disease.

Clinical Characteristics. Depending upon the site of inoculation, and therefore distance from the CNS, the incubation period can be as short as 10 days with head and neck wounds. Peripheral inoculation can result in delayed CNS manifestations for up to 2 years. Usually it is a matter of weeks to months. While a history of animal exposure may suggest the possibility of rabies, a patient may present with ascending paralysis or acute febrile CNS disease without suspicion of this infection.[47]

Pain or tingling at the original site of inoculation may be the significant clue. In contrast to most acute febrile encephalitides there may be a sequence of paresthesias and hyperesthesias associated with fever, particularly when the skin is stimulated by heat, cold or air movements. Hypersensitivity to noise and photophobia with pupillary dilatation may precede muscle spasms, particularly of those involving glutition. Such gagging at the sight of fluids or food is characteristic hydrophobia.

Another contrast to other viral encephalitides is the continued lucidity of the patient's awareness even though oral communication is difficult or impossible. Signs and written messages can often mark the perception of the patient. It is at this point that anxieties and muscular spasms must be treated.

Disease resulting from vampire bat rabies infection in tropical America is manifest by an ascending paralysis.

Treatment. The objectives can be divided into four categories of procedures.

1. Eliminate, diminish or inhibit virus replication at the bite site and prevent invasion of the peripheral nerve endings.

2. Institute systemic immunotherapy by:

   a. use of hyperimmune serum or immune human globulin to provide a humoral barrier to movement of virus by blood or across a tissue-nerve connection.

   b. administration of vaccines to stimulate systemic humoral and cellular immunity to block virus from entering the CNS.

3. Salvage the CNS by intensive administration of immunotherapy after early recognition of prodromal symptoms and signs. Such efforts are prohibitively costly, only rarely successful and may leave a patient in less than acceptable functional neurophysiologic condition.

4. Provide supportive relief and alleviation of suffering during the terminal hydrophobic, respiratory and cardiac failure, and encephalitic phases of the disease.

General guidelines for treatment are set forth in Table 1–7 that are the recommendations of the W.H.O. Expert Committee on Rabies.[48]

WOUND TREATMENT. Where there has been an animal bite penetration of the skin, or salivary contamination of a break in the integument, immediate treatment of the wound is essential to eliminate any virus or prevent its progression via the peripheral nerve ending. There is substantial evidence that wound treatment is the point where most human rabies is prevented.

This involves thorough washing of the wound by soap and water followed by thorough rinsing, with debridement where excess tissue might harbor virus or other microorganisms. Prophylaxis for tetanus is also indicated.

Viral disinfectants such as quaternary ammonium compounds, nitric acid cautery or tincture of iodine should be carefully and thoroughly applied to reach any remaining virus. Where soap has been used to clean wounds, all traces of it should be removed before the application of quaternary ammonium compounds because soap neutralizes the activity of such compounds. Antibiotics are used to treat any bacterial infection. Initially the wound should be kept open to the viricidal effects of air.

If available, after testing for sensitivity, hyperimmune rabies antiserum can be infiltrated into and around the wound for further antiviral effect. Since many persons are sensitive to sera of horse and goat in which most rabies antisera are prepared, it is imperative to test for this sensitivity prior to local or systemic administration of this substance.

POSTEXPOSURE TREATMENT. Under conditions of bite by a probable rabid dog or

Table 1–7. Rabies – Specific Systemic Treatment

Nature of Exposure	Status of Biting Animal Irrespective of Previous Vaccination: At Time of Exposure	During 10 Days*	Recommended Treatment
Contact but no lesions; indirect contact; no contact	Rabid	–	None
Licks of the skin; scratches or abrasions; minor bites (covered areas of arms, trunk, and legs)	Suspected as rabid†	Healthy	Start vaccine. Stop treatment if animal remains healthy for 5 days*‡
		Rabid	Start vaccine; administer serum upon positive diagnosis and complete the course of vaccine
	Rabid; wild animal,§ or animal unavailable for observation		Serum + vaccine
Licks of mucosa; major bites (multiple or on face, head, finger, or neck)	Suspect† or rabid domestic or wild§ animal, or animal unavailable for observation		Serum + vaccine. Stop treatment if animal remains healthy for 5 days*‡

Source: W.H.O. Expert Committee on Rabies, Sixth Report, 1973.[48]
*Observation period in this chart applies only to dogs and cats.
†All unprovoked bites in endemic areas should be considered suspect unless proved negative by laboratory examination (brain FA).
‡Or if its brain is found negative by FA examination.
§In general, exposure to rodents and rabbits seldom, if ever, requires specific antirabies treatment.

cat, or suspect wild animals, serotherapy is indicated with simultaneous initiation of daily vaccination. Antiserum is provided in vials of 1000 units and should be administered as 40 units per kg of body weight. Recently, rabies immune human globulin has become available and avoids the problem of serum sickness. It should be administered 20 units per kg of body weight.

Simultaneously the first dose of vaccine should be given at another site, usually subcutaneously over the abdomen, followed daily by inoculations on opposite sides never in the same site. A number of potency certified vaccines are available made from brains of sheep, goats, rats, rabbits and suckling mice. Those from rats, rabbits and suckling mice, while being more expensive, are less likely to cause allergenic neurologic complications.

Avianized rabies vaccine has been developed as a duck embryo tissue β-propiolactone-inactivated virus desiccate that is rehydrated and administered subcutaneously, as are the more traditional vaccines.

Unfortunately, the currently recommended course of rabies treatment, combined serotherapy and vaccination, cannot be considered universally effective. A variety of reasons, some supported by experimental data,[47] are given for failures of such treatment. Administration of hyperimmune antiserum against rabies interferes with the immunogenicity of the simultaneous and multiple injection of rabies immunizing antigen. So if the initial serum therapy passively interferes with the immunogenic vaccine, relict rabies virus can continue to replicate and progress to the CNS.

Also of some concern is the possibility

that the vaccine itself contains rabies virus. Use of vaccines prepared from rabies-infected brain material risks neuroparalytic complications resulting from an allergen attributed to a basic protein in myelin. While vaccine free of such allergen has been produced from suckling mouse brain prior to myelinization, duck embryo tissue growth of rabies antigen has been successfully accomplished as a means of bypassing the allergenic component in animal brain vaccines, but desiccated killed rabies virus duck embryo vaccines (DEV) are recognized to be less immunogenic than brain vaccines, although in recent years DEV has been improved by increasing its antigenicity. While no neurologic complications have been attributed to DEV, failure of DEV protection has been reported possibly owing to serotherapeutic interference with immunogenicity, or inadequate DEV immunogenicity due to insufficient duration of treatment or to insufficient antigen mass. This is the basis for recommending periodic DEV booster inoculations 10, 20 and 90 days after completion of a 14- or 21-day course of daily inoculations of DEV.

Neurologic complications following use of animal brain may be manifest as peripheral neuropathy, transverse myelitis, ascending paralysis, encephalitis and mimicry of rabies. While ascending paralysis may appear only a few days after vaccination was begun, peripheral neuropathy and transverse myelitis may not occur until 1 to 2 weeks after initiation of postexposure treatment. In such situations vaccination should be stopped immediately because these complications can progress to fatality. Since CNS signs can occur as a vaccine complication or as a manifestation of rabies, appropriate serologic and virologic procedures should be followed to establish a correct diagnosis.

Postclinical Onset Treatment. Since survival following heroic measures of serovaccine therapy has been reported, such attempts should be tried where adequate biologicals and facilities are available. This entails assignment of the patient to an intensive care unit where vital signs can be monitored, particularly by electrocardiogram, to treat signs of imminent cardiac failure. Muscle spasms causing pain and anxiety are the two most important clinical signs amenable to alleviation by analgesics, tranquilizers and sedatives.

The lucidity and hypersensitivity of the patient maintain an awareness of nerve stimuli that can cause suffering, for which palliative treatment may be applied. Preparations for maintaining respiration and tracheal patency should be made against the possibility of suffocation due to muscle spasm. Because of antagonism toward food and fluid, intravenous therapy responding to blood chemistry and urinary determinations will be part of good clinical management.

Although man-to-man transmission of rabies is rare, attending personnel should maintain isolation and precautions against exposure to saliva that may contain virus.

Diagnosis. History of exposure to a potential or actual rabid animal bite is an important element of medical management. The first step is to incarcerate the animal. If behavior is suspicious, treatment should be started. If the animal does not become rabid in 10 days, treatment can be suspended.

Attack by a wild animal such as a bat, skunk, raccoon, wolf or jackal is presumptive evidence of rabies. The animal should be killed and the brain examined as with rabid domestic animals. Exposure to the urine or scent of animals such as a skunk should not be considered infectious if the animal is not observed to be rabid. Virus has not been demonstrated in such secretions.

If the quarantined animal becomes rabid, specimens from several areas of the brain—cerebellum, temporal and parietal lobes, horn of Ammon, and basal nuclei—should be collected and submitted to the laboratory for examination. Classic intracytoplasmic inclusions called Negri bodies (Fig. 1–10) are pathognomonic of rabies. Even though these may not be visualized in stained sections, fluorescent antibody visualization can locate rabies virus in CNS tissues. Definitive diagnosis is accomplished by producing rabies encephalitis by intracerebral inoculation of CNS tissue into mice, or other laboratory animals, followed by definitive identification of the agent by mouse neutralization test using specific rabies immune serum.

Prevention. Availability of myelin-free vaccines such as DEV has provided a vaccine that can be used for protection of persons at high risk of exposure to potentially rabid animals. These include veterinarians, animal control personnel, wildlife trappers and collectors and laboratory workers. Two immunization schedules are suggested: (1) two 1.0 ml subcutaneous injections of DEV a month apart followed by a third 6 months later; (2) three 1.0 ml injections a week apart with a fourth dose 3 months later. Pre- and post-vaccination serum should be drawn to test for rabies antibody titer. These tests can be done by the Rabies Investigation Laboratory at the Center for Disease Control in Atlanta, Georgia. Those persons with low or absent titer should receive an additional course of immunization.

In those so immunized, a 1.0 ml booster should be administered every year or so with an additional inoculation after a presumptive exposure.

Control. Organized domestic animal control programs are credited with virtual elimination of human rabies due to exposure to rabid dogs and cats in the United States. Such programs consist of annual licensing of pets based upon evidence of valid certification of rabies vaccination—annual for killed virus vaccines and 2 to 3 years for avianized live attenuated Flury type vaccines. Systematic search for, collection of and disposal of unlicensed animals eliminates the collective reservoir of susceptibles. Facilities for quarantine holding of suspect animals following strange behavior or bites is an essential component of animal control.

Wildlife rabies, which is a constant potential source of rabies to susceptible domestic animals and human beings, has been the subject of various approaches to control. Elimination of skunks by continuous trapping has been effective. Other measures such as shooting have been used. Gonad sterilants to control potential wild reservoir populations and syringe guns for vaccination have also been considered. Chemosterilants have been used with demonstrable success against vampire bat-transmitted rabies.

Although of significant cost, animal control programs against rabies can be initiated and maintained within the health resources of developing countries. The ravages of rabies, particularly among the innocently exposed in tropical countries, need not be accepted as an indigenous condition with the variety of measures now available for prevention and control.

Transmissible Virus Dementias
Kuru

MICHAEL ALPERS

Synonym. "Laughing disease."

Definition. Kuru is a subacute familial degenerative disease of the central nervous system, characterized by cerebellar ataxia and a shivering-like tremor, which progresses to complete motor incapacity and death in about 12 months from onset. Kuru means shivering, or trembling, in the Fore language.[49]

Distribution. The disease is confined to a region of steep mountain valleys, ranging from 1000 to 2500 m above sea level and about 3000 sq km in area, in the Okapa subdistrict of the Eastern Highlands of Papua, New Guinea. People from ten contiguous linguistic groups have been affected;[50] over 80 per cent of the 2300 recorded cases have occurred in the Fore linguistic group, and the remainder in neighboring villages with a history of intermarriage with the Fore people. In all, 174 villages have been affected. Their total population, 36,000 in 1957 when case surveillance began, has grown to 50,000 in 16 years but the number of villages affected has diminished to less than half.

Etiology. Kuru has been transmitted to the chimpanzee, with an incubation period of 2 years after intracerebral inoculation,[51] and to other primate hosts. It is the prototype degenerative slow virus disease in man. It has been grouped with scrapie disease of sheep, mink encephalopathy and Creutzfeldt-Jakob disease in the subacute spongiform virus encephalopathies.[52] The kuru virus, though only partly characterized, resembles the scrapie virus in its unconventional properties. When associated with host cellular membrane it is unusually resistant to the physical and chemical agents that degrade more conventional viruses; it has not been seen by electron microscopy, and it is apparently nonimmunogenic. Yet it replicates to high titer and consistently produces the same clinicopathologic disease through many passages in different primate hosts.

It is probable that about 50 years ago the first case of kuru occurred sporadically, and from it the virus was transmitted to a uniquely large number of people through the practice of mortuary endocannibalism. Since cannibalism declined in 1956, the transmission of the disease has been broken, the continuing incidence being explained by an incubation period of the order of 20 years. The role of genetic susceptibility in the pathogenesis of kuru is still undetermined, but vertical transmission of the disease does not occur.

Epidemiology. Kuru is predominantly a disease of adult women, though children of both sexes were commonly affected. In the period 1957 to 1959, 60 per cent of patients were adult females, 31 per cent children (19 per cent female, 12 per cent male), 7 per cent adolescent (15 to 20 years) and 2 per cent adult males. Since then the disease has progressively disappeared in children. With a few exceptions from outlying hamlets, no person born since 1956 has developed kuru.

In 1957 kuru caused over half the female deaths in the villages with highest incidence, leaving about twice as many males as females in their populations. The highest village mortality recorded from kuru was 35 deaths per 1000 population per annum. Total annual mortality throughout the kuru region has declined from about 210 in 1957 to 1959 to about 70 in 1971 to 1973.

People of the kuru region continue to succumb to the disease even after years away from it in new environments. No case of kuru has occurred in any person migrating to the region since 1956 or in any person from outside of it who has been in contact with patients.

The epidemiologic findings have a ready explanation in the transmission of degenerative, noncontagious virus disease through the handling and ingestion of infected tissues during the practice of mortuary cannibalism. This was regularly performed by women but rarely by men, and the practice ceased abruptly in 1956 except in outlying hamlets. Recent studies are attempting to relate clustering of cases to particular mortuary feasts.

Pathology. Pathologic changes are confined to the central nervous system.[53] The principal change is widespread neuronal degeneration; this is found throughout the brain and spinal cord, but is always most severe in the cerebellum and associated nuclei. With the neuronal loss are found intense astroglial hypertrophy and proliferation, with associated gliosis. Very marked in some cases, though significantly absent in others, are anisotropic, PAS(periodic acid–Schiff)-positive plaques, with a uniform dark center and a rim of radiating filaments. Vacuolation occurs in the body of degenerating neurons and in cell processes, where it appears under light microscopy as status spongiosus. It is this feature that gives the subacute spongiform encephalopathies their name. Microglial proliferation and myelin degeneration are found as secondary features. Except for scattered perivascular mononuclear cuffing seen in some cases, inflammatory changes are conspicuously absent.

Clinical Characteristics. Kuru is characterized by a progressive and remarkably uniform course that divides itself naturally into three stages. There is no acute antecedent illness, but prodromal symptoms of headache and limb pains commonly usher in the disease. The first or ambulant stage begins with subjective unsteadiness of stance and gait and often of the voice, hands and eyes as well. Postural instability, with truncal tremor and titubation, and ataxia of gait are the first signs. A convergent strabismus often occurs early and persists throughout the disease (Fig. 1–11). Eye movements are ataxic but no true nystagmus occurs. Cerebellar ataxia, involving the midline and extremities, progresses rapidly and is associated with gross shivering-like tremors of the trunk and limbs, which are accentuated by cold or unstable posture. Dysarthria usually begins early and speech deteriorates as the disease progresses.

As complete support becomes necessary for walking, the patient passes into the second or sedentary stage. The ataxia and tremors become more marked. At this stage there is often rigidity of the limbs, with essentially normal reflexes and a negative Babinski response, associated with marked and widespread clonus. Muscular activity is poorly sustained. Emotional lability, leading especially to outbursts of pathologic laughter, is a feature of this stage, but does not occur in every case; it is this which has given rise to the inappropriate synonym for the disease. Mental deterioration and disorders of affect are, in general, conspicuously absent. No sensory changes have been detected. The fundi appear normal.

As the third or terminal stage is reached the patient becomes unable to sit up without support. Tendon reflexes may be exaggerated at this point. Ataxia, tremor and dys-

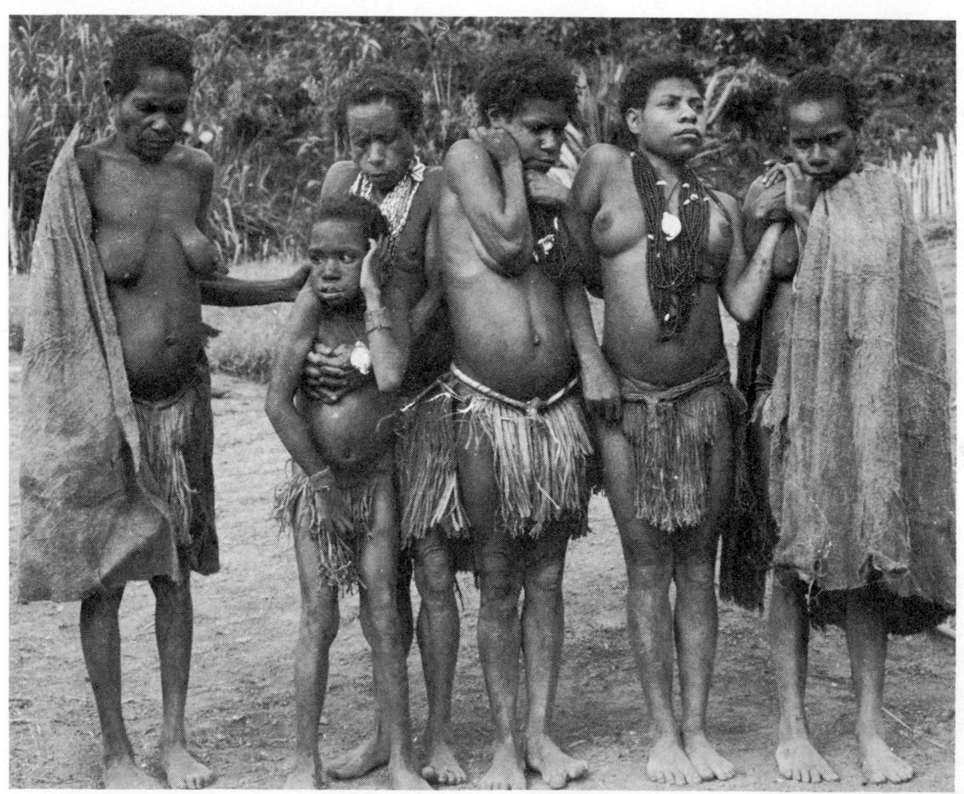

Figure 1–11. Six kuru patients from one village in the South Fore. Their postural instability may be seen from the activity of muscle groups in their legs and feet. To maintain their posture and also dampen down involuntary movements, their arms are held closely and firmly against each other. The girl shows a left convergent strabismus. (Courtesy of Dr. Carleton Gajdusek, N.I.N.D.S., National Institutes of Health, and Am. J. Med. *26*:447, 1959.)

arthria become progressively more severe and incapacitating. A grasp reflex may develop, and some cases show characteristic extrapyramidal defects of posture and movement. Terminally, urinary and fecal incontinence develop and dysphagia leads to starvation; flaccidity, inanition and signs of bulbar involvement supervene, and the mute and emaciated patient, often with gross decubitus ulceration and a hypostatic pneumonia, finally succumbs to the disease.

Diagnosis. In patients from the region, clinical progression through the stages described is diagnostic of kuru. Other tremor syndromes readily distinguishable from kuru occur in the New Guinea highlands. There is no biochemical or serologic test for the disease or its causative virus.

Prognosis. Kuru is a uniformly fatal disease. The duration from the first symptoms to death is normally about 12 months, with a range of 2½ months to 2 years or more. In general, the older the patient the longer the course. A few cases have shown a well documented remitting and exacerbating course but, despite many claims, no convincing case of recovery from the established disease has been found.

REFERENCES

1. Work, T. H. 1975. Introduction to Arthropod-Borne Viruses in Diseases Transmitted from Animals to Man. 6th ed. Charles C Thomas, Springfield, Illinois. pp. 922–928.
2. Theiler, M., and Downs, W. G. 1973. The Arthropod-Borne Viruses of Vertebrates (An Account of the Rockefeller Foundation Virus Program, 1951–1970). Yale University Press, New Haven. 578 pp.
3. Lehman-Grube, F. (ed.). 1973. Lymphocytic Choriomeningitis Virus and Other Arenaviruses. Springer-Verlag, Berlin. 339 pp.
4. Wildy, P. 1971. Classification and Nomenclature of Viruses. Monographs in Virology. Phiebig, Inc., New York. 81 pp.
5. Murphy, F. A. 1975. Arboviruses: Value of the New Taxonomy. Proc. 78th Annual Meeting, U.S. Animal Health Assoc. pp. 425–434.
6. Berge, T. O. (ed.). 1975. International Catalogue of Arboviruses, Including Certain Other Viruses of Vertebrates. 2nd ed. U.S. Department of Health, Education and Welfare No. CDC 75-8301 (For the Subcommittee on Information Exchange of the American Committee on Arthropod-Borne Viruses). 789 pp.
7. Work, T. H. 1971. On the Japanese B–West Nile virus complex or an arbovirus problem of six continents. Am. J. Trop. Med. Hyg. *20*:169–186.
8. Work, T. H. 1958. Russian spring-summer virus in India—Kyasanur Forest disease. Prog. Med. Virol. *1*:248–279.
9. Work, T. H. 1964. Arbovirus Impingement on the Natural History of Man. Occupational Diseases Acquired from Animals. The University of Michigan School of Public Health, Ann Arbor, Michigan. pp. 72–97.
10. Albrecht, P. 1968. Pathogenesis of neurotropic arbovirus infections. Curr. Top. Microbiol. Immunol. *43*:44–91.
11. Smith, C. E. G. 1970. Immunology and virus diseases. J. R. Coll. Physicians Lond. *5*:31–45.
12. Work, T. H. 1964. Isolation and identification of arthropod-borne viruses. *In* Lennette, E. H. (ed.): Diagnostic Procedures for Virus and Rickettsial Diseases. 3rd ed. American Public Health Association, New York. pp. 312–355.
13. Hanson, R. P., Sulkin, S. E., Buescher, E. L., Hammon, W. McD., McKinney, R. W., and Work, T. H. 1967. Arbovirus infections of laboratory workers. Science *158*:1283–1286.
14. Scientific Advisory Committee on Dengue (Periodical). Dengue Newsletter for the Americas. Pan American Health Organization, Washington, D.C. 1972 et seq.
15. Rosen, L., and Gubler, D. 1974. The use of mosquitoes to detect and propagate dengue viruses. Am. J. Trop. Med. Hyg. *23*:1153–1160.
16. Gajdusek, D. C. 1953. Acute Infectious Hemorrhagic Fevers and Mycotoxicoses in the Union of Soviet Socialist Republics. Med. Sci. Publ. 2, Walter Reed Medical Center, Washington, D.C. 140 pp.
17. Smorodintsev, A. A., Chudakov, V. G., and Churilov, A. V. 1959. Hemorrhagic Nephrosonephritis. Pergamon Press, New York. 124 pp.
18. Siegert, R., Shu, H.-L., and Slenczka, W. 1968. Isolierung und Identifizierung des "Marburg-Virus." Dtsch. Med. Wochenschr. *93*:604–612.
19. Strode, G. K. (ed.). 1951. Yellow Fever. McGraw-Hill Book Co., New York. 710 pp.
20. Smithburn, K. C., Durieux, C., Koerber, R., Penna, H. A., Dick, G. W. A., Courtois, G., de Souza Manso, C., Stuart, G., and Bonnel, P. H. 1956. Yellow Fever Vaccination. W.H.O. Monogr. Ser. No. 30, Geneva. 238 pp.
21. Halstead, S. B., and Nimmannitya, S. 1975. Technical Guide. 1. Clinical Diagnosis and Treatment of Dengue Hemorrhagic Fever. Pan American Health Organization, Washington, D.C. 17 pp.
22. Halstead, S. B. 1970. Observations related to pathogenesis of dengue hemorrhagic fever. VI. Hypothesis and Discussion. Yale J. Biol. Med. *42*:350–362.
23. Johnson, K. M., Webb, P. A., and Justines, G. 1973. Biology of Tacaribe Complex Viruses in Lymphocytic Choriomeningitis Virus and Other Arenaviruses. Springer-Verlag, Berlin. pp. 241–258.
24. Kuns, M. L. 1965. Epidemiology of Machupo virus infection. II. Ecological and control studies of hemorrhagic fever. Am. J. Trop. Med. Hyg., *14*:813–816.
25. Monath, T. P., Mertens, P. E., Patton, R., Moser, C. R., Baum, J. J., Pinneo, L., Gary, G. W., and Kissling, R. E. 1973. A hospital epidemic of Lassa fever in Zorzor, Liberia, March–April 1972. Am. J. Trop. Med. Hyg. *22*:773–779.
26. Troup, J. M., White, H. A., Fom, A. L. M. D., and

Carey, D. E. 1970. An outbreak of Lassa fever on the Jos Plateau, Nigeria, in January–February 1970. A preliminary report. Am. J. Trop. Med. Hyg. *19*:695–696.

27. Fuller, J. G. 1975. Fever. Ballantine Books, New York. 280 pp.
28. Leifer, E., Gocke, D. J., and Bourne, H. 1970. Lassa fever, a new virus disease of man from West Africa. II. Report of a laboratory acquired infection treated with plasma from a person recently recovered from the disease. Am. J. Trop. Med. Hyg. *19*:677–679.
29. Work, T. H. 1958. Russian spring-summer virus in India: Kyasanur Forest disease. Prog. Med. Virol. *1*:248–279.
30. Casals, J., Henderson, B. F., Hoogstraal, H., Johnson, K. M., and Shelokov, A. 1970. A review of Soviet viral hemorrhagic fevers, 1969. J. Infect. Dis. *122*:437–453.
31. Casals, J., Hoogstraal, H., Johnson, K. M., Shelokov, A., Wiebenga, N., and Work, T. H. 1966. A current appraisal of hemorrhagic fevers in the U.S.S.R. Am. J. Trop. Med. Hyg. *15*:751–764.
32. Chumakov, M. P. 1974. On thirty years of investigation of Crimean hemorrhagic fever. Medical Virology, Academy of Medical Sciences, U.S.S.R. *22*:5–18.
33. Siegert, R. 1972. Marburg Virus in Virology Monographs. Springer-Verlag, Berlin. 155 pp.
34. Morbidity and Mortality Weekly Report. 1975. Marburg Virus Disease, South Africa. *24*:89–90.
35. Monath, T. P. 1974. Lassa fever and Marburg virus disease. W.H.O. Chron. *28*:212–219.
36. Pan American Health Organization. 1972. Venezuelan encephalitis. P.A.H.O. Sci. Publ. No. 243, Washington, D.C. 416 pp.
37. Work, T. H. 1972. On the natural history of Venezuelan equine encephalitis: conclusions and correlations in Venezuelan encephalitis. P.A.H.O. Sci. Publ. No. 243, Washington, D.C. pp. 333–346.
38. Sudia, W. D., et al. 1975. Epidemic Venezuelan equine encephalitis in North America in 1971. Am. J. Epidemiol. *101*:1–13; 17–58.
39. World Health Organization. 1975. Japanese encephalitis in West Bengal. Weekly Epidemiological Record *23*:216.
40. Grossman, R. A., et al. 1973. Study of Japanese encephalitis virus in Chiengmai Valley, Thailand. Parts I, II and III. Am. J. Epidemiol. *98*:111–149.
41. Henderson, B. E., Pigford, C. A., Work, T. H., and Wende, R. D. 1970. Serologic survey for St. Louis encephalitis and other Group B arbovirus antibodies in residents of Houston, Texas. Am. J. Epidemiol. *91*:87–98.
42. Parkin, W. E., Hammon, W. McD., and Sather, G. E. 1972. Review of current epidemiological literature on viruses of the California arbovirus group. Am. J. Trop. Med. Hyg. *21*:964–978.
43. Watts, D. M., Pantuwana, S., DeFoliart, G. R., Yuill, T. M., and Thompson, W. H. 1973. Transovarial transmission of La Crosse virus (California encephalitis group) in the mosquito *Aedes triseriatus*. Science *182*:1140–1141.
44. van Bogaert, L., Radermecker, J., Hozay, J., and Lowenthal, A. (eds.). 1961. Encephalitides. Elsevier Publishing Co., New York. 718 pp.
45. Work, T. H. 1975. Tick-Borne Virus Diseases in Diseases Transmitted From Animals to Man. Charles C Thomas, Springfield, Illinois. pp. 994–1001.
46. Kaplan, M. M., and Koprowski, H. 1973. Laboratory Techniques in Rabies. 3rd ed. World Health Organization, Geneva. 367 pp.
47. Hattwick, M. A. W. 1974. Human rabies. Public Health Review *3*:229–274.
48. World Health Organization. 1973. W.H.O. Expert Committee on Rabies (Sixth Report). Tech. Rept. Ser. No. 523, World Health Organization, Geneva. 55 pp.
49. Gajdusek, D. C., and Zigas, V. 1959. Kuru: Clinical, pathological and epidemiological study of an acute progressive degenerative disease of the central nervous system among natives of the eastern highlands of New Guinea. Am. J. Med. *26*:442–469.
50. Gajdusek, D. C., and Alpers, M. 1972. Genetic studies in relation to Kuru. I. Cultural, historical, and demographic background. Am. J. Hum. Genet. *24*:S1–S38.
51. Gajdusek, D. C., Gibbs, C. J., Jr., and Alpers, M. 1966. Experimental transmission of a kuru-like syndrome to chimpanzees. Nature *209*:794–796.
52. Gibbs, C. J., Jr., and Gajdusek, D. C. 1973. Experimental subacute spongiform virus encephalopathies in primates and other laboratory animals. Science *182*:67–68.
53. Klatzo, I., Gajdusek, D. C., and Zigas, V. 1959. Pathology of kuru. Lab. Invest. *8*:799–847.

CHAPTER 2
Enteric Virus Diseases

TELFORD H. WORK

Unhygienic conditions fostered by climate and poverty produce and perpetuate fecal-oral transmission of enteric viruses. As with protozoal and metazoal parasites and enteric bacterial pathogens, these infections contribute substantially to morbidity and mortality of infants and children in tropical regions. Enteric virus infections confer a durable immunity that protects those who survive into later life. Maintenance of the fecal-oral pathogenic milieu often produces disease in newcomers and supports rapid transmission of enteric pathogens that are newly introduced.[1]

General Characteristics. While a number of enteric viruses produce infections of the respiratory tract with consequent respiratory disease, for sake of convenience these agents will be considered with those that are commonly found infecting the intestinal tract. Table 2–1 is a schematic classification of the clinical manifestations of enterovirus diseases; it relates specific virus types that have been found etiologically associated by virus isolation and serologic findings with the different syndromes. The usual mechanism for infection is by inhalation or ingestion.

Among the smallest pathogens of human disease are the *picornaviruses*—*pico* referring to the small size (17 to 30 nm diameter), and *rna* to the ribonucleic acid core constituent. Without appreciable lipid constituents and with no lipid envelope, this large group of viruses, except for the rhinoviruses, is chemically resistant to decomposition in acids of the stomach and in lipid digestive enzymes of the small intestine. These viruses therefore survive ingestion and journey through the alimentary tract to infect mucosal and subepithelial cells of the intestinal tract in manifesting their tropism for the enteric tissues of the anatomical organ system. As such, they constitute the major constellation of enteric virus infections, many of which result in diarrheal,

Table 2–1. ETIOLOGY OF CLINICAL SYNDROMES IN ENTEROVIRUS DISEASES

Characterized Disease Syndrome	*Coxsackievirus* *A*	*Coxsackievirus* *B*	*Echovirus*	*Poliovirus*
Upper Respiratory	21,24*	4,5	4,8,9,11,20,25,28	
Exanthem	9,16		4,6,9,16,18	
Herpangina	3,4,5,6,8,10			
Pleurodynia		1,2,3,4,5		
Pericarditis		1,2,3,4,5		
Myocarditis		1,2,3,4,5		
Nonparalytic Febrile Illness	2,3,4,5,6,7,8, 9,10,16,21,24	1,2,3,4,5,6		1,2,3
Aseptic Meningitis	2,4,7,9,10	1,2,3,4,5,6	2,3,4,5,6,7,9,11,14, 16,18,21,30,31	1,2,3
Meningoencephalitis		1,2,3,4,5		
Paralysis	7,9	2,3,4,5	2,4,5,6,9,11,20,25,28	1,2,3

*Types designated as etiologically associated.

influenzal, myositic, meningeal, neurologic and erythematous syndromes (Table 2–1). Individually or in various combinations, these syndromes result in the commonest febrile illnesses of the temperate summer seasons or of endemic tropical regions.

Epidemiology. Decades of research resulting in delineation of the basic mechanisms of the cause, spread and maintenance of poliomyelitis have established the fundamental concepts of all enterovirus infections that are generated and maintained by a fecal-oral means of transmission in which replication in the human intestinal tract occurs for extended periods of time.[2] This mode of transmission involves intermittent or continuous fecal excretion with direct person-to-person contact infection by inhalation or ingestion of effluvia, by ingestion of contaminated food which may result from fly or other arthropod-borne transfer of durable viruses from fecal deposits, or by intake of sewage-contaminated, unpurified water. Cationic, chemical and thermal stability of many enteroviruses allows for extended survival outside a living tissue system in the fecal-oral link in the chain of infection.

Not infrequently more than one enterovirus type may be isolated from a single specimen of throat swab, rectal swab or stool. This demonstrates that these agents can circulate continuously in environments where unsanitary conditions of inadequate sewage disposal, impure water supply and contaminated food are characteristic, as in extensive areas of the tropical and subtropical regions. Epidemiologic research relating to serology has established that 90 to 100 per cent of indigenes have been infected with the most prevalent types by age 5. In fecally contaminated communities that are isolated for long periods, introduction of a pathogenic enterovirus can have devastating consequences to the entire population. In contrast, individuals who travel into these areas from a highly sanitated community are subject to multiple infections and disease owing to the prevalent enterovirus pathogens circulating in the poorly sanitated indigenes. On numerous occasions high attack rates for paralytic poliomyelitis in military expeditionary forces and expatriate pregnant women have been reported.

Because of prolonged intestinal replication, physicochemical durability, and protective maintenance in excrement, enteroviruses are the most prevalent pathogens in environments of poor sanitation. Studies in virology by isolation from intestinal tracts, feces, water, milk, food and nasopharyngeal secretions, and those in serologic epidemiology have established that enteroviruses are the most widely disseminated pathogens among infants and children living in tropical areas. A close association with high attack rates of infant and child morbidity has been demonstrated for the enteroviruses, and it is probable that significant infant mortality is associated with these agents, but inadequate or improper nutrition may be a synergistic cause.

Serologic studies have shown that antibodies to a myriad of enteroviruses appear in such populations of infants and children very early in life. Although poliomyelitis is not generally considered a common disease in tropical regions, careful clinical observation has shown that it does result in significant paralytic disease in the very young; attack rates shift to older children and immigrant adults as improved sanitation develops, resulting in prolongation of susceptibility to three different polioviruses into later life when disease severity and case paralytic rates are significantly higher. The appearance of a child dragging a "polio limb" behind a throng of children in a tropical village is not an uncommon sight. The presence of a paralyzed child in an educated or affluent family in a developing country is also not uncommon. Enterovirus-caused clinical disease is expected to increase in many developing tropical countries. In fact, the increase in reported cases of poliomyelitis and other enterovirus diseases not only will reflect better disease surveillance but will serve as one measure of improved sanitation, particularly in association with the very young and with young adults and pregnant women.

Poliovirus Infections

Etiology. There are three antigenically distinct types of poliovirus. Reference strains named Brunhilde (I), Lansing (II) and Leon (III) and other prototypes have been identified in various virologic and epidemiologic studies. While perhaps only 2 or 3 per cent of poliovirus infections result in clinical symptoms and signs of nonparalytic or paralytic disease, it is theoretically possible to suffer poliomyelitis three times even though each infection confers lifelong immunity. It was this etiology by three types of pathogens, none of which readily produced experimental disease in other than expensive primate hosts, that created confusion in early attempts to associate paralytic disease with a single pathogen.[2]

Lack of an experimental animal of reasonable cost delayed emergence of epidemiologic and pathogenetic information that allowed elucidation of the cause of poliovirus infection. Determination of the oral-enteric-lymphatic-humoral-central nervous system chain of events led to an understanding of the mechanisms by which polioviruses reached the anterior horn cells or basal areas of the brain to produce lower and upper motor neuron lesions that resulted in paralytic disease.

Only after demonstration of a relatively long incubation period of a week to 35 days, which allowed development of antibodies in acute phase sera following a viremia, was it possible to conceive of active immunization against such blood dissemination of virus. This led to development of killed virus (Salk) vaccination followed by attenuated live virus immunization (Sabin) as the now generally recognized means for prevention of poliomyelitis.

Pathology. The pathogenesis of central nervous system involvement in poliomyelitis is only incompletely known. The mouth is probably the portal of entry, and primary virus multiplication takes place in the pharynx or in the intestines, or both. It is thought that possibly the virus multiplies in lymphoid tissue, for example in tonsils or in Peyer's patches, and that it then enters the blood. At this stage antibody is highly effective in preventing further spread. If there is sufficient viremia, however, the blood-brain barrier is overcome and the central nervous system is invaded. It is possible, therefore, to prevent the central nervous system manifestations of poliomyelitis infection if relatively small amounts of neutralizing antibody are present in the blood.

In the central nervous system, the anterior horn cells of the spinal cord are the classic location for lesions, but other areas of the cord and sometimes the dorsal root ganglia may be damaged. In the brain, the cortex is not usually involved, except for the precentral motor cortex. Neuronal destruction with neuronophagia is the classic neurologic lesion. If neurons are not completely destroyed, recovery of function is possible, and this is important clinically. Perivascular cuffing and invasion of areas of neuronal destruction by lymphocytes are characteristic of poliomyelitis. Poliomyelitis virus may attack muscle directly and may cause myocarditis.

It is now generally accepted that, on ingestion of one of the three types, the poliovirus can initially infect and replicate in the nasopharyngeal, mucosal and regional lymph nodes, followed by passage through the alimentary tract to the intestinal mucosa and lymphatic drainage where further viral replication occurs. The resulting virus spills into the blood for wide dissemination. Most often, the humoral antibody response blocks further invasion. However, in a small percentage of persons the poliovirus—of which there are strains of varying neurotropism and virulence—crosses the blood-central nervous system barrier with a proclivity for the anterior horn cells of the spinal cord. Destruction of these neurons produces a lower motor neuron lesion, which results in a flaccid paralysis. The poliovirus that invades the brain can cause destruction of cranial nerves and upper motor neurons in various areas of the brain. This often results in cleavage of central nervous system control of respiration and other vital functions, and is known as bulbar poliomyelitis because the lesions are in the base of the brain.

Maintenance of peripheral muscular tone by physical therapy allows regeneration of nerves to the skeletal muscles with varying resumption of function. Central nervous system lesions lack myelin so that recovery of function from brain centers rests upon utilization and re-education of accessory nerve pathways.

Clinical Characteristics. Poliomyelitis is a classic infection manifesting the entire spectrum of the process of infection from inapparent and subclinical to self-limited febrile prodrome, nonparalytic syndrome, overt paralytic disease and fulminating fatality.

Because such a small number of poliovirus infections result in overt signs of disease, the sporadic case in an endemic situation, or the index case preceding an epidemic, presents symptoms and signs that may not be readily diagnosed. Many infections produce fever, malaise, pharyngitis, possibly a stiff neck and muscle pains which constitute a self-limited episode that is passed off as a nonparalytic poliomyelitis, or other enterovirus infection, on the basis of a history of exposure within a period of 1 to 5 weeks, usually 7 to 21 days. A careful history or epidemiologic surveillance often reveals other cases, some of which present characteristic paralytic manifestations.

Overt poliomyelitis may follow the prodrome as continuous illness or as a recrudescence. There are fever, evidence of meningitis, muscle pains and muscle spasm followed by flaccidity in 1 or 2 days. Muscle involvement is related to the segmental level of anterior horn cell lesions in the spinal cord, and lower extremity paralysis is identified with lumbar segments. Upper extremity and respiratory paralysis reflects cervical and basal brain neuron destruction. Progression of paralysis usually ceases with decline of the fever. While cerebrospinal fluid may manifest a mild pleocytosis – usually lymphocytes numbering 5 to 500 – followed by a rise in protein, these changes are only supportive clues when abnormal, but are not diagnostic.

Significantly higher attack rates of paralytic poliomyelitis have been observed following tonsillectomy. Localization of paralysis in limbs traumatized by inoculations of vaccine and drugs has also been common. These are important considerations when such elective procedures are contemplated for the unimmunized, especially in the tropics where there is no safe winter season.

Diagnosis. Because of the variety of clinical manifestations, specific diagnosis depends upon a 4-fold or greater rise in serum neutralizing antibodies. Isolation of virus from the intestinal tract swab or stool, or an unusual number of clinically paralyzed cases, provides a high degree of suspicion. Such laboratory capability should be available through local, national or World Health Organization reference laboratories. Establishment of a clear virologic diagnosis is very important because it has been repeatedly demonstrated that effective administration of Sabin live attenuated virus vaccine has aborted epidemics.

Prognosis. The extent of paralysis corresponds to the febrile period. The cerebrospinal fluid findings may be diagnostically helpful but have no prognostic value. If paralytic signs are clearly of lower motor neuron lesions, persistent physical therapy will encourage return of function over periods of time as long as 2 years. However, involvement of medullary centers and cranial nerves constitutes a grave prognosis in regard to threat of death. Respiratory failure or permanent postinfection paralysis may be partially compensated by replacement training of other neural pathways and muscles.

Treatment. Symptomatic relief is provided by antipyretics and analgesics for fever, headache and pains of nonparalytic poliomyelitis. Bed rest prepares for the least stress or any further involvement that may occur.

Severe muscle pain of more serious disease, back pain and other discomfort may require narcotic analgesics. A hard mattress supported by boards may alleviate back and limb pain due to movement of the bed. Hot packs and other pain-relieving physical measures are indicated for severe muscle pain. As soon as this subsides a regimen of physical therapy should be initiated and developed to avoid atrophy of the paralyzed muscles. Supportive psychological as well as physical treatment is very important to encourage the patient to accept and undertake early and prolonged physical therapy and rehabilitation.

Once acute disease is manifest, there is no way to terminate progression of paralytic involvement. However, patients threatened with respiratory failure should be provided with an appropriate respirator and continuous nursing care to maintain an airway with frequent removal of accumulating oropharyngeal secretions.

Prevention. Besides provision for protection from fecal contamination, those considered at risk should receive at least three administrations of Sabin oral trivalent live virus vaccine. This is because only one poliovirus type may replicate in the intestinal tract at a time. The objective is to produce a humoral immune response to all three poliovirus types. Because of the high risk of exposure of infants to oropharyngeal and fecal excretions, such immunization should be initiated as early as 2 months of age. Oral poliovirus revaccination is recommended for all expected to visit, enter or live in a tropical or other questionably sanitated environment.

Coxsackievirus Infections

Etiology. The term coxsackievirus derives from the name of the small New York town on the Hudson River where in 1947 stool specimens were collected from two boys suffering apparent paralytic poliomyelitis. From these stools were isolated filterable agents that produced paralytic disease and death in suckling mice and suckling hamsters, but no disease in weanling mice and hamsters nor in rhesus monkeys inoculated according to the classic technique for isolation of poliomyelitis viruses.[3] It was noted that clinically there was no nuchal rigidity in the two juvenile patients, although muscular weakness of the back and lower extremities gave physiologic paralysis. Spinal fluid from one patient lacked abnormal cell count. Both boys recovered fully.

By various routes of suckling mouse inoculation (intracerebral, intraperitoneal, intramuscular) it was noted that the histopathologic lesions were inflammatory degeneration of the skeletal musculature, with no sign of nervous system damage. This became the classic histopathologic characterization of coxsackievirus A isolation infections in suckling mice.

Later isolation attempts from stool specimens of patients with nonparalytic and apparent paralytic poliomyelitis yielded agents with restricted pathogenicity for suckling mice. However, these agents produced spastic paralysis in suckling mice (in contrast to muscular weakness of coxsackie A), fat pad necrosis, necrosis of the acinar cells of the pancreas, and focal necrosis in myocardial and striated muscle. The agents also produced inflammatory degeneration in suckling mouse brain. These lesions characterized the coxsackie B group of agents, which may produce upper respiratory, nonparalytic febrile illness, aseptic meningitis, meningoencephalitis, and paralysis similar to that caused by some coxsackievirus A pathogens. Diagnosis therefore rests on characterization of virus isolates with significant rise in neutralizing antibody titer.

Epidemiology. That these agents and associated diseases emerged from presumptive summer epidemics of atypical, nonparalytic and paralytic disease, initially considered to be poliovirus infections, reflects a similar fecal-oral route of intestinal excretion, dissemination and infection. Epidemic curves, attack rates by age and sex in exposed communities, and a generally nonfatal outcome with complete recovery mark the usually recognized pattern of epidemics. Sporadic cases occur when nonimmune individuals enter environments where there is widespread dissemination of feces-borne pathogens.

Pathology. The pathogenesis of coxsackievirus infections in man has not been worked out completely, but is thought to resemble that of poliomyelitis in many respects. Viremia is more marked and more prolonged in coxsackievirus infections than in poliomyelitis. Whereas poliomyelitis virus can rarely be recovered from cerebrospinal fluid, coxsackieviruses of group B can be recovered from the cerebrospinal fluid of patients with aseptic meningitis with sufficient frequency to be useful diagnostically.

Although myositis is prominent in experimentally infected suckling mice, particularly in group A infections, and has also been demonstrated in a few human cases, there is still relatively little evidence that coxsackieviruses cause widespread or severe damage of skeletal muscle in man. However, both myocarditis and encephalitis are important manifestations of group B infections of humans. Myocarditis may be fatal to infants, and encephalitis may be followed by residual weakness of involved muscle groups. Poliomyelitis-like lesions of the spinal cord have been demonstrated in infected monkeys.

Clinical Characteristics. Because of the ubiquitous spread of coxsackieviruses and the variety of clinical consequences of infection associated with particular types of virus, as presented in Table 2–1, the different syndromes are briefly characterized. Suspicion rests not only on the clinical signs and symptoms but also on the epidemiologic association of infected patients. Clusters of cases may erupt within families or in various other human aggregations. It is important to remember that although the infecting pathogen may be of a single type, clinical cases may vary by syndrome or may present a combination of more than one type of clinical sign. Also, an epidemiologic situation that involves fecal dissemination may encompass fecal-oral transmission of more than one enterovirus ranging from poliomyelitis to several coxsackieviruses, and even echoviruses.

UPPER RESPIRATORY TRACT DISEASE. Symptoms and signs of the common cold, self-limited or including pharyngitis with fever, may appear.

EXANTHEM. When associated with a demonstrable erythema, or macular or maculopapular rash, coxsackie A virus infection must be considered. More commonly an echovirus is the cause.

HERPANGINA. This is the one clinical manifestation that suggests to the clinician an A coxsackievirus infection. It may be combined with a febrile illness involving muscular weakness that might be considered nonparalytic poliomyelitis.

While the sore throat may be only inflamed, careful examination will reveal papular and vesicular lesions, surrounded by reddened rings on the tonsillar fauces, uvula, palate and tongue. Although uncomfortable, the patient is not acutely ill and recovery occurs in 1 to 4 days.

Another, sometimes alarming, combination may be "hand, foot and mouth disease," with vesicles appearing not only in the oral cavity but also on the hands and feet.

PLEURODYNIA. This is almost exclusively caused by one of the coxsackie B viruses. Sometimes in multiple or clusters of cases it is called epidemic myalgia. Fever and pain are invariably present. A prodromal malaise may precede the characteristic abrupt onset by a few hours to several days. Adults complain commonly of headache and thoracic pain. This pain may be substernal or referred to either side of the chest. In single, sporadic or index cases differential diagnosis of angina pectoris or myocardial infarction must be considered.

In children the pain may be abdominal without thoracic involvement. Patient observation is important to differentiate from an acute abdominal condition. A superficial level of pain will indicate muscular involvement. Occasionally there will be associated neck or back stiffness but appropriate re-examination will establish that myalgia is present. While classic aseptic meningitis may occur, it is rare.

ORCHITIS. This condition is a significant complication in males, more commonly in the tropics. In contrast to mumps, complete recovery is the rule.

PERICARDITIS AND MYOCARDITIS. Suspicion of a coxsackie B virus as the cause of acute cardiac involvement stems from recognition of other syndromes attributable to coxsackie B virus, or isolation of coxsackie B viruses in an epidemic situation. Acute myocarditis is seen in infants who have a sudden onset of dyspnea, cyanosis, tachycardia, heart failure and general collapse. This often rapidly terminates in death.

Histologically, there is diffuse, patchy or focal cellular infiltration around degenerated muscle fibers of the myocardium. Coxsackie B viruses have been isolated from such necrotic tissue. Onset of a febrile illness with cardiac signs in infants, or physical signs of a pericardial pathologic condition such as pericardial rub or fluid, calls for electrocardiographic monitoring and cardiovascular support.

Because cardiac complications are not frequently considered in enterovirus infections, adequate clinical attention is not given to these potential complications until cyanosis, tachycardia and cardiac failure attract appropriate diagnostic and therapeutic measures, which are probably instituted too late. More careful application of clinical examination for cardiac complications should bring about earlier protective measures that will lessen what is now left to a postmortem diagnosis.

OTHER MANIFESTATIONS. *Nonparalytic Febrile Illness, Aseptic Meningitis, Meningoencephalitis, Paralysis.* These are clinical components of what is a summer seasonal collection in a large pediatric service with associated adult cases being admitted to the infectious disease wards. It has been established that the spinal fluid pleocytosis may be supportive but not diagnostic of poliomyelitis, and the same is true of coxsackievirus infections. Aseptic meningitis may show no abnormal cell count, whereas coxsackievirus meningoencephalitis may show a marked pleocytosis of the cerebrospinal fluid. While the term "aseptic meningitis" is not precisely correct, since the causative virus can often be isolated from spinal fluid, it refers to analysis of constituents of the fluid that do not present the appearance of a bacterial, fungal or parasitic infection. Except for myocarditis in infants, the rapid and complete recovery of these patients indicates that an enterovirus other than poliovirus is the responsible pathogen.

Diagnosis. It is obvious that with such a plethora of etiologic agents and multiple combinations of clinical syndromes, dependence for an accurate diagnosis rests upon the virus laboratory. Stool specimens must be inoculated into suckling mice and tissue culture must be undertaken. It should be remembered that isolation of a suckling mouse pathogen does not establish the diagnosis. Only after demonstration of rise in titer of specific neutralizing antibody between acute and convalescent sera can such a diagnosis be established.

Inoculation of stool or rectal swabs collected from normal populations in tropical areas, or during the summer season in temperate zone communities, will yield facultative enteroviruses unrelated to any particular disease syndrome that is occurring. On the other hand, recovery of a test pathogen from sewage samples may be necessary to obtain an antigen for which there will be a diagnostic rise in antibody titer in paired sera.

Such a diagnosis may be important in order to establish the epidemiologic source or mode of transmission which will govern measures to be applied for epidemic control.

Treatment. This is symptomatic and includes administration of antipyretics and analgesics with bed rest.

Prevention. This depends upon sanitary measures. There are no vaccines for coxsackievirus infections. Because there are so many agents, and the disease is usually self-limited with full recovery, there is little rationale for developing a large armamentarium of immunogens for these infections.

Echovirus Infections

Etiology. Following a principle similar to that which characterized the coxsackieviruses by their distinctive and almost exclusive pathogenicity for suckling mice, the echoviruses emergedwhen rhesus monkey kidney tissue cultures became a principal laboratory means for isolation of enteroviruses from fecal materal. Initially the viruses assigned to the echovirus group were those that produced cytopathogenic changes in monkey cell culture but were not pathogenic by intracerebral inoculation into rhesus monkeys like poliovirus, or into suckling mice like coxsackieviruses. Because they went only into tissue culture they were called *enteric cytopathogenic human orphan* viruses, the acronym *echoviruses* being applied for conservation of space.

Because most of these viruses were not associated with human disease when isolated, they were for some time known as "viruses in search of disease." Subsequent epidemic and clinical studies incriminated many, but by no means all, of the more than 30 echoviruses with human disease.

Epidemiology. As enteroviruses, echoviruses are propagated and transmitted by the fecal-oral route. Many are particularly infectious among small children where echovirus infections are predominant.

Clinical Characteristics. Because of the many manifestations of echovirus infections along with or exclusively as enterovirus pathogens, it is useful to list only clinical signs of echovirus disease that should lead the clinician to consider what specimens should be collected for and what tests run by the virus laboratory to establish a diagnosis. The following have been observed as disease manifestations associated with echovirus infections: aseptic meningitis, paralysis, encephalitis, ataxia, exanthem, enanthema, myalgia, pericarditis, myocarditis, diarrheal disease, and respiratory syndromes. For types incriminated, refer to Table 2–1.

Seasonal respiratory disease, summer exanthems, aseptic meningitis and paralytic disease are the most common manifestations of echovirus disease. Because they occur often in the very young they can be fatal. A virologic diagnosis is therefore important because these diseases may be involved in nursery and preschool epidemics or threaten susceptible infants with serious disease consequences.

Diagnosis. Isolation of virus from rectal swab, stool, throat swab, body fluids and cerebrospinal fluid in continuous live monkey cells followed by serologic demonstration of rise in titer to the isolate is the basis for a virologic diagnosis. Typing of the isolate may prove to be important in epidemiologic definition.

Because echoviruses, like other enteroviruses, are ubiquitous, association of a specific virus with a disease syndrome is based on four criteria:

1. Prevalence of virus type among diseased individuals greater than in healthy controls.
2. Development of antibodies during the course of the illness.
3. Negative evidence of concurrent infection by pathogens known to cause similar illness.
4. Isolation from body fluid or postmortem tissue of afflicted patients.

Treatment. Since symptoms and signs are manifestations of tissue invasion and destruction, there is no therapy known to inhibit such viral invasion. Therefore treatment is bed rest, antipyretics, analgesics and maintenance of fluid balance.

Prevention. This depends upon a sanitary environment and hygienic behavior. No vaccines have been developed.

Viral Hepatitis

Jaundice in the tropics is one of the most perplexing problems in differential diagnosis. Often there is not even a clinical laboratory capability sufficient to measure accurately serum glutamic oxaloacetic transaminase (SGOT) or serum glutamic pyruvic transaminase (SGPT), the enzymes that increase in serum as a clue to icteric or anicteric hepatitis virus infection.

Other infectious causes of jaundice frequently encountered in tropical regions are: yellow fever, infectious mononucleosis, leptospirosis, syphilis, brucellosis and malaria. Diagnosis rests on isolation of the causative agent or serologic demonstration of rise in titer of specific antibodies.

Noninfectious causes of jaundice are hepatocellular toxins such as carbon tetrachloride and various therapeutic drugs, extrahepatic biliary obstruction by bile duct calculi or neoplasm, and hemolytic conditions. Careful history to elicit information on solvent inhalation and drug consumption, and other environmental exposures, should establish the chemical nature of exposure. Blood biochemistry and the occurrence of light to white chalky stools associated with symptoms and signs of biliary obstruction should establish the cause. Hematologic studies would characterize the anemia.

Etiology. Results from experimental feeding of effluent filtrates from icteric patients to human volunteers have established the viral nature of the hepatitis pathogens. Failure to achieve repeatable cytopathic effects in any tissue culture system so far attempted indicates that infectivity and pathogenicity of hepatitis viruses are highly host-specific for human beings.

There are at least two different viruses that have been historically categorized as the etiologic factors in hepatitis A or infectious hepatitis (IH), and hepatitis B or serum hepatitis (SH). They are also clinically and epidemiologically referred to as short-incubation (A, IH) and long-incubation (B, SH, HBV) hepatitis viruses. Virologic and epidemiologic studies in recent years have characterized an antigen associated with hepatitis B. Persons with detectable hepatitis-associated antigen (HAA)—sometimes referred to as Australia antigen—are considered to be infected and their blood to be infectious. It has been established that long-incubation hepatitis B virus can be transmitted by means other than injection or transfusion.

Virologic studies have shown that a 42 nm structure called the Dane particle may be HBV. The 20 nm spherical and filamentous particle associated with it is a surface antigen and has been designated HB_sAg. The core antigen of the Dane particle is HB_cAg. Other antigens have been detected, demonstrating that the Dane particle is antigenically complex. Therefore, it is no longer acceptable to report HBV antibody (HBab), but necessary to designate more specifically which antibody, such as anti-HB or anti-Hb_c, is detected as evidence of HBV infection or circulation of HBV in a donor's serum.[4]

With such antigenic characterization of one type of viral hepatitis it has been possible to elucidate more precisely the public health implications of hepatitis B antigen in human blood.[5] A confirmed positive reaction is evidence of acute or chronic type B viral hepatitis, or of an asymptomatic carrier state. While presence of HBV antigen is usually transient, persistence beyond 3 months is indicative of a chronic carrier state. Presence of the antigen in pregnancy or the neonatal period is often followed by postpartum infection of the infant. Evidence of HBV antigen in potential donors eliminates them from consideration. However, there are no data yet that indicate these persons are of unusual risk in transmission as carriers by other routes.[6]

Efforts in the past quarter century to isolate hepatitis viruses in experimental animals and tissue culture systems have produced a sequence of reports that ultimately failed confirmatory study. Recent studies of marmosets injected with icterogenic specimens from human patients with type A infectious hepatitis produced serum enzyme evidence of disease. Characterization of the CR326 agent as an enterovirus related to the cause of type A hepatitis and its use in an immune adherence test provide a specific serologic diagnostic procedure as useful as those now available for HBV.[7] Isolation of agents from cases of hepatitis A, such as the CR69 (076) strain with acid pH requirements in tissue culture and unusual thermostability, may be the precursor of successful diagnostic isolation of the infecting viruses from blood and stool of patients with hepatitis A.[7a]. These agents, which have uncommon culture characteristics, may herald recognition of a new group of enteroviruses in the same way as coxsackie- and echoviruses emerged from new developments in virologic technology. As yet, however, identification of acute viral hepatitis rests primarily on clinical diagnosis and serum biochemistry demonstrating acute viral damage of the parenchymal cells of the liver, except where the specialized immunologic tests for antibodies to hepatitis A and B are available.

Neutralization of this effect appears to have been accomplished with convalescent serum collected from patients following acute infectious hepatitis in a series of marmoset protection tests mixing various doses of the icterogenic (virus-containing) suspension with acute and convalescent sera.[7]

Both hepatitis A and B viruses are highly thermostable. Infections do occur by use of needles and instruments that have been boiled for sterilization. It has been determined that hepatitis A virus withstands 56° C (132.8° F) for at least 1/2 hour, and hepatitis B 60° C (140° F) for more than 4 hours. Autoclaving and concentrated exposure to chlorine (Clorox) will inactivate the viruses. Intestinal contents and blood-contaminated secretions of inapparently or overtly infected persons are considered to be infectious by ingestion and possibly by inhalation.

Epidemiology. While clinical cases in children are milder than in adults, epidemics do occur with significant attack rates of icteric disease in children. In tropical regions and in temperate situations encompassing rural communities without sanitary disposal of human excrement, a milieu is maintained in which there is continuous fecal-oral transmission of enteric virus infections, including viral hepatitis. There are numerous reports of epidemics in the military such as occurred in the Mediterranean region in World War II. Of the 60 American Peace Corps volunteers in the initial contingent assigned to Colombia, 11 suffered clinical viral hepatitis during their 2-year residence in rural areas.

Accidental or occasional fecal contamination of an inadequately treated water supply results in widespread cases. Possibly the largest hepatitis epidemic ever to occur resulted from a sandbar blocking the Jamuna River water supply of New Delhi in 1955;[8] effluent from the Najafgarh Nulla was siphoned into the water plant intake. Even though the dose of chlorine was increased to a discomforting level, sufficient to inactivate all other pathogens, resistant hepatitis virus was delivered to three segments of a population of almost 2,000,000 people with what was estimated to be 40,000 cases resulting in significant mortality among notables and a particularly high death rate in pregnant women.[9]

That so many cases occurred in a population that has a high prevalence of protective antibodies indicates that prior exposure does not fully protect against subsequent massive infections. There is no cross-protection between hepatitis A and B viruses. It can be assumed that the unprotected and unaware entering such a milieu are at high risk of infection unless very careful precautions in eating and drinking are followed.

Outbreaks following consumption of raw shellfish (oysters and clams) have been documented in the United States.[10-12] Such shellfish from seafood bars in other countries have also been implicated as the source of infections that produce disease after return from travels or in geographic situations distant from the actual exposure. Because human beings are the primary host, encounters with the infection can occur anywhere in the world.

High attack rates have also been reported for animal handlers associated with primates, particularly chimpanzees, which indicates that these animals serve as a passage host, not necessarily from their sylvan origin but after contact with infectious persons.

Saliva is probably an important vehicle of infection in non-parenterally acquired type B hepatitis.[13] Arthropod transmission as by cockroaches and flies has not been proved. Intimate contact, such as that which occurs within families, is a common characteristic of transmission but theoretical transfer by the venereal route has not been proved.

Clinical Characteristics. While some

patients may suffer an acute onset at the time signs of jaundice appear, usually there is insidious onset of malaise, fever, marked anorexia, gastrointestinal signs and even diarrhea. This may be difficult to diagnose as hepatitis because overt jaundice is absent. It may be recognized only because of other cases with jaundice or a history of association with an earlier case or potential past exposure to sewage or other fecal contamination.

The incubation period varies greatly; type A has a shorter incubation of 2 to 7 weeks whereas type B has a long incubation period of 7 weeks to 5 months. The pathologic physiology is similar and consists of extensive destruction of the parenchymal cells of the liver.

Hepatitis in children is usually a milder disease than in adults and jaundice occurs less often. When it does occur, it appears at the end of the febrile anorexic and irritable phase; the child may present the anomalous picture of marked jaundice while feeling well and resuming a good appetite and substantial food consumption. Complications are rare.

On the other hand, adult hepatitis is marked by high frequency of jaundice with malaise, fever, anorexia, weakness, irritability and gastrointestinal symptoms. The first indication of the specific liver involvement may be dark or mahogany-colored urine which leads to closer scrutiny for clinical jaundice and to blood examination which shows abnormal serum transaminase levels.

Besides jaundice in light-skinned persons, evident sometimes only by yellowing of the conjunctivae, the liver and spleen may be enlarged. There may be epigastric and right upper quadrant and even focal abdominal pain that requires careful differential distinction from an acute surgical abdomen. Splenomegaly and generalized lymph node enlargement may require differential exclusion of infectious mononucleosis.

While an acute attack of what is referred to in the early and European literature as catarrhal jaundice (type A) and homologous serum jaundice (type B) may incapacitate the adult patient for several weeks, recovery is usually uneventful except for the rare complications discussed below. Jaundice usually lasts from 10 days to 2 weeks. If it lasts longer than a month, surgical consultation is in order.

Diagnosis. Establishment of a diagnosis of anicteric and icteric viral hepatitis rests initially on suspicion, which in turn results from a careful history or epidemiologic association with other cases and contacts in the community. Most often type A hepatitis virus infection is associated with contaminated water and food, the latter usually from an asymptomatic food handler excreting virus. Type B usually results from needle transmission related to (1) blood transfusion, (2) inoculation procedures where needles are inadequately sterilized *(boiling needles will not always kill hepatitis virus; autoclave* or *use disposable needles),* and (3) drug addiction using a single person-to-person needle transfer.

While a specific viral diagnosis cannot be established by usual laboratory procedures, a number of biochemical indicators can strengthen the clinical suspicion when a blood specimen collected in the preicteric or icteric phase of the illness is examined. There is often a leukopenia with atypical lymphocytes. With biochemical tests, abnormal liver function is first detected by positive cephalin flocculation and thymol turbidity tests, and shortly thereafter increases to abnormal levels are found in the serum glutamic oxaloacetic and serum glutamic pyruvic transaminases. Bromsulphalein retention is increased. Serum bilirubin rise reflects the level of jaundice. Of considerable importance is a direct van den Bergh reaction.

Sophisticated and sensitive methods exist for detecting hepatitis B antibody by radioimmunoassay, rheophoresis and direct hemagglutination. Immune adherence (IA)[14] and complement-fixation (CF)[15] tests for hepatitis A antibody in human serum have been developed, employing liver extract of marmosets infected with the CR326 strain of human hepatitis A virus. The IA test is more sensitive than the CF test. The IA test should be a valuable tool for diagnosis, for epidemiologic surveys, for identification of susceptible and immune persons, for quantitative assays of gamma globulin, and for identification of hepatitis A virus in attempts to propagate the virus in cell culture.[16]

Complications. While a feared nodular cirrhosis occurs, it is rare. Subacute or chronic pathologic changes may result in exacerbation of jaundice, particularly in the elderly. If cirrhosis does develop, ascites, edema, and hemorrhagic phenomena mark a long-term decline that terminates fatally. Massive damage to the liver parenchyma can cause hepatic coma and death.

Treatment. Once established, there is no specific inhibitor of the virus infection. Administration of human pooled gamma globulin to those intimately exposed to a case or at other high risk of infection can modify the infection sufficiently to produce mild or inapparent disease. Supportive therapy of bed rest and proper nutrition is the best that can be done to withstand the complex pathophysiology of the disease and to facilitate the reparative process that regenerates hepatic cellular structure to normal functional condition.

Anorexia inhibits food consumption. All categories of food should be encouraged according to the palate of the patient, including staples such as milk, butter and eggs. The objective is to reverse the weight loss and regain strength, which will significantly shorten convalescence. B-complex vitamin supplementation may benefit patients substantially.

Whereas those who are old, debilitated or physically exhausted may relapse if physical activity is resumed too soon, previously healthy individuals should be encouraged to get out of bed and resume light exercise, providing a rest period of an hour or so is taken after every meal.

For acute hepatic decompensation manifested by disorientation, coma, or hemorrhagic phenomena, daily intravenous administration of 10 per cent dextrose solution and 25 gm of low-salinity albumin is recommended.

Beneficial use of corticosteroids in adults suffering fulminating hepatitis and hepatic coma has been reported and is therefore a consideration in such cases. However, there is no clinical justification for such therapy in the usual clinical hepatitis with jaundice. Likewise, human immune pooled gamma globulin has no role in treatment of acute hepatitis with jaundice. Its effect is to convey passive-active immunity in prophylaxis against acute disease manifestation following infection with hepatitis viruses.

Prevention. Blocking intestinal-oral and humoral-parenteral transmission of virus is the hallmark of preventing infection. This focuses on adequate purification of water, proper postdefecation cleansing of hands, elimination of insect carriers of fecal contamination to food, sanitary disposal of sewage, and avoidance of physical oral contact. These are reasonable hygienic measures to be followed and enforced in rural situations and urban eating and drinking establishments.

There is evidence that usual daily contact with HB_sAg carriers does not increase risk of infection. High attack rates in military populations deployed in underdeveloped tropical and subtropical regions, American Peace Corps volunteers, foreign aid personnel, and travelers has led to the recommended prophylaxis by injection of pooled human gamma globulin (ISG). The collective antibody experience of the donors of plasma from which ISG is precipitated reflects enough infection-induced antibody to produce passive-active protection against overt disease following fortuitous hepatitis virus infection in a situation of high risk.

Because the protective capacity of immune serum globulin (ISG) varies from one lot to another, it has been necessary to establish a minimum recommended dose for differing situations. This is 0.02 ml per kg of body weight. A more general dosage schedule would be 0.5 ml ISG for children up to 25 kg, 1.0 ml ISG for persons weighing 26 to 50 kg, and 2.0 ml for those over 50 kg. ISG does not prevent infection; it modifies disease to a mild or inapparent form. Increase in the recommended dose will not increase the palliation of disease, but in a situation of prolonged exposure will extend the period of protection up to 4 months.

Viral Diarrheal Disease

Etiology. Although long suspected clinically and epidemiologically, demonstration of viral causation of diarrheal disease has awaited technological progress in visualization of pathogens in the intestinal tract and feces by negative stain and immune electron microscopy.[17] Orbivirus-like particles have been demonstrated in the duodenal mucosa of children acutely ill with diarrheal disease and in stool specimens.[18, 19] Because the virus is of double-shelled cuboid structure with the appearance of a wheel, it has been given the tentative name of rotavirus. Serologic association has been demonstrated by immune electron microscopy. Aggregates of antibody from convalescent sera are visualized, but acute serum controls do not form such conglomerates.

Epidemiology. Although rotavirus-associated diarrheal disease has been reported from many parts of the world,[19, 20] and type A hepatitis virus antigen identified in fecal specimens, there is no sound estimate of the number or variety of enteric viral agents responsible for diarrheal disease. The etiologic association of these viruses has been demonstrated in infants.

In contrast to many enteric infections, the seasonal incidence is not clear. Many outbreaks have occurred in winter months when infants and children are intimately exposed because of closed environments.

Clinical Characteristics. The incubation period appears to range from 2 to 5 days. Onset may include vomiting; diarrhea may persist for 15 days.

Diagnosis. Where electron microscopy is available, virus can be purified and concentrated by differential centrifugation designed to separate rotavirus from other enteroviruses. The sediment is then suspended in drops of distilled water and examined by electron microscopy after negative staining.[21]

Treatment. There is no evidence that any chemotherapy of antibiotics affects these pathogens. Standard treatment measures for dehydration are indicated as with other diarrheal diseases.

Prevention. This involves consumption of uncontaminated fluids and sanitary disposal of excrement. Because explosive epidemics have occurred in young children following close association or sequential exposure in closed environments, which may be fecally contaminated, unaffected children should be kept apart or cared for in separate rooms or facilities.

REFERENCES

1. Horsfall, F. L., and Tamm, I. 1965. Viral and Rickettsial Infections of Man. 4th ed. J. B. Lippincott Co., Philadelphia. 1282 pp.
2. Paul, J. R. 1971. A History of Poliomyelitis. Yale University Press, New Haven. 486 pp.
3. Dalldorf, G., Sickles, G. M., Plager, H., and Gifford, R. 1949. A virus recovered from the feces of "poliomyelitis" patients pathogenic for suckling mice. J. Exp. Med. *89*:567–582.
4. Committee on Viral Hepatitis of the National Research Council – National Academy of Sciences. 1974. Nomenclature of antigens associated with viral hepatitis type B. Morbidity, Mortality Weekly Report *23*:29.
5. Committee on Viral Hepatitis of the Division of Medical Sciences, National Academy of Science – National Research Council. 1974. The public health implications of hepatitis B antigen in human blood – a revised statement. Morbidity, Mortality Weekly Report *23*:125–126.
6. Alter, H. J., Chalmers, T. C., Freeman, B. M., Lunceford, J. L., Lewis, T. L., Holland, P. V., Pizzo, P. A., Plotz, P. H., and Meyer, W. J., III. 1975. Health care workers positive for hepatitis B surface antigen. Are their contacts at risk? N. Engl. J. Med. *292*:454–457.
7. Provost, P. J., Ittensohn, O. L., Villarejos, V. M., Arguedas-Gamboa, J. A., and Hilleman, M. R. 1973. Etiologic relationship of marmoset propagated CR 326 hepatitis A virus to hepatitis in man. Proc. Soc. Exp. Biol. Med. *142*:1257–1267.

7a. Pelon, W., Miller, J. H., and Deas, J. E. 1974. Hepatitis A: in vitro isolation of an agent with unusual growth requirements from a clinical case occurring in Costa Rica. Bull. P.A.H.O. *8*:212–220.

8. Viswanathan, R. 1957. Certain epidemiological features of infectious hepatitis during the Delhi epidemic, 1955–1956. *In* Hartman, F. W., Lo Grippo, G. A., Mateer, J. G., and Barron, J. (eds.): Hepatitis Frontiers. Little, Brown & Co., Boston. pp. 207–210.
9. Melnick, J. L. 1957. A water-borne urban epidemic of hepatitis. *In* Hartman, F. W., Lo Grippo, G. A., Mateer, J. G., and Barron, J. (eds.): Hepatitis Frontiers. Little, Brown & Co., Boston. pp. 211–225.
10. Hartman, F. W., Lo Grippo, G. A., Mateer, J. G., and Barron, J. 1957. *In* Hepatitis Frontiers. Henry Ford Hospital International Symposium, October

25–27, 1956, Detroit, Michigan. Little, Brown & Co., Boston, 169 pp.

11. Dougherty, W. J., and Altman, R. 1962. Viral hepatitis in New Jersey, 1960–1961. Am. J. Med. *32*:704–716.
12. Mason, J. O., and McLean, W. R. 1962. Infectious hepatitis traced to the consumption of raw oysters. An epidemiological study. Am. J. Hyg. *75*:90–111.
13. Villarejos, V. M., Visoná, K. A., Alvaro Gutiérrez, D., and Rodríguez, A. 1974. Role of saliva, urine and feces in the transmission of type B hepatitis. N. Engl. J. Med. *291*:1375–1378.
14. Miller, W. J., Provost, P. J., McAleer, W. J., Ittensohn, O. L., Villarejos, V. M., and Hilleman, M. R. 1975. Specific immune adherence assay for hepatitis A antibody. Application to diagnostic and epidemiologic investigations. Proc. Soc. Exp. Biol. Med. *149*:254–261.
15. Provost, P. J., Ittensohn, O. L., Villarejos, V. M., and Hilleman, M. L. 1975. A specific complement-fixation test for human hepatitis A employing CR326 virus antigen. Diagnosis and epidemiology. Proc. Soc. Exp. Biol. Med. *148*:962–969.
16. Krugman, S., Friedman, H., and Lattimer, C. 1975. Viral hepatitis A identified by complement-fixation and immune adherence. N. Engl. J. Med. *292*: 1141–1143.
17. Almeida, J. D., and Waterson, A. P. 1969. The morphology of virus-antibody interaction. Adv. Virus Res. *15*:307–338.
18. Middleton, P. J., Szymanski, M. T., Abbott, G. D., Bortolussi, R., and Hamilton, J. R. 1974. Orbivirus acute gastroenteritis of infancy. Lancet *1*:1241–1244.
19. Davidson, G. P., Bishop, R. F., Townley, R. R. W., Holmes, I. H., and Ruck, B. J. 1975. Importance of a new virus in acute sporadic enteritis in children. Lancet *1*:242–246.
20. Flewett, T. H., Bryden, A. S., and Davies, H. 1975. Epidemic viral enteritis in a long-stay children's ward. Lancet *1*:4–5.
21. Bishop, R. F., Davidson, G. P., Holmes, I. H., and Ruck, B. J. 1974. Detection of a new virus by electron microscopy of faecal extracts from children with acute gastroenteritis. Lancet *1*:149–151.

CHAPTER 3

Respiratory Virus Diseases

TELFORD H. WORK

Human aggregation fosters occurrence of person-to-person contact respiratory virus diseases. The variety of pathogenic viruses that initiate infections of the respiratory tract results in frequent individual episodes of coryza and fever. These viruses also cause family, community and institutional epidemics that deplete individual and organized endeavors. Such epidemics often overburden health care facilities. Secondary complications may result in significant mortality.

While presently accepted beliefs often associate respiratory virus diseases with temperate and colder climatic and geographic zones, it must be remembered that huge populations, between the Tropics of Cancer and Capricorn, reside at cooler, higher altitudes such as the Andes of South America and the uplands of Africa. Temperate effects producing human clustering for warmth are characteristic of tropical arid regions such as the Sahara and the Arabian and Rajasthan deserts where extremes of daily temperature change are great. Seasonal cold, which afflicts such tropical country cities as Cairo and Delhi, is marked by an early morning pall of smoke. This motionless blanket visually conveys the atmospheric congestion dynamics by which viruses are readily exhaled and inspired among people huddled in crude shelters or over coals and fires trying to keep warm. In low income communities in the most crowded urban area of Calcutta, for example, intense transmission occurs in contrast to much less transmission in isolated villages in the same district.[1]

While the viruses causing many clinical respiratory syndromes are ubiquitous, the diseases often reflect exotic situations in which people live.

Etiology. Clinical and virologic studies of the past 2 decades have provided a systematic approach to an etiologic diagnosis of respiratory virus disease by careful clinical examination. This not only enables the physician to suggest a suspect virus, but assists in prognosis, which is so important in anticipating diminution of productivity in a labor force or requirements for mobilization of health care resources. With a suspected source apparent, appropriate specimens can be collected for laboratory examination in order to characterize and identify specific viral etiology; this is of importance in managing respiratory disease, particularly in infants and children, and in the aged and debilitated.

Clinicians have logically divided the respiratory tree into upper and lower, divided at the larynx. The upper system involves mucous membranes and lymphoid tissues of the sinuses, nasopharynx, oropharynx and larynx. The lower respiratory infections are associated with the respiratory epithelium of the trachea, bronchi, bronchioles and alveoli. Different syndromes associated with particular respiratory viruses reflect their selective infectivity and pathogenesis.

In Table 3–1 the clinical manifestations of respiratory virus disease are arranged in anatomical sequence of signs and symptoms that relate to syndromes commonly associated with different causative viruses.

Table 3–1. Etiology of Clinical Syndromes in Acute Viral Respiratory Disease†

DIMENSIONS OF INVOLVEMENT	CHARACTERIZED DISEASE SYNDROME	MYXOVIRUSES				ADENO-VIRUSES	PICORNAVIRUSES					OTHER VIRUSES					
							Rhino-viruses 60 Types	ENTEROVIRUSES				REO-VIRUSES	HERPESVIRUSES			ZOONOTIC	
		Influenza	Para-Influenza	Respi-ratory Syncytial	Measles			Coxsackievirus A	Coxsackievirus B	Echo-Virus	Polio-Virus	1, 2, or 3	Herpes Simplex	Varicella Zoster	Cytomegalo Virus	Lymphocytic Chorio-meningitis	Psittacosis Ornithosis
GENERALIZED	INFLUENZA	A, B, C*	+					21, 24	+			?				+	
	PLEURODYNIA								+								
UPPER RESPIRATORY TRACT (SUPRA-LARYNGEAL)	HERPANGINA							2, 4, 5, 6, 8, 10					+				
	CORYZAL			+	+	1, 2, 3, 4, 5, 6, 7, 14, 21	+++	21		8, 11, 20, 25		?					
	PHARYNGITIS		1, 2, 3, 4			1, 2, 3, 4, 5, 6, 7, 14, 21		21		4, 6, 8, 9, 11, 16, 20	+		+				
	PHARYNGO-CONJUNCTIVITIS					8										+	
LOWER RESPIRATORY TRACT (INFRA-LARYNGEAL)	PULMONARY DUCT INFLAMMATION LARYNGOTRACHEO-BRONCHITIS – ACUTE EPIGLOTTITIS (croup)	+	1, 2, 3	+	+	1, 2, 3 4, 5, 6, 7, 14, 21	+?			+							
	ACUTE BRONCHIOLITIS	+	3	+++		+											
	PNEUMONITIS AND PNEUMONIA	+	3	+++	+	1, 2, 3, 4, 7, 14	+?							+	+	+	+

*Types designated where significant.
†Original; courtesy of Dr. Telford H. Work.

Influenza

This term is improperly applied to a variety of acute respiratory, gastrointestinal and generalized febrile illnesses in which the patient feels miserable. Generalized aches and pains, headache, myositis and malaise, with or without respiratory symptoms, characterize "influenza." Usually the disease is self-limited, with recovery within a few hours to a few days.

Etiology. Proper influenza results from lower respiratory tract infection with a specific myxovirus of type A, B or C. Influenza C is only occasionally recognized as the cause of clinical disease and appears to be antigenically stable. Antigenic change has been observed in type B over long periods of time but it has been associated usually with milder disease than type A, which causes severe attacks, most often in epidemics and periodically in pandemics originating in eastern Asia.

Continuous drift in antigenic character of type A is related to infectivity and pathogenicity of influenza in a particular population group at a particular time reflecting the profile of immunity to type A influenza.[2] About every 10 years it is the sudden mutation and shift in hemagglutinin and neuraminidase characteristics of the virus particle that prepare it for a new onslaught on human susceptibles who have insufficient cross-immunity from exposure or immunization with a previous antigenic type A.

The surface hemagglutinin constitutes the ability of the virus to attack the epithelial cells of the lower respiratory tract. There ensue an invasion, replication in the nucleus and formation of new whole particles by incorporation of the cell membrane into envelope constituents, which include hemagglutinins and neuraminidase. The neuraminidase is involved in the mechanism enabling the particle to leave the cell so that the hemagglutinin can attach to a new cell. These are the two key elements of the virus in the pathogenesis of disease. These virion envelope projections determine the antigenic character of the type A virus infecting the host. Serologic tests can determine the hemagglutinin-neuraminidase characteristics of the pathogen, in which important diagnostic and epidemiologic information lies.

Humoral (IgM) and secretory (IgA) antibodies are specific for these subunit components of the virion. Hence, in the face of a change of either hemagglutinins or neuraminidase or both in a new type A virus, existing antibody will no longer adequately protect.

Epidemiology. Influenza can cause sporadic cases, especially when a particular type A is passing through a population it has afflicted several times before. An epidemic is often recognized only by the sudden occurrence of many cases of characteristic clinical disease, possibly with an unusual number of fatalities in the debilitated and elderly from cardiac complications and pneumonia. This has led to utilization of excess influenza-pneumonia mortality, i.e. above that regularly observed, as an indication of epidemic influenza in a population subject to a continuous disease surveillance system. (See Fig. 3–1.)

Pandemics occur when there is a change in the antigenic characteristics that enable the new virus to infect and produce disease in a population that no longer has antibody suitable for inhibiting the new type. It is therefore of prime importance to isolate, characterize and constantly monitor the antigenic characteristics of type A influenza virus to warn of a new type in order to institute preventive measures, including a vaccine matching the new antigenic characteristics. This is done by a global network of World Health Organization Influenza Reference Laboratories.

The recently devised hemagglutinin-neuraminidase antigenic classification scheme has contributed to ease in classifying new isolates, definitive serologic epidemiology, and conceptual and practical advances in preparation of subunit vaccines.

By using characterized reference prototype strains isolated from epidemics of the past 40 years in antibody tests of various age groups bled in different decades, a retrospective panorama of antigenic changes in influenza A has been constructed (Fig. 3–2).

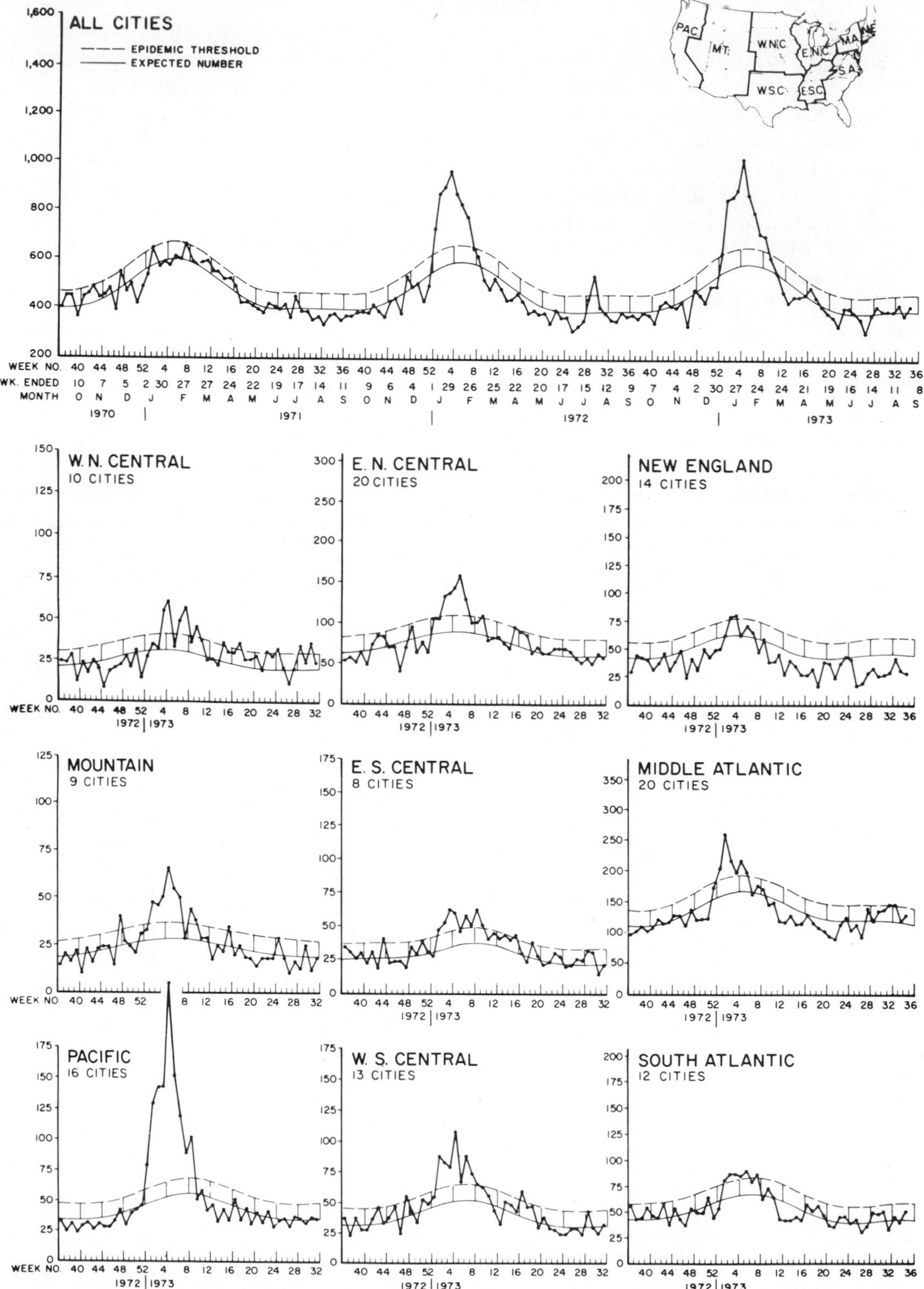

Figure 3–1. Pneumonia-influenza deaths in 122 United States cities. (From: Influenza–Respiratory Disease Surveillance. Center for Disease Control, U. S. Department of Health, Education and Welfare [Report 89], 1972–73. pp. 1–24.)

It explains the occurrence of the periodic pandemics. This has illuminated the need for methods of expeditious production of a vaccine specific for any new virus type.[3]

Clinical Characteristics and Pathology. Sudden onset of fever, headache, malaise, myalgia, nasal obstruction and prostration in a cluster of patients leads to suspicion of influenza. The fever will last from one to several days in uncomplicated cases. A dry cough occurs, which may continue after fever and myalgia subside. There may be substernal pain on inspiration, and even rales and increased breath sounds on auscultation because the primary lesion of influenza is necrosis of the respiratory tract epithelium, particularly of that lining the trachea. Although all cases do not manifest a leukopenia, this sign is indicative of classic viral influenza.

Complications. Two main complications can occur: interstitial viral pneumonia and secondary bacterial pneumonia.

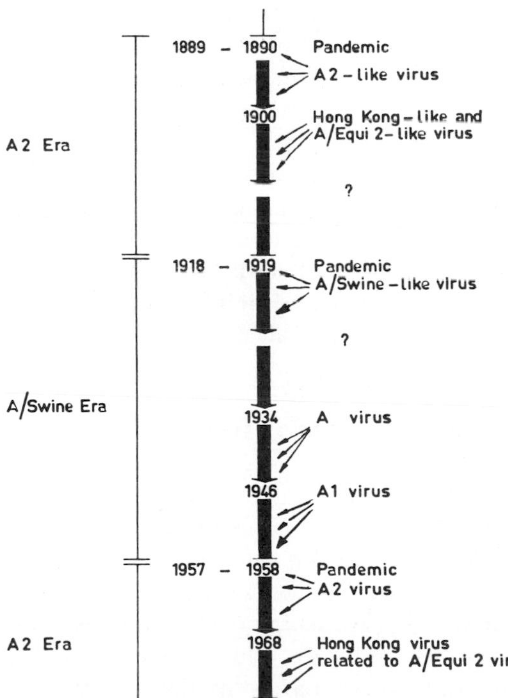

Figure 3–2. Serologically determined chronology of antigenic shifts in influenza A virus that have resulted in global pandemics. (From N. Mansurel. 1969. Serological characteristics of a "new" serotype of influenza A virus: the Hong Kong strain. Bull. W. H. O. *41*:461–468.)

Influenza viral pneumonia involves virus invasion of lower respiratory tract tissues. This is most often seen in patients with chronic lung disease or cardiac disease. Roentgen examination reveals increasing density of tissues, most pronounced around the hilus. The cough becomes productive of bloody sputum, severe dyspnea develops, and in contrast to the lassitude and prostration exhibited by the patient with self-limited influenza, those with viral pneumonia are anxious and apprehensive, ominous signs that commonly precede a fatal outcome.

Secondary bacterial pneumonia follows a regular course of acute influenza and even an apparent recovery. It is marked by the high fever and leukocytosis of a septic condition and the roentgenogram shows focal consolidation of a broncho- or lobar pneumonia. The most common secondary invaders of the accumulated detritus from ciliated epithelial sloughing are pneumococcus, hemolytic streptococcus, *Staphylococcus aureus* and *Haemophilus influenzae* bacteria, which respond to appropriate antibiotic therapy. There is no therapy for the viral pneumonia.

Viral pneumonia may be compounded by secondary bacterial complications, a situation with a poor prognosis.

Diagnosis. Only clinical symptoms and signs in other than a sporadic case can provide confidence in a diagnosis. Virus is recoverable from throat washings or other effluents of the respiratory tract when inoculated into the amnion of embryonated eggs or primary cell lines of human fetal or primate origin.

Humoral antibody develops about 10 days following onset so that by 2 weeks or later, testing a serum collected during the early phase of the illness and a convalescent serum will show a significant rise in titer of hemagglutination-inhibiting antibody to influenza virus antigen, homologous for the infecting virus.

Treatment. Amantadine hydrochloride has recently become commercially available for prophylaxis against infection by recent exposure to influenza A viruses. It is of no apparent value against types B and C.

Although it has no demonstrated value in shortening the shedding of virus by an acute case, diminution in severity and shortening of the febrile period have been observed in acutely ill patients who took 200 mg per day beginning early in the illness. The short period of effectiveness, cost, and limited distribution of amantadine hydrochloride class this chemotherapy as of academic interest. However, its use in larger doses in influenza viral pneumonia may be justified considering the otherwise poor prognosis.

The usual treatment for influenza is symptomatic, with aspirin for analgesia of the headache, malaise and myalgia. Codeine sulfate may be indicated for cough and substernal pain. Prostration automatically puts the patient to bed, where a light diet is in order, with provision for ample fluid intake.

In uncomplicated illness antibiotics are not of any value. Only in critical situations where there is a high risk of bacterial complications is antibiotic administration justified.

Bacterial pneumonia should be vigorously treated with penicillin or other antibiotics. The consequences of viral pneumonia on the bronchiolar and alveolar tissues substantially change the aerating capacity of the lung so that oxygen therapy or positive air pressure in a regulated breathing apparatus may prove beneficial.

Prevention. Elucidation of the antigenic characteristics of new influenza virus isolates has led to sophisticated and timely vaccine production. Modern vaccines contain antigen corresponding to the most recent H_3N_2 influenza A strains. Some vaccine available has type B component as well. These antigens are formalin-inactivated viruses grown in chick embryos and purified by density gradient centrifugation. While not universally protective, their use has significantly reduced the number of influenza cases compared to unvaccinated controls.

Another vaccine that may be of use is subunit hemagglutinin, which is less immunogenic but also less reactogenic in causing reaction to chick embryo vaccines, a serious problem for some people. The Russians use an attenuated live virus instilled by nasal spray. It causes illness in some recipients and is therefore not widely used elsewhere in the world.

For short-term protection of exposed individuals, amantadine hydrochloride has proved effective.

Because the protective effect of vaccination lasts no more than a year or one influenza season, mass vaccination is impractical.

Vaccination prophylaxis of 1.0 ml annually in the autumn is therefore directed toward reducing morbidity in essential servants of the community, such as police, medical care personnel, and key transportation employees; in those at higher risk because of institutional status, such as residents of barracks, armed forces and boarding schools; and in the elderly and debilitated, who have a higher risk of mortality.

Parainfluenza and Respiratory Syncytial Virus Infections

These agents cause laryngotracheobronchitis in children and upper respiratory tract illness in adults.[4] Because they directly attack the mucous membranes and ciliated epithelium of the respiratory tree, repeated infections occur with the same virus types during the life of an individual. Probably because of detectable circulating antibody, subsequent episodes caused by the same virus type are milder and self-limited.

Etiology. Human parainfluenza viruses are a subgroup of the paramyxoviruses with some characteristics of influenza virus. There are structural similarities with surface hemagglutinin and neuraminidase. They replicate in the cytoplasm with formation of eosinophilic inclusions. In contrast to influenza viruses, which can be isolated and rapidly multiply in embryonated chicken eggs, the human parainfluenza viruses are refractory to replication in chick embryos. They were not discovered until advances in tissue culture—human amnion, HeLa and primary monkey kidney cells—provided a system in which cytopathic effects and hemadsorption could be demonstrated. With new isolates, cultures of fresh material must be observed for long periods because these characteristics are slow to manifest the presence of parainfluenza viruses.

Respiratory syncytial viruses also produce cytopathic effects in continuous human cell lines and primary monkey kidney cell cultures in which they form characteristic syncytia and also eosinophilic cytoplasmic inclusions. However, hemadsorption does not occur, nor is any hemagglutinin produced.

The etiologic agent responsible for respiratory tract infections in tropical countries varies, during epidemics yielding to the agent concerned, usually a type A influenza virus variant. In a survey undertaken in Bangkok, a presumptive viral etiology was established in 40 per cent of patients having suggestive symptoms. In those cases in which the virus was identified, 40 per cent were infected with parainfluenza virus, and 13 per cent each with respiratory syncytial virus and adenoviruses.[5]

Epidemiology. Characteristic of most respiratory virus infections is the limited effect of humoral antibody in host protection, because infection occurs by direct invasion of the epithelial surfaces of the upper and lower respiratory tract. While humoral antibody may limit dissemination of the virus, the initial immunologic protection depends upon secretory IgA. This wanes in relation to time. Such transient protection puts the individual host at risk of repeated infections with the same or antigenically similar viruses.

Even though there may be prevalent and high titer humoral antibodies to parainfluenza, respiratory syncytial viruses and rhinoviruses in a population, these infections can remain endemic and circulate as milder adult disease; however, they can produce severe infant and childhood disease as a consequence of primary encounters with numerous different respiratory viruses.[6] These infections are also recognized as the frequent cause of family epidemics resulting from reintroduction of virus from childhood associations such as nursery enterprises, kindergartens and primary schools. Explosive epidemics in youth camps and similar aggregations are not uncommon.[7]

Clinical Characteristics. The clinical picture may differ in relation to age. Disease manifestations in infants and young children can be severe and even fatal, while infections in older, previously exposed persons may be self-limited owing to anamnestic recall of IgA and IgM, limiting disease to the upper respiratory tract.[8] Coryza, sore throat, or laryngitis are characteristic of parainfluenza infections in adults.

General physiologic decompensation of the elderly and debilitated exposes them to more severe consequences, with respiratory epithelial detritus in the bronchioles leading to secondary bacterial pneumonia and atelectasis with fatal outcome.

In nutritionally deprived and poorly housed populations high rates of infant mortality are common. A significant contributor is viral infection of the lower respiratory tract. Parainfluenza 1 and 2 and respiratory syncytial viruses in infants and young children are causes of bronchitis, bronchiolitis and pneumonia. A condition called croup, because of its distinctive sounds, is marked by hoarseness and spasmodic cough due to laryngeal obstruction. These signs are often associated with bronchospasm, accumulation of fluids, dyspnea, rales and rhonchi in the lower respiratory tract where they may be precursors of death in infants. Respiratory syncytial virus is the most common cause of croup in infants, while parainfluenza viruses cause this sign in young children.

Adenovirus Infections

Adenovirus infections also contribute significantly to respiratory illness in children, with a few specific types causing fatal pneumonia in early childhood. Three of these agents (3, 4, 7) have been commonly associated with acute respiratory disease in military recruits.

Etiology. The adenoviruses form a large group of at least 31 antigenically distinct but related DNA viruses. These have been further divided into three groups according to their ability to agglutinate monkey and rat erythrocytes. While this is an important screening mechanism for indicating what kind of adenovirus may have been isolated from a respiratory disease patient, most of the adenovirus types have not been attached to particular disease syndromes, and some to no disease at all. A few skip involvement of the respiratory tract and merely cause antibody-producing intestinal excretion from asymptomatic enteric infections. Thus large-scale serologic screening of juvenile populations has shown large antibody prevalence to a variety of adenoviruses with no associated illnesses.

While no human neoplastic disease has been established as due to an adenovirus, a variety of types (3, 7, 14, 16, 18, 21) has been found oncogenic for newborn rodents and as transforming agents in a number of tissue culture cell lines.

Epidemiology. Irregular lines and clusters of mothers with infants and children, awaiting attention from nurses and doctors at outpatient clinics, mark the level of present-day urban and rural health care delivery systems in many tropical countries. They also mark the environmental conditions in which airborne viruses are aerosolized and inhaled by susceptibles because the people composing these aggregations are unaware of the infectious milieu they create.

Experimental studies with a number of respiratory disease viruses have demonstrated the dispersion of viral pathogens by coughs, sneezes and personal contact. Other experiments have demonstrated dose-related severity of illness, with deep inhalation of aerosol-suspended viruses resulting in pneumonia from direct viral invasion of the epithelial cells of the bronchioles and alveoli.

Acute respiratory disease and pharyngoconjunctival fever were clinically characterized by community and military epidemiologic studies years before virologic technology—especially tissue culture—enabled isolation and characterization of etiologic adenoviruses. Acute respiratory disease is a frequent cause of epidemics in military recruits, who during early training under emotional and physical stress are housed in close association in barracks and tents. Adenoviruses 3, 4, 7 and 11 have been associated with these outbreaks.

Epidemiologic assessment indicates that high adenovirus morbidity occurs only in definable populations at special risk. Vaccination has so far been a practical measure only for such groups as ships' crews and military contingents living under conditions of close respiratory association.

Clinical Characteristics. In an assessment of respiratory disease etiology in the general population at any one time, adenoviruses would be of a low order. However, over a period of years the diversity of adenoviruses produces episodes that mimic almost every other respiratory virus disease syndrome.

ACUTE RESPIRATORY DISEASE. After an incubation period of 4 or 5 days the patient feels malaise, headache and sore throat. Fever and cough develop, with minimal nasal discharge and sputum. Often there is sternal pain. On examination there is usually pharyngitis and rhinitis. Cervical adenopathy is often palpated. Earache may occur. The fever may last up to a week but usually lasts only 3 or 4 days unless complicated by pneumonia.

PNEUMONIA. This is not an infrequent sequel to acute respiratory disease in adults. Auscultation detects rales and rhonchi with the roentgenogram showing mottling or patchy areas of density usually in the lower lobes. The cough produces little sputum, which contains high titer of adenoviruses and few or no bacterial invaders. This complication may keep the patient bedridden for several weeks.

PHARYNGOCONJUNCTIVAL FEVER. This entity is more commonly seen in children, who complain of malaise, headache and fever. The adenopathy may be evident in preauricular nodes, particularly on the side associated with unilateral conjunctivitis. This condition is often observed in summer or warm season epidemics of respiratory virus disease, particularly in camps and recreational aggregations of children.

AFEBRILE PHARYNGITIS. Adenovirus 1

and 2 infections in children are often observed in school epidemics of this condition. Complaints are malaise and sore throat, but with minimal physical signs that would prevent regular activity.

SEVERE LOWER RESPIRATORY DISEASE. This manifestation may simulate respiratory syncytial virus infection, producing not only upper respiratory symptoms but also signs of lower tree involvement. Bronchiolitis and pneumonia in infants are often fatal. Survivors may suffer chronic sequelae of obliterative bronchiolitis and bronchiectasis.

KERATOCONJUNCTIVITIS. This condition follows some trauma to the conjunctiva, either occupational or simply as a result of rubbing the eyes irritated by chlorinated swimming pool water or dry dust. It is a subepithelial inflammation of the conjunctivae. While it often appears in only one eye, the other eye may erupt a week to 10 days later. Self-limited to 10 days to 2 weeks, a small percentage may develop opacities as a result of healing, or a chronic keratitis may continue for months, ultimately causing visual defects.

Diagnosis. The history of association, incubation period, type of onset and clinical course can indicate a viral respiratory disease. Only the laboratory isolation from nasal and throat swabs and sputum can identify the specific causative virus.

Treatment. Other than the specific measures mentioned in relation to specific viral entities, the treatment of respiratory virus illnesses is essentially symptomatic and supportive. Little beyond antipyretics, analgesics, antihistamines, bed rest and forced fluids can be prescribed for the acutely ill. Antibiotics are abused almost universally, justified as prophylaxis for secondary bacterial diseases such as pneumonia. The risk of untoward reactions and problems of resistance exceed the risk of bacterial complications.

While perhaps increasing the confidence of the physician that he is doing something beneficial for the patient, such a regimen often costs the patient more than he can afford. There are situations where use of antibiotic prophylaxis may be indicated. In the face of recognized cases of bacterial infections, the aged and infants may be at high risk of secondary bacterial infection.

Prevention. Avoidance of crowds and other aggregations that maintain and transmit respiroviruses may be advisable, but in most situations is impractical. Hospitalized infants and the elderly ill can be protected by limiting visits from those who have symptoms of respirovirus illness and from children who are carriers of the many different agents from associations at school and other gatherings of youth.

Prophylactic vaccines are not available as yet for individuals because of difficulty of matching immunization to etiologic virus type. The frequency and high morbidity associated with adenoviruses 3, 4, 7 and 11 have stimulated research toward specific vaccines. First produced was a formalin-inactivated tissue culture harvest of types 3, 4 and 7, which was discontinued because it contained potentially oncogenic simian virus 40. The next development was oral administration of enteric-coated capsules containing live type 4 virus. This established an asymptomatic intestinal infection that produced antibody resulting in a significant decrease in acute respiratory disease morbidity. Because of the undesirable oncogenic potential of live adenoviruses, efforts were made to produce antigens free of viral nucleic acids. Hexon and fiber derivatives of types 1 and 5 produced neutralizing antibodies that appeared to be highly protective in early trials.

REFERENCES

1. Bang, F. B., Bang, M. G., and Bang, B. G. 1975. Ecology of respiratory virus transmission: a comparison of three communities in West Bengal. Am. J. Trop. Med. Hyg. *24*:326–346.
2. Behbehani, A. M. 1972. Human Viral, Bedsonial and Rickettsial Diseases. Charles C Thomas, Springfield, Illinois. pp. 274–278.
3. Stuart-Harris, C. H. 1970. Pandemic influenza: an unresolved problem in prevention. J. Infect. Dis. *122*:108–115.
4. Gardner, P. S. 1971. Acute respiratory virus infections of childhood. *In* Banatvala, J. E. (ed.): Current

Problems in Clinical Virology. Churchill Livingstone, Edinburgh. pp. 1–32.

5. Olson, L. C., Lexomboon, U., Sithisarn, P., and Noyes, H. E. 1973. The etiology of respiratory tract infections in a tropical country. Am. J. Epidemiol. *97*:34–43.
6. Hillis, W. D., Cooper, M. R., and Bang, F. B. 1971. Respiratory syncytial virus survey in four villages in West Bengal, India. Indian J. Med. Res. *59*:1354–1364.
7. McClelland, L., Hilleman, M. R., Hamparian, V. V., Ketler, A., Reilly, C. M., Cornfield, D., and Stokes, J., Jr. 1961. Studies of acute respiratory illnesses caused by respiratory syncytial virus. 2. Epidemiology and assessment of importance. N. Engl. J. Med. *264*: 1169–1175.
8. Gardner, P. S., McQuillin, J., and Court, S. D. M. 1970. Speculation on pathogenesis in death from respiratory syncytial virus infection. Br. Med. J. *1*: 327–330.

CHAPTER 4

Exanthematous and Other Virus Diseases

Smallpox

Synonyms. Variola (major and minor), alastrim, amaas.

Definition. Smallpox is an acute communicable virus disease, usually characterized by severe toxemia and a single crop of skin lesions that typically progress through macular, papular, vesicular and pustular stages. In the purpura variolosa variety of variola major, this skin eruption does not develop.

Distribution. The disease was endemic throughout the world, but the intensified program of smallpox eradication begun by the World Health Organization in 1967 has by 1975 limited transmission to three specific areas in three countries—Bangladesh, India and Ethiopia.[1] These remaining areas of transmission are in two districts of Bangladesh, in northeastern India almost entirely in Assam, Bihar, U.P., and West Bengal, and in contiguous mountainous portions of four northern provinces of Ethiopia (Begemdir, Gojjam, Shoa and Wollo). A few cases exported from these foci have been seen in neighboring countries.

Etiology. Smallpox is caused by the variola virus, *Poxvirus variolae* (the Paschen body), which is demonstrable in exudates of skin lesions as a roughly rectangular particle measuring 300 by 250 nm. Aggregates of the virus seen as epithelial cytoplasmic inclusions are known as Guarnieri bodies. *Poxvirus officinale,* the vaccinia virus, and *P. bovis,* the cowpox virus, are related to *P. variolae.* Provided the temperature does not exceed 25° C (77° F), the variola virus can survive in skin crusts for more than 1 year, and in the dried exudate from vesicles and pustules for 3 months or more. It is present in the upper respiratory tract of the patient or in the skin lesions, which retain the virus until they are healed. The two stable types of virus, variola major and variola minor, can be distinguished in most cases by the severity of the disease.

Epidemiology. The human is the natural host for variola virus, there being no animal reservoir. Transmission from person to person is generally through direct contact or by respiratory droplets, but indirect spread may occur from contact with contaminated clothing or bedding. The virus is destroyed if materials in which it is carried are kept at a temperature of 55° C (131° F) for 30 minutes.

Smallpox is highly contagious, its period of communicability extending from 1 to 2 days prior to the onset of symptoms until all scabs and crusts have been shed. In certain circumstances inapparent but nevertheless contagious infections have been identified serologically.[2] Everybody in the immediate environment must be considered a contact exposed to infection and susceptible to the disease unless immune by reason of a prior attack of smallpox or successful vaccination. Rapid air travel has increased the hazard of spread of smallpox. A traveler exposed to variola in an endemic region may pass asymptomatic and unsuspected into a country where smallpox is a rarity. This emphasizes the importance of proper vaccination techniques as well as the maintenance of a high index of suspicion among physicians.

Pathology. The virus enters the body through the upper respiratory tract and, in the susceptible individual, multiplies locally. Viremia follows, with dissemination of the virus to the viscera and particularly to the skin and certain other epithelial surfaces where multiplication continues.

The typical focal lesions develop in the skin. Degeneration and separation of cells of the epidermis and exudation result in vesicle formation. The vesicle is multilocular and umbilicated. The lesions are deeply situated within the skin. In the course of several days the vesicle fluid becomes cloudy and subsequently purulent, forming the pustule. This progression may be modified, however, by the use of antibiotics, and the lesions may develop from the vesicular to the desiccated stage without becoming pustular.

Other organs than the skin are also affected and show inflammatory reactions, cloudy swelling and, at times, focal hemorrhages.

In the severe fulminating hemorrhagic form of the disease, purpura variolosa, there are massive intracutaneous hemorrhages as well as mucosal hemorrhages in the kidney, gums and oral mucous membranes. In this form, the blood findings include thrombocytopenia, a high leukocytosis with many young granulocytes including blast cells, and anemia.

Clinical Characteristics. The incubation period is usually about 12 days, with extremes of 6 to 22 days. Ordinarily the onset is abrupt, with sharply rising temperature following chills or chilly sensations and accompanied by symptoms of severe toxemia, headache, nausea and vomiting, and severe general aching that is most pronounced in the back muscles. Marked prostration is common. This stage of invasion usually continues for 2 or 3 days, during which a prodromal flushing or rash may appear. During this period also, the generalized violaceous erythematous blush of purpura variolosa appears and is an exceedingly unfavorable prognostic omen. It is usually followed immediately by hemorrhagic phenomena, and death ensues before the appearance of the typical eruption.

The characteristic skin lesions commonly appear about the fourth day and are accompanied by subjective and objective improvement in the patient's condition. The lesions at first are macular, soon becoming papular and, within a few days, vesicular. In the absence of antibiotic therapy the pustular stage is reached in about 1 week. By the tenth day, or soon after, the contents of the lesions are absorbed and desiccation with crusting and scaling follows.

The character and distribution of the skin lesions have diagnostic and prognostic significance. In contradistinction to those of chickenpox, they are deep within the skin and even in the early stages have a hard "shotty" feel; the vesicles are multilocular, tough and difficult to break. All lesions tend to be at the same stage of development (whereas in chickenpox the spots appear in successive crops, and several stages may be seen together). Distribution of the lesions is peripheral (Fig. 4–1), the greatest concentration being on face and limbs, particularly the extensor surfaces of forearms, wrists, hands, lower legs and feet including the soles, with few on trunk or thighs (whereas in chickenpox mainly the face, abdomen, chest and back are affected).

When the skin lesions remain well separated, particularly on the face, the disease is referred to as "discrete" smallpox, and the fatality rate averages 10 to 15 per cent. When the lesions merge or appear to coalesce, the disease is spoken of as "confluent," and the mortality rate approaches 50 per cent. In hemorrhagic smallpox, in which there is appreciable hemorrhage into the

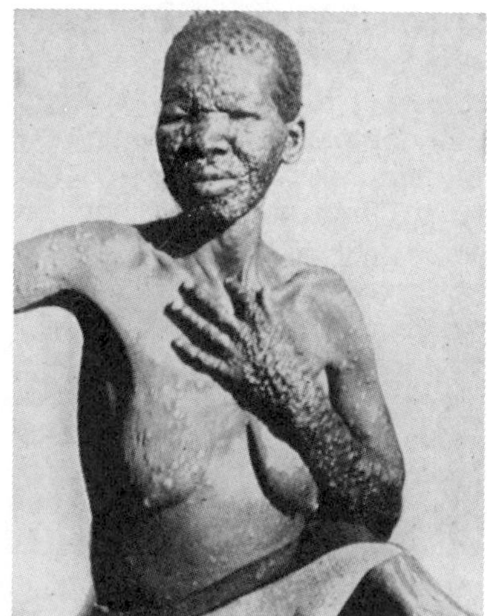

Figure 4–1. Smallpox (variola major): characteristic distribution of lesions. (Courtesy of Capt. L. D. Greentree, M.C., A.U.S.)

lesions, the fatality rate approximates 80 per cent. Purpura variolosa, in which the typical eruption fails to develop, is almost invariably fatal (Fig. 4–2).

Diagnosis. The differential diagnosis is concerned particularly with chickenpox and to a much lesser extent with generalized vaccinia. Despite the characteristic differences between the eruptions of smallpox and chickenpox, either of the alternative diagnoses is hazardous to make in adults, particularly in areas where smallpox is known to be endemic. In such circumstances a presumptive diagnosis of smallpox is safer.

The variety of laboratory aids useful in diagnosis is perhaps greater for smallpox than for any other virus disease.[3] The demonstration of characteristic cytologic lesions was mentioned previously as a helpful technique for the confirmation of certain virus infections as is the detection of virus antigen in lesions. These two approaches, together with isolation of the virus and demonstration of specific antibody response in the patient, are available to confirm a clinical diagnosis of smallpox.

In the early macular and papular stages of the eruption, smears from skin lesions contain demonstrable virus if specimens are obtained carefully and stained properly. A presumptive diagnosis can sometimes be made within an hour. While a positive report is of real value, failure to find virus does not rule out the diagnosis of smallpox. An essential method for the differentiation of varicella virus from variola virus is electron microscopy, which is highly diagnostic for varicella-herpes but less dependable for vaccinia; the latter, being less abundant in test specimens, is often not visualized. An attempt should be made to identify the virus by isolating it in chick embryo chorioallantoic membrane (CAM), particularly important for the identification of vaccinia, or in tissue cultures, and by detecting specific antigen in a complement-fixation test. After the pustular stage, microscopic examination of smears from skin lesions is no longer of value, but infectious virus is still present. Attempts to isolate virus from crusts by inoculation of chick embryos and to detect antigen in complement-fixation tests should be made. During convalescence, specific antibody appears in the serum, and comple-

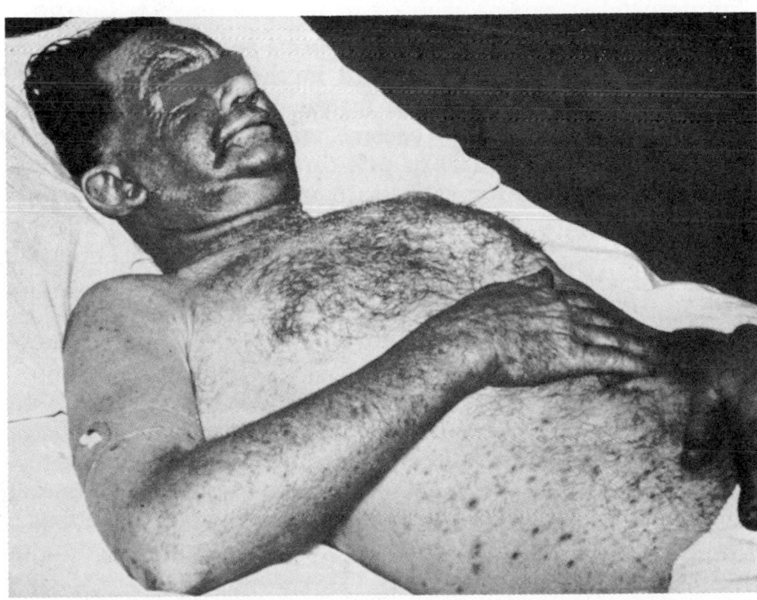

Figure 4–2. Smallpox (purpura variolosa): showing skin hemorrhages but no other lesions. (Courtesy of Col. A. P. Long, M.C. and 406th Medical General Laboratory.)

ment-fixation tests or agglutination-inhibition tests should be performed with serum specimens from both the acute and the chronic phase.

Recombinations between variola and vaccinia viruses may produce atypical cases of pox disease, usually of lessened severity. The aberrant characteristics of the causative agent are determined by virologic testing, the ceiling temperature on CAM and the mortality rate in chick embryos being particularly useful.

Treatment. Of primary importance in the treatment of smallpox is general supportive care and isolation from other patients. Attendants must have been vaccinated successfully, and all contact materials must be sterilized. Thiosemicarbazone (Marboran, Isatin B), rifampicin and idoxuridine may prevent development of smallpox in contacts if administered promptly after exposure. The dosage of thiosemicarbazone is 200 mg per kg initially, followed by 50 mg per kg every 6 hours for 8 doses, and the drug should be given as a syrup after meals to minimize vomiting. Vaccinia immune globulin (VIG) or convalescent serum will also prevent or modify smallpox if given within 24 hours after exposure. Once the lesions are manifest there is no specific effective treatment, but symptomatic treatment of the fever and its adverse effects, and of the itching of the rash, are important. Antibiotics and sulfonamides are useful to prevent complicating bacterial infections but have not materially improved the prognosis in severe cases.

Prophylaxis. Meticulously performed vaccination with potent vaccine is the only effective method for the prevention of smallpox, both variola major and minor, and forms the basis of the worldwide campaign organized by the World Health Organization. This campaign has since 1967 eliminated smallpox from the Americas and most of Africa, and is progressively restricting the disease in Asia. Indeed, in 1971 the United States Public Health Service ceased to recommend the routine vaccination of preschool children, advising instead that only those people at risk of encountering smallpox should be vaccinated. In the remaining areas of prevalence, particularly where virulent forms of the virus occur, vaccination should be repeated frequently, probably at least yearly or every second year rather than at the 3-year intervals generally accepted as adequate. In the presence of an outbreak of the disease, all known and possible contacts must be vaccinated to prevent spread.

Vaccine must be stored according to directions or it will lose activity. It will protect the person only if it is infectious and induces vaccinia. Correct inoculation of potent vaccine produces a major reaction in nearly 100 per cent of primary vaccinees, and in 70 to 100 per cent of revaccinees depending on the number of previous vaccinations and the time elapsed since the last major reaction. A jennerian vesicle develops 6 to 8 days after vaccination (occasionally longer) in nonimmune vaccinees, while an erythematous or indurated area surrounding a small ulcer or scab occurs in people with residual immunity. During the ensuing week a crust covers the jennerian vesicle. Revaccinations in individuals immunized in the past should be examined at 4 to 7 days, since an accelerated recall (vaccinoid reaction) may occur. People who have previously been vaccinated develop hypersensitivity to antigenic components of smallpox vaccine and will respond to inactive vaccine by developing a typical delayed hypersensitivity response at the site of inoculation. This should never be misinterpreted as an effective vaccination; only if there is other evidence of a "take" should vaccination be considered successful. Failure makes revaccination mandatory. The techniques of vaccination now in use include use of jet injectors, or multiple pressure or single scratch through a drop of lymph placed on the cleansed, dry skin.[4]

If eczema, impetigo, or other forms of dermatitis are present, vaccination is contraindicated since a widespread dangerous vaccinia infection (eczema vaccinatum) may ensue. However, an eczematous individual who must travel to smallpox areas may receive smallpox vaccination followed by vaccinia immune globulin (VIG), the latter in a prophylactic dose of 0.3 ml per kg body weight. This does not interfere with the development of the jennerian vesicle. Vaccination of women in the first two trimesters of pregnancy has been considered hazardous, owing to the rare possibility of inducing fatal generalized vaccinia in the fetus.[5] However, a pregnant woman may receive VIG at the time of vaccination if she has not had a vaccination "take" (successful reaction) within 10 years. Infants may receive VIG when they are vaccinated, as a protection against postvaccinial encephalitis. Patients with coincidental chickenpox and vaccinia should not receive VIG unless the chickenpox lesions are widely superinfected by the vaccinia.

Adverse reactions to vaccination are generally best treated with VIG, the prophylactic dose being doubled and repeated in 24 hours if necessary. Other products that may prove useful are thiosemicarbazone, rifampicin, idoxuridine and cytosine arabinoside, but steroids are contraindicated since they suppress developing immunity. The principal adverse reactions to vaccination are:

1. Vaccinia necrosum (progressive vaccinia, vaccinia gangrenosa). This condition depends on an immunologic defect in the patient, resulting in the lesion's continuing to spread for more than 2 weeks after vaccination. The high mortality makes immediate treatment necessary; this should include VIG, surgical debridement, maintenance of fluid and electrolyte balance, and treatment of secondary infection.

2. Eczema vaccinatum. The development of vaccinial lesions away from the inoculation site indicates a need for treatment with VIG, repeated if new lesions appear after 24 hours. Should additional lesions develop 48 hours after the initial dose of VIG has been given, thiosemicarbazone or idoxuridine should be administered.

3. Generalized vaccinia. This generalized maculopapular rash, with multiple lesions resembling the normal vaccination lesion, may be treated with VIG if the patient develops systemic symptoms.

4. Ocular vaccinia, and other accidental implantations of vaccine, mainly in infants, may be treated with VIG although a watch should be kept for secondary infection.

5. Postvaccinial encephalitis does not respond to VIG, but requires measures directed against cerebral edema, including the use of steroids.

Immunity as a result of vaccination develops more quickly than does immunity to smallpox infection itself. Contacts must be vaccinated as promptly as possible, however, since smallpox has occurred in previously unvaccinated people who were vaccinated after contact.

Monkeypox And Related Conditions

Synonyms. None. Tanapox is a closely related but less virulent disease.

Definition. A simian poxvirus disease transmissible to, but not between, humans.

Distribution. In western and central Africa, vigorous vaccination campaigns resulted in the disappearance of smallpox by May 1970. Since then, however, a few unvaccinated individuals, mainly children, have been seen with illness indistinguishable from smallpox. No source of human infection could be identified. The disease differed from smallpox in that no secondary cases developed from person-to-person contact in unvaccinated people.

The first case was diagnosed in Zaire in 1970.[6] More cases were seen during the ensuing 12 months in Liberia, Nigeria and Sierra Leone. Vaccination of the convalescent patients produced doubtful reactions. Their numerous unvaccinated household contacts did not develop the disease, and subsequently responded with a primary reaction to vaccination. A similar but less severe condition, Tanapox, has been described from Kenya, and is believed to have been responsible for epidemics in 1957 and 1962.[7]

Surveys undertaken among nonhuman primates suggest that monkeypox in the natural environment is rare and probably focalized. It was first identified in 1958 in *Cynomolgus* monkeys imported into Denmark from Southeast Asia, and outbreaks have been observed in captive monkeys and apes in Europe and North America since then.

Etiology. Monkeypox virus produces a smallpox-like disease in monkeys and apes, transmissible to man through direct contact or mechanically by mosquito bite. The virus is closely related to variola and vaccinia viruses, but transmission from human to human does not occur.

Epidemiology. The occasional cases in humans living in western and central Africa have probably been caused by direct transfer of monkeypox virus from the skins and possibly other organs of monkeys during the process of handling captured or shot animals, which are prized as a dietary delicacy in many remote African communities. Tanapox of Kenya may have arisen through mechanical transfer of the virus from monkeys to humans by biting mosquitoes.

Pathology. The pathology of monkeypox is assumed to be similar to that of smallpox (p. 81).

Clinical Characteristics. The western and central African form of monkeypox in humans has the clinical appearance of smallpox, whereas Kenyan Tanapox is considerably milder, being characterized by a fever of 3 or 4 days' duration and the presence of one or two umbilicated vesicles resembling modified smallpox lesions.

Diagnosis. Hemagglutination-inhibition tests with homologous and heterologous antisera serve to differentiate monkeypox from vaccinia and cowpox, but not from variola. The following virologic laboratory tests are diagnostic.[8]

DERMAL REACTION IN RABBITS. This is the best screen for differentiating human monkeypox virus from variola virus. Monkeypox virus produces large necrotic, hemorrhagic lesions at the site of intradermal inoculation, and generalized illness and secondary perifocal exanthemas occur. Variola virus produces virtually no visible reaction, and vaccinia a reaction only just visible. Monkeypox, in contrast to variola, can be transmitted through rabbits by intradermal passage.

POCK MORPHOLOGY ON CHICK EMBRYO CHORIOALLANTOIC MEMBRANE CULTURE. The virus of monkeypox produces small white pocks with pinpoint necrosis and hemorrhage. Variola shows no central necrosis or hemorrhage, and vaccinia pocks are much larger. With Tanapox virus, no pocks developed. The maximum temperature for monkeypox virus growth on this membrane is 39.0° C (102.2° F), whereas variola and vaccinia will grow at 39.5° C (103.2° F).

PLAQUE MORPHOLOGY IN VERO CELL LINE. Monkeypox and vaccinia viruses produce large plaques with clear centers. Variola virus causes hyperplastic clumping of cells followed by formation of small plaques. The viruses may also be distinguished in kidney continuous cell line culture.

CHICK EMBRYO LETHALITY. Monkeypox and vaccinia viruses are 1000 times more lethal than variola virus for chick embryos.

SUCKLING MICE VIRULENCE TEST. Monkeypox virus is much more lethal than variola or vaccinia when inoculated intracerebrally or into footpads in suckling mice.

Treatment. Treatment of monkeypox is symptomatic and supportive.

Prophylaxis. Since monkeypox occurs in areas of Africa from which smallpox has been eradicated, and has been seen extremely infrequently, vaccination need not be considered. The most effective preventive measure is to discourage the contact of monkey hunters and zoo personnel with the skins of obviously infected monkeys.

Care must be taken in handling monkeys that have skin lesions of any description. Transmissible viruses other than monkeypox may be present, of particular danger being those of the simian herpes group. One group, biologically similar to herpes simplex, includes *Herpesvirus simiae* ("B virus") from Asian monkeys, SA8 virus from African monkeys, *Herpesvirus tamarinus,* and KM 322 virus from the owl monkey, *Aotus trivirgatus.* These viruses may remain latent in dorsal root spinal sensory ganglia of apparently healthy but seropositive monkeys for at least 2 years, and may be reactivated by cortisone treatment or the stress of experimentation.[9] When this happens, virus returns to the relevant skin areas, producing herpes lesions (small erythematous papules) that shed virus infective, indeed highly lethal, to humans. On grounds of safety, the experimental use of monkeys found to be seropositive for this group of viruses is questionable.

Measles

Synonym. Rubeola.

Definition. An acute infectious viral disease of humans affecting epithelial tissues including the skin, the bronchial and intestinal mucosae, the larynx, mouth and conjunctivae.

Distribution. Measles occurs worldwide. Although it is becoming well controlled in some countries, it continues to be a serious problem and common cause of death in others, particularly in Africa and South America. In the latter, control measures are being undertaken in several countries where the maximum morbidity and mortality is in infants. In Chile, following a combined measles and smallpox vaccination campaign in 1964 and 1965, with subsequent routine vaccinations, by 1969 morbidity had fallen by 78 per cent and mortality by 91 per cent. In West and Central Africa in 1966 a coordinated measles vaccination campaign, supported by technical assistance from the United States Agency for International Development, was undertaken by 20 countries, children aged 6 months to 5 years (later reduced to 3 years) receiving the vaccine. By 1970, 20 million children had been vaccinated, with a 60 per cent reduction in measles incidence.

Etiology. The measles virus is a paramyxovirus structurally resembling the mumps and parainfluenza viruses.

Epidemiology. The introduction of measles to tropical communities in which the disease was not previously prevalent has resulted in severe epidemics, with case fatality rates ranging up to 40 per cent. Children aged 6 months to 3 years are the most severely affected, whereas in temperate climates older children are attacked and the disease is generally milder, tending to occur in 2- to 4-year cycles as new groups of susceptible children accumulate. In the tropics measles is one of the most serious of the acute infectious diseases, and its adverse effects are enhanced when it attacks malnourished children or is combined with whooping cough, falciparum malaria, sickle cell anemia, tuberculosis, fibrocystic disease or leukemia.

In tropical countries, the disease is often spread during the prodromal, catarrhal stage at family and tribal gatherings and celebrations. The customs of some regions tend to enhance its effects. In Mali, where these have been well documented, food and water may be withheld in the belief that these are detrimental during the illness, the child may not be washed but is plastered with local mixtures containing dung with the object of bringing out the rash, and solutions often of a caustic nature may be applied to the eyes.[10]

Pathology. The measles virus produces catarrhal inflammation of the dermal, respiratory and intestinal epithelium, which focally degenerate with exfoliation of the affected cells. When this destruction is widespread or confluent, particularly in the alimentary tract, mucosal atrophy may occur. The mouth, larynx and conjunctivae are affected. Children with protein energy malnutrition may show a modified rash or none at all. It is believed that the rash is a manifestation of cell-mediated immunity, in the absence of which giant cell pneumonia is prone to develop and be fatal. In Africa pulmonary complications account for the majority of deaths due to measles, but protein energy malnutrition, particularly kwashiorkor, is a principal factor in the mortality, most deaths from measles occurring in children with weights below the tenth centile for age.

The ocular complications in measles, including subepithelial punctate keratitis, xerosis of the conjunctiva, ulcerating keratomalacia, formation of staphyloma, and ultimately perforation and phthisis bulbi, are primarily those of xerophthalmia dependent upon vitamin A deficiency, which becomes manifest under the stress of the diarrhea and dehydration of a measles attack.[11]

Immunity to measles is passively transferred from mother to infant, but antibody decay (measured by hemagglutination-inhibition testing) is marked after 3 months of age. Infections acquired during this period of decreasing immunity may be sufficiently modified to be unnoticed, as approximately 30 per cent of children in later life possess antibodies and pass through epidemics unscathed without a history of having had measles.

Primary tuberculosis may be reactivated by an attack of measles. Malnourished children and those suffering from leukemia are at most serious risk from measles.

Clinical Characteristics. The clinical course of measles in tropical countries resembles that seen elsewhere, an asymptomatic incubation stage of about 10 days' duration being followed by a prodromal stage with an enanthem (Koplik's spots—grayish white dots with a red areola) on the mucosa of mouth and pharynx, some temperature elevation, and coryza and cough. The exanthem appears 3 to 4 days later, in the form of a maculopapular rash erupting first on face and neck and then on the body and limbs, and is accompanied by high fever. The rash may become confluent. Desquamation commences 2 to 4 days later, and may result in a patchy depigmentation lasting several weeks and accompanied by a widespread pyoderma due to secondary infection. Similar changes occurring in the respiratory and intestinal tracts are made apparent by stomatitis and sometimes cancrum oris with an inability to eat, by laryngitis and sometimes laryngeal obstruction, by bronchitis and frequently bronchopneumonia with its high mortality, and by diarrhea with passage of mucus and blood resulting in dehydration, often severe.

The occurrence of conjunctivitis may produce irreversible damage and result in blindness, although it should be noted that xerophthalmia is the primary cause of this blindness.[11] Infection of the middle ear may develop. The systemic disease may result in or be complicated by cerebral manifestations and convulsions, or myocarditis, with a correspondingly poor prognosis.

The relationship of measles to malnutrition is particularly important. Not only are the adverse effects of measles enhanced in malnourished children, but the oral and intestinal pathologic changes of the disease lead to inability to eat and excessive loss of tissue fluids, thus precipitating protein energy malnutrition.

Diagnosis. The clinical diagnosis of measles is made from the characteristics of the prodromal Koplik's spots and the rash. It may be confirmed by demonstration in the nasopharyngeal mucus of multinucleate giant cells, which are excreted only during the first week in mild attacks but to the end of the fourth week in severe attacks.

Measles is distinguished from rubella (German measles) clinically and by serologic testing, specific hemagglutination-inhibition antibodies developing. Use of this method in parts of Mexico and Paraguay revealed that 65 to 71 per cent of children aged 7 years had antibody to measles virus; however, seroconversion to rubella virus was much slower among the Paraguayan than the Mexican children, respectively 17 versus 76 per cent.[12] These results for measles in preschool children are similar to those reported for Costa Rica, Guatemala and other Central and South American countries. Rubella is much more variable, but in most places in the tropical and subtropical Americas rubella antibody seropositivity rates have always been considerably lower than those of measles.[13] Rubella may also be differentiated from rubeola by tissue culture of virus isolated from the pharynx. Because of the very serious risk of congenital malformations of the fetus in women contracting rubella early in pregnancy, such women should be serologically tested and, if still susceptible to the disease, should receive immune serum globulin. If not pregnant, they should be actively vaccinated against rubella.

Treatment. There is no specific therapy for measles, and immune globulin does little to modify the severity of the attack. In the early stages of the disease steroids are valuable. Because of the generally toxemic state of the severely affected patient, the loss of tissue fluids through intestinal mucosal damage, and the difficulty in swallowing due to buccal lesions, parenteral fluid replacement is highly desirable. Milk is the most useful dietary ingredient. Bacterial complications, particularly pulmonary, should be countered with antibiotics: a combination of penicillin and streptomycin has been recommended in tropical practice,[14] and penicillin has proved superior to chloramphenicol.

Since low levels of vitamin A contribute to eye damage that is often related to xerophthalmia, treatment with 300,000 IU of vitamin A daily is advisable in areas where that dietary deficiency exists.

Prophylaxis. Measles virus vaccines were introduced in the United States in 1963, and in Britain the following year. In the United States 385,156 cases of measles were reported during 1963, the subsequent dramatic reduction resulting in 22,231 cases being reported in 1968. Thereafter an increase occurred, largely owing to a premature slackening of the vaccination campaign, but also because measles occasionally developed, usually subclinically, in previously vaccinated children. Resurgent vaccination in the United States has again reduced the incidence, 22,085 cases being reported in 1974 (provisional total).

Large-scale measles immunization campaigns, using the intradermal jet injector (the dermojet), have proved remarkably effective in reducing the incidence of the disease in many tropical countries, particularly those of West and Central Africa. It has, however, been pointed out that to maintain an interepidemic state for measles (no more than 4 per cent of susceptibles aged less than 4 years becoming infected annually), 40 to 50 per cent of infants must be vaccinated; if the natural measles rate falls lower, 80 to 90 per cent of infants would have to be vaccinated to make up for the lack of naturally induced immunity, until eradication is achieved.[15] For West Africa it is estimated that the level of acceptance and performance of vaccination will not exceed 60 per cent, and continued campaigns even at this reduced level are financially unattainable. To reduce the cost of the campaigns the individual dose of vaccine has been halved (from 1000 $TCID_{50}$ [median tissue culture infective dose] to 500 $TCID_{50}$), and the target limited from country-wide measles eradication to protection of small areas and children at particular risk.[16] The latter are now defined as aged 6 months to 3 years (when likelihood of malnutrition declines), preeminently if they are malnourished or suffering from sickle cell anemia, tuberculosis or fibrocystic disease.

The immunizing agent consists of live attenuated substrains of the Edmonston strain of measles virus, injection of which is followed several days later by a generally mild febrile reaction. Seroconversion occurs in 97 per cent of children aged 1 year or more, and the high degree of protection that develops probably lasts for several years since antibody persists for at least 8 years. Vaccination with live attenuated virus of children aged 9 to 10 months is given principal credit for the overall reduction in mortality and malnutrition of preschool children in West Africa.[14]

Because measles vaccination may stimulate a primary tuberculosis focus, tuberculosis should be treated before vaccination is undertaken. Leukemia is a contraindication to this vaccination.

Killed measles virus vaccine does not provide adequate immunity, but in special cases may be given 1 month before inoculation of live vaccine, the reaction to which it mitigates. Passive immunization using pooled plasma or placental gamma globulin (or, less effectively, pooled adult or convalescent serum) is prophylactic if undertaken within 5 days of exposure.

Epidemic Hemorrhagic Fever

David P. Earle

Synonyms. The common designation in the Soviet Union is now hemorrhagic fever with renal syndrome. Other currently used synonyms include Far Eastern hemorrhagic fever, hemorrhagic nephrosonephritis, Korean hemorrhagic fever, Songo fever, Kokka disease, Korin fever, Nidoko disease.

Definition. Epidemic hemorrhagic fever is an acute infectious disease of still unproved etiology that is characterized by fever, prostration, a variety of hemorrhagic phenomena, shock, proteinuria and renal failure.[17, 18]

Distribution. The disease was first described in 1913 in Vladivostok.[19] It was extensively studied by the Russians and Japanese in the 1930s when it was recognized in the Amur River Basin between Siberia and Manchuria. It first appeared among United Nation troops in Korea above the 38th parallel in the summer of 1951. Subsequently the disease, or one very similar, has been recognized in Scandinavia, the Upper and Middle Volga Basins and Bashkiria. Apparently it has not occurred in Siberia between Sverdlovsk and Lake Baikal (Fig. 4–3). Other hemorrhagic fevers in the Soviet Union appear to be different entities.[20]

Etiology. The causative agent is filtrable and is transmissible by inoculation of blood, urine or tissues obtained early in the disease. Neutralizing antibodies appear in the serum in convalescence. Susceptible animals have not been found. Nevertheless, the responsibile virus appears to have been propagated in tissue culture, and combinations of immunofluorescence counterstain and indirect hemagglutination techniques have demonstrated antibodies in patients from a number of endemic regions.

Epidemiology. The lack of a susceptible laboratory animal and of a specific diagnostic laboratory test limits epidemiologic study, since dependence must be placed

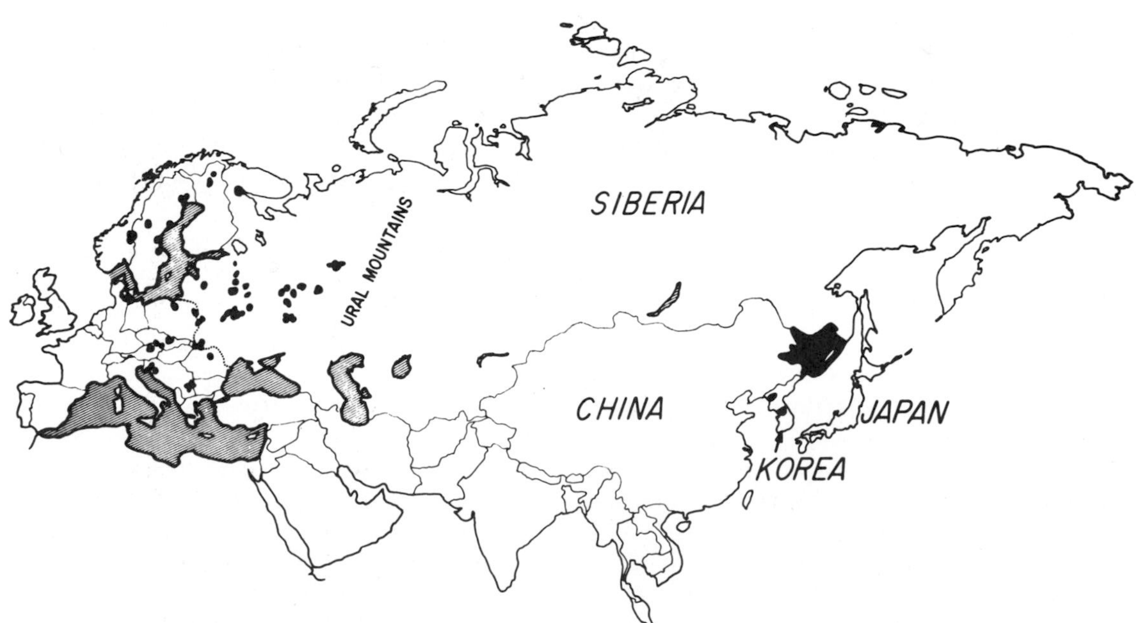

Figure 4–3. Geographic distribution of epidemic hemorrhagic fever. (Courtesy of Dr. J. Casals, J. Infect. Dis. *122*:437, 1970, and the University of Chicago Press.)

upon those human infections that are clinically recognizable. The disease occurs chiefly in rural areas. Entomologic and epidemiologic evidence suggests that the disease is transmitted to man probably by the bite of mites that infest the ground vole or perhaps, in some areas, field mice.[19] In many areas outbreaks occur when rodents move into human habitats from the fields or forests in the late fall and winter. In Korea the disease occurs with two peaks of incidence, one in May and June, the other in October and November. Ninety per cent of infections are isolated events as regards time, place and person. The remaining 10 per cent, however, consist of sharply defined outbreaks limited to a company, platoon or squad. The disease is not communicable from person to person by ordinary contacts.

Since cessation of active military operations, epidemic hemorrhagic fever has continued to occur in the Korean armed forces stationed in the endemic area. The seasonal occurrence and other epidemiologic features remain unchanged.

Pathology. Three-fourths of all deaths occur within the first 10 days of the disease. Shock is the most common cause of death, particularly in the early period, although not limited to it. Later in the disease, acute renal failure, pulmonary edema, or secondary infections also are responsible for fatal outcomes. The basic morphologic changes observed are (1) evidence of capillary dysfunction, (2) necrosis probably resulting from ischemia, and (3) a mononuclear cellular response.[18, 21] The kidney is invariably involved, the medulla being greatly congested. Necrosis in the same region varies from involvement of the tubular epithelium only to extensive necrosis of all pyramids.[22] The heart characteristically exhibits a hemorrhagic appearance of the right atrium. On careful study this again reflects marked capillary congestion. A similar process is almost universally encountered in the anterior pituitary and adrenal medulla. Focal myocarditis and cellular infiltration of the endocardium are common but not extensive. Retroperitoneal edema is marked early but disappears later in the disease. Edema of areolar tissue, particularly in the retroperitoneum, is striking early in the disease.

Clinical Characteristics. The incubation period is usually 14 days, with extremes of 9 days to 5 weeks. The disease varies widely in its severity, the greater number of cases taking the form of a mild febrile illness with proteinuria and minimal symptoms of infection. One-fourth of the clinically recognized cases can be classed as moderate or severe, and in these the progression of symptoms is relatively uniform.[18] For descriptive purposes this relatively typical clinical picture may be divided into phases, each arbitrarily named for an obvious clinical feature. However, some degree of overlap between the phases is common.

FEBRILE PHASE. The onset is acute, with fever, malaise, anorexia and thirst. The temperature rises rapidly to 37.8 to 40.6°C (100 to 105°F), persists for 3 to 7 days, and usually falls by rapid lysis by the sixth day. During this period the face, neck and throat are flushed, and the conjunctivae are suffused. Evidence of beginning increased capillary permeability or frank leakage of plasma may be manifested by chemosis, periorbital edema and proteinuria. Abdominal or lumbar pain may possibly indicate developing retroperitoneal edema. Petechiae may be found in the axillary folds, the conjunctivae or elsewhere. Hematuria is common, Rumpel-Leede's test is positive, and thrombocytopenia may be present. The blood count, which earlier was normal or slightly leukopenic, often shows a leukemoid leukocytosis by the third day.

HYPOTENSIVE PHASE. At or about the time of defervescence, hypotension may appear. In severe cases, faintness, anxiety and apprehension are signals of the approach of shock in which the pulse becomes rapid and the blood pressure undemonstrable. Warm extremities at this time indicate arteriolar dilation. The hematocrit increases rapidly and the plasma volume decreases, reflecting loss of plasma from damaged capillaries. This period, characterized by hypotension, lasts from several hours to a few days. Shock merges with the phase of renal failure but is not necessarily a causative factor for the renal failure.

OLIGURIC PHASE. Hematuria continues and proteinuria is pronounced. Even in the absence of preceding shock, some signs of renal failure appear, heralded by a diminishing urinary output and rising levels of nitrogenous products in the blood. The degree to which each of these functions is impaired is quite variable and not necessarily parallel. Oliguria of some degree is common in severe cases, and even anuria may develop. Mild azotemia or severe uremia may be seen. During this oliguric period hypotension disappears, arterioles apparently regain their tone, capillary leakage ceases, extravasated plasma returns to the vascular compartment, and the elevated hematocrit decreases. Apparently the dilated capillary channels, which were packed with erythrocytes during the period of shock, do not rapidly return to a functional state. The restoration of blood volume combined with the reduced capillary space produces a "relative hypervolemia."

At this time blood pressure increases, sometimes to hypertensive levels. Peripheral veins are distended despite normal venous pressure; circulation time is reduced, but renal plasma flow is diminished. Hemorrhages become more frequent or marked, and symptoms appear that are ascribed by some to "relative hypervolemia" and considered by others to be typical of uremia. Furthermore, there appears to be a hemodynamic inflexibility in which minor variations in fluid balance result in pulmonary edema or dehydration and shock. Hyperkalemia may be a threat during this period.

DIURETIC (RECOVERY) PHASE. Following a 1- to 5-day period of mild or marked urinary suppression, diuresis occurs. There follows a relatively rapid readjustment of hemodynamics, fluid balance, electrolyte equilibrium and azotemia. Urinary excretion may reach 6 or 8 liters per day. If adequate fluid replacement is not maintained, the patient may suffer secondary shock. Pulmonary infection is a serious complication during this phase.

CONVALESCENCE. Symptoms and signs rapidly disappear, except polyuria, and concentrating functions of the kidney return more slowly to normal over the next few weeks. Residua are rarely seen, and long-term sequelae are almost unknown.

Diagnosis. The diagnosis is suspected with the acute onset of fever in a person who has been exposed to rural conditions in a known endemic area. No single, early finding is diagnostic. Appearance of the flush, petechiae, hematuria, proteinuria and leukemoid leukocytosis offer strong supporting evidence. Progressive defervescence, shock and renal failure in the absence of other obvious causes establish the diagnosis.

DIFFERENTIAL DIAGNOSIS. At various stages before the full progression of the disease is apparent it may be confused with leukemia, thrombocytopenic purpura, infectious mononucleosis, leptospirosis, acute glomerulonephritis, scarlet fever, the typhus fevers, encephalitis, purpura variolosa and an acute surgical abdomen.

Treatment. No specific chemotherapeutic agent is known to date. Sulfonamides, antibiotics, vitamins, antihistaminics, pituitary and adrenal hormones, convalescent serum and whole blood have had little or no effect on the course of the disease.[18, 23] At present, treatment is primarily supportive, as follows:

Early hospitalization is recommended, since the severity of the disease cannot be prophesied on the basis of early symptoms. The tendency toward hemorrhage and shock is reduced by gentle handling, avoidance of trauma and physical activity and institution of early bed rest.

Maintenance of fluid balance must begin early to avoid the overhydration that can result from the patient's attempts to satisfy the thirst which is prominent early in the disease. In fact, if hospitalization is delayed and careful intake-output records have not been kept, it is often wise to allow only minimal fluid requirements. Until convalescence begins, it is of prime importance to set fluid requirements on the basis of the volume lost in urine and vomitus, with an allowance of no more than 500 ml per day. Fluids above minimal requirements merely leak through the damaged capillaries, accentuating the clinical symptoms in the early phases and precipitating pulmonary edema or hemorrhages in later stages. At the same time, dehydration must be avoided. When intravenous administration of fluid is required because of severe nausea and vomiting, 5 per cent dextrose is recommended. Saline solutions are contraindicated during the hypotensive and oliguric phases. However, during the diuretic phase, replacement with saline may become essential.

Hypotension must be watched for by recording periodic blood pressure readings early in the disease in order to avoid the insidious and often sudden appearance of severe shock. Mild degrees of medical shock may be handled by the simple measures such as the Trendelenburg position and elastic bandaging of the extremities. If shock is more severe, continuous intravenous pressor therapy is usually required. For this purpose, *l*-arterenol *l*-norepinephrine (Levophed) or other pressor agents may be administered in 5 per cent glucose, using an indwelling catheter in the femoral vein. The diastolic pressure should not be raised to 90 mm of mercury or above, since such pressures result in reduced blood flow through the kidney. When plasma volume has been greatly reduced, as indicated by hematocrit levels above 55 to 60 per cent, the administration of salt-free albumin is indicated. After capillary leakage has ceased, albumin is contraindicated. Blood transfusions are contraindicated at all stages except in the rare instances of massive gastrointestinal hemorrhage. With the hypertension of the late renal phase, a phlebotomy of 500 ml may be effective in relieving the uremic or "hypervolemic" symptoms, particularly if improvement has been noted on a preceding trial of bloodless phlebotomy using pneumatic cuffs about the extremities.

Electrolyte imbalance must be corrected when possible by replacement of deficits. Administration of insulin and 5 per cent dextrose in water may control hyperkalemia for 12 to 18 hours. Retention enemas of cation exchange resin to remove potassium have also been useful, but care must be taken to avoid inspissation and impaction in dehydrated patients.

Sedation is effective in allaying or reducing many of the symptoms that disturb the patient or aggravate the physiologic imbalance. Barbiturates may be sufficient, but there should be no hesitation in employing meperidine hydrochloride (Demerol) if required. In the presence of severe shock and impaired circulation, repeated intravenous doses of 10 mg of this drug are more effective than larger doses by other routes and are less likely to result in overdosage.

Close *medical observation* and good nursing care are essential.

Ambulation during convalescence should be based on return of renal tubular function as determined by concentration tests. When a concentration to 1.012 is reached, bathroom privileges are permitted; free ambulation on the ward is allowed with a concentrating power of 1.014; and full activity when specific gravity reaches 1.023.

Prognosis. With close observation and sound supportive care, the case fatality rate can be held to 5 per cent. Recovery is usually rapid and apparently complete, although rarely a patient may show evidence of persistent renal tubular damage for some months. Sequelae are almost unknown.

Prophylaxis and Control. In view of the suggested implication of trombiculid mites as vectors of the disease, the control measures applicable to scrub typhus are advisable. These methods include impregnation of clothing with miticides, use of insect repellents on exposed body surfaces, rodent control measures, and burning or bulldozing of camp sites. (See Table 72-1).

REFERENCES

Smallpox

1. Anonymous. 1975. Smallpox in 1974. W.H.O. Chron. *29*:134–139.
2. Heiner, G. G., Fatima, N., Daniel, R. W., Cole, J. L., Anthony, R. L., and McCrumb, F. R., Jr. 1971. A study of inapparent infection in smallpox. Am. J. Epidemiol. *94*:252–268.
3. Downie, A. W., and Kempe, C. H. 1969. Poxviruses. *In* Lennette, E. H., and Schmidt, N. J. (eds.): Diagnostic Procedures for Viral and Rickettsial Infec-

tions. 4th ed. American Public Health Association, New York. pp. 281–320.

4. Anonymous. 1968. Smallpox eradication. W.H.O. Tech. Rep. Ser. No. 393, Geneva. 52 pp.
5. Kaplan, C. 1969. Immunization against smallpox. Br. Med. Bull. *25*:131–135.

Monkeypox and Related Conditions (Tanapox, Simian Herpes Virus Infections)

6. Ladnyj, I. D., Ziegler, P., and Kima, E. 1972. A human infection caused by monkeypox virus in Basankusu Territory, Democratic Republic of the Congo. Bull. W.H.O. *46*:593–597.
7. Downie, A. W., Taylor-Robinson, C. H., Caunt, A. E., Nelson, G. S., Manson-Bahr, P. E. C., and Matthews, T. C. H. 1971. Tanapox: a new disease caused by a pox virus. Br. Med. J. *1*:363–368.
8. Lourie, B., Bingham, P. G., Evans, H. H., Foster, S. O., Nakano, J. H., and Herrmann, K. L. 1972. Human infection with monkeypox virus: laboratory investigation of six cases in West Africa. Bull. W.H.O. *46*:633–639.
9. McCarthy, K., and Tosolini, F. A. 1975. Hazards from simian herpes viruses: reactivation of skin lesions with virus shedding. Lancet *1*:649–650.

Measles

10. Imperato, P. J. 1969. Traditional attitudes towards measles in the Republic of Mali. Trans. R. Soc. Trop. Med. Hyg. *63*:768–780.
11. Frankeln, S. 1974. Measles and xerophthalmia in East Africa. Trop. Geogr. Med. *26*:39–44.
12. Golubjatnikov, R., Elsea, W. R., and Leppla, L. 1971. Measles and rubella hemagglutination-inhibition antibody patterns in Mexican and Paraguayan children. Am. J. Trop. Med. Hyg. *20*:958–963.
13. Dowdle, W. R., Ferreira, W., De Salles Gomes, L. F., King, D., Kourany, M., Madalengoitia, J., Pearson, F., Swanston, W. H., Tosi, H. C., and Vilches, A. M. 1970. W.H.O. collaborative study on the sero-epidemiology of rubella in Caribbean and Middle and South American populations in 1968. Bull. W.H.O. *42*:419–422.
14. Morley, D. 1969. Severe measles in the tropics. Parts I and II. Br. Med. J. *1*:297–300; 363–365.
15. Sutherland, I., and Fayers, P. M. 1971. Effect of measles vaccination on incidence of measles in the community. Br. Med. J. *1*:698–702.
16. Stanfield, J. P., and Bracken, P. M. 1975. Evaluation of methods designed to reduce cost of measles vaccine programmes. Trans. R. Soc. Trop. Med. Hyg. *69*:26–28.

Epidemic Hemorrhagic Fever

17. McNinch, J. H. 1953. Far East Command conference on epidemic hemorrhagic fever. Ann. Intern. Med. *38*:53–60.
18. Earle, D. P. (ed.). 1954. Symposium on epidemic hemorrhagic fever. Am. J. Med. *16*:617–709.
19. Casals, J., Henderson, B. E., Hoogstraal, H., Johnson, K. M., and Shelokov, A. 1970. A review of Soviet viral hemorrhagic fevers, 1969. J. Infect. Dis. *122*:437–453.
20. Gajdusek, D. C. 1953. Crimean Hemorrhagic Fever, pp. 61–79. *In* Acute Infectious Hemorrhagic Fevers and Mycotoxicoses in the Union of Soviet Socialist Republics. Med. Sci. Publ. 2, Walter Reed Army Medical Center, Washington, D.C. 140 pp.
21. Hullinghorst, R. R., and Steer, A. 1953. Pathology of epidemic hemorrhagic fever. Ann. Intern. Med. *38*:77–101.
22. Oliver, J., and MacDowell, M. 1957. The renal lesion in epidemic hemorrhagic fever. J. Clin. Invest. *36*:99–223.
23. Katz, S., Leedham, C. L., and Kessler, W. H. 1953. Medical management of hemorrhagic fever. J.A.M.A. *50*:1363–1366.

SECTION II
Rickettsial Diseases

CHAPTER 5
Introduction

WILLY BURGDORFER

Description of Rickettsiae

Rickettsial diseases are caused by rickettsiae of the family *Rickettsiaceae.* According to the eighth edition of *Bergey's Manual of Determinative Bacteriology,* this family includes the following three genera: (1) *Rickettsia,* consisting of the agents of the typhus, spotted fever and scrub typhus groups; (2) *Coxiella,* represented by a single species, *Coxiella burnetii,* the etiologic agent of Q fever; and (3) *Rochalimaea,* which includes *Rochalimaea quintana,* the agent of trench fever.[1] Thus, the former *Rickettsia quintana* has been placed into a separate genus because of its extracellular development in the arthropod host and its cultivation on host cell-free medium.

Rickettsiae are fastidious bacteria with obligate intracellular parasitism and independent metabolic activities. Like viruses, they require, with exception of *Rochalimaea quintana,* living host cells for growth. On the other hand, they resemble bacteria by virtue of their morphology, growth characteristics and visibility by conventional light microscopy (Fig. 5–1). They are pleomorphic, ranging from coccoid to rod-shaped, even threadlike forms, and are bounded by a multilayered cell wall (Fig. 5–2); as many as five cell wall layers have been observed. They possess both ribonucleic and deoxyribonucleic acids and multiply by binary fission. Their internal structure consists of electron-dense ribosomes and fine strands of deoxyribonucleic acid (DNA). They are gram-negative and stain poorly with aniline dyes. Staining methods used include those of Giménez, Macchiavello and Giemsa.[2] Fluorescent antibody staining has been shown to be of great value, especially for distinguishing rickettsiae from rickettsia-like nonpathogenic microorganisms in arthropod tissues.

Rickettsiae are maintained in nature in a primary cycle between various bloodsucking arthropods, such as ticks, mites, fleas and lice, and a large variety of small host animals. Thus, most rickettsial diseases are zoonoses acquired by man only through accidental intrusion into the natural cycle of infection. However, man is considered the reservoir of *Rickettsia prowazekii,* the etiologic agent of epidemic typhus. Patients who recover from this disease retain the rickettsiae for many years and may experience a recrudescence (Brill-Zinsser disease) with renewed infectivity of the blood for lice.

With the exception of *R. prowazekii* which invariably kills its arthropod host, the louse, rickettsiae are well adapted to their arthropod vectors. Transovarial passage of the spotted fever group rickettsiae in ticks and of *Rickettsia tsutsugamushi* in mites represents an important means by which these agents are maintained and distributed in nature.

Although a large variety of small mammals are used in rickettsial research, male guinea pigs, mice and, more recently,

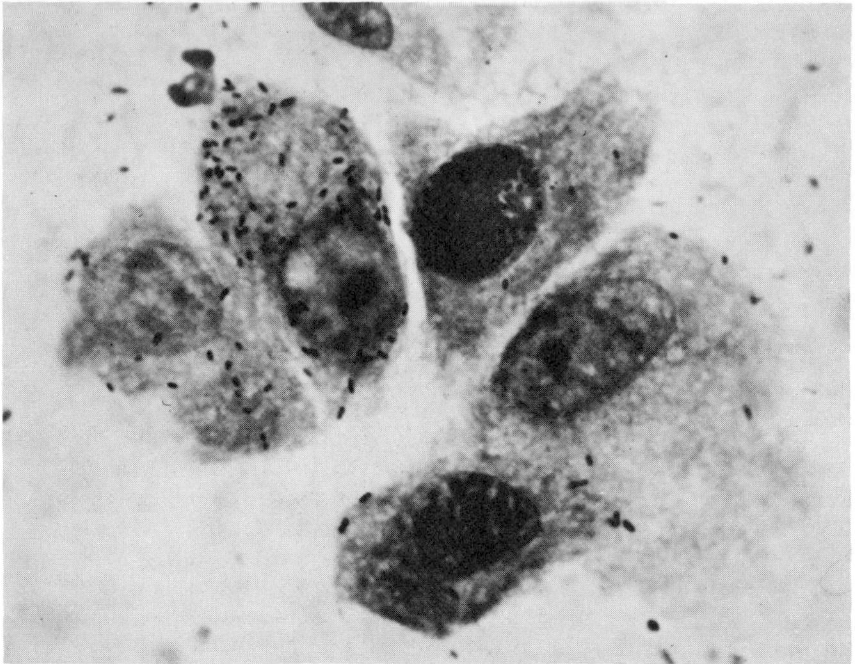

Figure 5–1. *Rickettsia rickettsii* in tunica vaginalis smear of infected meadow vole. Note intranuclear growth in cell at upper right. (Giménez stain, × 1500. Courtesy of Dr. W. Burgdorfer, Rocky Mountain Laboratory.)

meadow voles *(Microtus pennsylvanicus)* have been found of particular value for isolation and differentiation of rickettsial species. In susceptible experimental animals, rickettsiae accumulate in cells of mesothelial origin, especially the lining cells of serous cavities and those of the intima and media of blood vessels. The rickettsiae of epidemic, murine, and scrub typhus and of Q fever grow intracellularly, whereas those of the spotted fever group may appear both in the cytoplasm and in the nucleus (Fig. 5–1). Intracellular and intranuclear growth have been established also for *Rickettsia canada,* a recently discovered member of the typhus group. Most species of rickettsiae, including *C. burnetii,* have been cultivated successfully in yolk sacs of developing chick embryos and in a variety of primary and established arthropod and vertebrate cell lines.

Coxiella burnetii differs in many respects from members of the genus *Rickettsia.* Most important, it appears to have become independent of its arthropod vectors. Although occasionally transmitted by ticks and other hematophagous arthropods, it is capable of surviving as an aerosol because of its resistance to the external environment. Q fever is the most ubiquitous rickettsial disease in the world today.

The rickettsioses of man, by virtue of their epidemiologic and immunologic characteristics, have been separated into the following distinct groups:

1. *Typhus group,* including epidemic (louse-borne) and murine (flea-borne) typhus.
2. *Spotted fever group,* including the tick typhus fevers (spotted fevers from Canada south through Latin America to Colombia and Brazil, boutonneuse fever [including Kenya tick typhus, South African tick bite fever, and Indian tick typhus], North Asian tick typhus, and Queensland tick typhus) and rickettsialpox.
3. *Scrub typhus.*
4. *Q fever.*
5. *Trench fever.*

Data pertaining to the rickettsial agent, vectors and reservoir hosts of each disease are summarized in Table 5–1. There is serologic evidence that *R. canada,* a new member of the typhus group, causes severe febrile disease in the United States.[3] The agent has been recovered only once from the tick *Haemaphysalis leporis-palustris* but not from man.

Additional information about the rickettsiae and the diseases they cause is available.[4–7]

Diagnostic Features of the Rickettsial Diseases

Diagnosis of rickettsial diseases is based on (1) occurrence of clinical features, such as rash and lymphadenopathy; (2) isolation of the specific agent in experimental animals; and (3) demonstration of an increase of specific antibodies in a patient's serum during infection and convalescence (Table 5–2).

Clinical Features. Certain clinical features are of value in the diagnosis of rickettsial diseases. In scrub typhus, fièvre boutonneuse, Queensland tick typhus and rickettsialpox, a characteristic local reaction develops at the site of the arthropod bites—an ulcer often covered by a black adherent crust (eschar, tache noire). This is followed by local or regional lymphadenitis.

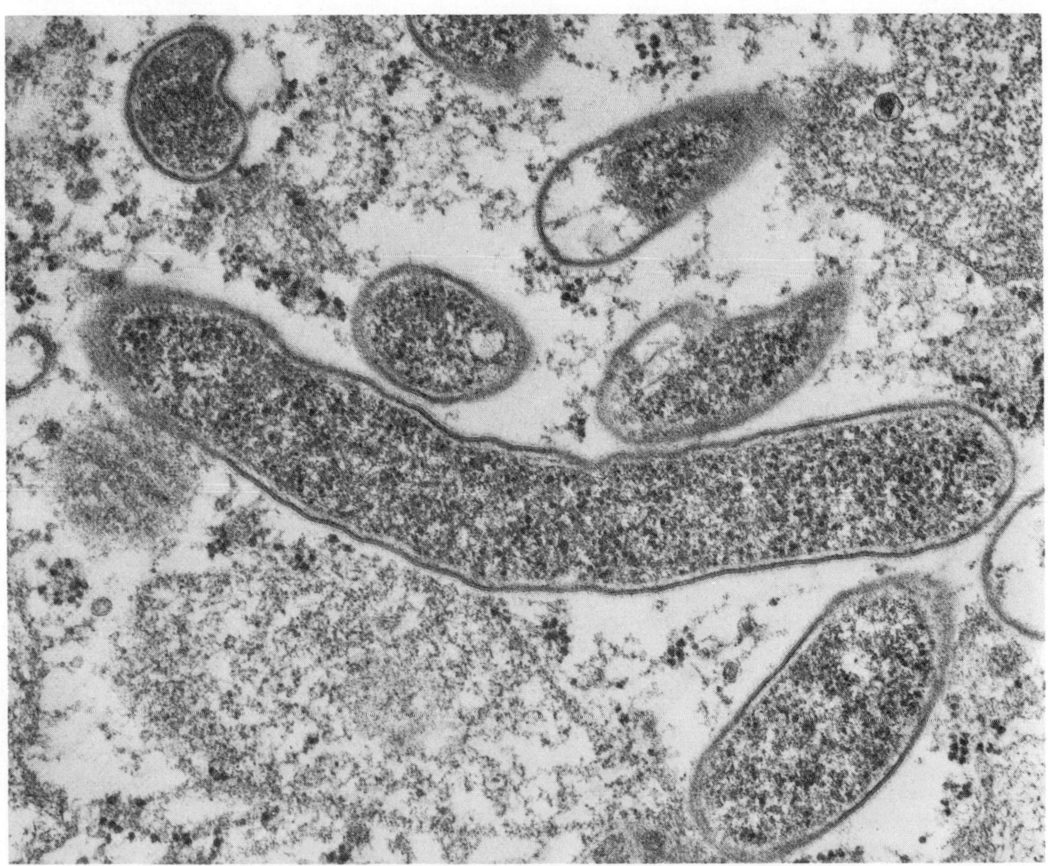

Figure 5–2. The causative agent of Rocky Mountain spotted fever, *Rickettsia rickettsii,* in ovarian tissue of *Dermacentor andersoni.* (Electron micrograph, × 48,000. Courtesy of Dr. L. P. Brinton, Rocky Mountain Laboratory.)

Table 5–1. RICKETTSIAL DISEASES OF MAN

Disease	*Etiologic Agent*	*Usual Vector to Man*	*Reservoir*
Typhus group			
A. Epidemic (Brill-Zinsser disease)	*Rickettsia prowazekii*	*Pediculus humanus humanus*	Man
B. Murine	*R. typhi*	*Xenopsylla cheopis*	Rats
Spotted fever group			
A. American spotted fevers (including spotted fevers from Canada south through Latin America to Colombia and Brazil)	*R. rickettsii*	*Dermacentor andersoni, D. variabilis* and *Amblyomma americanum* (U.S.A.). *Rhipicephalus sanguineus* (Mexico). *A. cajennense* (South America and (?)Mexico).	Ticks, small mammals, particularly rodents, dogs
B. Fièvre boutonneuse (including Kenya tick typhus, South African tick bite fever and Indian tick typhus)	*R. conorii*	*Rhipicephalus sanguineus* in Mediterranean basin and India. *R. evertsi, A. hebraeum, Haemaphysalis leachi* in South Africa and Kenya.	Ticks, dogs, small mammals
C. Siberian tick typhus	*R. sibirica*	*D. silvarum, D. nuttalli, D. marginatus, D. pictus, H. concinna, H punctata*	Ticks, rodents
D. Queensland tick typhus	*R. australis*	*Ixodes holocyclus* (?)	Unknown (complement-fixation antibodies in rats, bandicoots and other small mammals)
E. Rickettsialpox	*R. akari*	Mites: *Liponyssoides* (=*Allodermanyssus*) *sanguineus*	House mice (*Mus musculus*)
Scrub typhus (*Tsutsugamushi* disease)	*R. tsutsugamushi*	Trombiculid mites: *Leptotrombidium deliense* group	Mites, field rats and mice and small mammals
Q fever	*Coxiella burnetii*	Infection of man probably by inhalation of contaminated airborne droplets or dust.	Ticks, cattle, sheep, goats and certain wild animals
Trench fever	*Rochalimaea quintana*	*P. humanus humanus*	Man

Initial distribution of the rash likewise is helpful in differential diagnosis.

In epidemic typhus, murine typhus, scrub typhus and trench fever, the rash first appears on the trunk and later spreads to the extremities. In diseases of the spotted fever group, the rash appears first on the extremities, ankles and wrists, and may then spread over the entire body, except the palms and soles. In Rocky Mountain spotted fever the rash also includes palms and soles. The rash in rickettsialpox is characteristic and resembles that seen in chickenpox; individual lesions begin as small erythematous papules that acquire a centrally located vesicle as they increase in size.

Isolation of Rickettsial Agents in Experimental Animals. Adult guinea pigs, white mice and male meadow voles *(Microtus pennsylvanicus)* are the animals of choice for primary isolation of rickettsiae. The trench fever agent, *Rochalimaea quintana,* is the only rickettsial agent that can be isolated on artificial medium (blood agar). For isolation of typhus and spotted fever group rickettsiae and *Coxiella burnetii,* male guinea pigs weighing 550 to 750 gm are used. Recovery of rickettsiae from a patient's blood, from ticks, or from bloods and tissues of wild animals is usually accompanied by fever in the inoculated guinea pigs. Virulent strains of *R. rickettsii* and other tick-borne typhus rickettsiae produce scrotal swelling that is reducible on pressure and which may be followed by typical hemorrhagic and necrotic lesions and death. The primary pathologic change is endothelial proliferation followed by thrombosis and necrosis. In smears of the tunica vaginalis, rickettsiae may be seen in both the cytoplasm and the nucleus of large mononuclear cells. Many strains of spotted fever rickettsiae are avirulent for guinea pigs and do not evoke fever or scrotal reactions; their infectivity has to be demonstrated by serologic procedures.

Rickettsia typhi produces a nonreducible scrotal swelling in guinea pigs with erythema of the scrotum appearing on the first or second day of fever, i.e. the Neill-Mooser reaction, which essentially is an inflammatory reaction of the tunica vaginalis. The inflammatory exudate consists of large serosal cells filled with intracytoplasmic rickettsiae. These cells are referred to as "Mooser cells" (Fig. 5–3). In contrast to tick typhus rickettsiae, *R. typhi* does not grow in the nucleus.

Rickettsia prowazekii and *Coxiella burnetii* do not produce visible scrotal reactions.

Adult white mice are considered the animal of choice for recovery of *R. tsutsugamushi* and *Rickettsia akari,* and suckling mice have been shown highly susceptible to *Rickettsia australis,* the etiologic agent of Queensland tick typhus. Recently it was found that all rickettsial agents pathogenic for man produce microscopically detectable infections in male meadow voles, particularly in the tunica vaginalis.[8]

Serologic Diagnosis. The Weil-Felix

Table 5–2. RICKETTSIAL DISEASES—DIAGNOSTIC FEATURES IN MAN

Disease	*Weil-Felix*	*Specific Complement-Fixation**	*Early Distribution of Rash*	*Primary Ulcer—Local Adenopathy*
Typhus group				
A. Epidemic (Brill-Zinsser disease)	OX–19	*Rickettsia prowazekii*	Trunk	0
B. Murine	OX–19	*R. typhi*	Trunk	0
Spotted fever group				
A. American spotted fevers (including spotted fevers of U.S.A., Canada, Mexico, Panama, Colombia and Brazil)	OX–19	*R. rickettsii*	Extremities	0
B. Fièvre boutonneuse (including Kenya tick typhus, South African tick bite fever and Indian tick typhus)	OX–19	*R. conorii*	Extremities	+
C. Siberian tick typhus	OX–19	*R. sibirica*	Extremities	+
D. Queensland tick typhus	OX–19 OX–2	*R. australis*	General	+
E. Rickettsialpox	Occas. OX–19	*R. akari*	Trunk, varicelliform rash	+
Scrub typhus (*Tsutsugamushi* disease)	OX–K	*R. tsutsugamushi*	Trunk	±
Q fever	None	*C. burnetii*	No rash	0
Trench fever	None	*Rochalimaea quintana*	Trunk	0

*It is only by the use of washed rickettsial suspensions and by comparison of serum titers that specific complement-fixation may be observed in the typhus group and in the spotted fever group.

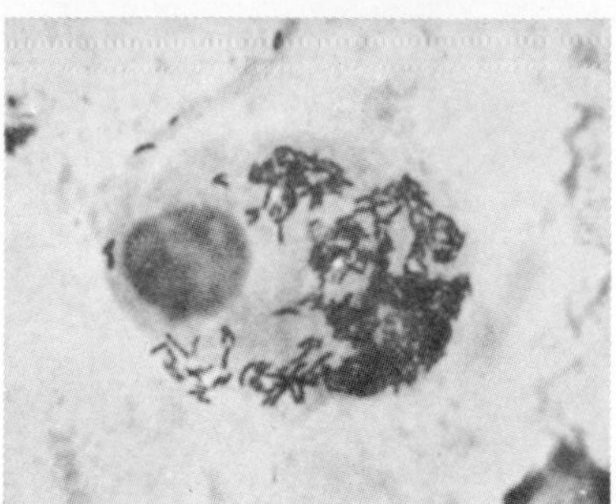

Figure 5-3. Murine typhus. Mooser cell. Intracytoplasmic rickettsiae in large serosal cell of tunica vaginalis. (Courtesy of U.S.A. Typhus Commission.)

reaction and the complement-fixation test are most commonly used because the reagents needed for these tests are commercially available. The indirect fluorescent antibody test may eventually become a valuable tool for detection of rickettsial antibodies. Numerous other tests,[2] including a variety of agglutination and neutralization procedures, have been developed; however, because the necessary reagents are difficult to prepare and cannot be obtained commercially, these tests are not adapted to routine serologic diagnosis.

THE WEIL-FELIX REACTION. This test is based on the fact that certain rickettsiae of the typhus and spotted fever groups and of scrub typhus produce nonspecific agglutinins for the "O" antigens of certain nonmotile strains of *Proteus.* Serial 2-fold dilutions of serum are mixed equally with suspensions of *Proteus vulgaris* OX–19 and OX–2, and *Proteus mirabilis* OX–K. The tubes are then incubated at 37.5° C (99.5° F) for 2 hours, followed by overnight storage at 4° C (39.2° F) or at 52° C (125.6° F) for 16 to 18 hours. Paired sera, i.e. one as soon as possible after onset of the disease and another during convalescence, should be included in the same test. A 4-fold or greater increase of antibodies in the second specimen is considered positive. The Weil-Felix reaction is *nonspecific,* and a positive test should be considered only presumptive evidence of rickettsial infection. It does not differentiate typhus group and spotted fever group infections, since OX–19 titers may occur in all of these diseases. Also, a negative Weil-Felix test does not exclude rickettsial etiology because patients with rickettsialpox, Q fever or trench fever do not develop *Proteus* agglutinins, and those suffering with Brill-Zinsser disease do so only rarely. Strain OX–K is the only one that is agglutinated in scrub typhus, and a rising titer of agglutinins for this strain is considered diagnostic, provided *Proteus* urinary tract infection, leptospirosis and relapsing fever, all of which give positive reactions, are ruled out.

COMPLEMENT-FIXATION (CF) TEST. The CF test, using respective group-specific soluble antigens, provides a means for identifying rickettsiae of the typhus and spotted fever groups. A soluble antigen has also been demonstrated for the agent of Q fever, but it is of no diagnostic value. Soluble antigens for *R. tsutsugamushi* do provide an etiologic diagnosis but are not considered satisfactory for routine use because of the antigenic diversity among isolates of this rickettsia.

For within-group differentiation of spotted fever and typhus group agents, it is necessary to use type-specific antigens prepared by removing the soluble antigens from the rickettsial organisms. Such type-specific, highly purified rickettsial antigens have been prepared by a variety of methods, including differential centrifugation plus ether extraction, use of anion exchange resins in chromatographic columns, density gradient sedimentation and other procedures.[2] Such antigens, however, are not available commercially.

INDIRECT FLUORESCENT ANTIBODY (FA) TEST. Indirect staining of rickettsial antigens has been used to detect typhus group, spotted fever group, scrub typhus and Q fever infections. The test is group-specific but not species-specific, although it has been applied to distinguish between epidemic and murine typhus after antibody absorption of soluble antigens. Because the test permits detection of rickettsial agglutinins (IgM) present early in the course of the disease and of agglutinins (IgG) persisting long after convalescence, it is considered of value in differentiating primary epidemic typhus from recrudescent typhus (Brill-Zinsser disease). Patients suffering from the latter disease possess IgG immunoglobulins only. Like many other serologic procedures, the indirect FA test is of value only to experienced investigators.

Treatment. All pathogenic rickettsiae are susceptible to broad spectrum antibiotics, chloramphenicol and the tetracyclines. Dangerous side effects of chloramphenicol, notably blood dyscrasias, have been observed. Regimens for therapy are provided under the individual rickettsioses.

Prophylaxis. Rickettsioses are controlled (1) by preventive measures against the source of infection and (2) by vaccination of exposed personnel. Control practices depend upon the epidemiology of the specific disease. However, in general, they include sanitary measures; insecticides directed against arthropod vectors (Table 72–1, p. 794); extermination of animal "reservoirs," such as rats and other rodents; destruction of rat harborages; and use of protective clothing and insect repellents (Table 72–1, pp. 800 and 793) to reduce exposure to contaminated animal and arthropod fomites.

Practical vaccines against epidemic typhus and Rocky Mountain spotted fever have been developed commercially through use of infected chicken embryo yolk sacs as sources of antigen. Attempts at producing vaccines against other rickettsioses have had varied results, such as vaccines against murine or endemic typhus and scrub typhus. Effective vaccines against Q fever are now imminent. Others have not been attempted or are not needed.

REFERENCES

1. Weiss, E., and Moulder, J. W. 1974. Rickettsia, Coxiella, Rochalimaea. *In* Buchanan, R. E., and Gibbons, N. E. (eds.): Bergey's Manual of Determinative Bacteriology. 8th ed. The Williams & Wilkins Co., Baltimore. pp. 882–893.
2. Elisberg, B. L., and Bozeman, F. M. 1969. Rickettsiae. *In* Lennette, E. H., and Schmidt, N. J.: Diagnostic Procedures for Viral and Rickettsial Infections. Am. Pub. Hlth. Assoc., Inc., New York. pp. 826–868.
3. Bozeman, F. M., Elisberg, B. L., Humphries, J. W., Runcik, K., and Palmer, D. B., Jr. 1970. Serologic evidence of *Rickettsia canada* infection of man. J. Inf. Dis. *121*:367–371.
4. Horsfall, F. L., Jr., and Tamm, I. 1965. Viral and Rickettsial Infections of Man. 4th ed. J. B. Lippincott Co., Philadelphia. 1282 pp.
5. Zdrodovskii, P. F., and Golinevich, E. H. 1960. The Rickettsial Diseases. 2nd ed. Pergamon Press, London. (English ed.) 630 pp.
6. Ormsbee, R. A. 1969. Rickettsiae. Ann. Rev. Microbiol. *23*:275–292.
7. Weiss, E. 1973. Growth and physiology of rickettsiae. Bact. Rev. *37*:259–283.
8. Burgdorfer, W. Susceptibility of the meadow vole *(Microtus pennsylvanicus)* to the rickettsiae pathogenic to man (manuscript in preparation).

CHAPTER 6

Epidemic (Louse-Borne) Typhus

WILLY BURGDORFER

Synonyms. Classic, historic, human, or European typhus; jail fever, ship fever, war fever, Fleckfieber; typhus exanthématique, tifus exanthemático, tabardillo.

Definition. Epidemic (louse-borne) typhus is an acute infectious disease caused by *Rickettsia prowazekii* and transmitted by the body louse, *Pediculus humanus humanus*.[1] It is characterized by fairly abrupt onset, continuous fever of about 2 weeks' duration accompanied by severe headache and marked prostration, a characteristic rash appearing about the fifth day, first in the axillae, on the loins, abdomen and back, and terminating by crisis or rapid lysis. The case fatality rate in untreated patients rises sharply with age and deficient nutrition, and usually exceeds 50 per cent in middle-aged and older persons.

Distribution. Epidemic typhus occurred in most parts of the world, except Australia, and is still prevalent in cooler areas, including higher altitudes of the tropic zone. The disease has been part of man's history as far back as medical historians are able to determine. It appeared often along with typhoid and plague wherever mankind was struck by war, famine or other misfortunes. Europe has been the great epidemic center, although one of the most devastating epidemics occurred during the sixteenth century in the highland of Mexico where 2 million people fell victim to the disease. During World War I, typhus killed thousands of soldiers on various European battlefields, especially in Serbia. During the postwar years of 1918 to 1922, as many as 30 million cases with about 3 million deaths are believed to have occurred in Russia.

Before 1939, small outbreaks of typhus were reported each winter in several European and North African countries. However, with the advent of World War II and its disastrous effects on human populations, the disease recurred in epidemic proportions in Morocco, Algeria, Tunisia, Egypt, Iran, Turkey, Yugoslavia and Poland. In 1945 in Germany and Austria more than 90 per cent of all typhus cases occurred among inmates of Nazi concentration camps. Since 1945 the number of reported typhus cases has steadily declined in certain areas of the world. However, endemic centers still exist in mountainous regions of Mexico, South America, Africa, numerous countries in Asia and some parts of eastern Europe. According to W.H.O. statistics, in the years 1967, 1968 and 1969, 11,757, 12,335 and 25,264 cases, respectively, were reported with the most occurring in Africa, especially Burundi and Ethiopia.[2] The true incidence of louse-borne typhus throughout the world is unknown because there is no information about large areas, such as the People's Republic of China, the Democratic People's Republic of Korea, Vietnam and the U.S.S.R. In the United States and Canada, primary typhus has not been reported in recent years, although recrudescent cases (Brill-Zinsser disease) have occurred occasionally in immigrants from Central Europe or other endemic areas.

Etiology. Although *R. prowazekii* is one of the larger rickettsiae, it cannot be distinguished morphologically from *R. typhi*, the agent of murine (flea-borne) typhus with which it shares certain antigenic characteristics, or from rickettsiae of the spotted fever group. Highly pleomorphic, *R. prowazekii* may vary from minute coccoid and rod-shaped organisms to chain or threadlike structures, particularly in the louse. Unlike spotted fever group rickettsiae, it does not invade the cell nucleus. It is relatively labile and does not survive temperatures above 56° C (132.8° F) for more than 30 minutes.

However, in louse feces, *R. prowazekii* remains viable for several months, especially at lower temperatures and humidity.

Natural infections occur only in man and in the body louse, *Pediculus humanus humanus*. Experimentally, a variety of animals, including monkeys, guinea pigs, cotton rats, mice, and voles, developing chick embryos, fleas, and other species of lice can readily be infected. Antibodies against *R. prowazekii* in sera of domestic animals (camels, cattle, donkeys, sheep, goats and others) in certain African countries, and isolation of several strains from such animals and from ticks led to the hypothesis that epidemic typhus may exist in nature in an animal-tick cycle.[3] However, efforts in recent years to find additional support for this hypothesis were unsuccessful.[4, 5]

Epidemiology. Man, the reservoir of

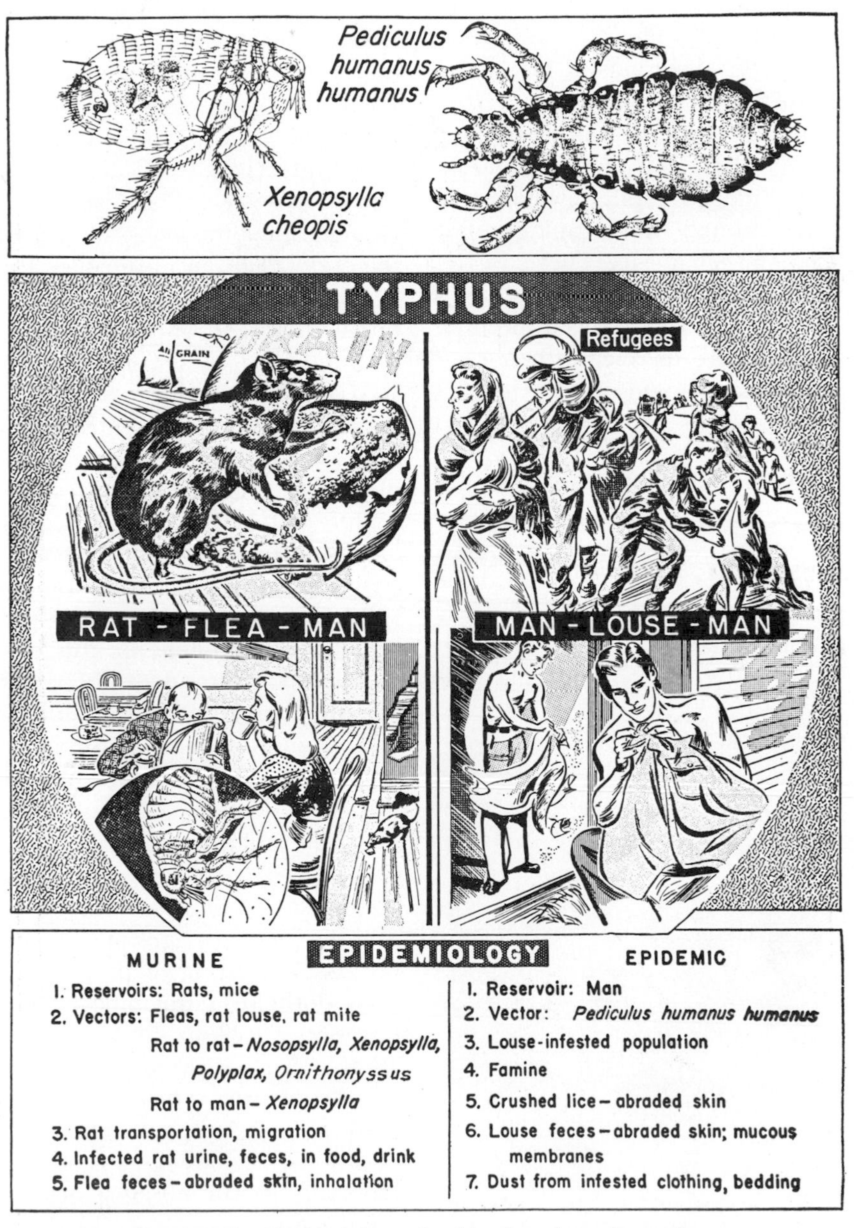

Figure 6–1. Epidemiology of epidemic and murine typhus.

R. prowazekii, and the body louse, *P. humanus humanus*, are the basic factors in the epidemiology of this disease (Figs. 6–1 and 6–2). Occurrence of typhus in its epidemic form usually follows increased levels of lousiness—as may occur among human populations affected by war, famine or other disasters, among persons in jails or refugee camps, or among people in cooler climates who live under crowded conditions with poor bathing and laundering facilities and therefore wear the same garments day and night for long periods.

Infection of *P. humanus humanus* depends on the concentrations of rickettsiae that circulate in the blood of a patient from early in the disease to about the tenth day, occasionally later. Ingested with the blood, the rickettsiae undergo rapid development not only in the lumen of the midgut but especially in its epithelial cells. There, in the cytoplasm, multiplication of rickettsiae takes place to such an extent that the cells become distended and rupture to release their contents into the gut lumen and into the insect's excrements. As early as 5 to 8 days after its infectious blood meal, the louse excretes after each feeding massive quantities of rickettsiae in its fecal material. With the digestive processes no longer functioning properly, the infected louse dies after about 10 days. Because the louse thrives best at 37° C (98.6° F), it tends to leave a febrile patient in search of a new host—a phenomenon explaining the rapid dissemination of the disease during epidemics.

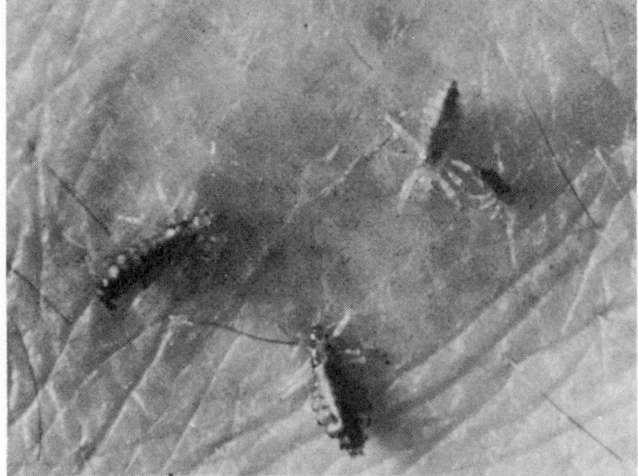

Figure 6–2. *Pediculus humanus humanus* feeding on human skin. (Courtesy of John P. Fox, Tulane University School of Medicine, New Orleans.)

Transmission of *R. prowazekii* to the new host does not occur by bite but from contamination of abraded skin (caused by scratching irritated bite wound) with fluids from the crushed louse feces. Infection may also result from conjunctival contact with, or inhalation of, dried feces from clothing or bedding (Fig. 6–1).

Because the louse dies as a result of rickettsial infection and does not pass rickettsiae transovarially to its progeny, it is not considered a reservoir. This important role is attributed to man, in whom *R. prowazekii* may persist over long periods and may lead to a recrudescence with renewed blood infectivity (Brill-Zinsser disease).

Pathology. The specific pathologic change of typhus consists of proliferation of the endothelium of arterioles and capillaries, which leads to thrombosis, hemorrhage, secondary necrosis and gangrene. There is an accompanying perivascular round cell infiltration. These changes affect particularly vessels of the skin, central nervous system and myocardium. In some areas they resemble early miliary tubercles, the Fraenkel typhus nodules of the skin, whereas in the brain the perivascular cell accumulations resemble those of encephalitis. Thrombosis of larger blood vessels is rare (Fig. 6–3).

Cloudy swelling of the myocardium is frequently observed. The spleen may be slightly enlarged, is often extremely friable, and commonly shows diminution of lymphoid elements. The liver and kidneys likewise show cloudy swelling. In the brain numerous miliary lesions are frequently observed in the basal ganglia, medulla oblongata and cerebral cortex. These present varying stages of the basic pathologic process, consisting of proliferation of vascular endothelium, thrombosis, perivascular infiltration, necrosis and neuroglia proliferation.

Bronchitis, bronchopneumonia and nephritis are frequent and often fatal complications. Secondary parotitis is common, especially in the absence of proper care of the mouth.

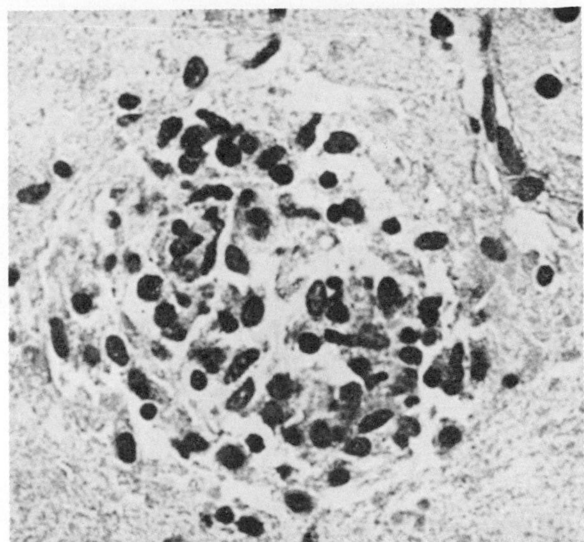

Figure 6–3. Typhus nodule in brain showing necrosis and accumulation of mononuclear phagocytes. (Courtesy of U.S.A. Typhus Commission.)

The rash is often evident after death, and hemorrhagic areas in the skin and subcutaneous tissues are common, especially in sites that have been subjected to pressure and trauma. Areas of skin necrosis or gangrene are frequently present.

Clinical Characteristics. After an incubation period varying from 5 to 15 days (usually 12 to 14 days), the classic disease either occurs abruptly or, more commonly, begins with a prodromal period of 1 to 2 days in which headache, vertigo, backache, anorexia and general malaise are prominent. Usually body temperature rises rapidly by the end of the second day, reaching 39.5 to 40° C (103 to 104° F) by the third or fourth day, and then remains continuously elevated. With the rise of temperature the face becomes flushed, the conjunctivae injected, the expression apathetic, and the headache usually severe. Conjunctivitis is frequent in the early stages. Consciousness is commonly dulled, and there is marked prostration. Early and persistent circulatory weakness is usual.

The characteristic skin eruption appears on the third to the seventh day, first in the axilla and on the flanks, then extends to the abdomen, chest and back and, later, to the extremities. It is most marked on the back. The palms and soles are rarely affected, and the face remains clear. Initially, the eruption consists of slightly raised rose spots that blanch on pressure, but these soon become permanent and later are purpuric. During convalescence the rash fades to a brownish pigmentation which gradually disappears (Fig. 6–4).

With the appearance of the rash, prostration and cardiac depression become more evident. Headache is severe; the patient becomes stuporous, sometimes as markedly as in plague. The mouth is foul, and a cough frequently develops. Constipation is usual. Temperature remains elevated except for slight morning remissions. Pulse is weak and irregular and blood pressure is low. White blood cell count is not characteristic, rarely exceeding 12,000 with a differential count of about 80 to 85 per cent polymorphonuclear leukocytes.

At about the end of the second week, in nonfatal cases, a critical change occurs in the apparently grave condition of the patient. The fever subsides, and this change is accompanied by marked sweating. Stupor disappears, consciousness clears, and the urinary output improves. Circulatory weakness may continue, however, for some time during convalescence. In other instances, the decline in temperature is followed by severe and increasing signs of involvement of the

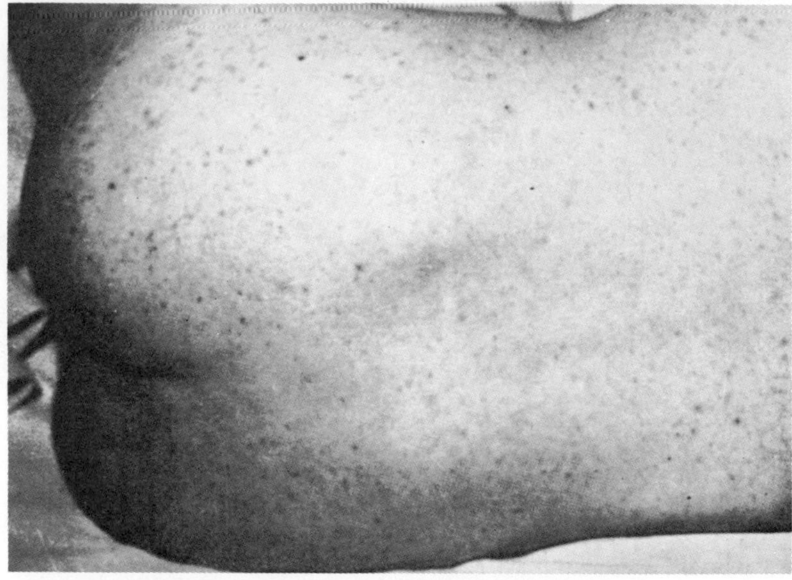

Figure 6–4. Erythematous and petechial rash, epidemic typhus. (Courtesy of U.S.A. Typhus Commission.)

central nervous system, which progress to death.

Bronchitis, bronchopneumonia and nephritis are common complications, and parotitis and otitis media are not infrequent. Gangrene of the toes, less often of the fingers, and of the skin over the sacrum is common.

In uncomplicated cases convalescence is usually rapid and complete. Recovery is followed by long-standing, probably lifelong, immunity.

Previous immunization with an effective vaccine may greatly modify the clinical picture of classic typhus fever. The rash may be absent or of very short duration, the symptoms are less severe, and fever may be present no more than 3 to 5 days.

In addition to vaccination, age and perhaps racial or other genetic factors may influence the course of infection. Among patients with fairly classic illness, case fatality rates rise sharply with age. Studies in Peru indicate further that, at least among the Andean Indians, who apparently have lived in contact with *R. prowazekii* for several centuries, many infections are either subclinical or so benign as to escape recognition, especially in persons younger than 20. In this group it was estimated that about 27 infections occur for each clinically recognized case of typhus.

Diagnosis. The clinical diagnosis of typhus is often difficult in children and in the early stages of an epidemic. During the prodromal period, as well as in the pre-eruptive days following onset, a variety of acute infectious diseases may be considered. Among these are typhoid fever, relapsing fever, malaria, influenza, and Rocky Mountain spotted fever or scrub typhus. The exanthem and subsequent course, however, make clinical differentiation from nonrickettsial diseases possible. Murine typhus, although generally a milder disease, can be ruled out definitely only by isolation and identification of the rickettsiae or by careful serologic tests. Lice, if detected on the patient or in his clothes, should cause early suspicion of relapsing fever or epidemic typhus.

In all isolated cases, or in the absence of a recognized epidemic, the clinical diagnosis should be confirmed by serologic tests. The Weil-Felix reaction becomes positive in 50 per cent of cases by the eighth day of the disease, and by the thirteenth day it is positive in all infected persons. This test provides the earliest presumptive evidence, although it does not exclude murine typhus or the spotted fever group. To have diagnostic significance, a rise in antibody titer of the patient's serum is necessary. A single positive test is only suggestive. The reaction becomes negative in late convalescence and, therefore, cannot be used to determine past infection.

With suspensions of washed rickettsiae, the complement-fixation (CF) test is highly specific. Such antigen is not commercially available and requires skilled use. With the available antigens, which contain much "soluble" antigen, considerable crossing with murine typhus antibody is observed. Fortunately, if both epidemic and murine antigens are used, the differences in titer are usually sufficient to permit specific diagnosis. With the customary two units of complement-fixing antigen, antibody usually appears between 7 and 14 days after onset. Recent observations suggest that detection of this early appearing antibody is facilitated by using eight units of antigen. Peak titers are reached after 2 or 3 weeks of convalescence, but because of the relatively long persistence of such antibody, the complement-fixation test is useful to identify past infections.

Other serologic tests include mouse-toxin neutralization tests, rickettsial agglutination, and agglutination of sheep red cells sensitized with rickettsial antigen. Because of cost and the hazard of working with highly infectious material, the neutralization test remains a research procedure. This is also true for the sensitive method of rickettsial agglutination, for which antigen is not commercially available. The red cell agglutination method remains to be confirmed as a satisfactory routine diagnostic test.

Isolation of *R. prowazekii* from the patient's blood may be accomplished during the acute phase by inoculating clot suspensions intraperitoneally into guinea pigs or cotton rats. Classically a febrile response with little or no scrotal swelling (tunica reaction) is observed in guinea pigs, whereas, in contrast, murine typhus results in marked scrotal swelling. In cotton rats, death may occur. In both kinds of animals, infection can also be demonstrated by presence of antibody in sera from surviving animals.

Treatment. Good nursing care is extremely important. Symptomatic management should be directed primarily to the control of toxemia by administration of ample fluids, the maintenance of bowel function by enemas, strict oral hygiene, great care to protect the skin against bed sores, and protection of the circulatory system. Delirium may be controlled by sponge baths and application of ice bags to the head, although severe cases may require hyoscine with or without morphine. Lumbar drainage may be useful in some instances. Circulatory changes must be watched for carefully; cardiac stimulants are often indicated.

The foregoing limited measures were the only ones available before the advent of broad spectrum antibiotics and are still to be used when patients first come for treatment late in the disease or when antibiotics are not available. Drugs of the tetracycline group (Terramycin, Achromycin, Aureomycin) and chloramphenicol are apparently equally effective. Recommended for adults is an initial dose of 2 gm followed by 2 gm daily in divided doses. Treatment should result in defervescence within 48 to 72 hours but should be continued until at least the tenth day from onset and for a minimum of 48 hours after the patient becomes afebrile. During recent studies of typhus in Burundi, a single dose of 200 mg of doxycycline (Vibramycin), a derivative of tetracycline, given to adult patients on the first day of the disease or later, regularly effected a cure without relapse.[6] This represents a dramatic turn in treatment of this disease because it requires only a single contact between medical personnel and patients.

Prophylaxis. All persons entering a typhus area should be immunized with an effective vaccine made from killed *R. prowazekii.* The Cox-type yolk sac vaccine was extensively used during World War II. Although it did not completely prevent infection among exposed personnel, the course of the disease among vaccinated persons was much shorter and milder, the incidence of serious complications greatly reduced, and mortality practically nil. It is now recommended that one dose of 1.0 ml be given subcutaneously. This should be followed by a booster dose of 0.1 ml before exposure in an area where the disease is endemic. Since this vaccine contains egg material, it must be administered with caution to egg-sensitive persons.

It must be remembered that, whereas a clinical attack of epidemic typhus confers protection against murine typhus, immunization with the killed rickettsiae of epidemic typhus does not produce such cross-immunity.

Vaccine containing a living attenuated strain of *R. prowazekii* (strain E) has been under evaluation since 1951, especially in the U.S.S.R.[7] A single intramuscular injection of proper dosage (between 10^4 and 10^5 egg infective doses) induces, with a tolerable level of reaction, solid immunity to later challenge with virulent organisms. This immunity has been observed to endure for at least 5½ years. The vaccine also induces lesser but significant resistance to challenge with virulent murine typhus rickettsiae.

Medical personnel and health officials working in an epidemic area must exercise great care to avoid infection. Louse-infested clothing should be removed and sterilized, and the patient should be deloused. Attendants should wear clothing impregnated with a lousicide, and in view of the infectiousness of dried louse feces, they should wear protective masks, goggles and gloves while in a potentially infected environment.

When typhus epidemics occur, the protection of population groups involves extensive application of delousing measures with adequate police support to insure treatment of all members of the community and to prevent ingress of louse-infested persons into treated areas (Table 72–1, p. 796). Immediate delousing of all contacts of acute cases is of utmost urgency. This in turn entails an effective case finding and reporting mechanism. The first spectacular demonstration of the efficacy of this procedure occurred early in World War II during a civilian epidemic in Naples, Italy, where disinfestation, easily and rapidly accomplished by the use of louse powders containing 10 per cent DDT in an inert base such as talc or pyrophyllite, blown into each individual's clothing by hand or power dusters, proved very effective. Where DDT-resistant strains of lice were encountered, as happened in Korea, lindane, 1 per cent in inert dust, was substituted (Table 72–1, p. 796).

In both instances, mass application of an effective insecticide was used as a short-term measure to interrupt transmission and to control the outbreak. Once the population in these areas had recovered from the effects of war, conditions conducive to a high level of lousiness and to typhus transmission had essentially disappeared, and the use of insecticides for louse control was no longer required. However, a completely different situation exists in areas where lousiness and conditions for typhus transmission are found throughout the year, or where the affected populace is spread over large geographic areas with limited access. Here, an insecticide program would result only in spotty and temporary reduction of lousiness, and with the termination of such a program, louse populations would again proliferate to original levels. It is under such conditions that resistance of body lice to DDT, lindane and even malathion has developed.

Body louse infestations persist in most parts of the world, and infestation rates remain very high in some areas of low socioeconomic development and poor sanitary facilities. Concern about resurgence of louse-borne diseases, particularly epidemic typhus, appears justified, especially in view of widespread resistance of lice to insecticides and the questions raised concerning environmental contamination and toxicity of insecticides to man. Until new, more efficient means of louse-control are found, it is hoped that through subsidiary measures—including improvement of living conditions, provisions for adequate bathing and laundering, and the dispensation of adequate supplies of clothing and food to underdeveloped nations—the degree of lousiness can be held below the threshold figure necessary for the occurrence of epidemics.

BRILL-ZINSSER DISEASE

As first suggested by Zinsser, Brill-Zinsser disease, once confused with murine typhus in the southern United States, is a recrudescence of infection with *R. prowazekii.* Proof of Zinsser's hypothesis has been established by serologic studies and by the recovery of *R. prowazekii* from patients affected with Brill-Zinsser disease and from lymph nodes obtained by biopsy from two healthy persons who had typhus several years previously. Recrudescent typhus occurs sporadically throughout the year in adults or elderly people who had experienced typhus 10 to 15 years earlier. Factors that provoke recrudescence in man remain to be defined. The clinical picture is usually that of mild epidemic typhus with mortality being rare. There is no familial spread in the absence of lice. Cases of primary typhus may occur, however, if a Brill-Zinsser case develops in a milieu of severe lousiness. In Bosnia (Yugoslavia), for instance, more than 800 cases of Brill-Zinsser disease have been reported since 1963.[8] Only seven of these were infested with lice in sufficient numbers to cause transmission to a susceptible person. Experimental data show that the percentage of lice becoming infected while feeding on a patient affected with Brill-Zinsser disease usually is low and rarely exceeds 5 per cent. In the United States, Brill-Zinsser disease occurs sporadically in persons who have immigrated from Central Europe where they had experienced a primary attack of typhus many years before.

The Weil-Felix agglutination test with *Proteus* OX–19, which is of great value in the diagnosis of epidemic typhus, is of no diagnostic value. The CF test, microagglutination test, and particularly the indirect fluorescent antibody (FA) test with conjugates against IgM and IgG antibodies are recommended.

Epidemiologically, the phenomenon of long-enduring latent infection with recrudescence and renewed infectivity for lice constitutes an important reservoir mechanism for *R. prowazekii.*

REFERENCES

1. Snyder, J. C. 1965. Typhus fever rickettsiae. *In* Horsfall, F. L., Jr., and Tamm, I.: Viral and Rickettsial Infections of Man. 4th ed. J. B. Lippincott Co., Philadelphia. pp. 1059–1094.
2. Tarizzo, M. L. 1973. Geographic distribution of louse-borne diseases. *In* Proceedings of the International Symposium on the Control of Lice and Louse-borne Diseases. P.A.H.O. Sci. Publ. No. 263, Washington, D. C. (1972). pp. 50–59.
3. Philip, C. B. 1968. A review of growing evidence that domestic animals may be involved in cycles of rickettsial zoonoses. Zb1. Bakt. Abt. I. Orig. *206*:343–353.
4. Ormsbee, R. A. 1973. The hypothesis of louse-borne infections: Possible extrahuman reservoirs. *In* Proceedings of the International Symposium on the Control of Lice and Louse-Borne Diseases. P.A.H.O. Sci. Publ. No. 263, Washington, D. C. (1972). pp. 104–109.
5. Burgdorfer, W., Ormsbee, R. A., and Hoogstraal, H. 1972. Ticks as vectors of *Rickettsia prowazeki*—a controversial issue. Am. J. Trop. Med. Hyg. *21*:989–998.
6. Wisseman, C. L., Jr. Personal communication.
7. Golinevich, E. M., and Iablonshaia, V. A. 1963. [Live exanthematous vaccine from Strain E of *R. prowazekii.*] *In* Zdrodovskii, P. F.: Problems of Infectious Pathology and Immunology. (In Russian.) Medgiz. pp. 199–211.
8. Murray, E. S., and Gaon, J. A. 1973. Louse-borne typhus: Major categories of control problems. *In* Proceedings of the International Symposium on the Control of Lice and Louse-borne Diseases. P.A.H.O. Sci. Publ. No. 263, Washington, D. C. (1972). pp. 270–272.

CHAPTER 7

Murine (Flea-Borne) Typhus

WILLY BURGDORFER

Synonyms. Endemic typhus, flea or rat typhus, urban or shop typhus of Malaya.

Definition. A relatively mild febrile disease of about 14 days' duration, characterized by chills, severe headaches, generalized body pains and a macular rash. The etiologic agent, *Rickettsia typhi* (syn. *R. mooseri*), is transmitted to man by introduction of infectious flea feces either into the bite wound or into skin abrasions caused by scratching.

Distribution. Murine typhus occurs in areas of warmer climates throughout the world.

Etiology. *Rickettsia typhi* is morphologically indistinguishable from *R. prowazekii*, with which it also shares various antigenic characteristics. Its host range is rather broad and includes various species of small rodents and other mammals. Infection of male guinea pigs results in adhesions so the testes can no longer be pushed into the abdomen. This "Neill-Mooser" reaction is associated with large masses of rickettsiae in the cytoplasm of mesothelial cells of the tunica vaginalis (Fig. 5–3).

Epidemiology. Commensal rats, especially *Rattus norvegicus*, constitute the chief reservoirs of *R. typhi*. Acute infection in these rodents results in only slight overt disease, but rickettsiae circulate in the peripheral blood for 6 to 8 days. During this period, various rat ectoparasites become infected and are presumed to spread infection from rat to rat. These include the tropical rat mite, *Ornithonyssus bacoti;* the rat louse, *Polyplax spinulosa;* and fleas, *Nosopsyllus fasciatus* (rarely bites man), and *Xenopsylla cheopis*, the tropical rat flea. The last named is considered the classic vector of *R. typhi*, both from rat to rat and from rat to man.

Undisturbed by the infection, the flea remains infectious for its entire adult life. Salivary glands and reproductive tissues are not invaded by *R. typhi*. Therefore, transovarial infection does not occur, and transmission to man takes place chiefly through rubbing rickettsiae-laden flea feces into the skin either through the bite wound or through abrasions caused by scratching. There is also evidence that the disease is contracted by inhalation of dry flea feces and by ingestion of food contaminated by the urine of infected rats.

Although *X. cheopis* is considered the classic vector, other species of fleas (*Leptosylla musculi, Ctenocephalides canis* and *Ctenocephalides felis)* and the human body louse, *Pediculus humanus humanus*, are highly susceptible to *R. typhi*. Spread of murine typhus via the body louse has long been speculated, particularly in areas of Mexico, Ethiopia and China where louse infestations and *R. typhi* may coexist. Recently, *C. felis* and one of its hosts, the opossum *(Didelphis marsupialis)*, have been shown to be involved in a natural cycle in an area of southern California where *X. cheopis* was absent and where seropositive rats could not be found.

Murine typhus in man is influenced largely by season and by occupational exposure (food warehouses, granaries and poultry farms). This latter factor explains why, in the southern United States, incidence in men is twice that in women. In the United States, murine typhus reached its peak incidence in 1944 and 1945 with 5401 and 5193 reported cases, respectively, plus an estimated 20,000 unreported cases each year. Since then there has been an abrupt decline; since 1961 the number of annually reported cases has been below 50.

Pathology. In general, the pathologic findings in murine typhus are similar to those in epidemic typhus (p. 104). However, they are not known in detail because death is uncommon (less than 5 per cent in the United States). It is probable that there are histopathologic changes in small vessels similar to those seen in epidemic typhus. Cutaneous petechiae are infrequent, and large areas of skin necrosis have not been reported.

Clinical Characteristics. Except in persons over 50, murine typhus is a milder disease than the epidemic variety. Onset follows an incubation period of 6 to 14 days and may be either abrupt or gradual. In the latter case, the body temperature rises to 38.9 to 40.5° C (102 to 105° F) during the first week and remains elevated until about 2 weeks after onset. The rash, usually limited to the chest, abdomen and inner surfaces of the arms, resembles that of epidemic typhus, except that petechiae are rare. The macules, appearing about the fifth day, at first fade on pressure but soon lose this characteristic. After 2 to 10 days they disappear. Fever usually recedes by rapid lysis, and recovery is complete, although convalescence may be delayed. Abnormal symptoms are not marked and complications are rare.

Diagnosis. The diagnosis of murine typhus presents problems similar to those connected with epidemic typhus. Serologic procedures described for epidemic typhus, including the Weil-Felix test, are equally applicable, as are the methods for agent isolation and identification (pp. 106, 107). In addition, a characteristic scrotal swelling may develop in inoculated guinea pigs (without the necrosis seen with virulent strains of Rocky Mountain spotted fever rickettsiae), and Mooser bodies (aggregates of rickettsiae) may be demonstrated in smear preparations of mesothelial cells of the tunica vaginalis. Isolation may be accomplished by direct inoculation of uncontaminated homogenized blood clot into the yolk sacs of 7-day chick embryos.

Treatment and Prophylaxis. Treatment of murine typhus is the same as that of epidemic typhus (p. 107).

Because rats constitute the primary reservoir in nature, poisoning, trapping and rat-proofing are logical procedures for control. Rat-proofing is the only measure of permanent value. Particular attention should be paid to granaries and storehouses, thereby depriving rats of their major food supply.

Control of fleas by the use of DDT for dusting rat runs is considered by most workers the best modern method of controlling murine typhus. (See Table 72–1, p. 797, for other insecticides for flea control.)

Effective experimental vaccines have been prepared, but a practical vaccine has not been needed.

CHAPTER 8
American Spotted Fevers

RICHARD A. ORMSBEE

Synonyms. Rocky Mountain spotted fever, exanthematic typhus of São Paulo, Tobia fever, Choix fever, pinta fever.

Definition. An acute febrile disease caused by *Rickettsia rickettsii* (Fig. 8–1) and transmitted by the bite of certain ticks. It is characterized by a rash that appears first on the wrists and ankles and later, in some cases, over the entire body, including the face, palms of the hands and soles of the feet.[1–4]

Distribution. Formerly thought to be restricted to certain areas of the Rocky Mountain states, the disease has since been reported from British Columbia, Alberta and Saskatchewan (Canada), from 46 states (U.S.A.), and from Brazil, Colombia, Mexico and Panama. In Brazil the disease was originally reported as exanthematic typhus of São Paulo and in Colombia as Tobia fever. Choix or pinta fever in northern Mexico has also been identified with spotted fever.

Etiology. *Rickettsia rickettsii* cells are slightly larger than those of *R. prowazekii,* but possess similar staining properties. Like other members of the spotted fever group, of which it is the prototype, *R. rickettsii* differs from members of the typhus group by its ability to invade nuclei of host cells. The spotted fevers of the Western Hemisphere apparently represent a single disease entity, as indicated by serologic tests and other laboratory studies. *Rickettsia canada,* a newly described species isolated from a pool of *Haemaphysalis leporis-palustris* ticks in Ontario, Canada, also invades cell nuclei. It possesses antigens in common with rickettsiae of both spotted fever and typhus groups, but has not yet been unequivocally associated with human disease.

Epidemiology. Spotted fever is essentially a rural disease, occurring in areas where ticks and their rodent hosts are prevalent. In the eastern United States, dogs have carried infected vector ticks into human habitations and their environs, thereby establishing foci of infection in some suburban areas. Increasing use of parks and similar recreational areas probably has been a factor in the increasing incidence of spotted fever during the past 10 years. Because ticks are not habitual parasites of man, the disease does not, as a rule, occur in epidemic form. However, in some heavily tick-infested areas in Colombia, it has reached almost epidemic proportions, and in other areas multiple infections within a family are not infrequent.

The severity of spotted fever may vary greatly in areas separated only by short distances. For unknown reasons, the degree of virulence of the rickettsia in a given area appears to remain relatively constant.

Tick vectors may be considered in two groups: (1) those which feed both on wild rodents and on man; and (2) those which serve as vectors among wild rodents but do not feed on man or seldom come in contact with him.[4] Ticks are believed to furnish the chief reservoir mechanism in nature because they remain infected for life and transmit the infection transovarially with high efficiency, although they themselves appear to be little affected by the infection. *R. rickettsii* has not been observed to survive longer than a month in small animals. However, recovery of the rickettsia from lymph nodes of a man convalescent for a year has been reported.

The common vectors of the human disease are: in western Canada and the western United States, the wood tick, *Dermacentor andersoni* Stiles (Fig. 8–2); in the eastern United States, the dog tick, *Dermacentor variabilis* (Say); and in Texas and Oklahoma, the Lone Star tick, *Amblyomma americanum* (Linn.). As a rule, only the adults of the two species of *Dermacentor* feed on man; nymphs, however,

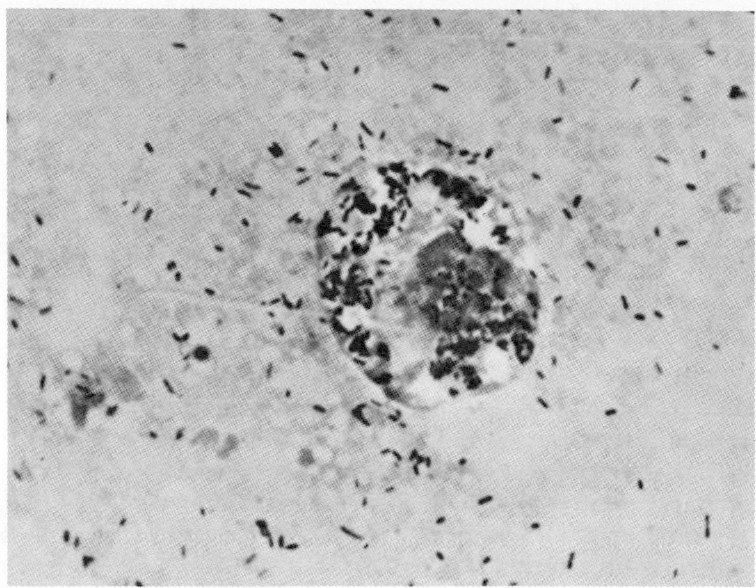

Figure 8–1. *Rickettsia rickettsii,* causative agent of Rocky Mountain spotted fever, in stained smear of infected yolk sac of chick embryo. Extracellular and intracellular bodies and possibly some intranuclear (see halos around some organisms) are depicted. (Courtesy of Rocky Mountain Laboratory; photo by N. J. Kramis.)

may in rare instances feed on children. On the other hand, larvae, nymphs and adults of *A. americanum* have been found on man. In Mexico, *Rhipicephalus sanguineus* (Latr.) is the only proved vector to man, but *Amblyomma cajennense* (Fabr.), *Ornithodoros nicollei* (Mooser) and *Otobius lagophilus* Cooley and Kohls have also been found naturally infected there. In Colombia and Brazil, *A. cajennense* is the accepted vector, and all active stages likewise attack man. Several other species of ixodid ticks and at least three species of argasid or soft ticks are efficient experimental vectors.

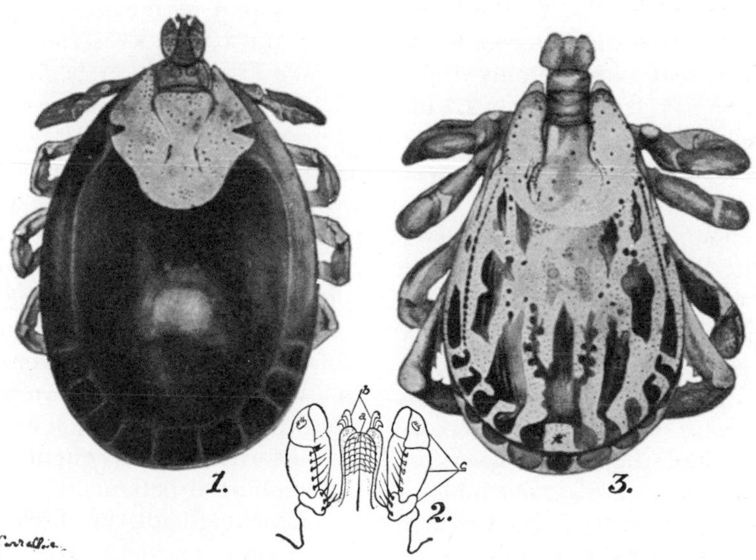

Figure 8–2. *1,* Female *Dermacentor andersoni* Stiles. *2,* Mouthparts showing (*a*) hypostome, (*b*) chelicerae, (*c*) palps. *3,* Male. (Strong: Stitt's Diagnosis, Prevention and Treatment of Tropical Diseases. The Blakiston Co.)

The rabbit tick, *Haemaphysalis leporis-palustris* (Packard), an important vector of *Francisella tularensis* among rabbits, is also considered an important vector of spotted fever rickettsiae among these animals. It is found over most of the United States and in southern Canada. This tick does not feed on man. Rabbits, however, are hosts also to *D. andersoni,* a common vector of *R. rickettsii* to man. The argasid tick, *Ornithodoros parkeri* Cooley, may play an equally important role in nature in nine western states. It has several hosts in common with *D. andersoni,* and transmission through the egg to the fourth generation with no reduction in the virulence of the rickettsiae over a period of 5 years has been demonstrated. This tick feeds readily on man but seldom comes in contact with him. Many of the small animal hosts of immature ticks are considered to be important in the maintenance of spotted fever rickettsiae in nature. *Rickettsia rickettsii* has been isolated from six species of wild rodents and an opossum in Virginia and from three species of wild rodents in Montana. Spotted fever complement-fixing antibodies have been found in sera of 15 species of wild mammals, including *Carnivora,* and in sera from 18 species of birds.[5] The ticks *H. leporis-palustris, Ixodes dentatus* and *A. americanum* are commonly found on both wild animals and birds and may be important links in the spread of infection between these two groups.

Although *R. rickettsii* is commonly transmitted to man by tick bite, infections with this organism have resulted from handling ticks incident to their removal from domestic animals.

Pathology. Pathologic changes in Rocky Mountain spotted fever resemble those of typhus in that the chief lesions are found in small blood vessels. There are distinct differences, however, in the histopathologic findings and in the structures affected. In Rocky Mountain spotted fever there is greater destruction of the deeper layers of the vessel walls and less perivascular infiltration. The rickettsiae invade both the vascular endothelium and smooth muscle fibers of the vessel wall, causing endothelial proliferation, necrosis of the wall, thrombosis and infarction with hemorrhage into surrounding tissues (Fig. 8–3). These lesions occur predominantly in the skin and subcutaneous tissues, the voluntary muscles and the testes, with resulting areas of necrosis. There are no distinctive changes in the viscera; the spleen is commonly much enlarged, firm and dark red. Lesions of the central nervous system are uncommon.

In fatal cases, the rash is hemorrhagic, and necrosis of the scrotum or vulva is frequent. There may likewise be necrosis of the prepuce, fingers, toes, lobes of the ears, or soft palate. Hemorrhages into the muscles and subcutaneous tissues are widespread, with frequent confluence of the rash at points of bed pressure, such as the buttocks.

Clinical Characteristics. Both mild and virulent strains of *R. rickettsii* are well known, and, contrary to former belief, both are found in all regions where Rocky Mountain spotted fever occurs. Depending on the virulence of the strain, the incubation period varies from 3 to 14 days. In severe disease the onset is sudden, with headache, chills, marked pains in the joints and generalized body pains. The fever rises gradually or fairly rapidly to about 40° C (104° F) and remains elevated without morning remissions. On the third or fourth day the rash makes its appearance. At first it closely resembles that of measles, but unlike this exanthem, it remains discrete in its subsequent course. The eruption begins as macules on the forearms and ankles, spreading within 12 hours inward along the extremities to the trunk and forehead (Fig. 8–4). There is a still later spread to the palms, soles and scalp; mucous membranes may also be involved. By the fourth day, the rash (now maculopapular) may become petechial and fail to fade on pressure. There is a moderate leukocytosis, and the differential count is not characteristic. Thrombocytopenia occurs in almost 50 per cent of patients and coagulation disorders are frequent in the more severely affected patients.

The height of the disease is reached in the second week. At this time the pulse becomes rapid and weak, and neurologic signs, especially delirium, may appear. It is

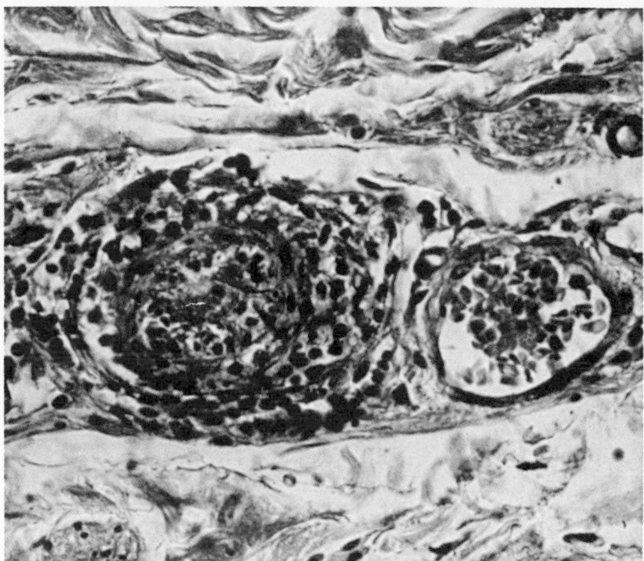

Figure 8–3. Rocky Mountain spotted fever: lesion of skin showing thrombosis, necrosis of vessel wall and perivascular infiltration.

during this period that necrosis of the skin and death usually occur. If the patient survives the fourteenth day, his chances for recovery are excellent.

The fever gradually recedes during the third week. Areas in which the rash was petechial or purpuric often show scaly exfoliation or, occasionally, castlike desquamation. There may be residual cicatrices in such areas of the skin. Complications, such as deafness and visual disturbances, may follow severe attacks, but they are not permanent. Convalescence is rapid in uncomplicated cases.

Severity of spotted fever may vary with the geographic locality, presumably because of differences in virulence of the rickettsiae established in particular areas. Case fatality rates are low in children (5 per cent) but are much higher in adults, particularly in those over 50 years of age. The advent of broad spectrum antibiotics in the 1940s was coincident with a great decrease in the reported

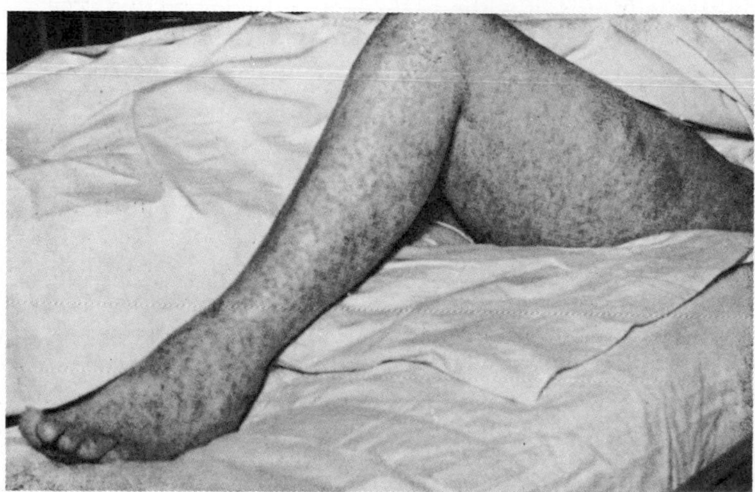

Figure 8–4. Generalized rash of Rocky Mountain spotted fever. (Courtesy of Rocky Mountain Laboratory.)

morbidity and mortality from spotted fever in the United States. Since 1960, however, continued increase in the number of reported cases has occurred, and in 1973 the number was the largest ever recorded. Case fatality ratios have remained under 10 per cent since effective antibiotics became available, although there has been a small but definite increase since 1960.

Diagnosis. Clinical and epidemiologic features, combined with a history of tick bite or contact with ticks, should immediately suggest the possibility of Rocky Mountain spotted fever, although purely clinical distinction between it and murine or epidemic typhus may be difficult.

Available laboratory tests are of limited help in early stages of the disease. Although the Weil-Felix test with OX–19 and OX–2 antigens has been widely employed, it may give false negative as well as false positive reactions. In a recent study of 504 cases of Rocky Mountain spotted fever,[6] sera from only 60 per cent of patients tested gave a positive (≥1:80) Weil-Felix reaction, and a 4-fold increase occurred in only 52 per cent of the patients when paired sera were tested. The complement-fixation (CF) test is much more reliable, although significant CF antibody levels may not occur until 10 to 12 days after onset of disease. The CF test is highly effective in differentiating this disease from murine and epidemic typhus. Weil-Felix agglutinins tend to appear slightly earlier than CF antibody. In both tests, it is the *rise* in titer in second and subsequent blood samples which is significant. Agglutination tests with purified particulate antigen and immunofluorescence tests are more sensitive, but requisite antigens are not commercially available. Early antibiotic treatment may partially suppress antibody rises which otherwise occur in convalescent patients.

The organism can be isolated from the blood of patients by inoculating embryonated chicken eggs or guinea pigs with specimens taken during the febrile course of the disease and before broad spectrum antibiotics have been given. Strains isolated by these methods are identified by appropriate immunologic and serologic procedures. Examination of tick hemolymph by direct immunofluorescence test performed with specific antiserum has been employed successfully to demonstrate the presence of *R. rickettsii* in an infected tick.

Isolates of *R. rickettsii* highly pathogenic for guinea pigs typically produce a characteristic scrotal necrosis, whereas less pathogenic strains usually do not. However, pathogenicity of a given isolate for man bears no necessary relation to pathogenicity in the inoculated guinea pig. A strain of rickettsiae that is highly pathogenic in man may be of low pathogenicity in the laboratory animal and, conversely, a strain that produces mild disease in man may produce severe disease in the guinea pig.

Treatment. When death occurs, it is usually about 10 days after onset. Antibiotic therapy, therefore, should be initiated on the basis of clinical diagnosis without waiting for laboratory confirmation. The broad spectrum antibiotics tetracycline, oxytetracycline and chlortetracycline are highly effective and will arrest most clinical manifestations of the disease within 2 to 3 days. Chloramphenicol is also effective, although its use is not recommended because of the attendant danger of causing blood dyscrasias.

Therapeutic regimens are similar for the various drugs and depend upon body weight of the patient. For a 70 kg adult, an initial oral dose of 2 gm may be given, followed by an oral dose of 250 mg given every 6 hours. Antibiotic therapy may be discontinued safely after defervescence is complete.

Sole reliance should not be placed upon antibiotics in seriously ill patients late in the disease. Symptomatic treatment including transfusions of saline, glucose, plasma and whole blood may be vital for support of the seriously embarrassed circulatory system.

Prophylaxis. In areas where Rocky Mountain spotted fever commonly occurs, it has been found practicable to immunize large groups of the population by the inoculation of a killed suspension of the specific rickettsiae. Such vaccination reduces the incidence of disease and also lessens the severity of those attacks which may subsequently occur. The injections should be repeated yearly in persons likely to be exposed.

Tick-infested areas should be avoided, if possible; if not, clothing treated with repellent, such as diethyltoluamide, should be worn (Table 72–1, p. 794). Careful inspection of the body and head should be made every few hours to remove any ticks that may be present. Ticks usually attach in hairy areas of the body. Infected wood ticks may inoculate a person within 6 hours after attachment; hence, regular removal of ticks is an important measure in avoiding infection. Ticks should be removed with forceps or a piece of paper rather than by grasping them between unprotected fingers. Hands should be washed with soap and water after contact with ticks.

Numerous insecticides are effective in providing temporary control of ticks in localized areas and on vegetation along roadsides, pathways, and other places where ticks concentrate (Table 72–1, p. 794).

REFERENCES

1. Woodward, T. E., and Jackson, E. B. 1965. Spotted fever rickettsiae. *In* Horsfall, F. L., Jr., and Tamm, I.: Viral and Rickettsial Infections of Man. 4th ed. J. B. Lippincott Co., Philadelphia. pp. 1095–1129.
2. Parker, R. R., and Oliphant, J. W. 1950. Rocky Mountain spotted fever. *In* Pullen, R. L.: Communicable Diseases. Lea & Febiger, Philadelphia. pp. 719–752.
3. Price, W. H. 1954. Variation in virulence of "*Rickettsia rickettsii*" under natural and experimental conditions. *In* The Dynamics of Virus and Rickettsial Infections. Blakiston Co., Inc., New York. pp. 164–183.
4. Kohls, G. M. 1948. Vectors of rickettsial diseases. *In* The Rickettsial Diseases of Man. Am. Assoc. Advance. Sci., Washington, D. C. pp. 83–96.
5. Bozeman, F. M., Shirai, A., Humphries, J. W., and Fuller, H. S. 1967. Ecology of Rocky Mountain spotted fever. II. Natural infection of wild mammals and birds in Virginia and Maryland. Am. J. Trop. Med. Hyg. *16*:48–59.
6. Hattwick, M. A. W., Peters, A. H., Gregg, M. B., and Hanson, B. 1973. Surveillance of Rocky Mountain spotted fever. J.A.M.A. *225*:1338–1343.

CHAPTER 9

Related Spotted Fevers and Rickettsioses

RICHARD A. ORMSBEE

Fièvre Boutonneuse

Synonyms. Boutonneuse fever, fièvre exanthématique de Marseille, escarronodulaire (French).

Definition. A disease of the spotted fever group[1–5] caused by *Rickettsia conorii* which is transmitted in the Mediterranean area and probably in India chiefly by the tick *Rhipicephalus sanguineus* (Latr.). A tache noire (eschar) is present. The rash appears on the trunk and may subsequently involve the entire body.

Distribution. First reported from Tunis in 1910, fièvre boutonneuse is now known to be endemic in most countries of the Mediterranean Basin and in the Crimea. Serologic and clinical evidence, as well as the character of the disease in experimental animals, suggests that infections caused by *R. conorii,* or members of a very closely related complex of strains of *R. conorii,* occur in South Africa (South African tick-bite fever), Kenya (Kenya tick typhus), Ethiopia, Republic of Congo, Pakistan and India (Indian tick typhus).

Etiology. *Rickettsia conorii* is the etiologic agent, although this designation may include a variety of strains which differ slightly in antigenic composition and in other biologic characteristics. Intranuclear rickettsiae have been reported, but *R. conorii* is much less regularly seen in this location than is *R. rickettsii.*[2,5]

Epidemiology. The usual host of *Rhipicephalus sanguineus* is the domestic dog, which may be the chief animal reservoir of the disease. The epidemiology of the disease in areas where this tick is involved is therefore comparable to that of spotted fever in many areas in eastern United States, where dogs are prominent hosts of the adult tick vector. In Kenya, *Rhipicephalus simus, Haemaphysalis leachi* and *Amblyomma hebraeum* are also reported as vectors, so the infection is contracted in rural as well as in urban environments.

In South Africa, infections occur more often in fields or veld than in urban areas. The larvae of *Rhipicephalus evertsi* and *A. hebraeum* are common vectors in some rural areas, whereas the dog tick *H. leachi* appears to play an important role in dissemination of the disease into the suburbs. The latter tick, in which transovarial transmission of the infection occurs, constitutes a natural reservoir of this rickettsia. In South Africa, *Rhipicephalus appendiculatus* and *Hyalomma rufipes,* formerly referred to as *H. aegyptium* in South Africa, have also been found to be carriers of *R. conorii.* A strain of rickettsia antigenically closely related to, or identical with, *R. conorii* was isolated from *R. sanguineus* ticks collected on the premises of a former tick-typhus patient in Kashmir. This rickettsia has also been isolated from *H. leachi* and *Ixodes ricinus* in India.

Similar strains of rickettsiae have been isolated from *Amblyomma variegatum, Amblyomma cohaerens* and *Amblyomma gemma* in Ethiopia.

Pathology. Detailed pathologic findings in fièvre boutonneuse, Kenya typhus and South African tick-bite fever have not been reported because of the low mortality. They differ from the spotted fever of the

Americas in the frequent occurrence of a primary lesion (tache noire), supposedly at the site of the infective tick bite. This is a granulomatous process which frequently ulcerates and which is accompanied by regional lymphadenitis.

The basic lesion may be widely distributed in the body as in spotted fever. It consists of localized thrombosis of capillaries, small arteries and veins, and development of perivascular infiltration by mononuclear leukocytes and plasma cells in areas surrounding thromboses. Earliest changes occur in vascular endothelium and include swelling, proliferation and degeneration of endothelial cells.

Clinical Characteristics. After an incubation period of about a week, there is an abrupt onset of fever, headache, malaise and conjunctival injection.[1, 5] At this time, the characteristic primary eschar (tache noire) consisting of a small ulcer with a black, necrotic center, and a surrounding erythematous area accompanied by regional lymphadenitis is usually present. Except for severe headache, persistent insomnia and myalgia, the febrile course is accompanied by less intense symptoms than those seen in spotted fever. Prostration and delirium are not marked, and the febrile course usually lasts less than 2 weeks. Mortality is low.

On the second to fifth day a macular or maculopapular rash appears, usually first on the forearms. It rapidly involves the trunk and extremities, including palms, soles and face, and may become hemorrhagic and markedly papular.

Diagnosis. Clinical diagnosis is simplified by a history of tick bite and presence of an eschar with its associated regional adenopathy. The rash and typhus-like clinical course of the disease are diagnostically significant. Geographic considerations help to distinguish it from other similar rickettsioses, such as North Asian or Siberian tick typhus and Queensland tick typhus.

The Weil-Felix test with *Proteus* OX–19 or OX–2 antigens becomes positive in 12 to 14 days but does not serve to distinguish *R. conorii* infections from other rickettsial infections except Q fever. The complement-fixation (CF) test with group-specific soluble antigens can be used to distinguish between diseases of the spotted fever group and the typhus group. With carefully prepared, washed, particulate antigens, the CF test can differentiate between *R. conorii* infections and those caused by other members of the

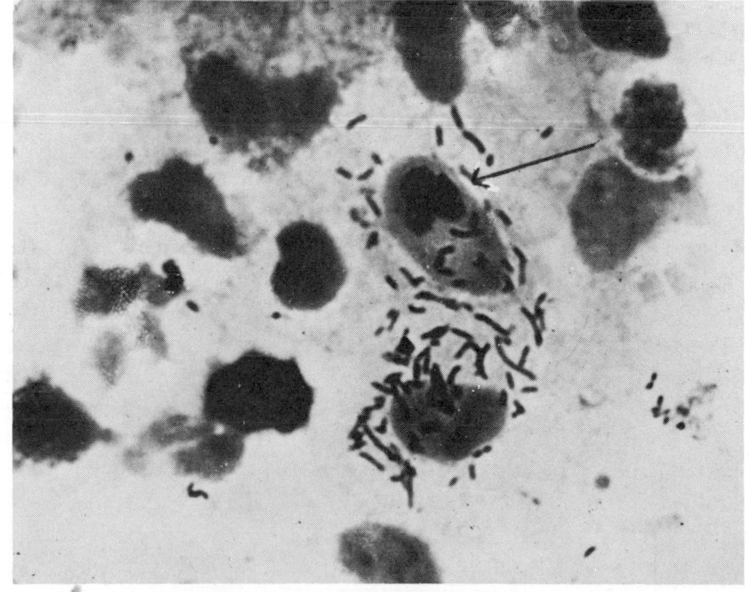

Figure 9–1. *Rickettsia sibirica,* causative agent of Siberian tick typhus showing clump of organisms inside nucleus and scattered in cytoplasm of cells from scrotal sac of infected guinea pig. (Courtesy of P. F. Zdrodovskii.)

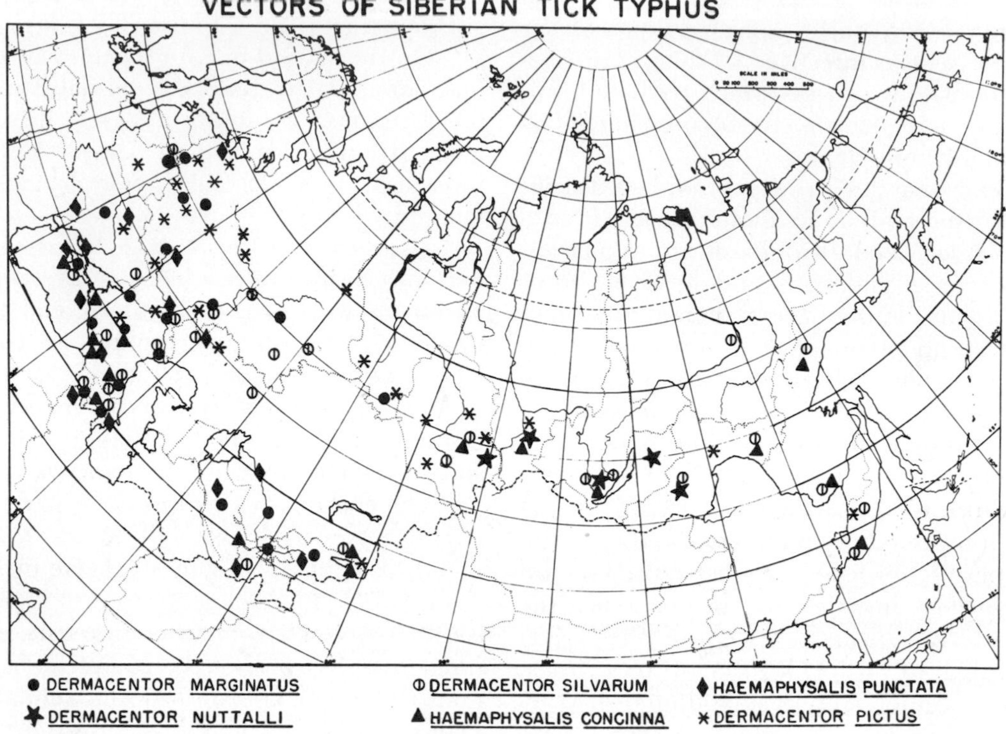

Figure 9–2. Distribution of known vectors of Siberian tick typhus. (Courtesy of Cornelius B. Philip.)

spotted fever group.[4] Because CF antibodies may persist in patients' sera for many years, it is important to examine both early acute and convalescent serum to demonstrate a rise in titer, which will distinguish between current and past rickettsial infection. Agglutination tests with purified specific antigen will often detect antibodies before the CF test becomes positive, but may not serve to identify the particular disease as certainly as the CF test.

Inoculation of guinea pigs with blood from febrile patients causes nonfatal, febrile disease which cannot be distinguished from that caused by many strains of *R. rickettsii,* except that the animals' early agglutinins may be much more species-specific than those found in human serum.

Treatment. The tetracycline group of broad spectrum antibiotics are the drugs of choice. Treatment is the same as described for American spotted fevers (p. 116). Patients generally become afebrile after 2 to 3 days of treatment. As in other rickettsioses, good nursing care and symptomatic treatment are important, particularly in severe cases.

Prophylaxis. Ticks and tick-infested areas should be avoided when possible. Since dogs are the usual hosts of several tick vectors of fièvre boutonneuse and related diseases, special care should be exercised in preventing tick infestation of such pets and of human habitations. Effective tick repellents and insecticides for such purposes are available. (Table 72–1, p. 794.) A short-haired dog might be considered a more desirable domestic animal in endemic areas. Stray or feral dogs should be exterminated. The preventive measures advocated for Rocky Mountain spotted fever apply also in the prevention of this disease. Immunizing vaccines have been reported only for the American spotted fevers, but vaccines against these diseases do not confer protection against fièvre boutonneuse.

Siberian Tick Typhus

Siberian tick typhus or North Asian tick typhus is a tick-borne rickettsiosis of the spotted fever group caused by *Rickettsia sibirica* and encountered in western, central and eastern Siberia (Fig. 9–1). The disease is characterized by a mild, acutely febrile course, a lesion at the site of tick bite, and a maculopapular rash.[1, 2] Complement-fixation tests with type-specific antigens and toxin neutralization tests indicate that *R. sibirica* is a distinct entity within the spotted fever group.[3–5]

Six species of ticks have been implicated in the transmission of this disease: *Dermacentor nuttalli* (Olenev), *Dermacentor silvarum* (Olenev), *Dermacentor marginatus* (Sulzer), *Dermacentor pictus* (Herm.), *Haemaphysalis concinna* (Koch) and *Haemaphysalis punctata* (Can. and Fanz.) (Fig. 9–2). Natural infection with *R. sibirica* and its transovarial transmission have been demonstrated in most of these tick species. Clinically, the disease is relatively mild and resembles fièvre boutonneuse, but epidemiologically it is closer to American spotted fever, with its natural cycle between native rodents and their immature tick parasites. Man is bitten by adult ticks encountered in open areas of the steppes, grassy meadows or brush-covered hillsides as he accidentally interrupts the natural cycle.

Spotted fever group antibodies which can be detected by CF and Weil-Felix tests result from infection with *R. sibirica*. Guinea pigs inoculated intraperitoneally with a patient's blood taken early during the febrile phase become febrile for 4 to 6 days and have scrotal swelling; rickettsiae may be found in the mesothelium of the tunica vaginalis. In this animal, Siberian tick typhus cannot be distinguished from fièvre boutonneuse; both produce similar reactions and cross-immunize with each other in guinea pig tests. However, strains established in guinea pigs can be identified by appropriate CF and toxin neutralization techniques.

REFERENCES

1. Zdrodovskii, P. F., and Golinevich, E. H. 1960. The Rickettsial Diseases. 2nd ed. Pergamon Press, London. 630 pp.
2. Cox, H. R. 1959. The spotted fever group. *In* Rivers, T. M., and Horsfall, F. L., Jr.: Viral and Rickettsial Infections of Man. 3rd ed. J. B. Lippincott Co., Philadelphia. pp. 828–868.
3. Bozeman, F. M., Humphries, J. W., Campbell, J. M., and O'Hara, P. L. 1960. Laboratory studies of the spotted fever group of rickettsiae. *In* Symposium on the Spotted Fever Group of Rickettsiae. WRAIR, Walter Reed Army Medical Center, Washington, D.C. U.S. Government Printing Office, Med. Sci. Publ. No. 7, pp. 7–11.
4. Lackman, D. B., Bell, E. J., Stoenner, H. G., and Pickens, E. G. 1965. The Rocky Mountain spotted fever group of rickettsias. Hlth. Lab. Sci. *2*:135–141.
5. Woodward, T. E., and Jackson, E. B. 1965. Spotted fever rickettsiae. *In* Horsfall, F. L., Jr., and Tamm, I.: Viral and Rickettsial Infections of Man. 4th ed. J. B. Lippincott Co., Philadelphia. pp. 1095–1129.

CHAPTER 10

Queensland Tick Typhus

WILLY BURGDORFER

Definition. Queensland tick typhus is a mild rickettsial disease of man that resembles boutonneuse fever.[1] History of tick exposure and development of an eschar at the site of tick bite suggest that the disease is tick-borne. *Ixodes holocyclus* (Neumann) is assumed to be the vector, although the etiologic agent, *Rickettsia australis,* has been recovered only from blood of patients.

Distribution. The disease has been reported since 1946 from both northern and southern areas of Queensland, Australia.

Etiology. Antigenic and biologic (intranuclear growth) characteristics suggest *R. australis* to be a member of the spotted fever group rickettsiae, from which, however, it can be distinguished by specific complement-fixation and other laboratory tests.

Epidemiology. The first described infections occurred among troops undergoing training in heavily tick-infested areas in North Queensland. Most affected persons were known to have been bitten by ticks; they developed typical eschars at the sites of bites. *Ixodes holocyclus,* the suspected vector, has been taken from several patients. In serologic surveys of animals trapped in areas where human cases were reported, complement-fixing antibodies were detected in four species of small marsupials and in one rat, suggesting a natural cycle of *R. australis* between *I. holocyclus* and a variety of small animals.

Clinical Characteristics. After an incubation period of 7 to 10 days, the disease begins gradually with general malaise and headache. The eschar, if present, resembles that of scrub typhus. Fever is moderate, continuous or remittent, and subsides gradually after 2 to 12 days. Regional lymphadenopathy is always present; lymph nodes draining the eschar are enlarged, painful and tender. The rash that appears from 1 to 6 days after onset of illness varies in color, size and distribution from patient to patient. Individual lesions may be small and scattered, or may consist of large pink papules. In some cases the lesions become confluent on the trunk; large purplish blotches of a generalized rash may also involve the face, scalp and palms. Usually, the rash disappears after defervescence.

Diagnosis. Presence of the eschar associated with regional lymphadenopathy, together with characteristic rash and clinical course, aids diagnosis. For cases without eschar or rash, diagnosis must be made serologically with either the Weil-Felix test, in which all patients show titers against *Proteus* OX–19 and OX–2, or the complement-fixation (CF) test. Guinea pigs and mice, especially suckling mice, are recommended for isolating *R. australis* from the blood of febrile patients.[2] Sera of recovered adult mice contain specific CF antibodies which distinguish *R. australis* from other spotted fever group rickettsiae.

Both murine (flea-borne) and scrub typhus occur in the same area as Queensland tick typhus. In murine typhus, however, eschar and lymphadenitis do not occur. Scrub typhus is usually a more serious disease with complications.

Treatment. Procedures are the same as those outlined previously for other rickettsioses. (See pp. 101, 107 and 116.)

REFERENCES

1. Cox, H. R. 1959. Rickettsialpox. Queensland tick typhus. *In* Rivers, T. M., and Horsfall, F. L., Jr.: Viral and Rickettsial Infections of Man. 3rd ed. J. B. Lippincott Co., Philadelphia. pp. 852–858.
2. Campbell, R. W., and Pope, J. H. 1968. The value of newborn mice as sensitive hosts for *Rickettsia australis.* Austral. J. Sci. *30*:324–325.

CHAPTER 11

Rickettsialpox

WILLY BURGDORFER

Synonym. Kew Gardens spotted fever.

Definition. Rickettsialpox is a relatively mild disease caused by *Rickettsia akari,* a member of the spotted fever group rickettsiae.[1,2] It is accompanied by a varicelliform rash, lymphadenopathy and leukopenia. In over 90 per cent of the cases, an initial lesion or eschar occurs at the site of attachment of the transmitting rodent mite, *Liponyssoides* (= *Allodermanyssus) sanguineus.*

Distribution. Most cases have occurred in urban communities in the northeastern United States. Following its recognition during a small epidemic in New York City, sporadic cases occurred in Boston, Philadelphia, Cleveland, Pittsburgh, West Hartford (Connecticut) and Utah. A disease indistinguishable from rickettsialpox has been described in the U.S.S.R.,[3] and cases resembling this disease have been reported under the name "rickettsiose vésiculeuse" from French Equatorial Africa and from South Africa.

Etiology. The etiologic agent, *Rickettsia (Dermacentroxenus) akari,* like all other rickettsiae of the spotted fever group, develops not only in the cytoplasm but also in the nucleus of infected cells. Its relationship to the spotted fever group rickettsiae is also indicated by cross-reactions in the complement-fixation test. In addition to man, wild and laboratory mice, guinea pigs and embryonated hen's eggs are susceptible (Fig. 11–1).

Epidemiology. Rickettsialpox is an urban disease associated with large numbers of house mice *(Mus musculus)* and bloodsucking mites, although there is evidence of its occurrence in natural cycles not involving commensal mice.

The natural vector, *L. sanguineus,* is a widespread, though not a common, parasite of mice. Unlike the trombiculid vectors of scrub typhus, all developmental stages, except the larva, are hematophagous and leave their hosts between blood meals (Fig. 69–6, p. 723).

Patients are not aware of attachment of the rapidly feeding mites and are probably attacked while asleep. In residents of endemic foci, prevalence of the disease is influenced by age, sex and occupation. Ages of patients have ranged from less than 1 to over 50 years. Epidemiologic findings in the U.S.S.R. are almost identical to those in the United States.

Pathology. Reports of pathologic changes in persons are confined to biopsy studies of primary and secondary cutaneous lesions. During the fastigium of the disease, the initial lesion at the site of attachment of the infected mite consists of a shallow ulcer about 0.5 to 1.5 cm in diameter. It is covered with a brown to black crust and is surrounded by an erythematous area about 2.5 cm in diameter. The lesion may occur on any part of the body.

Clinical Characteristics. The incubation period varies from 10 to 24 days. Usually an initial lesion resembling that of a primary vaccinia reaction develops at the site of infectious mite bites. Five to 10 days later the clinical syndrome appears suddenly. It is characterized by fever, chills, sweating, headache, backache and lassitude. These persist for a week or 10 days. Regional or generalized lymphadenopathy and a maculopapular and papulovesicular rash, usually appearing early in the course of disease but occasionally not until the fifth or sixth day, are nearly constant features. The cutaneous lesions may be scanty or profuse. They never become confluent. They do not involve the soles of the feet or the palms of the hands, and seldom the mucous membranes. Body temperature becomes elevated, especially in the afternoons, and frequently fluctuates be-

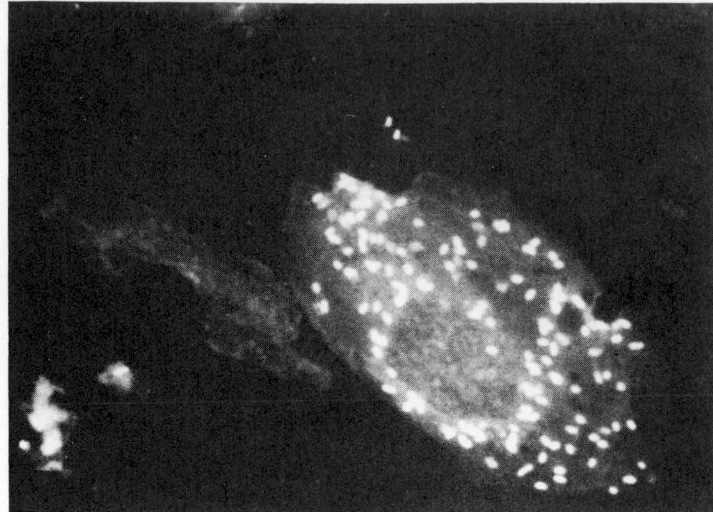

Figure 11-1. *Rickettsia akari* in macrophage from mouse peritoneum. (Fluorescent antibody staining, ×1000; Courtesy of Dr. Willy Burgdorfer, Rocky Mountain Laboratory.)

tween 36.7 and 40° C (98 and 104° F) in the course of a day. Photophobia is common.

The symptoms subside by lysis, generally from 1 to 2 weeks after onset. Convalescence may be protracted in severe cases. A lasting immunity is produced, since second attacks have not been reported and recovered laboratory animals resist reinfection.

Diagnosis. The clinical syndrome accompanied by eschar, rash and lymphadenopathy, together with history of residence in murine-infested premises, should direct attention to this disease. The geographic distribution eliminates the clinically similar fièvre boutonneuse and scrub typhus. The occurrence of the primary lesion, a vesicular rash, and vector determination will aid in differentiation from other rickettsioses. The rash of chickenpox is more superficial, and the vesicles are thin and easily broken. Lesions of smallpox, though initially quite similar to those of rickettsialpox in their deeper, firmer character, have a different maturation, usually becoming pustular with eventual scar formation.

Leukopenia is the only significant blood change.

Recovery of the infectious agent by intraperitoneal inoculation of blood from the patient into white mice or via yolk sac into chick embryos is desirable for laboratory diagnosis of sporadic cases. A specific antigen prepared from yolk sacs fixes complement in higher dilutions of convalescent serum than of sera prepared against other spotted fever group rickettsiae. Because of its rich growth, *R. akari* is often used as a common antigen for this group. There is no cross-fixation with the typhus group rickettsiae. A rising complement-fixation titer against spotted fever group antigens will differentiate rickettsialpox from other conditions with which it might be confused. The Weil-Felix test is of no value.

Treatment. Oxytetracycline (Terramycin), Aureomycin, and chloramphenicol (Chloromycetin) have been beneficial against infections with *R. akari.* Only 2.5 gm of Terramycin administered early in the disease (an initial dose of 0.5 gm and 0.25 gm thereafter every 6 hours) induce defervescence in about 24 hours without relapse.

Prophylaxis. Prevention of infection is dependent upon elimination of mice from infested buildings.

REFERENCES

1. Woodward, T. E., and Jackson, E. B. 1965. Spotted fever rickettsiae. *In* Horsfall, F. L., Jr., and Tamm, I.: Viral and Rickettsial Infections of Man. 4th ed. J. B. Lippincott Co., Philadelphia. pp. 1122–1129.
2. Lackman, D. B. 1963. A review of information on rickettsialpox in the United States. Clin. Pediat. *2*:296–301.
3. Zdrodovskii, P. F., and Golinevich, E. H. 1960. Vesicular and varioliform rickettsiosis (rickettsialpox). *In* The Rickettsial Diseases. 2nd ed. Pergamon Press, London. 630 pp.

CHAPTER 12

Scrub Typhus (Chigger-Borne Rickettsiosis)

CHARLES L. WISSEMAN, JR.
ROBERT TRAUB

Synonyms. Tsutsugamushi disease, Japanese river or flood fever, Shichito disease, kedani fever, mite typhus, rural typhus, tropical typhus, Mossman fever.

Definition. An acute, febrile, typhus-like disease transmitted by larval trombiculid mites (chiggers). The site of infection is usually marked by an eschar accompanied by regional lymphadenitis.[1,2]

Distribution. Scrub typhus has a wide distribution in eastern and southern Asia and the islands of the western and southern Pacific. It is known to occur in suitable habitats within the following limits: in Japan, Korea and the Primorye region of the U.S.S.R. and the islands adjacent to those areas; southern China and Tibet; the Indian subcontinent; Tadzhikistan; Indochina; the Philippines; New Guinea and adjacent islands; coastal North Queensland; Ceylon; the Nicobars and atolls of the Indian Ocean as far as the Chagos Archipelago. Endemic infection is unknown in the New World, Europe and the rest of Asia, while its occurrence in Africa is conjectural and doubted. Cases, imported during the incubation period following infection in an endemic area, have been recognized in the United States.

Etiology. *Rickettsia tsutsugamushi (=R. orientalis)* is a small obligate intracellular bacterial parasite. Its ultrastructure resembles that of a gram-negative bacterium. It grows free within host cell cytoplasm. Multiple serotypes exist. Virulence for white mice varies among strains from avirulent to highly lethal.

Epidemiology. Chigger-borne rickettsiosis is a zoonosis whose main constant elements constitute a tetrad: (1) *R. tsutsugamushi;* (2) chiggers of the *Leptotrombidium deliense* group (Fig. 12–1); (3) wild rats, especially of the subgenus *Rattus;* and (4) transitional vegetation. Man is not essential to maintenance of the infection cycle and acquires the disease by the bite of the infected chigger when he intrudes into an endemic focus. The characteristic epidemiologic features of chigger-borne typhus, such as a marked focal distribution of cases and sudden outbreaks among field personnel, are explained by attributes of the vector chiggers. In temperate zones, most vector chiggers are active sometime during the warm months and, hence, the disease is seasonal here. However, on the Izu islands of Japan *Leptotrombidium scutellare* transmits the disease in the winter.[3] In tropical and subtropical regions, the disease may be more prevalent at one time of the year than another,

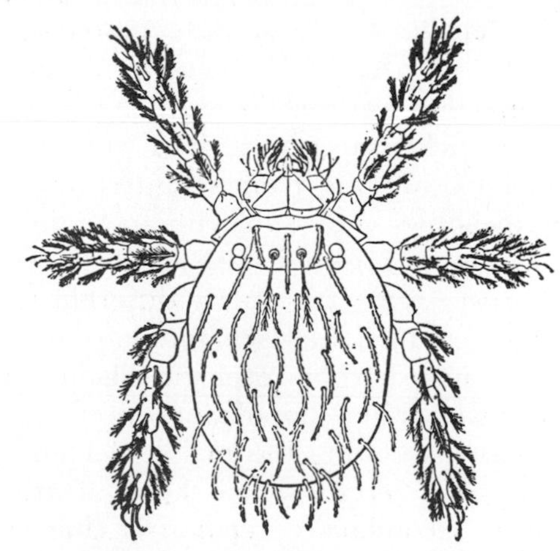

Figure 12–1. *Leptotrombidium akamushi* larva (greatly enlarged), vector of scrub typhus. (Nagayo et al.: Am. J. Hyg. *1*:569–591, 1921.)

depending on rainfall, flooding and other factors. Chigger-borne rickettsiosis is transmitted by the bite of the infected larval mite. Since the chigger is the only parasitic stage of the mite and usually feeds only once, if infected, it must have acquired the organism from its mother. Naturally infected chiggers presumably constitute the main reservoirs of *R. tsutsugamushi* in nature, maintaining and perpetuating the cycle of infection by transovarian transmission of rickettsiae from mother to progeny. Chiggers of the *Leptotrombidium deliense* group are the main vectors to man and perhaps to other hosts as well; *L. deliense, L. akamushi, L. fletcheri, L. arenicola, L. pallidum, L. pavlovskyi* and *L. scutellare* are known vectors. *Rickettsia tsutsugamushi* infections also occur in areas where none of the known vectors is present. The role of other kinds of chiggers is unclear, but members of the genera *Neotrombicula, Gahrliepia* and others may prove to serve as minor vectors to man, or be important as intrazootic vectors. Infected chiggers often occur in very circumscribed foci or "islands."[4]

Rats, particularly wild rats of the subgenus *Rattus,* serve as prime hosts of *Leptotrombidium* throughout their native ranges. Other small mammals (e.g. field mice, voles, shrews) often serve as secondary hosts. Although these chigger hosts readily acquire *R. tsutsugamushi* from infected chiggers and harbor the organism for long periods of time, it has not yet been possible to demonstrate that *R. tsutsugamushi* acquired from them by uninfected chiggers establishes a true infection transmissible to progeny.

The rickettsiosis exists in a wide variety of habitats, ranging from semideserts to alpine meadows and subarctic scree in the Himalayas, and from disturbed rain forest to seashores. Areas with utterly different topographic features, well separated by natural barriers, may harbor "ecologic islands" and "oases" with relict populations of the geologic past exhibiting the major elements of the zoonotic tetrad. Some kind of transitional or secondary vegetation is characteristic of all terrain where outbreaks occur, and is present in some form in all known foci of chigger-borne rickettsiosis, even if only as fringe habitat along streams in deep forest. All known foci are characterized by changing environmental conditions, whether induced by man (e.g. clearing of forest) or by nature, either suddenly (e.g., landslides) or cyclically (tidal zones, spring floods, glacial run-off). Just as new endemic foci may appear when the ecologic features of a habitat are modified and members of the zoonotic tetrad become predominant in consequence, so may endemicity in existing areas wax or wane as local conditions affect the rodent and chigger fauna, and the flora, with the passage of time.

Pathology. A primary local ulcer with regional lymphadenitis and, later, generalized lymphadenitis and acute splenitis with congestion and enlargement are common. Rickettsial pericarditis, pleuritis, peritonitis and perisplenitis, with or without effusion, may occur. The main histologic lesion, as with epidemic typhus and Rocky Mountain spotted fever, is a widespread, focal endangiitis, vasculitis and perivasculitis with accumulations of lymphocytes, plasma cells and macrophages. Vascular thrombosis is less frequent than in epidemic typhus and Rocky Mountain spotted fever, but inflammatory lesions of larger arteries are more common. Focal and diffuse myocarditis with round cell infiltration is common; necrosis of myocardial fibers is rare (Fig. 12–2). Interstitial pneumonitis is a constant feature. The brain shows a mononuclear leptomeningitis and a focal encephalitis with typhus nodules, perivascular cuffing of arteries, focal hemorrhages and some degeneration of ganglion cells (Fig. 12–3). Lesions are more frequent in the pons and medulla. The kidneys regularly show focal interstitial lesions and cloudy swelling of tubular epithelium, and less frequently glomerular injury and severe vascular damage. The liver may or may not be enlarged and shows no constant histologic features, but often shows mild cloudy swelling and fatty degeneration, swollen and prominent Kupffer cells, and numerous mononuclear cells scattered in the sinusoids and portal spaces. Other organs also show lesions related to the vasculitis.

Clinical Characteristics. The spec-

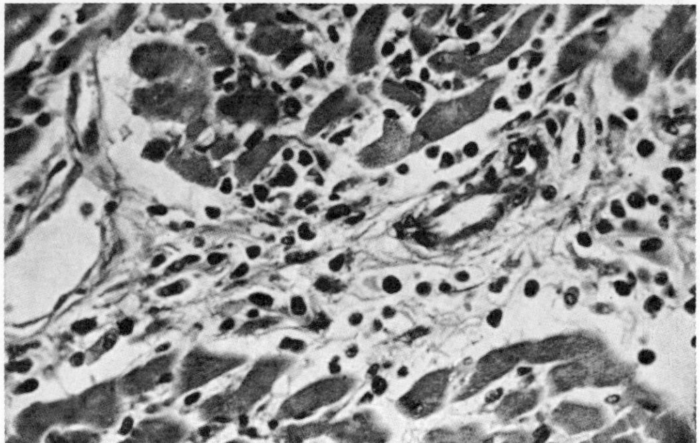

Figure 12-2. Scrub typhus, monocytic infiltration of heart muscle.

trum of clinical severity of untreated scrub typhus ranges from inapparent or mild to severe or mortal, with mortality rates varying from 0 to more than 30 per cent in different places and outbreaks.[3] The following description pertains to a classic, relatively severe untreated case of scrub typhus.

The bite of the infecting chigger, which may be on any part of the body, is usually unnoticed, but in roughly 60 per cent of the cases a small painless papule develops during the 6- to 18-day (usually 9- to 12-day) incubation period. It enlarges, undergoes central necrosis and crusts to form the eschar or primary lesion which is well developed at the onset of disease (Fig. 12-4). The regional lymph nodes are enlarged and tender. Prodromes of headache, malaise, anorexia and weakness may occur. The onset is usually acute. The fever rises progressively during the first few days, sometimes accompanied by chills after about the third day, to 39.5 to 40.5° C (103 to 105° F). Fever is accompanied by severe headache, ocular pain, conjunctival injection, anorexia, generalized aches, malaise, apathy and cough. Physical signs of pneumonitis are common. The pulse remains relatively slow. Toward the end of the first week, a macular rash, later sometimes papular, often appears, first on the trunk and

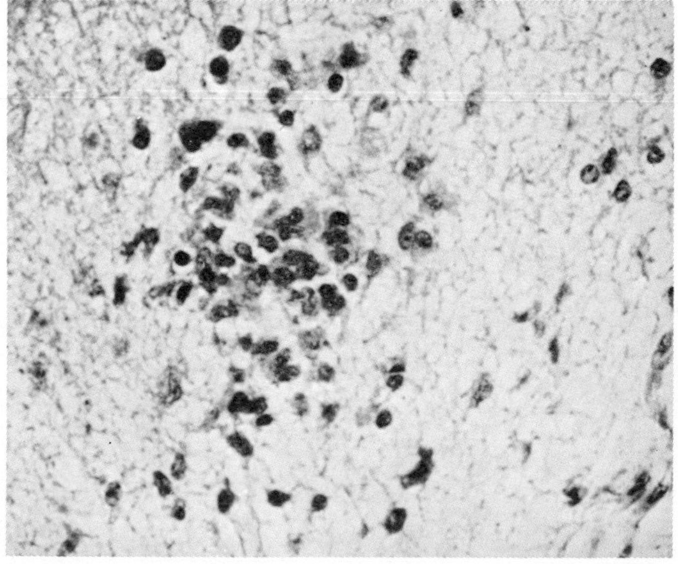

Figure 12-3. Scrub typhus, nodule in brain showing edema, degeneration and monocytic infiltration.

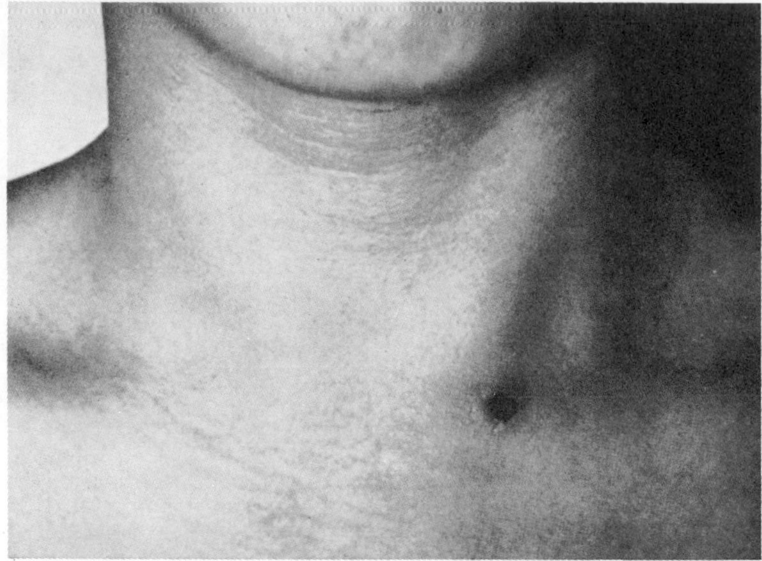

Figure 12–4. Eschar or primary lesion of scrub typhus. (Courtesy of U.S.A. Typhus Commission.)

then on the extremities (Fig. 12–5). About this time there is generalized lymphadenopathy, soft splenic enlargement and sometimes hepatomegaly.

During the second week of disease, the temperature remains elevated and signs of complex multiple organ system involvement appear. Apathy may give way to more pronounced signs of meningoencephalitis: delirium and restlessness, stupor, coma, convulsions, muscular weakness, hyperesthesias and coarse intention tremors. Cranial nerves are selectively involved: varying degrees of nerve deafness and papilledema and congestion of retinal vessels are common; dysarthria and dysphagia, less frequent. Signs of diffuse and focal myocarditis may appear: soft first heart sound, systolic murmurs, ectopic beats, occasional cardiac enlargement, transient gallop rhythm and minor abnormalities of the electrocardiogram (prolonged P-R interval, inverted T waves). Classic

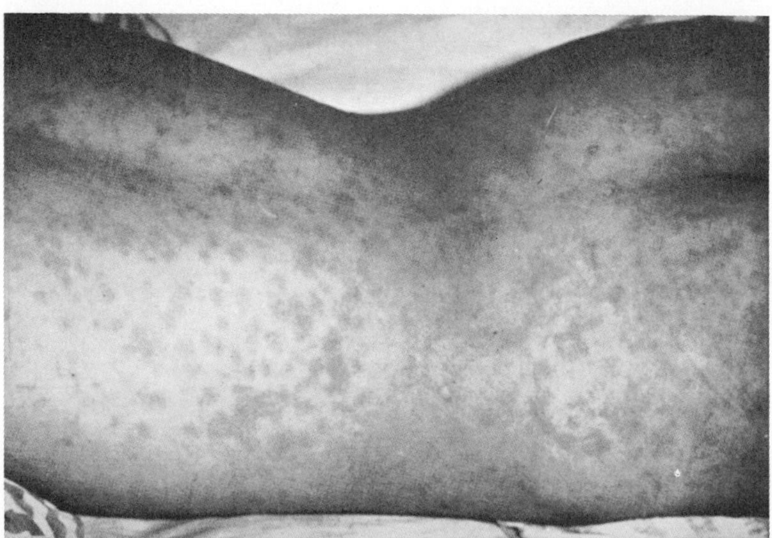

Figure 12–5. Rash of scrub typhus. (Courtesy of U.S.A. Typhus Commission.)

congestive failure is rare, but varying degrees of circulatory failure may appear: increasing pulse rate, falling blood pressure (commonly below 100 mm Hg systolic), rapid shallow respirations, cyanosis, sweating and cold clammy skin. Gangrene is rare, but edema may be overt in severe cases. Clinical evidence for renal insufficiency is often absent, but oliguria or anuria occur in some. Spontaneous diuresis is fairly common late in the febrile course or in early convalescence.

In untreated cases, defervescence is by lysis usually after about 10 to 14 days (21 or more days in severe cases). Convalescence is prolonged. However, in nonfatal cases, all abnormalities appear to be completely reversible, though some, such as cardiovascular instability, personality changes and deafness, may occasionally persist for weeks to months. Long-term (10 or more years) follow-up of United States servicemen who survived scrub typhus in World War II failed to reveal any significant residuum.

Laboratory Findings. An early leukopenia (1000 to 5000 white blood cells per cu mm) gives way to slightly depressed or normal total white blood counts which may become somewhat elevated late in the disease. Total serum proteins are usually normal or low, but the albumin-globulin (A/G) ratio is often reversed. The sedimentation rate may rise as the disease progresses and remain elevated well into convalescence. Occasional clotting disturbances have been reported recently, including disseminated intravascular clotting syndrome. Jaundice is rare but serum glutamic oxaloacetic transaminase (SGOT) and serum glutamic pyruvic transaminase (SGPT) enzyme levels may be elevated. Albuminuria is common. Isosthenuria, oliguria and azotemia may occur.

Diagnosis. Differential diagnosis may be difficult in some endemic regions where the clinical picture may suggest other rickettsial infections (especially tick-borne typhus, which may also have an eschar), dengue, infectious hepatitis, typhoid and malaria. Often malaria, newly acquired or activated latent, is a concurrent infection. However, in endemic areas the association of a primary lesion or eschar with regional lymphadenitis, headache, prostration, disproportionately low pulse rate, fever, leukopenia and, later, rash is highly suggestive. Definitive diagnosis must be based on laboratory tests.

The Weil-Felix test remains useful because it is generally available. Titers against *Proteus* OX-K, but not OX-2 or OX-19, begin to rise in the second week of disease, reach peak values at 3 to 4 weeks, and decline thereafter. The test may not be positive in all cases of chigger-borne typhus; moreover, it may be positive in some other diseases, e.g. relapsing fever. An indirect fluorescent antibody test, with a mixture of Karp, Gilliam and Kato strains of *R. tsutsugamushi* as antigen, proved useful and specific for the diagnosis of scrub typhus in United States servicemen in Vietnam. The organism can be isolated by inoculating white mice intraperitoneally with blood or tissue homogenates.

Immunity. Immunity to homologous strains is long-lasting. However, to heterologous serotypes immunity is transient, often lasting no more than 1 to 3 months.

Treatment. In most instances, prompt treatment with an antirickettsial antibiotic (a tetracycline or chloramphenicol) causes prompt defervescence (usually within 24 to 48 hours) and rapid resolution of the disease processes, and essentially eliminates mortality. Usually, only severe cases, especially those treated late, may require special attention to correct fluid and electrolyte imbalance, disturbances in clotting mechanisms or other physiologic disturbances, and specific treatment of secondary bacterial infections. Because of generalized vascular damage, electrolyte solutions should be given cautiously. Albumin is preferred as a plasma expander to combat shock; washed erythrocytes, to correct anemia if necessary. Severe cases may benefit from cortisone as an adjunct to antimicrobial therapy to speed defervescence and reduce manifestations of encephalitis.

Antirickettsial chemotherapy may be intermittent or continuous. Since the antibiotics presently in use are primarily rickettsiostatic, rickettsemia may persist for 48 hours after start of treatment and relapse may occur if therapy is discontinued before an adequate immune response develops. Drugs of the tetracycline series constitute treatment of choice, but chloramphenicol is an effective alternate. The usual precautions should be observed with respect to age and physiologic development, renal and hepatic disease, bone marrow depression, hypersensitivity, staining of developing teeth, and to other conditions.

For the average adult, intermittent oral therapy with tetracycline hydrochloride consists of a loading dose of 2.0 to 3.0 gm followed by an additional 2.0 to 3.0 gm given over the next 24 hours. Relapse, more frequent in patients treated in the first 3 days of disease, can usually be prevented with an additional 2.0 to 3.0 gm given 5 days after the initial dose. Continuous therapy consists of a loading dose of 2.0 gm followed by 2.0 gm per day in divided doses until the patient has been afebrile for at least 48 hours. The dosage regimens for chloramphenicol are the same. Though not tested yet, a single 100 to 200 mg dose of doxycycline or minocycline may be as effective for scrub typhus as it is for epidemic typhus. In patients unable to swallow, treatment may be initiated with parenteral tetracycline (1 to 2 gm per day) or chloramphenicol (2 gm per day).

Prophylaxis. Killed vaccines have not been effective. Transient broad, and more persistent strain-specific, immunity follows combined living virulent vaccine and intermittent chemotherapy. Chemoprophylactic regimens with intermittent chloramphenicol dosage (3.0 gm every 4 to 7 days continued 21 to 28 days after last exposure) have been established; though as yet unproven, small weekly doses of doxycycline or minocycline probably would be effective.

Treatment of clothing with emulsions of benzyl benzoate, dibutyl phthalate or dimethyl phthalate, which withstand several launderings, provides personal protection against vector chiggers. Spraying clothing and exposed skin areas with diethyltoluamide preparations ("OFF," "DEET") is also effective, but they readily wash away. (See Table 72–1, p. 794.)

Control of chiggers is feasible for small areas, e.g. campsites, by clearing vegetation (bulldozing, burning, herbicides), rodent control and spraying with acaricides (particularly dieldrin or lindane). (See Table 72–1, p. 795.) Logistic and ecologic considerations determine choice of method and substances.[5,6]

REFERENCES

1. Smadel, J. E., and Elisberg, B. L. 1965. Scrub typhus rickettsia. *In* Horsfall, F. L., Jr., and Tamm, I.: Viral and Rickettsial Infections of Man. 4th ed. J. B. Lippincott Co., Philadelphia. pp. 1130–1143.
2. Tamiya, T. 1962. Recent Advances in Studies of Tsutsugamushi Disease in Japan. Medical Culture, Inc., Tokyo. 309 pp.
3. Philip, C. B. 1964. Scrub typhus and scrub itch. *In* Coates, J. B., Jr., et al. (eds.): Preventive Medicine in World War II. Vol. III. Washington, D.C., Office of the Surgeon General, Department of the Army. pp. 275–347.
4. Traub, R., and Wisseman, C. L., Jr. 1974. The ecology of chigger-borne rickettsiosis (scrub typhus). J. Med. Entomol. *11*:(3): 237–303.
5. Traub, R., and Wisseman, C. L., Jr. 1968. Ecological considerations in scrub typhus. 3. Methods of area control. Bull. W.H.O. *39*:231–237.
6. Department of the Army TB MED 31. 1962. Scrub Typhus (Mite-borne Typhus Fever, Tsutsugamushi Disease). U.S. Government Printing Office, Washington, D.C. pp. 1–16.

CHAPTER 13

Q Fever

RICHARD A. ORMSBEE

Synonyms. Nine mile fever (United States), Balkan grippe (Greece).

Definition. An acute systemic disease of rickettsial origin clinically characterized by abrupt onset, malaise, myalgia, severe headache, chills, remittent fever, pneumonitis and absence of rash.

Distribution. Worldwide, except Finland, Sweden and Denmark.

Etiology. *Coxiella burnetii (=Rickettsia burnetii, Rickettsia diaporica)* is similar to other rickettsiae in morphology and most staining reactions, and in possessing the attributes of obligate intracellular parasitism, transmission by biting arthropods, and division by binary fission. It also possesses some distinguishing features.[1] Its surprising resistance to inactivation by a broad spectrum of chemical and physical agents makes it one of the most resistant nonsporogenic microorganisms known.[2] In distilled water, milk, and tick feces, it remains viable for months and even years. Infectious aerosols have been generated from organic mixtures, contaminated with *C. burnetii,* which have been exposed out-of-doors in fields and pastures for many months. *Coxiella burnetii* is also one of the most infectious microorganisms known. The infectious dose of many wild strains for man and guinea pig is one organism, although strains may vary in pathogenicity. This agent typically is transmitted as an aerosol, but can be transmitted to man by infected ticks. It does not invade nuclei of host cells, as does *Rickettsia rickettsii,* but grows in cytoplasmic vacuoles. These as well as other differences from other pathogenic rickettsiae have resulted in *C. burnetii* being placed in a separate genus. Antigens of *C. burnetii* are unique and vary in composition only slightly from strain to strain. There are no known antigens in common with other pathogenic rickettsiae or any other known microorganism. The disease, in contrast to typhus and spotted fevers, is not accompanied by a rash.

Epidemiology. Man usually contracts Q fever by inhaling dust particles contaminated with rickettsiae originating from livestock. The agent has been isolated from air samples taken from environs of infected sheep, cattle and goats. Exposure to infected livestock or their products, residence near contaminated premises, and household use of raw milk are factors predisposing to infection.[3] Use of infected milk has been connected with at least one explosive outbreak.[4] Rarely, secondary cases have occurred among persons having contact with patients. In North America, Q fever chiefly affects males of working age. Seasonal distribution is uniform in areas where cattle are the major source of infection, but a peak of cases during the post-lambing season where sheep are a common source of infection is characteristic. From serologic evidence, inapparent and unrecognized infections with *C. burnetii* are common and widespread.

Coxiella burnetii has been isolated from milk of cattle, sheep and goats, but placentas of these animals are principally responsible for gross environmental contamination. Infected bovine placentas have been found to contain up to 10^6 guinea pig infectious doses per gram of tissue. In Australia the disease is associated particularly with sheep shearers and abattoir workers. Experimental studies indicate that the agent is disseminated among livestock by the airborne route. *Coxiella burnetii* infects other hosts (geese, pigeons, dogs, donkeys), but their epizootiologic roles have not been determined.[2]

Natural infection has been demonstrated in at least 40 species of ticks, but tick transmission of the agent to man is rare. In Australia, Africa and North America, the organism has been isolated from wild mammalian hosts of infected ticks (*Haemaphysalis, Ixodes, Boophilus* and other genera; see Chapter 69). Several species of wild birds also have been found to be naturally infected. These findings suggest that *C. burnetii* has a separate cycle in nature, but the relationship of this cycle to that in livestock remains obscure.

Pathology. Death usually has been ascribed to diffuse lobar pneumonia.[5] Gross appearance of the consolidated lung resembled that seen in pneumococcal pneumonia, but the histologic picture was more like that of viral and psittacosal pneumonia. In areas of red hepatization, intense congestion of blood vessels was prominent. Alveolar exudate contained relatively few cells, which were predominantly large mononuclear macrophages, many of which exhibited degenerative changes. In areas of gray hepatization, alveolar walls were thickened by infiltration of macrophages and smaller numbers of other cells, and areas of necrosis and septal breakdown were apparent. Alveolar exudates composed of vacuolated, degenerate macrophages were present. Bronchioles showed loss of epithelium and mucosal necrosis. Interlobular and subpleural connective tissue exhibited edema and round cell infiltration. Lesions of the spleen, kidney, brain, testis and liver were also found. Liver disease, characterized by miliary granulomas throughout the parencyma, has been found in liver biopsy specimens. Liver involvement appears to be more common in Australia than in North America.

Occasionally, *C. burnetii* causes a fatal progressive endocarditis[6] characterized by either vegetative valvular lesions or thromboangiitis obliterans or both. Aortic and mitral valves are most frequently involved. Old lesions, consisting of dense collagen deposits with mild infiltrates of lymphocytes and plasma cells, and superficial patches of loose granulation tissue containing intense mononuclear infiltrates are present on affected heart valves. Masses of extracellular rickettsiae may be found in the collagen matrix, and microcolonies of *C. burnetii* may be seen in mast cells found in active lesions. In thromboangiitis obliterans, rickettsiae are usually found intracellularly in the adventitia and outer media of affected vessels.

Clinical Characteristics. Symptoms appear suddenly after an incubation period of about 18 days (range from 12 to 30 days). The clinical syndrome varies considerably in severity and duration, and is characterized by remittent fever, chills, sweating, headache, muscle pains, malaise and anorexia. Pneumonitis demonstrable only by x-ray and attended by cough, scanty expectoration, and chest pain occurs in about one-half of the patients. In Australia, many cases present themselves as hepatitis. Roentgenographic findings, which resemble those of primary atypical pneumonia, first appear on the third or fourth day and usually persist after the febrile period. Evidence of pulmonary involvement may accompany mild or inapparent infections. Although sequelae (phlebothrombosis and pleural effusions) occur infrequently, and the mortality is less than 1 per cent, relapses and protracted convalescences are not uncommon.

Chronic rickettsial endocarditis has been recognized as a sequel of Q fever, chiefly among persons who have had rheumatic fever.[6] After a latent period of several months to a year, the patient begins to show signs of valvular insufficiency, which progress until either treatment or death supervenes. This chronic disease is characterized by fever, loss of weight, finger clubbing, joint pains, increasing heart murmur and eventual heart failure. *Coxiella burnetii* can be isolated from peripheral blood of the patient and can be found readily in histologic sections of damaged heart valves. Elevated serum levels of both IgM and IgG are found.

Diagnosis. Q fever should be suspected in febrile patients whose history includes direct or indirect contact with livestock. Because Q fever may resemble other acute febrile illnesses—including other rickettsial diseases, malaria, dengue, brucellosis, leptospirosis, infectious hepatitis, and typhoid or paratyphoid fevers—diagnosis can best be established by demonstrating a 4-fold or greater rise in complement-fixing (CF) antibodies in paired sera taken early in the course of the disease and 3 to 4 weeks later. Specific agglutinins against both phase I organisms (animal-adapted) and phase II organisms (egg-adapted) appear within the first week of illness in 50 per cent of the patients and in over 90 per cent during the second week. In contrast, phase I CF antibodies are found in very low titer, if at all, late in convalescence, although phase II CF antibodies appear in 65 per cent of patients within the second week of illness, and in 90 per cent or more within 4 weeks. The CF test with phase II antigen is recommended as the method of choice for diagnostic laboratories because this antigen is most easily obtained from commercial sources. A variety of agglutination tests which give reliable results are used in research laboratories and diagnostic reference centers. Until the necessary antigens become commercially available, however, these tests are of no practical value to the laboratory diagnostician.

Coxiella burnetii may be isolated by intraperitoneal inoculation of guinea pigs or hamsters with blood, sputum, urine and spinal fluid taken from febrile patients. In infected animals, specific CF antibodies appear within 2 to 5 weeks. Infection is usually accompanied by fever and splenomegaly, and rickettsiae can readily be found in stained smears of spleen tissue and exudate from the intact surface of the spleen. Isolation procedures present a severe hazard of infection, however, and should not be undertaken in the absence of adequate isolation facilities and rigidly enforced safeguards.

Antibodies against *C. burnetii* are highly specific; cross-reactions with other microorganisms are unknown. Positive cold hemagglutination and Weil-Felix tests are never elicited by Q fever.

Treatment. The tetracyclines usually cause remission of fever, reduction of splenomegaly and hepatomegaly, and amelioration of headache and chills in most patients affected with Q fever. However, these antibiotics are much less effective against Q fever than they are in treatment of other rickettsial diseases. Some patients may not respond even to large doses, and relapses have been noted in patients treated with chlortetracycline. Chloramphenicol also has been employed with beneficial effect but is not recommended because of risk of blood dyscrasias. Penicillin, streptomycin, erythromycin, and sulfonamides are ineffective.

Treatment with tetracyclines of patients with rickettsial endocarditis has proved to be relatively ineffective in the past. However, recent information indicates that use of a combination of tetracycline and lincomycin may have resulted in cure of the disease.[7]

Prophylaxis. Theoretically, Q fever can be controlled by eliminating the infection in livestock, which are the principal sources of *C. burnetii* for man. Such control is presently not feasible, although sources of infection and infection rates can be reduced by destruction of placentas at parturition and by vaccination of dairy cattle. Immunization of high-risk occupation groups with inactivated vaccines can be done safely if persons hypersensitive to *C. burnetii* antigen are excluded on the basis of a positive prevaccination skin test. Household use of raw milk has been shown to be the source of infections and clinical disease. Domestic use of infected, unpasteurized milk in modern food blenders that produce aerosols may be particularly hazardous, because a most effective means of infection is inhalation of aerosols containing *C. burnetii*. Pasteurization of milk and other dairy products is strongly recommended.

REFERENCES

1. Ormsbee, R. A. 1965. Q fever rickettsiae. *In* Horsfall, F. L., Jr., and Tamm, I.: Viral and Rickettsial Infections of Man. 4th ed. J. B. Lippincott Co., Philadelphia. pp. 1144–1163.
2. Babudieri, B. 1959. Q fever. A zoonosis. *In* Advances in Veterinary Science. Academic Press, Inc., New York. pp. 81–182.
3. Beck, M. D., Bell, J. A., Shaw, E. W., and Huebner, R. J. 1949. Q fever studies in southern California. II.

An epidemiological study of 300 cases. Pub. Hlth. Rept. *64*:41–56.
4. Brown, G. L., Colwell, D. C., and Hooper, W. L. 1968. An outbreak of Q fever in Staffordshire. J. Hyg. (Camb.) *66*:649–655.
5. Lillie, R. D., Perrin, T. L., and Armstrong, C. 1941. An institutional outbreak of pneumonitis. III. Histopathology in man and rhesus monkeys of the pneumonitis due to the virus of Q fever. Pub. Hlth. Rept. *56*:149–155.
6. Marmion, B. P. 1962. Subacute rickettsial endocarditis: an unusual complication of Q fever. J. Hyg. Epidemiol. Microbiol. Immunol. *6*:79–84.
7. Turck, W. P. G., Howitt, G. H., Turnberg, L., Fox, H., Mathews, M. B., Longson, M., and Wade, E. G. 1974. Personal communication.

CHAPTER 14

Trench Fever

WILLY BURGDORFER

Synonyms. Wolhynian fever, His-Werner disease, shin bone fever, quintan or five-day fever.

Definition. Trench fever is a self-limited louse-borne rickettsial disease characterized by intermittent fever, generalized aches and pains, negligible mortality and multiple relapses.[1]

Distribution. Epidemics have occurred during World Wars I and II in eastern, central, and western Europe. From there the disease was transferred to other areas, such as northern Europe (Norway, Finland, Sweden). By recovery of infected lice or by serologic surveys, foci have also been detected in Africa (Egypt, Algeria, Ethiopia, Burundi), Asia (Japan, China), and the Americas (Mexico, Bolivia).

Etiology. The causative agent, *Rochalimaea quintana,* is transmitted from man to man by the body louse, *Pediculus humanus humanus* (Fig. 6–2, p. 104). Unlike other pathogenic rickettsiae, *R. quintana* grows extracellularly and can be readily cultivated on cell-free blood agar.[2] On the basis of this and other distinctive characteristics, including antigenic dissimilarities, *R. quintana* was set apart from the other pathogenic rickettsiae by classifying it in the genus *Rochalimaea. Rochalimaea quintana* produces an inapparent infection in monkeys but fails to infect the usual laboratory animals. It has been cultivated in yolk sacs of embryonated hens' eggs and in vitro cell cultures. In lice it grows extracellularly in the digestive system only. It is nonpathogenic for its vector, which once infected, remains so for life. *R. quintana* is fairly resistant to the usual environmental factors; dried louse feces may remain infectious for several months.

Epidemiology. Transmission of trench fever from man to man takes place by contamination of abraded skin with infective louse feces. Man, who usually experiences a long-term rickettsemia, is the reservoir of the agent; *R. quintana* has been recovered from the blood of convalescents up to 8 years after acute illness. In nearly all patients, the rickettsiae are present in blood during the illness and for a few weeks afterward. Their subsequent presence in this tissue may be periodic, in which case the organisms appear for a few weeks at a time at various intervals one or more times a year. Latent infections, manifested by either frank illness or merely an active blood carrier state, have been reported following introduction of some unrelated stimulus, such as other infections or injection of antityphus or antityphoid vaccines.

Pathology. Because of the negligible incidence of mortality, necropsy reports on trench fever patients do not exist. The exanthematic lesions reveal perivascular infiltration, principally of lymphocytes, but the vascular intima is normal and there is no thrombotic process. It is not known whether the rickettsiae develop only extracellularly, and only in the blood, or whether invasion of cells and tissues takes place.

Clinical Characteristics. The symptoms of trench fever are extremely variable, making clinical diagnosis of many cases difficult or impossible, although circumstantial evidence is a provisional help. Headache, malaise and body pains may appear as prodromes toward the close of the 10- to 30-day incubation period. Nevertheless, the actual onset is sudden. Headache, vertigo, pain in the back and legs, especially in the shins, postorbital pain on movement of the eyes, often nystagmus on lateral gaze, and injection of the eyes accompany a rapid rise of temperature to 39.5 or 40° C (103 or 104° F). The primary fever continues for several days to a week, less often for several weeks. The leukocyte count is variable, some cases presenting a leukocytosis; in others the count is normal or a leukopenia may be present. Albuminuria is usual and polyuria common.

The initial febrile episode is followed in about 50 per cent of cases by a regularly or irregularly relapsing type of febrile curve. Three to five such relapses are usual, although as many as seven may occur.

A distinctive, typhus-like rash is a fairly constant feature of the disease but is irregular in the time of its appearance. It is usually associated with an acute febrile phase, however, manifesting itself early in the initial attack or in a relapse. The rash consists of small erythematous macules—occasionally papules—that blanch on pressure. They are relatively few and often disappear within 24 hours. Their distribution is characteristic, involving particularly the chest, back and abdomen.

Convalescence is frequently prolonged and complicated by a variety of clinical signs, including functional derangements of the circulatory system and neurasthenia.

Immunity appears to be variable in duration, although its actual development is a controversial matter in view of the relapsing character of the disease, the periodic nature of the blood carrier state in some persons, and the evidence for existence of latent infections with *R. quintana.*

Diagnosis. The differential diagnosis of trench fever includes influenza, dengue, the dengue-like fevers, malaria and brucellosis. Laboratory tests present the best diagnostic aid and include isolation of the agent and specific serologic tests. Until 1961, the only reliable method of diagnosis for trench fever was through isolation of *R. quintana* from blood of a patient by the louse test (xenodiagnosis). This consisted of either feeding lice on a patient or injecting lice intrarectally with the patient's blood. A positive test revealed rickettsiae in the louse excreta within 4 to 12 days after the blood meal or within 2 to 4 days after inoculation.

The in vitro cultivation of *R. quintana* permitted preparation of antigens and application of the complement-fixation test, which has been shown to be very specific although titers, in general, are low.[3] The more sophisticated microagglutination technique has been found of value in serologic surveys in Bolivia, Mexico, Ethiopia and Burundi.[4] However, the indirect immunofluorescence test appears even more sensitive and may become the laboratory method of choice for diagnosing this disease.[5] The Weil-Felix reaction is negative.

Treatment. The use of broad spectrum antibiotics therapeutically has been reported.[6] Symptoms were ameliorated with tetracyclines in the total amount of 16 gm administered over a period of 5 to 8 days.

Prophylaxis. Prophylaxis of trench fever depends upon effective measures for louse control. (See Table 72–1, p. 796.) The infectious agent is present in the patient's urine during the acute stages of the disease, hence suitable precautions in the disposal of excreta must be emphasized. Because of the long persistence of this agent, persons who have recovered from this disease should not be blood donors.

REFERENCES

1. Zdrodovskii, P. F., and Golinevich, E. H. 1960. Wolhynian or five-day fever (febris *Wolhynica s. quintana*). *In* The Rickettsial Diseases. 2nd ed. Pergamon Press, London. 630 pp.
2. Vinson, J. W., and Fuller, H. S. 1961. Studies on trench fever. I. Propagation of rickettsia-like microorganisms from a patient's blood. Swiss J. Gen. Path. Bact. *24*: (Suppl.): 152–166.
3. Weyer, F., Vinson, J. W., Mannweiler, E., and Mohr, W. 1972. Serologische Untersuchungen bei Wolhynischem Fieber. Ztschr. Tropenmed. Parasit. *23*:187–196.
4. Myers, W. F., and Wisseman, C. L., Jr. 1973. Serologic studies of trench fever employing a microagglutination procedure. *In* Proceedings of the International Symposium on the Control of Lice and Louse-borne Diseases. P.A.H.O. Sci. Publ. No. 263, Washington, D.C. (1972). pp. 79–81.
5. Vinson, J. W., and Cooper, M. D. 1973. Detection of trench fever. Abstract, 9th Internat. Congr. Trop. Med. Mal., Athens, 14–21, October 1973, *1*:100.
6. Mohr, W., and Weyer, F. 1964. Spätrückfälle bei Wolynischem Fieber. Deut. Med. Wschr. *89*:244–247.

SECTION III
Spirochetal Diseases

CHAPTER 15
The Relapsing Fevers

WILLY BURGDORFER

Synonyms. Tifo recurrente, fiebre recurrente, febris recurrens, fièvre récurrente, Rückfall Fieber, Rückfall Typhus, garapata disease, kimputu, o'mushyiza gw'ebibo, spirillum fever, famine fever, tick fever.

Definition. Relapsing fevers are acute arthropod-borne diseases characterized by alternating febrile and afebrile periods, caused by spirochetes transmitted through the agency of the louse *Pediculus humanus humanus* and by ticks of the genus *Ornithodoros.*

Distribution. Louse-borne relapsing fever has been reported from all continents. It has disappeared from the United States but frequently occurs in parts of South America, Europe, Africa and Asia. Isolated cases in recently arrived immigrants in Cuba, Brazil and Australia are said to be louse-borne.

Tick-borne relapsing fevers are widely distributed throughout the Eastern and Western Hemispheres. In the Americas, endemic centers are known in southern British Columbia, Canada; in western United States; in Aguascalientes in the plateau regions of Mexico; in Guatemala and Panama in Central America; and in South America, chiefly in Colombia, Ecuador, Venezuela and northern Argentina.

Tick-borne relapsing fever is present throughout Africa, with the exception of the Sahara and the rain forest belt. In Europe it is reported from Spain, Portugal and the Caucasus. In Asia it occurs in Cyprus, Israel, Syria, Turkey, Iraq, Iran, southern Russia, as far east as the western border of China, Afghanistan, in Kashmir, and in Jammu, India. Indigenous tick-borne relapsing fever has not been reported from Australia, New Zealand or Oceania.

Etiology. Relapsing fever spirochetes are corkscrew-shaped microorganisms 8 to 16 μm long with coarse, shallow, irregular spirals that taper terminally into fine filaments (Fig. 15–1). They multiply by binary fission. Ultrastructural studies reveal an outer layer ("the coat") surrounding a central cytoplasmic core to which is attached laterally an evagination containing from 16 to 25 locomotory fibrils. The core is surrounded by a cytoplasmic membrane and contains mesosomes, ribosomes and, in the center, nuclear DNA formerly referred to as axial filament.

Taxonomically, relapsing fever spirochetes form the genus *Borrelia* in the family TREPONEMATACEAE.[1] They differ from the other two genera in this family, *Treponema* and *Leptospira,* by their staining reactions, growth conditions, and the fact that most of them are transmitted by arthropods. Whereas louse-borne relapsing fever has a single agent, *Borrelia recurrentis* (syn. *B. obermeyeri* and *B. novyi*), the tick-borne types are caused by various *Borrelia* species. Because of the close relationship between these agents and their tick vectors, the "tick-spirochete specificity" has been used as a criterion for classification and has led to the creation of numerous *Borrelia* species. However, in view of exceptions to this concept, and because various species of tick-borne *Borrelia* were shown to develop in experimentally infected

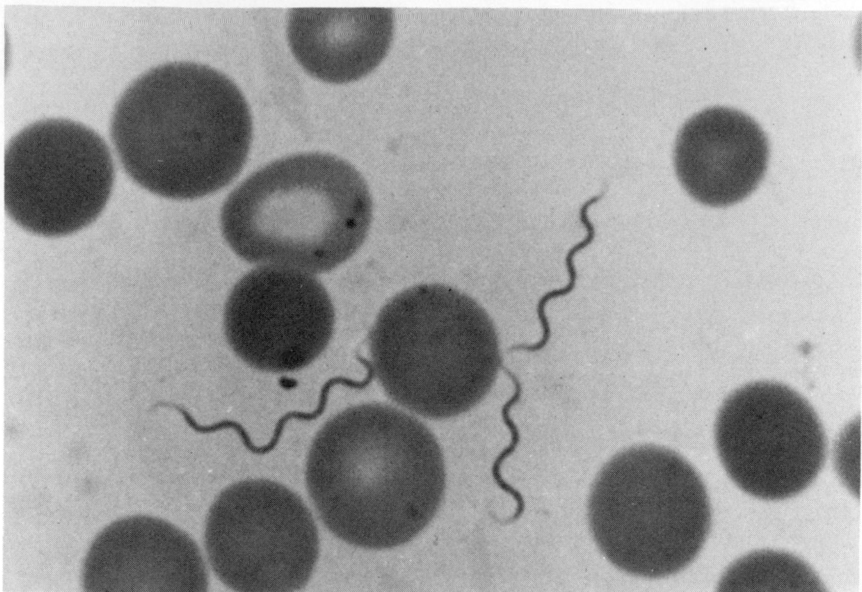

Figure 15–1. Relapsing fever spirochete, *Borrelia hermsii,* in mouse blood. Organism at right in process of binary fission. (Giemsa × 2700; courtesy of Dr. Willy Burgdorfer, Rocky Mountain Laboratory.)

P. humanus humanus, various investigators suggest that tick-borne spirochetes do not represent genetically distinct "strains" but derivatives of a single taxonomic entity, *B. recurrentis.*[2] The "tick-spirochete specificity" continues to be used as a classification concept at least until results of newer and more sophisticated research justify its re-evaluation.

Borrelia species stain readily with aniline dyes, especially with the Giemsa-Romanowsky blood stains. Cultivation of relapsing fever spirochetes has been possible only in susceptible animals, in embryonated hens' eggs, and in specific arthropod vectors. Recently, primary growth and serial subculture over a period of 1 year with no loss of virulence to laboratory animals was reported for *Borrelia hermsii.*[3]

Epidemiology. Epidemicity or endemicity of the relapsing fevers is determined by the arthropod vectors. Louse-borne relapsing fever is always associated with a high degree of louse infestations and is typically epidemic; the tick-borne disease is endemic (Fig. 15–2).

LOUSE-BORNE RELAPSING FEVER. This disease occurs under the same conditions as epidemic (louse-borne) typhus; in fact, both diseases frequently appear together. Its prevalence depends upon ecologic and sociologic conditions that favor rapid multiplication and frequent transfer of the louse *P. humanus humanus* (Figs. 6–2, p. 104, and 70–2, p. 733). Overcrowding and low standards of personal hygiene, especially in bathing and changing clothes, are contributing factors. The disease is seasonal, occurring most generally during cold winter months when clothing and living habits lead to a high degree of lousiness. Among the scantier-clothed populations of equatorial Africa, louse-borne relapsing fever is rarely seen. Outbreaks of the disease are difficult to explain because no animal reservoir, except man, has been established for the causative agent, *B. recurrentis.* The louse itself cannot be considered a reservoir because it does not transmit the spirochetes transovarially and it has a relatively short life span. Because louse-borne relapsing fever usually occurs in areas where ticks also are present, one of several hypotheses suggests that the louse may represent a secondary vector that acquired the spirochetes through feeding on patients originally infected by ticks.[4] That many strains of tick-borne relapsing fever spirochetes can be maintained and transmitted by the louse suggests this view. On the other hand, after World War II, louse-borne relapsing fever appeared in many places where the presence of *Borrelia* could not be established in indigenous ticks. More recently a similar situation existed in the Democratic People's Republic of Vietnam.

Infection of lice occurs during feeding on a spirochetemic patient. Ingested spirochetes pass through the esophagus to the midgut. A few spirochetes survive long enough to invade the gut epithelium and eventually penetrate into the hemocele where they multiply. Except for the central ganglion, other tissues, such as salivary glands and genital organs, are not invaded. Thus, transmission by bite, i.e. via saliva, or passage through the eggs to the progeny of

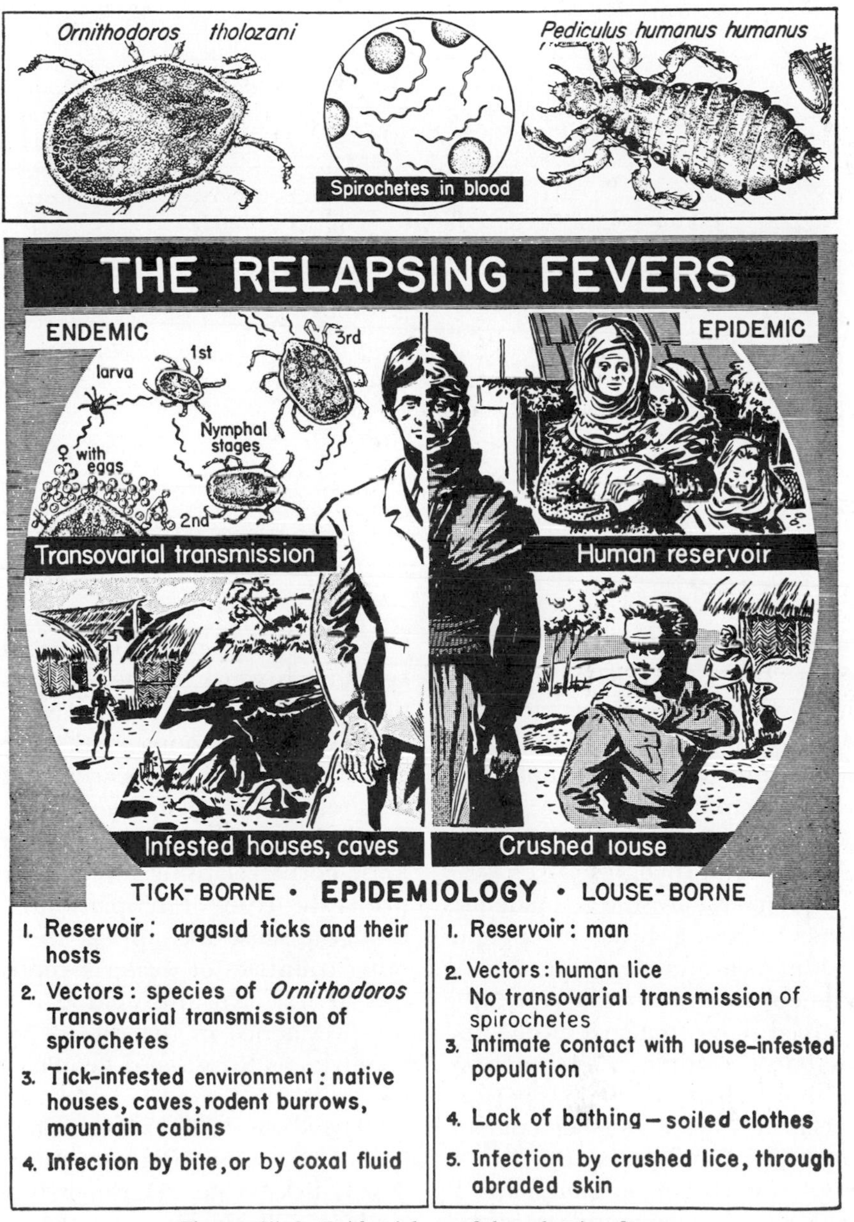

Figure 15–2. Epidemiology of the relapsing fevers.

Table 15–1. Distribution and Characteristics of Louse– and Tick–borne Relapsing Fevers

	Cosmopolitan	***African Tick-borne Relapsing Fevers***		
	LOUSE-BORNE RELAPSING FEVER	EAST AFRICAN RELAPSING FEVER	HISPANO-AFRICAN RELAPSING FEVERS	*Crocidurae* GROUP RELAPSING FEVERS
Vectors	*Pediculus humanus humanus*	*Ornithodoros moubata*	*Ornithodoros erraticus* (large variety)	*Ornithodoros erraticus* (small variety)
Etiologic Agent	*Borrelia recurrentis* syn. *B. obermeyeri, B. novyi*	*Borrelia duttonii*	*Borrelia hispanica*	*Borrelia crocidurae* *B. merionesi* *B. microti* *B. dipodilli*
Animal Hosts	Man	Man (?)	Wild rodents, rabbits	Rodents, hedgehog, lizards, toads
Geographic Distribution	Africa: Ethiopia, Sudan, Kenya, Nigeria, Chad, Zaire, Burundi, Tanzania; South America; Bolivia, Colombia; North Vietman, U.S.S.R. (?), People's Republic of China (?)	Africa: Ethiopia, Kenya, Uganda, Tanzania, Somalia, Ruanda, Burundi, Central and Eastern Congo, Malawi, Zambia, Rhodesia, South Africa	Southern Spain, Portugal, Morocco, Algeria, Tunisia	Morocco, Libya, Egypt, Iran, Turkey, Senegal, Kenya (*B. dipodilli*)

infected lice do not occur. Once infected the louse remains so throughout its entire life.

Transmission of spirochetes to man takes place through contamination of the bite wound with infectious hemolymph from lice crushed by scratching. There is also ample evidence that *Borrelia* species are capable of penetrating normal, unbroken skin.

Medical history records large epidemics of louse-borne relapsing fever throughout Europe, Africa, Asia and America. During the Rumanian epidemic of World War I, the disease occurred concomitantly with epidemic (louse-borne) typhus, and it is estimated that more than 1,000,000 persons contracted relapsing fever. Smaller epidemics took place in Edinburgh, Dublin, in coastal cities of eastern United States, and at Oroville, California. The extensive epidemic that appeared in French Guinea in 1921 spread eastward to the western border of Sudan and southward into Nigeria and the Gold Coast. In some areas, it resulted in a case mortality rate of nearly 75 per cent, and it is estimated that over a 2-year period 80,000 to 100,000 persons died. Since 1967, louse-borne relapsing fever is being reported primarily from Ethiopia and Sudan, although disease foci appear to be present in other countries of western, central and eastern Africa.[5] No information is available on the prevalence of the disease in such large countries as Russia and People's Republic of China.

Tick-borne Relapsing Fevers. Distribution and main characteristics of the endemic tick-borne relapsing fevers are included in Table 15–1. Of the vectors listed

Table 15–1. DISTRIBUTION AND CHARACTERISTICS OF LOUSE- AND TICK-BORNE RELAPSING FEVERS *(Continued)*

Asiatic Tick-borne Relapsing Fevers			
Ornithodoros tholozani syn. *O. papillipes, O. crossi(?)*	*Ornithodoros verrucosus*	*Ornithodoros tartakovskyi*	*Ornithodoros hermsi*
Borrelia persica	*Borrelia caucasica*	*Borrelia latyschewii*	*Borrelia hermsii*
Rats, mice, hedgehog, badger, porcupine	Rodents, birds, reptiles, foxes	Rodents, toads, lizards, turtles	Rodents (chipmunks and tree squirrels)
Cyrenaica, western Egyptian desert, Cyprus, eastern Mediterranean, Iran, Iraq, U.S.S.R. eastward to western border of China, India (*O. crossi* ?)	Caucasus, Ukraine, Iraq, Mesopotamia	Iran, Central Asia	Arizona, California, Colorado, Idaho, Kansas, Montana, New Mexico, Nevada, Oklahoma, Oregon, Utah, Washington, British Columbia (Canada)

Table 15–1 continued on following page

for the Eastern Hemisphere, *Ornithodoros moubata, Ornithodoros erraticus* (large variety), *Ornithodoros tholozani* and *Ornithodoros verrucosus* are important in the transmission of their respective spirochetes to man. The *Borrelia* species associated with *O. erraticus* and *Ornithodoros tartakovskyi* are either only moderately pathogenic or nonpathogenic for man. In the Western Hemisphere there are three important vectors: *Ornithodoros hermsi, Ornithodoros turicata* and *Ornithodoros rudis.* Only one human case has been attributed to *Borrelia parkeri. Ornithodoros talaje* has been linked to human infections in Panama, but many "strains" of this species are known not to bite man. There are numerous tick-spirochete associations that are not mentioned in Table 15–1 because their significance in relation to human disease is still unknown. Thus, *Ornithodoros brasiliensis* has been found infected with *Borrelia brasiliensis* in Brazil, *Ornithodoros zumpti* with *Borrelia tillae* in South Africa, and *Ornithodoros alactagalis* with *Borrelia armenica* in Armenia. *Ornithodoros dugesi* may be an alternate vector of *Borrelia mazzottii* in Mexico, and *Ornithodoros gurneyi* may be involved in maintaining *Borrelia queenslandica* in Australia. In Kenya, *Ornithodoros graingeri* has been shown to be a vector of *Borrelia graingeri,* which has been the cause of one experimentally induced human infection.

Most foci of tick-borne relapsing fever exist in nature in rather closed tick biotopes, such as burrows, nests or caves. Man becomes part of this biocenotic system only accidentally while visiting such areas or using them as a refuge in inclement weather. How-

Table 15-1. DISTRIBUTION AND CHARACTERISTICS OF LOUSE- AND TICK-BORNE RELAPSING FEVERS *(Concluded)*

American Tick-borne Relapsing Fevers

Vectors	*Ornithodoros turicata*	*Ornithodoros parkeri*	*Ornithodoros talaje*	*Ornithodoros rudis* syn. *O. venezuelensis*
Etiologic Agent	*Borrelia turicatae*	*Borrelia parkeri*	*Borrelia mazzottii*	*Borrelia venezuelensis* syn. *B. neotropicalis*
Animal Hosts	Rodents, rabbits, owls	Rodents, rabbits, owls	Rodents, domestic animals	Rodents, rabbits
Geographic Distribution	Arizona, California, Florida, Kansas, New Mexico, Oklahoma, Utah, Texas, Mexico	California, Colorado, Idaho, Montana, Nevada, Oregon, Utah, Washington, Wyoming	Arizona, California, Florida, Kansas, Nevada, Texas, and southward to Guatemala, Panama, Colombia	Panama, Colombia, Ecuador, Venezuela, Paraguay

ever, human dwellings (log houses, cabins, shacks and animal shelters) built near such foci invariably attract rodents (rats, mice, squirrels) leading to new foci which often become established within the homes, especially if these are poorly constructed and maintained. Thus, the ticks become closely associated with man, whom they will readily attack once their rodent hosts have become exterminated as a result of either man-initiated control measures or naturally occurring diseases. Two large outbreaks of *O. hermsi*–borne relapsing fever, one with more than 50 cases, have recently been recorded in western United States among people occupying tick-infested log cabins.

The African relapsing fever tick, *O. moubata,* occurring chiefly in East and West Africa, is considered a domestic ectoparasite that lives in dirt and in cracks of mud floors or in mud and grass walls of native huts. It, too, was originally confined to the closed biotope of warthogs and porcupines and was transferred by man to human dwellings where it became well adapted and acquired anthropophilia.

Rodents are considered the main sources for spirochetal infections for all *Ornithodoros* vectors, except *O. moubata* which in nature has never been observed to feed on such animals. Indeed, the origin of *Borrelia duttonii,* the causative agent of East African relapsing fever, is still a matter of conjecture. Spirochetes have never been detected in field-collected ticks or in the primary tick host, the warthog, which appears to be refractory to experimental infection with *B. duttonii.*

Endemicity of tick-borne relapsing fevers is closely related to the biology of the various vectors. *Ornithodoros* ticks (Fig. 69–3, p. 718) are intermittent, mostly nocturnal, fast feeders (5 to 20 minutes) that spend most of their life underground in dust and dirt of rodent burrows (e.g. *Ornithodoros parkeri, O. turicata),* in crevices of old tree stumps (e.g. *O. hermsi),* between logs of rodent-infested cabins, or in dirt and mud of native huts (e.g. *O. moubata)* or animal shelters *(O. tholozani*). Adult ticks feed repeatedly and mated females lay from 50 to several hundred eggs after each blood meal. All species go through one larval and four to six nymphal stages before reaching maturity. With the exception of *O. moubata* whose larvae develop to nymphs without a blood meal, all stages require a blood meal before developing further. Adult *Ornithodoros* ticks are noted for their ability to survive prolonged starvation; in fact, storage of ticks from 5 to 13 years without feeding has been noted.

Development of *Borrelia* in *Ornithodoros*, thoroughly explored in the case of *B. duttonii* in *O. moubata*, differs from development in the body louse in that the spirochetes once in the hemocele invade all the tick tissues including those of the salivary glands and, in most instances, those of the female genital organs from where they may be passed via eggs to the progeny. This phenomenon, called "transovarial infection," is an important mechanism for the survival and distribution of certain relapsing fever spirochetes. It has been demonstrated in *O. moubata*, *O. erraticus* (both varieties), *O. tholozani*, *O. tartakovskyi*, *O. verrucosus*, *O. turicata* and *O. hermsi*; it does not occur in *O. parkeri*, *O. talaje* and *O. rudis*.

The percentage of infected female ticks passing spirochetes via eggs varies greatly, as does the percentage of infected filial ticks. Filial infection rates from 2 to 98 per cent have been reported for *O. moubata*, and from 35 to 100 per cent for *O. turicata*.

Transmission of tick-borne relapsing fever spirochetes takes place either via secretions of infectious saliva or via coxal fluid. Most *Ornithodoros* species transmit via saliva, although their bites may not always be infective. This is particularly true for adult ticks, especially for *O. moubata* whose salivary gland tissues usually are only moderately or not at all infected. During its feeding process, however, this tick vector secretes a large amount of spirochete-containing coxal fluid. Thus, the *Borrelia* may enter the host's blood stream either through the bite wound or directly through the intact skin. Other species of *Ornithodoros* leave their hosts before secreting coxal fluids. *Ornithodoros hermsi* secretes only a minute amount of this fluid which crystallizes immediately on the tick before getting in contact with the host. This tick, like *O. turicata*, is very efficient in transmitting its spirochetes; feedings of less than 1 minute have resulted in infections.

Pathology. The most striking and constant pathologic changes are found in the spleen and liver; less often lesions are present in the kidneys, myocardium and central nervous system.[1] Jaundice is common. Numerous small hemorrhages may be seen in the skin, stomach, intestine and kidneys. The spleen is usually enlarged and soft and often has multiple infarcts. Characteristic miliary lesions are commonly visible macroscopically (Fig. 15–3). These consist of a zone of congestion and cellular infiltration in which spirochetes are particularly numerous around the lymphoid follicles. The liver may be enlarged and may present parenchymatous degeneration. Usually, spirochetes cannot be demonstrated in reticuloendothelial cells. Areas of degeneration may likewise be found in the kidney and myocardium. Rarely, hemorrhagic meningitis is present, and spirochetes may be demonstrable in the brain. Death most often is caused by complications, particularly pneumonia.

Clinical Characteristics. Relapsing fever is characterized clinically by recurring periods of fever and toxemia, each of a few days' duration, and separated by afebrile intervals of about 1 week or 10 days.[1] Two to ten or more relapses may occur in untreated or improperly treated patients.

The louse-borne and tick-borne forms of the disease are indistinguishable clinically, although, in general, the louse-borne variety reportedly has a lesser tendency to multiple relapses. Mortality, usually from 2 to 5 per cent, reached nearly 75 per cent in a serious West African epidemic outbreak.

There seem to be rather characteristic variations in the severity of the disease in different areas. These variations have led to the consideration of the relapsing fevers in terms of specific geographic regions. However, great variations in severity of the disease occur from one person to another even within a given area.

Thus, certain special types have been described, such as African tick fever, and North African, Persian, Indian, European and American relapsing fevers. In North Africa the disease is said to have a relatively short course, but it is frequently complicated by involvement of the central nervous sys-

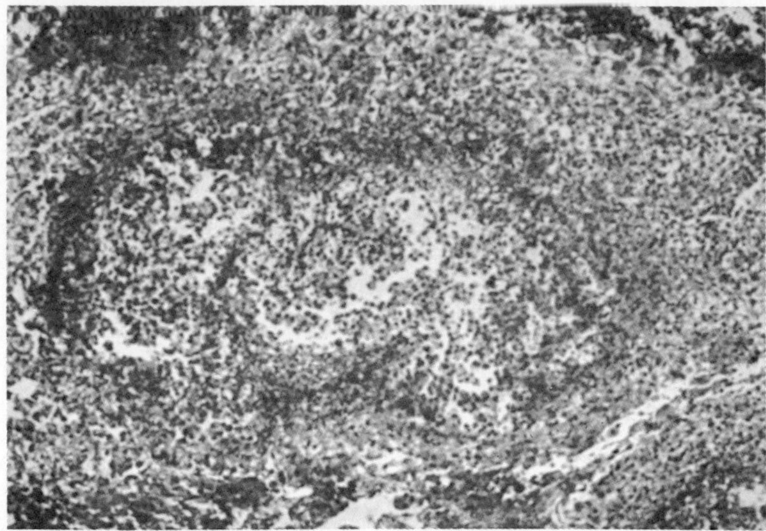

Figure 15–3. Miliary lesion in spleen with central necrosis and mononuclear exudate. Spirochetes in surrounding zone of infiltration.

tem. Facial and ocular palsies are said to be common in this form. Jaundice and a somewhat high mortality rate are rather frequent in the Indian form. The Persian type is characteristically mild and relapses are few. Relapsing fever in Europe and the Americas is commonly a moderately severe disease; however, there are seldom more than two or three relapses.

The incubation period varies from 2 to 10 days, but may be as long as 2 to 3 weeks. Onset is usually sudden, associated with vertigo, headache, myalgia, and fever, which develops rapidly to 40 to 40.5° C (104 to 105° F) or higher. Temperature remains elevated, with slight daily remissions throughout the primary febrile period. Vomiting is common. A slight icteric tint of the sclerae is usual. In severe cases marked jaundice may occur by the time of the crisis. A diffuse bronchitis is frequently present, especially in the first febrile episode. Transitory erythematous or petechial eruptions are quite common during the initial fever; characteristically, they are most pronounced about the neck and shoulder girdle, and later extend to the chest and abdomen. Herpes and epistaxis also are not unusual. The spleen is often somewhat enlarged and tender. A polymorphonuclear leukocytosis is present from the onset and may be marked in patients experiencing high fever and bronchitis. The liver is enlarged and tender, especially in severe cases. The urine commonly contains albumin and casts, and in severe cases hematuria may occur. Spirochetes are usually demonstrable in the blood during febrile periods but not in the afebrile intervals.

After 4 or 5 days of severe illness the temperature falls by crisis, accompanied by profuse sweating and not infrequently by prostration and signs of cardiac weakness. The afebrile period lasts 3 to 10 days, during which time there is usually marked clinical improvement.

Relapse sets in acutely, and the subjective and objective phenomena are quite similar to those of the initial attack. Conjunctivitis and iritis are often seen during relapses, and there may be transitory or permanent cranial nerve palsies. Deafness is not uncommon and may persist. Uterine hemorrhage is not unusual, and pregnant women frequently abort. Again, after a few days of illness, the attack terminates by crisis.

There are usually four or five such recurrences, although occasionally there may be ten or more. Late in the course of the disease peripheral neuritis may be persistent and troublesome.

Diagnosis. In differential diagnosis,

relapsing fever may have to be distinguished particularly from malaria, dengue and typhus. When jaundice is present, it may be confused with that of yellow fever and leptospirosis.

The clinical picture and leukocytosis may be suggestive. Definitive diagnosis, however, depends upon detection of the spirochetes. These are demonstrable in the blood only during the febrile periods. In some instances they may be seen easily in Giemsa-stained thick and thin blood films. In others, when the organisms are scanty, intraperitoneal inoculation of blood into young white mice or young white rats is useful. Spirochetes are found easily in their blood within 48 to 72 hours. With some strains spirochetemia may continue for many days. Spirochetes may be recovered from the brain of some experimental animals several months after initial infection.

The disease produced in monkeys and guinea pigs resembles that in man. Although guinea pigs are resistant to infection with some strains of *Borrelia,* other strains produce typical febrile relapses with disappearance of spirochetes from the peripheral blood during afebrile periods and their reappearance at the time of the rise in temperature. Hemoperitoneum has been reported as a constant reaction with some tick strains from northern Africa.

Demonstration of spirochetes in infected lice or ticks can readily be accomplished by dark field examination of hemolymph or tissues, or by injection of tissue suspensions into adult or suckling white mice. These techniques are also used for examination of field-collected ticks or ticks found in human dwellings. At times, the Wassermann reaction is positive during the acute stage of the disease.

Treatment. Susceptibility of the relapsing fever spirochetes to certain drugs and antibiotics varies widely, and treatment is complicated by serious reactions. The treatment of choice, tetracycline intravenously, is highly effective in louse-borne relapsing fever but less so in the tick-borne type. In the former, a single intravenous dose of 0.25 gm rapidly clears spirochetes.[6] Relapses do not occur if a second dose of 0.5 gm is given the next day. In tick-borne relapsing fever, prolonged oral treatment to a total amount of 6.0 to 8.0 gm may be necessary. The crisis type reaction to this treatment is, however, severe.

Penicillin 600,000 units as a single intramuscular injection, or in divided doses to a total of 1,000,000 units, is less effective in preventing relapses, but the adverse reaction is less severe than following tetracycline. For this reason, penicillin may be recommended for the treatment of louse-borne relapsing fever,[7] but is relatively ineffective against the tick-borne disease. Individual patients may be sensitive to penicillin.

Chloramphenicol 1.0 gm (given in divided doses, by mouth) is also effective against louse-borne relapsing fever, but the usual reaction occurs. Cases of the tick-borne disease in widely separated geographic areas have been successfully treated with other antibiotics, especially streptomycin. Combinations of the tetracyclines Aureomycin and Terramycin have been used. In one series of patients infected with *B. hispanica,* 0.25 gm of Aureomycin was administered at 6-hour intervals for a total dose of 3.0 gm. In another series of *B. persica* infections, 0.5 gm of streptomycin was given twice daily for 2 days. However, in the evaluation of any treatment it should be remembered that in untreated cases the number of relapses varies from one to as many as 14.

Arsenical compounds have proved useful, but have not prevented relapse. Neoarsphenamine was administered intravenously during a rise in temperature as a single dose of 0.3 to 0.9 gm for adults, and 0.005 to 0.01 gm per kg of body weight for children. The treatment was sometimes repeated the next day. Administration of the drug was frequently followed by vomiting, elevation of temperature, and aggravation of other symptoms. The treatment was instituted as early as possible and limited to the early hours of one of the paroxysms. If given late in the febrile episode reactions were more severe, and if given in the apyrexial intervals the drug was ineffective.

The reaction that begins an hour or so

following initiation of parenteral therapy with these drugs and antibiotics is of the Jarisch-Herxheimer type, and may be extremely severe. An initial rigor lasting 1/4 to 1/2 hour is followed by sweating and elevation of temperature, at which time marked leukopenia is evident. The spirochetes disappear from the blood at this time. Pulmonary and cardiac strain is severe, sometimes constituting a graver danger to the patient than the crisis that precedes spontaneous remission of the untreated illness. Collapse due to hypotension may occur, for which reason complete bed rest is essential for 48 hours after treatment. Nevertheless, the greatly reduced mortality following treatment, despite the reaction, fully justifies employment of one of these regimens.

Prophylaxis. Avoidance of lice and rigid louse control constitute the best prophylaxis against louse-borne relapsing fever. (See Table 72–1, p. 796.)

Measures in the control of *Ornithodoros* ticks vary depending on the habits of the various species. In the Western Hemisphere, where rodents are the ticks' primary host animals, all dwellings should be rodent-proofed. Rodents in immediate surroundings should be exterminated or kept at low level. Old tree stumps and snags that may harbor or may have harbored nests of squirrels, chipmunks and other rodents should be removed and burned; and firewood, the cracks of which offer excellent harborage for ticks, should not be stored in homes. Tick-infested dwellings should become subjects of rodent eradication and tick control efforts (Table 72–1, p. 794). Because ticks (e.g. *O. hermsi, O. turicata)* are often hiding in practically inaccessible places such as cracks and crevices of floor boards and walls, periodic application of acaricides (chlordane 2 to 3 per cent, DDT 5 per cent spray, Diazinon 0.5 per cent, dichlorvos 0.5 per cent, dieldrin 0.5 per cent spray or 1 per cent dust, lindane 0.5 per cent, and malathion 2 to 3 per cent spray or 4 to 5 per cent dust) is recommended. It should be emphasized that these control measures offer only temporary relief, for rodents and their ticks will eventually return unless their ingress is prevented by rodent-proofing the dwellings.

In Africa, 1 per cent lindane (BHC) applied as dust directly onto the floor of *O. moubata*–infested huts has proved effective for about 4 weeks. In Iran and Russia, BHC, 2 gm per sq m in houses, and 6 to 8 gm per sq m in animal sheds gave favorable results in controlling *O. tholozani.*

REFERENCES

1. Felsenfeld, O. 1971. Borrelia: Strains, Vectors, Human and Animal Borreliosis. Warren H. Green, Inc., St. Louis, Missouri, 180 pp.
2. Walton, G. A. 1973. Possible extrahuman reservoirs of the relapsing fever spirochete *Borrelia recurrentis. In* Proceedings of the International Symposium on the Control of Lice and Louse-borne Diseases. P.A.H.O. Sci. Publ. No. 263, Washington, D.C. (1972). pp. 117–128.
3. Kelly, R. 1971. Cultivation of *Borrelia hermsi.* Science *173*:443–444.
4. Geigy, R. 1968. Relapsing Fevers. *In* Weinman, D., and Ristic, M. (eds.): Infectious Blood Diseases of Man and Animals. Vol. 2. Academic Press, New York. pp. 175–216.
5. Tarizzo, M. L. 1973. Geographic distribution of louse-borne diseases. *In* Proceedings of the International Symposium on the Control of Lice and Louse-borne Diseases. P.A.H.O. Sci. Publ. No. 263, Washington, D.C. (1972). pp. 50–59.
6. Bryceson, A. D. M., Parry, E. H. O., Perine, P. L., Warrell, D. A., Vokotich, D., and Leithead, C. S. 1970. Louse-borne relapsing fever. A clinical and laboratory study of 62 cases in Ethiopia and a reconsideration of the literature. Q. J. Med. *39*:129–170.
7. Knaack, R. H., Wright, L. J., Leithead, C. S., Kidan, T. G., and Plorde, J. J. 1972. Penicillin vs. tetracycline in the treatment of louse-borne relapsing fever. Ethiop. Med. J. *10*:15–22.

CHAPTER 16
Syphilis

MERLIN L. BRUBAKER

Synonyms. Venereal syphilis, sporadic syphilis, lues.

Definition. Syphilis is a chronic infectious disease caused by *Treponema pallidum.* It is usually transmitted by direct contact with an infectious lesion, but may be passed from the untreated mother to the fetus in utero. The disease may produce varied manifestations depending upon the organ attacked. It may occur with florid signs and symptoms, but it is also noted for long periods of symptomless latency.

Distribution. Syphilis is worldwide in its distribution and occurs mostly in urban areas, where the more concentrated population results in a greater reservoir of infection and opportunity for spread. Venereal syphilis was less frequently diagnosed in the tropical areas before the World Health Organization started programs of eradication of the treponematoses other than venereal syphilis, i.e. yaws, pinta and endemic syphilis, soon after 1950. Since then, however, venereal syphilis appears to have increased considerably, and in some instances enormously, as these diseases have declined. Indeed, venereal syphilis has been reported in rural areas of some countries where yaws was previously endemic, e.g. Western Samoa, Thailand and New Guinea.[1]

Etiology. The causative agent of syphilis is the spirochete *Treponema pallidum,* a slender spiral organism measuring from 6.0 to 14.0 μm in length and 0.1 to 0.2 μm in width. Its morphology and type of movement are distinctive and distinguish it from the borreliae and leptospirae. It stains pink with Giemsa though with difficulty, and appears black when stained by the silver impregnation method. While alive it is best seen by the use of dark field illumination. The treponema organisms other than *Treponema pallidum* include: *Treponema pertenue,* the causative agent of yaws; *Treponema carateum,* the causative agent of pinta; and the treponemae that cause bejel and other nonvenereal syndromes. These treponematoses have the following characteristics in common:

1. caused by members of the *Treponema* group of spirochetes;
2. subacute and chronic course with intervals of clinical quiescence and relapse;
3. lesions of the skin and bones;
4. presence of the same type of serum antibodies;
5. prompt response to penicillin; and
6. predominant occurrence among persons living in poor hygienic conditions.[2]

Treponema pallidum is extremely susceptible to physical and chemical agents such as heat, drying, soap and water, and even storage at standard refrigerator temperatures. It can be kept frozen at dry ice temperature (−78.5° C; −110° F) for years, however, and still retain its infectiveness. It has not been successfully grown in vitro, but can infect certain animals such as the rabbit, which appears to retain the infection the rest of its life. Monkeys and chimpanzees are also susceptible to *T. pallidum* infections.

Epidemiology. It was estimated in 1948 that at least 2 million cases of syphilis were caused each year by sexual contact. It was further estimated that the annual prevalence was as high as 20 million cases in the world population over 15 years of age.[3] Based on population increases since 1948 and the increasing incidence since 1950 of not less than 3 million cases (with a prevalence of 30 million), a cautious prediction for the present decade is an annual incidence of 4 million cases of early syphilis.[4]

The true incidence of syphilis is not known, however, because of failures to recognize it early and to report it even when diagnosed. Despite the difficulty of obtaining accurate statistical data, it appears that syphilis has been generally decreasing over the past century. Following World War II both syphilis and gonorrhea increased, as often happens during times of stress and social upheaval. The introduction of penicillin, extremely effective in the treatment of syphilis, produced a notable effect on the global incidence of the disease, which decreased in many countries during the decade 1950 to 1959. Toward the end of that period, an increase in early syphilis led to the stated goal of eradication of infectious syphilis in the United States of America. This policy appeared to be succeeding until about 1968, when increasing eradication program costs were not matched by budgetary increases, and program reductions followed. Many factors may have contributed to the increase in early syphilis as 1970 approached. A general complacency toward venereal disease control by the public as well as by health officials was noted, and large movements of people between and within countries and from rural to urban areas, as well as other socioeconomic factors, led to social unrest. These and other factors, coupled with increasing sexual permissiveness and opportunities for sexual encounter, have provided the basis for increased early syphilis. An expected increase in late syphilis as a result of the post–World War II increase in early syphilis did not occur. This was probably due to the excessive use, and misuse, of penicillin to treat other diseases; nevertheless, it affected early or incubating syphilis. Congenital syphilis has also shown a general decrease which reflects the effectiveness of maternal and child health programs – in particular, the serologic screening of pregnant women for syphilis.[5]

In the United States of America, the epidemiology of syphilis has had a more limited scope. Control procedures emphasize treatment and prevention of spread rather than the details of infection in the usual sense of epidemiologic surveillance. Epidemiology in this sense begins with the diagnosed case of infectious syphilis. Using patient interviews by specially chosen and trained interviewers as a method of identifying each contact, all possible persons exposed are located and brought to treatment to prevent disease of the contacts and its spread by them, and to seek the source of the infection. Because of the relatively slow incubation time of syphilis – 10 to 90 days – appropriately timed interviews, contact tracing, and treatment of all contacts can effectively reduce disease incidence.

Pathology. A patient acquires syphilis by direct contact with an infectious lesion. The spirochete is capable of passing through the mucous membrane and the abraded skin and possibly the unbroken skin, as through a hair follicle. The infection remains local and also disseminates throughout the body in a few hours. The pathologic changes of syphilis are primarily of the blood vessels, with resulting endarteritis and periarteritis. The immunologic response of the host determines the scope and severity of the pathologic picture following the introduction of infection. Serologic tests, therefore, will be negative for a week or more after the introduction of the disease.

In primary syphilis a chancre develops at the site of infection as the spirochetes multiply and pass into the lymphatic and perivascular spaces and blood stream. Thus, the disease is systemic from the beginning. Locally and later, as other tissues are involved, mononuclear cells, i.e., lymphocytes and plasma cells, accumulate. The capillaries and lymphatics proliferate, as do all coats of the larger vessels, accompanied by invasion of the walls by the inflammatory infiltrate. The endarteritic process may be so marked as to lead to obliteration of the lumen with resulting thrombosis and small areas of necrosis. *Treponema pallidum* can be identified in the lesions when appropriately stained.[6]

As local healing occurs, the spirochetes survive elsewhere in the body, and from 2 weeks to 6 months later a generalized macular or papular rash develops as a result of the vascular changes described. Changes in the epidermis vary considerably, producing acanthosis with broadening and elongation of the rete ridges, intracellular and intercellular edema of the rete cells, or migration of neutrophils through the epidermis in extreme cases. These changes in secondary syphilis are brought about by the marked endothelial swelling. The lesions are surrounded by a pronounced infiltrate of monocytes, plasma cells and lymphocytes. *Treponema pallidum* may be identified through appropriate staining. The more severe obliterative endarteritis of late syphilis may produce a gumma as a result of extensive tissue destruction accompanied by giant cells and classic granulomatous inflammation. In other instances, the low-grade inflammatory changes accompanied by degeneration and fibrosis are characteristic of cardiovascular or neurologic syphilis.[6, 7]

Immunology. Although predicted histopathologically for some time, the explanation of the immunologic response is now being studied by modern immunologic techniques. Early in the disease (primary and secondary stages) there is a humoral (B-cell) response, as evidenced by the serologic tests for syphilis, but apparently no tissue hypersensitivity. Late syphilis, however, produces a cell-mediated immunologic response (T-cell), as typified by the gumma which is an example of granulomatous inflammation histopathologically.

Clinical Characteristics. PRIMARY SYPHILIS. The characteristic lesion of primary syphilis is the chancre (Figs. 16–1, 16–2). Following introduction of infection there is a 3- to 4-week incubation period which may, however, vary from 10 days to 3 months. The chancre characteristically appears at the portal of entry as a single eroded papule a few mm to 1 to 2 cm in diameter; it is firm, indurated and painless unless secondarily infected. The border is raised and firm. Extragenital lesions occur in about 10 per cent of cases and may be tender (Fig. 16–3). The regional lymph nodes are frequently enlarged and hard, but painless (satellite bubo). Dark field examination of the aspirate of a lymph node may aid in the diagnosis when adequate material is not obtainable from the chancre itself. Most lesions appear on the penis or the vulva. In females, however, lesions of the vagina and cervix may be missed unless looked for. Extragenital lesions in both sexes appear mostly on the lips but may occur in the mouth or on the tongue, tonsils, breasts, fingers or anus. As a result of homosexual activity, anorectal syphilis is increasingly noted. Because syphilis is a systemic disease from the beginning, it is not

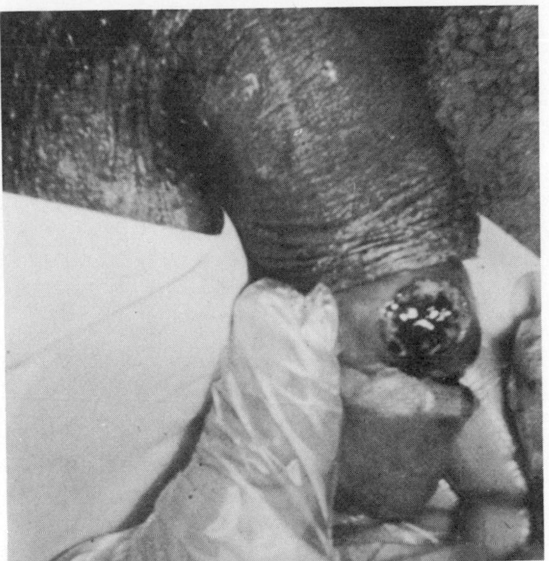

Figure 16–1. Primary syphilis. Typical chancre located at the coronal sulcus. (Courtesy of Public Health Service. 1968. Publication No. 1660; Syphilis – A Synopsis. p. 46.)

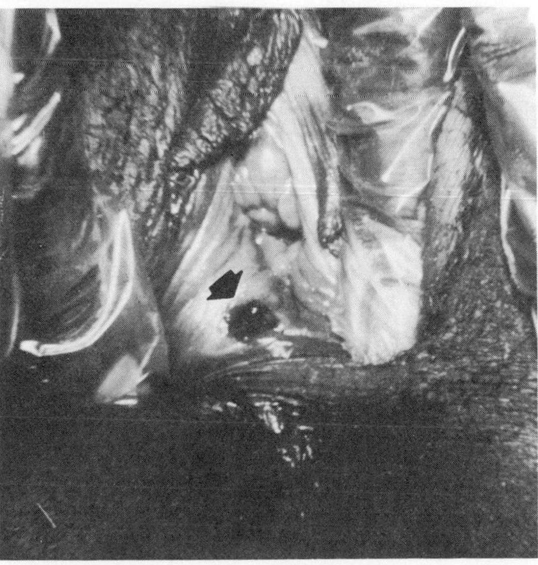

Figure 16–2. Primary syphilis. Chancre of fourchette. (Courtesy of Public Health Service. 1968. Publication No. 1660: Syphilis – A Synopsis. p. 46.)

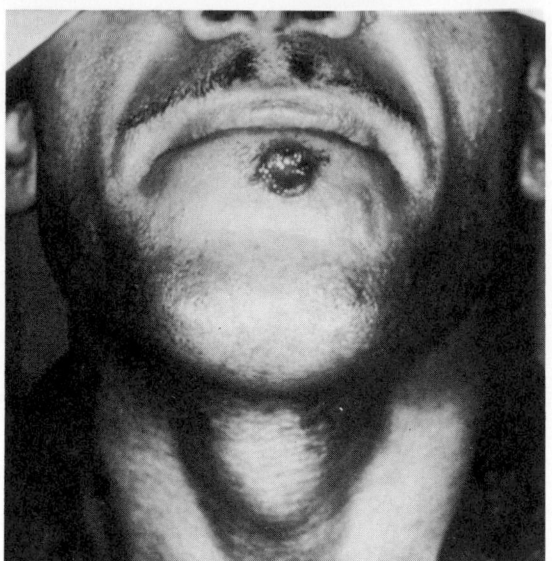

Figure 16–3. Primary syphilis. Typical Hunterian chancre on lower lip. (Courtesy of Public Health Service. 1968. Publication No. 1660:Syphilis—A Synopsis. p. 51.)

surprising that about 25 per cent of patients, especially women, have associated systemic symptoms such as headache, pyrexia, joint pains, malaise and anemia. After 1 to 5 weeks the lesion heals spontaneously, and because there is no tissue hypersensitivity, residual damage is minimal.[7]

SECONDARY SYPHILIS. A cutaneous eruption occurs approximately 6 weeks (2 weeks to 6 months) after the chancre heals, although it may occur before then. Secondary syphilis may be suspected on the basis of the skin and mucous membrane lesions. Such lesions may never be clinically apparent, or may vary from minimal and transient even to the characteristic symmetric eruption, which may be macular, papular, follicular, papulosquamous or pustular but never vesicular or bullous (Fig. 16–4). The lesions are usually dry and do not itch. Moist lesions may occur around the genitalia, anus, mouth, or moist folds of the skin such as the axillae and breasts; these lesions may become fleshy and vegetative (condylomata lata). A generalized lymphadenopathy is an important clinical sign in secondary syphilis and there may be associated splenomegaly. *Treponema pallidum* is more easily identified in the moist lesions, but diagnosis for all practical purposes may be made on the basis of the characteristic skin and mucous membrane lesions and high-titer serologic reactivity. A history of a chancre-like lesion is most indicative. After 2 to 6 weeks, the eruption heals spontaneously and enters a quiescent or latent stage in which there are no clinical signs or symptoms. In about 25 per cent of cases there is at least one cutaneous relapse after the secondary eruption heals, determined by the immunologic response of the host. During this period, serologic testing is always reactive.[6]

LATENT SYPHILIS. This stage is characterized by the absence of syphilitic signs and symptoms, which does not imply the absence of disease activity or progression of the disease. The spinal fluid and serologic tests for syphilis are reactive. This stage may last the rest of the patient's life, progress to manifes-

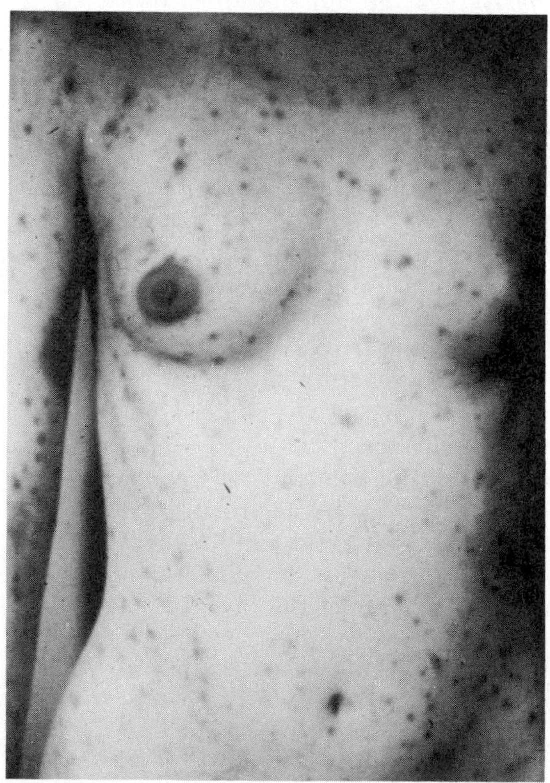

Figure 16–4. Secondary syphilis. Extensive papulosquamous rash on body. (Courtesy of Public Health Service. 1968. Publication No. 1660: Syphilis—A Synopsis. p. 58.)

tations of late syphilis, or end in spontaneous cure. Diagnosis of latent syphilis is usually the result of screening procedures such as job physicals, hospital and clinic admissions, blood donor, or emigration, prenatal or premarital examinations. The World Health Organization defines latent syphilis in two stages: (1) early latent for cases which react serologically in less than 4 years; and (2) late latent for those which react after 4 years. Studies in syphilis epidemiology, however, indicate that only early latent cases of under 1 year's duration produce sufficient infectious syphilis to warrant patient and contact interviewing.[6]

LATE SYPHILIS. Because late syphilis is essentially a vascular disease which may attack any tissue or organ, clinical manifestations may simulate almost any disease. It has thus earned the reputation of the "Great Imitator." Late syphilis was at one time more associated with severe cutaneous and bone lesions, but today cardiovascular and central nervous system manifestations are more frequent.[8] In contrast to the vascular changes of obliterative endarteritis of terminal arterioles and small arteries and the resulting inflammatory and necrotic changes, gumma formation is probably the result of hypersensitivity. When neurosyphilis is suspected, a spinal tap and reagin determination are indicated. The serologic tests for syphilis (VDRL) will be positive, and in late benign syphilis with gumma the serologic test will probably be positive and usually of high titer.[6]

SYPHILIS AND PREGNANCY. Unfortunately, syphilis in the pregnant woman can seriously affect the fetus. Whereas syphilis after 1 year in the nonpregnant patient is not considered infectious and is therefore epidemiologically insignificant, the fetus becomes infected in pregnant females who have had syphilis for more than 1 year. However, the longer the duration of the untreated infection before the pregnancy, the less likely it is that the fetus will be stillborn or infected (Kassowitz's law). Pregnancy that occurs while the mother is in the primary or secondary stages of infection frequently ends in stillbirth; however, when pregnancy occurs during the late stages, it may result in fulminating fatal congenital syphilis. Treponemae are seldom if ever found in fetal tissue before the fourth month of pregnancy. Therefore, treatment before that time will prevent any fetal involvement. Routine serologic testing of prenatal patients has remarkably reduced fetal wastage and congenital syphilis. Testing must be carried out both early and late in pregnancy, in order to insure treatment of infection in the mother occurring during her pregnancy. A serologic reaction in the newborn, if due to passive transfer from the mother, should revert to nonreactive by 3 to 4 months of age. If it does not, active infection of the newborn is strongly indicated. A rising titer is diagnostic.[6]

Diagnosis. PRIMARY SYPHILIS. Positive diagnosis of primary syphilis is made by finding *T. pallidum* through dark field examination of serum from the chancre or of aspirate from a regional lymph node. A presumptive diagnosis can be made from the presence of a genital or other suspicious lesion with regional lymphadenopathy, a reactive serologic test, and a history of sexual activity within the previous 1 to 3 months. The longer the chancre has been present, the more likely the serology will be positive.[6]

SECONDARY SYPHILIS. Secondary syphilis should be suspected on the basis of the skin and mucous membrane eruption described. *Treponema pallidum* may not be demonstrated in dry lesions by dark field microscopy, but may be present in moist lesions. These lesions, combined with a high-titer seroreaction, are diagnostic for all practical purposes. A history of a chancre-like lesion may be helpful.[6]

Treatment. With the introduction of penicillin for the treatment of syphilis, the possibility of cure was realized and the ideas of control or eradication became meaningful for the first time. Penicillin continues to be the drug of choice in the treatment of syphilis. The following schedule has been recommended.[6]

For primary, secondary and latent syphilis, a total of 2.4 million units of benzathine penicillin G is administered by intramuscular injection (1.2 million units in each buttock).

If procaine penicillin G in oil with aluminum monostearate (PAM) is used, a dose of 2.4 million units should be given in two sites on the first visit and 1.2 million units should be given on each of two subsequent visits 3 days apart (total, 4.8 million units).

Aqueous procaine penicillin G (APPG) may also be given, for a total of 4.8 million units (600,000 units daily for 8 days).

Erythromycin, 500 mg orally 4 times daily for 20 days (40 gm total dose), may be substituted when the patient is allergic to penicillin. Tetracycline hydrochloride, 500 mg orally 4 times daily for 15 days (30 gm total dose), may also be substituted.

Late syphilis requires the administration of 6 to 9 million units of benzathine penicillin G, 3 million units initially and once or twice thereafter at weekly intervals. PAM and APPG may be given in a similar total dose at the rate of 1.2 million units every 3 days (PAM) or 600,000 units a day (APPG). Congenital syphilis should be treated with proportionate dosages according to age and weight.

Prognosis. If left untreated, approximately one-third of the people with syphilis will develop late destructive lesions of syphilis. Up to 23 per cent of the entire group can be expected to die primarily as the result of the disease. Approximately two-thirds of the cases, though infected, will experience minimal or no physical inconvenience. Over one-half of this latter group will remain serologically positive for life. Occasionally, late manifestations occur but show no reactivity in standard blood tests.[6]

Treatment, however, alters both the clinical course and the serologic pattern of syphilis. No seropositivity should result if treatment is instituted before appearance of the chancre. Treatment given in the secondary stage leads to seronegativity within 18 months in 90 to 95 per cent of cases. Treatment administered after 2 years or more of disease may leave the patient seropositive for life despite clinical cure.[6]

Prophylaxis and Control. Individual prevention, other than sexual abstinence, has not been demonstrated to be of routine value. In the absence of an effective vaccine against syphilis, the use of a condom by the male and washing thoroughly with soap and water after sexual contact may be of some value. A therapeutic injection of penicillin should prevent the development of syphilis in some cases. Treatment of acute gonorrhea has been shown to be effective in preventing incubating syphilis from developing. In any event, individual prevention will be determined by the person's knowledge and understanding of the potential of the disease and his willingness to seek medical attention. Health education at some stage of his life will thus have been of benefit.

Syphilis is a controllable disease, and can sometimes be considered an eradicable one. The total and effective execution of all components of an ideal program will vary from country to country and depend on the available resources. The elements of a control program are listed below.[9]

1. *Evaluation of the problem.* This is the determination of the actual situation based on information from hospitals, private and public clinics, and laboratories; from examination of workers, police, military, students and others; and from screening programs carried out in maternal and child health units and family planning clinics.

2. *Diagnosis and treatment services.* This component is the basis of any syphilis control program. Such services should be conveniently organized for the patient as well as the staff, and free or within the reach of all needing care. The stereotype concept of the "V.D. Clinic" should be encouraged to pass from sight.

3. *Laboratories.* These must be convenient for patient and doctor for the early and accurate diagnosis of syphilis. There should be at least a central laboratory for confirmatory tests such as the FTA-ABS or TPHA (*Treponema pallidum* hemagglutination) test when the cardiolipin antigen (VDRL) test is in question. A central laboratory must also carry out quality control tests of the other laboratories, and all should be actively engaged in providing service for syphilis screening programs.

4. *Data registry system.* Such a system is necessary for individual patient care, for cross reference to prevent reduplication of diagnoses, and for consolidation of information of all cases and all contacts.

5. *Serologic case finding.* This part of the program is essential if the infectious reservoir is to be more precisely defined. It should be carried out continually among persons who are frequently at risk, especially pregnant women, military personnel, seamen, homosexuals and prostitutes.

6. *Health education.* This must be directed to the general public, high-risk groups, and professional personnel involved in the diagnosis, treatment and prevention of the disease.

7. *Case reporting.* Directed at all physicians, laboratories and medical care centers, the goal of case reporting is to improve the statistical basis of subsequent epidemiologic studies, disease control and program evaluation.

8. *Case interview and contact tracing.* These activities are carried out by specially selected and trained persons for the purpose of early case finding in order to reduce, through preventive treatment, the infectious reservoir.

9. *Periodic program evaluation.* Only through evaluation of programs and the transmission of their results to management can changes be implemented which can continually improve the total program effort.

REFERENCES

1. Guthe, T., Ridet, J., Vorst, F., D'Costa, J., and Grab, B. 1972. Methods for the surveillance of endemic treponematoses and sero-immunological investigations of "disappearing" disease. Bull. W.H.O. *46*:1–14.
2. Turner, T. B. 1965. The Spirochetes. *In*: Dubos, R. J., and Hirsch, J. G. Bacterial and Mycotic Infections of Man. 4th ed. J. B. Lippincott Co., Philadelphia. pp. 573–609.
3. Guthe, T., and Hume, J. 1948. Quoted by Llopis, A. 1971. The Problem of the Venereal Diseases in the Americas. P.A.H.O./W.H.O. Sci. Publ. No. 220. pp. 20–21.
4. Llopis, A. 1971. The Problem of the Venereal Diseases in the Americas. P.A.H.O./W.H.O. Sci. Publ. No. 220. p. 21.
5. Guthe, T. 1971. Worldwide Epidemiological Trends in Syphilis and Gonorrhea. P.A.H.O./W.H.O. Sci. Publ. No. 220. p. 4.
6. U.S.P.H.S. 1968. Syphilis: A Synopsis. P.H.S. Publ. No. 1660. U.S. Government Printing Office, Washington, D.C., 1967. 133 pp.
7. Schofield, C. B. S. 1972. Sexually Transmitted Diseases. Churchill Livingstone, Edinburgh and London. pp. 46–47.
8. Olansky, S., and Shaffer, L. W. 1968. Syphilis. *In*: Top, F. H., Sr. Communicable Diseases. 6th ed. The C. V. Mosby Co., St. Louis. pp. 604–619.
9. Miranda, D. M., Latimer, K. P., and Brubaker, M. L. 1973. Alternative designs and methods for venereal disease control programs. Bull. P.A.H.O. *3*:1–8.

CHAPTER 17

Yaws and Endemic Syphilis

MERLIN L. BRUBAKER

Yaws

Synonyms. Framboesia, pian, bouba parangi, domaria, domaru khahu.

Definition. Yaws is an acute and chronic relapsing, infectious, contagious, nonvenereal, spirochetal disease caused by *Treponema pertenue.* It is characterized by three stages: an initial ulcer or granulomatous cutaneous lesion, the "mother yaw"; nondestructive secondary lesions of the skin, bones and periosteum; and, finally, destructive deforming lesions of the skin, bones and periosteum. Onset is rare before the age of 18 months. The disease may extend over 40 years or more, causing ill health and disability. Infection produces a slowly developing relative immunity.[1]

Distribution. Yaws is restricted to the tropical zones, where it has been widely distributed in many areas of the world. It is especially prevalent in hot, moist, lowland countries. It has been common in the Caribbean Islands, tropical America, throughout equatorial Africa, Sri Lanka, Malaya, Burma, Thailand, Laos, Cambodia, Vietnam, Indonesia, and in the Philippines, Samoa, and other Pacific islands. It is also present in northern Australia but is relatively uncommon in India and China. The incidence of yaws has been markedly altered in some of these areas by eradication campaigns conducted by national governments and the World Health Organization.

Etiology. The etiologic agent, *T. pertenue,* is a rigid, spiral organism with attenuated extremities which is morphologically indistinguishable from *T. pallidum.* Infection is accompanied by positive serologic reactions, as in syphilis. The organism has not been grown in artificial culture media. It is present in great numbers in the discharges from open primary and secondary lesions.

Epidemiology. For many years there was a sharp difference of opinion as to the identity of yaws and syphilis. The generally accepted view, however, holds that yaws is due to infection by a different but closely related organism. It has frequently been observed that syphilis is rare or unknown among populations in which yaws is prevalent.

There are important clinical and epidemiologic differences between the two diseases. Yaws is not a venereal disease; it is not congenital and is predominantly a disease of childhood. Transmission from child to mother by contact reportedly is frequent.[2] The primary lesion of yaws is almost invariably extragenital and is similar to the lesions of the secondary stage of the disease. In moist skin areas, however, the "mother yaw" may closely resemble a chancroid.

Yaws is a disease strictly of the tropical zones. In the colder climates within the tropics it occurs in modified form, and it does not spread when introduced into the temperate zones. The incidence is highest among native populations whose level of personal hygiene is low, and Europeans are rarely infected. It is more common in men than in women.

The spirochetes are unable to penetrate unbroken skin, and infection occurs directly through contact of cuts, abrasions or other cutaneous lesions with an open yaws lesion on another individual, or indirectly through soiling of the broken skin with contaminated material. It is commonly communicated by person to person contact, and primary yaws in an adult is usually confined to nursing mothers who are infected by their infants.

Flies, especially species of *Hippelates,* may be mechanical vectors in some areas. In general, however, insects are of minor importance in transmission.

Yaws tends to be a seasonal disease. Cases presenting the lesions of the primary and the secondary stages are much more numerous during the rainy season than at any other time of year.

Climate and environment influence the clinical forms of yaws. The spottiness of yaws, especially in its late stage (rhinopharyngitis militans), known as gangosa, is remarkable. In the highlands of the Philippines, Assam, Sumatra, South Africa, and other regions, polypapillomas on the naked skin are rare. On the other hand, condylomas caused by yaws are frequently encountered in folds of the skin where it is moist, warm and slightly irritated by perspiration and attrition.

The disease is favored by situations where huts are crowded, clothing scant, feet bare and soap absent. The cases decrease with improvement in socioeconomic standards.[3]

Based upon immunologic studies, the belief has been expressed that *T. pertenue* infection exists in baboons and monkeys in West Africa.[4]

Pathology. The most characteristic pathologic feature of yaws is the predominant involvement of the skin. The organisms are most abundant in the epidermis.

The cutaneous lesions consist of granulomatous papules and macules. In the papules, or framboesiform lesions, the epidermis is greatly thickened by epithelial hyperplasia, by cellular infiltration, and by exudation of serum. The papillae are elongated and infiltrated, and hyperplasia and thickening of the interpapillary pegs often occur. The infiltration consists of plasma cells, lymphocytes, polymorphonu-

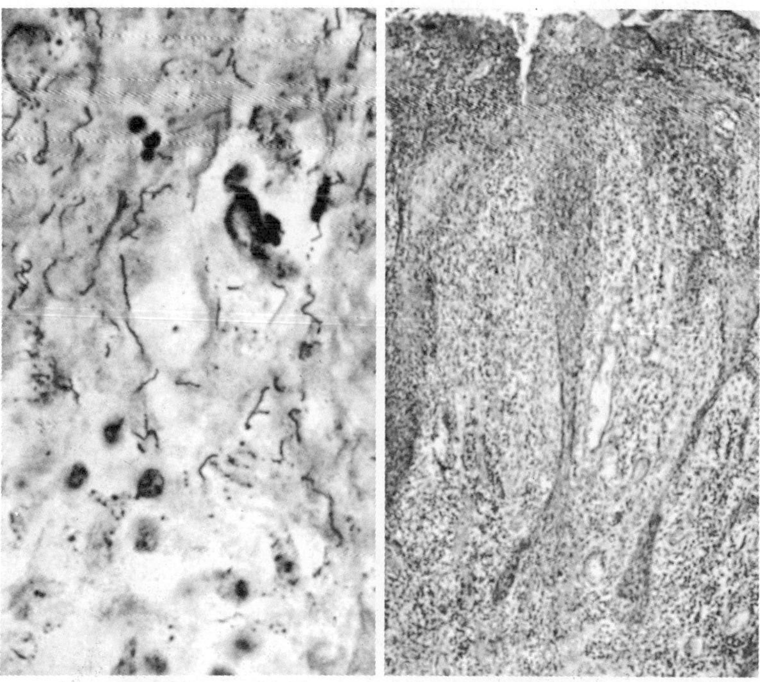

Figure 17-1 **Figure 17-2**

Figure 17-1. *Treponema pertenue* in epidermis.

Figure 17-2. Papular lesion of yaws showing thickening of epidermis, elongation and infiltration of papillae and hyperplasia of interpapillary pegs.

clear leukocytes, eosinophils and some increase of large mononuclear cells and fibroblasts. Perivascular cell accumulations in the corium are not so characteristic as in syphilis (Figs. 17–1, 17–2).

This process, leading to the formation of a smooth papule, may be followed by hyperkeratosis of the overlying epithelium and by superficial erosion. The eroded lesion exudes a yellowish secretion which dries to form a crust. The underlying ulcer is shallow and sharply defined, and the floor of granulation tissue bleeds easily. Progressive overgrowth of granulation tissue then produces the characteristic fungating, more or less ulcerated framboesiform lesion, which is covered with a dirty yellow crust of dried exudate. The epidermis at the margin of the granuloma is thickened and contains many spirochetes.

The later lesions of the disease include ulcerating granulomatous nodules of the skin and subcutaneous tissues and indolent ulcers (Fig. 17–3). Invasion of skeletal tissues produces osteitis and periostitis leading to bone deformities. Less often there may be extensive destructive lesions of the nose and hard palate, producing the condition known as gangosa (Fig. 17–4). A spindle-cell carcinoma, regarded as malignant degeneration of an old yaws ulcer, has been reported.[5]

Clinical Characteristics. After an incubation period of 2 to 8 weeks, the initial lesion appears at the site of implantation of the spirochete, usually at some pre-existing break in the skin. This "mother yaw" resembles the typical granulomatous secondary lesion, except that it is often larger and spontaneous healing is less rapid. It is frequently present when the secondary eruption appears. When it is superimposed on a pre-existing ulcer, a more extensive and ulcerating lesion is produced. The development of the primary yaw is accompanied by moderate systemic symptoms, aching of the limbs and joint pains, and often there is irregular fever. There may be enlargement of the regional lymph nodes.

The secondary or generalized stage of the disease begins a few weeks to 4 months after the appearance of the initial lesion. Secondary lesions usually appear as elevated, apparently granulomatous, papules scattered over the surface of the body. These vary from a few to 50 mm or more in diameter and tend to be round or oval. At first the

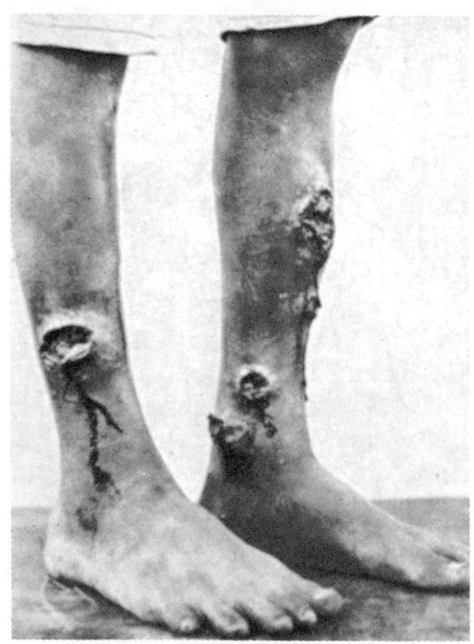

Figure 17–3

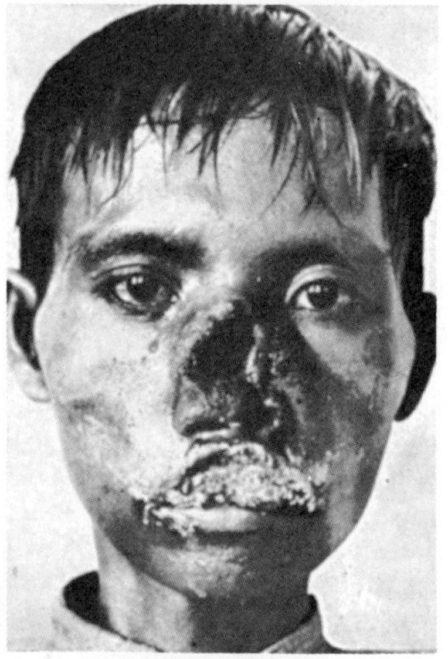

Figure 17–4

Figure 17–3. Yaws: chronic ulcers and periostitis.
Figure 17–4. Gangosa.

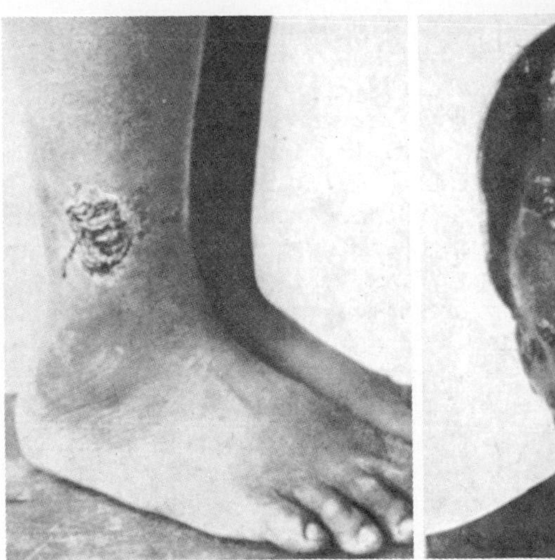

Figure 17–5

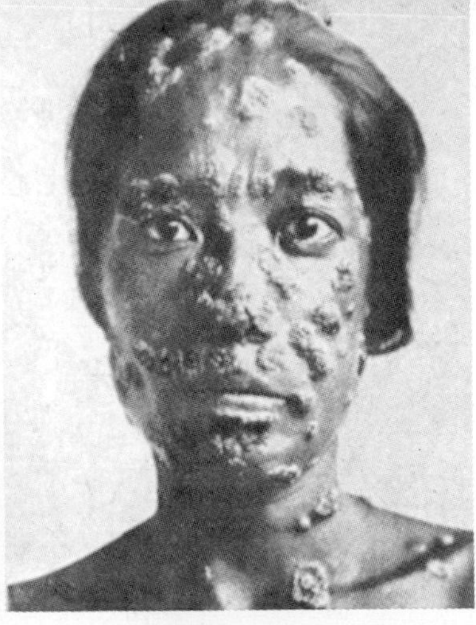

Figure 17–6

Figure 17–5. The primary lesion or mother yaw.
Figure 17–6. Yaws: framboesiform lesions in a Filipino.

surface is composed of greatly proliferated epithelium exuding clear serum which contains great numbers of spirochetes. Later, a crust develops, yellow at first but becoming discolored by debris. In young children suffering from anemia or malnutrition the lesions may not be elevated but appear as erosions with bright pink borders and whitish centers. The eruption may involve the palms of the hands or the soles of the feet. The plantar lesions are painful and disabling.

Successive eruptions often appear before the preceding ones heal. The later lesions tend to be most numerous about the lips, axillae, genitalia and anus. Although typical generalized secondary lesions probably do not occur more than 2 to 3 years after the primary eruption, secondary lesions about the lips or on the soles of the feet may recur after many years (Figs. 17–5, 17–6).

In cooler environments the skin lesions may be restricted to condyloma-like processes limited to the perianal, perineal and axillary regions. Healing of the secondary lesions leaves only slight scarring, and the scars are never permanently atrophic and pigmented.

Nondestructive lesions of the bones are frequent in the secondary stage. The characteristic changes are focal rarefactions – rarefying osteitis and periostitis. These develop rapidly and usually resolve spontaneously in a few weeks or months. The rarefaction disappears, but the periosteal reaction may lead to thickening of the bone. Goundou and saber shin may be the result of this process (Fig. 17–7).

The tertiary stage of yaws commonly does not appear until after a relatively or completely symptom-free interval of several years. A negative VDRL test during this quiescent period indicates termination of the infection. A positive reaction is an indication of latency.

The appearance of tertiary lesions is the only evidence of the beginning of the final stage. These destructive changes do not occur in the presence of the secondary eruption. Although they may develop within a few years after infection, they reach their highest incidence in the third and fourth decades of life. In this stage resolution and spontaneous cure may occur, or the disease may again become latent, with the subsequent appearance of relapsing tertiary lesions.

The lesions of the skin are characteristically of three types. There may be extensive, spreading, superficial, and relatively clean ulceration, ultimately healing from the

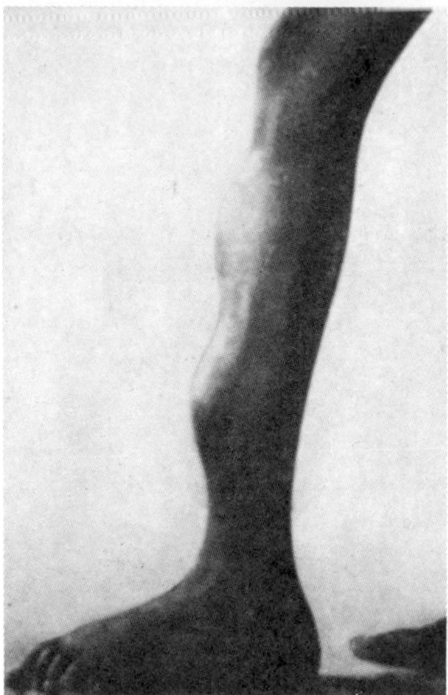

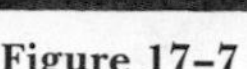

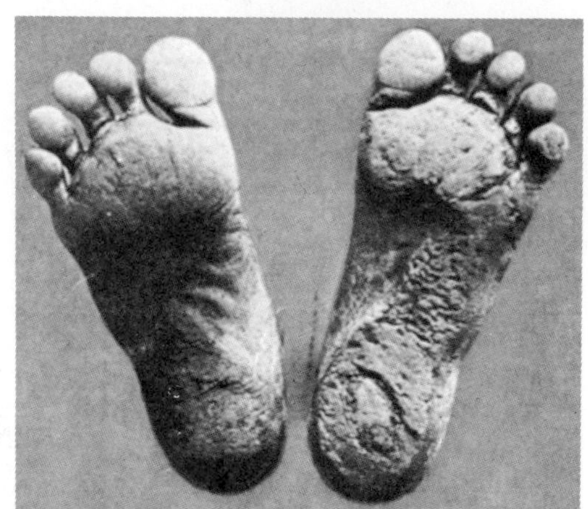

Figure 17–7 Figure 17–8

Figure 17–7. Saber shin of late yaws. (Courtesy of Dr. Alan Fisher, for the Office of the Coordinator of Inter-American Affairs.)

Figure 17–8. Yaws: hyperkeratosis with fissuring of the soles of feet; "crab yaws."

center. Cutaneous and subcutaneous nodules develop, which break down to form deep indolent ulcers with irregular bases. Spirochetes cannot usually be demonstrated. Healing proceeds from the margin and from isolated islands in the base, producing atrophic scars. These may be unpigmented in the early stages but later are often deeply pigmented and may cause severe contractures. Hyperkeratotic lesions of the soles of the feet and less commonly of the palms of the hands cause extensive thickening of the skin with fissuring and ulceration. These "crab yaws" are painful and the source of severe disability (Fig. 17–8). In different parts of the world they constitute from 40 to 90 per cent of all yaws cases. They are most common in young adults, particularly men, and develop especially during the rainy season and after trauma.

Destructive bone and periosteal lesions are frequent. They resemble the gumma of syphilis and are usually single or few in number. These lesions develop slowly and may extend through the subcutaneous tissues and the skin to produce chronic ulceration which responds only slowly to treatment. They are accompanied by local swelling, tenderness and pain. The tibia, other long bones and the bones of the hands are most commonly involved. Less frequently lesions occur in the tarsal and carpal bones, the skull, clavicles, scapulae and sternum. Involvement of the hard palate leads to perforation, and the process may progress, causing extensive destruction of the structures of the nose to produce gangosa (Fig. 17–4). Joint lesions are not uncommon, and fibromatous tumors in the vicinity of the appendicular joints—juxta-articular nodules—are often associated with the late lesions of yaws. The nodules are painless, symmetrically placed and higher in incidence in males over 30 years than in younger men. The differentiation of juxta-articular nodules of yaws from those due to *Onchocerca volvulus* does not present a problem except when the lesions occur in the region of the sacrum, trochanters and knees.[6]

Diagnosis. The diagnosis of yaws may often be made on clinical grounds, as the typical generalized lesions are not easily confused with other diseases. Confirmation is made by the demonstration of spirochetes in a dark field examination of exudate from the lesion, or by a smear stained by Giemsa's method. Spirochetes may likewise be demonstrated by India ink preparations. The serologic tests for syphilis, i.e. VDRL, FTA–ABS, TPI and TPHA, are positive, but such tests of the cerebrospinal fluid are usually negative.[7]

The lesions of mucocutaneous leishmaniasis may be confused with the nasopharyngeal manifestations of yaws. Similarly, ulcerating lesions of leprosy and tuberculosis may present differential diagnostic problems, the solution of which will depend upon demonstration of the specific etiologic agents. The accurate differentiation of yaws from other conditions becomes increasingly important as eradication campaigns approach success. Many cases reported as failures proved to be due to infections other than yaws.[8]

The differential diagnosis between late lesions of yaws and syphilis, especially those affecting bony structures, may be extremely difficult if not impossible, especially when the serology is positive and the patient comes from an endemic or formerly endemic area. The history and presence of a scar from a healed "mother yaw" are important.

Treatment. The response of early infectious yaws to antibiotic therapy is dramatic, and total eradication of the disease is now possible. The use of arsenical drugs and bismuth is no longer recommended.

PRIMARY AND SECONDARY YAWS. Penicillin is the drug of choice in the treatment of infectious yaws. One injection of procaine penicillin in 2 per cent aluminum monostearate and oil (PAM), in doses of not less than 1,200,000 units for adults and proportionately less for children, is recommended for treatment of the usual case. Benzathine penicillin can also be used. The response to this therapy is very rapid. The infectious lesions become dark-field negative within 48 hours, and healing is complete within 1 week. Serologic titers decline rapidly, but a substantial group of patients may show a low titer for several months following therapy. Serologic tests should be repeated at 3-month intervals and the treatment repeated if the serologic findings remain positive after 6 months.

TERTIARY YAWS. The late lesions of yaws are much more resistant, and repeated therapy may be required to accomplish healing and render the patient serologically negative. In addition to penicillin, the broad spectrum antibiotics may be effective.

Oxytetracycline and chlortetracycline have been found to be of great value in the treatment of indolent ulcerations, gummas and deforming osteoperiostitis. These drugs are given orally, 2 gm daily for 5 to 10 days in adults and proportionately smaller doses in children. Oxytetracycline, given intramuscularly 150 mg once daily, may be of value when extensive lesions are resistant to penicillin, or the broad spectrum antibiotics may be given orally in such cases.

Ulcerations of late yaws should be treated concomitantly with local antiseptic dressings. The hypertrophied nasal bones of goundou must be excised surgically. Other deformities, such as contractures or chronic osteitis, may also necessitate surgical relief, either plastic operations or amputation, although the response of such advanced lesions to chemotherapy alone is sometimes satisfactory if the pathologic process is still in an active stage.

Control. The primary objective of yaws control campaigns is to eliminate the infectious primary and secondary lesions from the population; it is not necessarily to effect radical cure of the disease. A single injection of penicillin has proved to be completely effective for such control operations, and should include all contacts of a known case. Epidemiologic surveillance in the latter stages can then assure the eradication of yaws.

Prophylaxis. The prevention of yaws consists essentially of avoidance of infected contacts and the adequate protection of open infectious lesions. In areas where the disease is endemic, mass therapy constitutes an important control measure. No methods of artificial immunization are available.

Endemic Syphilis

Synonyms. Bejel (Syria), bishel (Iraq), belesh (Arabia), dichuchwa (Bechuanaland), njovera (Rhodesia), skerljevo or frenga (Bosnia), nonvenereal syphilis.

Definition. Endemic syphilis is an infectious, chronic, nonvenereal treponemal infection of the intermediate tropical and temperate climates. Lesions are concentrated on moist areas such as the mouth, axilla, inguinal area and rectum.[9] Onset is during early childhood and spread is by direct body contact. Primary lesions are seldom observed. The late stage may be evident within a few years after onset or may be delayed for many years. Inflammatory and destructive lesions of the skin, long bones and nasopharynx are late manifestations; the nervous and cardiovascular systems are rarely involved. Congenital transmission is almost unknown. Endemic syphilis has a negligible case fatality. The disease is known by a variety of names, depending upon the geographic area. Previously some of these have been considered as distinct disease entities but are now generally accepted as endemic or nonvenereal.

It is the firm conviction of some authorities that venereal syphilis and endemic (nonvenereal) syphilis are the same disease. However, these two forms of syphilis constitute distinct and easily distinguished syndromes.

Distribution. Endemic syphilis occurs in localized areas in backward regions where socioeconomic levels are low and advanced education is lacking. It is present in the Balkans, Turkey, the eastern Mediterranean countries, and along the desert borders (dry savannahs) of northern Africa. A similar, if not identical, nonvenereal treponematosis has been reported from India. The dry areas where endemic syphilis is present are in contrast to the moist jungle areas where yaws is endemic. Endemic syphilis has not been positively identified in the Western Hemisphere. The number of persons affected by nonvenereal syphilis may be higher than those affected by venereal syphilis; hence, the importance of venereal syphilis would be surpassed, if based upon the number of cases.[10, 11]

Etiology. The etiologic agent, a *Treponema* (presumably *T. pallidum*), is a rigid, spiral organism with attenuated extremities and is morphologically indistinguishable from *T. pertenue,* the causative agent for yaws. As in venereal syphilis, infection is accompanied by positive serologic reactions. *Treponema pallidum* (?) may be recovered from lesions and wound aspirates.

Epidemiology. As in venereal syphilis, man is the reservoir of infection for the endemic form. Nonvenereal syphilis is usually a disease of childhood, spread by direct body contact among children and adults in primitive areas where few, if any, clothes are worn and soap is unknown. Every member of the family may be infected eventually, or even entire communities in backward regions where crowded housing and poor personal hygiene exist. The common drinking cup has been incriminated in mechanical transmission because the buccal mucous junctions are frequently infected. Incidence of endemic syphilis decreases as socioeconomic standards are improved. When modern civilization reaches endemic areas through the construction of a highway or the development of an oil field, endemic syphilis disappears and venereal syphilis appears.[10]

Pathology. The most characteristic pathologic feature is the predominant involvement of the skin. It is characterized by the destructive gummas of the skin and bones. Late plantar and palmar lesions, patchy pigmentation of the skin, and destructive lesions of the long bones, nose and throat are common. Eyes are rarely affected. Cardiovascular lesions occur with some frequency; involvement of the central nervous system is rare; tabes and paresis are virtually unknown.[11] Primary lesions consist of eruptions of the skin or mucous membranes, though they are seldom recognized. Eruptions in the mouth are usually first, followed by moist papules in folds of skin. Primary skin lesions often resemble those of venereal syphilis in being hypertrophic, circinate, and even maculopapular. Genital, perineal and perianal condylomas are very common. Periostitis commonly occurs, and adenopathy of the superficial chains invariably occurs.[11] The late stage may appear within a few years after onset or may be delayed for many years, when inflammatory and destructive lesions of skin, long bones, and nasopharynx are evident. Plantar and palmar hyperkeratoses are associated with painful fissuring and patchy depigmentation or hyperpigmentation of the skin. Juxta-articular nodules have been noted frequently in late cases.

Diagnosis. Diagnosis is made on clinical grounds and may be confirmed by demonstrating the organism in wound aspirates. While the serologic tests for venereal syphilis are positive in the endemic form, the results of spinal fluid examination are normal.

Treatment. Treatment with long-acting penicillin is curative, using the same dosage schedules as for yaws (p. 159).

Control. Measures for control and eradication of yaws should be effective for the control of endemic syphilis. Control measures should be on a family and a communitywide basis.[11]

REFERENCES

1. Anonymous. 1963. Bibliography of Yaws. 1905–1962. World Health Organization, Geneva. 106 pp.
2. Lees, R. E. M. 1973. A selective approach to yaws control. Can. J. Public Health *64*:52–56.
3. Saxena, V. B., and Prasad, B. G. 1963. An epidemiological study of yaws in Madhya Pradesh. Indian J. Med. Res. Pt. I, Historical and geographical, *51*:768–783; Pt. II, Social and cultural aspects, *51*:784–804; Pt. III, Economic aspects, *51*:805–820.
4. Mollaret, H. H., and Fribourg-Blanc, A. 1967. Le singe serait-il réservoir du pian? Méd. Afr. Noire *14*:397–399.
5. Furtado, T. A., and Battista, G. 1962. Karzinomatöse entartung alter frambösie-ulcera. Ztschr. Tropenmed. Parasit. *13*:198–201.
6. Browne, S. G. 1961. Juxta-articular nodules in yaws. A clinical study of 210 cases. Ann. Trop. Med. Parasit. *55*:309–313.
7. Garner, M. F., Backhouse, J. L., Cook, C. A., and Roeder, P. J. 1970. Fluorescent treponemal antibody absorption (FTA-ABS) test in yaws. Br. J. Vener. Dis. *46*:284–286.
8. Hackett, C. J., and Loewenthal, L. J. A. 1960. Differential diagnosis of yaws. W.H.O. Monogr. Ser. No. 45, Geneva. 88 pp.
9. Cahill, K. M. 1964. Treponematosis and rickettsiosis. N.Y. State J. Med. *64*:647–650.
10. Koch, R. A. 1964. Late syphilis: modern concepts and treatment. J. Am. Geriatr. Soc. *12*:255–261.
11. Hudson, E. H. 1961. Endemic syphilis – heir of the syphiloids. Arch. Intern. Med. *108*:1–4.

CHAPTER 18

Pinta

MERLIN L. BRUBAKER

Synonyms. Mal del pinto, carate, azul, boussarole, tina, lota, empeines.

Definition. Pinta is an acute and chronic nonvenereal treponematosis caused by *Treponema carateum.* The disease is characterized by a superficial nonulcerative primary lesion, a secondary eruption and late depigmentation and hyperkeratosis of the skin. Pinta is limited almost exclusively to dark-skinned races, but light- or dark-colored persons can acquire it if they live in close contact with infected persons. The hands and wrists are involved most frequently, although other common sites are the feet and ankles.

Distribution. Pinta is a disease primarily of the Western Hemisphere, occurring in many parts of the American tropics. It has been especially prevalent in parts of tropical America such as Mexico, Colombia, Venezuela, Bolivia, Brazil, Peru, Ecuador, Chile, Central America and Cuba.

Etiology. Formerly thought to be a superficial mycosis, pinta is now known to be caused by a spirochete morphologically identical with that of syphilis. The organism, *Treponema carateum* Brumpt *(Treponema herrejoni* León y Blanco), has not been cultivated (Fig. 18–1). Recently the disease has been successfully inoculated into chimpanzees.[1]

Epidemiology. The method of spread is unknown. *Treponema carateum* has been found in the fluid oozing from fissures in hyperkeratotic lesions of the disease, so that direct contact is suggested as the means of infection. Flies feeding on open sores have been suspected of carrying the spirochetes from person to person. There is some evidence which suggests that species of *Simulium* and *Hippelates* may be involved in the transmission of pinta. No evidence of congenital transmission has been reported.

The disease is most frequent in the young and, when the prevalence is high, begins during the first 2 years of life, even in infants a few months old. It occurs most frequently in low-lying and wooded areas,

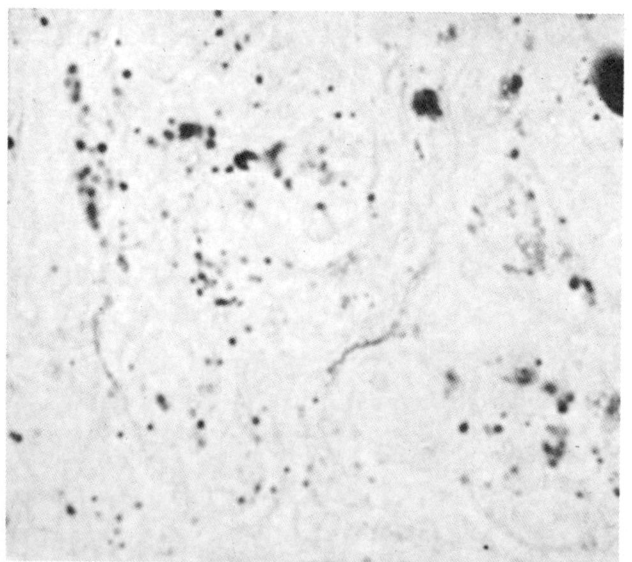

Figure 18–1. Pinta: *Treponema carateum* in epidermis.

usually near to the banks of rivers where temperatures average 26 to 30° C (79 to 86° F) and the relative humidity is 80 per cent or more. The way of life of these people existing in small groups in primitive conditions and wearing few clothes appears to promote the conditions necessary for them to contract pinta. The importance of close prolonged contact of healthy persons with infected persons as in a family situation is supported by experimental observation. It is possible to live in a highly endemic area and not get pinta if contact with infectious persons is avoided.[2]

Pathology. The epidermis and corium are both involved in a low-grade inflammation that results in (1) a disturbance of the melanophores and (2) a thickening of the corium. Spirochetes have been demonstrated in histologic sections of early skin lesions. The liver is normal in size in patients with the late disseminated form of pinta. Spirochetes have not been demonstrated in biopsies of this organ.[3] Neurologic and cardiovascular involvement is reported to be fully as significant in pinta as in venereal syphilis.[4] This is denied by others,[2] however, and it may be impossible to prove these changes are not due to late syphilis. Other visceral lesions or involvement of the long bones have not been observed.

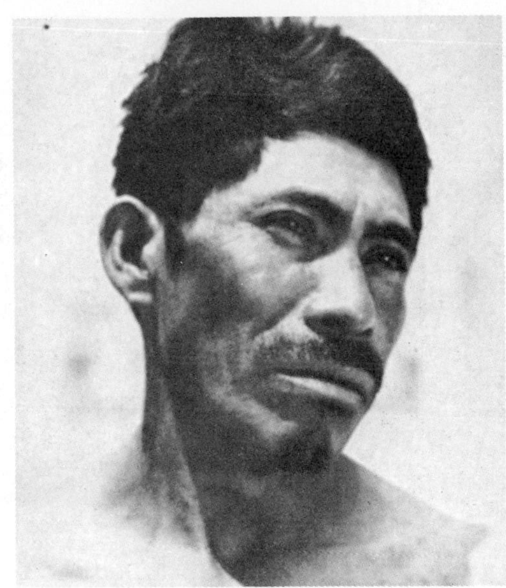

Figure 18-2. Secondary lesion or pintid on right cheek.

Clinical Characteristics. In human volunteers inoculated with lymph from infected areas, the incubation period ranged from 6 to 122 days. Three stages have been described. The first is that of the initial papular lesion. It occurs on the lower extremities in 80 per cent of cases and on the upper extremities in another 10 per cent. The second is characterized by a spreading

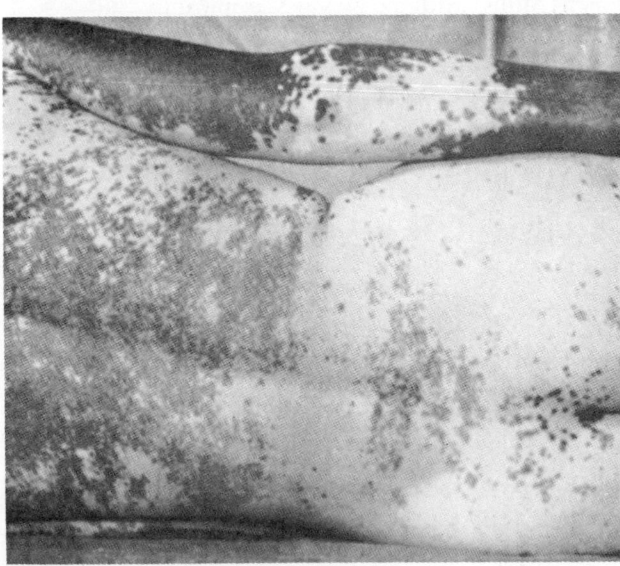

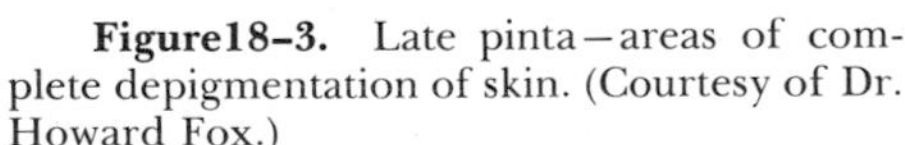

Figure18-3. Late pinta—areas of complete depigmentation of skin. (Courtesy of Dr. Howard Fox.)

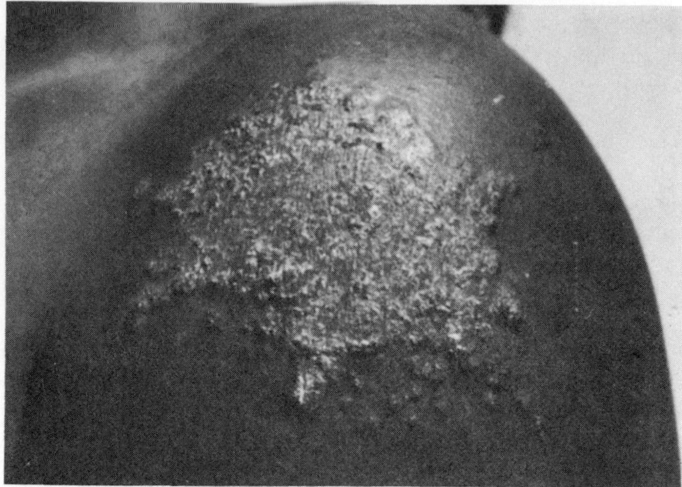

Figure 18-4. Experimental pinta. (Courtesy of Dr. Rafael Medina.)

eruption of flat erythematous lesions known as pintids (Fig. 18-2). In the tertiary stage, which develops in 1 to 2½ years, pigmentary disturbances become manifest, often consisting first of variously colored patches and progressing, finally, to leukoderma (Fig. 18-3). Not infrequently these are symmetrically distributed. Hyperkeratoses appear simultaneously on the palms and soles, causing inconvenience if fissuring occurs. Pinta resembles yaws in having a predilection for the palmar surfaces but not for the mucous membranes. The disease rarely causes disabling illness or death.

Syphilis and early yaws apparently do not confer immunity to pinta. Persons with late yaws reportedly could not be so easily infected with *T. carateum* as in the early stage. Volunteers with pinta appear to develop a certain degree of protection against syphilis[5] (Fig. 18-4).

Diagnosis. Symmetric vitiligo of the hands and possibly of the feet in a dark-skinned native of tropical America is probably pinta. The Wassermann reaction, VDRL, Kolmer and Reiter tests are positive in the tertiary stage.[5] Late pinta may have spinal fluid changes similar to those of venereal syphilis.[4] Eosinophilia is often present. The Chediak test, with a drop of blood and cardiolipin antigen, has proved useful for rural surveys, as has the use of "rondelles" (dried fingerprick blood absorbed by blotting paper disks for FTA testing of the eluent).[6, 7]

Treatment. Penicillin, administered as in syphilis, is specific in the treatment of this disease. Early papular and late pigmented lesions heal promptly, and often the vitiliginous spots, if present less than 5 years, regain pigment after antibiotic therapy.

Prophylaxis. Although the epidemiology of pinta has not been fully studied, it is probable that the measures applicable to yaws are efficient in the control and prevention of this disease.

REFERENCES

1. Kuhn, U. S. G. III, Varela, G., Chandler, F. W., Jr., and Osuna, G. G. 1968. Experimental pinta in the chimpanzee. J.A.M.A. *206*:829.
2. Medina, R. 1965. Pinta, an endemic treponematosis of the Americas. Unpublished W.H.O. Document (INT/VDT/204.65).
3. Sosa Camacho, B. 1960. Exploración histopatológica y treponémica de higado en el mal de pinto. Dermatología *4*:104-112.
4. Koch, R. A. 1964. Late syphilis; modern concepts and treatment. J. Am. Geriatr. Soc. *12*:255-261.
5. Medina, R. 1963. El carate en Venezuela. Dermat. Venezolana *3*:160-230.
6. Varela, G., and Zavala, J. 1961. Microreacción de Chediak con gota de sangre para encuestas de mal de pinta. Rev. Inst. Salubridad y Enfermedades Trop. *21*:41-43.
7. Vaisman, A., Hamelin, A., and Guthe, T. 1963. La technique des anticorps fluorescents pratiquée sur sang desséché et élué. Bull. W.H.O. *29*:1-6.

CHAPTER 19

Leptospirosis

J-J. GUNNING

Synonyms. Weil's disease, pretibial (Fort Bragg) fever, swineherd's disease. The use of eponyms and synonyms is discouraged because they perpetuate the confusion incident to the varied epidemiologic and clinical manifestations of leptospirosis.

Definition. Leptospirosis is an acute, febrile, biphasic illness characterized by abrupt fever, chills, headache, conjunctival suffusion and considerable muscle tenderness. Nephritis, hepatitis, gastroenteritis and meningitis of varying severity are frequent accompaniments.

Distribution. Leptospirosis is a global zoonosis more prevalent in the tropics and in areas where rats are known to abound.

Etiology. Leptospirae belong to the order SPIROCHAETALES, family TREPONEMATACEAE, along with the borreliae and treponemae with which they have little in common except a spiral form. Electron microscopy reveals a cylindrical body wound in a helix about a rigid axial filament (Fig. 19–1). Ordinary stains and light microscopy are not useful in detecting the organisms. They are visible in tissue by silver impregnation stains. Leptospirae are 4 to 20 μm long and 0.1 to 0.2 μm wide. One end usually terminates in a hook and there is a generically distinct, rotational motility easily seen by dark field examination.

Leptospirae are easily cultivated aerobically at 28 to 30° C (82 to 86° F) in buffered, alkaline, 2 per cent nutrient agar containing peptone or serum enrichment. (See p. 834, Fletcher's medium.) Growth may be slow and cultures should be examined weekly and kept at least 28 days. The addition of 200 μg of 5-fluorouracil per ml to primary isolations, especially from urine, reduces contamination by other bacteria.

The genus *Leptospira* contains one species which is *L. interrogans.*[1] It is convenient to retain the concept of a biflexa complex, which includes the saprophytic and presumably nonpathogenic members, and an interrogans complex comprising some 130 zoonotic serotypes. The serotype is the basic taxon and correct terminology is *L. interrogans* serotype *louisiana,* not *L. louisiana.* The letter "L" should be omitted before all serotypes. Serotypes are currently arranged into 18 serogroups which by convention are capitalized and not italicized. They are: Icterohemorrhagia, Javanica, Celledoni, Canicola, Ballum, Pyrogenes, Cynopteri, Autumnalis, Australis, Pomona, Grippotyphosa, Hebdomadis, Bataviae, Tarassovi, Panama, Shermani, Semaranga and Andamana.

Epidemiology. Leptospirosis was first diagnosed in the United States of America in 1922. By 1948 a total of 299 cases had been reported and 286 were caused by serotype *icterohemorrhagiae.* The majority of patients were jaundiced and 25 per cent died.[2] During 1972 only 103 cases of human leptospirosis were reported to the U.S. Center for Disease Control (USCDC). Nine different serogroups were involved. Most patients were not jaundiced and only 6 per cent died.[3] Experience in the rest of the world has shown that fatality is the exception and that jaundice is rare.[4] In Southeast Asia as many as 20 per cent of fevers of unknown origin are caused by anicteric leptospirosis.[5] The paucity of cases reported to the USCDC probably indicates that many cases are not being subjected to serologic scrutiny, since the clinical picture may not be sufficiently distinctive to suggest the diagnosis. The true incidence of the disease will not be known until extensive serologic studies are undertaken.

Leptospirosis is perhaps the most prevalent contemporary zoonosis. Small rodents, especially rats, are the natural hosts and es-

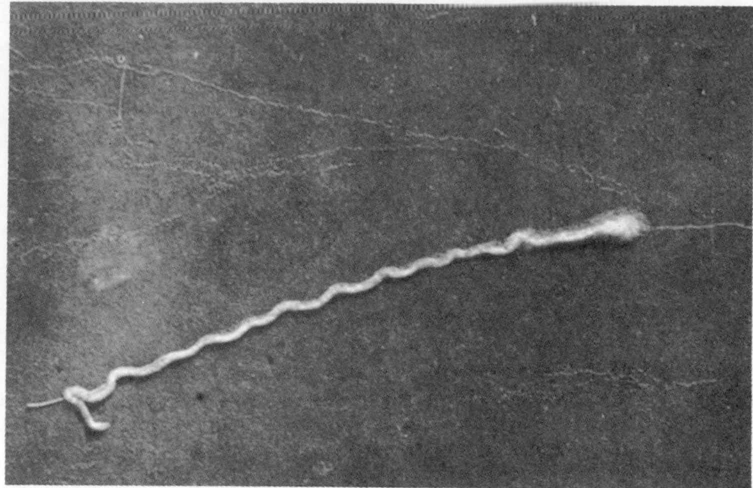

Figure 19-1. Electron photomicrograph of *Leptospira hyos*, chromium shadowed, showing typical spiral shape and axial filament entwined along the central cell mass (10,600 ×). (Courtesy of Breese, Gochenour and Yager in Proc. Soc. Exp. Biol. Med. *80*:185–188, 1952.)

sential reservoirs. *Rattus norvegicus* and *Mus musculus* are ubiquitous and carry a wide array of serotypes, insuring ample dissemination to man and other mammals.[6] Rodents do not usually succumb to leptospiral infection and have a urine and renal tissue pH of sufficient alkalinity to permit what may be lifelong colonization and urinary shedding. Leptospirae are frequently isolated from urine, blood and brain of seronegative rats. An explanation may be that transplacental infection prior to fetal thymic maturity may render the offspring incapable of developing antibodies at least to the cultured serotype. Leptospirae may infect any animal but some serotypes have not yet been isolated from rats.

Soil or surface waters that are shaded, of ideal temperature and alkalinity, and free of competing microorganisms or toxic chemicals are receptive to leptospirae. It is not known whether *L. interrogans* can multiply in these environs, but it must at least persist a sufficient time to allow infection of other rats and mammals including man. These latter probably constitute aberrant hosts and are less well suited as urinary carriers. The ecosystem may be so complex as to further involve fish, amphibians, reptiles, cloaca of aquatic birds, and ticks.

Penetration is presumed to be through broken skin or mucous membranes. Certain occupations by virtue of proximity to infected animals, their urine or contaminated surface waters have traditionally yielded a greater incidence of infection. These are sewer and abattoir workers, stevedores, dairy farmers, rice farmers, cane field workers, and soldiers exposed to jungle swamps and rice fields notably in Southeast Asia. Summer vacationers, during swimming and camping, have a great potential for becoming infected.

Pathology. Diffuse inflammatory lesions occur in many organs. Cell damage may be caused by direct action of a toxin, tissue anoxia secondary to hypotension or vasculitis, and immunologically mediated damage. Hemolysins, various endotoxins and lipolytic substances have been identified.[1] Complement-fixing IgM antibodies which may initiate cellular injury have been demonstrated during at least the second week of illness and coincide with the appearance of IgM agglutinating and opsonizing antibodies. Concentrations of C3 complement have remained within the normal range.[7] Leptospiral antigen has been demonstrated in muscle by fluorescent antibody technique.

Hemorrhages may involve most organs and tissues. There is no evidence for disseminated intravascular coagulation and it appears that capillary vasculitis is the principal lesion.

Focal necrotic changes are widespread in skeletal and cardiac muscle. There is swelling, vacuolization, and subsequent hyaline deposition. Healing by formation of new muscle fibers takes place and very little fibrosis is seen.

Interstitial nephritis may be an invariable and basic lesion in leptospirosis.[8, 9] Capillary loops are normal. The interstitial infiltrate shows histiocytes, lymphocytes and a few eosinophils and neutrophils. There is focal tubular damage which varies from simple dilatation to degeneration and necrosis of cells. Electron microscopy has revealed some mesangial hyperplasia and irregular foot processes with focal fusion. The tubules show thickening of the basement membranes and loss of the brush border or microprojections from the brush border.[8]

The lobular architecture of the liver is intact and findings are restricted to the central zone where enlarged hepatocytes with clear cytoplasm, a few mitotic figures and multinucleated cells are seen. A few necrotic cells and acidophilic (Councilman-like) bodies similar to those in viral hepatitis are seen. Trabecular arrangement is normal. Cholestasis is marked and characterized by bile granules in the cytoplasm of the liver cells and by bile thrombi. Electron microscopy shows total or partial disappearance of sinusoidal and bile ductule microvilli. Severe cases show definite mitochondrial pathology. Cell necrosis is not prominent and this is in keeping with the low levels of serum transaminase seen in this disease. The basic pathology appears to be a defect of bile transport.

Very minimal polymorphonuclear leukocyte infiltration is seen in the brain and meninges. There is hemorrhagic pneumonitis[10] and myocarditis. Silver impregnation stains have revealed the presence of leptospirae in various tissue.

Clinical Characteristics. The severity ranges from asymptomatic acquisition of seropositivity to fatality. Leptospirosis is a flu-like illness on which may be superimposed one or several manifestations such as hepatitis, nephritis, meningitis, pneumonitis, skin rashes (at times pretibial), and hemorrhagic features. Singly or in combination these features have accounted for the various synonyms and syndromes credited to one or another serotype. Some serotypes have a proclivity for specific mammalian hosts, clearly defined geographies and the development of specific syndromes. However, virtually any serotype can be found anywhere in the world and cause any of the disease manifestations. This variable expression appears related to the virulence of the offending serotype and host susceptibility.

The incubation period is usually between 1 and 2 weeks following exposure. It may be as short as 2 days or as long as 3 weeks. Leptospirosis is frequently a biphasic illness with an abrupt beginning. The initial phase lasts from 4 to 7 days during which leptospirae can be cultured from blood or cerebrospinal fluid and, less frequently, from the urine. There is an unrelenting frontal headache, severe myalgias, chills, rapidly rising temperature and prostration may supervene. Photophobia, sore throat, cough, nausea, vomiting and diarrhea are frequent. There is considerable cutaneous hyperesthesia and myalgia especially on deep palpation of the thigh, calf, lumbar and cervical muscles. Prominent conjunctival suffusion is evident. Petechiae and maculopapular skin rashes occur. Less frequently there may be hepatosplenomegaly, lymphadenopathy or jaundice. Chest pain is frequent and pneumonitis is present in about 15 per cent of patients.[4] Atrial and ventricular disturbances in cardiac rhythm have been noted.

The fever disappears, symptoms improve and leptospirae leave the blood and spinal fluid. This hiatus may last 1 to 3 days.

The second phase is not always clinically apparent and the patient may reflect this stage only by the appearance of antibodies. Fever and any of the foregoing symptoms may recur. Signs of meningeal irritation are not infrequent. During this phase cerebrospinal fluid pleocytosis is present in 85 per cent of patients. Other neurologic problems such as encephalitis, myelitis and peripheral and cranial nerve palsies may be present.

Iridocyclitis and optic neuritis may also occur. Resolution of all symptoms within 3 or 4 days without sequelae is the rule but some patients may be ill for several weeks. Leptospirae usually can be cultured from the urine during this stage.

Several reported series from the tropics have emphasized the extreme variability of leptospirosis. One-half of patients failed to demonstrate a biphasic fever. Few patients were jaundiced. Meningitis, nephritis and skin rashes were rare.[4] This is in contrast to the experience reported from the temperate zones of America and Europe where *icterohemorrhagiae* and *canicola* are more frequent. Hepatorenal involvement (Weil's disease) is more common, but this probably constitutes the major criterion for the diagnosis of leptospirosis and results in skewed statistics.

Prognosis. Most patients recover completely. Mortality is greater in the elderly and is not seen in the absence of jaundice. Renal lesions are reversible. A few patients are left with a permanent renal tubular concentrating defect and iridocyclitis may persist many years.

Laboratory Features. The total leukocyte count may vary from levels below 5000 to over 50,000 cells per cu mm. Usually it is between 5 and 12 thousand with an absolute granulocytosis of 70 per cent or greater. Anemia is infrequent in anicteric cases. Platelets are seldom depressed. Urinalysis reveals proteinuria, a few red and white cells and granular casts. Blood urea nitrogen, creatinine or creatinine clearance tests may be abnormal even in the absence of hepatic involvement. When jaundice is present, levels of transaminase are lower than would be expected in viral hepatitis and this may provide a useful diagnostic clue. Mild transaminase elevation in the absence of jaundice occurs in about one-half of all cases.

Cerebrospinal fluid pleocytosis from 10 to 1500 lymphocytes occurs in 50 per cent of patients examined after the sixth day of illness; protein is elevated and glucose is normal.

Diagnosis. The clinical diagnosis of leptospirosis is difficult because the disease mimics so many others. Knowledge that the disease exists in a given area and an illness presenting with fever, muscle tenderness, conjunctivitis and gastrointestinal complaints are helpful clues. Reliable diagnosis is made by isolation of leptospirae from inoculations of blood, spinal fluid or urine into Fletcher's medium. If this medium is not readily available, leptospirae can remain viable in oxalated blood for up to 10 days. Animal inoculations into guinea pigs or Syrian hamsters are also useful.

Antibodies appear from about the sixth to the twelfth day of illness and are usually detected by macroscopic slide agglutination tests utilizing four or five pools of antigens. These are commercially available but are not optimally sensitive. Microscopic agglutination tests are relatively serotype-specific and routinely used in reference laboratories.[3] Differential testing by single antigen microscopic agglutination lysis (MAL) using live serotypes is highly specific; although not infallible, the highest titer closely corresponds to the recovered leptospira.[4] A 4-fold or greater rise in titer during the course of illness is diagnostic. An absolute MAL titer of 1:400 is acceptable for diagnosis but less exact.

Treatment. Various antimicrobials such as penicillin, streptomycin, tetracyclines, chloramphenicol and erythromycin are effective in experimental animals and in vitro. Penicillin is probably the drug of choice. Evidence concerning the influence of these drugs on the outcome of leptospirosis in man is very conflicting. To be effective it is thought that they must be administered before the fourth day of illness. Since the detection of organisms in blood or urine is difficult and since diagnostic antibodies are not immediately present, prospective studies are nonexistent. Some experience gained in Vietnam suggests that aqueous penicillin 10 to 20 million units per day intravenously given during the first 4 days of illness may favorably alter the course of the disease. Jarisch-Herxheimer reactions may occur. Tetracycline administered without respect to the onset of symptoms does not alter the course of the disease.[4]

An antiserum against serotype *icterohemorrhagiae* is commercially available but not much is known about its therapeutic value. It is doubtful that its effective valency would extend to other serogroups or even serotypes within the same group.

Severely ill patients with azotemia and jaundice require meticulous attention to fluid and electrolyte balance. Because complete hepatic and renal recovery usually occurs, supportive measures such as peritoneal or hemodialysis should be used when indicated.

Prevention. Nearly 130 serotypes, many of which do not elicit cross-immunity, render vaccines impractical unless specifically tailored for areas with few serotypes. Vaccines have been effective in preventing disease in animals. Even so, animals immunized against leptospirae have been shown to be asymptomatic urinary carriers although they were seropositive.[11]

Laboratory workers accidentally exposed should take immediate antibiotic prophylaxis using full therapeutic doses.

Elimination of rat infestation, avoidance of contaminated water for drinking, bathing and wading, and the wearing of protective clothing for high-risk groups such as sewer, dairy and poultry workers are important preventive measures.

REFERENCES

1. W.H.O. Technical Report Series No. 380. 1967. Current problems in leptospirosis research. 32 pp.
2. Edwards, G. A., and Domm, B. M. 1960. Human leptospirosis. Medicine *39*:117–156.
3. Center for Disease Control. Leptospirosis Annual Summary, 1972. Issued February 1974. 11 pp.
4. Berman, S. J., Tsai, C. C., Holmes, K., Fresh, J. W., and Watten, R. H. 1973. Sporadic anicteric leptospirosis in South Vietnam. Ann. Intern. Med. *79*:167–173.
5. Berman, S. J., Irving, G. S., Kundin, W. D., Gunning, J-J., and Watten, R. H. 1973. Epidemiology of the acute fevers of unknown origin in South Vietnam. Effect of laboratory support upon clinical diagnosis. Am. J. Trop. Med. Hyg. *22*:796–801.
6. Van der Hoeden, J., and Szenbirg, E. 1962. Infections with *Leptospira mini szwajizak* in man and animals in Israel. Zoonosis Research (N.Y.) *1*:251–276.
7. Tong, M. J., Rosenberg, E. B., Votteri, B. A., and Tsai, C. C. 1971. Immunological response in leptospirosis. Report of three cases. Am. J. Trop. Med. Hyg. *20*:625–630.
8. De Brito, T., Freymuller, E., Penna, D. O., Santos, H. S., Soares De Almeida, S., Ayroza Galvao, P. A., and Pereira, V. G. 1965. Electron microscopy of the biopsied kidney in human leptospirosis. Am. J. Trop. Med. Hyg. *14*:397–403.
9. Sitprija, V., and Evans, H. 1970. The kidney in human leptospirosis. Am. J. Med. *49*:780–788.
10. Tong, M. J., Youel, D. B., and Cotten, C. L. 1972. Acute pneumonia in tropical infections. Am. J. Trop. Med. Hyg. *21*:50–57.
11. Feigin, R. D., Lobes, L. A., Jr., Anderson, D., and Pickering, L. 1973. Human leptospirosis from immunized dogs. Ann. Intern. Med. *79*:777–785.

SECTION IV
Bacterial Diseases

CHAPTER 20
The Diarrheal Diseases and Food-Borne Illnesses

DAVID M. WEBER

The diarrheal diseases constitute significant illnesses of high prevalence in the tropics. Indeed, in certain parts of the world diarrhea produces more illness and causes death of more infants and children than all other diseases combined.[1] The etiologies of tropical diarrheas are manifold. Infectious agents are responsible for the majority of instances, while other diarrheas relate to noninfectious, obscure, or multiple etiologies. In many areas lack of sanitary facilities, lack of refrigeration, prevalence of flies and intense heat all combine to provide a milieu conducive to the endemicity and spread of diarrheal disease.

Pathophysiology of Diarrhea. Diarrhea may be defined as a situation in which an adult's daily stool exceeds 200 gm and contains 60 to 95 per cent water.[2] Since intestinal water absorption is due to passive forces arising secondarily to transport of solute, one might implicate malabsorption or secretion of fecal solute as being responsible for increased fecal water. Diarrhea occurs when the colon is overloaded by discharge of organic anion and electrolyte solution from the small bowel. Thus, diarrhea can be explained in terms of increased excretion of solute, a factor that cannot be ignored in physiologic replacement therapy. The principal cations in stools consist of sodium and potassium. Diarrheal exudate, especially of the infectious type, may contain much mucus, desquamated cells and bacteria, all of which contribute to the passive excretion of potassium. Organic anions (acetate, propionate, butyrate and other substances produced by the action of bacterial enzymes on carbohydrate) comprise well over 50 per cent of fecal anions, while bicarbonate and chloride make up a lesser proportion.

Morbidity in diarrheal diseases varies in a wide range. At one extreme, dehydration and toxemia may be life-threatening, while in other instances frequent, watery stools may be merely an annoyance to an otherwise healthy individual. The direct infection of the intestinal mucosa by enteric pathogens (such as shigellae, salmonellae, protozoa and viruses), or the action of bacterial enterotoxins (cholera, certain strains of *Escherichia coli,* bacterial food poisonings), and a wide variety of other poisonous substances are capable of producing diarrhea through the above mechanism. The heat of tropical climates aggravates dehydration from insensible water loss.

Differential Diagnosis. Enteric diseases caused by bacteria constitute the most important tropical diarrheas and these will be discussed as specific entities. In the clinical evaluation of a patient suffering from a diarrheal illness acquired in the tropics, special attention should be given to a number of considerations which will both aid the medical management of the patient and, perhaps, facilitate the early detection of an outbreak of disease toward which some specific pre-

Table 20–1. SUMMARY OF COMMON DIARRHEAL DISEASES*†

Disease	*Causative Agent(s)*	*Mode of Onset—Duration*
Amebiasis See Chapter 37	*E. histolytica*	Insidious; course may be chronic
Shigellosis	*Shigella* spp. *S. sonnei* *S. flexneri* *S. boydii* *S. dysenteriae*	Acute; often with high fever; explosive diarrhea; tenesmus; acute course
Typhoid (Paratyphoid)	*Salmonella typhi* *S. paratyphi*—A and B	Begins as septicemia; no gastrointestinal symptoms until second week of illness; untreated disease lasts 3–4 weeks
Other Salmonella enteritides	*Salmonella* spp.; over 1200 serotypes have been described	Variable
Cholera See Chapter 21	*Vibrio cholerae;* also see *V. parahaemolyticus* (p. 181)	Usually sudden; acute course
Enteric viruses	See Chapter 2	
Other bacteria associated with diarrheal illness	Bacteria of genera: *Arizona* *Edwardsiella* *Providencia*	Variable
Diarrhea of travelers	Not known; possibly related to changes in bowel flora or pathogenic strains of *E. coli*	Variable onset; loose stool usually commences within 14 days after arrival in new environment; duration variable
Lactase deficiency	Deficiency of intestinal lactase	Onset variable; chronic course
Tropical sprue	Not known	Insidious onset; chronic course
Food-borne illness See Table 20–2	Table 20–2	Rapid onset

*It is of note that in the majority of instances the exact etiology of tropical diarrheas cannot be determined. No attempt has been made to list *all* of the diarrheal diseases.

†It is also of note that the above diarrheal diseases are often difficult to differentiate from one another and that tropical diarrheas may be due to multiple factors.

Table 20–1. Summary of Common Diarrheal Diseases*† *(Continued)*

Helpful Distinguishing Clinical Symptoms and Signs	*Helpful Laboratory Aids*	*Definitive Diagnosis*
History of bloody diarrhea; low-grade fever; weight loss	Macrophages predominate in diarrheal exudate; rectosigmoid lesions tend to be circumscribed; complement-fixation for *E. histolytica* is positive	Identification of trophozoites of *E. histolytica* in stool
Patient often appears "toxic"	Leukocytosis; predominance of polymorphonuclear leukocytes in diarrheal exudate (See Fig. 20–2)	Isolation of *Shigella* spp. from stool
Spiking fever that does not return to baseline; relative bradycardia; splenomegaly	Leukopenia; rising antibody titers to somatic (O) and flagellar (H) antigens	Isolation of *S. typhi, S. paratyphi* A and B from blood or stool
Nonspecific; fever; diarrhea; may be mild to severe	Important to exclude other etiologies of diarrhea	Isolation of *Salmonella* spp. from stool
In classic instances stool is relatively odorless and massive in quantity; this may rapidly cause severe dehydration	See Chapter 21; biotype *eltor* may cause milder disease (pp. 174, 183)	Isolation of *V. cholerae* from stool
Variable; nonspecific	Exclude other etiologies of diarrhea	Isolation of suspect species from stool
No fever; patient generally does not appear clinically ill	Stool contains inflammatory cells; type specific sera for enteropathogenic *E. coli*	Not available; exclude other etiologies of diarrhea
Diarrhea following ingestion of milk or milk products	Stool gives acid reaction	"Flat" glucose tolerance curve after ingestion of standard dose of lactose
Evidence of malnutrition; steatorrhea	Stool fat determination; intestinal biopsy	Response to antibiotic and folate therapy; see Chapter 58
Multiple persons often affected by same batch of poisoned food	Table 20–2	Table 20–2

ventive measures may be directed. An acute onset of chills, fever and explosive diarrhea (often dysentery, i.e. bloody diarrhea) associated with cramps and tenesmus suggests a diagnosis of shigellosis, whereas a more insidious, milder and protracted fever with dysentery is more consistent with amebic colitis. Food poisoning, while abrupt in onset and characterized by severe nausea, vomiting and diarrhea, is generally not associated with fever or with blood in the stools. Salmonellae can produce febrile diarrheal illnesses which, with the possible exception of typhoid fever, usually do not present with easily recognizable clinical syndromes (Table 20–1).

Cholera is characterized by massive "rice water" fluid loss, and is discussed elsewhere (Chapter 21). Cholera caused by the classic Inaba and Ogawa strains is not likely to be confused clinically with the other diarrheal diseases, particularly in the presence of an epidemic. Cholera caused by the biotype *eltor* produces a spectrum of disease from mild to severe, with many asymptomatic carriers. Since 1961, *eltor* has been producing a pandemic from which thus far only the Western Hemisphere has been spared.

In performing the physical examination of any person with diarrhea it is imperative to assess the degree of dehydration. This is especially important in infants and children in whom dehydration can rapidly lead to lethal complications, such as shock or intracranial venous thrombosis.

Proctosigmoidoscopy offers an opportunity to inspect the mucosa for characteristic lesions (e.g. the generalized erythematous swelling of shigellosis, in contrast to the circumscribed ulcers of amebiasis). This procedure also provides the best fresh material for bacterial culture (*Salmonella spp., Shigella spp.*) and microscopic diagnosis *(Entamoeba histolytica)*, and a chance to observe other lesions that may be responsible for rectal or bowel symptomatology.

Stool examination, both gross and microscopic, can be very useful. The presence of pus (Figs. 20–1 and 20–2) is suggestive of bacillary dysentery, whereas mononuclear cells are more consistent with amebiasis or chronic colitis. In examining stools it is important not to confuse macrophages with nonmotile trophozoites of *E. histolytica.* (See page 334.) The diarrhea of travelers ("turista") and that of "irritable colon" may be less watery and contain only few inflammatory cells. The discovery of intestinal parasites in the stool does not necessarily implicate these as causative agents of diarrhea.

Shigellosis – Bacillary Dysentery

Definition. Bacillary dysentery is an acute, self-limiting disease of man caused by organisms of the genus *Shigella*, family ENTEROBACTERIACEAE. Clinically, it is characterized by fever and diarrhea usually containing pus and blood. There is inflammation of the colon, particularly in the distal portion.

Etiology. Four species of *Shigella* are known to cause disease in man. These are *S. boydii, S. dysenteriae, S. flexneri,* and *S. sonnei.* Although the prevalence of these species varies in different parts of the world, all four species have been identified as disease agents in major areas studied.

Epidemiology. Shigellosis occurs almost exclusively in man. The disease is prevalent wherever local conditions permit contamination of food and water by the feces of infected individuals. Human carriers are the only important source of shigellosis. The most important means of transmission are contamination of food by infected food handlers, the transfer of the bacilli by houseflies, and fecal pollution of water supplies.

The organisms are easily killed by chemical agents and direct sunlight. They survive, however, for considerable periods in water, ice, and mucoid discharges from active infections. The disease is highly contagious and can be spread by contact with infected people, bed linens or other contaminated objects. Following clinical recovery, the major-

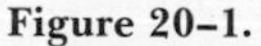

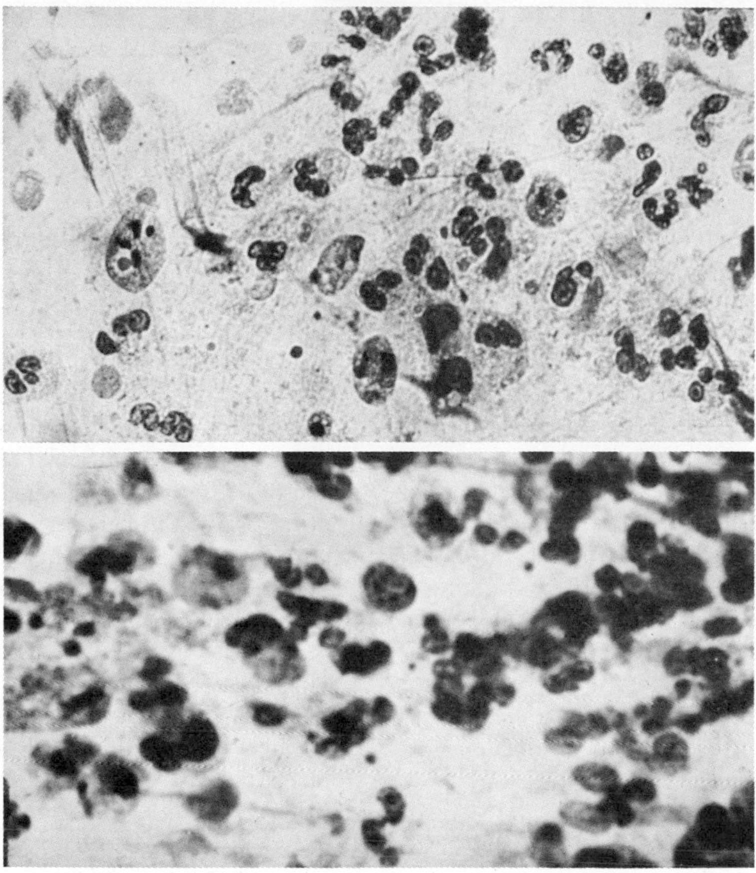

Figure 20–1.

Figure 20–2.

Figure 20–1. Bacillary dysentery (shigellosis). Early exudate in stool showing polymorphonuclear leukocytes and macrophages, one of which resembles an ameba with extruded pseudopod.

Figure 20–2. Exudate in later stage of illness: macrophage cells and many polymorphonuclear leukocytes and erythrocytes.

ity of patients continue to shed shigellae for only several days. The carrier state rarely persists for more than 3 months.

Pathology. The pathologic findings of bacillary dysentery are essentially an acute diffuse inflammation of the mucosa of the colon with the formation of a diphtheritic type of membrane, followed by necrosis and ulceration. This process is reflected by the presence of an inflammatory cellular exudate in the patient's stool.

In the early stage there is a rapidly spreading hyperemia of the mucosa, often accentuated in the lymph nodules, followed by edema, hemorrhage, and infiltration with granular leukocytes and macrophages. This process frequently extends into the submucosa, producing marked phlegmon-like thickening of the intestinal wall. The necrosis and desquamation of the epithelium with the formation of a diphtheritic type of membrane on the surface are followed by ulceration, beginning on the summits of the intestinal folds and often extending deep into the submucosa and sometimes into the muscularis. This process usually is not distributed uniformly throughout the colon, tending to be most marked in the distal portion. It may involve the lower ileum. Perforation is rare. With the development of the ulcerated lesions, secondary bacterial infection occurs and may enhance the pathologic process, especially in a subsequent chronic stage of the disease.

In cases of long duration, adjacent ulcers may be connected by ulcerating channels beneath bridges of more or less hyperplastic mucosa. In chronic recurrent cases there is much fibrosis of the mucosa and submucosa, the epithelium losing its normal glandular structure. Epithelial cystlike structures may be formed in the mucosa as the result of imperfect healing. These mucus retention cysts retain the bacilli, and may be responsible for the intermittent discharge of organisms characteristic of the chronic carrier state.

Clinical Characteristics. Following an incubation period of 1 to 7 days there is rather abrupt onset of fever, which may reach 40°C (104°F). Tachycardia is generally present. Although diarrhea usually follows promptly, there may be a delay of up to 24 hours leading to initial difficulty in establishing the diagnosis. The stools are frequent, watery, and often contain gelatinous blood-stained material (Figs. 20–1 and 20–2). In severe instances profound dehydration may be present with evidence of toxemia and vascular collapse.

Diagnosis. Examination of the peripheral blood generally reveals leukocytosis with a preponderance of polymorphonuclear leukocytes. Definitive diagnosis is established by the isolation of *Shigella* species from the stool. One may have to sample more than one specimen to isolate the organism. It is important to sample fresh stool, since shigellae survive only a short time in feces. (It would thus appear that shigellae are more easily inoculated into humans than onto laboratory media.) Since shigellae are non-fermenters of lactose, standard SS agar may be employed for initial isolation. Desoxycholate citrate agar may also be used. At proctoscopic examination the rectal and colonic mucosa appears diffusely reddened and exuding blood. Purulent exudate is usually present. Serologic tests are of little or no diagnostic value at present, the antigenic structure of shigellae being extremely complex.

Treatment. Severe dehydration when present, particularly in children, requires emergency corrective measures and must take precedence over all other modalities of treatment. Intravenous administration of electrolyte solutions should be initiated promptly and vigorously.

Clinical study of United States servicemen with shigellosis in Vietnam demonstrated that ampicillin significantly shortened the duration of diarrhea and fever while having no significant effect on the elimination of shigellae from the stools.[3] The dosage of ampicillin for adults of 250 to 500 mg 4 times a day, orally, is usually adequate; the parenteral route is preferable for children. Tetracycline hydrochloride 2.0 gm in a single dose orally (adult), or minocycline or doxycycline in appropriate lesser quantities, generally suffices to eradicate *Shigella* species, but the antibiotics of this group may be administered in smaller amounts during a 4-day period. Chloramphenicol is generally effective but should be employed only in severe instances in which other agents cannot be used. Other antibiotics, such as kanamycin and neomycin, do not appear to ameliorate the course of the disease significantly or to alter the shedding of shigellae in the stool. However, there is some evidence of emerging resistance of shigellae to ampicillin and tetracycline.

Symptomatic therapy with antidiarrheals tends to be of value. Orally administered drugs that reduce intestinal motility include diphenoxylate (Lomotil), 2.5 or 5.0 mg from 1 to 4 times a day, or camphorated tincture of opium (paregoric), 1 to 2 teaspoons 4 times a day. The parenteral use of anticholinergic compounds such as propantheline bromide 15 mg or atropine sulfate 0.4 to 0.6 mg, either drug given every 4 to 6 hours, may be helpful. The avoidance of oral carbohydrate in all diarrheal illnesses appears to be warranted for reasons discussed under Pathophysiology of Diarrhea.

It should be noted that there is evidence in cases of enteric bacterial infections due to invasive pathogens such as the shigellae that diarrhea may be a protective mechanism, and that treatment with drugs such as belladonna or opium alkaloids may cause a more severe disease through increasing the time of contact between the pathogen and intestinal mucosa where penetration occurs.[4]

Prophylaxis. Although patients need

not be completely isolated, their bedding and clothing should be sterilized. Disinfection and disposal of their stools are essential. Control of food handlers, the establishment of clean water and milk supplies, sanitary sewage disposal and the elimination of flies are of fundamental importance. The sequence of feces to flies or fingers to mouth must be interrupted.

Ice manufactured from untreated water is an important factor in the transmission of the pathogenic intestinal bacteria. In areas where a safe water supply is not available, all drinking water should be boiled. Under field conditions chemical sterilization with iodine or chlorine is reasonably effective for small quantities. For this purpose 1 or 2 tablets of Globaline, or 1 drop of 7.5 per cent tincture of iodine, or 2 or more tablets (130 mg each) of Halazone (*p*-sulfondichloramidobenzoic acid) should be added to each quart of water, the solution being insured by thorough shaking. After a contact period of 30 minutes the taste of chlorine may be removed by addition of 35 mg of sodium sulfite followed by thorough shaking. "Candle" filters, unless carefully cleaned at frequent intervals, are unreliable.

The Salmonelloses

INVASIVE SALMONELLOSES

Definition. Diseases caused by bacteria of the genus *Salmonella* are prevalent in the tropics where poor sanitation results in contamination of food and water with these organisms. More than 1200 serologic types of salmonellae have been identified. Although there is striking variation in the pathogenicity of the various serotypes, most are capable of causing human disease involving multiple organ systems, e.g. osteomyelitis, endocarditis or abscess. Only the enteric disease produced by *Salmonella* will be considered here. *Salmonella* species have been isolated from the gastrointestinal tract of man and many other mammals and lower animals. These are probably not zoonoses but rather part of the animals' intestinal flora. Humans will generally contract disease after ingesting large numbers of these organisms. Children tend to be affected more severely than adults.

Distribution. Salmonellae are worldwide in distribution.

TYPHOID AND PARATYPHOID FEVERS

Typhoid fever caused by *Salmonella typhi* is a disease that is unique to man.[5] It is spread by the contamination of water or food by infected human feces, often from an asymptomatic typhoid "carrier." Natural disasters such as floods and earthquakes have been known to precipitate epidemics, but typhoid is endemic throughout the tropics.

Pathogenesis. Following oral ingestion, *S. typhi* may multiply in the intestine to the point where it overwhelms commensal flora and invades the intestinal mucosa. A septicemic phase then follows, and this usually lasts for about 1 week. The elaboration of an endotoxin may have a role (though generally not a major one) in producing the systemic manifestations. Following the septicemic phase, there is invasion and ulceration of Peyer's patches and solitary lymphoid follicles of the ileum during the second week of the disease. At this time, organisms have disappeared from the blood and may be recovered from the stool and (rarely) from the urine. During the third week, severe complications such as bowel perforation or hemorrhage may occur.

Patients passing the bacilli in feces and urine constitute the principal source of infection, salmonellae being conveyed either directly from man to man or indirectly through contaminated water or food or by flies. People who have recovered from the disease may continue to excrete bacilli for many years, the organisms finding a haven in chronically inflamed gallbladders more often of women than of men. Occasionally a chronic carrier has no history of salmonellosis.

Clinical Characteristics. At the onset of the illness, fever rises in a stepwise fashion over a period of 2 to 3 days. The temperature then fluctuates in the 39.5 to 41.2° C (103.1 to 106.2° F) range and there is relative bradycardia. At this time headache and abdominal pain are commonly present, and there may be tenderness to palpation in the lower quadrants of the abdomen. Chills and sweats are not prominent features of the illness. The spleen often becomes palpable as the disease progresses. The presence of "rose spots" (hyperemic papules on the trunk, measuring 2 to 4 mm) is a helpful aid in clinical diagnosis, but these are present in only about 10 per cent of patients with typhoid. During the second week, gastrointestinal manifestations dominate the clinical picture. These variably include constipation, diarrhea, nausea and vomiting. During the third week (in an untreated individual), severe complications including intestinal hemorrhage and perforation of the bowel may occur. Extreme toxicity resembling "gram-negative shock" has been described following antibiotic treatment. Between 5 and 15 per cent of patients will have a relapse regardless of the duration of treatment.

Paratyphoid fever produced by *S. paratyphi* A or B is clinically indistinguishable from typhoid fever, although the disease tends to be milder. In some localities a third paratyphoid organism, *S. paratyphi* C, occurs.

Diagnosis. Isolation of *S. typhi* from the blood, stool or urine of a patient with appropriate clinical manifestations constitutes the only definitive diagnosis of typhoid. Examination of the peripheral blood reveals moderate leukopenia (3000 to 5000 white blood cells per cu mm). Specific agglutinins appear in the serum after about 7 to 10 days of illness, and are of diagnostic value (the Widal reaction) provided the patient has not had a previous attack or received protective inoculation. The titer of the antiflagellar (H) antibody is generally higher than that of the antisomatic (O) antibody. Measurement of the antibody to the superficial (Vi) antigen has been employed with some success in identifying the carrier state. The latter, of course, must be confirmed by bacterial isolation. Of the antigens, H and Vi are heat labile and O is heat stable.

In general, measurement of the O antibody is more valuable than that of the H antibody inasmuch as the O titer rises more quickly and is eliminated faster than the H antibody. The O titer will decline after about 6 months, while the H titer will persist from 2 to 3 years. A 3- to 4-fold rise in antibody titer is considered to be significant.

Treatment. Although salmonellae are sensitive in vitro to many antibiotics, a number of these same antibiotics fail to cure typhoid. Chloramphenicol is considered to be the agent of choice. An initial dose of 50 mg per kg of body weight is recommended. An additional 50 mg per kg daily is administered in divided doses at 8-hour intervals over the ensuing 3 days. The dosage may then be halved. The total period of antibiotic treatment should be 14 days. When possible, chloramphenicol should be administered orally. If vomiting precludes the oral route, intravenous treatment may be given in doses not exceeding 3 gm per day. Ampicillin is less effective than chloramphenicol in acute cases, although it is preferable for the treatment of chronic carriers and can be administered at a dosage of 100 mg per kg of body weight daily for 2 weeks or longer. In certain instances, patients may develop severe toxicity and a syndrome resembling "gram-negative shock" following the institution of antibiotic therapy. Such patients should benefit from the daily administration of cortisone 200 to 300 mg, or its equivalent. Relapses may occur within several weeks of completion of antibiotic therapy. These should be treated by 1 week of specific antibiotic therapy.

Hemorrhage and perforation of the bowel constitute serious complications of typhoid. These may occur in the enteric phase of the disease, usually in the third week. The treatment of bowel perforation has been the subject of some controversy. Some physicians consider the treatment of choice to be laparotomy with efforts at surgical closure of perforations. This is associated with high risk and the procedure is technically difficult owing to the friability of the infected bowel. Others prefer intubation and vigorous antibiotic therapy without surgical intervention. The course of treatment must be guided by the condition of the patient and availability of facilities. Both "medical" and "surgical" managements are associated with high mortality.

Prophylaxis. Immunization was, until recently, generally undertaken with triple vaccine, TAB, containing killed typhoid bacilli and paratyphoid A and B bacilli. In some areas this vaccine was enhanced by the addition of paratyphoid C. However, the protective effect against paratyphoid has been questionable, and present immunization practice is increasingly restricted to typhoid alone. Primary immunization is undertaken with 2 doses of vaccine, given subcutaneously 4 weeks apart. Booster doses may be given subcutaneously or intradermally at least every 3 years, but preferably annually. Reactions, consisting of pain at the injection site, persistent pyrexia and malaise, occur in many individuals. Alcohol-killed vaccine is superior to the heat-killed product. The Vi antigen of *S. typhi* remains potent only in the former preparation.

INFECTION BY OTHER SALMONELLAE

As mentioned above, numerous other species of *Salmonella* have produced disease in man, including diarrheal illnesses or septicemias or both. In patients with schistosomiasis, salmonella septicemias may persist for strikingly long periods of time. Patients infected with *Schistosoma haematobium* often excrete *Salmonella* in the urine. The high incidence of salmonella septicemia in patients with bartonellosis (Carrión's disease) has led to the use of chloramphenicol as an adjunct to treatment of this disorder (Chapter 30, p. 259). Probably, in patients presenting with a clinical picture characterized by fever and diarrhea, and in whom *Salmonella* is isolated from the stool, a cause and effect relationship may be considered (although not proven). As in typhoid fever, chloramphenicol is the antibiotic of choice. The recommended dosage (adult) is 3 gm per day for 2 weeks. Ampicillin may also be effective at 6 to 8 gm per day for 2 weeks. A rapid defervescence of fever (within 48 hours) might suggest that the illness was salmonella food poisoning, described below, rather than invasive salmonellosis. Also, it is conceivable that a person shedding salmonellae may contract diarrhea from some other, unrelated cause.

Food-Borne Illnesses

A wide variety of food-borne agents can produce acute gastrointestinal disorders. These include chemicals, poisonous plants and animals, certain living microorganisms, and poisons produced by microorganisms growing in food prior to its consumption. A number of these are more prevalent in tropical regions as a consequence of either climate or local prevailing conditions and customs or both. Some of these will be discussed briefly; others are listed in Table 20–2.

When an outbreak of food-borne illness occurs, it is important to associate it with the food conveying the causative agent as soon as possible. The pattern of the outbreak, relating time of onset of symptoms to the ingestion of the food, is significant; for example, illness occurring from 15 minutes to 1 hour after ingestion of food is frequently attributable to chemical agents causing metallic poisoning. Such poisoning occurs in food with high acid content stored in metal containers. Examples of such chemical poisoning include those due to antimony, cadmium and zinc (Table 20–2).

STAPHYLOCOCCAL FOOD POISONING

Though not by any means restricted to the tropics, this disorder is more common

Table 20-2. CAUSATIVE AGENTS OF FOOD-BORNE ILLNESSES*

Agent	*Food*	*Symptoms*	*Onset*
Chemicals			
Antimony	Acid foods cooked in gray-enameled or galvanized utensils	Vomiting	A few minutes to 1 hour
Cadmium	Acid foods stored in cadmium-plated refrigerator trays, pitchers and other utensils	Vomiting, abdominal cramps, diarrhea	15–30 minutes
Sodium fluoride	Roach powder mistaken for baking powder or soda or powdered milk	Vomiting, abdominal pain, diarrhea, convulsions, paresis	A few minutes to 2 hours
Zinc	Acid foods or drink (apples, lemonade) prepared in galvanized iron utensils	Astringent taste, pain in mouth and throat, gastric distress, vomiting, abdominal pain, diarrhea	A few minutes, or symptoms may be delayed as in food infections
Poisonous plants			
Akee fruit: Glucoside (saponin) toxic; the arils of the unripe fruit and the cotyledons of both ripe and unripe fruit have shown toxicity	Akee fruit (*Blighia sapida*)	Hyperemia, vomiting, convulsions, coma	2–3 hours; frequently fatal within 3–4 days
Ergot in rye: Alkaloid, ergosterol, ergothioneine	Food made with rye flour in which ergot fungus has grown	Gangrene of ears, toes, fingers; headache, convulsions, itching	Gradual, after several meals
Poisonous mushrooms: Alkaloids from 80 species	Toadstools, and others	Vomiting, abdominal pain, diarrhea, convulsions	6–15 hours
Snake root: Trematol—unsaturated alcohol $C_{16}H_{22}O_3$	Milk from cows which have eaten snakeroot, the poison of which was not destroyed by pasteurization	Vomiting, abdominal pain, constipation	Variable, after repeated use
Water hemlock: Cicutoxin (alkaloid) $C_{19}H_{26}O_3$, Mol. wt.: 302.40	Plant frequently mistaken for edible variety (leaves and root)	Vomiting, convulsions	1–2 hours
Poisonous animals			
Shellfish: $C_{10}H_{17}N_3O_8.2\ HCl$	Mussels and clams feeding on dinoflagellates (*Gonyaulax catenella*)	Numbness of lips and fingertips; respiratory and motor paralysis	½–3 hours
Fish: Ciguatera (poisg.) Toxin not clearly defined; insoluble in HOH; soluble in 90% ethanol, acetone and diethyl ether; withstands boiling (can be extracted with absol. alcohol and chloroform)	Barracuda, snappers, sea bass, groupers, and all toxic fish in the Pacific area and West Indies	Tingling sensation around lips and tongue, general malaise, profuse sweating, chills, abdominal pain, diarrhea, vomiting	1–30 hours
Tetraodontoxin: $C_{11}H_{17}N_3O_8$ Soluble in water and insoluble in ether	Puffer or globe fish (fugu); Tetraodons	Hypersalivation, vomiting, prickling sensation around lips and tongue, numbness, headache, vertigo, abdominal and lumbar pain, diarrhea, rapid pulse	½–3 hours
Microbial infections			
Clostridium botulinum: Exotoxin; antigenically different toxins types A, B, C, D, E and F; types A, B and E most common in man	Usually underprocessed canned vegetables and fruits, meat, dairy products, fish and seafoods	Vomiting and diarrhea may precede the neurologic symptoms, such as difficulty in swallowing, double vision, aphonia, respiratory paralysis	8–20 hours
Staphylococcus: Exotoxin; *Staph.* enterotoxins A, B and others	Custards, ham, mayonnaise, meat products, potato salad, dairy products	Vomiting, diarrhea, abdominal cramps, prostration	1–6 hours
Salmonella: Infection with one or more of approximately 1200 serotypes of *Salmonella*	Unheated eggs and egg products, poultry, swine, bakery goods, dairy products, bone meal, feather meal, fish meal	Abdominal pain, chills, fever, diarrhea, vomiting	7–72 hours
Halophilic *Vibrio parahaemolyticus*	Fish (raw and cooked), salad, meat, vegetables	Headache, chills, abdominal pain, diarrhea, fever, vomiting	8–24 hours
Alpha-type *Streptococcus* (in large numbers)	Heated meat products, turkey dressing, evaporated milk, charlotte russe allowed to stand without refrigeration	Abdominal cramps and diarrhea	5–18 hours
Large numbers of *Cl. perfringens* enteropathogenic Type A in food	Heated meat dishes, gravy, fried fish paste, poultry, fish, cooked and allowed to stand without refrigeration	Abdominal cramps, diarrhea	8–20 hours
Large numbers of *Bacillus cereus, B. subtilis*	Turkey meat, vanilla pudding cooked and allowed to stand without refrigeration	Abdominal cramps, diarrhea	8–16 hours

*Modified from G. M. Dack.

where warm climate and lack of adequate refrigeration create an increased risk. Food poisoning due to *Staphylococcus aureus* is caused by ingestion of preformed enterotoxin. The staphylococci are generally introduced into food from pyogenic lesions in food handlers. Outbreaks have involved ham, corned beef, potato salad, custard-filled baked goods, and milk products. Wholesome foods contaminated with staphylococci may become toxic within 7 hours at temperatures of approximately 29.5° C (85° F).

The symptoms, increased salivation followed by nausea, vomiting, abdominal pain and watery diarrhea, occur from 1 to 6 hours after ingestion of the contaminated food. Fever is generally absent. Recovery takes place within 24 hours. Death occurs only when dehydration is excessive, particularly in infants and the debilitated. Severe dehydration requires treatment with intravenous fluid and electrolytes.

The etiology can be established only if specimens of ingested food can be shown to contain large numbers of enterotoxin-producing staphylococci.

SALMONELLA GASTROENTERITIS

Following the consumption of contaminated food, gastroenteritis caused by *Salmonella* occurs after an incubation of 8 to 14 hours, which is generally shorter than that of staphylococcal food poisoning. The onset is nearly always sudden and may be characterized by headache, chills and abdominal pain. Nausea, vomiting and diarrhea follow. There is often an associated low-grade fever. The illness lasts from 1 to 4 days and tends to be more severe in infants and young children. Blood cultures are negative but frequently organisms can be isolated from the feces, and occasionally from the vomitus. Antibiotics probably do not alter the course of the illness. Supportive measures such as rehydration and electrolyte replacement are indicated. Salmonella gastroenteritis should be distinguished from invasive *Salmonella* infections.

Less commonly encountered food-borne illnesses include those caused by *Vibrio parahaemolyticus*, an organism which proliferates on raw or cooked seafood, raw vegetables, and meat. The organisms produce an illness which is pathophysiologically similar to cholera, though less severe. It is of interest that in Japan, where raw fish is served fresh in restaurants, *V. parahaemolyticus* has no opportunity to proliferate on the surface of fish and hence does not produce disease. However, when the fish is ordered for the home during the summer months, and allowed to stand for several hours, this disease occurs. Diarrheal disease produced by this organism has also been described in various parts of the United States. *Vibrio parahaemolyticus* has been isolated from the sea in the Bay of Panama, and more recently disease by this organism has been documented in Panama.

LACTASE DEFICIENCY

Since the inhabitants of certain tropical regions tend to have diets deficient in protein, efforts have been directed toward providing high-protein supplements. Prominent among these is powdered milk, which is both high in nutritional value and resistant to spoilage. It has been discovered, however, that as many as 80 to 90 per cent of populations long unaccustomed to dairy products have poorly developed production of lactase (the intestinal enzyme that splits lactose into glucose and galactose). The feeding of milk products therefore results in a high level of intestinal lactic acid which, in turn, causes an acid diarrhea with associated abdominal discomfort and weight loss. The diagnosis of lactase deficiency should be considered in individuals whose diarrhea occurs following the ingestion of milk or milk products. The diagnosis may be established by demonstrating a "flat" blood glucose curve following ingestion of a standard dose (100 gm) of lactose. For proper evaluation of the lactose tolerance test, malabsorptive states such as tropical sprue must be excluded by appropriate diagnostic measures.

Tropical sprue, another disorder characterized by diarrhea and malnutrition, is discussed elsewhere. (See Chapter 58.)

DIARRHEA OF TRAVELERS

Travelers' diarrhea ("turista") has been characterized as a disease that afflicts new arrivals in a foreign country, usually within 14 days. Reports in recent years have indicated that enteropathogenic strains of *Escherichia coli* may be implicated in a significant number of these diarrheas.[6] The only difference between diarrhea-causing *E. coli* and the normal intestinal varieties is that the former contain certain antigenic substances which permit them either to invade the intestinal mucosa or to elicit an enterotoxin. The diarrhea of travelers is popularly thought to affect individuals from highly sanitary environments when they travel in areas where standards of sanitation are less rigid. This view is incorrect, since approximately one-third of tourists from the United States traveling in Mexico contract the illness while an equal proportion of Mexicans coming to the United States acquire an identical illness.

Antibiotics are of no value in the treatment of this disorder. Specifically not recommended is the use of Entero-Vioform, since this agent has been associated with subacute myelo-optic neuropathy (SMON).[7] Symptomatic antidiarrheal medications should suffice.

OTHER BACTERIA ASSOCIATED WITH DIARRHEAL ILLNESS

Bacteria of the genus *Arizona* may cause gastroenteritis, and quite often are involved in localized lesions both in man and in lower animals. In some areas serotypes of *Arizona* also are very important economically because of their disease role in turkeys.

Scattered reports in the medical literature have implicated bacteria from the genera *Edwardsiella* and *Providencia* as causative agents in infectious diarrhea, but there is insufficient evidence that these organisms are pathogens. It is not known under what circumstances they might become pathogenic. Nonetheless, there are sufficient clinical and epidemiologic data to warrant further investigation in this area. The genera *Edwardsiella* and *Arizona* have been isolated from the gastrointestinal tracts of various animals. The associated diarrheal disease in man may range from mild to severe.

Several viruses have been implicated as causal agents of diarrhea. Attention is invited to the section dealing with the viral diseases, on page 69.

REFERENCES

1. Gordon, J. E. 1968. Weanling diarrhea. *In* Scrimshaw, N. S., Taylor, C. E., and Gordon, J. E. (eds.): Interaction of Nutrition and Infection. W.H.O. Monograph No. 57, Geneva. 329 pp.
2. Phillips, S. F. 1972. Diarrhea: a current review of the pathophysiology. Gastroenterology *63*:459–518.
3. Tong, M. J., Martin, D. G., Cunningham, J. J., and Gunning, J-J. 1970. Clinical and bacteriological evaluation of antibiotic treatment in shigellosis. J.A.M.A. *204*:1841–1844.
4. DuPont, H. L., and Hornick, R. B. 1973. Clinical approach to infectious diarrheas. Medicine *52*:265–270.
5. Hornick, R. B., Greisman, S. E., Woodward, T. E., DuPont, H. L., Dawkins, A. T., Jr., and Snyder, M. J. 1970. Typhoid fever: pathogenesis and immunologic control. N. Engl. J. Med. *283*:686–691; 739–746.
6. Rowe, B., Taylor, J., and Battelheim, K. A. 1970. An investigation of travellers diarrhoea. Lancet *1*:1–5.
7. Wolfe, M. S., and Mishtowt, G. I. 1972. Entero-Vioform in travelers' diarrhea. J.A.M.A. *220*:275–276.

CHAPTER 21

Cholera

CHARLES C. J. CARPENTER

Synonyms. Asiatic cholera, Indian cholera.

Definition. Cholera is an acute illness caused by an enterotoxin elaborated by *Vibrio cholerae* which have colonized the small bowel. It is characterized in the more severe cases by extreme saline depletion, shock and acidosis, resulting from the rapid gastrointestinal loss of massive quantities of fluid and electrolytes. Although the mortality rate may be extremely high in untreated cases, excellent therapeutic results can be obtained by prompt replacement of lost water and electrolytes by either the intravenous or the oral route.[1-3]

Distribution. Throughout the first 6 decades of the twentieth century cholera was largely confined to Asia, with a major endemic focus in the common delta of the Ganges and Brahmaputra rivers. However, the three major North American epidemics of 1832, 1848 and 1867 had shown that the potential distribution of cholera was worldwide. The period 1961 to 1974 has witnessed a seventh major pandemic spread of cholera from Indonesia westward throughout South and Central Asia to Western Europe and the entire African continent. Serious outbreaks of cholera occurred in Spain in the summer of 1972, and in Italy in the summer of 1973, and isolated cases have been identified in travelers returning from these areas to most of the other nations of Western Europe. The ultimate limits of the recent pandemic have not yet been delineated.

Etiology. *Vibrio cholerae (V. comma)* Neisser, 1893 is a short, curved, motile, gram-negative rod possessing a single polar flagellum.

Cultural Characteristics. *Vibrio cholerae* grows aerobically on ordinary media having a pH from 7.0 to 9.0; acid but not gas is produced from dextrose under anaerobic conditions. Acid is also produced from sucrose, mannose, mannitol and lactose (delayed 2 to 4 days), but not from arabinose or xylose. Nitrates are reduced to nitrites; indole is produced from tryptophan; and gelatin is liquefied by *V. cholerae.* The tests for urease and hydrogen sulfide production are negative. The organisms are agglutinated by vibrio O group I antibodies. Differentiation between classic *V. cholerae* and *V. cholerae* var. *eltor* is based upon the ability of the latter variant to lyse sheep erythrocytes, agglutinate chick erythrocytes and resist lysis by Mukerjee's type IV cholerophage.

Many other noncholera vibrios, which are ubiquitous in nature, have been found in man. These may exhibit the same morphologic and cultural characteristics as true *V. cholerae;* they do not, however, agglutinate in O group I antisera. Certain strains of nonagglutinating vibrios produce an enterotoxin similar to that produced by *V. cholerae,* and have been implicated in less severe outbreaks of diarrheal disease.[4]

Epidemiology. Man is the only documented natural host and victim of *V. cholerae,* although a carrier state in other species remains a possibility. Most major epidemics of this disease appear to have been waterborne, and water plays the major role in transmission of *V. cholerae* in endemic rural areas. During major epidemics, however, the direct contamination of food with infected excreta may also be important. Persons with mild or asymptomatic infections (contact carriers) play a major role in the dissemination of epidemic disease. A prolonged gallbladder carrier state may develop in 3 to 5 per cent of patients convalescing from cholera caused by the *eltor* biotype. The gallbladder carrier state is more common in older convalescents, and it has never been observed in the pediatric age group. The role of such convalescent carriers in the transmission of disease is not yet clarified. In the endemic areas of Bangladesh and West Bengal, cholera is predominantly a disease of children. Attack rates are 10 times greater in the 1 to 5 age group than in those above 20 years of age. However, when the disease spreads to previously uninvolved areas, the attack rates are initially at least as high in adults as in children.[5]

Pathogenesis and Pathology. All symptoms, signs and metabolic derangements in cholera result from the rapid loss of fluid and electrolytes from the gut. These losses result from increased secretion of isotonic fluids by all segments of the small bowel. The increased electrolyte secretion is caused by a protein enterotoxin with a molecular weight of 84,000 which is elaborated by all pathogenic strains of *V. cholerae.* This enterotoxin rapidly binds to the gut mucosal epithelial cells and causes, after a lag period of about 30 minutes, an increase in adenyl cyclase activity in the gut epithelial cells. This results in an increase in intracellular cyclic adenosine 3′, 5′-monophosphate level which leads, in turn, to secretion of isotonic fluid by all segments of the small bowel. Precise studies have demonstrated that the adult cholera stool is nearly isotonic, with sodium and chloride concentrations slightly less than those of plasma, a bicarbonate concentration of approximately twice that of plasma, and a potassium concentration 3 to 5 times that of plasma (Table 21–1).[2] Disease caused by all known strains of *V. cholerae* results in the same stool electrolyte pattern. The loss of large quantities of intestinal fluids results in severe extracellular fluid depletion, with resultant hypovolemic shock, base deficit acidosis and progressive potassium depletion. There is no evidence that the cholera vibrio invades any tissue, nor has the enterotoxin been shown, in the naturally occurring disease, to have any direct effect on any organ other than the small intestine.

Clinical Characteristics. All signs and symptoms of cholera result directly from the gastrointestinal fluid and electrolyte losses. The initial symptom is that of painless, watery diarrhea, which may be abrupt in onset. The stool volume varies greatly; in the more severe cases the initial loss may be in excess of 1500 ml. At varying intervals after the onset of diarrhea, vomiting ensues; this is also characteristically effortless and productive of rice-watery material. In fulminant cases, severe muscle cramps, most commonly involving the gastrocnemius group, almost invariably develop. Prostration occurs at varying intervals after the onset of symptoms, in direct relationship to the magnitude of the fluid loss.

When first seen by the physician, the typical severe cholera patient presents a characteristic appearance: collapsed, cyanotic, with no palpable peripheral pulses, pinched facies and scaphoid abdomen. Although the patient is usually conscious, the voice is very weak, high-pitched and often nearly inaudible. Vital signs include tachycardia, varying degrees of tachypnea, hypopyrexia and hypotension, often with no obtainable blood pressure. Heart sounds are faint or inaudible, and bowel sounds are hypoactive or entirely absent. Laboratory abnormalities are those which would be expected to result from the massive gastrointestinal loss of an isotonic, alkaline, virtually protein-free fluid. They include elevated hematocrit, increased plasma and whole blood specific gravity, elevated plasma protein, de-

Table 21–1. Mean Electrolyte Concentrations in Cholera Stool

	mEq/L of H_2O			
Sample	Na^+	Cl^-	HCO_3^-	K^+
On admission	128	120	43	26
After rehydration	138	112	41	19

creased plasma bicarbonate, low arterial pH, normal plasma sodium, slightly increased plasma chloride and moderately elevated plasma potassium. Since the bicarbonate loss is proportional to stool volume, the decrease in whole blood pH is roughly proportional to the increase in plasma specific gravity at all stages of the untreated disease (Table 21–2).

The illness may last from 12 hours to 7 days, and later clinical manifestations depend on the adequacy of therapy. With adequate fluid and electrolyte repletion, recovery is remarkably rapid. If hypertonic replacement fluids are used, an almost intolerable thirst and agitation develop; thirst is not, however, a prominent presenting feature of this disease. If therapy is inadequate, the mortality is quite high; the most common causes of death are hypovolemic shock, uncompensated metabolic acidosis (which may be aggravated by the administration of saline without alkali) and uremia. In the latter cases, the characteristic picture is that of acute tubular necrosis secondary to prolonged hypotension.

In the presence of an epidemic of cholera, a wide variety of clinical types may be encountered. These may vary from ambulatory cases with only mild diarrhea to fulminating cases in which death occurs, in the absence of appropriate treatment, within 2 to 3 hours after onset of diarrhea.

Diagnosis. Although cultural techniques are relatively simple, in endemic or epidemic areas the diagnosis should be made on the basis of the clinical picture and therapy instituted immediately. Although a cholera-like illness may be caused by organisms other than *V. cholerae,* the resulting metabolic abnormalities are essentially the same, so that the same therapeutic approach should be used in all such cases.

The most reliable technique for identification of *V. cholerae* consists in direct plating of the cholera stool on the bile-salt or gelatin-tellurite-taurocholate (G-T-T) agar. Typical translucent colonies appear in 18 hours; use of oblique lighting technique makes it possible to identify one vibrio colony among several hundred colonies of other organisms. Final identification requires agglutination with type-specific antiserum and demonstration of the characteristic biochemical reactions. In mild or convalescent cases, recovery of vibrios may be improved by initial enrichment for 6 hours in alkaline (pH 9.0) peptone water, followed by subculture on bile salt or G-T-T (monsur) agar.

Diagnosis may also be confirmed by demonstration of rises in agglutinating or vibriocidal antibody titers or both. Significant rises in both titers are present by the seventh to tenth day of illness in over 90 per cent of cases with bacteriologically proved *V. cholerae* infection.[6]

Treatment. Successful therapy demands only prompt replacement of the gas-

Table 21–2. Serial Studies in Cholera Patients Treated by 2:1 Saline: Lactate Regimen (Average Values, 40 Patients)

	On Admission	*4 Hours*	*24 Hours*
Sodium*	152	156	153
Chloride*	117	118	113
Potassium*	5.7	3.3	3.1
Bicarbonate*	7.4	21.0	24.5
Arterial pH	7.21	7.43	7.46
Plasma specific gravity	1.043	1.026	1.026

*Plasma electrolyte values are expressed in milliequivalents per liter of plasma H_2O.

trointestinal losses of fluid and electrolytes.[1-3] In adults isotonic saline solution and isotonic sodium bicarbonate (either isotonic sodium acetate or sodium lactate can replace the bicarbonate) in a 2:1 ratio should be infused intravenously and rapidly—50 to 100 ml per minute—until a strong radial pulse has been restored. An equally effective alternative isotonic intravenous solution is that obtained by adding 5 gm of sodium chloride, 4 gm of sodium bicarbonate and 1 gm of potassium chloride to a liter of sterile distilled water. After the initial correction of hypovolemic shock, this same intravenous fluid should be infused in quantities equal to the gastrointestinal losses. If these losses cannot be measured accurately, intravenous fluid should be given at a rate sufficient to maintain a normal radial pulse volume and normal skin turgor. Overhydration can be avoided by careful observation of the veins in the neck and by auscultation of the lungs. Close observation of the patient is mandatory during the acute phase of the illness. An adult patient can lose as much as 1 liter of isotonic fluid an hour during the first 24 hours of the disease. Inadequate or delayed restoration of electrolyte losses results in a very high incidence of acute renal insufficiency. Serious hypokalemia is rare in the adult, and potassium replacement can be carried out either intravenously (by using the 5:4:1 solution delineated above) or orally by giving approximately 15 milliequivalents (mEq) of potassium chloride for each liter of feces that is produced.

In children complications are both more frequent and more severe.[7] The most serious complications include stupor, coma and convulsions (unique to the pediatric patient), pulmonary edema and cardiac arrhythmias that occasionally lead to cardiac arrest. The central nervous system complications may be due to hypoglycemia (observed only in pediatric patients); to hypernatremia resulting from the administration of isotonic fluid to the pediatric patient who, unlike the adult patient, produces feces with a sodium concentration significantly less than that of plasma; or to cerebral edema, presumably secondary to rapid fluid shifts during the administration of intravenous fluids. Pulmonary edema may result if the fluids are given intravenously at too rapid a rate, especially in the presence of severe metabolic acidosis. Cardiac arrhythmias are usually secondary to hypokalemia. Serious arrhythmias are observed with less severe degrees of potassium depletion in children than in adults with cholera.

Each of the above complications can be avoided by the careful administration of intravenous fluids that are designed especially to replace the fecal losses of children with cholera. The following solution has been used successfully to correct hypokalemia and hyperglycemia without provoking hypernatremia: sodium 90 mEq per liter, chloride 60 mEq per liter, potassium 15 mEq per liter, bicarbonate 45 mEq per liter, and glucose 20 gm per liter. Administration of this solution must be carefully monitored, with frequent auscultation of the lungs and inspection of venous filling in the neck in order to avoid overhydration. The outcome in pediatric cholera should be essentially as favorable as that in the adult disease—an overall mortality rate of less than 1 per cent.

If intravenous fluids are in short supply, oral replacement of water and electrolytes is effective in adults and in those children who are alert and able to retain orally administered solutions. Since the cholera enterotoxin does not alter glucose-facilitated sodium absorption, fluid repletion can be effected by the oral administration of glucose-containing electrolyte solutions. Since the limiting factor in the treatment of cholera in both epidemic and endemic situations is often the lack of adequate quantities of intravenous fluids, the availability of an oral treatment regimen has greatly reduced mortality from cholera during the recent pandemic spread of this disease. A solution containing glucose 20 gm per liter, sodium bicarbonate 4 gm per liter, sodium chloride 4 gm per liter, and potassium chloride 1 gm per liter can be readily prepared and should be satisfactory for the treatment of all age groups. This solution, administered orally at a rate equal to the stool losses, can be given to mild cholera cases throughout the course of illness, and is also satisfactory in the more severe cases, once the hypovolemic shock has been corrected by initial rapid intravenous fluid therapy. Oral therapy does not decrease the rate of gut fluid loss, but provides an electrolyte solution which can be absorbed at a rate sufficient, in most cases, to counterbalance the continuing fluid losses. Therefore, successful management of the cholera patient with oral therapy requires just as close supervision, with careful monitoring of pulse volume, skin turgor and neck veins, as does management with intravenous solutions. Supplemental intravenous fluids must be administered whenever the clinical signs of saline depletion recur.

Adequate fluid and electrolyte therapy alone results in rapid recovery in virtually all cholera patients. However, adjunctive therapy with antibiotics dramatically reduces the duration and volume of diarrhea, and results in early eradication of vibrios from the feces. Tetracycline in a daily oral dose of 30 to 40 mg per kg of body weight, given in divided doses every 6 hours for 2 days, has been consistently successful. Furazolidone and chloramphenicol are of value, but they are slightly less effective than tetracycline.[8]

Prognosis. Under ideal conditions and with prompt and adequate fluid replacement, mortality approaches zero and significant sequelae are rare. With oral glucose-electrolyte therapy, successful treatment can be effective even under primitive conditions, as was recently demonstrated in the management of cholera in Bangladesh refugees in West Bengal.[9] Unfortunately, death rates as high as 60 per cent were still being reported in certain cholera outbreaks in 1973, especially during the initial phases of the epidemic. This high mortality reflects the lack of pyrogen-free intravenous fluids in remote areas, the difficulties of initiating the treatment promptly when large numbers of cases are occurring in poverty-stricken populations, and the compromises which may have to be made under emergency conditions.

Prophylaxis. Immunization using the standard commercial vaccine (containing 10 billion killed organisms per milliliter) provides 60 to 80 per cent protection for 3 to 6 months. Immunization with toxoid provides highly significant protection in experimental animals, but has not yet been tried extensively in man. At present, only careful hygiene provides sure protection against cholera. Ultimate control of cholera will depend upon adequate sanitary factors, sewage disposal and water supply in the areas in which endemic disease persists.

Additional information on a wide range of aspects of cholera is presented in the recent book *Cholera* edited by Barua and Burrows.[10]

REFERENCES

1. Watten, R. H., Morgan, F. M., Songkhla, Y. N., Vanikiati, B., and Phillips, R. A. 1959. Water and electrolyte studies in cholera. J. Clin. Invest. *38*:1879–1889.
2. Carpenter, C. C. J., Mondal, A., Sack, R. B., Mitra, P. P., Dans, P. E., Wells, S. A., Hinman, E. J., and Chandhuri, R. N. 1966. Clinical studies in Asiatic cholera. II. Bull. Johns Hopkins Hosp. *118*:174–196.
3. Pierce, N. F., Sack, R. B., Mitra, R. C., Banwell, J. G., Brigham, K. L., Fedson, D. S., and Mondal, A. 1969. Replacement of water and electrolyte losses in cholera by an oral glucose-electrolyte solution. Ann. Intern. Med. *70*:1173–1181.
4. Zinnaka, Y., and Carpenter, C. C. J. 1972. An enterotoxin produced by noncholera vibrios. Johns Hopkins Med. J. *131*:403–411.
5. Woodward, W. E., and Mosley, W. H. 1972. The spectrum of cholera in rural Bangladesh. 2. Comparison of eltor Ogawa and classical Inaba infection. Am. J. Epidemiol. *96*:342–351.
6. Sack, R. B., Barua, D., Saxena, R., and Carpenter, C. C. J. 1966. Vibriocidal and agglutinating antibody patterns in cholera patients. J. Inf. Dis. *116*:630–640.
7. Carpenter, C. C. J., and Hirschhorn, N. 1972. Pediatric cholera: current concepts. J. Pediat. *80*:874–882.
8. Wallace, C. K., Anderson, P. N., Brown, T. C., Khanra, S. R., Lewis, G. W., Pierce, N. F., Sanyal, S. N., Segre, G. V., and Waldman, R. H. 1968. Optimal antibiotic therapy in cholera. Bull. W.H.O. *39*:239–245.
9. Mahalanobis, D., Choudhuri, A. B., Bagchi, N. G., Bhattacharya, A. K., and Simpson, T. W. 1973. Oral fluid therapy of cholera among Bangladesh refugees. Johns Hopkins Med. J. *132*:197–205.
10. Barua, D., and Burrows, W. (eds.) 1974. Cholera. W. B. Saunders Co., Philadelphia. 458 pp.

CHAPTER 22

Brucellosis

WESLEY W. SPINK

Synonyms. Undulant, Malta, Mediterranean, Gibraltar, rock, Neapolitan, or Cyprus fever; Mediterranean phthisis; melitensis septicemia; abortus fever; fièvre caprine; febris melitensis.

Definition. Brucellosis is an infectious disease transmitted to man from animals, principally cattle, sheep, goats and swine, and caused by microorganisms belonging to the genus *Brucella.* The acute form is a febrile illness that simulates many other diseases and is characterized by few or no localized findings. Chronic disease occurs with and without abnormal physical findings. Death occurs rarely and with modern antibiotic therapy the complications have been reduced considerably.

Distribution. The genus *Brucella* occurs in naturally infected animals in all parts of the world, and human brucellosis, in consequence, has a cosmopolitan distribution. The clinical types and the severity of the disease will vary in different areas in accordance with the relative preponderance of the three species of the genus in these regions.

Etiology. Brucellosis is a disease primarily of animals. The bovine species, *Brucella abortus* (Schmidt and Weis, 1901) Meyer and Shaw, 1920, occurs in cattle; the caprine species, *Brucella melitensis* (Hughes, 1892) Meyer and Shaw, 1920, in goats; and the porcine form, *Brucella suis* Huddleson, 1929, in hogs. Atypical strains have been isolated in various parts of the world that do not conform strictly to the pattern of one of the three basic species. Because of certain metabolic patterns, the International Committee on Nomenclature has designated several subtypes of brucellae within each of the three species: *Br. abortus* with nine, *Br. melitensis* and *Br. suis* each with three.[1] Four other groups are considered separately; one is *Brucella neotomae,* which was isolated from the desert wood rat (*Neotoma lepida* Thomas), and resembles *Br. suis;* the second is *Brucella ovis,* which was cultured from the ram and considered a rough variant of *Br. melitensis;* the third is *Brucella rangiferi tarandi,* recovered from reindeer in northern Russia and from Eskimos in Alaska and Canada, resembling *Br. suis,* type 3; and the fourth is *Brucella canis,* recovered from dogs in the United States, which is a rough variant of *Br. suis. Brucella abortus strain 19* is stable, has attenuated virulence and, consequently, is widely used in bovine vaccination programs.

Brucellosis is a serious cause of abortion in bovines, less so in sheep, goats and swine. Human abortions do not result from the disease any more frequently than from other systemic microbial infections.

The members of the genus *Brucella* are small, gram-negative, nonmotile, non-spore-forming coccobacilli. The species of *Brucella* are exceedingly difficult to differentiate in stained preparations. Identification must be made by means of metabolic studies and serologic methods.

Cultural Characteristics. These organisms do not grow well on ordinary laboratory media. Primary blood stream isolations are not easily accomplished, probably owing to the paucity of organisms in the circulation. Furthermore, it has been demonstrated that certain peptones in the isolation media may be toxic to the *Brucella* organisms. Trypticase soy broth or agar, Albini *Brucella* media or liver infusion agar or liver infusion broth with a pH of 6.8 to 7.4 should be used, especially for primary isolation. Growth is slow, requiring up to 14 days. On solid media the colonies are small, usually smooth and opaque. In liquid media they produce diffuse turbidity.

Brucella melitensis and *Br. suis* are aerobic. For primary isolation and a varying number of subsequent generations, *Br. abortus* requires a carbon dioxide content 10 per cent by volume over that of atmospheric air. Such increased carbon dioxide tension does not inhibit growth of *Br. melitensis* or *Br. suis.*

Differentiation among the three species of the genus *Brucella* is difficult. Metabolic and serologic procedures that aid in the differentiation of the species are summarized in Table 22–1. Bacteriophage for *Br. abortus* has been identified and lytic tests for smooth cultures of this species are also helpful in differentiation, but such tests are not available for *Br. melitensis* and *Br. suis.*

Epidemiology. The genus *Brucella* is widely distributed throughout the world and produces natural infections in horses, dogs, sheep, cattle, goats, swine, wild deer and wild buffalo. The human disease is acquired from direct or indirect contact with goats, cattle or hogs. The tissues and discharges of infected animals contain the organisms. *Brucella* species are commonly present in the milk of infected cattle and goats.

The organisms are present in large numbers in the vaginal discharge of animals which have aborted. They are present less commonly in the urine and feces. The frequent association of *Br. abortus* with both fistulous withers and abortion of horses provides a source of potential infection for individuals in contact with such animals.

Brucellae are not easily destroyed under natural conditions except by temperatures above 55° C (131°F) or by exposure to direct sunlight. They will survive in dry soil for 40 to 60 days, in sterile tap water for 42 days, in meat-curing brine for 40 days, and in milk at 10° C (50° F) for 10 days. They have been reported to remain viable in unpasteurized cheese for periods up to 2 months.

The majority of human infections are acquired through direct contact with infected animals, or through exposure to the secretions and infected products of parturition. The organisms gain entrance into the body through abrasions of the skin and through the conjunctivae. Rarely, if ever, is infection acquired through the respiratory tract. Brucellosis is properly called an occupational disease, since it usually involves farmers, livestock producers, meat packing plant employees, veterinarians and laboratory workers.[2]

Brucellosis is also caused by the ingestion of fresh, unpasteurized milk and milk products (cheese and butter) obtained from infected goats, sheep or cattle. Brucellae do not survive in ripened, aged cheeses.

On rare occasions, infants have been infected through maternal milk. In utero infections of fetuses have been recorded.

In the United States, where the majority of infections are due to *Br. abortus,* the disease is uncommon in infants and children. However, in those areas of the world in which *Br. melitensis* infections predominate, the disease is common in the young, probably related in part to the increased invasive capacity of *Br. melitensis* strains.

Although an attack of brucellosis does confirm immunity, recovery is associated with the acquisition of *Brucella* hypersensitivity of the delayed type. This hypersensitivity can be expressed in a febrile state upon subsequent contact with *Brucella* antigen and

Table 22–1. Differential Tests for Brucella Cultures

			Growth		*Agglutination in Nonspecific Sera*	
Species	*CO_2 Requirement*	*H_2S Production*	Thionin	Basic Fuchsin	Abortus	Melitensis
Br. abortus	+	+4 days	0	+	+	0
Br. melitensis	0	0	+	+	0	+
Br. suis	0	+5 days	+	0	+	0

is most commonly seen in veterinarians who are repeatedly exposed to the *Brucella* organisms.

Pathology. A characteristic feature of brucellosis is the intracellular localization of the organisms in the cells of the reticuloendothelial system, with the formation of granulomas in which little or no necrosis occurs. These lesions simulate those of sarcoidosis and are found primarily in the lymph nodes, liver, spleen and bone marrow. Brucellae also localize in the spine, meninges, endocardium and testes. Suppurative lesions can occur with any one of the three species, but caseation, simulating tuberculosis, is most frequently caused by *Br. suis*.[2, 3]

Clinical Characteristics. The incubation period is usually 1 to 3 weeks, but several months can elapse between the time of exposure and the onset of symptoms. The severity and duration of the illness depend upon the species of *Brucella* causing illness. In general, disease due to *Br. abortus* is less severe than that caused by the other two species, and *Br. abortus* has been responsible for at least three-fourths of the cases that have occurred in the United States. *Brucella melitensis* causes a more severe illness with a higher incidence of complications; *Br. suis* has a tendency to cause chronic illness with suppurative lesions and remains a serious menace in the United States.

Brucellosis can have an acute onset, with chills, fever, sweats, headache, backache, anorexia and weakness. These features are not specific, and the most frequently mistaken diagnoses are influenza or viral infections. The onset is often insidious; patients exhibit a low-grade fever and complain of weakness, easy fatigability and insomnia, somatic aches and pains, and mental depression. They usually feel better in the morning than later in the day. Frequently, under these circumstances, the correct diagnosis is either completely overlooked or delayed.

In a study of several hundred cases of brucellosis the major symptoms in order of frequency were: weakness, chills, sweats, anorexia, generalized aches, headache, nervousness and backache. Brucellosis does have a severe impact upon the nervous system, the most significant complaints being mental depression, nervousness, insomnia and sexual impotence. It is not surprising that occasionally patients have been designated as suffering from severe neurotic tendencies. In fact, even in recognized cases there is a serious overlay of neuroses that occur in relatively unstable individuals.

The majority of patients with acute brucellosis usually recover completely within 6 to 9 months, and more rapidly with the aid of antibiotic therapy. Experience has shown that over 80 per cent of the cases recover within a year, leaving about 10 per cent with definite chronic illness and 10 per cent with questionably active disease. The patient with chronic illness usually exhibits no abnormal physical findings, except in those rare cases in which suppuration of the long bones or spine, liver, spleen and kidneys occurs. In the chronic cases with involvement of the liver and spleen, x-ray films of the abdomen may reveal calcification.[3]

The pertinent physical findings of acute brucellosis include lymphadenopathy and splenomegaly. Hepatomegaly occurs occasionally. Other features found in both acute and chronic brucellosis are cited in the following discussion.

Complications. The most common complication relates to neuropsychiatric disorders ranging from acute psychoses to chronic reactive depressions. Organic neurologic disturbances include chronic encephalomeningitis and peripheral neuritis. Pain distributed over the course of the sciatic nerve is very common and is associated with *Brucella* spondylitis of the lumbar spine. Spondylitis is the second most common complication and often simulates the complaints and findings in herniation of intervertebral disks. Involvement of the lumbar spine is most common, but localization in the thoracic and cervical areas also occurs. While painful joints occur in acute brucellosis, rarely with suppuration, rheumatoid arthritis cannot be considered a complication of the disease. An interesting complication is chronic synovitis with effusions into the knee joints.

Cardiovascular complications include

subacute bacterial endocarditis. However, no evidence has accumulated to indicate that idiopathic aortic stenosis is due to brucellosis. Thrombophlebitis is a rare complication. Pulmonary complications rarely, if ever, occur.

Although brucellae localize in the liver, serious hepatic complications, such as cirrhosis and suppuration, rarely occur. Jaundice is rare. Hypersplenism is associated with splenomegaly due to brucellosis and has led, on rare occasions, to thrombocytopenia or hemolytic anemia.

Epididymitis and orchitis occur in about 5 per cent of the cases, and cystitis and prostatitis have been reported rarely. Pyelonephritis does occur and is a serious complication, simulating the course of tuberculosis of the kidneys.

Ocular complications include iritis, choroiditis, uveitis and nummular keratitis. Visual disturbances are due primarily to involvement of the optic nerve.

Diagnosis. The diagnosis of brucellosis in a highly endemic area is not difficult because the disease is considered in the differential diagnosis of febrile conditions. However, the problem in many areas, including the United States, revolves about the sporadic, unrecognized case. A helpful diagnostic point is to recall that brucellosis is largely an occupational disease, and the occupational history of a febrile patient will often lead to successful laboratory confirmation of the disease. The symptoms and signs of brucellosis simulate those of many other conditions, including typhoid, malaria, infectious mononucleosis and anicteric viral hepatitis.

There are no specific features in the examination of the urine. Leukopenia and lymphocytosis are helpful aids. Atypical lymphocytes, such as those occurring in infectious mononucleosis, are frequently present. The erythrocyte sedimentation rate may be normal or accelerated and is of no diagnostic help.

The most helpful laboratory test for screening suspected cases of brucellosis is the tube-dilution agglutination test done with a dependable *Brucella* antigen, such as described by the Committee on Brucellosis of the National Research Council.[4] A titer of 1:100 or above is usually considered significant when associated with the clinical features consistent with brucellosis. On occasion, lower titers may indicate the presence of blocking antibodies, which may be detected by centrifuging the tubes after 48 hours of incubation at 37° C (98.6° F) at 3000 rpm for 30 minutes. Blocking antibodies are usually present in the more chronic cases. The *Brucella* agglutination test is not specific, since a common antigenic factor is shared with *Vibrio cholerae* and *Francisella tularensis*. Individuals recently immunized with cholera vaccine, as well as patients with tularemia, may acquire *Brucella* agglutinins. Patients recovering from brucellosis may have a low titer of agglutinins extending beyond a year, but rarely above 1:100. The detection of 7S agglutinating antibody even in a titer less than 1:100 indicates active infection.[5]

At least three blood cultures should be completed with Albini *Brucella* broth or trypticase soy broth. Ten per cent of the air in the culture bottles should be replaced with carbon dioxide. Cultures usually will reveal growth of brucellae within 10 days to 2 weeks, but should not be discarded until an elapse of 30 days. Rarely have brucellae been recovered from patients in the absence of *Brucella* agglutinins.

Various other diagnostic procedures have been recommended. Dermal sensitivity tests have the same significance as the tuberculin test and consequently are of no assistance in diagnosis but may be of value in epidemiologic surveys. Their use is often followed by a high titer of agglutinins, which may confuse the interpretation of the agglutination reaction.

Treatment. There is no significant difference in the therapy of acute or chronic brucellosis.[6] In either case, the patients should be assured that the vast majority of patients recover completely after proper antibiotic therapy. The most appropriate antibiotic is a tetracycline drug given orally in a dose of 0.5 gm 4 times daily for 21 days. For the more severe cases some recommend the simultaneous use of 0.5 gm streptomycin given intramuscularly twice daily for 14 days. Therapy with tetracycline as above may be repeated once in the case of relapse, but should rarely be given a third time. Further drug therapy is of little or no benefit.

For the seriously ill and toxic patient, adrenocorticoids can be used concurrently with a tetracycline agent. Cortisol in a dose of 100 mg 3 times daily or prednisone 20 mg 2 to 3 times daily for 3 to 5 days is recommended.

In addition, patients should be placed at rest and given sedation when needed. Salicylates will frequently control the somatic aches and pains.

Prophylaxis. The widespread geographic distribution and the occurrence of *Brucella* in a variety of animals provide many opportunities for contact. However, human infection in most instances is acquired by direct contact with infected animal tissues or discharges. Important factors in prophylaxis are a properly protected water supply and avoidance of unpasteurized milk and milk products.

REFERENCES

1. Stableforth, A. W., and Jones, L. M. 1963. Report of the subcommittee on taxonomy of the genus *Brucella*. Speciation in the genus *Brucella*. Int. Bull. Bact. Nomen. Tax. *13*:145–158.
2. Buchanan, T. M., et al. 1974. Brucellosis in the United States, 1960–1972: An abattoir-associated disease. Parts I, II, and III. Medicine *53*:403–439.
3. Spink, W. W. 1964. Host-parasite relationship in human brucellosis with prolonged illness due to suppuration of the liver and spleen. Am. J. Med. Sci. *247*:129–136.
4. Spink, W. W., McCullough, N. B., Hutchings, L. M., and Mingle, C. K. 1954. A standardized antigen and agglutination technic for human brucellosis: Report No. 3 of the National Research Council, Committee on Public Health Aspects of Brucellosis. Am. J. Clin. Path. *24*:496–498.
5. Reddin, J. L., Anderson, R. K., Jenness, R., and Spink, W. W. 1965. Significance of 7S and macroglobulin brucella agglutinins in human brucellosis. N. Engl. J. Med. *272*:1263–1268.
6. Spink, W. W. 1956. The Nature of Brucellosis. University of Minnesota Press, Minneapolis. 464 pp.

CHAPTER 23

Tuberculosis

GUY P. YOUMANS

Synonyms. Consumption, phthisis.

Definition. Tuberculosis is a chronic infectious disease in human beings caused by *Mycobacterium tuberculosis.* (Zopf, 1883), Lehmann and Neumann, 1896.

Etiology. The above definition is too restrictive because it is now known that *Mycobacterium bovis, Mycobacterium avium, Mycobacterium kansasii* and *Mycobacterium intracellulare* all may produce pulmonary disease in man indistinguishable from that caused by *M. tuberculosis.* Certain types of disease caused by *M. tuberculosis,* e.g. infection of the skin and the lymph glands, can also be produced by other microorganisms such as *Mycobacterium marinum, Mycobacterium ulcerans* and *Mycobacterium scrofulaceum.*

It has long been recognized that acid-fast microorganisms different from *M. tuberculosis* sometimes were associated with pulmonary disease in human beings. Until recently, little thought had been given to the possibility that some of these might be etiologically related to the pulmonary pathology, in spite of descriptions in the earlier literature of cases which supported this possibility. During about the last 20 years, however, it has become established that a significant proportion of cases diagnosed as tuberculosis may be caused by acid-fast microorganisms so different from *M. tuberculosis* that they represent separate mycobacterial species.

The reasons for this tardy recognition of the role of other mycobacteria in latent infection and pulmonary disease are several. First, for many years following the initial isolation by Koch in 1882 of *M. tuberculosis,* pulmonary disease due to *M. tuberculosis* was so prevalent that the relatively few cases which may have been caused by other mycobacteria were not apparent. Therefore, the doctrine became firmly established that tuberculosis was caused only by one fairly characteristic microbe, *M. tuberculosis.* Later it was found that *M. bovis* also could cause pulmonary disease in man. Second, this state of obscurity of the other pathogenic mycobacteria was maintained, in part, by the failure of workers in diagnostic laboratories routinely to isolate and cultivate the acid-fast bacteria present in the sputum or infected tissue of persons suffering from pulmonary disease; smears and Ziehl-Neelsen stain were considered adequate bacteriologic control procedures. Third, the recognition of the pathogenic propensities of other mycobacteria has been hindered by the fact that most of them are not pathogenic for guinea pigs as are *M. tuberculosis* and *M. bovis.* Finally, pigmented and nonpigmented acid-fast organisms are widely distributed in nature, e.g. soil and water, and may be found in association with tubercle bacilli in sputum or gastric washings. It is not surprising that when microorganisms of similar appearance have been encountered alone their etiologic significance has been regarded with skepticism.

It has been traditional to refer to mycobacteria which differ appreciably from *M. tuberculosis* and which were found in association with disease in man as atypical mycobacteria. Most of these now have been given species names; these names together with other characteristics are listed in Table 23–1.

The role of mycobacteria other than *M. tuberculosis* and *M. bovis* in the production of pulmonary and other diseases in man probably could not have become apparent until the two following conditions existed. First, it would be necessary for the prevalence of infection and disease caused by *M. tuberculosis* to be very low as compared with that during

---

Portions of this chapter have also appeared in *The Biologic and Clinical Basis of Infectious Diseases,* W. B. Saunders Co., 1975.

Table 23–1. CHARACTERISTICS OF MYCOBACTERIA

Legitimate Name	*Relative Patho-genicity for Man*	*Runyon Group*	*Acceptable Common Name*	*Names Without Legitimate Standing and Comments*
M. avium	+++	Group III Nonphotochromogen	Avian tubercle bacillus	Closely related to *M. intracellulare*
M. bovis	++++		Bovine tubercle bacillus	
M. chelonei	+	Group IV Rapid Grower		*M. abscessus*
M. fortuitum	+	Group IV Rapid Grower		Only rapid growing mycobacterium pathogenic for man
M. gastri	0	Group III Nonphotochromogen		Not known to be pathogenic for man
M. intracellulare	+++	Group III Nonphotochromogen	Battey bacillus	*M. batteyi*
M. kansasii	+++	Group I Photochromogen		Rare, nonpigmented and scotochromogenic strains
M. marinum	+++	Group I Photochromogen (Nonpigmented when grown in the dark, pigmented when exposed to light during growth)		*M. balnei* *M. platypoecilus* (skin infections)
M. scrofulaceum	++	Group II Scotochromogen		*M. marianum* (scrofula)
M. gordonae	0	Group II Scotochromogen (Pigmented when grown in the dark)	"Tap-water" scotochromogen	*M. aquae*—not known to be pathogenic for man
M. terrae	Rare?	Group III Nonphotochromogen	Radish bacillus	
M. tuberculosis	++++		Human tubercle bacillus	
M. triviale	0	Group III Nonphotochromogen	V bacillus	Similar to *M. terrae*
M. ulcerans	++++			Associated with skin infections
M. xenopi	++	Group III Nonphotochromogen		Formerly spelled *M. xenopei* *M. littorale*
M. leprae	++++		Hansen's bacillus	Causes leprosy (Hansen's disease)

the earlier years of this century. Second, it also would be necessary for the isolation, cultivation and characterization of the microorganisms found in pathologic material from cases of chronic pulmonary disease to be widely, even if not routinely, practiced. Both of these situations fortuitously prevailed in the United States in the early 1950s, both as a result of a half-century of intensive effort to control tuberculosis by public health measures, and because of the impact of chemotherapy. Chemotherapy played a dual role. Not only did it contribute significantly to the decrease in the incidence and prevalence of tuberculous disease, but once it was realized that *M. tuberculosis* could readily develop a high degree of resistance to the antimicrobial drugs in use, there was a marked increase in the routine use of procedures for the isolation, cultivation and characterization of the acid-fast bacteria present in the pathologic material obtained from patients. Initially, these procedures were carried out primarily to permit the determination of the sensitivity of the microorganisms to chemotherapeutic agents, but they functioned equally well to reveal the presence of other mycobacteria.

Epidemiology. TUBERCULOSIS *(Mycobacterium tuberculosis).* The distribution of tuberculosis is worldwide. The prevalence of the disease, though, varies widely. In the more developed countries, and in particular in the United States, the incidence has been reduced dramatically. In many developing and tropical countries tuberculosis is a major problem.[1]

Tuberculosis is primarily a disease of man. The major reservoir of *M. tuberculosis* is man, and the disease is transmitted from man to man principally by droplet nuclei which form when infectious material is discharged into the air by coughing. The portal of entry for the infection is usually the lower respiratory tract; the major site of initial infection, therefore, is the lung. With the development of pulmonary disease and particularly with the formation of cavities, large numbers of virulent tubercle bacilli may be excreted. The transmission of the disease, then, is from active case to susceptible persons by infected droplet nuclei. Indirect transmission can occur from contaminated objects (fomites) handled by both diseased persons and susceptible persons, but is relatively uncommon.

Infection with virulent tubercle bacilli can also take place through the skin. This is called inoculation tuberculosis and rarely occurs under natural conditions, but is not infrequently seen in pathologists, medical students and laboratory workers as a result of handling infectious materials.

Tuberculosis can also be acquired by way of the gastrointestinal tract. This is the principal way in which infection with *M. bovis* occurs. This microorganism may be excreted in large numbers in the milk of infected cows. Ingestion of such milk by human beings may result in extensive tuberculous disease. In some areas of the world this is still a major source of infection. In the United States, control of tuberculosis in cattle and the pasteurization of milk have virtually eliminated tuberculosis in man caused by *M. bovis.*

Although man is the major reservoir of infection for *M. tuberculosis,* other reservoirs of infection may be established under special circumstances. For example, cattle, dogs, cats and pet monkeys can become infected if they are exposed to a master who has active pulmonary tuberculosis. Such animals, if they develop active disease, can serve as reservoirs of infection and transmit the disease to susceptible human beings with whom they may come into close contact. Such situations are rare and the disease apparently does not maintain itself readily in such animals.

ATYPICAL MYCOBACTERIAL INFECTION AND DISEASE. The epidemiology of pulmonary or other atypical mycobacterial disease is quite different from that of tuberculosis.[2] For example, pulmonary disease caused by *M. kansasii* and *M. intracellulare* is not transmitted from open cases to contacts, and the disease is seen most frequently in white males over 40 years of age. Patients excreting these mycobacteria need not be isolated. The lack of contagiousness is especially puzzling because a high degree of contagiousness is one of the outstanding features of the disease caused by *M. tuberculosis.* The low degree of pathogenicity of these microorganisms for experimental animals, even though viable cells may persist in the tissues of these animals for extended periods, may provide an explanation. If pathogenicity is also very low for human beings, a situation might exist in which large numbers of human beings become infected with atypical mycobacteria at some period in their lives, without developing clinically recognizable disease. However, an occasional infected person might develop disease under conditions which would so lower local or general resistance that the atypical mycobacteria already in the body would begin to proliferate. Once a focal area of necrosis appeared, the disease might become slowly progressive. This situation would be analogous to that seen in certain mycotic diseases, e.g. coccidioidomycosis, blastomycosis and histoplasmosis.

The production of disease by the mycobacteria found in Runyon's groups I, II, III and IV (Table 23–3) emphasizes the importance of host susceptibility. It is probably safe to postulate that progressive disease due to these other mycobacteria will occur only in the abnormal host. The abnormality may be caused by other local or systemic disease, or by one or more of the factors which are known to reduce cellular immunity to infection. In general, the mycobacteria included within the Runyon groups should be regarded as opportunists, rather than as primary pathogens capable of producing progressive disease in the normal host; *M. tuberculosis* and *M. bovis* would fall in the latter category.

Thus, certain features of the epidemiology of atypical mycobacterial pulmonary disease in man become clearer. There is apparently a broad base of latent subclinical infection in the human population with one or more of these microorganisms. This is revealed by skin-testing surveys (Table 23–2). It would be reasonable to propose that in certain persons later in life when immunity wanes, either naturally or because of some as yet unknown predisposing factor or factors, disease might result; hence, the observed pattern of greater prevalence of disease in older people, and the lack of relationship between cases. No explanation is currently available, however, for the predominance of pulmonary disease due to these microorganisms in white males. This may represent a racial predisposition, an occupational hazard not shared by colored races, or merely a higher incidence of initial infection.

The appreciably larger prevalence of latent infection due to the Group II scotochromogens is most probably a reflection of their greater ubiquitousness in nature. The very low prevalence of actual disease due to Group II microorganisms is probably, in turn, a reflection of their much lower pathogenicity for man. The low prevalence of latent infection due to *M. kansasii* but the relatively high incidence of pulmonary disease may indicate a higher degree of pathogenicity of *M. kansasii* for man than of Group III or Group II mycobacteria.

The source of infection for man with these atypical mycobacteria has not been firmly established. Contact with Group II scotochromogenic atypical mycobacteria undoubtedly is frequent because of their wide

Table 23–2. Frequency and Mean Size of Reactions Among Navy Recruits to 0.0001 mg of PPD Antigens Prepared From Various Strains of Mycobacteria*

PPD Antigen	*Prepared From*	*Number Tested*	*Reactions of 2 mm or More* Percentage	Mean Size (mm)
PPD–S	*M. tuberculosis*	212,462	8.6	10.3
PPD–F	*M. fortuitum*	3,415	7.7	4.8
PPD–240	Unclassified; group 3	3,729	12.0	5.8
PPD–Y	*M. kansasii*	13,913	13.1	6.2
PPD–63	Unclassified; group 3	9,473	17.5	7.0
PPD–sm	*M. smegmatis*	14,239	18.3	5.7
PPD–ph	*M. phlei*	15,229	23.1	6.4
PPD–216	Unclassified; group 2	10,060	28.4	9.0
PPD–A	*M. avium*	10,769	30.5	6.7
PPD–B	Unclassified; (Battey type)	212,462	35.1	7.7
PPD–269	Unclassified; group 3	8,402	39.0	7.2
PPD–G	Unclassified; group 2	29,540	48.7	10.3

*Reprinted from L. B. Edwards, 1963. Current status of the tuberculin test. Ann. N.Y. Acad. Sci. *106*:32–43.

distribution, e.g. in water and soil. These microorganisms have also been isolated from secretions of the upper respiratory tract of man, so they may, under certain conditions, be normal microbial inhabitants of this area. However, it should be emphasized that the high degree of tuberculin sensitivity to purified protein derivative (PPD) prepared from these organisms indicates actual infection. Such infection might occur following their ingestion in water or food; following inhalation of the organism in dust or in droplets; or as a consequence of invasion from a habitat in the upper respiratory tract by way of the regional lymphatics. No clarifying information is available on this point.

There is a close relationship between Group III nonphotochromogenic atypical mycobacteria and *M. avium.* This suggests that man may become infected with these microorganisms from sources where one would expect to find *M. avium.* Infected fowl are known to distribute this bacterium widely in their environment, and it is known also that these microorganisms may persist for long periods in the soil in which they may even multiply. Although pulmonary infection in man caused by *M. avium* is rare, swine are frequently infected. Low-grade infection can occur in cattle and possibly in sheep. The greater prevalence of tuberculin sensitivity to PPD-B (Table 23–2) in rural areas has added support to the possibility that humans may become infected directly from domestic animals, or indirectly from soil contaminated by infected domestic animals, although the lack of pathogenicity of the Group III nonphotochromogenic atypical mycobacteria for experimental animals does not lend support to this hypothesis. Many of the atypical mycobacteria may reside in soil and be carried from there to water supplies and hence to man or animals by either inhalation or ingestion. Microorganisms similar to the "Battey" bacillus (Table 23–1) also have been isolated from the secretions of the upper respiratory tract of healthy humans, so human beings also might serve as a source of infection.

Mycobacterium kansasii, on the other hand, has not been found in association with any disease of lower animals. There have been no reports of it being found in the upper respiratory tract of man.

Pathogenesis. Since infection usually takes place by way of the lower respiratory tract, the lung is the first organ involved and it is here that the initial major manifestations of disease occur. *Mycobacterium tuberculosis* can produce infection and disease in almost every tissue and organ in the body, but such disease is usually the result of dissemination from an initial pulmonary focus.[1,3] There is evidence which suggests that the predilection of *M. tuberculosis* for pulmonary tissue is directly related to its requirement for molecular oxygen for growth. Although, as mentioned before, the process of infection and multiplication of the microorganisms will take place in other tissues, it proceeds most rapidly in the lung. Therefore, the sequence of events which follows infection of the lung with *M. tuberculosis* can be used as an example of what may occur following infection of any organ or tissue.

In following the progress of tubercu-

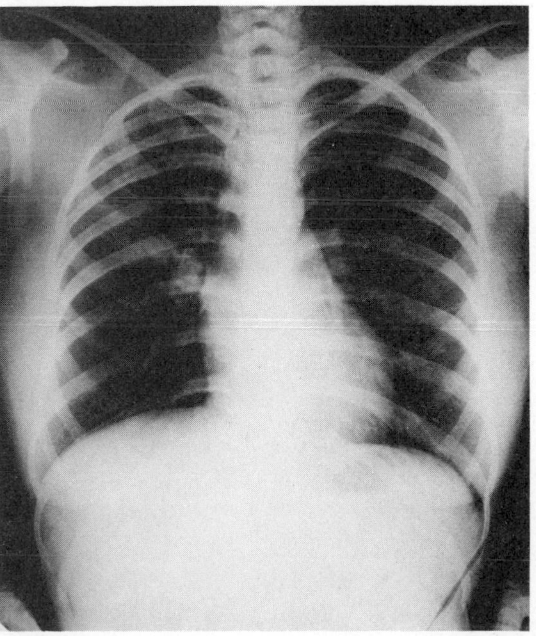

Figure 23–1. Progressive primary pulmonary tuberculosis in an adult Negro. The disease appeared first in the apex of the right lower lobe. The right hilar nodes are enlarged, and progression can be seen in the first and second anterior interspaces of the right upper lobe. (Courtesy of Dr. John H. Seabury, Louisiana State University School of Medicine, New Orleans.)

lous infection it is important to differentiate between that which occurs following infection of a person who has had no previous experience with *M. tuberculosis* (Fig. 23–1), and the process in a person who has previously been infected (Fig. 23–2). In the former person there develops primary infection or primary disease. In primary infection one or more mycobacterial cells lodge within an alveolus where they are rapidly phagocytosed, most likely by alveolar macrophages. Because of their resistance to destruction, these virulent mycobacteria multiply within these macrophages almost as rapidly as they do in an artificial culture medium. However, since the maximum rate of multiplication still is slow, the numbers of virulent tubercle bacilli increase slowly. Therefore, the appearance of symptoms or pathologic changes due to the infection may require several weeks.

When the tubercle bacilli reach a significant number, an inflammatory cellular exudate appears. Therefore, primary tuberculous infection is characterized by being pneumonic in character. In spite of the cellular reaction there is little resistance to the multiplication of the tubercle bacilli and soon dissemination of infection from this focus will occur. This spread is primarily by way of the lymphatics and there is early extensive involvement of the regional (hilar) lymph nodes. At the same time there is spillover from the lymphatics into the blood stream with a seeding of virulent tubercle bacilli in all of the organs and tissues of the body. In a small proportion of such persons this process proceeds until widespread tuberculous disease occurs, and possibly death provided treatment is not given. In the majority of such persons, however, after a period of a few weeks the following dramatic changes will occur. The rate of multiplication of the tubercle bacilli markedly decreases, the pneumonic process resolves and the dissemination of tubercle bacilli to other organs ceases. The same changes will occur also in all other tissues where tubercle bacilli may reside. Resolution of the disease process may proceed to a point such that, in many people so infected, little or no residue of the infection remains. In some, particularly in infants and children, only the Ghon complex, a small calcified nodule in the lung and enlarged hilar lymph nodes, may remain.

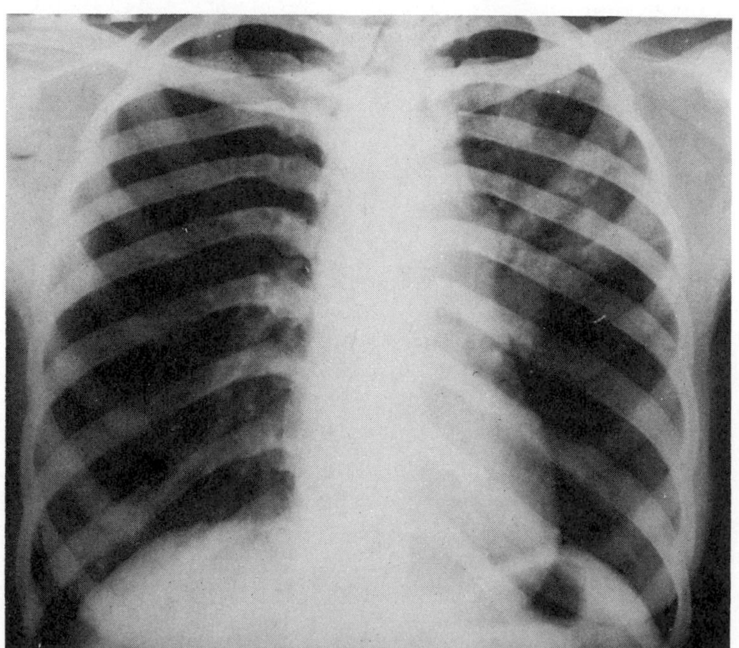

Figure 23–2. Postprimary progressive pulmonary tuberculosis in an adult Negro. The primary pulmonary component was in the base of the left lower lobe and healed. An enlarged left hilar lymph node ruptured several months later, discharging into the upper lobe bronchus. Tuberculous pneumonia is present with cavitation in the second interspace and overlying the second rib anteriorly. (Courtesy of Dr. John H. Seabury, Louisiana State University School of Medicine, New Orleans.)

Coincident with the changes described above, two immunologic manifestations will appear. First, the affected individual becomes tuberculin-positive and will show reactions of delayed hypersensitivity to certain low molecular weight proteins or polypeptides which are found in the tubercle bacillus. Second, the macrophages within which the tubercle bacilli previously were able to multiply so readily now have acquired the ability to inhibit markedly the multiplication of virulent tubercle bacilli. Therefore, the disease process is arrested and with time many of the virulent cells are destroyed. The diseased person has thus become immunized as a consequence of the reaction of his immunologic system to the infection, an example of acquired cellular immunity.

It is of critical importance at this point to examine the relationship between tuberculin hypersensitivity and acquired cellular immunity. Tuberculin hypersensitivity is a specific immunologic response to tuberculoprotein or polypeptide. This hypersensitivity does not involve circulating antibody, cannot be passively transferred by serum, but can be passively transferred using lymphocytes obtained from tuberculin-sensitive animals. Such lymphocytes in the presence of tuberculoprotein apparently elaborate a substance or substances (lymphotoxin) which destroy tissue cells and may be responsible, in part, for the destructive inflammatory reaction. On the other hand, the acquired cellular immunity to infection manifests itself as the intracellular inhibition of multiplication of virulent tubercle bacilli. This immunity also cannot be transferred with serum, i.e. circulating antibodies are not involved, but it can be transferred with lymphocytes. Thus, there are some parallels between these two phenomena, and, because of these parallels, the majority of investigators take the position that tuberculin hypersensitivity is responsible for acquired cellular immunity. This appears reasonable when one realizes that when a tuberculin reaction occurs, macrophages accumulate and will become activated. Thus, they are better able to prevent the multiplication of virulent tubercle bacilli. This explanation requires that immunity to tuberculosis be specifically engendered (since the tuberculin reaction is specific for tuberculoprotein), but that the immune process itself (the inhibition of multiplication of virulent tubercle bacilli) must be nonspecific because it depends only on macrophage activation, and activated macrophages will be more capable of handling all bacteria.

There are a number of findings which make it difficult to accept this relationship between tuberculin hypersensitivity and immunity to tuberculosis. First, animals can be rendered highly tuberculin-sensitive by injecting them with Wax D together with tuberculoprotein, both extracted from tubercle bacilli. These animals do not show any increased resistance over animals which have not been rendered tuberculin sensitive. Second, certain RNA-protein complexes can be isolated from mycobacterial cells which will induce high degrees of increased resistance to infection with tuberculosis but which do not induce any detectable tuberculin hypersensitivity. Finally, there is strong evidence indicating that the acquired immune state in tuberculosis is specific. Since these two phenomena, tuberculin hypersensitivity and acquired cellular immunity, can be dissociated and since there is a specific element in resistance to tuberculosis, it would appear more reasonable to take the position that tuberculin hypersensitivity is not responsible for acquired immunity. It is more likely that, while macrophage activation, regardless of how it occurs, may play a role in resistance to tuberculous infection, this role is a minor one compared to the specific resistance which develops and which recently has been shown probably to be lymphocyte mediated.

Another reason for being skeptical of the role of tuberculin hypersensitivity in immunity to tuberculosis is the fact that tuberculin hypersensitivity is largely responsible for the destructive lesions, i.e. necrosis and cavity formation, which occur in tuberculous disease. This is illustrated by looking at the sequence of events in secondary, or reinfection, tuberculosis.

Primary tuberculosis is the disease that occurs in persons who have never been exposed to tubercle bacilli and who, therefore, are not tuberculin-sensitive, nor do they have any acquired cellular immunity. Until tuberculin hypersensitivity and acquired immunity develop, primary tuberculosis is for the most part a nondestructive disease process with rapid dissemination of the infecting microorganism. On the other hand, reinfection tuberculosis is a disease that occurs in the presence of tuberculin hypersensitivity and in spite of the presence of acquired cellular immunity. Secondary tuberculosis may occur as a result of recrudescence of an old infection (endogenous) or by reinfection from an active case (exogenous). Regardless of source, the initial lesion is characterized by necrosis and by being circumscribed (localized). The necrosis is the result of the destructive nature of the inflammatory reaction of tuberculin hypersensitivity. The lesion is circumscribed and localized because of cellular immunity, which, operating in all of the adjacent tissues and within the lymphatic system which drains the lesion, will prevent multiplication of tubercle bacilli and spread of the disease. Initially, the tubercle bacilli will multiply only in or near the necrotic area where cellular immunity has been reduced or is absent. The disease may progress, however, by extension as adjacent tissues develop necrosis as a consequence of allergic inflammation. Spread also may occur in the lung if a bronchus is eroded and infected material enters (bronchogenic spread), or by the blood stream if a blood vessel is eroded (hematogenous spread).

The reasons for the local breakdown of resistance which leads to a necrotic focus and disease are not well known. It is known that any factor, e.g. age, degenerative disease or immunosuppressive therapy, which lowers resistance to infection will promote the development of tuberculous disease in previously infected people. Therefore there must be a breakdown in cellular immunity which permits growth of the tubercle bacilli to the point where enough tuberculoprotein is produced to elicit a local necrotizing allergic reaction. Since necrosis is the outstanding feature of the reinfection tuberculosis, the resolution of the disease process becomes far more difficult than is the resolution of a primary infection, which frequently is overcome by the acquired cellular immunity before the allergic state develops to the point where extensive necrosis will occur.

It is important to realize that tubercle bacilli may remain viable but dormant within the tissues of human beings for many months, or years, or even a lifetime. This follows from the fact that the acquired immune response inhibits the multiplication of tubercle bacilli but apparently does not confer upon the cells the capability to destroy all of the tubercle bacilli. Therefore tubercle bacilli within macrophages located in a small tubercle in a lymph node or in the lung may be held in check for long periods but be perfectly capable of again beginning to metabolize and divide if local resistance is lowered. Evidence for this type of infection is provided by the fact that tuberculin hypersensitivity will persist in many persons for years following a primary infection even though all signs of tuberculous disease have disappeared. Differentiation must be made between tuberculous infection, which can be defined as the presence of viable and frequently nonmultiplying virulent tubercle bacilli within the cells or tissues of a host, and tuberculous disease, which is due to viable multiplying tubercle bacilli within cells or tissues or necrotic foci which produce overt manifestations of disease.

Clinical Characteristics. Many primary infections are asymptomatic or accompanied by minor constitutional manifestations of low-grade fever and lassitude. If pleuritic involvement accompanies the primary infection or the primary infection becomes progressive, localizing symptoms of cough, chest pain and subsequent increase in fever may be observed. Infantile primary infections not only may be progressive but also may result in acute dissemination with meningeal or other localizing manifestations.[1,4]

The only clue to the establishment of primary infection may be found in chest roentgenograms or the conversion of the tuberculin test from negative to positive.

Most primary infections, especially in children, tend to regress and heal or become inactive. Progressive primary disease is more likely to be symptomatic.

Postprimary progression and reinfection tuberculosis may also be asymptomatic, but constitutional manifestations of some degree can usually be elicited by careful history taking. Fatigability, anorexia, weight loss, malaise, fever and night sweats are manifestations which are more common than all the localizing symptoms except cough. Unfortunately, these are common to many illnesses, and in the tropics the people most afflicted with tuberculosis frequently are those who never have known the feeling of good health. Patients who have a relatively acute onset, with fever and localizing symptoms, are more likely to seek medical attention.

Local symptoms depend upon the sites of involvement, the responsiveness of the tissue or organ to inflammation and the patient's psychological orientation to illness. It is important to remember that localizing symptoms may be absent in the presence of extensive disease. The lung is the organ most commonly involved and cough the most frequent symptom. The latter may not be recognized as a complaint unless accompanied by hemoptysis, abundant sputum production, or pleuritic pain.

Tuberculous lymphadenitis, most easily recognized in the neck or mediastinum, is chiefly seen in childhood and, with lesser frequency, in primary infection in adults. Its overall incidence varies considerably from one population group to another, but it is relatively frequent in Negroes. Although often associated with infection by *M. bovis*, this form of tuberculosis continues to be rather common in areas where bovine infection is very rare, e.g. East and West Africa. More recently it has been found that *M. scrofulaceum* (Group II, scotochromogen) frequently produces lymphadenitis in children.

Abdominal tuberculous infection may accompany the primary tuberculous infection in childhood, principally as tuberculous lymphadenitis. Intestinal involvement in adults is usually associated with extensive pulmonary involvement or acute progressive primary infection. Tuberculous peritonitis with ascites may be only a part of polyserositis or a separate expression of hematogenous or lymphogenous dissemination.

Serositis due to tuberculosis is serious and is often followed by clinically apparent extrathoracic tuberculosis; it is more frequent in the Negro than the Caucasian. Although serositis may appear subsequent to bacillemia, it is more often an expression of extension from lymph node involvement.

In infants, central nervous system tuberculosis may appear as a consequence of bacillemia during the primary infection; it usually occurs as an acute disease with meningitis. Central nervous system tuberculosis in the reinfection state may develop insidiously, with behavioral and neurologic changes due to submeningeal reactivating granulomas; it may also appear as an acute meningitis during miliary dissemination.

Tuberculosis of the skeletal system usually presents with localizing symptoms and signs. Pain of vertebral origin may be diffuse or segmentally referred and is easily misinterpreted unless there is careful x-ray examination.

Although renal tuberculosis may produce constitutional manifestations and decreased renal function, it usually remains asymptomatic until the lower urinary tract is involved. Pyuria in the absence of organisms which can be cultured on ordinary blood agar plates should provoke a study for urinary tract tuberculosis.

Clinically, pulmonary or other disease produced by atypical mycobacteria cannot be distinguished from that caused by *M. tuberculosis.*

Diagnosis. The diagnosis of active tuberculosis can be made with certainty only by showing that viable virulent tubercle bacilli are associated with a lesion or an affected organ. This association, in turn, can be revealed only by the isolation of virulent tubercle bacilli.[2,4] Tuberculosis usually is a pulmonary infection; therefore, sputum is the specimen most commonly examined for the presence of tubercle bacilli. However, other materials, such as urine, spinal fluid or tissue biopsies, may need to be examined.

When adequate laboratory facilities and

personnel are available, attempts should always be made to isolate the offending mycobacterial species. Certain principles and procedures essential for the successful performance of this task are given below.

Emphasis must be placed upon the obtaining of a suitable specimen for bacteriologic examination. This is of particular importance in the case of sputum, since it is always contaminated with microorganisms from the oral cavity. In the laboratory, such contaminated specimens must be decontaminated and then inoculated upon media selective for the growth of mycobacteria. In the decontamination process, advantage is taken of the fact that tubercle bacilli are much more resistant to deleterious agents such as acids and alkali than most other bacteria. Treatment of the sputum sample with alkali, for example, will markedly reduce the non-mycobacterial microbial population without seriously affecting the tubercle bacilli. Not all of the contaminating bacteria are killed in this manner, however, so the treated sputum specimens should be inoculated upon a medium containing an inhibitory dye such as malachite green. Although growth of the mycobacteria will be retarded somewhat, multiplication of a wide variety of other bacteria will be inhibited almost completely.

It follows that a sputum specimen which contains the fewest contaminating microorganisms will be the best material for the isolation of *M. tuberculosis.* Therefore, the collection of 24-hour sputum specimens, as is commonly done, is not always an appropriate procedure. This specimen, much of which will sit around at room temperature for hours, will have a heavy growth of oral bacteria and the decontaminating procedures used in the laboratory may not be adequate to dispose of them. The preferred procedure is to nebulize the patient early in the morning in order to take advantage of the presence of overnight pooled bronchial secretions. These specimens should then immediately be taken to the microbiology laboratory for prompt processing and inoculation upon suitable media. It is important not to use propylene glycol in the nebulizer, for this substance may inhibit the growth of, or even kill, tubercle bacilli.

Gastric contents are sometimes aspirated in order to obtain material from which tubercle bacilli may be isolated. Since bronchial secretions are automatically swallowed, the stomach may become a repository for virulent tubercle bacilli in patients suffering from pulmonary tuberculosis. This procedure should be avoided unless absolutely necessary because such specimens are frequently contaminated with saprophytic mycobacteria which, as noted previously, may be found in water and soil and therefore be ingested with food. The presence of such saprophytic mycobacteria makes the isolation and identification of virulent tubercle bacilli more difficult. However, at times gastric aspiration may be necessary in children and in adults from whom bronchial secretions, for one reason or another, may not readily be obtained.

It is important to recognize that several specimens (not less than three and preferably not more than six) of sputum, urine or other material should be collected from each patient with suspected tuberculosis. This is essential because the number of tubercle bacilli excreted may be small and in many cases not every sample collected will contain tubercle bacilli. This arises from the fact that there may be only occasional release of tubercle bacilli from subepithelial bronchial abscesses. Single, early morning urine specimens are better than specimens collected over a 24-hour period for the same reasons as given above for sputum.

It is also important to recognize that in most cases, because of the slow multiplication rate of virulent tubercle bacilli, growth will not be detected on a medium inoculated with material containing tubercle bacilli until 3 to 6 weeks have elapsed. In some cases from 2 to 3 months may be required for growth to appear. When large numbers of tubercle bacilli are present, e.g. in a sputum sample, growth will be evident in a shorter time than when specimens are inoculated which contain very few tubercle bacilli.

Therefore, the result of the microbiologic examination of sputum samples will not be forthcoming rapidly.

Once growth has appeared, *M. tuberculosis* can be identified by virulence for animals, or by certain chemical tests (Table 23–3).

Microscopic examination of sputum specimens also is frequently employed. Advantage here is taken of the fact that mycobacteria are acid-fast and can be revealed as red rodlike organisms against a blue background in the material placed upon the microscopic slide. Unfortunately, acid-fast staining does not distinguish virulent tubercle bacilli from contaminating saprophytic bacteria or from atypical mycobacteria. Therefore, the presence of acid-fast bacteria in the sputum specimen from a person suspected of having tuberculosis does not provide a definitive diagnosis. The presence of large numbers of acid-fast rods in the sputum of a patient with gross manifestations of pulmonary involvement may be suggestive but must be confirmed by isolation and identification of virulent tubercle bacilli. One exception to this rule, however, should be noted. In certain underdeveloped areas of the world, active pulmonary tuberculosis is common and laboratory facilities which can be used for the isolation and identification of mycobacteria are almost nonexistent. In such areas, many of them tropical, the finding of numerous acid-fast rods in sputum samples by the Ziehl-Neelsen technique can be considered sufficient evidence of the presence of active pulmonary tuberculosis to justify the initiation of treatment with antituberculous drugs. The effect of chemotherapy on the course of the disease in such cases can also be followed by the use of the acid-fast stain. Of course, such an assumption cannot be made in the United States where tuberculous disease, relatively speaking, is uncommon and where adequate facilities can be found for the isolation and identification of the offending microorganisms. Furthermore, the isolation of tubercle bacilli by culture upon a suitable medium is a far more sensitive and reliable method than the demonstration of acid-fast microorganisms by smear and staining.

THE TUBERCULIN TEST. It has already been noted that persons who develop tuberculous disease or become infected with tubercle bacilli develop delayed-type hypersensitivity to certain low molecular weight proteins or polypeptides of the tubercle bacillus. This hypersensitivity, when detected, can serve as an indication of the presence of tuberculous disease or infection.[1,4] Such hypersensitivity can readily be detected by introducing small amounts of tuberculoprotein (tuberculin) into the skin; then, if hypersensitivity is present, a delayed indurated inflammatory reaction will occur at the site of the injection. This procedure is feasible and practical and is known as the tuberculin test. There are two major types of tuberculin. One, called old tuberculin (OT), was introduced by Robert Koch many years ago and consists essentially of a concentrate of a culture medium upon which tubercle bacilli have grown. The material is concentrated by evaporating the fluid by boiling. Old tuberculin, however, contains many impurities and is difficult to standardize. It is not used very often today. The other material, purified protein derivative (PPD–S), is prepared from culture filtrates of tubercle bacilli by ammonium sulfate precipitation. PPD is much purer, is easier to standardize and gives fewer nonspecific reactions. However, PPD should not be regarded as being pure, since preparations contain a heterogeneous population of protein molecules and also polysaccharides derived from the tubercle bacillus. PPDs can also be prepared from other mycobacterial species, and reactions in persons to these PPDs can be very helpful in defining the infecting species (Table 23–2).

When tuberculin-testing human beings who may have tuberculous disease, care must be taken not to introduce too much tuberculin into the skin, since severe and damaging local and systemic reactions may occur. The whole forearm may become swollen, red and tender. The axillary lymph nodes may become enlarged and tender and fever with a temperature as high as 40° C

Table 23-3. CHARACTERISTICS OF MYCOBACTERIA

Organism	Best Isolation Temperature	Rate of Growth	Colony Color Grown In:		Niacin Test	Nitrate Reduction	Catalase		Tween 80 Hydrolysis (in days)	Arylsulfatase (3 days)	Tellurite Reduction (days)
			LIGHT	DARK			SEMI-QUANTITATIVE	pH7 68° C (154.4° F)			
M. tuberculosis	37° C (98.6° F)	12–25 days	buff	buff	+	3.5+	40	–	6	–	9
M. bovis	37° C (98.6° F)	24–40 days	buff	– –		–	20	–	6	–	9
M. ulcerans	32° C (89.6° F)	14–21 days	buff	buff	+	–		+	6	–	
GROUP I											
M. kansasii	37° C (98.6° F)	10–20 days	yellow	buff	∓ (rare)	3.5+	50	+	5	–	–
M. marinum (balnei)	32° C (89.6° F)	3–11 days	yellow	buff	+(occas.)	–	40	–	5	–	–
GROUP II											
M. scrofulaceum	37° C (98.6°F)	10+ days	deep yellow	yellow	–	–	50	+	6	–	9
M. gordonae "tap-water" scotochromogen	37° C (98.6° F)	10+ days	orange	yellow	–	–	50	+	5	–	–
GROUP III											
M. intracellulare	37° C (98.6° F)	10–21 days	buff to yellow	buff to yellow	–	–	40	–	21	–	3
M. terrae ("radish")	37°C (98.6°F)	10–21 days	buff	buff		1.5+	50	+	5	–	9
M. gastri	37°C (98.6°F)	10–21 days	buff		–	–	40	–	5	–	9
M. triviale	37°C (98.6°F)		buff		–	1+	50	+	5	±	9
M. xenopi	42°C (107.6°F)	12–25 days	buff to yellow	buff to yellow	–	–	40	+	–		9
GROUP IV											
M. fortuitum	37°C (98.6°F)	3–5 days	buff	buff	–	3.5+	50	+	variable	2–3+	3
M. chelonei	37°C (98.6°F)	5–7 days	buff	buff	–	–	50			2–3+	

+ = more than 84 per cent of strains positive; ± = between 50 and 84 per cent of strains positive; ∓ = between 16 and 49 per cent of strains positive; – = less than 16 per cent of strains positive.

(104° F) may occur. The site of the injection of tuberculin will become necrotic and eventually slough. With the fever the patient experiences considerable malaise and may be prostrated for several days. In addition, complications such as pleural effusions may occur.

Three doses of PPD are generally recognized as being suitable. These are: first strength PPD, which consists of 0.00002 mg (1 tuberculin unit); intermediate strength PPD, which contains 0.0001 mg (5 tuberculin units); and second strength PPD, which contains 0.005 mg PPD (250 tuberculin units). When testing persons strongly suspected of having active tuberculosis, the first strength PPD is the dose of choice; certainly no dose higher than the intermediate strength should be used. When making tuberculin surveys in healthy people to determine the presence only of tuberculous infection, the intermediate strength is the dose of choice. The second strength PPD should be used only in persons who are negative to the intermediate strength test dose and, therefore, is of value only for the detection of rather low levels of hypersensitivity to tuberculoprotein. In Table 23–4 the various doses of OT and PPD are summarized and their relationship to each other is given.

A variety of techniques can be employed to introduce either OT or PPD into the skin of human beings. These include (1) the Mantoux test procedure, in which the desired amount of PPD or OT is injected directly into the skin in a volume of 0.1 ml; (2) the Vollmer Patch test, in which tuberculin is merely placed on a piece of gauze which is held in contact with the skin by a strip of adhesive; and (3) the Tine test, in which OT is dried upon the points of several small tines and, using a standard device, punctures are made in the skin so that small amounts of tuberculin are introduced.

All of these procedures have a certain usefulness but by far the best is the Mantoux procedure, since it permits the introduction directly into the skin of a standard volume and amount of tuberculin. More reliable and reproducible skin-test reactions will be obtained by this procedure than by any of the others. The Patch test, for instance, is sometimes particularly useful where skin-testing infants and children may be difficult, and the Tine test provides a rapid and easy procedure for use in large population groups. It is sometimes worthwhile to sacrifice some sensitivity for the number of skin tests that can be done. When testing individual patients, however, the Mantoux is the only really acceptable procedure.

After the Mantoux test has been performed by the intradermal injection of 0.1 ml of diluent containing the desired amount of PPD, the ensuing reactions must be read and interpreted with care. The major reaction which occurs is one of delayed hypersensitivity; therefore, the inflammatory reaction will be visible only after a matter of hours and will reach a peak at 48 to 72

Table 23–4. Comparable Doses of OT and PPD*

Dilution of OT	*Tuberculin Injected (mg)†*	*PPD Injected (mg)‡*	*Tuberculin Units (TU)*	*Strength*
1:100,000	0.001		0.1	
1:10,000	0.01	0.00002	1.0	First
1:2000	0.05	0.0001	5.0	Intermediate
1:1000	0.1		10.0	
1:100	1.0	0.005	250.0	Second

*Modified from D. T. Smith, 1968. *Mycobacterium tuberculosis* and tuberculosis. *In* Smith, D. T., Conant, N. F., and Willett, H. P. (eds.): Zinsser – Microbiology. 14th ed. Appleton-Century-Crofts, New York. p. 541.

†Based on 1 ml of concentrated OT = 1000 mg.

‡Based on mg of protein.

hours. These reactions in human beings are characteristically erythematous and indurated. The area of induration should be outlined and the diameter of the induration measured. Some people measure the erythema because there usually is a direct relationship between the amount of erythema and the amount of induration. However, since this correlation is not absolute, the amount of induration should be recorded either in terms of the diameter of the induraation in millimeters or by calculation of the area of induration. Arthus reactions, probably due to antibody specific for the polysaccharides found in tuberculin preparaations, may be seen. These reactions appear earlier, reach a peak at about 24 hours, and frequently are nearly gone at 48 hours; they are inflammatory and edematous and therefore soft to the touch, and are not regarded as true tuberculin reactions. In addition, occasionally atypical wheal-flare reactions may occur. These, of course, subside rapidly and will not be confused with a true tuberculin reaction. Rarely, persons who show no reaction whatsoever within 72 hours may in approximately 7 to 10 days develop an erythematous reaction at the site of the injection of tuberculin. These undoubtedly represent Arthus-type reactions which develop because antibodies are produced to some ingredient of the PPD. The latter reaches a level that, when it combines with antigen retained at the injection site, will be sufficient to produce an inflammatory reaction. This type of reaction should never be regarded as evidence of tuberculous infection or disease.

Since nonspecific reactions do occur, either as a result of the trauma of the injection or because of sensitization by infection with mycobacteria other than tubercle bacilli, small indurative or erythematous tuberculin reactions are not regarded as positive.

To be truly positive a tuberculin reaction following the intradermal infection of PPD should be 10 mm or more in diameter. The size of the tuberculin reaction to a given dose of PPD is rough indication of the degree of sensitivity. A person showing a reaction over 15 mm has a substantially greater degree of hypersensitivity to tuberculin than the person who shows a reaction of less than 15 mm. A person who reacts negatively to first strength and intermediate strength, but shows a positive reaction to second strength, probably may never have been infected with *M. tuberculosis* but may have been infected with one or more atypical mycobacteria. A reaction of less than 10 mm of induration to either first or intermediate strength PPD also, in many cases, probably represents infection with one or more atypical mycobacteria. Positive reactions in adults to first strength or intermediate strength PPD in the absence of any other signs or symptoms of what might be tuberculous disease are regarded as indications of infection with *M. tuberculosis,* but cannot be regarded as an indication of tuberculous disease. On the other hand, strong reactions in adults to first strength or intermediate strength PPD in the presence of evidence of pulmonary involvement definitely suggest but do not prove the presence of the tuberculous disease. Infants and young children who have not lived long enough to become infected with other mycobacteria and have had no time to control an active tuberculous infection and set up a dormant infection, but do show strong reactions to first or intermediate strength PPD, are regarded as probably having an active tuberculous process.

Reactions to PPD also have some prognostic significance because the incidence of active tuberculous disease is significantly greater in those persons who have reactions greater than 15 mm in diameter. These large reactions indicate a high degree of tuberculin hypersensitivity and this, in turn, probably reflects some, possibly very slight, active disease. Therefore, a high degree of tuberculin sensitivity is associated with less immunity and progressive disease is more probable. On the other hand, small reactions, or a reaction only to the second strength PPD, represent little or no mycobacterial activity because of a high degree of acquired immunity.

For another reason positive tuberculin reactions must be interpreted with caution. In view of the widespread use of bacille Calmette-Guérin (BCG) vaccine in some parts of the world, tuberculin hypersensitivity may exist in people so vaccinated.

Perhaps the greatest value of tuberculin-testing resides in its negative implications. A properly executed negative tuberculin test, even in the presence of pulmonary disease, constitutes strong evidence against the existence of active tuberculous disease in the majority of cases. Two points, discussed below, deserve emphasis in considering negative tuberculin tests.

First, a dilute PPD solution may lose potency rapidly owing to adsorption of PPD to the glass surface of the vial or syringe within which it is contained. This can be prevented by dissolving the PPD in a solution containing a small amount of an antiabsorbent such as Tween 80. All available PPD products are now prepared in this manner.

Second, increasing evidence suggests that patients with active tuberculosis may exhibit two patterns of altered delayed hypersensitivity responses. An occasional patient will appear to be completely anergic, giving negative skin-test responses to PPD as well as to other skin-test antigens (mumps, trichophyton, streptococcal streptokinase-streptodornase and monilia) routinely employed to assess overall cutaneous reactivity of the delayed type. More commonly, patients will exhibit a negative tuberculin test while simultaneously giving positive responses to one or more of the other test reagents. While both cutaneous anergy and specific PPD-negativity are known to be associated with far advanced tuberculosis, especially the miliary form of the disease, both types of altered cutaneous reactivity may be observed in patients with active disease confined to one pulmonary segment or lobe. Furthermore, these patients do not appear seriously ill by the usual clinical criteria. After instituting effective antituberculous therapy, positive responses to PPD, or to other test antigens in those subjects with anergy, can be anticipated to occur within 2 to 4 weeks. The occurrence of PPD-positivity may antedate isolation of *M. tuberculosis* from sputum or other specimens and, especially in patients with negative acid-fast smears, provide welcome indirect support for the clinical diagnosis of active tuberculosis.

Treatment. The treatment of tuberculosis is a large and complex subject and cannot be dealt with completely here.[1,4-7] The modern therapeutic era began in 1944 with a discovery by Schatz and Waksman of streptomycin, which then was found to be effective for the treatment of tuberculosis in lower animals and in man by Feldman and Hinshaw in 1945. Since that time a number of other antimicrobial agents suitable for treatment of this disease in humans have been developed.

At the present the first-line drugs—those used most commonly for initial treatment—consist of isoniazid, rifampin, ethambutol and streptomycin. Second-line drugs—those used for retreatment or whenever first-line drugs are not suitable—are, when given orally, ethionamide, cycloserine, pyrazinamide and para-aminosalicylic acid (PAS). When parenteral use is required, capreomycin, viomycin and kanamycin are available.

The foundation of therapy of tuberculosis rests upon the use of isoniazid plus a companion drug, usually either ethambutol or streptomycin. Rifampin can also be used but, while it is a highly effective drug even when used alone, a significant number of patients will show signs of hepatotoxicity. This appears to be especially noticeable when rifampin is given together with isoniazid. Isoniazid itself alone can result in serious liver disease in a small proportion of patients. Therefore, since the incidence of liver disease is higher when using rifampin together with isoniazid, this combination of drugs should be avoided.

Streptomycin is an effective drug. However, it should be used with care in persons over 50 years of age because of its ototoxicity.

The rationale for the use of two drugs instead of a single highly effective drug such as isoniazid or rifampin is that drug-resistant tubercle bacilli will emerge fairly rapidly when only a single drug is employed. The use of a companion drug such as ethambutol or PAS will markedly reduce the likelihood of the emergence of drug-resistant virulent tubercle bacilli. The use of as many as three drugs is indicated for serious tuberculous disease, such as far advanced pulmonary disease, miliary tuberculosis, tuberculous meningitis and tuberculous disease of the genitourinary system.

Treatment of tuberculosis must be prolonged. Even minimal, and certainly moderately advanced disease without complications, will require isoniazid and ethambutol treatment for at least 2 years. For advanced or disseminated disease, not only may three drugs be given but drug therapy can be continued for as long as 3 years.

It is not always necessary to give tuberculous drugs in multiple daily doses. Most of the orally administered antituberculosis drugs may be given in a single dose daily rather than in multiple doses. Divided doses, however, should be used with drugs such as cycloserine, ethionamide and PAS in order to reduce the likelihood of toxic reactions and gastrointestinal side effects.

In populations where it is difficult to supervise administration of drugs, intermittent therapy can be given. For example, after a period of several months of daily treatment the doses of isoniazid, 15 mg per kg orally, and streptomycin, 20 to 25 mg per kg intramuscularly, can be given twice weekly. The therapeutic effect is not as great as with daily administration, but significant improvement will be found in most patients so treated. Rifampin, though, should not be given intermittently. It has been found that there is a high proportion of allergic reactions in patients who receive rifampin once or twice a week only. Reactions may occur in such a large number of patients and be of such severity that rifampin therapy must be discontinued. The incidence of such reactions is greatly reduced when rifampin is given daily.

The treatment of disease caused by the atypical mycobacteria will pose special problems because of the generally greater natural drug resistance of these microorganisms. *Mycobacterium kansasii,* however, is highly susceptible to rifampin and only slightly more resistant to isoniazid. Regimens using three drugs are usually employed.

Mycobacterium intracellulare is quite resistant to all of the antituberculous drugs. Best treatment should consist of at least four drugs chosen from isoniazid, rifampin, ethambutol and ethionamide, and, in addition, either streptomycin, capreomycin or kanamycin.

All of the other atypical mycobacteria tend to be more resistant to the antituberculous drugs. They may pose special therapeutic problems.

Advantage is taken of the antimicrobial potency of isoniazid and its low toxicity to treat recent tuberculin converters. This is usually referred to as chemoprophylaxis but should more properly be called treatment. The appearance of tuberculin hypersensitivity in previously tuberculin-negative persons indicates recent infection with *M. tuberculosis.* It also means that the tubercle bacilli have multiplied and may still be multiplying even though no overt signs of disease may have appeared. Therefore, the drug is being used to treat an active process and this constitutes therapy. This is an effective way of preventing the development of serious disease in people who, because of the development of tuberculin hypersensitivity, are known to have been recently infected with *M. tuberculosis.*

Some physicians recommend treatment of all persons with a high degree of tuberculin hypersensitivity regardless of whether the infection was acquired recently or many years before. As pointed out earlier, there is a direct relationship between the degree of tuberculin sensitivity as indicated by the size of the reaction obtained following injection of the low or the intermediate dose of PPD and the eventual occurrence of grossly evident tuberculous disease. It would appear logical, therefore, to reduce the risk of the development of destructive disease by the administration of isoniazid when a high degree of tuberculin hypersensitivity is present in persons undergoing treatment with immunosuppressive drugs, or in those persons whose acquired cellular immunity may be compromised by other disease.

Prevention. Tuberculosis is transmitted from a person with active pulmonary disease to a susceptible person who inhales infected droplet nuclei generated from the bronchial secretions of the diseased person. The prevention of tuberculosis will revolve, then, around procedures that prevent contact between susceptible persons and the diseased carrier.[1,4] Since tuberculosis develops slowly, tubercle bacilli may be excreted long before a person is aware that he is ill. Therefore the prevention of spread of tuberculosis will depend upon the early detection of pulmonary disease, then the isolation of the diseased person, and finally the treatment of the diseased person to the point where tubercle bacilli are no longer being excreted. Over this century in the United States, intensive efforts have been made to control tuberculosis by these means. In addition to the cases of tuberculosis that have been found in persons examined by physicians because of some illness, mass x-ray screening programs have been conducted in order to detect persons with a pathologic pulmonary condition. Such people then have been checked to see whether they have tuberculosis. When active cases are discovered in this manner, the family, and contacts, of the patient are examined in order to reveal possible sources for the infection and to determine whether the person has infected others. In this way many cases of tuberculosis have been located. These diseased persons are then intensively treated with chemotherapeutic agents to render them noninfectious. This frequently can be accomplished without confining the patient to a hospital or sanatorium.

In many communities tuberculin-testing surveys of populations, particularly school children, have been conducted. Those found to be tuberculin-positive to the intermediate strength PPD are then examined by x-ray for the presence of pulmonary disease; if found, the contacts are investigated to reveal possible sources of infection. Intensive application of these procedures for the detection, isolation and treatment of tuberculosis in the more developed countries has resulted in a steady drop in the incidence and prevalence of and mortality from tuberculosis. There is little doubt that the complete application of these procedures to an entire population would result in the reduction of tuberculosis in human beings to an insignificant level.

The preventive programs described above, however, are enormously expensive and it is impossible to obtain the full cooperation of every person. Although tuberculosis in the United States has been reduced to a very low level in most rural areas, there still remain large endemic foci in certain population groups found in the large cities. As might be expected from the mode of transmission, most tuberculosis is found in those areas of the cities where there is overpopulation, overcrowding and lower standards of personal hygiene and sanitation.

The application of the above-mentioned methods for the prevention of tuberculosis is also difficult, if not impossible, in many of the underdeveloped and tropical areas of the world. Here, in conditions of low level of education, lack of sanitation and crowding, tuberculosis is a major problem. In these areas the facilities for the detection of tuberculosis and the isolation and treatment of cases do not exist, nor is there money available to provide them, while the low level of both education and understanding limits the required degree of cooperation of a large portion of the population. Therefore other means for the control of tuberculosis in such population groups must be found.

Fortunately another approach to this problem is available. It is well recognized that if the level of resistance of a population to an infectious disease can be increased, and maintained to the point where the number of susceptible persons is reduced to a small proportion of the population, the disease cannot maintain itself readily and may eventually disappear. This end has been realized in certain parts of the world as the result of vaccination against such diseases as diphtheria and smallpox. A potent vaccine against tuberculosis could be expected to reduce markedly the incidence of tuberculosis in susceptible persons even though there are factors which make the elimination of this disease by vaccination very improbable. A vaccine against tuberculosis would also be of particular usefulness in areas where the conventional procedures of detection, isolation and treatment of cases cannot be applied. Such a vaccine is available in the form of BCG (bacille Calmette-Guérin). The bacillus Calmette-Guérin is an attenuated mutant of a virulent strain of *M. bovis* developed by the French scientists Calmette and Guérin in the early years of this century. The vaccine, which consists of living cells of this attenuated strain, when injected in very small numbers into the skin of susceptible persons will induce a high degree of resistance to infection with virulent tubercle bacilli. There have been a number of field trials with this vaccine which have conclusively shown that when small numbers of properly prepared living BCG cells are injected in this manner into human beings, the incidence of tuberculosis can be reduced by as much as 80 per cent. Furthermore, this degree of protection will persist for many years.

In the United States, BCG vaccination of human beings has not been widely practiced. The majority of medical opinion has held that BCG vaccine was neither safe nor effective. Furthermore, since vaccination with BCG will induce hypersensitivity to tuberculin in the recipient, a valuable diagnostic tool may be lost. Only the last reason has any validity, and even here the importance of this as a contraindication to vaccination is frequently overestimated. As for safety, the vaccination of hundreds of millions of people in various parts of the world with the appearance of few untoward reactions attests to the safety of the vaccine. BCG vaccination is the preventive measure of choice in the developing nations of the world where other methods cannot be applied.

Finally, attempts have been made to prevent tuberculosis by chemoprophylaxis. It has been demonstrated that isoniazid administered in appropriate daily doses to populations at risk of infection will significantly reduce the occurrence of active tuberculosis as compared with similar populations not so treated. Isoniazid chemoprophylaxis usually is employed in any child who develops a positive tuberculin test before 4 years of age; in tuberculin-positive individuals found to be or to have been in close contact with cases of tuberculosis; or in clinically well persons in special settings (e.g. physicians, nurses, hospital attendants) whose tuberculin tests have recently turned positive. The worried medical student or house officer often asks how soon he might be expected to exhibit positive tuberculoprotein reactivity or pulmonary abnormalities in chest x-rays, should intimate contact with a patient with tuberculosis lead to active disease. Although considerable individual variation might well obtain, 3 weeks and 6 weeks, respectively, would appear to be reasonable time periods to consider from the practical standpoint of tuberculin skin-testing and securing of chest x-rays.

Chemoprophylaxis also is often employed for patients known to have a positive tuberculin test and either to be afflicted by disease or receiving drugs, or both, which alter host resistance and predispose to activation of subclinical or apparently healed tuberculosis. These diseases include leukemia, lymphoma or lymphosarcoma. The drugs include corticosteroids and any of the immunosuppressive agents (e.g. those routinely used in patients receiving renal or heart allografts). However, chemoprophylaxis is a completely unsatisfactory method for the prevention of tuberculosis on a community basis and particularly in the underdeveloped nations. The requirement that a pill be taken daily over periods of months or years cannot be met by the majority of the people who are in the greatest need of protection. BCG vaccination, which needs to be given only once and which will provide protection for years, is the prophylactic method of choice for large numbers of people.

REFERENCES

1. Des Prez, R., and Goodwin, R. 1971. Tuberculosis. *In* Beeson, P. B., and McDermott, W. (eds.): Cecil-Loeb Textbook of Medicine. 13th ed. W. B. Saunders Co., Philadelphia. pp. 609–650.

2. Fogan, L. 1970. Atypical mycobacteria: their clinical, laboratory and epidemiologic significance. Medicine *49*:243–255.
3. Rich, A. 1951. Pathogenesis of Tuberculosis. 2nd ed. Charles C Thomas, Springfield, Illinois. 1028 pp.
4. Harris, W. H., and McClement, J. H. 1972. *In* Hoeprich, P. D. (ed.): Infectious Diseases. Harper & Row, Hagerstown, Maryland. pp. 351–388.
5. Lester, W. 1972. Rifampin: a semisynthetic derivative of 1589 rifampicin—a prototype for the future. Ann. Rev. Microbiol. *26*:85–102.
6. Anonymous: Tuberculosis Chemotherapy Centre, Madras. 1959. A concurrent comparison of home and sanatorium treatment of pulmonary tuberculosis in South India. Bull. W.H.O. *31*:51–131.
7. Gordon, C. G. I. 1961. A method of controlled home treatment of pulmonary tuberculosis in Tanganyika. Tubercle *42*:148–158.

CHAPTER 24
Leprosy

Merlin L. Brubaker

Synonyms. Lepra; la lèpre; Aussatz; spedalskhed; Hansen's disease.

Definition. Leprosy is a chronic infectious disease primarily of the skin, nerves and certain mucous membranes caused by *Mycobacterium leprae.* It is one of the least infectious of all the infectious diseases. The incubation period varies from less than a year to many years, but probably averages 3 to 5 years. Several variants of the disease are demonstrable, but the disease can be divided generally into two polar types: tuberculoid and lepromatous. A transitional or dimorphous (borderline) type may show a variable degree of similarity to the tuberculoid or the lepromatous, depending upon which pole it approximates. Nonlepromatous cases exhibit resistance to the infection evidenced by paucity of bacilli in the lesions and their tissue response. In the lepromatous type there is obvious lack of resistance, with an abundance of bacilli in the lesions.

Distribution. The disease is widely distributed in tropical and subtropical regions. It occurs throughout most of Asia, with a high prevalence in India and other countries of southeast Asia, southern China, and in some of the Pacific islands. It is particularly widespread in central Africa and has become endemic in much of the Western Hemisphere, especially in certain South and Central American countries except Chile. The disease occurs widely in Mexico. In the continental United States leprosy is indigenous but of low incidence in southern California, Florida (chiefly in Key West, Miami and Tampa), Louisiana and southeastern Texas. It is estimated that at least 10,700,000 people in the world have leprosy. About 4,000,000 of these suffer from some form of disablement as a result of the disease.[1]

Etiology. In spite of the failure to fulfill Koch's postulates, it is generally accepted that *Mycobacterium leprae* (Hansen, 1874) Lehmann and Neumann, 1896, is the etiologic agent of leprosy. *Mycobacterium leprae* is an acid-fast, gram-positive, non-spore-forming, nonmotile, pleomorphic bacillus. It has certain morphologic resemblances to *Mycobacterium tuberculosis* but shows less affinity for an acid-fast stain. The organisms present considerable variation in morphology from slender rod-shaped bacteria staining irregularly with a resultant beaded appearance to a shorter cigar-shaped organism, or they may appear granular. These differences appear to be consistent with the healing effect. Electron microscopy has helped to demonstrate the cell wall and internal structure in greater detail. The Ziehl-Neelsen method of staining and the electron microscope have made it possible to ascertain that it is the cytoplasm and not the cell wall which takes the stain.[2] The leprosy bacillus has not been cultivated in vitro. Until very recently, attempts to produce leproma-like lesions in experimental animals have failed completely. The leprosy bacillus has been successfully cultivated in the foot pads of mice.[3] More recently, the armadillo *(Dasypus novemcintus* and *Dasypus sabiniola)* has been introduced as an animal model for the study of leprosy and a source for *M. leprae* heretofore in extremely scarce supply. The full extent of this animal's unique contribution to leprosy research is being developed in research centers at Carville, Louisiana; New Iberia, Louisiana; and Caracas, Venezuela.[4] In the patient's lesions the bacilli are mostly intracellular; they multiply abundantly in the cells of the lepromatous lesions. In the "lepra cell" or "Virchow cell," the mass or group of bacilli may lie in a matrix or *gloea,* the combination composing the *globus.*

Epidemiology. The traditional, and

simplest, explanation of the spread of leprosy is by the close, prolonged contact of the susceptible individual with the infectious (open) case. The source of the infection is often not found. Nonetheless, if sufficient time and effort were expended, it is probable that the source could be uncovered somewhere in the history of the patient.

Host susceptibility is important in understanding the epidemiology, natural history and clinical classification of leprosy. Probably all cases go through an indeterminate phase, whether the portal of entry is through the broken or unbroken skin, or both.[5] At this point, if the subject possesses adequate immunity, the process may be limited to the nerve endings without manifestation in the dermis. If the process progresses, and the body reacts immunologically (cell-mediated immunity), the characteristic lesion of the tuberculoid type may develop. If there is no tissue response, the disease proceeds toward the lepromatous pole. If the virulence of the disease and the antagonism of the immunologic forces of the host are not so decisive, the transitional or dimorphous case develops. Inherent susceptibility of the host, opportunity for exposure and community experience with the disease are far more important to the epidemiologic understanding of leprosy than race, sex, age per se or environmental factors such as climate, altitude or nutrition. Leprosy occurs more frequently in children and young adults and in adult males more frequently than in females. The lepromatous rate varies geographically and reflects the community experience with the disease. A lepromatous rate of 15 per cent in West Africa is considered high, while in Asian areas the lepromatous rate is often about 50 per cent.

Pathology. Gross pathologic aspects of leprosy are the manifestations of the effect on the skin, its cutaneous appendages and local nerve endings, or the marked disability manifested when larger nerves such as the ulnar, median, radial, tibial, peroneal and saphenous are involved. Anesthesia is associated with the cutaneous lesion of leprosy; the loss of eyebrows is associated with lepromatous leprosy. Many of the injuries and deformities of leprosy, such as serious burns and neglected infections, result from the effects of the anesthesia rather than direct effects of the infection itself. Skin lesions of leprosy vary from the simplest well defined macule to thick patches of the major tuberculoid variety; from the multifarious, poorly defined macules to the nodular or furrowed infiltrations of lepromatous leprosy. The peripheral nerve trunks are involved in both the benign and malign forms. This involvement is one of the most important elements of the disease.

Sometimes bacteria may be demonstrated in the blood during severe reactions (lepra fever); they have also been found in the liver, spleen and bone marrow without causing any dysfunction. However, gynecomastia may result from involvement of the testes. In lepromatous leprosy the superficial lymph nodes, upper respiratory tract and eyes are often conspicuously involved.

Histologically, the infiltrates in the skin, of whatever type, affect primarily the zones of vascular areolar tissue. Initially, there is

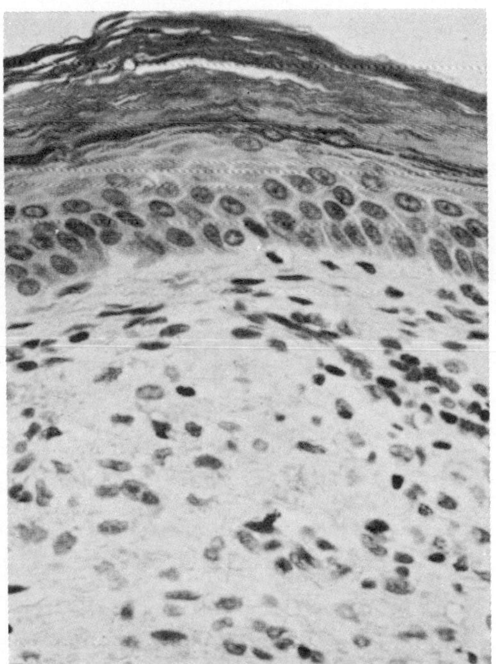

Figure 24-1. A marked lepromatous infiltration, showing flattening of the epidermis with hyperkeratosis and the characteristic free zone below. The infiltrate is a solid mass of lepra cells with many small globus spaces. Note beginning of change to the foamy condition.

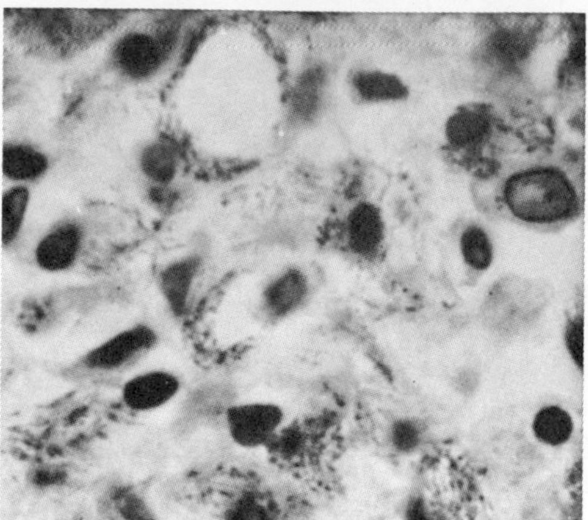

Figure 24–2. Lepra cells in a skin lesion of lepromatous leprosy. Large mononuclear phagocytes with many *M. leprae*, some exhibiting different degrees of vacuolation due to globus formation from the spaces of which most bacilli have escaped during preparation.

always a nonspecific inflammatory response. Involvement of dermal nerve branches is unique among cutaneous infections and virtually constant. Lesions in other structures, including those in the nerve trunks (except when caseation occurs in tuberculoid nerve lesions), correspond to the different types occurring in the skin.

The only distinctive lesion of leprosy is the *leproma*. This is a granuloma composed mainly of massed macrophages, altered to form the lepra cells of Virchow, lying in a well vascularized supporting stroma (Fig. 24–1). These cells harbor many bacilli, and in the classic lesion they become vacuolated by the formation of globi (Fig. 24–2, top and center). "Giant globi" are often found within foreign body giant cells or ensheathed in a sort of syncytium, and at times they constitute veritable microcolonies. However, some lepromas may be composed of massed spindle-shaped cells loaded with bacilli in which globus formation is absent. As the lesions gradually age, the lepra cells become foamy, multivacuolated and often multinucleated. They then contain few bacilli but much acid-fast lipidic material.

As the infiltrate in the skin increases, it disrupts the normal architecture and seriously affects the accessory structures. These persist, however, even in massive lesions, except in the tumor-like secondary nodules which are pure lepromas. The subcutis is commonly invaded, and subcutaneous nodules may develop.

The lepromatous infiltrate in the peripheral nerve trunks involves the endoneurium, but, despite its intensity, functional disturbance is long delayed unless reactional inflammation supervenes.

The tissue-reactive *tuberculoid* lesions are nonspecific in character, presenting focal masses of epithelioid cells with variable degrees of lymphoid cell accumulation and giant cell formation (Fig. 24–3). The epithelioid cells ingest and destroy the bacilli. When bacilli are demonstrable, they are usually in other cells or other structures, especially the nerves. The more marked lesions of the skin resemble noncaseating tuberculosis or Boeck's sarcoid, except for the involvement of the nerve branches. Extension of the process may be seen in the nerves of the subcutis, and caseation necrosis occasionally occurs.

In the milder cases of clinically tuberculoid lesions, the epithelioid foci tend to be correspondingly smaller and more isolated. In their simplest form "pretuberculoid" groups occur clinically as simple flat macules, while under more advanced conditions the lesions are massive and less orderly. When such cases evolve to the dimorphous stage, the picture is even more atypical and confused. When both tuberculoid and lepromatous changes coexist, the condition is sometimes called dimorphous.

Simple chronic inflammatory round cell infiltration is found in many pale, flat macules and often in the peripheral nerves in the classic "neural leprosy." The cells are mostly lymphoid, but larger cells of the monocyte type may also be present. Bacilli are seldom demonstrable. The amount of infiltration in the nerve trunks is much less than in lepromatous leprosy, yet nerve fiber degeneration and fibrosis occur earlier.

Clinical Characteristics. CLASSIFICATION. The grouping of leprosy cases is based on clinical and bacteriologic features primarily, aided by immunologic and histopathologic criteria. This important subject is one of interminable

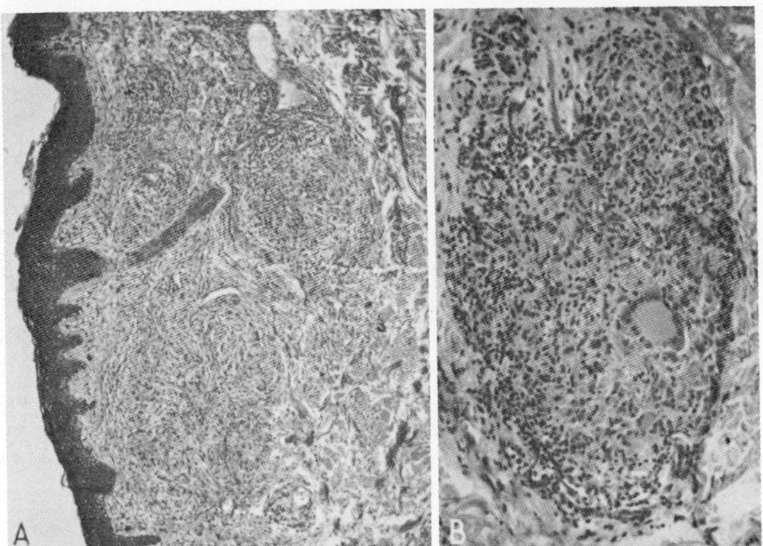

Figure 24–3. Tuberculoid lesions of leprosy. *A*, Multiple epithelioid foci, in one place in contact with the epidermis, in a clinically minor tuberculoid lesion of moderate degree (80 ×). *B*, A sarcoid-like focus, showing massed epithelioid cells and a Langhans' giant cell, with lymphoid cell accumulation on one side (150 ×). (Courtesy of Dr. H. W. Wade.)

discussion and dispute. However, in the spectrum of forms and varieties there is general recognition of two types, lepromatous (malign) and tuberculoid (benign), so far apart and dissimilar clinically that they are often called "polar." As the clinical types are determined by the immunologic response of the host, the lepromin test can be expected to be positive in the tuberculoid type of leprosy and negative in the lepromatous form. The dimorphous transitional form may be lepromin-positive or -negative, depending upon which pole it approaches in clinical and histologic characteristics. The indeterminate form is an early, macular, benign stage of the disease which as yet has not established itself and may be either lepromin-positive or -negative. The relatively uncommon neuritic subtype of leprosy, which shows only neural signs clinically and has no visible cutaneous lesions or scars of previous cutaneous lesions, has been described frequently enough to establish it as a clinical entity.[6] This form must be distinguished from neuritic forms of tuberculoid, dimorphous and lepromatous leprosy.

General. The onset of leprosy is usually insidious. There are no definite prodromes, although some patients may complain of early sensory disturbances or neuritic pain. Occasionally, the disease appears abruptly in a spectacular reactional form.

Early leprosy is often difficult to recognize, and examination in the direct sunlight can be helpful. Typically, there are one or a few small, well defined, simple, indeterminate macules. These are anesthetic and hypopigmented. It is probable that in all cases of leprosy, anesthesia is the first presenting sign.[6] Some cases, apparently lepromatous from the outset, present diffusely outlined, erythematous macules with little, if any, perceptible infiltration, no marginal thickening or differentiation between margin and center, little or no anesthesia, but positive bacteriologic findings. These lesions may be found on the extremities, on the body, more commonly on the back than anteriorly, often on the buttocks, and not infrequently on the face (Fig. 24–4). In advanced cases, whatever the form, there are naturally immune areas: the cubital and popliteal fossae, the axillary and inguinal regions, the retroauricular area and, generally, the scalp.

The evolution of the indeterminate cases is variable. Some clear up spontaneously; others persist and progress indefinitely as "maculoanesthetic"; in still others, increase of tissue reactivity leads to the development of the tuberculoid form or, conversely, absence or loss of resistance results in development into the lepromatous type. Tuberculoid cases may persist as such for long periods. There may be wide extension of the lesions, but ultimately they tend to subside spontaneously. On the other hand, they may change to the borderline type, and from that they occasionally become frankly lepromatous. Lepromatous cases seldom change in type and are almost invariably progressive if not effectively treated.

The color of the lesions may vary considerably, apart from the influence of racial characteristics. Because involvement of the nerves and cutaneous appendages produces the clinical manifestations of the disease, in the macular lesions there is dissociation of sensation. Discrimination between heat and cold is lost first, then sensitivity to pain and, finally, tactile sense. Perception of pressure remains intact. In most lesions there is little or no sweating, and hairs are usually absent. Atrophy of the skin may occur in resolved lesions or parts of lesions; on the other hand, the texture and even the color may return to normal. Ichthyosis of the legs is common, and there may be marked thickening of the skin of the lower extremities in advanced lepromatous cases.

Frequently there is thickening and often tenderness of the peripheral nerve trunks at the points of flexure, the ulnars above the elbows, the external peroneals at the knees, and also the great auriculars. These are important diagnostic signs.

Degeneration of the trunk nerves leads to anesthetic, paralytic and trophic changes of the extremities, followed by mutilations often aggravated by trauma. Muscle atrophy of the hands becomes conspicuous, contractures slowly develop, and the bones of the phalanges gradually undergo absorption, or become necrotic, infected and extruded (Fig. 24–5). The soft tissues of the fingers are absorbed, leaving distorted residua of the nails on the stumps of the hands. Wristdrop is occasionally seen. Similar changes occur in the feet, and troublesome trophic ulcers develop on the plantar surfaces. There are seemingly "pure neural" or "polyneuritic" cases which present only such changes.

In its ordinary course leprosy is a nontoxic disease despite the immense numbers of bacilli in the lepromatous lesions. The ultimate deterioration of such cases, producing indolent bacillus-discharging ulcerations and other changes, comes on very gradually. However, acute episodes of "lepra reaction," with or without fever, apparently allergic in nature and which may be analogous to the Herxheimer reaction, occur in many cases. These reactions, which differ greatly in the different types, may be harmful.

Death from leprosy itself is infrequent. Pulmonary tuberculosis and nephritis are common terminal events, although the

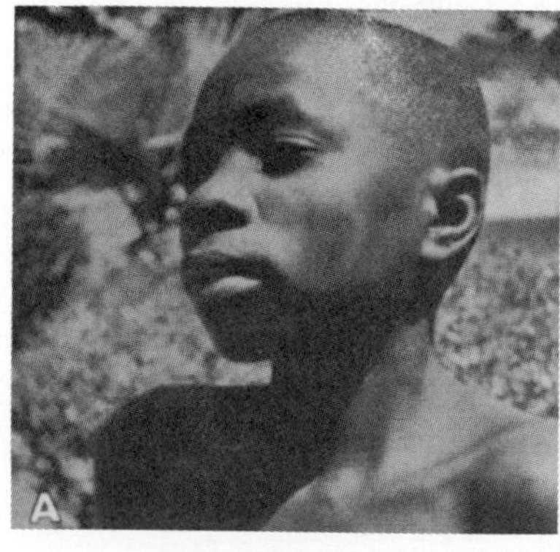

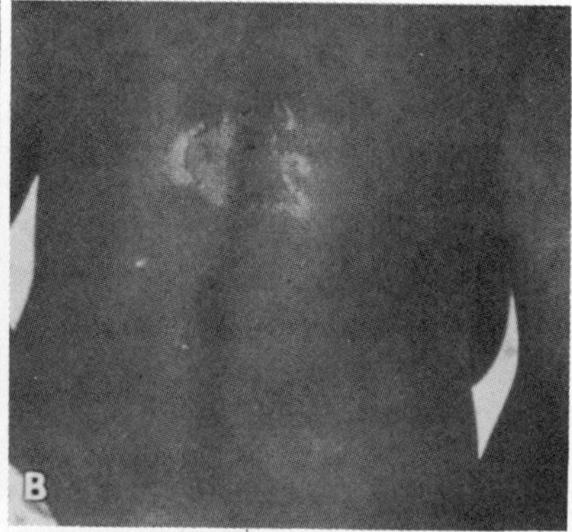

Figure 24–4. Tuberculoid lesions of leprosy. *A*, Lesion of the face often seen where children are carried on the mother's back. Note healed center with minimal activity remaining on periphery. *B*, Minor tuberculoid lesion of the back. Note beaded edge with ameboid border. (Courtesy of Dr. M. L. Brubaker.)

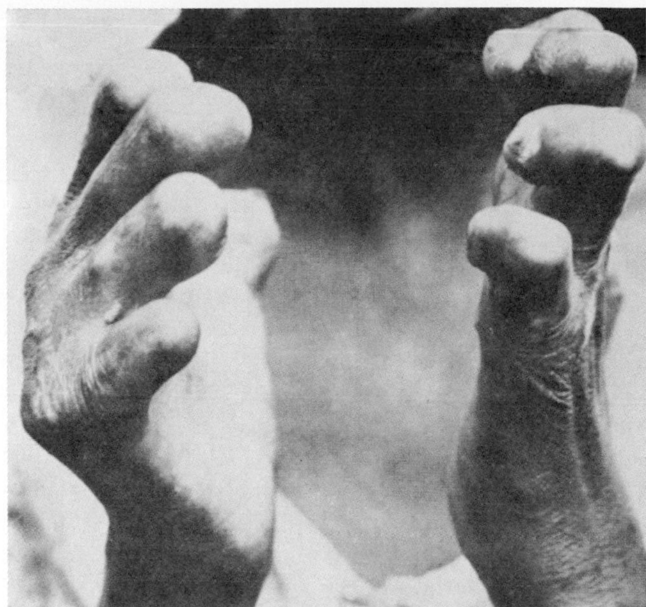

Figure 24–5. Advanced trophic changes of the hands due to severe nerve damage, with muscular atrophy, contractures and progressive absorption of the digits, on some of which residua of the nails can be seen.

frequency of tuberculosis has greatly diminished since the advent of sulfone treatment. Amyloidosis is often found at autopsy and may have led to death because of renal involvement.

LEPROMATOUS LEPROSY. Symmetric distribution of the lesions is typical. The brownish red lepromatous macules or infiltrations often appear first on the face but may be on other parts of the body. Thickening of the earlobes is sometimes an early development. As the disease progresses, the lesions increase in number and size, and the macule may develop into the infiltrated lepromatous lesion. Infiltrations become smooth and tense and discrete nodulations or the leonine furrowing of the face may appear (Fig. 24–6). The loss of the eyebrows is often significant in type diagnosis. A peculiar type of diffuse lepromatosis *(Lepra manchada)* has been described as occurring only on the American continent, especially Central America and Mexico. When this form progresses, small red lesions appear which ultimately darken in the center, crust and drop off. This has been called the Lucio phenomenon.[7]

In advanced cases, ulceration of the nasal mucosa may lead to perforation of the cartilaginous septum and to falling of the nose. Infiltration of the vocal cords causes the characteristic raucous voice, and occasionally leads to severe stenosis. The eyes may be involved either by extension of infiltration from the conjunctiva to the cornea or by involvement of the uveal tract.

Mild lepra reactions of the erythema nodosum type often suggest favorable response to therapy.[6] If they are severe and repeated, however, they are harmful; ulcerations of the skin may occur, especially on the extremities, and also acute neuritis, iridocyclitis or orchitis. Erythema nodosum reaction occurs with the appearance of small acute nodules which typically are tender, often bacteriologically negative in smears, and usually of short duration. Should this condition become chronic, producing dense indurations on the extremities, it is doubtful that the reaction is beneficial. Rather, when progressive lepra reaction develops, the patient's condition tends to deteriorate; ultimately, the patient dies of general debilitation or an intercurrent infection.

MACULOANESTHETIC LEPROSY. This benign group comprises many of the cases having simple macules and, in the older sense, many of those of the lesser tuberculoid type.

In these cases the skin lesions persist, increase in numbers and spread centrifugally, at times with fusion of adjacent lesions.

If the process is not arrested, involvement of peripheral nerves becomes evident sooner or later. Typically, there is less thickening of the nerve trunks than occurs in lepromatous leprosy. In some instances, attacks of acute neuritis hasten and intensify the nerve damage. In many cases, the skin lesions will disappear spontaneously, and neural manifestations, if present, may be so slight that the recovered patients appear practically normal. Often, however, they are crippled and deformed (Fig. 24–5).

Paralysis of the lower eyelids results in lagophthalmos, and traumatic corneal damage is apt to follow. There may be paralysis of the orbicularis oris muscles and even of the masseters. Occasionally, nasal ulcers develop, in which case the bacilli can be demonstrated in this lesion but not elsewhere.

TUBERCULOID LEPROSY. This variety of the benign form is characterized primarily by distinctive skin lesions which may be slightly elevated (Figs. 24–7, 24–8). In the common minor variety the elevation, which usually has an irregular or micropapular surface, occurs only in the outer advancing margin of the lesion or in a part of it. In the less common major form there is more marked thickening and elevation of the margin zone, which is broader, and the process tends to show deeper extension. Recent lesions of this sort may show incomplete central resolution, and those of reactional origin may be solid plaques. Hyperesthesia is often found in the active outer zones of the tuberculoid macules, and anesthesia in the central areas. The sharply defined borders, whether macular, papular or plaquelike, characterize this lesion.

Thickening of the cutaneous nerve cephalad to a lesion, especially of the major variety, is found. It may extend to, and involve, the corresponding nerve trunk. This condition is typically asymmetric and unilateral, which is distinctive. Massive thickening,

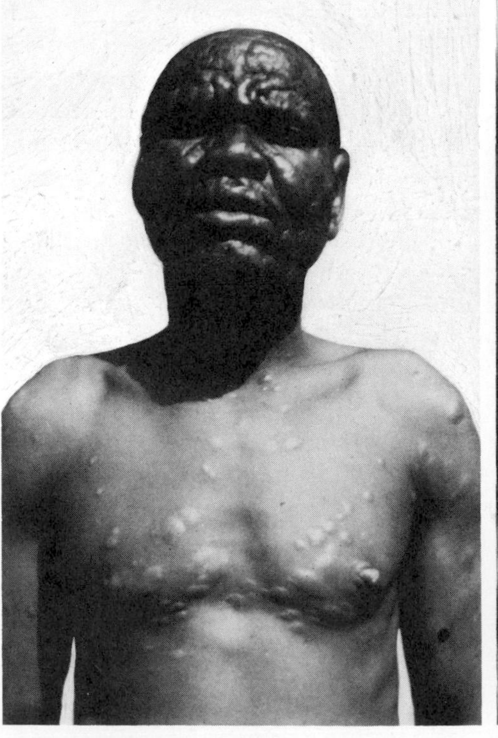

A

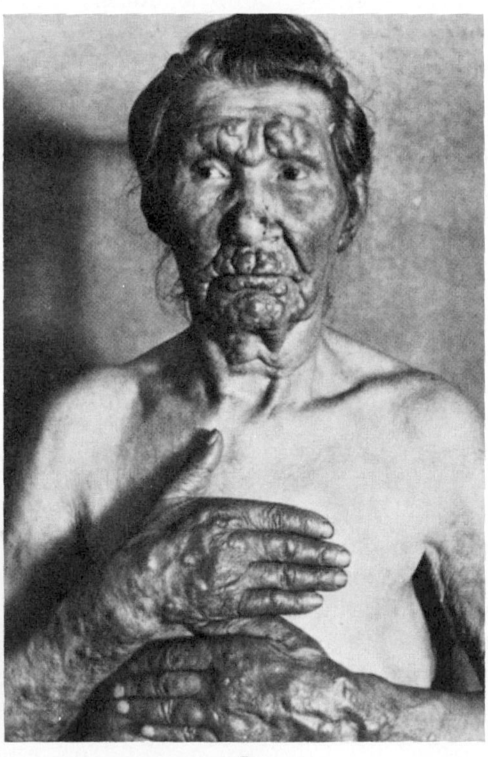

B

Figure 24–6. *A,* Earlier case of definite lepromatous leprosy with developing characteristics of *B.* (Courtesy of Dr. M. L. Brubaker.) *B,* An advanced lepromatous case with leonine face, both furrowed and nodulate, and with marked involvement of the forearms and hands, less of the upper arms and still less of the body.

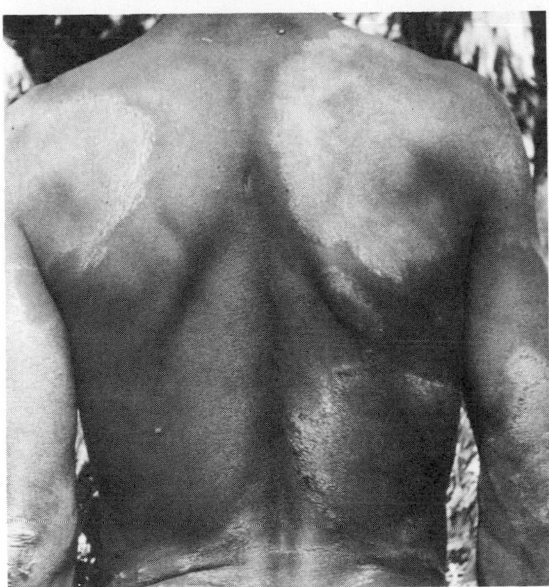

Figure 24–7. Reactional borderline tuberculoid subsiding. Note depigmented, healing scapular lesions and active elevated border of right lumbar lesion. (Courtesy of Dr. M. L. Brubaker.)

especially if it is irregular, signifies caseation necrosis which may undergo liquefaction to produce a nerve abscess.

The reactional lesions of the skin in this type are often spectacular. They may be mistaken for lepromatous lesions, especially when there are disseminated metastatic nodules. Severe reactions in the true tuberculoid type, though distressing, usually are beneficial. Crippling due to nerve damage may result, however, unless the condition is promptly recognized and adequately treated. It is sometimes wise to suppress the reactional phenomenon by the use of large doses of corticosteroids.

Dimorphous Leprosy. These cases belong to the malign group and may progress to become truly lepromatous. In the past, they have usually been classed as lepromatous, sometimes called atypical because of the asymmetry of the lesions and other peculiarities (Fig. 24–9). However, if not too far advanced, they may regress to the original dimorphous tuberculoid form. In general, they respond better to treatment than do real lepromatous cases.

Diagnosis. Bacteriologic Diagnosis. The cardinal diagnostic signs are the presence of anesthetic macular lesions or thickening and tenderness of peripheral nerve trunks and the demonstration of bacilli. Search should be made for suspicious macules or infiltrations of the skin and for thickening of the earlobes and the eyebrows. The peripheral nerves should be palpated carefully. As stated earlier, the patient should be examined in bright sunlight to appreciate fully, indeed even to find, certain lesions of leprosy.

Smears for bacilli should be made from several sites: skin lesions, earlobes and the nasal septum. Since bacilli are usually obtainable only from lepromatous and dimorphous lesions, many cases must be diagnosed on the basis of clinical appearance and the presence of anesthesia in simple macular or tuberculoid lesions. In such lesions, loss of sensitivity to light touch and absence of pain on pinprick justify the diagnosis. Tests for histamine flare and for sweating afford confirmatory evidence. In the absence of skin lesions, muscular weakness of the face or areas of numbness on the extremities should be regarded as suspicious. Polyneuritic anesthesias, stocking and glove distribution, almost certainly will be due to leprosy, especially if the nerve trunks are thickened.

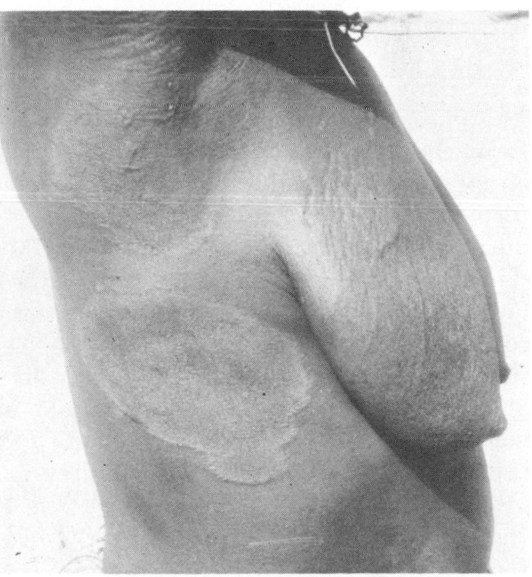

Figure 24–8. Active tuberculoid leprosy with elevated, ameboid border and healed central plaque demonstrating centrifugal spread. (Courtesy of Dr. M. L. Brubaker.)

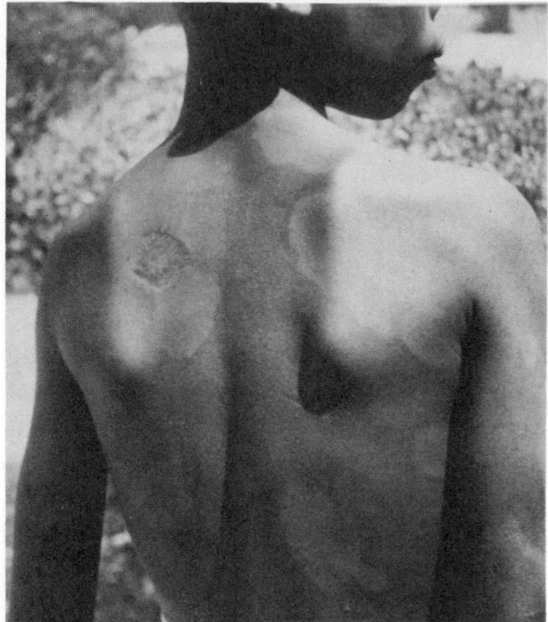

Figure 24–9. Dimorphous leprosy with multiple lesions of more or less symmetrical distribution. This shows the sharp border of tuberculoid type, but less dry and crusting lesions than found in lepromatous cases. (Courtesy of Dr. M. L. Brubaker.)

The histamine flare test is performed by making a needle puncture into the skin through a drop of 1:1000 histamine acid phosphate solution. The test is positive if there is no erythema flare when the puncture is made within the lesion area, or if the flare stops at the margin of the lesion when the puncture is made a little to the outside of it. The sweating tests are seldom used.

Smears for bacteriologic examination from the skin should be obtained by the scraped incision method, which can be performed at any point in the lepromas and at the active marginal zone of leprids. A fold of skin is compressed between thumb and forefinger, an incision is made well into the corium, and material is scraped from the cut surface with as little blood as possible. Smears from the nasal mucosa should be made under direct observation using a speculum, searching the septum for infiltrations or ulcers. In lepromatous cases bacilli may be very numerous (Fig. 24–10). The Bacterial Index (BI) is a measure from 1+ to 6+ of the number of bacilli present in an oil immersion. field. The Morphological Index (MI) is the percentage of solid-staining bacilli divided by the total counted per field. Puncture and aspiration of an enlarged lymph node or thickened ulnar nerve is rarely necessary. A biopsy should be performed for positive diagnosis as confirmation of clinical interpretation which is so basic to proper treatment.

IMMUNOLOGY. There is no diagnostic test for leprosy, serologic or other, and what was known of its immunology was derived largely from studies of the lepromin (Mitsuda) test. The antigen of this test is a heat-killed suspension of bacillus-rich lepromas. Intradermal injection into a fully reactive person elicits (1) the early (48-hour) Fernandez reaction, and (2) the late (3-week) Mitsuda reaction. The former is an allergic reaction analogous to the tuberculin reaction but too inconstant even among contacts to be of diagnostic value. The latter is a papulonodular lesion which appears in most nonlepromatous cases and also in many apparently normal persons. Lepromatous cases are by definition nonreactive to lepromin. The positive Mitsuda reaction demonstrates the presence of a reactivity which signifies a degree of resistance to the disease. This host resistance may prevent infection or determine the course of the disease. The test has significance with respect to classification (page 215) and prognosis.

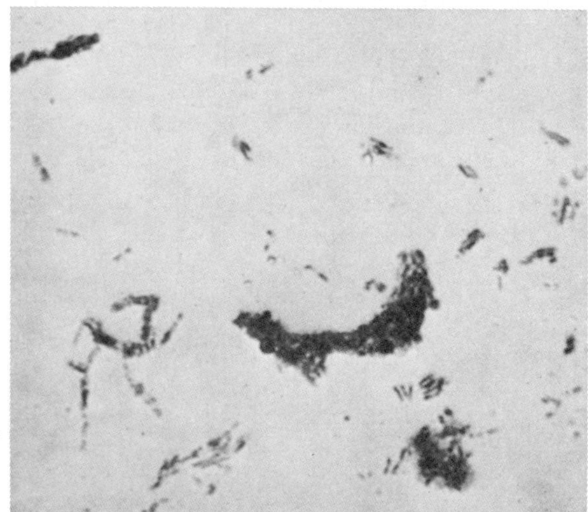

Figure 24–10. *Mycobacterium leprae* in stained smear from the nasal septum of an advanced lepromatous case, with typical grouping but without globi or lepra cells.

Biopsy of the lepromin nodule, and the type of cellular response observed, has been useful to determine the type of response one would develop if he should contract leprosy. Recently a modification of this test has demonstrated a variation in the bacilli clearance ability by the cellular response to injection of 640×10^6 heat-killed acid-fast bacteria per milliliter after 4 weeks.[8] This test—the Bacillus Clearance Competency Test (CCB Test)—is used, therefore, to determine the type of disease to expect in early indeterminate leprosy, or in a contact should disease develop. Other newer tests of cell-mediated immunologic response, i.e. macrophage migration inhibition and lymphocyte blast transformation, are consistent with the response measured by the CCB Test.

The abnormal proteins which develop in leprosy may cause false positive reactions in laboratory tests which depend upon protein fractions, such as the cephalin flocculation test. Serologic tests, i.e. those for syphilis, may also be positive in this disease.

Differential Diagnosis. The lesions of leprosy are protean in character and resemble those of many other conditions. Simple macular leprids must be distinguished from such conditions as tinea versicolor, leukoderma (vitiligo), hypochromia of yaws, pale birthmarks and scars and certain lichenoid lesions. In these conditions anesthesia is absent and the histamine and sweating tests are negative. Syringomyelia, Raynaud's disease, Bernhardt's syndrome and other peripheral neuritic conditions may be confused with neural (polyneuritic) leprosy without skin lesions.

Various lesions of tuberculoid leprosy, which is often misdiagnosed, must be distinguished from Boeck's sarcoid (Fig. 24–11), granuloma annulare, lupus vulgaris, lupus erythematosus, tinea circinata, psoriasis and certain lesions of secondary syphilis and yaws. With respect to the first two, the confusion may even extend to the histologic findings.

In lepromatous leprosy, infiltrations and nodules may have to be distinguished from such conditions as dermal leishmaniasis, mycosis fungoides, leukemia cutis and neurofibromatosis. Smears of such lepromas will always be found positive. If bacilli are not obtained from the reactional lesions of the erythema nodosum type, they should be demonstrable elsewhere in the patient's skin.

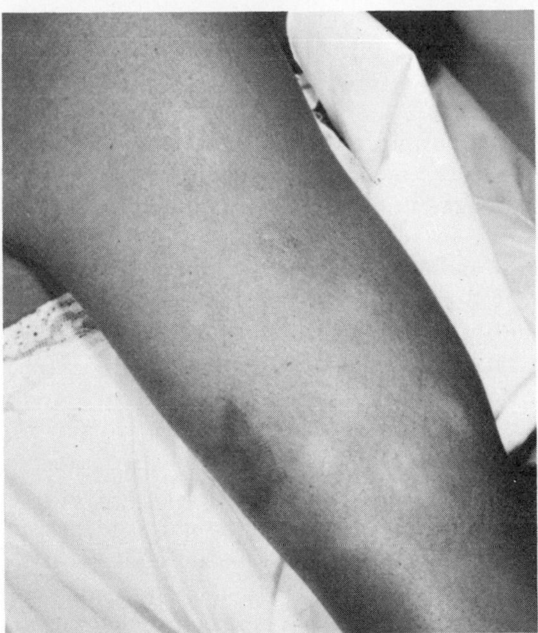

Figure 24–11. Dermal sarcoidosis in an American Negro resembling the macules of an early leproma. (Courtesy of Dr. M. L. Brubaker.)

Treatment. General treatment, including personal and environmental hygiene, an ample well balanced diet and the correction of concomitant conditions, is important. With such measures even severe lepromatous cases may show some degree of amelioration, at least for a time.

Introduction of the sulfones revolutionized the treatment of leprosy and also opened new possibilities for the control of the disease by mass treatment. Chaulmoogra preparations are virtually in disuse in most areas of the world. In advanced lepromatous cases sulfones are conspicuously useful in the rapid healing of skin ulcers and lesions of the upper respiratory tract; tracheotomies are now rare. Early lepromatous cases clear up relatively rapidly as a rule. If the skin lesions are well established, however, they recede slowly, and the reduction of the bacterial index is still slower. As a result, even responsive cases may require 3 or more years before smears become negative. The importance of early recognition and diagnosis is thereby emphasized. Improvement often seems to be slower at first in the nonlepromatous forms of the disease. The sulfones do not alleviate the effects of nerve damage; in fact, neural sequelae often develop in sulfone-treated patients as skin lesions subside.

Because of the toxicity of the parent substance, 4,4′-diaminodiphenyl sulfone (DDS), relatively expensive derivatives (Promin, Diasone, Sulphetrone) were used exclusively at first. When it was found that the much cheaper DDS could be used satisfactorily in proper dosage, the new treatment became much more generally available, including extensive use on an outpatient basis.

Dosage schedules of DDS vary considerably, by physician's choice or depending on the tolerance of the individual patient, but the maximal dose is generally up to 400 mg a week in divided dosage: 200 mg twice weekly by mouth. When well tolerated for a month, the dose can be increased to 100 mg daily for 6 days each week. In all cases the maximal dosage is attained gradually beginning with 25 mg weekly, or a smaller dose if indicated. In some places DDS in depot preparations is given by injection at intervals of a week or longer. With the derivatives, doses are aimed at attaining blood levels similar to those with the parent substance.

There is an active search for drugs that may be more regularly or rapidly effective than the sulfones, or that might be given in combination with them, or that could be substituted when patients are not responsive or cannot tolerate the sulfones. When DDS is not tolerated because of repeated reactions, or when the organism has become sulfone-resistant, clofazimine (B663), Lamprene, is a good second-line drug. Though somewhat slower in effect, clofazimine has been shown to be as effective as DDS and useful in the treatment of reactions, for which it was originally introduced. The diphenyl thioureas (thiambutosine and thiocarbonylimide) have produced good therapeutic results in small groups of lepromatous patients. However, difficulties posed by their cost, utilization problems, and the tendency of infections to develop resistance have made them second-choice drugs for leprosy treatment.

Clinical trials using 4, 4′-diacetyldiaminodiphenyl sulfone (DADDS) were recently reviewed.[9] Earlier studies using 225 mg of DADDS by injection every 77 days were comparable to those produced by standard doses of DDS. Use of twice the dose, given at a shorter interval, is now under consideration. The advantage of a long-term drug by injection is apparent by insuring that the patient is taking his drug. Studies using DADDS on an entire population have demonstrated its value as a public health measure by reducing the infectious reservoir of the disease.[10]

The most recent and perhaps the most promising antileprosy drug is the new semisynthetic antibiotic rifampin, belonging to the group of rifamycins. This drug is the most rapidly bactericidal of leprosy drugs tested and has produced much more rapid clearance from the skin than any drug to date. The use of rifampin in combination with other drugs is currently being studied at the Pan American Health Organization/World Health Organization Center for Training and Research in Leprosy and Related Diseases in Caracas, Venezuela, and elsewhere; the results are so far impressive.

Treatment of Reactional States. Because reactions in leprosy can cause more damage to the patient than the disease itself, it is important to deal with them properly and adequately. Erythema nodosum leprosum (ENL), when not severe, is best treated symptomatically with analgesics and antipyretics and perhaps chloroquine. When ENL is severe, and especially if there is associated neuritis, use of corticosteroids and adrenocorticotropic hormone (ACTH) in adequate doses is indicated. Thalidomide has been shown to be very effective in severe ENL; however, because of its teratogenic effects it must be carefully administered to selected patients—never when pregnancy is possible.

Prognosis. The prognosis of untreated lepromatous and dimorphous leprosy is generally unfavorable. In the self-healing benign cases, crippling deformities often develop before the disease is overcome. Lepromatous cases almost always deteriorate intermittently. With modern treatment many benign cases are arrested before the development of neural sequelae, and many of the lepromatous type are rendered bacteriologically negative. It must always be assumed, however, that deep-seated bacilli still persist and that relapse may occur after treatment is suspended. With modern treatment of secondary or concurrent conditions the death rates in leprosy institutions have decreased greatly.

Prophylaxis and Control. Until an effective vaccine or other immunotherapy is available, the control of leprosy depends upon the early diagnosis and treatment of cases. When effectively carried out, the disease can thus be cured or arrested, deformity and disability prevented and, from a public health standpoint, the infectious reservoir reduced. Most cases today can and should be treated on an outpatient basis. The existence of special leprosy laws is deplored, as is the continued and costly institutionalization of leprosy patients.

The use of bacille Calmette-Guérin (BCG) inoculation is indicated for persons who are nonreactive to lepromin and are known to have had, or may possibly have had, contact with a leprosy case. Prophylactic sulfone is probably indicated in those high-risk groups who have had contact with infectious, nontreated leprosy.

REFERENCES

1. Bechelli, L. M., and Martínez Domínguez, V. 1966. The leprosy problem in the world. Bull. W.H.O. *34*:811–826.
2. Waters, M. F. R., and Rees, R. J. W. 1962. Changes in the morphology of *Mycobacterium leprae* in patients under treatment. Int. J. Lepr. *30*:266–275.
3. Shepard, C. C. 1962. Multiplication of *Mycobacterium leprae* in the foot-pad of the mouse. Int. J. Lepr. *30*:291–306.
4. Kirchheimer, W., and Storrs, E. 1971. Attempts to establish the armadillo *(Dasypus novemcinctus* Linn.) as a model for the study of leprosy. Int. J. Lepr. *39*:693–702.
5. Doull, J. A. 1962. The epidemiology of leprosy—present status and problems. Int. J. Lepr. *30*:48–66.
6. Cochrane, R. G., and Davey, T. F. 1964. Leprosy in Theory and Practice. 2nd ed. John Wright & Sons, Ltd., Bristol. 659 pp.
7. Latapi, F., and Zamera, A. C. 1948. The "spotted" leprosy of Lucio—An introduction to its clinical and histological study. Int. J. Lepr. *16*:421–430.
8. Convit, J., Avila, J. L., Goihman, M., and Pinardi, M. E. 1972. A test for the determination of competency in clearing bacilli in leprosy patients. Bull. W.H.O. *46*:821–826.
9. Brubaker, M. L. 1972. Leprosy: Fifty years of progress. Bol. Of. Sanit. Panam. *4*:1–14.
10. Russell, D. A., Shepard, C. C., McRae, D. H., Scott, G. C., and Vincin, D. R. 1971. Treatment with 4,4′-diacetyldiaminodiphenylsulfone (DADDS) of leprosy patients in the Karimui, New Guinea. Am. J. Trop. Med. Hyg. *20*:495–501.

CHAPTER 25

Plague

ROBERT E. BLOUNT, JR.

Synonyms. Oriental plague, pest, black death.

Definition. Plague is an acute, febrile, infectious, highly fatal disease which is characterized by inflammation of the lymphatics, septicemia, and petechial and diffuse hemorrhages into the skin, subcutaneous tissues and viscera. It is frequently characterized by buboes, less often by secondary plague pneumonia and rarely by primary pneumonia or meningitis.

Distribution. In the course of the last pandemic, which is believed to have originated in Yunan on the Tibetan border of China, nearly every important country in the world was invaded. The more important present endemic centers appear in Table 25–1 and Figure 25–1.

Etiology. *Yersinia pestis* (Yersin and Kitasato, 1894) Holland is a member of the group producing hemorrhagic septicemias in animals. It is a short, nonmotile, gram-negative, bipolar-staining bacillus which exhibits marked pleomorphism and is often encapsulated. A potent endotoxin is produced. Three general forms may be seen:

1. Short, rounded or oval, often appearing as diplococci.
2. Longer rods.
3. Large, oval or pear-shaped, or club-shaped involution forms.

Specific identification is based upon the morphology, staining reactions, cultural characteristics, the results of animal inoculation, and fluorescent antibody and phage testing.

Epidemiology. Although plague is a disease primarily of rats and other rodents, in man it is one of the most fatal of all infectious diseases. It occurs in three forms—bubonic, primary septicemic and primary pneumonic. Age, sex, race and occupation play no role in susceptibility. Epidemics are usually bubonic but always include a small number of primary septicemic cases and cases of secondary plague pneumonia.[1-3]

The reservoirs of infection are rats and other rodents in which the disease occurs in acute, subacute and chronic or latent forms. Domestic rodents belonging to the family MURIDAE are primarily concerned in the infection of man. Plague infection among the rat population is referred to as murine or rat plague, and among wild rodents as sylvatic, campestral or wild rodent plague.[4]

Meteorologic conditions exert an important influence upon the epidemiology of the disease. The gross climate is important in determining the survival of plague bacilli and the types of disease which they may produce in man. Primary pneumonic plague epidemics rarely if ever occur in the absence of constantly low temperatures and high relative humidity. Microclimate—the immediate environment of the flea—is of extreme importance in determining the life of the vectors.

Extreme heat and dryness are inimical to the spread of plague. The disease is more commonly seen in the Temperate Zone in the summer and autumn months when fleas are most numerous, and human disease in consequence often takes the bubonic form. In India and other parts of the tropics the plague season frequently prevails during the cooler months of the year.

Dissemination from one area to another may occur in a variety of ways but is usually by the transportation of infected rats on ships. Occasionally, it may be by the importation of fleas in bales of material containing the infected, living insects. Sometimes an ambulatory or more severe human case may be responsible. In areas where sylvatic plague is present, migrations of the rodent population may extend the endemic area.

Murine or rat plague is disseminated

Table 25-1. Principal Endemic Foci of Plague in Rodents

Type	*Locality*
Murine plague: (domestic rodents)	India China, Manchuria, Mongolia Burma Indonesia East Africa West Africa Malagasy Republic South America: Brazil, Bolivia, Peru, Ecuador
Sylvatic plague: (wild rodents)	United States: western states Argentina, Mexico China, Mongolia Transcaucasia South Africa

primarily by the brown sewer rat, *Rattus norvegicus,* to the smaller domestic black house rat, *R. rattus rattus.* The infected sewer rat not infrequently will enter the lower parts of buildings and die. Immediately after its death the fleas leave the carcass in search of a new host, to whom the infection is transmitted.

Rodents may frequently be found infected with bipolar-staining bacilli which are difficult to differentiate from *Y. pestis.* The more important of these are *Yersinia pseudotuberculosis rodentium* and *Yersinia avicada.*

Rattus r. rattus is rare in Europe today but widespread and common in the tropics where it lives in close association with man. *Rattus norvegicus* has a worldwide distribution. *Rattus r. alexandrinus* has been important in the epidemiology of plague in Egypt in the past and has been reported to be present in the South Pacific islands. *Rattus hawaiiensis* is the reservoir in the Hawaiian

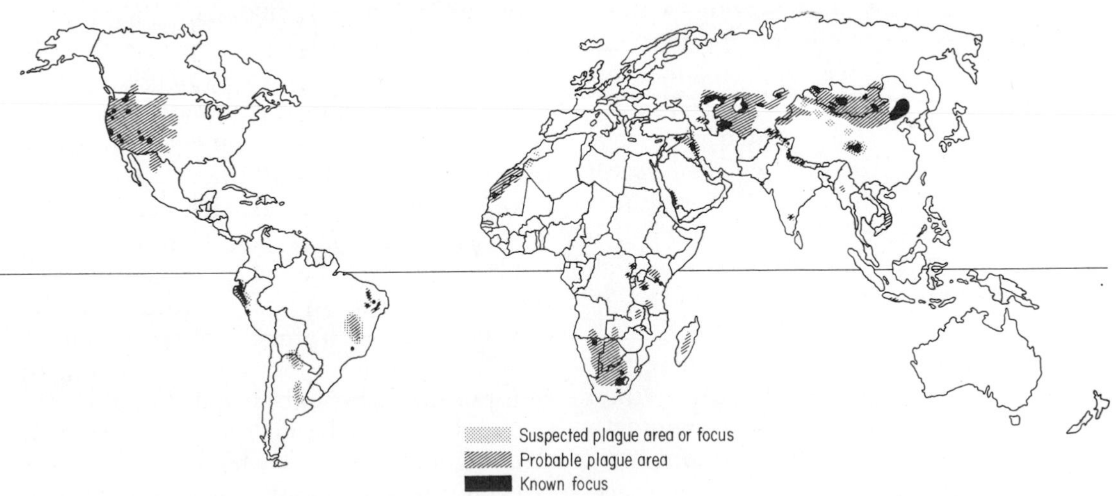

Figure 25-1. Known and probable foci and areas of plague, 1969. (Redrawn and updated by Don Alvarado from W.H.O. Technical Report Series 447, 1970. 4th Report. 25 pp.)

Islands. Rats in different areas apparently possess varying degrees of resistance to infection by the plague bacillus. The disease is transmitted from rat to rat and from rat to man by fleas.

SYLVATIC (CAMPESTRAL) PLAGUE. This epidemiologic entity refers to the nondomestic character of the reservoir host; the organism is the same as in murine plague. More than 70 rodents, of which the ground squirrel (western United States) and the gerbil and the multimammate mouse (South Africa) are the most important, may act as reservoirs of the infection. Sylvatic plague in wild rodents occurs in areas sparsely inhabited by man. The rarity of human infections in the United States, even in the presence of marked epizootics, implies a weakness in the flea link of the transmission chain, since man is rarely infected unless directly exposed to fleas from rodent burrows or, more often, to contamination by handling infected animals. The spread to a domestic rodent population, that is to say translation from sylvatic to murine plague, is most apt to occur when uncontrolled rodent populations come into contact and freely exchange their ectoparasites (Fig. 25–2).

THE VECTOR. Various fleas are immediately responsible for transmission of the infection from the reservoir to man. These insects may live for 1 to 2 years under favorable conditions of temperature and moisture. They survive several months without food in cool and moist environments but die quickly in a hot dry climate. In moderate temperatures they may remain infective for prolonged periods. The Indian rat flea, *Xenopsylla cheopis,* is the most efficient vector of plague; however, it is readily transmitted by the common rat flea of Europe and North America, *Nosopsyllus fasciatus. Pulex irritans* also can transmit plague.[5] (See Chapter 70 and Fig. 70–12, p. 744.)

A flea feeding upon its infected rodent host ingests the plague bacilli, which then multiply in its gut, sometimes becoming so numerous as to block the lumen. Man may be infected by the bite of such an insect, since *Y. pestis* is regurgitated from the esophagus and proventriculus as the flea attempts to feed. The organisms are likewise passed in the feces of the flea and may infect man either through the bite wound or through a minute abrasion of the skin. It is possible that the body louse, *Pediculus humanus humanus,* and, more remotely, the bedbug, *Cimex lectularius,* may occasionally transmit the infection directly from man to man (Table 25–2).

OTHER MEANS OF TRANSMISSION. Transmission of plague to man by other means is less common. A small proportion of cases of bubonic plague may be traced to entry of the bacilli through abraded skin of the feet, as in cowdung-floored houses in India, or of the hands in the performance of an autopsy or in handling or skinning infected animals.

Primary septicemic plague may result from the entry of the bacilli through mucous membranes, especially those of the mouth, throat and conjunctivae.

PREDISPOSING FACTORS. Bubonic plague is commonly acquired through the bite of an infected rat flea or human flea. Important contributory factors are an overcrowded human population housed in unsanitary buildings which provide adequate food and harborage for an uncontrolled rodent population. Epidemics of bubonic plague are associated with a high incidence of the disease in rats, with great mortality among them. When the rodent population is sufficiently reduced, many of the infected fleas migrate to man.

A few severe epidemics of plague have been of the primary pneumonic type, which is transmitted directly from man to man by droplet infection from the cough. Meteorologic conditions, particularly temperature, are exceedingly important factors in determining the spread or failure to spread of the pneumonic type of the disease. Freezing temperatures with high relative humidity favor transmission, since pulverized and frozen sputum and cough droplets retain infective and virulent bacilli for long periods of time. Communities in which there is overcrowding of the population with close contact between sick and well and in which unsanitary conditions and practices are usual provide a fertile field for this type of the disease. Isolated cases of secondary plague pneumonia occurring as a complication of bubonic or of primary septicemic plague often constitute the immediate origin of such an outbreak. Such secondary pneumonia, however, is not as infectious as is primary pneumonic plague, and unless the conditions for respiratory transmission are wholly suitable it is less apt to initiate large epidemics.

Pathology. The pathology of plague is essentially that of lymphangitis, lymphadenitis or bubo formation and bacteremia with metastatic localization.

In bubonic plague the lymph nodes draining the site of infection are swollen, edematous, congested and hemorrhagic,

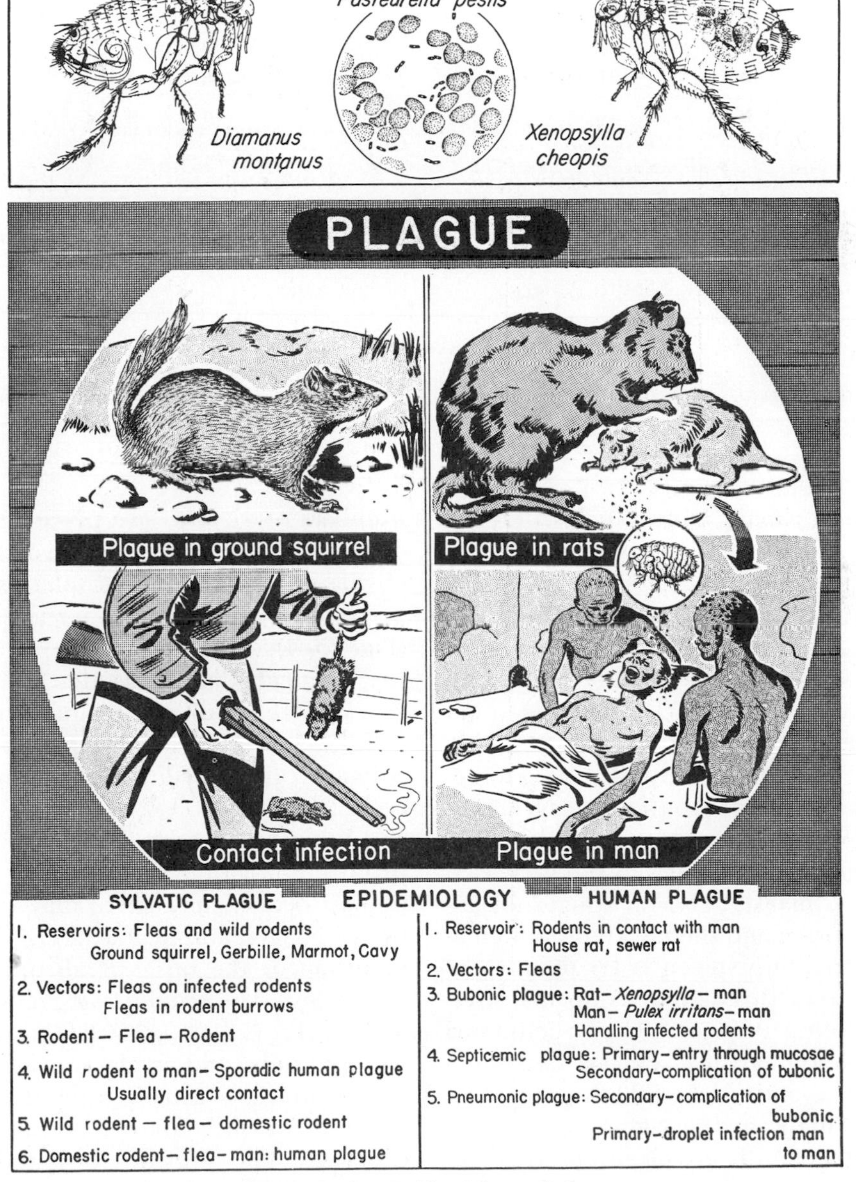

Figure 25–2. Epidemiology of plague.

Table 25–2. Some Important Flea Vectors of Yersinia pestis

Flea	Distribution	Reservoir Hosts	Transmits Primarily To:
Xenopsylla cheopis	Widely disseminated	*Rattus r. rattus* *R. norvegicus*	Rats and man
X. brasiliensis	Uganda, Kenya, Nigeria	Rats	Rats and man
X. astia	India, Ceylon, Burma, Mesopotamia, Mombasa	Rats	Rats
X. nubicus	Tropical East and West Africa	Rats	Rats
X. eridos	South Africa	Wild rodents	Wild rodents
Pulex irritans	Nearly cosmopolitan	Man, swine, rodents	Man, rodents
Nosopsyllus fasciatus	Temperate Zone	*R. norvegicus*	Rats
Diamanus montanus	Western United States	Ground squirrels	Ground squirrels
Rhopalopsyllus cavicola	South America	Cavies	Cavies
Ceratophyllus tesquorum	Russian steppes	Ground squirrels	Ground squirrels
Oropsylla silantiewi	Manchuria	Rodents	Rodents

forming the primary bubo which often undergoes necrosis. Adjacent nodes are matted together and there is much edema and hemorrhage in the surrounding tissues (Fig. 25–3).

There are often secondary inflammatory changes, similar in character, in other lymph nodes in the body. There is extensive damage to vascular and lymphatic endothelium which contributes to this process and to the development of cutaneous petechiae and hemorrhages in many parts of the body.

There is marked visceral congestion involving the brain and the meninges as well as other organs. The spleen is frequently enlarged to two or three times its normal size.

Pneumonic Plague. The pneumonia of plague is lobular in character, extending to involve the entire lobes. There is intense congestion of the air passages, with hemorrhagic exudate in the alveoli and bronchi but with little or no fibrin formation. Great numbers of *Y. pestis* are present. The bronchial and hilar nodes are involved, and ecchymoses and fibrinous pleurisy may be present over the affected portion of the lung (Fig. 25–4).

Clinical Characteristics. The incubation period of bubonic plague is usually 2 to 4 days, less often as long as 10 days. In primary pneumonic plague it may not exceed 2 to 3 days.

Bubonic Plague. Usually there is no prodromal period in bubonic plague, although occasionally there may be a day or two of malaise and headache. In the majority of instances the onset is abrupt, with chill and followed by rapidly rising temperature to 39.5 or 40° C (103 or 104° F), accompanied by rapid pulse and accelerated respiration. A severe attack is usually attended by mental dullness, which is followed by anxiety or excitement. The eyes are injected, the face congested, the tongue coated, and nausea

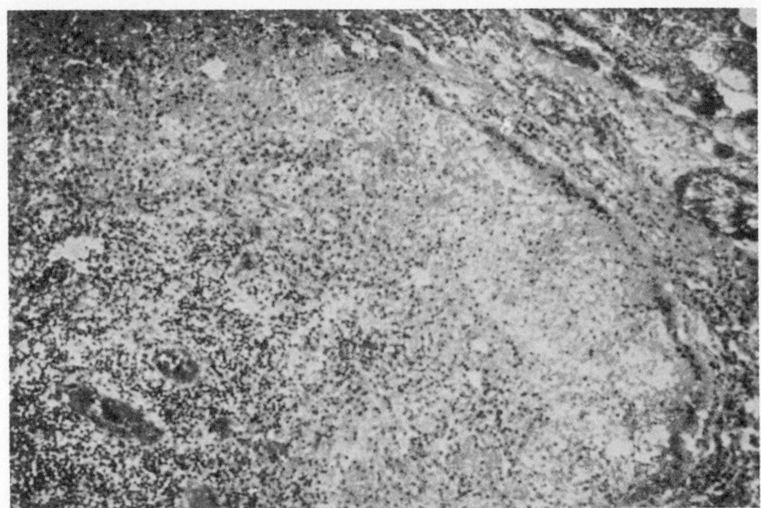

Figure 25-3. Section through plague bubo showing necrosis and beginning abscess formation, capsule of lymph node and surrounding edema and infiltration.

and vomiting may be present. Constipation is usual; the urine is scanty, with moderate albuminuria. An expression of intense anxiety is very characteristic of the disease. In some instances, maniacal delirium may occur, in others lethargy or coma; convulsions are common in children. The acute stage with high fever commonly lasts 2 to 5 days, following which, in favorable cases, the temperature falls by slow lysis, reaching normal in about 2 weeks.

Definite bubo formation occurs in 75 per cent of cases, usually appearing from the second to the fifth day and preceded by local pain. When fully developed the bubo may be the size of an egg and is hard and tender. In fatal cases it remains indurated; in others, suppuration is common. Incision, especially prior to the appearance of definite fluctuation, is hazardous because of the risk of initiating blood stream infection. The common sites of the bubo are as follows:

Inguinal	65 to 75 per cent
Axillary	15 to 20 per cent
Cervical	5 to 10 per cent

The acute stage is accompanied by a high leukocytosis which may reach 40,000 per cu mm with a corresponding increase in the polymorphonuclear cells. Positive blood culture is obtained in about 45 per cent of cases. Death may occur within 5 days.

PESTIS MINOR. Mild ambulatory cases of plague with little or no fever or toxemia may be encountered. Frequently there is a bubo in one groin, less commonly on one side of the neck or in one axilla. These may suppurate or may gradually be resorbed (Fig. 25-5).

PRIMARY PNEUMONIC PLAGUE. The onset of primary pneumonic plague is usually abrupt, with fever rising to 39.5 or 40°C (103 or 104°F) within 24 to 36 hours. True rigor is rare. Painless cough and dyspnea appear within the first 24 hours. The sputum at first is mucoid, becoming blood-tinged but not tenacious; in the fully developed case it is thin and bright red, and contains enormous numbers of *Y. pestis*. Physical signs are often not marked even in advanced cases. There is usually a high leukocytosis.

PRIMARY SEPTICEMIC PLAGUE. Septicemic plague can occur as a form of primary infection. However, a secondary septicemia occurs invariably in primary pneumonic cases and may occur in the course of bubonic plague. In primary septicemia cerebral symptoms frequently develop with great rapidity and intensity, rapidly progressing to coma. Peripheral vascular collapse due to the endotoxin as well as all the complications of gram-negative septicemia, including disseminated intravascular coagulation, may be seen. This form of the disease, if untreated, is fatal. Death occurs usually within 3 days of onset and frequently before there is demonstrable enlargement of superficial lymph nodes.

Diagnosis. The clinical picture of sudden onset of high fever, marked toxemia, lymphadenitis, extreme anxiety and high leukocytosis is suggestive. The appearance of a bubo is important supporting evidence. However, in primary septicemic plague there may be no significant clinical signs, and in primary pneumonic plague physical signs over the chest may be trivial even in the presence of enormous numbers of bacilli in the sputum.

The definitive diagnosis depends upon the demonstration and identification of *Y. pestis*. In bubonic cases, material aspirated from the bubo should be stained by Gram's method and examined for the characteristic bipolar pleomorphic bacilli. In septic and pneumonic cases, smears of blood and sputum should be examined similarly. Phage sensitivity and fluorescent antibody (FA) tests for *Y. pestis* in aspirates or culture may yield confirmation of specific diagnosis. However, the results of these tests and of culture and animal inoculation are too delayed to permit the early diagnosis essential for effective treatment.

All material suspected of containing *Y. pestis* must be handled with extreme care. Inoculated animals must be free from fleas and maintained under strict quarantine in insect-free cages. All individuals handling infected material, such as cultures, inoculated animals or cages, should wear gowns, rubber gloves and masks. All procedures must be carried out with the strictest possible aseptic technique.

Cultural Characteristics. *Yersinia pestis* grows equally well at 30 to 37° C (86 to

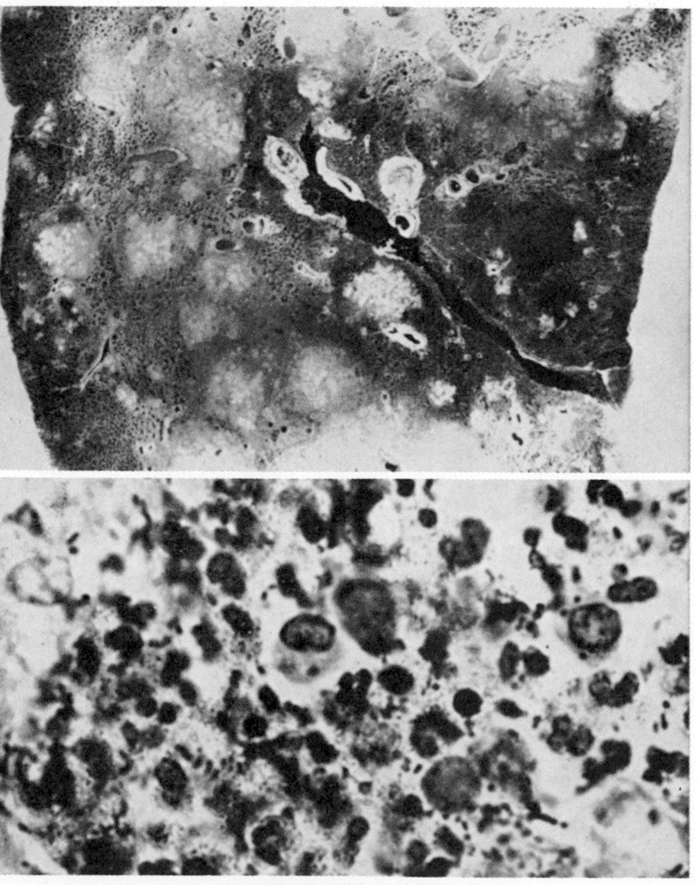

Figure 25–4. Primary pneumonic plague. *A*, Confluent lobular pneumonia. *B*, Bacilli and exudate in alveolus.

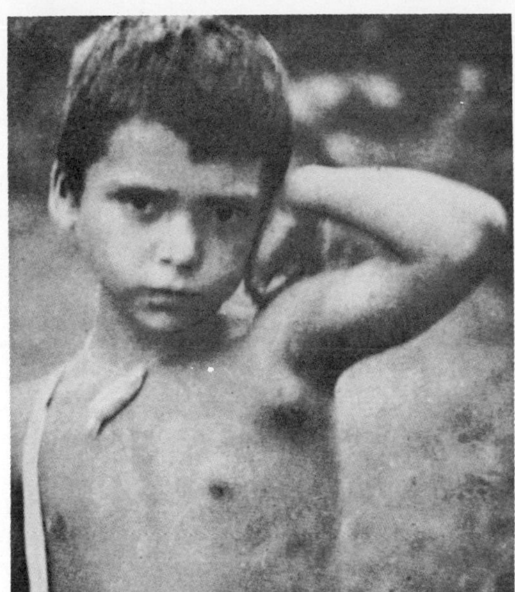

Figure 25–5. Pestis minor; case of ambulatory plague showing axillary bubo. (Courtesy of Dr. A. Macchiavello.)

98.6° F). This is of value for its isolation in pure culture and for identification. On alkaline agar small translucent dewdrop colonies appear in 18 to 24 hours. Acid without gas is formed from glucose, maltose, mannite and salicin. Lactose is not fermented; milk is not coagulated. There is no indole production. In bouillon under oil there is a characteristic stalactite growth extending downward from the surface. Salt agar, 2.5 to 3.5 per cent, is useful for the production of involution forms which are of value in diagnosis.

ANIMAL INOCULATION. The guinea pig is the best laboratory animal for the recovery of these organisms, since a single virulent bacillus produces fatal infection. Inoculation should be made by rubbing into the shaved scarified skin of the abdomen. If the inoculum contains plague bacilli, death results in 3 to 5 days with the following characteristic findings:

1. Marked subcutaneous edema, congestion and hemorrhage about the site of inoculation.

2. Buboes in one or both inguinal regions.

3. Numerous yellowish white necrotic foci in the spleen and at times in the liver.

4. Hemorrhages in the lungs and other tissues and occasionally in the heart muscle due to diffuse endotoxin injury to the vasculature.

5. Smears from the lesions and from the heart blood revealing large numbers of typical bipolar-staining bacilli.

Yersinia pestis is easily killed by drying in sunlight and by ordinary disinfectants. Its viability varies greatly in different environments: in putrefying animal matter, 4 days; in buried bodies, 3 to 30 days, depending upon the temperature; in the cowdung floors of houses in India, 48 hours; in grain and meal if there is sufficient moisture, 13 days; and in dried flea feces, 4 weeks. In frozen sputum or in frozen corpses the bacilli remain viable for prolonged periods.

DIFFERENTIAL DIAGNOSIS. In the early stages of the disease certain of the clinical types may be confused with typhus fever, relapsing fever, malaria, dengue, tularemia and, rarely, with typhoid.

Prognosis. Untreated, or inadequately treated, primary pneumonic and septicemic plague are generally fatal diseases. In the past, the mortality from bubonic plague has varied from 60 to 90 per cent. Since the introduction of the antibiotics, the mortality has been reduced remarkably. In India, streptomycin alone lowered the fatality rate of bubonic and septicemic plague to 10 per cent initially. Unfortunately, resistant strains of *Y. pestis* have since emerged. In severe cases endotoxin injury to the peripheral vasculature may result in death in spite of prompt and vigorous antibiotic therapy.

Treatment. Therapy should be instituted as soon as the diagnosis of plague is suspected. Early treatment is extremely important and its initiation should not await laboratory confirmation. Streptomycin is the drug of choice for the treatment of all forms of plague. It should be administered intramuscularly in the following dosage: 0.5 gm every 3 or 4 hours until the temperature becomes normal, thereafter 1.0 gm daily in divided doses until a total of 15.0 gm has been given.

Because of the increasing resistance of strains of *Y. pestis* to streptomycin, it is recommended that a second antibiotic be used in combination until the definitive sensitivities of the organism can be obtained from the laboratory. Chloramphenicol, tetracycline, gentamicin, cephalothin and kanamycin are all highly effective against sensitive strains. Some authorities advocate combined therapy with sulfadiazine.

The usual management of gram-negative septicemia and its complications should be instituted promptly when applicable, but should not delay antibiotic treatment of the underlying infection.

Simultaneous antitoxin administration is recommended in more than minimally ill patients. Since a generalized Shwartzman reaction can be elicited by administration of antibiotics, this point should be considered carefully in spite of the well recognized risk assumed when using any antitoxin.

Sulfadiazine and sulfamerazine are also recommended for use in large outbreaks or when the antibiotics are not available. The following dosages are advised: sulfadiazine initial dose 4.0 gm followed by doses of 1.5 to 2.0 gm every 4 hours for 10 days.

SURGICAL TREATMENT OF BUBO. Hot wet applications may hasten localization. Incision should be avoided until frank fluctuation occurs.

Prophylaxis. Prophylaxis against plague is accomplished: (1) by strict isolation of the sick, (2) by appropriate sanitary measures, and (3) by protection of the individual.

ISOLATION OF THE SICK. Strict isolation of the patient in a separate insect-proof room is essential. All waste articles possibly contaminated and all discharges from the patient should be burned or otherwise satisfactorily disinfected. Bodies of humans and animals dead from plague should be disposed of with extreme sanitary precautions. A room previously occupied by a patient with plague must be completely and thoroughly cleaned and treated with residual spray or powder insecticide. Either Diazinon or Gammexane is recommended where DDT resistance may be suspected or the use of DDT is discouraged (Table 72–1, p. 797).

In the presence of pneumonic plague or when its presence is suspected, physicians, nurses and any others in contact with the patient or entering the patient's room must have protection against potential infection through both aerosol and insect vector routes. Contacts or suspected contacts should be treated with insecticides and should be segregated. Their temperatures should be recorded daily. Sulfadiazine or sulfamerazine, 3.0 gm daily, should be given for at least 5 days after the last exposure. Streptomycin is not recommended for prophylactic purposes because of the rapid excretion and the difficulties of repeated dosage. It should, however, be given immediately if suggestive symptoms develop.

SANITARY MEASURES. The general sanitary measures directed toward the prevention or control of plague are concerned primarily with rat and rat flea eradication.

Importation of rats from an endemic area should be guarded against by rat-proofing of ships, application of measures to prevent rats from leaving ships, and appropriate fumigation by cyanide gas.

In towns and cities, buildings should be rat-proofed and natural harborages, especially rubbish, refuse and garbage, eliminated. Trained personnel should be utilized in well organized programs to distribute the highly effective rodenticides sodium fluoroacetate ("1080") and warfarin (Coumadin). Other poison baits using red squill, thallium sulfate, zinc phosphide or barium carbonate may be used, but these are generally considered less effective than "1080" or warfarin.

All rats obtained should be systematically examined for the presence of *Y. pestis* in their ectoparasites and in their viscera. Examination of rats found dead is of great importance, since rodent epizootics commonly precede the appearance of plague in man.

In the control of outbreaks or epidemics of human plague, the elimination of rat fleas is of major importance. The insecticide should be sprayed or dusted extensively in and around houses, as well as in clothing, bedding and house furnishings (Table 72–1). The eradication program must be energetic and prompt and must be directed by personnel who are familiar with current epidemiologic control measures.

Clothing and personal effects of passengers at ports of departure from an active plague area, and departing vehicles and aircraft, should be thoroughly dusted with insecticide.

PERSONAL PROPHYLAXIS. When human plague represents a potential hazard, the first line of defense is vaccination.[6] In the presence of an outbreak or prior to entering an area where human plague is known to occur with any regularity, all potentially exposed persons should be vaccinated. Both heat-killed and virulent live vaccines are available and have been observed to reduce the attack rate markedly, though in both methods periodic revaccination is necessary to maintain immunity.

Personnel engaged in rat control programs should be immunized and should wear flea-proof insecticide-dusted clothing, with particular attention given to high boots, tight wristbands and tight collars. This insures maximum protection against fleas found on the rodents and present abundantly in their burrows and nests.

REFERENCES

1. Pollitzer, R. 1954. Plague. W.H.O. Monogr. Ser. No. 2, Geneva. 698 pp.
2. Pollitzer, R. 1960. A review of recent literature on plague. Bull. W.H.O. No. 23. pp. 313–400.
3. Meyer, K. F. 1957. The natural history of plague and psittacosis. Pub. Hlth. Rept. *72*:705–719.
4. Sandoval, D., Pérez-Miravete, A., and Barrera, A. 1962. Hallazgo de una cepa de *Pasteurella pestis* en *Microtus* capturado en la cuidad de México. Rev. Latino-amer. Microbiol. (Mexico) *5*:55–60.
5. Baltazard, M. 1961. La peste; état actuel de la question. Acta Med. Iranica *4*:1–19.
6. W.H.O. Tech. Rept. Ser. No. 447. 4th Rept. 1970, Geneva. 25 pp.

CHAPTER 26

Gonococcal Infections

MERLIN L. BRUBAKER

Synonyms. Blennorrhagia, clap, dose, strain.

Definition. Gonorrhea is a specific infection of the genitourinary tract caused by the gonococcus, *Neisseria gonorrhoeae.* Extragenital infections (rectal, oropharyngeal, joint-dermal manifestations of disseminated infection and ocular infection of the newborn) do occur, but rarely in comparison to the urogenital disease. Gonococcal infection is almost always sexually transmitted. In young girls, vulvovaginitis may be caused by an infectious discharge on bed clothing, linens, or towels or through actual sexual contact.

Distribution. Gonorrhea is worldwide in its distribution—the disease certainly is not limited to the tropics. It occurs frequently in countries situated at 60° latitude as well as at the equator. Opportunities for sexual contact and conditions that favor movements of people have contributed to the present worldwide increase in gonorrhea. The distribution and prevalence of this infection is therefore determined by the frequency of sexual contact with more than one partner, promiscuity being the most effective modus vivendi for spread of the disease. Since gonococcal infections are important infectious disease entities encountered in the practice of medicine in the tropics, they are included and discussed here.

Etiology. The infectious agent of gonorrhea is *Neisseria gonorrhoeae,* a gram-negative, nonmotile, non-spore-forming intracellular diplococcus, which measures 0.6 to 1.0 μm in diameter. The organism may occur singly, or in pairs with flattened sides where they are in contact, producing a coffee bean–shape appearance. Early in the disease, or when the disease has become chronic, the organism may be extracellular—appearing perhaps as a single coccus. *Neisseria gonorrhoeae* is fastidious and dies rapidly outside the body, unless careful attention is paid to primary isolation and appropriate culture media. Within the body it can apparently continue to live for many years. Man is the only reservoir for gonococcal infection. The disease has, however, recently been successfully transmitted experimentally to the chimpanzee.[1]

Epidemiology. Gonorrhea is spread by sexual intercourse. Because of the intimate nature of this relationship, the epidemiology of gonococcal infections is different from that of any other diseases, except those also transmitted sexually.

According to a 1964 estimate by the World Health Organization, there are 65,000,000 new cases of gonorrhea each year in the world.[2] In the period 1964 to 1972, there has been a 17.5 per cent increase in the world population, from 3,220,000,000 in 1964 to 3,787,000,000 in 1972. All things being equal, a proportional increase in gonococcal infections should also have occurred. This has taken place, but because all conditions have not been equal, the world population and venereal disease incidence have increased geometrically instead. Of special note is the increase in the number of young people, which is translated by an increase in the number of susceptibles at the age of greatest sexual activity. Fifty per cent of the cases occur in patients under 25 years of age. These factors have led to the dissemination of gonorrhea and the disease has reached epidemic proportions in most countries of the world. Gonorrhea has become the most prevalent reportable disease, in places where reporting is actively practiced by health authorities.

Reporting of gonorrhea, however, is notoriously poor. In the United States of

America where probably less than 10 per cent of cases are reported, it has been estimated that more than 85,000 new cases per month are occurring—exceeding 1 million per year.[3]

Several factors peculiar to this disease lead to very rapid spread of infection when the conditions are right, especially when promiscuity of sexual activity is practiced. The incubation time of gonococcal infection is extremely short—2 to 5 days (range 1 to 31 days). Promiscuous encounters can thus lead to rapid and even widespread dissemination before infection becomes apparent. Of great importance is the large hidden reservoir in infected women, who are asymptomatic in 80 per cent of the cases or more. Of lesser degree, but equally significant, is the fact that 5 to 30 per cent of men may be asymptomatic. Both, nonetheless, are infectious. Infection appears to give little if any protection from future infections.

Throughout the world, traditional views on sexual activity are changing. This change of attitude has created much greater sexual freedom and provides increasing opportunity for sexual encounter.

The reported frequency ratio of male to female for this infection is about 3:1. This ratio, which varies from country to country, is probably an indicator more of reporting activity and accuracy than of the real ratio. It may be seen from the foregoing that gonococcal disease in the asymptomatic patient (usually the female) will not be diagnosed as often as in the male, who is more likely to have obvious and often quite painful infection.

Pathology. Without an experimental animal model, the study of the histopathology of gonorrhea has been limited. The gonococcus appears unable to penetrate stratified epithelium, but possesses an affinity for columnar, and less so for transitional epithelium, as found in the urethra and female cervix. Within a few days the gonococcus can be found in the subepithelial spaces with accumulation of polymorphonuclear leukocytes. Soon, these leukocyte-contained bacteria pass into the lumen of the urethra and the combination of the numerous polymorphonuclear white cells, desquamated epithelium, and serum produces the characteristic profuse urethral discharge of gonorrhea. In the male, the urethra, Littre's and Cowper's glands, seminal vesicles, epididymis and prostate may become involved. In the female, Skene's and Bartholin's glands, the urethra and its glands, the cervix and fallopian tubes are susceptible organs in the natural history of untreated gonorrhea. Many of the former complications have been reduced since the advent of antibiotics. Other features of gonococcal infection depend upon the spread to and involvement of other parts of the body, including the joints, skin and eye.[4]

Clinical Characteristics. Gonorrhea is primarily an acute infection of the anterior urethra, especially in the male. With the exception of ophthalmia neonatorum and the vulvovaginitis of young girls, gonorrhea is transmitted by sexual intercourse. The locus of infection varies according to the site of inoculation, such as the rectum in the passive homosexual or the oropharynx when fellatio is practiced. The latter is being increasingly observed (in about 5 per cent of all gonococcal infections).

ACUTE INFECTION IN THE MALE. After exposure (2 to 7 days, average 3 days), a transient mucoid urethral discharge develops which becomes a profuse, thick, greenish, purulent urethral excretion. Painful urination is the outstanding symptom; it may be severe, moderate or even absent. Both discharge and symptoms of dysuria may be minimal or absent. Recent studies have indicated that 10 per cent of cases or more may have no signs or symptoms, diagnosis having been established by urethral scraping technique with a platinum loop. Therefore, *N. gonorrhoeae* appears to have established a carrier state, as in other *Neisseria* infections. Rectal infection is most often asymptomatic, and the result of direct implantation of infection by homosexual activity in almost all instances.

ACUTE INFECTION IN THE FEMALE. Gonococcal infection in the female is, more often than not, silent. Up to 80 or 90 per cent of the female patients have no signs or symptoms of infection, but continue to be an infectious reservoir for occasional spread or local outbreak of epidemic disease.

In the infected female, dysuria or vaginal discharge are the most frequent presenting symptoms or signs of disease. These may be so mild as to go unnoticed, unless previous experience suggests gonorrhea. Rectal infection, which may occur by contamination from a cervical discharge but which more likely results from rectal intercourse, is usually asymptomatic, and must therefore be thought of and looked for when suspected.

Complications. MALE. Before the advent of antibiotics, approximately 25 per cent of gonorrhea cases produced complications in the male. The incidence is now less than 3 per cent.[5] In acute infection, the inflammatory response appears to be largely caused by the endotoxin liberated by the gonococcus.[6] The resulting characteristic discharge consists of numerous polymorphonuclear leukocytes, desquamated epithelium and serum. Many phagocytosed gonococci appear within the leukocytes in the acute phase. The discharge may become serosanguineous when infection is heavy. When left untreated, small abscesses may form in Littre's glands which, before the use of antibiotics, frequently resulted in fistulas. Ultimately, in chronic infection, fibroblasts replace the polymorphonuclear infiltration in the subepithelial layer and a fibrous band develops producing a urethral stricture, formerly a frequent complication of gonorrhea.

Left untreated, the infection may spread via the lymphatic and blood vessels to produce a mildly painful inguinal lymphadenitis. This spread continues and may produce a seminal vesiculitis, epididymitis or prostatitis.

FEMALE. Because the female is so often asymptomatic, the acute cervical, rectal, or even urethral infection may spread locally to produce a bartholinitis or salpingitis or both. This spread may continue from the fallopian tubes into the peritoneal cavity and up the right colonic gutter to produce a perihepatitis, the so-called Fitz-Hugh–Curtis syndrome.[5]

Both males and females, but usually females, may have disseminated gonococcal infection spread from the primary site via the blood. Disseminated infection may be the first apparent manifestation of disease and may present in many and varied ways depending on the organ attacked. Most commonly observed are arthritis (the most frequent systemic manifestation of gonococcal infection), skin eruptions, meningitis, endocarditis, or conjunctivitis (via the blood or by contamination from genital secretions). Other rarer metastatic infections may include myocarditis, pericarditis, uveitis, cystitis, perihepatitis, hepatic abscess, glomerulonephritis, osteomyelitis, myositis and pneumonia.[4] These may occur in conjunction with the typical arthritis-dermatitis syndrome.

Pharyngeal involvement in gonococcal infections has been receiving increasing attention, leading to some very interesting and important observations. Infection of the pharynx is seen in about 5 per cent of the total number of patients infected at any site.[7] The incidence increases to 10 per cent among heterosexual females and to 21 per cent among homosexual males. The relationship to fellatio is clear. Cunnilingus has not been found to be associated with pharyngeal gonococcal infection, nor has mouth-to-mouth contact been demonstrated to be a source of transmission.[8]

Diagnosis. In the male with signs and symptoms suggestive of gonorrhea, a presumptive diagnosis may be made when gram-negative intracellular diplococci are found in the smear of the urethral discharge. The definitive diagnosis rests, however, on the culture (Thayer-Martin) of the organism from material taken from the suspected site. Unfortunately, a negative Gram-stained smear does not rule out the diagnosis of gonococcal infection, and mistakes can be made in identifying as gonococci those gram-positive cocci that have been overdecolorized, or gram-negative "diplobacilli." When the urethral discharge is scanty or absent, material for smear and culture should be obtained by the use of a platinum loop inserted about 1 cm into the urethral meatus and scraped along the wall as it is withdrawn. A prostatic massage may also produce material for culture and a definitive diagnosis.

In the female, the greatest yield of positive results comes from cultures of material from the cervix, vagina, urethra and rectum. The greatest single yield comes from the cervix alone in about 85 per cent of cases, and when rectal culture is added the yield will be about 95 per cent.[3] Gram stain smears are unreliable and should not be used except perhaps in rural clinics where bacteriologic culture or transport media are not available. In this latter instance, false negative findings have been obtained in 54.9 per cent, as compared with results obtained with cultures made on selective media.[5] Fluorescent antibody procedures, especially the delayed technique, though time-consuming and requiring skilled laboratory personnel, have improved diagnostic ability to a point approaching the results with the selective culture medium technique.[3] The use of Transgrow and Stuart's media has increased the availability of cultures for definitive diagnosis to even remote areas. After growth has been observed on selective culture media, the oxidase test and sugar fermentation reactions should differentiate the *Neisseria*. *Neisseria gonorrhoeae* ferments only glucose, but *N. meningitidis* ferments both glucose and maltose.

Using a radioimmunoassay procedure, serum tested for antibody to gonococcal pili has shown an apparent sensitivity when gonococcal infection of the cervix in the asymptomatic female is present. This finding has rekindled interest in the serologic diagnosis of gonococcal infection and hope for its use as a screening tool. Its future is currently being determined in several clinics in Sweden, England and the United States of America.

The etiologic agents of other sexually transmitted diseases are shown in Table 26-1. Some of these infections should be considered in the differential diagnosis of gonococcal infections.

Treatment. The treatment of gonorrhea has come a considerable distance since the days of sandalwood oil and, later, at the end of the nineteenth century, the introduction of potassium permanganate solution. The advent of the sulfonamides marked the beginning of a new era for this previously unsuccessfully treated disease. The sulfonamides soon lost their effectiveness owing to

Table 26-1. SEXUALLY TRANSMITTED DISEASES IN MAN*†

	Organism ‡	***Disease***
Spirochetes	*Treponema pallidum*	Syphilis
Bacteria	*Neisseria gonorrhoeae*	Gonorrhea
	Hemophilus ducreyi	Chancroid
	Calymmatobacterium (= Donovania) granulomatis	Granuloma inguinale
	Chlamydia spp.	Nongonococcal urethritis
		Lymphogranuloma venereum
Viruses		Herpes simplex
		Molluscum contagiosum
		Condylomata acuminata
Protozoa	*Trichomonas vaginalis*	Trichomoniasis
Fungi	*Candida albicans*	Candidosis
	Epidermophyton floccosum	Tinea cruris
Parasites	*Sarcoptes scabiei*	Scabies
	Phthirus pubis	Pediculosis

*From Willcox, R. R. 1972. A world look at the venereal diseases. Med. Clin. North Am. 56:1061.

†See the respective chapters of this book for additional information on the organisms listed in this table.

‡Other sexually transmitted organisms whose roles in relation to venereal disease are not yet clear include mycoplasmas, diphtheroids, mimeae (moraxellas), *Herellea vaginicola*, cytomegalic virus.

resistant organisms, but the introduction of penicillin for the first time in the long history of the chronic and painful complications of gonorrhea gave justified hope for cure, for prevention of the disabling effects, and for a real possibility of control. The optimism as to effective treatment of gonorrhea was justified; but complacency by health authorities and the public led to reduced effort by all and allowed for the ultimate resurgence of gonorrhea throughout the world.

In the beginning, the response to penicillin therapy for gonorrhea was dramatic even with comparatively small doses. Over the years, however, a relative resistance to penicillin has been developed by the gonococcus, and higher and higher doses have become necessary in order to be effective. In spite of this, penicillin remains the preferred form of treatment. It must, however, be used in adequate dose and in a form that produces rapid and sufficiently high blood levels; the peak serum level of penicillin attained is more important than the length of time of the treatment. Only 6 to 12 hours are required to eliminate the gonococci.[9] The peak serum level of penicillin is further increased 2- to 4-fold by the addition of 1 gm of probenecid prior to injection. The following schedule has recently been recommended.[10]

Uncomplicated Gonococcal Infection of Men and Women. Aqueous procaine penicillin G(APPG) 4.8 million units intramuscularly divided into at least two doses injected at different sites at one visit, together with 1 gm of probenecid by mouth just before the injections. Alternate regimens include:

1. Ampicillin 3.5 gm by mouth, together with 1 gm of probenecid by mouth administered at the same time. There is evidence that this regimen may be slightly less effective than the recommended APPG regimen.

2. For patients who are allergic to the penicillins or probenecid: tetracycline hydrochloride, 1.5 gm initially by mouth, followed by 0.5 gm by mouth 4 times per day for 4 days (total 9.5 gm). Other tetracyclines are not more effective than tetracycline hydrochloride, and none is effective as single dose therapy. Postgonococcal urethritis is less common after tetracycline therapy, probably because of its effects on the chlamydia (or the mycoplasma). When nongonococcal urethritis occurs after gonorrhea treatment with other forms of therapy, it should be treated with tetracycline hydrochloride 0.5 gm 4 times per day by mouth, for at least 7 days.

Pharyngeal infection may be more difficult to treat than urogenital and rectal infections, and both ampicillin and spectinomycin as recommended are ineffective for pharyngeal infection with the gonococcus. Therefore, if 4.8 million units of APPG with 1 gm of probenecid added are inadequate to eradicate the gonococcus from the pharynx, the patient should be treated with 9.5 gm of tetracycline hydrochloride as recommended.

Acute salpingitis (pelvic inflammatory disease) should be suspected in women with acute lower abdominal pain and adnexal tenderness on pelvic examination. Cervical cultures should be taken, but therapy should be started without waiting for the culture results. The patient should be hospitalized when necessary for adequate work-up, observation and treatment. If not hospitalized, treatment can be given with tetracycline hydrochloride 1.5 gm as a single oral dose followed by 0.5 gm orally 4 times daily for 10 days. Aqueous procaine penicillin G 4.8 million units in divided doses in different sites or oral ampicillin 3.5 gm may be used in place of tetracycline. One gram of probenecid is given along with either penicillin or ampicillin. Both are followed by 0.5 gm of ampicillin orally 4 times per day for 10 days.

Hospitalized patients with pelvic inflammatory disease may be treated with aqueous crystalline penicillin G 20 million units intravenously each day until clear-cut improvement is noted, followed by 0.5 gm ampicillin orally 4 times per day to complete 10 days of treatment. Aminoglycoside therapy is sometimes indicated because of difficulty in distinguishing gonococcal from nongonococcal salpingitis. Tetracycline hydrochloride 0.5 gm intravenously 4 times per day until improvement occurs, followed by 0.5 gm orally 4 times per day to complete 10 days of therapy, may also be administered except in pregnant patients or those with renal failure.

Disseminated gonococcal infection may be treated in a similar fashion to that of pelvic inflammatory disease, but with 10 million units of aqueous crystalline penicillin for 3 days or until improvement occurs, followed by ampicillin for 7 days. Ampicillin with probenecid, tetracycline or erythromycin, 0.5 gm intravenously every 6 hours for at least 3 days, may be substituted for penicillin. At least 3 to 4 weeks of treatment is needed for endocarditis.

Follow-up cultures are necessary in the male and female to insure cure of the patient and to prevent further spread of the infection. Cultures from appropriate sites (urethral, rectal, cervical and pharyngeal) should be carried out 7 to 14 days after completion of therapy, and repeated in the female after at least the next two menses. Two grams of spectinomycin intramuscularly can be used when treatment failure occurs with penicillin, ampicillin or tetracycline.

Because syphilis can be acquired at the same time as gonorrhea, a serologic test for syphilis should be done at the initial visit (baseline) and monthly thereafter until the patient is discharged as cured (about 4 months).

Prophylaxis. Individual prevention of gonorrhea is different from that of almost any other disease because the chance for exposure is largely voluntary and the alternative—abstinence—is generally unacceptable. The use of a condom offers the best mechanical means of protection and studies are currently going on as to the prophylactic as well as contraceptive effectiveness of products currently available for contraception. Many of the latter, including the condom, have diminished in current usage because of the convenience and availability of the contraceptive pill and intrauterine device. Both the pill and the intrauterine device have contributed to an increase in venereal diseases (especially gonorrhea): the pill, by altering genital secretions toward alkalinity; the intrauterine device, by mechanically promoting the spread of the disease; both by reducing the fear of pregnancy, and permitting greater ease for sexual intercourse.

Antibiotic prophylaxis after known exposure is of value in selected instances. On a wider application it has considerable public health benefit.

Control of gonorrhea is a public health problem. In the absence of an effective vaccine, control rests firmly on the base of clinical services. These services should be convenient and acceptable to both patients and staff, and they should be free or within the reach of everyone needing them. Although the contact tracing and interviewing as carried out for syphilis is not practical, every effort must be made to identify the source of the disease for the index case as well as all possible contacts of either. When all possible contacts have been identified, they should be treated. Some will be treated unnecessarily, but all should be prevented from developing gonococcal infection. The infectious reservoir will thus be reduced. It has been shown further that adequate gonorrhea therapy will also treat incubating syphilis. From a public health standpoint, therefore, prophylactic treatment of contacts is necessary to break the chain of infection and to reduce the reservoir. Many features of gonococcal infection, for example the short incubation period, make this a less than completely effective approach.

One of the most dramatic efforts to get at the hidden reservoir in the asymptomatic female (and now the asymptomatic male) has been the program of culture screening promoted by the United States Public Health Service. This country-wide effort produced 345,090 positive cultures from females in the United States of America during the period July 1973 to June 1974, from 8,016,879 tests, with an average from all sources (private, public, venereal disease and nonvenereal disease clinics) of 4.3 per cent positives.[11] Though costly, this effort has demonstrated the need to do such screening whenever possible if the true reservoir of infection is to be exposed and treated.

REFERENCES

1. Brown, W. J., Lucas, C. T., and Kuhn, U. S. G. 1972. Gonorrhea in the chimpanzee: Infection with laboratories–passed gonococci and natural transmission. W.H.O. Unpublished Document 72.62.
2. World Health Organization. 1963. W.H.O. expert committee on gonococcal infections. First Report. W.H.O. Tech. Rept. Ser. No. 262. 70 pp.
3. Brown, W. J., Donohue, J. F., Axnick, N. W., Blount, J. H., Ewen, N. H., and Jones, O. G. 1970. Syphilis and Other Venereal Diseases. Harvard University Press, Cambridge, Massachusetts. pp. 87–97.
4. Brown, W. J., and Lucas, J. B. 1967. Gonorrhea. *In:* Tice's Practice of Medicine. Vol. 3. Harper & Row, Hagerstown, Maryland. pp. 5–7.
5. Wiesner, P. J. 1973. Diagnostic problems in gonorrhea. Proc. Third Internat. Vener. Dis. Symp., New Orleans. pp. 39–41.
6. Thayer, J. D., Sparling, P. F., and Carson, W. 1965. The gonococcus. *In* Dubos, R. J.: Bacterial and Mycotic Infections of Man. J. B. Lippincott Co., Philadelphia. pp. 451–467.
7. Juhlin, L. 1973. Personal communication.
8. Holmes, K. K. 1972. Pharyngeal gonorrhea. Proc. Sec. Internat. Vener. Dis. Symp., St. Louis, Missouri. pp. 27–29.
9. Sparling, P. F. 1973. Resistance and reactions in the treatment of gonorrhea. Proc. Third Internat. Vener. Dis. Symp., New Orleans, Louisiana. p. 56.
10. United States Public Health Service. 1974. Venereal disease control advisory committee. C.D.C. Morb. Mort. Wk. Rept. *23*:341–348.
11. United States Public Health Service. 1974. Results of screening for gonorrhea–U.S.A. 12-month period ending June 30, 1974. C.D.C. Morb. Mort. Wk. Rept. *23*:363.

CHAPTER 27

Granuloma Inguinale

MERLIN L. BRUBAKER

Synonyms. Granuloma venereum, granuloma pudente tropicum, chronic venereal sore, donovanosis, granulomatosis, granuloma contagiosa, sclerosing granuloma.

Definition. Granuloma inguinale is usually considered to be a venereal infection characterized by destructive, granulomatous, ulcerated, autoinoculating and painful lesions generally involving the genitalia and adjacent tissues. Occasionally, invasion of the lymphatics and the blood stream produces metastatic foci accompanied by serious systemic disturbances that may result in marked destruction of the genital organs and spread to other parts of the body. There is little tendency to spontaneous healing.

Distribution. The disease is widespread in the tropics of Africa, the West Indies, South America, the Pacific Islands, New Guinea, north Australia, southern China and India. It is not uncommon among Negroes in the southern United States.

Etiology. The etiologic agent is an encapsulated bacillus, *Calymmatobacterium granulomatis,* Aragao and Vianna 1913, formerly *Donovania granulomatis,* the Donovan body. It occurs intracellularly in large mononuclear phagocytic cells and is constantly present in the lesions. It can be cultivated only in embryonated eggs or embryonic yolk medium. Isolated capsular material gives positive precipitin tests and fixes complement with sera of patients suffering from the disease (Figs. 27–1, 27–2).

Epidemiology. Granuloma inguinale occurs in both sexes but is more common in men. It has not been observed before puberty and appears predominantly between the ages of 20 and 40 years. Transmission is apparently by sexual contact, though this is doubted by some because it is often not transmitted to the sexual partner.

Pathology. The pathologic changes are essentially those of a granulomatous lesion of the skin, with superficial ulceration extending by continuity to adjacent areas, especially on the genitalia, the groins and the thighs. Although the disease is usually restricted to the genital region, involvement of the face, mouth, nose, neck, back and legs has been reported. In these regions it is probably the result of autoinoculation or metastasis. Metastatic lesions may occur in the

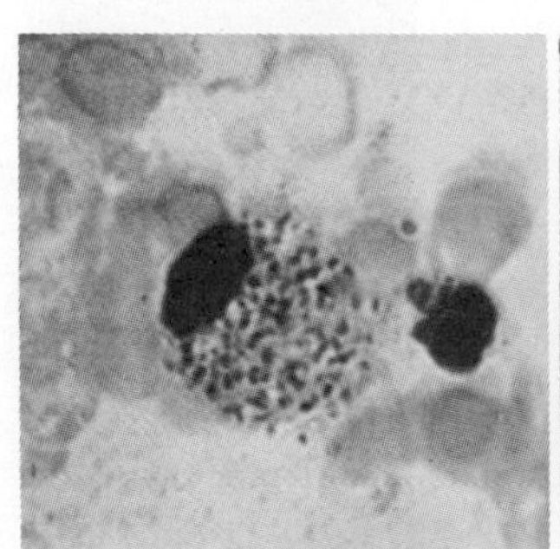

Figure 27–1

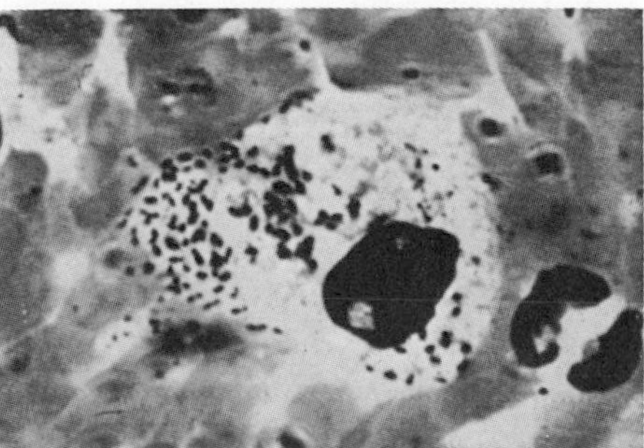

Figure 27–2

Figure 27–1. Granuloma inguinale: Donovan bodies in large mononuclear phagocytic cell in stained smear from lesion. (Courtesy of Dr. Donald C. A. Butts.)

Figure 27–2. Biopsy of lesion: Donovan bodies in large mononuclear phagocytic cell. (Courtesy of Dr. Donald C. A. Butts.)

bones and internal organs. Healing is accompanied by extensive fibrosis.

Histopathologic examination reveals a prominent round cell infiltration of the corium, with swelling, degeneration and ultimate disappearance of normal connective tissue elements. A surrounding infiltration of polymorphonuclear leukocytes, lymphoid and plasma cells and reticuloendothelial cells occurs. Many swollen mononuclear phagocytes containing numerous Donovan bodies are present in the lesion. There is marked formation of new connective tissue in which focal areas of inflammation and necrosis are commonly seen.

Clinical Characteristics. The incubation period is variable, extending from a few days to 2 to 3 months. The initial lesion may be a vesicle, papule or nodule commonly on the penis or the labia minora. This becomes eroded and superficially ulcerated, with new nodule formation at the periphery as the lesion extends. The ulcer, though painless in the beginning, may later become painful. There is little systemic effect.

In severe cases there may be extensive superficial destruction of the genitalia and the skin of the groins and thighs. Severe involvement of the vagina is followed occasionally by rectovaginal fistula. Concurrently with extension of the process there is marked scar tissue formation and epithelialization often presenting areas of secondary involvement and breakdown (Fig. 27–3). Elephantiasis of the genitalia in either sex may be a late complication. Massive enlargement of the labia may develop even after the ulcers have healed. Granuloma inguinale reportedly predisposes to development of cancer of the vulva.[1-3] This disease has been frequently associated with rectal intercourse.[4]

An awareness of this venereal disease, which does not respond to penicillin or to sulfonamides, is essential when dealing with genital and anal ulceration. It must also be remembered that it can coexist with syphilis and other sexually transmitted diseases. The lesions may simulate cancer and may occur in buccal mucosa or on the cervix.[5]

Diagnosis. The diagnosis is based upon demonstration of the characteristic Donovan bodies. These are found within large mononuclear phagocytes in smears of scrapings from the margins of the lesions, stained by Wright's or Giemsa's stains. Biopsy may also be indicated to establish the diagnosis. A long and careful search may be required to detect the diagnostic forms in some cases.

Treatment. The tetracyclines given orally 500 mg every 6 hours for 10 to 15 days are effective, as is streptomycin. The latter is usually given in 4 gm daily doses (at 6-hour intervals) for 5 days. Larger doses, 40 gm over 20 days, to insure cure, have been recommended.[4]

Erythromycin and chloramphenicol are also effective though toxicity with the latter makes its use limited. Penicillin and the sulfonamides are not effective against granuloma inguinale.

Troleandomycin (triacetyloleandomycin) has been used with good results and appears to lack the disadvantages of streptomycin or chloramphenicol.[4, 6]

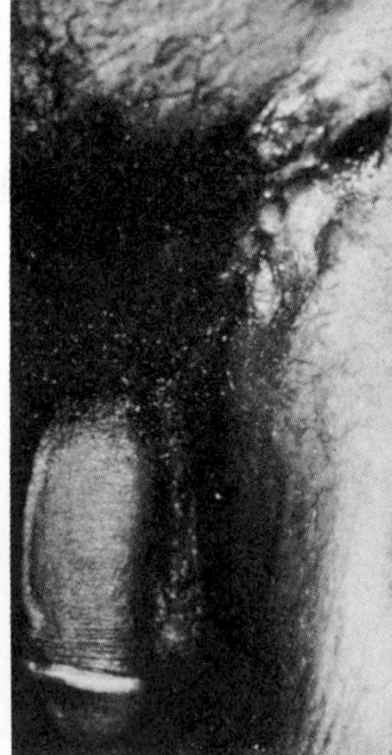

Figure 27–3. Granuloma inguinale: involvement of skin of inguinal region. (Courtesy of Dr. Donald C. A. Butts.)

REFERENCES

1. McDaniel, W. E. 1964. Four lesser venereal diseases. J. Kentucky Med. Assoc. *62*:281–283.
2. Douglas, C. P. 1962. Lymphogranuloma venereum and granuloma inguinale of the vulva. J. Obstet. Gynaecol. Br. Commonw. *69*:871–880.
3. Stewart, D. B. 1964. The gynecological lesions of lymphogranuloma venereum and granuloma inguinale. Med. Clin. North Am. *48*:773–786.
4. Medina, R. 1974. Personal communication.
5. Ayyanger, M. C. 1961. Granuloma venereum: a statistical study of 50 cases. J. Indian Med. Assoc. *37*: 70–74.
6. Kerdel-Vegas, F., Convit, J., and Soto, J. M. 1961. Treatment of granuloma inguinale with triacetyloleandomycin. Report of a case. Arch. Dermatol. *84*: 248–255.

CHAPTER 28

Cutaneous Diphtheria

JOHN P. O'BRIEN

Distribution. This infection is widespread and has been reported from North Africa, India, Burma, New Guinea, the Caribbean and the southern United States.

Clinical Characteristics. Cutaneous diphtheria may be secondary or primary. Secondary invasion by diphtheria bacilli may occur in wounds (wound diphtheria) and in any other skin lesion, such as a burn, insect bite, pyoderma,[1] tropical ulcer or even an eczematoid rash. The clinical features are pleomorphic. The infection should be suspected, even in the absence of exacerbation, necrosis or membrane formation. Children are more prone to infection than adults.[2]

Primary cutaneous diphtheria is more characteristic. It principally affects the extremities, although it is not confined to them. The scrotum is a common site. There may be a history of mild trauma. The most typical lesion is a round or oval ulcer measuring 1 to 3 cm in diameter. Vesicles or pustules are sometimes seen in early stages.

The ulcer is shallow with rolled, bluish, tender edges and characteristically is covered by an adherent membrane or, more often, by a hard, dark scab (eschar). An adjacent bulla may be present. Within a week or more the eschar separates and leaves a shallow punched-out ulcer with a flat unhealthy floor. Multiple lesions are common.

Pain is generally present at first, but later there may be anesthesia, a helpful point in diagnosis. Healing takes place from the periphery and is exceedingly slow. The resulting scar is thin and depressed; it may break down repeatedly before healing is complete. Infection (or the carrier state) in the throat or nose may be present. During the prolonged course of 4 months or more, one should watch for neurologic and cardiac complications. Weekly electrocardiographs should be taken.

Diagnosis. Confirmation is determined by bacteriologic examination, with culture on selective media. The inoculum must be taken from the deep aspect of the eschar or membrane. Virulence tests are necessary for confirmation of cultures. Distinction needs to be made between definite infections and simple contamination.[2]

Treatment. For definite infections, immediate isolation, bed rest and nursing care in a hospital are essential. After intracutaneous testing for sensitivity, and desensitization if required, diphtheria antitoxin should be given intramuscularly in doses of 20,000 to 40,000 units. Resuscitation equipment and drugs should be available in case of anaphylaxis. Supportive measures include use of penicillin and of simple antiseptics locally for control of secondary pyogenic infections. Convalescence is slow and may take weeks.

Carriers are treated with erythromycin (250 mg 4 times daily, between meals, for 7 days). In a serious outbreak, active immunization on a wide scale, preferably preceded by Schick testing, is recommended.

Prophylaxis. Contacts should be kept under observation and have throat, nose, and skin lesions checked for the presence of diphtheria bacilli. Active immunization with toxoid should be considered.

REFERENCES

1. Belsey, M. A., Sinclair, M., Roder, M. R., and LeBlanc, D. R. 1969. *Corynebacterium diphtheriae* skin infections in Alabama and Louisiana: a factor in the epidemiology of diphtheria. N. Engl. J. Med. *280*: 135–141.
2. Bray, J. P., Burt, E. G., Potter, E. V., Poon-King, T., and Earle, D. P. 1972. Epidemic diphtheria and skin infections in Trinidad. J. Inf. Dis. *126*:34–40.

CHAPTER 29

Rat-Bite Fevers

J-J. Gunning

Although linked historically by virtue of similar transmission and casual clinical mimicry, the rat-bite fevers are two distinct diseases deserving separate consideration.

Spirillum minus Infection

Synonym. Sodoku (Japanese: *so,* rat; *doku,* poison).

Definition. *Spirillum minus* infection is an acute, relapsing, febrile illness occurring about 2 weeks after the bite of a rodent. Recurrence of local inflammation or chancre-like ulceration at the site of the wound, regional lymphadenitis and a macular rash accompany the onset of fever.

Distribution. Rats infected with *S. minus* are found worldwide, but predominantly in Asia.

Etiology. *Spirillum minus* is a gram-negative, rigid, polar-tufted, two- to five spiral organism. Its length is from 1.5 to 6 μm. Dark field examination reveals darting motility. Despite claims to the contrary, the organism has never been cultivated and animal inoculation is required for isolation. Other members of this genus, however, have been cultivated and infrequently cause human disease.[1]

Epidemiology. Because infections in rodents may be inapparent, it is difficult to assess the extent of the zoonosis. The organism is found in the blood and infected eye discharges in up to 25 per cent of rats. Cats, pigs and other carnivores feed on rats and can transmit the disease by bite or scratch. Children inhabiting crowded urban slums and laboratory workers are at greatest risk.

Pathology. *Spirillum minus* infection provokes edema, mononuclear leukocyte infiltration and necrosis at the site of inoculation. Regional lymph nodes are hyperplastic. The relapsing course of the disease is characterized by cyclic reactivation of the initial lesion with invasion of the blood by the spirilla. Toxic, hemorrhagic, and necrotic changes have been noted in the liver and renal tubules. Hyperemia, edema and cloudy swelling occur in the myocardium, spleen and meninges.

Clinical Characteristics. One to 4 weeks after a healed animal bite, fever, chills and other systemic signs may occur. The site of the original inoculum becomes swollen and painful. A chancre-like ulceration usually ensues along with lymphangitis and regional adenopathy. The fever reaches 40° C (104° F) in a stepwise fashion in 2 to 4 days and falls by crisis. A hiatus of 3 to 7 days, during which all symptoms may disappear, usually separates up to six or eight regularly occurring relapses. A blotchy macular rash appears. In protracted, untreated cases complications such as meningitis, myocarditis, hepatitis and nephritis may be present and the mortality is approximately 6.5 per cent. Spontaneous cures in 4 to 8 weeks are the rule, but several untreated cases have lasted more than a year.[2]

Diagnosis. A compatible clinical course preceded by a rat bite may suggest the diagnosis. Clinical differentiation from other relapsing fevers such as malaria, *Borrelia* infection, Pel-Ebstein fever, Charcot's intermittent biliary fever and some urinary tract infections may be difficult. Demonstration of the spirillum by dark field or Giemsa-stained examination of blood or aspirates from the infected bite, lymph node or skin lesion may yield the diagnosis. Injection of these same materials into guinea pigs or mice may be needed to amplify the organism. Leukocytosis is variable. Biologic false positive tests for syphilis occur in about 50 per cent of patients. Specific serologic tests and culture methods are unavailable. (See Table 29–1.)

Streptobacillus moniliformis Infection

Synonym. Haverhill fever, erythema arthriticum epidemicum.

Definition. *Streptobacillus* infection is an acute febrile illness transmitted by an animal bite or by ingestion of contaminated food or milk (Haverhill fever) characterized usually by a remittent fever, polyarthritis and a discrete macular rash.

Distribution. Up to 50 per cent of both wild and laboratory rats harbor the streptobacillus. Other rodents and carnivores also carry the organism.

Etiology. *Streptobacillus moniliformis* (necklace-like) is a non-acid-fast, gram-negative, microaerophilic, highly pleomorphic bacillus. Cottonlike colonies, consisting of long, branching, filamentous, beadlike and fusiform shapes, can be cultivated in standard blood culture media and even on blood agar plates.[3] Stable L-forms have been isolated from human blood, or may develop spontaneously after passage to solid media. As a rule growth is slow but aided by increased carbon dioxide tension.

Epidemiology. *Streptobacillus moniliformis* is commonly recovered from the saliva of apparently healthy rodents. Epizootics of respiratory, arthritic and septicemic illnesses, with a high rate of abortion, have been described in rats and mice.

Although the disease is usually contracted by the bite of wild or laboratory rats, milk-borne epidemics have occurred. Turkeys are a potential food-borne source of the infection.

Pathology. Very few autopsies have been recorded. Bronchopneumonia and endocarditis with septic splenic and renal infarcts predominate in fatal cases. Hyperplasia of the spleen, myocarditis, hepatitis and nephritis with focal infiltration of predominantly mononuclear cells are seen.

Clinical Characteristics. Following a short incubation period an abrupt onset of a viral-like illness consisting of chills, fever, headache and myalgias is followed in 2 to 3 days by a peripheral macular rash and polyarthritis. The rash may cover the entire body, including the palms and soles, and may be confluent and purpuric. The arthritis may present as simple arthralgia or asymmetric large and small joint septic effusions. The knees are frequently involved. In untreated cases signs and symptoms usually resolve in about 2 weeks. Persisting bacilli or possibly L-forms on heart valves or in abscesses may occasion recurrences. Endocarditis is rare.

Diagnosis. A history of a rodent bite or an association with a food-borne outbreak coupled with appropriate signs and symptoms leads to a presumptive diagnosis. The differential diagnosis should include rickettsial, coxsackie B or arbovirus infections, meningococcemia, rheumatic fever and other infectious articular disease. An increased percentage of polymorphonuclear leukocytes is usually present and the total count may vary from 6000 to 30,000 per cu mm. *Streptobacillus moniliformis* can be cultured from blood and joint aspirates. Specific agglutinin titers in excess of 1:80 may appear at about 10 days, reach a maximum in 1 to 3 months and persist up to 2 years. Fluorescent antibody and complement-fixing tests are also available.[3] (See Table 29–1.)

Treatment. Parenteral penicillin G 600,000 units every 12 hours for 2 weeks appears adequate for either disease. Tetracycline, erythromycin, chloramphenicol and cephalothin seem to be effective alternate drugs.

Defervescence in *Spirillum minus* infections can occur in as little as 24 hours. Jarisch-Herxheimer reactions have been observed.[2]

In streptobacillary fever the duration of treated illnesses is about 6 days. After clinical response oral phenoxymethyl penicillin may

Table 29–1. Distinguishing Features and Similarities of Rat-Bite Fevers

Spirillum minus	*Similarities*	*Streptobacillus moniliformis*
Sodoku		Haverhill Fever
Inoculation	Rat Bite	Inoculation or ingestion
Chancre-like lesion	Wound	Heals permanently
Prominent with lymphangitis	Regional Lymphadenitis	Mild
Regularly relapsing Onset 5–30 days, usually about 15	Remittent Fever Chills Nausea Vomiting	Rarely relapsing Onset 1–10 days, usually about 2
Macular, confluent, reddish purple	Rash	Morbilliform to purpuric
Arthralgia and severe myalgia	Muscle and Joint Pain	Polyarthritis with effusion
Meningitis Hepatitis Nephritis	Headache Delirium Stupor Prostration	Endocarditis Pneumonia Septic infarcts and abscesses
6.5 per cent mortality	10 per cent mortality untreated	12.7 per cent mortality
False positive 50 per cent	Positive STS	False positive 25 per cent
No resistance apparent	Responds to penicillin	May develop resistant L-forms

be given to complete a 14-day course. Higher doses of intravenous penicillin may be used in more acutely ill patients. Endocarditis requires that serum bactericidal levels be determined and that treatment be continued a minimum of 4 weeks. Streptomycin may be included for added bactericidal and anti–L-form activity.[4, 5]

Prophylaxis. Rat eradication as outlined under plague control is effective (p. 232). Laboratory workers should wear gloves while handling animals.[6] Rodent bites must be cleansed meticulously and penicillin should be given in amounts sufficient to assure prevention.[4]

REFERENCES

1. Kowal, J. 1961. Spirillum fever. Report of a case and review of literature. New Engl. J. Med. *264*:123–128.
2. Roughgarden, J. W. 1965. Antimicrobial therapy of ratbite fever. A review. Arch. Intern. Med. *116*:39–54.
3. Carbeck, R. B., Murphy, J. F., and Britt, E. M. 1967. Streptobacillary rat-bite fever with massive pericardial effusion. J.A.M.A. *201*:703–704.
4. Yoshikawa, T. T., and Guze, L. B. 1974. Rat-bite fever. *In* Conn, H. F. (ed.): Current Therapy. W. B. Saunders Co., Philadelphia. pp. 53–54.
5. McCormack, R. C., Kaye, D., and Hook, E. W. 1967. Endocarditis due to *Streptobacillus moniliformis*. J.A.M.A. *200*:77–79.
6. Cole, J. S., Stoll, R. W., and Bulger, R. J. 1969. Ratbite fever. Report of three cases. Ann. Intern. Med. *71*:979–981.

CHAPTER 30

Miscellaneous Microbial Diseases

Introduction

Included in this chapter on miscellaneous microbial diseases are the chlamydial infections trachoma, inclusion conjunctivitis and lymphogranuloma venereum. To these is appended an unusual infection—bartonellosis, with its two clinical forms, the severe Oroya fever and the benign verruga peruana.

The uncertain and shifting taxonomic position of the chlamydial disease agents requires description. Psittacosis (ornithosis) of birds and mammals, and trachoma, inclusion conjunctivitis and lymphogranuloma venereum of humans, collectively known as the PLT group, were once thought to be caused by viruses, but were uncharacteristically responsive to antibiotics. More recent studies revealed that the causative organisms are small intracellular agents that possess both deoxyribonucleic and ribonucleic acid and rudimentary enzyme systems, together with a cell wall. The binary fission expressed in their development as diagnostic cytoplasmic inclusion bodies is inhibited by chloramphenicol and tetracyclines. Some are also sensitive to sulfonamides and penicillin.

Taxonomic Position of Chlamydiae. Once shifted to a genus known as *Bedsonia,* this complex, also known as TRIC (trachoma and inclusion conjunctivitis) and LGV (lymphogranuloma venereum) agents, now is classified in Bergey's *Manual of Determinative Bacteriology* (eighth edition) as CHLAMYDIACEAE. Because of similarities to rickettsiae, they have been placed in the order RICKETTSIALES. It has been proposed that within the genus *Chlamydia* Jones, Rake and Stearns 1945, two species be established, *Chlamydia trachomatis* (Busacca) Rake 1957 and *Chlamydia psittaci* (Lillie 1930) Page 1968, the differentiation being based on morphologic and chemical characteristics of the organisms.[1] *Chlamydia trachomatis* is responsible for the diseases trachoma, inclusion conjunctivitis, and lymphogranuloma venereum; *C. psittaci* is responsible for ornithosis (psittacosis).

Ornithosis (Psittacosis). Ornithosis is common in feral birds, notably parrots, and occurs often in epidemic form among domestic fowl, ducks, geese and turkeys in all of which it presents a major economic problem, and among mammals, particularly ruminants such as sheep, in which abortion is an important effect. An anthropozoonosis, *C. psittaci* infections represent an occupational hazard principally to people working with poultry, and to pigeon fanciers. In the United States, turkey breeders have been particularly affected, and in Europe, owners of ducks and geese.[2] The disease in humans ranges in severity from a mild influenza-like condition, often undiagnosed, to a fatal pneumonic and systemic infection.

Identification of Chlamydiae. The chlamydial organisms grow within the cytoplasm of host cells as basophilic inclusions (typical viruses appear acidophilic), 0.3 to 1.5 μm in size. These enlarge to fill the cytoplasm in the form of a cap-shaped body, the Halberstaedter-Prowazek inclusion, often indented by the host cell nucleus. The mature inclusion body is composed of elementary bodies, staining purple with Giemsa and enclosed in a glycogen matrix that stains with iodine. About 48 hours after it has been infected, the host cell bursts to release elementary bodies. Staining of conjunctival cell scrapings with Giemsa or iodine is diagnostically less sensitive for TRIC agents than direct immunofluorescent staining. Identification of the organisms has been improved by their cultivation in embryonated chick egg yolk sac or in HeLa–229 or irradiated McCoy cells. TRIC agents may be differentiated from LGV agents by cultivation in

HeLa–229 cells pretreated with DEAE-dextran, when TRIC but not LGV cultures will show greatly enhanced infectivity.[3]

Since these organisms are often present in a latent state, the number of people diagnosed as being infected is a small proportion of the whole, and many asymptomatic carriers exist.

Trachoma

PHILLIPS THYGESON

Synonym. Granular conjunctivitis.

Definition. Trachoma is a specific infectious disease of the conjunctiva and cornea. It is caused by *Chlamydia trachomatis* and is characterized by the presence of Halberstaedter-Prowazek cytoplasmic inclusion bodies in the conjunctival and corneal epithelial cells. It sometimes heals spontaneously, is subject to reinfection, runs a chronic course, and often displays acute or subacute exacerbations, due sometimes to the chlamydial activity and sometimes to superimposed bacterial infection. Visual damage is the result of corneal opacification due to scar tissue formation.

Distribution. Trachoma has a worldwide distribution with its greatest prevalence in Egypt and the Middle East where 90 to 100 per cent of the population in some villages may be affected. It was formerly very common along the entire Mediterranean littoral and in the Balkans, Africa and Asia, but recent control programs have been at least partially successful. There are important foci in Argentina, Brazil, Venezuela, and in certain of the Pacific Islands, Korea, China and Japan; minor foci still exist in the white population of the United States and Canada. Among the American Indians of the southwestern United States, the recrudescence of the disease that occurred in the 1950s has been largely brought under control, although a very low-grade trachoma is still widespread.

Etiology. Trachoma is caused by a large, pleomorphic organism, *Chlamydia trachomatis.* Strictly epitheliotropic, *C. trachomatis* affects the corneal and conjunctival epithelial cells, in which it appears as intracellular cytoplasmic agglomerations (inclusion bodies). In acute trachoma the agent can be seen free in the exudate in the form of elementary and initial bodies. Cultivation in series and in quantity (on the yolk sac of the developing chick embryo) was accomplished in 1957, but tissue culture on irradiated McCoy and other cells has recently proved to be more useful.[4]

Epidemiology. The infectivity of *C. trachomatis* is low in the chronic stage of the disease but may be high during an acute onset, during an acute exacerbation, or in the presence of secondary infection with bacteria. This is particularly true when the secondary invader is the gonococcus or *Haemophilus aegyptius* (Koch-Weeks bacillus), both of which are so commonly associated with trachoma in Egypt and the Middle East. For the most part transmission requires close personal contact, with transfer from mother to child a characteristic route. Physicians and nurses have been infected accidentally during surgical procedures.

Pathology. The earliest recognizable pathologic sign of trachoma is the cytoplasmic inclusion body, which develops in conjunctival and corneal epithelial cells and has been recognized in the incubation period of the experimental disease in human volunteers. The next observable changes are subepithelial infiltration with inflammatory cells, particularly plasma cells, and the development of lymphoid follicles. Follicular hypertrophy, principally of the tarsal conjunctiva, fornix and upper limbus, is characteristic of the chronic disease. Necrotic changes develop slowly but steadily in the subepithelial tissues and result in the conjunctival scars so characteristic of the disease.

Clinical Characteristics. Trachoma may start acutely, especially in adults, with dense conjunctival infiltration, papillary hypertrophy and considerable exudate. More

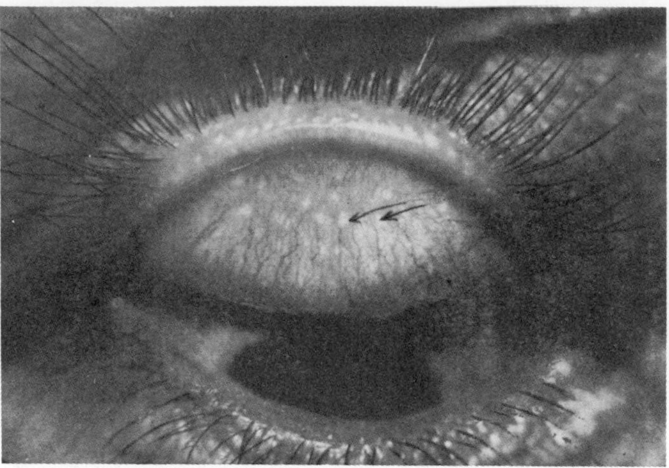

Figure 30–1. Trachoma: characteristic follicles, early infection. (Courtesy of Dr. Phillips Thygeson.)

often, especially in children, the onset is insidious, and there are few external signs other than slight ptosis; only when the upper lids are everted are the characteristic follicles of Stage I (MacCallan's classification) observed (Fig. 30–1). The cornea is always affected simultaneously with the conjunctiva, but the first epithelial changes, consisting of minute fluorescein-staining erosions and infiltrates, are recognized only with the biomicroscope. The later changes—pannus, corneal ulceration and scarring—are grossly visible. Unlike pannus from other causes, the pannus of trachoma begins in the upper quadrants and is always more extensive there.

Regardless of the mode of onset, the disease progresses over a period of months or years through Stage II, in which the hypertrophy is predominantly follicular (Fig. 30–2), to cicatricial trachoma (Stage III) (Fig. 30–3), whose features include lid deformity and corneal opacification. In severe Stage III trachoma there may also be loss of tear function and resultant cornification of the conjunctival and corneal epithelium. Healed trachoma (Stage IV) is characterized by a smooth, cicatrized conjunctiva and a scarred

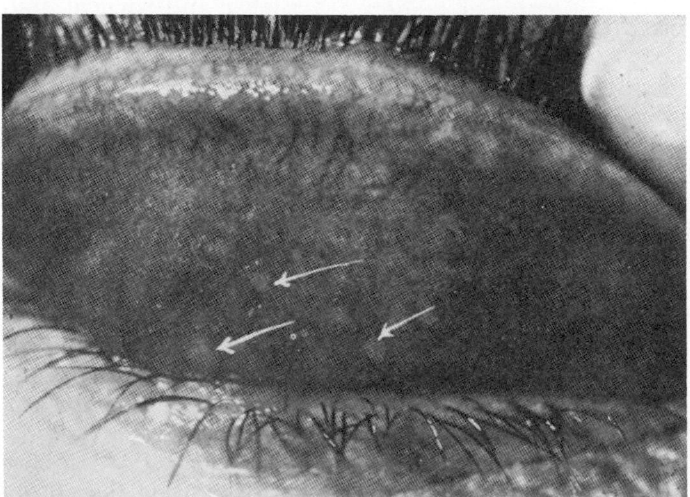

Figure 30–2. Trachoma: follicular hypertrophy. (Courtesy of Dr. Phillips Thygeson.)

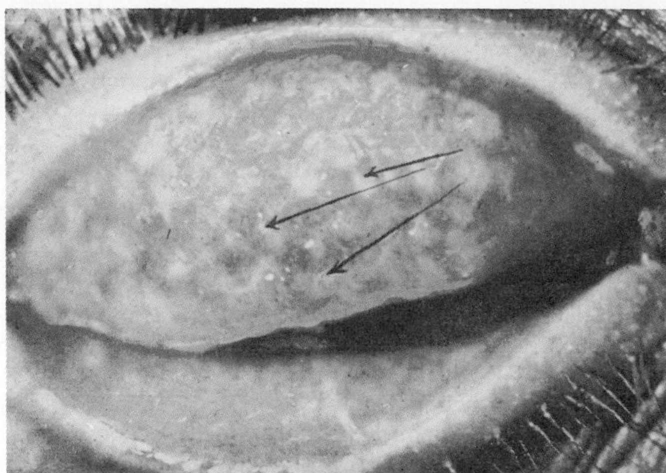

Figure 30-3. Trachoma: late scarring and deformity of lid. (Courtesy of Dr. Phillips Thygeson.)

but uninfiltrated cornea. Mild cases may be symptom-free, but the complications of trichiasis and secondary infection usually produce persistent irritation.

Diagnosis. Trachoma is usually diagnosed on the basis of clinical data alone, but the finding of cytoplasmic inclusion bodies in scrapings, or of the characteristic microscopic changes (cell necrosis, macrophages) in expressed follicular material, may be useful in early and atypical cases. A clinical diagnosis of trachoma may be made when follicular hypertrophy or scars involving predominantly the conjunctiva of the upper tarsus and fornix occur in association with the characteristically patterned pannus. With the aid of the biomicroscope these diagnostic changes can be recognized early in the disease.

The rare cases of acute trachoma at onset, seen sporadically in adults, must be differentiated from the various types of acute follicular conjunctivitis, especially inclusion conjunctivitis and epidemic keratoconjunctivitis (adenovirus type 8). For this purpose examination of the cornea is often helpful; inclusion conjunctivitis does not produce gross pannus, and the keratitis in epidemic keratoconjunctivitis is characterized (after 8 to 10 days) by coin-shaped subepithelial opacities without pannus formation. Laboratory methods of differentiation (cultivation and indirect immunofluorescence) are available but rarely needed.[5]

Chronic trachoma is readily differentiable from chronic follicular conjunctivitis (Axenfeld type) on clinical grounds: in the Axenfeld disease there is never any keratitis, and healing without scars occurs in 1 or 2 years. Severe cicatricial trachoma is occasionally confused with ocular pemphigoid and with the other types of severe cicatrizing conjunctivitis that follow erythema multiforme, membranous conjunctivitis due to *Corynebacterium diphtheriae,* and hemolytic streptococcic infection. However, trachoma can be easily differentiated from these conditions if the history of the infection is taken into account and a careful examination made; trachoma scars and trachoma pannus are distinctive.

Treatment. Prior to the introduction of the sulfonamides and broad spectrum antibiotics, the treatment of trachoma was highly unsatisfactory. Cures were obtained only rarely. The usual method consisted of cauterization of the conjunctiva with chemical agents such as copper sulfate ("blue stone"), combined with mechanical expression of the follicles. Sulfonamides and antibiotics supplanted cauterizing and surgical procedures and are effective in a high percentage of cases. Sulfonamide or antibiotic resistance is rarely encountered.

Although sulfonamide therapy is effective,[6] it has fallen into disfavor because erythema multiforme, associated with cicatrizing conjunctivitis (Stevens-Johnson syndrome), has been an occasional complication. As a result, the tetracyclines or erythromycin, given systemically, are now preferred. Topical therapy with the sulfonamides, tetracyclines, or erythromycin is effective only if the drugs (in ointment form) are used frequently enough (4 times a day or more) to maintain a constant concentration over the entire treatment period. Sustained release methods (e.g. with "ocusert") are under study, but for the present the recommended treatment is a 3-week course of orally administered tetracycline or erythromycin (or of a sulfonamide for young children and pregnant women) in the doses considered optimal for systemic infections. Severe cases of trachoma respond promptly to this regimen. Mild cases sometimes require retreatment, however, and if tarsal follicles or active keratitis are still in evidence 2 months after the treatment period, a second course is given.

Prevention. There is no specific prophylaxis, and vaccination research has been peculiarly disappointing. In endemic areas the control of the acute bacterial ophthalmias, particularly Koch-Weeks *(Haemophilus aegyptius)* conjunctivitis, reduces both primary infections and reinfections with the trachoma agent. Control of these bacterial ophthalmias can be accomplished by the use of 1 per cent tetracycline or erythromycin ointment twice daily during the fall and spring epidemics.

Trachoma is a disease that tends to disappear from a population as socioeconomic conditions improve. It is essentially a disease of the family, and the worst trachoma is found in poor families with low levels of personal hygiene and no running water in their houses. Malnutrition may contribute to the severity of individual cases by reducing the victim's defense mechanisms.

Inclusion Conjunctivitis

Definition. Inclusion conjunctivitis is an acute purulent conjunctivitis of the newborn and a follicular conjunctivitis of the adult that never progresses to corneal involvement or scarring.

Distribution. The disease has a worldwide distribution.

Etiology. The agent causing inclusion conjunctivitis is now classified as *Chlamydia trachomatis* (Busacca) Rake 1957. Its usual habitat is the human genital tract, and venereal transmission occurs.[7]

Epidemiology. Inclusion conjunctivitis is fundamentally an infection of the adult human genital tract. In the female the organism grows in transitional epithelium of the cervix. These cells contain typical inclusions, and occasionally a mild cervicitis is present. In the male a mild urethritis may result from genital infection. The organism enters the eye of the baby during passage through the birth canal, and after an incubation period of 3 to 15 days (usually about 1 week) produces acute purulent conjunctivitis. Occasionally, adults may be infected by eye-to-eye transfer of infectious agents from the newborn, but adult eyes are infected most commonly by contact with genital secretions, occasionally in contaminated swimming pools. The disease of the adult eye is an acute follicular conjunctivitis with epithelial keratitis and subepithelial opacities. The frequency with which inclusion conjunctivitis is diagnosed depends on the index of suspicion and on the intensity of the search for typical inclusions in conjunctival scrapings.

Clinical Characteristics. Most commonly inclusion conjunctivitis is observed as an acute, purulent conjunctivitis of the newborn. The onset is usually between the fifth and the fourteenth days of life, in contrast to gonococcal ophthalmia which generally begins on the second day of life. After 1 or 2 weeks of intense inflammation of the conjunctiva (particularly of the lower lids), purulent exudate and occasional pseudomembrane formation, the disease gradually subsides and the conjunctiva becomes normal within a few weeks to a year. Pannus or scarring never develops in infants, in marked contrast to trachoma, and the infection tends to be self-limited. In the adult, inclusion conjunctivitis is an acute follicular conjunctivitis with little discharge and some preauricular adenopathy. Follicular hypertrophy is most noticeable in the conjunctiva of the lower lid and tends to persist for weeks or months, occasionally accompanied by epithelial keratitis and subepithelial infiltrates. Adult inclusion conjunctivitis tends to resolve completely even without treatment, but the occasional production of pannus has been claimed. Adult cervicitis and urethritis are often asymptomatic or produce slight discharge and discomfort.

Diagnosis. The diagnosis of inclusion conjunctivitis rests on finding typical inclusions in purulent conjunctivitis of the newborn or in follicular conjunctivitis of the adult without scarring. In the differential diagnosis, bacterial and chemical conjunctivitis in the newborn must be considered, and in adults the types of follicular conjunctivitis. Early trachoma can be differentiated in the adult only with difficulty by the absence in inclusion conjunctivitis of cellular necrosis in lymphoid follicles and of pannus by biomicroscopic examination.

The causative agent may be isolated by inoculation of conjunctival scrapings into chick embryo yolk sac, provided that the patient has not already received antibiotics. The specimen should be treated with streptomycin, neomycin or polymyxin B to destroy contaminating bacteria. Using cell-cultured organisms, several immunologic types may be distinguished by the methods of (1) protection of immunized mice from toxic death following challenge by the organisms, and (2) indirect micro-immunofluorescence.[8] Indirect immunofluorescence testing is more specific and sensitive for the serum antibodies, which appear to be confined primarily to immunoglobulin G, than is the group-reactive complement-fixation test; but in both tests titers increase in untreated cases and reach a peak 4 to 6 weeks after infection occurred.

Treatment. Topical administration of tetracycline 4 times a day for 2 to 3 weeks usually controls the infection. Even without specific therapy the disease is self-limited. However, the best result is obtained by the use systemically of sulfonamides for at least 7 days—in adults, for example, sulfadiazine being given in doses of 2 to 4 gm daily. Systemic use of tetracyclines is also effective.

Prophylaxis. Inclusion conjunctivitis in the adult is most commonly contracted in water contaminated with genital secretions. Proper chlorination of the water probably prevents transmission. Because there is no simple method available for the detection of the infection in the pregnant woman, infection of the newborn cannot be readily prevented. Silver nitrate or penicillin instillation soon after birth does not prevent inclusion conjunctivitis. A newborn baby with the disease should be isolated to prevent spread of the organism, although in fact nursery cross-infection is very uncommon.

Lymphogranuloma Venereum

Synonyms. Climatic bubo, tropical bubo, Durand-Nicolas-Favre disease, lymphogranuloma inguinale.

Definition. Lymphogranuloma venereum is a specific infectious venereal disease characterized by transient, often unnoticed, primary lesions followed by superficial and deep lymphadenitis with eventual suppuration and fistula formation. The pelvic colon and rectovaginal septum are frequently involved in the female, producing proctitis, stricture of the rectum and rectovaginal fistula.

Distribution. The disease is widespread throughout the world, in both tropical and temperate regions. The infection is particularly prevalent among prostitutes and other sexually promiscuous individuals. In some areas it is an important public health problem.

Etiology. The lymphogranuloma venereum agents,[9] now classified as *Chlamydia trachomatis* (Busacca) Rake 1957, may be recovered from the primary genital lesions, affected lymph nodes, inflamed tissue of the rectum, inflammatory lesions of the colon and cerebrospinal fluid of patients with meningoencephalitis. Isolates from different cases have shown a wide variety of properties when tested for inclusion type, sulfonamide sensitivity and mouse virulence, ranging from typical LGV characteristics to those of the TRIC and even the psittacosis agents.[10] Large elementary bodies may be demonstrated within the leukocytes in Giemsa-, Macchiavello- or Castaneda-stained smears of pus from inguinal buboes.

The agent may be propagated by intracerebral inoculation in mice and upon the chorioallantoic membrane or in the yolk sac of the developing chick embryo, from which rich suspensions may be obtained. These are suitable for preparation of antigen for the Frei skin test and for the complement-fixation reaction.

Epidemiology. Although the disease is transmitted principally by sexual contact, accidental laboratory infections indicate that it may be acquired by other routes and without apparent localization or tissue reaction at the portal of entry. Cases have been reported in which invasion occurred apparently through the mucous membrane of the upper respiratory tract and through the skin of the hands. It is evident from surveys that mild, unrecognized infections are not infrequent. The disease is found particularly among lower social classes. The age incidence is that of greatest sexual activity. Sex differences are not pronounced and all races are affected.

Pathology. The pathologic changes of lymphogranuloma venereum vary with the duration and the severity of the infection. The primary lesion, which is seldom seen, is a transitory small papule, vesicle, or ulcer. From this site invasion of the lymphatics occurs. Different routes are followed in the two sexes with resultant differences in the pathologic process and the clinical phenomena. In the male the inguinal nodes are involved, with further extension to the deep iliac nodes. In the female, invasion of the inguinal nodes is uncommon; the usual pathologic findings are a pelvic lymphadenitis affecting the rectovaginal septum and producing inflammatory lesions of the rectum and rectosigmoid region.

Accompanying the acute adenitis in either sex there is inflammation of surrounding tissue, with matting of the lymph nodes, necrosis and stellate abscesses (which cannot be histologically differentiated from tularemia), and the development of chronic fistulas that may drain for a considerable time. Healing is accompanied by extensive scar tissue formation, which may lead to elephantiasis of the genitalia and rectal stricture. The microscopic picture of the involved lymph nodes and adjacent tissues is that of a subacute or chronic infectious granuloma. In the rare instances in which the upper respiratory tract has apparently been the portal of entry, there has been involvement of the cervical lymph nodes.

Clinical Characteristics. The incubation period frequently lasts only a few days. The primary lesion may or may not be noticed and usually consists of a small painless papule, vesicle or ulcer, often disappearing within a week or 10 days, situated on the penis in the male and commonly on the vaginal wall or cervix in the female.

The secondary stage of the disease is characterized by the appearance of lymphadenitis. It begins insidiously and runs a chronic indolent course in the male. Enlargement of the inguinal nodes of one or both sides is often the presenting symptom. At first they are discrete, later becoming considerably enlarged, matted, adherent to the skin and finally fluctuant. The overlying skin becomes discolored, and ultimately sinus formation occurs with the discharge of a seropurulent exudate, which may continue for weeks or months. In the female there are often no localizing symptoms prior to invasion of the rectum and the appearance of blood and pus in the stools. This stage may be accompanied by constitutional symptoms, such as malaise, anorexia, headache and fever. In the rare instances in which infection occurs through the respiratory tract, there may be acute disease with chills, sweating, septic fever and articular rheumatism. Severe meningoencephalitis has been reported in a few patients. It can occur in individuals who exhibit minimal or negligible evidence of this infection on the genitalia or lymph nodes. Untreated, it may last for many weeks.

The third stage of the disease is most striking in the female. It is characterized by chronic proctitis and, occasionally, by the development of rectovaginal fistula, fistulous tracts about the rectum, and perirectal abscess. The extensive fibrosis often leads to marked rectal stricture. In both sexes the disorganization of the lymphatic structures may lead to elephantiasis of the genitalia.

Diagnosis. In the differential diagnosis the inguinal bubo of lymphogranuloma venereum must be distinguished particularly from that of mild ambulant plague (pestis minor), from syphilis, from pyogenic lesions of the lower extremities, and from chancroidal infection. In plague the affected lymph nodes are much more painful and tender, and stained smears of material aspirated from them will reveal *Yersinia pestis.* In the adenitis of syphilis the lymph nodes are discrete, not matted or adherent, and the primary lesion or scar is usually demonstrable. The bubo occurring in the course of a chancroidal infection should seldom cause confusion because of the extensive ulceration usually accompanying it. The rectal and colonic lesions may be confused with fistulas due to other causes, perirectal abscess and chronic infections of the rectum and colon of other types.

Meningoencephalitis due to the agent of lymphogranuloma venereum must be differentiated especially from tuberculous or influenzal meningitis. In the early stages of central nervous system infection there is a lowered sugar content in the cerebrospinal fluid. Unusually high values for protein (250 to 3570 mg per 100 ml) are characteristic. Pleocytosis may be as high as 4000 leukocytes per cu mm, with as many as 75 per cent polymorphonuclear cells, during the early stages, and it may persist at lower levels, with a predominance of mononuclear leukocytes, for many months after clinical improvement.

The complement-fixation test is most useful for diagnosis, especially when a 4-fold or greater rise in titer can be demonstrated by two successive tests early in the disease. A rise may not be demonstrable when the first test is performed more than a month after onset. A titer of 1:32 or more in patients exhibiting clinical manifestations compatible with lymphogranuloma venereum may be accepted as confirmatory of the diagnosis, except in the presence of early syphilis.

The Frei test, performed with yolk sac antigen, is more specific than formerly and may be positive 7 to 10 days after onset of adenitis. However, a positive Frei test may not be noted for 5 to 6 weeks. The complement-fixation test may become positive before the Frei test, and is more reliable.

Treatment. Like other infections of the PLT group, this disease responds to antimicrobial therapy. Both rapidity of cure and ultimate prognosis are determined by the stage of the disease in which treatment is initiated. Good results may be expected in early cases. Later, in the presence of extensive damage with fistula formation and fibrosis, repeated courses of treatment may be required. Enlarged fluctuant lymph nodes should be aspirated but not incised. Rectal stenosis and rectovaginal fistula may require surgical intervention.

Although the tetracyclines and chloramphenicol are effective during early infection, they do not necessarily eradicate the organism and some therapeutic failures occur. Therapeutic response to sulfonamides tends to be superior to that to the antibiotics, but also may be incomplete. Treatment with either group of drugs must be continued for 3 to 6 weeks in early cases and for several months in patients suffering from chronic disease. The recommended dose of tetracycline compounds is 500 mg 4 times a day at first, later reduced to 250 mg 4 times daily.

Sulfamerazine, sulfadiazine and sulfisoxazole (sulfafurazole) are the sulfonamides of choice. The dose is 3 or 4 gm daily for 3 to 6 weeks; if further treatment is needed, the dose should be decreased to 2 gm daily. Sufficient fluid must be given to maintain a urinary output of 1500 ml per day to avoid precipitation of sulfonamide within the kidney. Inadequate treatment may give rise to resistant strains. Although a combination of tetracycline and sulfonamide therapy may be optimal, in some cases in which these drugs have failed a combination of penicillin and ampicillin has produced regression of the disease.

The antimonials are not recommended. It is probable that the value ascribed to these preparations in the past has been due to confusion of diagnosis with granuloma inguinale or chancroid, or to an effect on secondary bacterial infection.

Bartonellosis

Aristides Herrer

Synonyms. Verruga peruana, Oroya fever, Carrión's disease.

Definition. Bartonellosis is a specific infection caused by *Bartonella bacilliformis,* presenting two clinical types of disease. The severe form, Oroya fever, is characterized by fever, a rapidly developing macrocytic anemia, and frequently intercurrent infection with high mortality. The benign form, verruga peruana, is characterized by a verrucous eruption of hemangioma-like nodules and by a negligible mortality (Fig. 30–4).[11]

Distribution. The disease is restricted to the western portion of South America between latitudes 2° North and 13° South, occurring especially in Peru, Ecuador and Colombia. Its distribution is further restricted to narrow river valleys and canyons at altitudes between 800 and 3000 meters above sea level. It has been reported from both sides of the Andes.

Etiology. *Bartonella bacilliformis* Strong, Tyzzer and Sellards, 1915 is a minute gram-negative, rod-shaped or rounded organism found in varying numbers within both the red blood cells and cells of the reticuloendothelial system, especially those of the lymph nodes, spleen, liver, and kidney. *Bartonella bacilliformis* may be classified among bacteria.

In stained preparations of blood, both rod-shaped and rounded forms are seen. The rods are often slightly curved, occurring singly or end-to-end in pairs or in chains. Frequently, they lie parallel or are arranged in V's or Y's. The rod forms when stained by Giemsa's method commonly show a deep red or purplish granule at one end suggestive of chromatin, the remainder taking a bluish stain (Fig. 30–5).

They may be cultivated best in semisolid nutrient agar containing 10 per cent rabbit serum and 0.5 per cent rabbit hemoglobin. Proteose peptone produces high-intensity growth.[12]

Epidemiology. The disease is endemic in certain arid river valleys of the Andes region and is coextensive with the distribution of the sandflies *Lutzomyia verrucarum* and *Lutzomyia noguchii* in Peru. However, the latter does not bite humans and only rarely enters houses. At the present time only *L. verrucarum* has been incriminated as a vector. Other species are reported from the endemic areas in Colombia. The disease is especially prevalent at the close of the rainy season when these flies are most numerous.

Proboscis infections with *Bartonella* have been found in wild-caught female *Lutzomyia.* The source of these infections is unknown since there is no known reservoir host.

The disease is often mild among people of endemic areas, and latent infections without significant symptoms are observed in adults. Immunity is believed to follow both Oroya fever and verruga peruana.

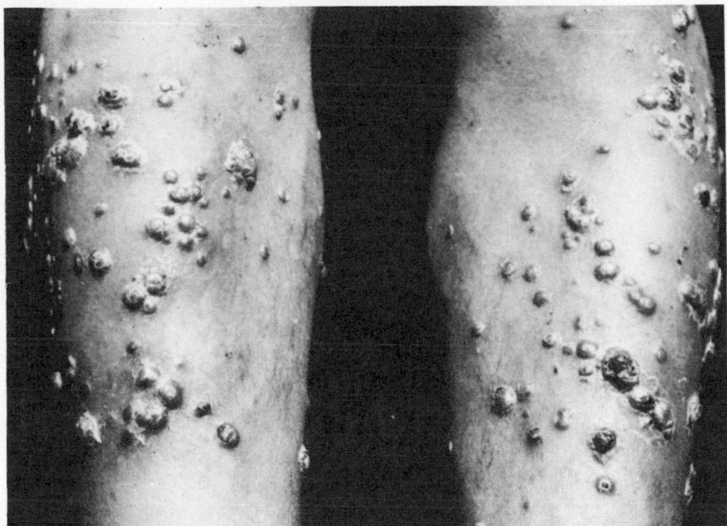

Figure 30–4. Miliary hemangiomatous lesions of verruga peruana. (Courtesy of Dr. Olga Palacios.)

Pathology. In the severe form of the disease the lymph nodes and the spleen are enlarged, the latter containing melanin-like pigment and sometimes showing areas of infarction. The liver is likewise increased in size, contains pigment, and may present areas of degeneration. On microscopic examination the reticuloendothelial cells of the lymphatic system and of the viscera are seen to be packed with organisms. The bone marrow is megaloblastic and hyperplastic. Patients who survive show hemangioma-like nodules.

The benign form, verruga peruana, is characterized by hemangiomatous nodules in the skin and subcutaneous tissue. The early lesion consists of newly formed blood vessels within edematous connective tissue. There are marked proliferation of the endothelial lining and pronounced capillary dilatation. Late lesions may resemble fibrosarcomas. The causative organisms are often

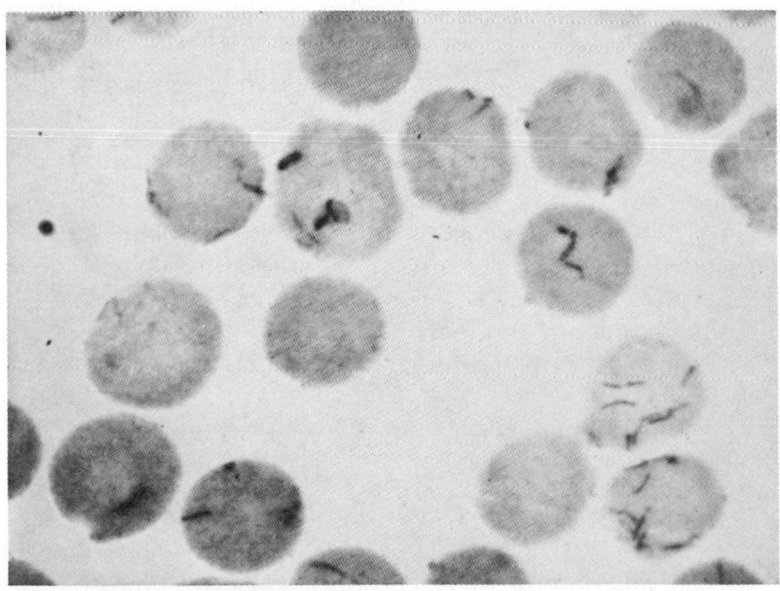

Figure 30–5. *Bartonella bacilliformis* in stained blood film.

demonstrable in the endothelial cells, although they are usually much less numerous than in acute Oroya fever.[13]

Clinical Characteristics. Bartonellosis presents four stages: incubation, invasion, the pre-eruptive and the eruptive. An incubation period of from 19 to 30 days, rarely up to 100 days, precedes the gradual onset of Oroya fever.

OROYA FEVER. The early symptoms are frequently vague and indefinite. In the invasive period, fever is usually moderate and is accompanied by the characteristic progressive anemia and slight jaundice. Although the organisms are commonly not demonstrable microscopically early in the course, they can be recovered by blood culture. Subsequently, great numbers of the bacillary forms appear in the erythrocytes.

The anemia progresses with great rapidity. Within 2 weeks the hemoglobin may fall to 20 or 30 per cent and the erythrocyte count to 1 or 2 million. There is marked evidence of new blood formation with reticulocytosis, at times up to 50 per cent. The erythrocytes are macrocytic, frequently hypochromic, and normoblasts and megaloblasts may be numerous. The mechanical fragility of the red corpuscles is increased in the majority of cases. No agglutinins or hemolysins have been demonstrated.[14] Leukocytosis is variable, apparently depending upon the presence or absence of intercurrent infection.

The "critical stage" is characterized by the apparent beginning of convalescence. The *Bartonella* change from bacillary to coccoid forms, the parasitized red cells become less numerous, and there are fewer organisms within the cells. Macrocytosis diminishes, the erythrocyte and reticulocyte counts rise; lymphocytosis and reappearance of monocytes and eosinophils occur, and there is a shift of the polymorphonuclear series to the right.

Intercurrent infections accompanied by high fever, diarrhea, splenomegaly and marked leukocytosis are prone to occur at this time. They are associated with mortality rates well above 50 per cent. It is thought that *Bartonella* anemia predisposes to fatal septic invasion by organisms from the gastrointestinal tract. In the presence of *Salmonella* and *Entamoeba histolytica* infections and of pulmonary tuberculosis, the prognosis is very grave. Deaths likewise occur from complicating thrombocytopenic purpura.

VERRUGA PERUANA. This is the benign form of bartonellosis. It usually runs a course of 2 to 3 months and is characterized by miliary and nodular hemangiomatous lesions which have a definite tendency to hemorrhage and occasionally to ulcerate; in the absence of intercurrent infection it is almost never fatal.

The incubation period is thought to be 30 to 60 days. The onset is usually accompanied by joint pains and fever seldom exceeding 37.8° C (100° F). The fever commonly subsides shortly after the onset of the eruptive stage.

The miliary type of eruption is more common and is most abundant on the face and the extensor surfaces of the extremities, appearing first as pink macules, later becoming bright red, nodular and bleeding easily (Fig. 30–4). The mucous membranes of the eye, nose and throat may be involved. The eruption disappears without scar formation.

The nodular subcutaneous lesions develop slowly and may reach 1 to 2 cm in diameter. Not infrequently they break down, producing an ulcerating and fungating process which may be a source of danger from hemorrhage. They do not occur in the mucous membranes and are commonly confined to the regions of the appendicular joints. They tend to appear in successive crops. Scarring varies with the extent of tissue destruction.

Diagnosis. The strictly limited geographic distribution and the distinctive clinical features of the infection almost eliminate any diagnostic difficulties. Definitive diagnosis depends upon the demonstration of *Bartonella* in Giemsa-stained blood films or on culture (Fig. 30–5).

Treatment. Patients with acute bartonellosis show dramatic clinical response when treated with penicillin, streptomycin, chloramphenicol or the tetracyclines. Fever disappears in 4 to 8 hours or less, and the organisms diminish markedly. Even though satisfactory clinical response is obtained, the patient may continue to have positive blood cultures and develop verrugas, but death will not result from the disease. Presumably the antibiotics control the acute infection and allow low-grade infection and the development of a protective immunity. The choice of an antimicrobial drug should depend on the presence of secondary bacterial infection. The high incidence of salmonella septicemia in patients with bartonellosis has led to the use of chloramphenicol as an adjunct to treatment of this disease (p. 179). Transfusions of whole blood are recommended for symptomatic relief of the acute anemia.

After the development of cutaneous lesions the response to antibiotic therapy is minimal. Excision of the large, necrotic, secondarily infected nodules may be indicated.

Prophylaxis. The prophylaxis of bartonellosis consists of control of or protection against *Lutzomyia*.[15] Residual spraying of buildings and adjacent potential breeding areas with 5 per cent DDT in kerosene gives excellent results that persist for several months. Temporary individual protection may be obtained by the use of insect repellents (p. 800).

REFERENCES

1. Page, L. A. 1968. Proposal for the recognition of two species in the genus *Chlamydia* Jones, Rake, and Stearns, 1945. Int. J. Systemat. Bacteriol. *18*:51–66.
2. Storz, J. 1971. Chlamydia and Chlamydia-Induced Diseases. Charles C Thomas, Springfield, Illinois. 358 pp.
3. Kuo, C. C., Wang, S. P., and Grayston, J. T. 1972. Differentiation of TRIC and LGV organisms based on enhancement of infectivity by DEAE-dextran in cell culture. J. Infect. Dis. *125*:313–317.
4. Darougar, S., Kinnison, J. R., and Jones, B. R. 1971. Simplified irradiated McCoy cell culture for isolation of *Chlamydiae. In* Nichols, R. L. (ed.): Trachoma and Related Disorders Caused by Chlamydial Agents. Excerpta Medica. Amsterdam. pp. 63–70.
5. Schachter, J., Mordhorst, C. H., Moore, B. W., and Tarizzo, M. L. 1973. Laboratory diagnosis of trachoma: a collaborative study. Bull. W.H.O. *48*:509–515.
6. Bietti, G. B., and Werner, G. H. 1967. Trachoma: Prevention and Treatment. Charles C Thomas, Springfield, Illinois. 227 pp.
7. Schachter, J., Rose, L., and Meyer, K. F. 1967. The venereal nature of inclusion conjunctivitis. Am. J. Epidemiol. *85*:445–452.
8. Wang, S. P., Kuo, C. C., and Grayston, J. T. 1973. A simplified method for immunological typing of trachoma-inclusion conjunctivitis-lymphogranuloma venereum organisms. Infect. Immun. 7:356–360.
9. Meyer, K. F. 1965. Lymphogranuloma venereum agents. *In* Horsfall, F. L., and Tamm, I.: Viral and Rickettsial Infections of Man. 4th ed. J. B. Lippincott Co., Philadelphia. pp. 1024–1041.
10. Schachter, J., and Meyer, K. F. 1969. Lymphogranuloma venereum. II. Characterization of some recently isolated strains. J. Bacteriol. *99*:636–638.
11. Hennemann, H. H. 1963. Oroya-fieber (carriónsche Krankheit): eine akute erworbene hämolytische Anämie. Deut. Med. Wschr. *88*:1759–1767.
12. Méndez Mondragón, M. 1974. Verruga peruana. Evaluación de nutrientes de la *Bartonella bacilliformis* en gel. Rev. Lat. Am. Microbiol. *16*:1–7.
13. Urteaga-Ballon, O. 1967. Verruga peruana o enfermedad de Carrión. Arch. peruanos Patol. Clin. *21*:107–136.
14. Reynafarje, C., and Ramos, J. 1961. The hemolytic anemia of human bartonellosis. Blood *17*:562–578.
15. Reynafarje, C. 1972. Enfermedad de Carrión. Acta Méd. peruana *1*:139–144.

SECTION V
Mycotic and Actinomycotic Diseases

JOHN W. RIPPON

CHAPTER 31
Introduction

The superficial and systemic mycoses form a group of diseases that result from infection of skin or viscera by pathogenic fungi (Table 31–1). The ability of these fungi to cause disease, however, is an accidental phenomenon. With the exception of a few dermatophytes, pathogenicity among the molds is not necessary for the maintenance or dissemination of the species. The dermatophytes are a closely related group of keratinophilic soil fungi. A few of these species have evolved into a constant association with man and animals so that a soil reservoir for them probably no longer exists. They depend on man to man or fomite to man transmission for survival. These species remain "specialized saprophytes," however, as they do not invade living tissue but utilize only the dead cornified structures of skin, hair, claws and nails.

The systemic infecting fungi are all soil saprophytes with the unique ability to adapt to the internal environment of the host and cause disease. This is a blind alley as far as the fungus is concerned; when the infected host expires, the infecting agent dies with it as these are not contagious diseases. The ability to adapt to existence in host tissue varies among the fungi. Those that adapt readily are the so-called pathogenic fungi that cause systemic disease, e.g. *Coccidioides* and *Histoplasma.* They are dimorphic in that they grow as spore-producing mycelial elements in soil but convert to spherules or budding yeasts during parasitic existence. This morphogenesis is controlled by temperature, carbon dioxide tension or other factors. Infection is acquired by inhalation of spores.

Most of the agents of the subcutaneous mycoses show some ability to adapt to a parasitic existence. The clinical entities known as chromomycosis and mycetoma are caused by a diverse group of soil organisms. Following entrance into the host, usually as a result of traumatic implantation, these organisms go through what may be termed a tissue-induced dimorphism to form grains, granules or sclerotic bodies. These infections are usually very long and chronic and develop very slowly.

Another category of fungous diseases is caused by the so-called "opportunistic fungi." These organisms are not able to infect the normal host but cause disease only in the debilitated patient. The debilitations include diseases such as diabetes and neoplasias or are iatrogenically produced by the presence of steroids, antibiotics or cytotoxins. The organisms involved do not show an adaptive dimorphism to parasitic existence; if they are mycelial in the soil, they are mycelial in tissue.

Other differences exist between the etiologic agents of the several groups of mycoses. The dimorphic pathogenic fungi are usually geographically restricted to a particular environment. Infection with these fungi is common among the endemic population but clinical disease is rare; the infection usually results in granuloma formation (Table 31–2). The agents of the subcuta-

Table 31–1. Clinical Types of Fungous Infections*

Type	*Disease*	*Causative Organism*
Superficial infections	Pityriasis versicolor	*Pityrosporum orbiculare (Malassezia furfur)*
	Piedra	*Trichosporon cutaneum* (white) *Piedraia hortai* (black)
Cutaneous infections	Ringworm of scalp, glabrous skin, nails	Dermatophytes (*Microsporum, Trichophyton, Epidermophyton* spp.)
	Candidosis of skin, mucous membranes and nails	*Candida albicans* and related species
Subcutaneous infections	Chromomycosis	*Fonsecaea pedrosoi* and related forms
	Mycotic mycetoma	*Allescheria boydii, Madurella mycetomii* and others
	Subcutaneous phycomycosis	*Basidiobolus haptosporus* *Entomophthora coronata*
	Rhinosporidiosis	*Rhinosporidium seeberii*
	Lobomycosis	*Loboa loboi*
	Sporotrichosis	*Sporothrix schenckii*
Systemic infections	Dimorphic pathogenic fungous infections	
	Histoplasmosis	*Histoplasma capsulatum*
	Blastomycosis	*Blastomyces dermatitidis*
	Paracoccidioidomycosis	*Paracoccidioides brasiliensis*
	Coccidioidomycosis	*Coccidioides immitis*
	Opportunistic fungous infections	
	Cryptococcosis	*Cryptococcus neoformans*
	Aspergillosis	*Aspergillus fumigatus* and others
	Mucormycosis	*Mucor* sp., *Absidia* sp., *Rhizopus* sp.
	Candidosis, systemic	*Candida albicans* *Candida tropicalis*

*Modified from J. W. Rippon. 1973. *In* Burrows, W.: Textbook of Microbiology. 20th ed. W. B. Saunders Co., Philadelphia. p. 683.

neous mycoses are often restricted geographically but some are of worldwide distribution; the tissue reaction is usually a mixed pyogenic and granulomatous response. The opportunistic fungi are of worldwide distribution; their occurrence in a disease process depends upon a susceptible debilitated host. The tissue reaction in such infections reflects the immune status of the patient, varying from little or no response to a pyogenic or granulomatous reaction. The dermatophytes do not invade living tissue. The pathology that is induced in the skin is the result of toxic products produced by the fungi and allergy to them. The tissue reaction seen in dermatophytosis is a nonspecific toxic or allergic dermatitis or both.

Also included in this section are diseases caused by actinomycetes. By tradition these infections were grouped with the mycoses because they were long chronic diseases, and the etiologic agents involved were thought to be a "link" between fungi and bacteria. The actinomycetes, like bacteria, are prokaryotic, contain muramic acid in their cell wall and are susceptible to antibacterial antibiotics. The fungi are eukaryotic, have true chromosomes and nuclei, follow Mendelian

Table 31–2. Tissue Reactions in Fungous Diseases*†

Disease Responses and Histologic Picture	*Fungous Diseases and Agents*
Chronic inflammation Lymphocytes, plasma cells, neutrophils, and fibroblasts; occasionally giant cells	*Rhinosporidium seeberii* Entomophthoromycosis
Pyogenic reaction Acute or chronic, suppurative neutrophilic infiltrate (see also at right)	*Actinomyces israelii:* sulfur granules, also lipid-laden peripheral histiocytes *Nocardia asteroides* Acute aspergillosis Acute candidosis
Mixed pyogenic and granulomatous reaction Neutrophilic infiltration and granulomatous reaction, lymphocytes, plasma cells (see also at right)	*Blastomyces dermatitidis* *Paracoccidioides brasiliensis* *Coccidioides immitis:* neutrophils, especially at broken spherule *Sporothrix schenckii:* organism rarely seen in tissue Chromomycosis: chronic pyogenic and inflammatory reaction, epithelioid cell nodules and giant cells Mycetoma: in addition may be large foamy giant cells similar to xanthoma
Pseudoepitheliomatous hyperplasia Following chronic inflammation in the skin, hyperplasia of epidermal cells, hyperkeratosis, extension of rete pegs	*Blastomyces dermatitidis* *Paracoccidioides brasiliensis* Chromomycosis *Coccidioides immitis*
Histiocytic granuloma Histiocytes frequently with intracellular organisms, sometimes becoming multinucleate giant cells	*Histoplasma capsulatum* Meningeal *Cryptococcus neoformans*
Granuloma with caseation Granulomatous reaction, Langhans' giant cells (LGC), central necrosis	*Histoplasma capsulatum* *Coccidioides immitis* Sometimes pulmonary blastomycosis Rarely pulmonary cryptococcosis
Granuloma "sarcoid" type Nonnecrotizing	*Cryptococcus neoformans* Occasionally *Histoplasma capsulatum*
Fibrocaseous pulmonary granuloma; "tuberculoma" (see also at right)	*Histoplasma capsulatum:* thick fibrous wall surrounding epithelioid and LGC organisms in soft center, often calcification *Coccidioides immitis:* thin fibrous wall, occasionally calcified *Cryptococcus neoformans:* poorly defined but occasionally encapsulated, fibrosed and calcified
Thrombotic arteritis Thrombosis, purulent coagulative necrosis, invasion of vessel	Aspergillosis Mucormycosis
Fibrosis Proliferating fibroblasts, deposition of collagen—resembles keloid	*Loboa loboi* (lobomycosis)
Sclerosing foreign body granuloma In paranasal sinuses or following viral infection (see also at right)	*Aspergillus* spp.: bizarre hyphae in giant cells

*From J. W. Rippon. 1973. *In* Burrows, W.: Textbook of Microbiology. 20th ed. W. B. Saunders Co., Philadelphia. p. 685.

†A Gram stain is used for actinomycosis, nocardiosis, actinomycotic mycetoma, and candidosis; otherwise a periodic acid–Schiff stain is recommended.

laws of inheritance, contain chitin in their cell walls and are not susceptible to antibacterial antibiotics. There remains at least one good reason for including the pathogenic actinomycetes in a study of medical mycology: the clinical entity mycetoma may be caused by several soil-inhabiting actinomycetes or true fungi. The treatment of the disease depends on the category of the etiologic agent.

The true fungi are divided into several classes depending on type of sexual reproduction: Zygomycetes, Ascomycetes, Basidiomycetes and Deuteromycetes (Fungi Imperfecti). This latter group is composed of fungi whose sexual stage is as yet unknown. The dermatophytes and some of the agents of the systemic mycoses *(Histoplasma, Blastomyces)* are Ascomycetes. Most of the others are retained in the Fungi Imperfecti. Often the imperfect stage was known before a sexual stage was discovered. For this reason some species have two names: one describing their imperfect stage and one their sexual, e.g. *Trichophyton mentagrophytes* (imperfect), *Arthroderma benhamii* (sexual).

Sources of additional information are given in the chapter references.[1-3]

REFERENCES

Textbooks of Medical Mycology

1. Rippon, J. W. 1974. Medical Mycology: The Pathogenic Fungi and the Pathogenic Actinomycetes. W. B. Saunders Co., Philadelphia. 587 pp.
2. Conant, N. F., Smith, D. T., Baker, P. D., and Callaway, J. L. 1971. Manual of Clinical Mycology. W. B. Saunders Co., Philadelphia. 755 pp.
3. Emmons, C. W., Binford, C. H., and Utz, J. P. 1970. Medical Mycology. Lea & Febiger, Philadelphia. 508 pp.

CHAPTER 32

Actinomycotic Diseases

This is a group of diseases caused by various Actinomycetes. By tradition some actinomycotic infections, such as tuberculosis and leprosy, were studied with other bacterial diseases, whereas nocardiosis and actinomycosis were more "mycotic" diseases. They are all caused by gram-positive, nonmotile bacilli that may branch to form mycelial-like threads 1 μm in diameter. *Nocardia asteroides* and *Nocardia brasiliensis* are, like the tubercle bacillus, acid-fast. *Actinomyces* are anaerobic; *Nocardia, Actinomadura* and *Streptomyces* are aerobic (Table 32–1).

Actinomycosis

Synonyms. Lumpy jaw, leptothricosis, streptothricosis.

Definition. A chronic, suppurating, granulomatous infection characterized by multiple abscesses and fistula formation; characteristic granules of the bacteria are present in the drainage from these lesions; infection is produced by *Actinomyces israelii* and related species.

Distribution. The causative organism is an obligate parasite of man. It is found in the absence of disease on the mucous membranes of the mouth, around carious teeth and in tonsillar crypts, and probably also in the large intestine. Because of this association, the disease has a worldwide distribution.

Etiology. Actinomycosis in man is caused by *Actinomyces israelii* and rarely by *Actinomyces naeslundii, Arachnia propionica,* and *Bifidobacterium eriksonii.* In animals (cattle) it is caused by *Actinomyces bovis.* They are all fastidious anaerobic organisms that are difficult to grow. In tissues, sputum or pus, *A. israelii* is visible to the naked eye as the characteristic "sulfur granule" composed of a mass of tangled, branching, mycelial threads, which at the periphery of the granule may show radially arranged, club-shaped swellings, giving rise to the term "ray fungus" (Fig. 32–1).

Pathology. The fundamental lesion is a granulomatous process in which the colonies of the bacteria (granules) are surrounded by mononuclear cells, with occasional giant cells, and numerous polymorphonuclear leukocytes in the areas of necrosis. There are marked new connective tissue formation and fibrosis producing hard tumor-like masses or indurations. In these are multiple abscesses interconnected by sinus tracts, often with multiple external fistula formations, which discharge sanguinopurulent material containing the granules. Extension of the infection is by continuity, rarely by the blood stream or lymphatics.

Clinical Characteristics. The clinical types of actinomycosis fall into three general groups:

	Up to 1950 per cent of cases	***1950–67 per cent of cases***
Cervicofacial	50	24
Abdominal	20–30	13
Pulmonary	15	63

In the *cervicofacial type* the portal of entry appears to be the mucous membrane of the mouth or pharynx following an injury, especially tooth extraction. Marked induration is produced, and direct extension may lead to involvement of the bones of the skull, or of the skin with the formation of multiple fistulous tracts. Pain is not marked, and there may be little or no systemic reaction.

The *abdominal* or *intestinal type* usually originates in the region of the appendix and cecum, with the formation of a gradually

Table 32–1. THE PATHOGENIC ACTINOMYCETES AND THEIR DISEASES*

Disease	*Organism*	*Geographic Distribution*
Actinomycosis	*Actinomyces israelii* (man) *Actinomyces bovis* (cattle) *Bifidobacterium eriksonii* *Actinomyces naeslundii* *Arachnia propionica*	Ubiquitous
Nocardiosis (pulmonary and systemic)	*Nocardia asteroides* *Nocardia brasiliensis*	Ubiquitous Mexico, South America, Africa, India
Mycetoma (actinomycotic)	*Actinomadura madurae* *Streptomyces somaliensis* *Actinomadura pelletierii*	Ubiquitous Africa, Brazil, Mexico Africa, South America, Mexico
Erythrasma	*Corynebacterium minutissimum*	Ubiquitous
Cracked heel	*Nocardia keratolytica* (?)	India, United States, Southeast Asia
Trichomycosis axillaris	*Corynebacterium tenuis*	Ubiquitous
Epidemic eczema	*Dermatophilus congolensis*	Australia, Africa, United States

*From J. W. Rippon. 1973. *In* Burrows, W.: Textbook of Microbiology. 20th ed. W. B. Saunders Co., Philadelphia. p. 687.

enlarging mass in the right lower quadrant, followed by internal and external sinus formation. Extension occurs to adjacent structures, often with involvement of the liver and spleen and, subsequently, the lung. Abdominal actinomycosis may be accompanied by toxemia, fever, chills and other evidence of an intra-abdominal inflammatory process.

The *pulmonary type* may be primary, or secondary to a cervicofacial lesion with ex-

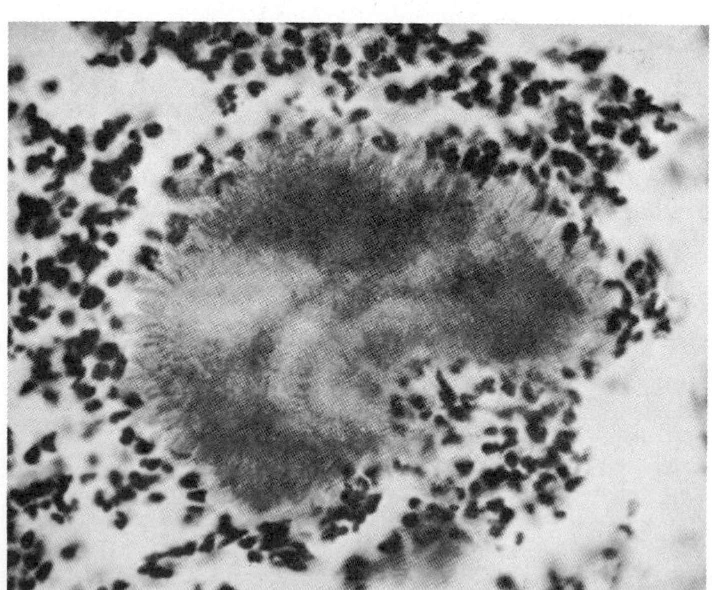

Figure 32–1. Actinomycosis. Sulfur granule in pus from sinus tract.

tension through the mediastinum. It is characterized by cough, sputum, hemoptysis, fever, dyspnea and night sweats. Invasion of the pleura is accompanied by pain, and empyema is not unusual. This is frequently followed by invasion of the chest wall with the development of areas of induration, abscess formation and multiple external sinuses (Fig. 32–2). Involvement of the mediastinum may be followed by invasion of the esophagus or pericardium. *Actinomyces* species are particularly notorious for invading bony structures. Involvement of the ribs and vertebrae is quite common. Bone involvement is rare in nocardiosis, which may have some presenting features similar to actinomycosis.

Diagnosis. The combination of the clinical picture and the demonstration of characteristic sulfur granules in the tissues, or in pus, is characteristic. Microscopic examination of a granule crushed beneath a coverglass, revealing the characteristic structure and the presence of branching mycelial threads, permits specific diagnosis of infection by a member of the family ACTINOMYCETACEAE. The material should be cultured on suitable media under both anaerobic and aerobic conditions.

Treatment. Penicillin, Aureomycin and chloramphenicol (Chloromycetin) have been used successfully. Penicillin, however, is the drug of choice. Associated organisms may necessitate concurrent treatment with sulfonamides or streptomycin or both.[1] In patients who are allergic to penicillin, lincomycin can be used.[2] Very high doses of penicillin (10 to 20 million units per day) may be necessary and treatment, especially of abdominal disease, may continue for 16 to 18 months.

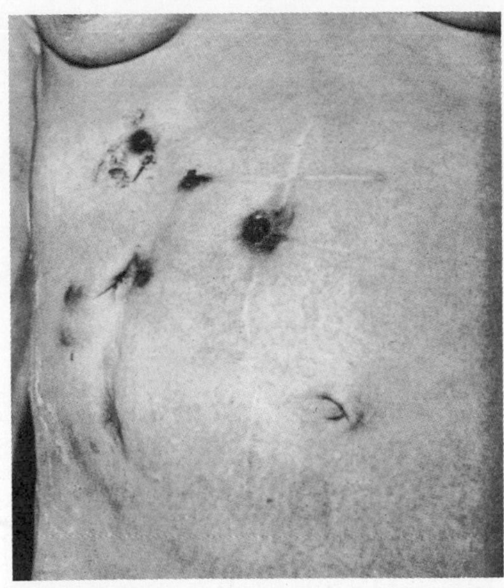

Figure 32–2. Actinomycosis of chest wall with draining sinuses. Ribs involved and sinus tracts extending through abdominal wall. (Courtesy of Dr. D. T. Smith.)

Nocardiosis

Synonym. Systemic nocardiosis.

Definition. A primary pulmonary infection which may later become systemic with a particular predilection for the brain.[1,3] The protean symptoms may resemble tuberculosis, bacterial pneumonia, meningitis or brain abscess.

Distribution. Nocardiosis caused by the ubiquitous *Nocardia asteroides* is usually an opportunistic infection and thus may occur in almost any geographic area. The highly virulent *Nocardia brasiliensis* produces disease in agricultural workers in Mexico, Central America and South America. A few cases have been caused by *N. caviae.*[4]

Etiology. Infection with *N. asteroides* is particularly associated with use of steroids and cytotoxins (Table 32–1). The highly virulent *N. brasiliensis* causes chronic pulmonary disease. Sinuous-branching, gram-positive, partially acid-fast filaments are seen in sputum, spinal fluid and tissues. Granules such as those found in actinomycosis are rarely seen. *Nocardia brasiliensis* and very rarely *N. asteroides* are also agents of actinomycotic mycetoma.

Pathology. The primary pulmonary disease resembles tuberculosis in any stage of its pathology. A mixed pyogenic and granulomatous response is present. Systemic no-

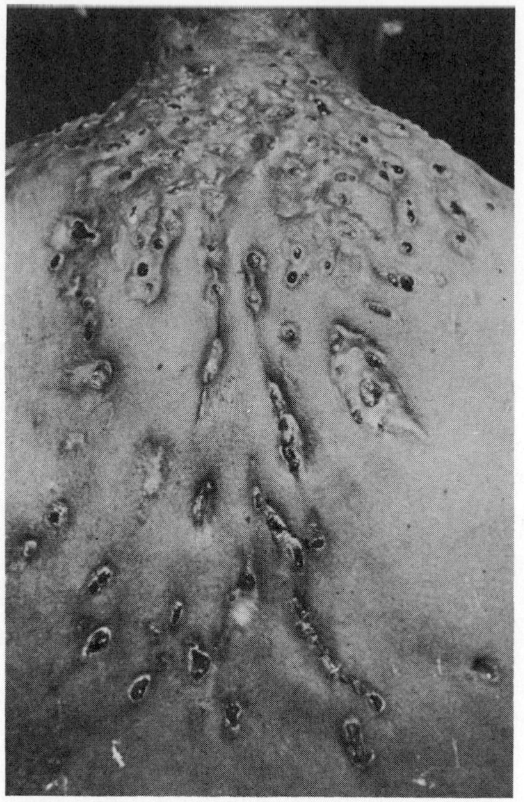

Figure 32–3. Nocardiosis. Multiple perforations of a chest infection by *Nocardia brasiliensis.* (Courtesy of Dr. R. Mayorga, Universidad de San Carlos, Guatemala.)

cardiosis is the result of hematogenous spread from a primary pulmonary infection, resulting in generalized pyemia with abscesses and granulomatous lesions found in many organs. The organism occurs as sinuous, beaded, branched, hyphal elements and is seen in materials stained by Gram's method or methenamine silver.

Clinical Characteristics. Systemic infection follows a primary pulmonary disease which may simulate tuberculosis or a malignant neoplasm. Hematogenous spread resulting in abscess formation in many organs, including the brain, causes protean symptoms, which make a differential diagnosis difficult.[1] In pulmonary nocardiosis caused by *N. brasiliensis,* sinus tracts with granules may perforate the chest wall (Fig. 32–3).

Diagnosis. Observation of delicately branched, gram-positive, partially acid-fast filaments 1 μm in diameter with little tendency to form granules seen in sputum, spinal fluid or fistula exudate constitutes a presumptive diagnosis of nocardiosis. *Nocardia asteroides* and *N. brasiliensis* are aerobic and nonfastidious, and grow on almost all laboratory media not containing antibiotics. The colonies consist of coccoid bodies and branching filaments and are variable in color (white to orange to cream or rarely pink or brown).

Treatment. The sulfonamides offer specific therapy for both the localized and systemic infections caused by *Nocardia.* Treatment with sulfadiazine alone, or in combination with sulfamerazine to obtain higher serum concentrations, has proved effective. The drugs should be administered in such quantity as to obtain blood levels of 10 to 20 mg per 100 ml; therapy should be continued for 3 to 4 months following an apparent cure.[5] Sulfamethoxazole at a dosage of 2.5 gm per day with 480 mg per day of trimethoprim has also been used successfully.[6]

Mycetoma

Synonyms. Madura foot, maduromycosis.

Definition. Mycetoma is a clinical syndrome of localized, indolent, deforming swollen lesions and sinuses involving cutaneous or subcutaneous tissues, fascia and bone.[7, 8] The foot or the hand may be involved. The lesions are composed of suppurating abscesses, granulomas and draining sinuses containing grains or microcolonies of the etiologic agents. The clinical disease is the result of traumatic implantation of soil actinomycetes (actinomycotic mycetoma) or fungi (mycotic mycetoma).

Distribution. Mycetoma is encountered through the tropical and subtropical regions of the earth. Each geographic area may have a predominant agent as *Madurella mycetomii* in the trans-Africa belt (from Senegal and Mauritania to the Sudan and So-

Table 32-2. MYCOTIC MYCETOMA (TISSUE DIMORPHIC FUNGI)*

Species	Grain	Histology (H and E)	Colonial and Microscopic Characteristics	Physiologic Profile†						
				ST	GEL	G	GAL	L	M	S
Allescheria boydii	White, soft, oval to lobed, < 2 mm	Hyaline hyphae. 5 μm; huge swollen cells, < 20 μm; no cement; red border; pink periphery	Rapid growth (30–37° C; 86–98.6° F); fluffy mouse-fur gray. Large 7 μm unicellular aleuriospore conidia on simple conidiophore; black cleistothecia	+	+	+		0	0	
Madurella grisea	Black, soft to firm, oval to lobed, < 1 mm	Little dark cement in edge; polygonal cells in periphery; center hyaline mycelium	Very slow growth (30° C; 86° F); leathery tan-gray, later downy. Diffusible pigment	+	−	+	+	0	+	+
Madurella mycetomii	Black, firm to brittle, oval to lobed, < 2 mm	Compact type with brown-staining cement; vesicular type with brown cement only at edge; swollen cells, < 15 μm; center hyaline mycelium	Very slow growth (37°C; 98.6°F); downy, velvety, smooth or ridged; cream apricot to ochre. Diffusible brown pigment; black sclerotia, < 2 mm; rare conidia, phialids	+	±	+	+	+	+	0
Acremonium kiliense	White, soft, irregular, < 1.5 mm	No cement; hyaline hyphae > 4 μm; swollen cells, > 12 μm	White glabrous colony (30° C; 86° F); later downy. Violet pigment diffusible; curved septate; conidia arranged as head on simple conidiophore	0	±					
Phialophora jeanselmei	Black, soft, irregular to vermicular	Helicoid to serpiginous; center often hollow; no cement; vesicular cells, < 10 μm; brown hyphae	Slow growth (30° C; 86° F); leathery black moist, later velvety. Reverse black; toruloid yeast cells, moniliform cells, long tubular phialids	0	0	+	+	0	+	+
Leptosphoeria senegalensis	Black, soft, irregular, ~ 1 mm	Black hyphae; cement in periphery; center hyaline	Rapid growth; downy gray. Reverse black–rare rose pigment diffusible; black perithecia, < 300 μm; septate ascospores, 25 × 10 μm							

*From J. W. Rippon. 1973. *In* Burrows, W.: Textbook of Microbiology. 20th ed. W. B. Saunders Co., Philadelphia. p. 696.
†Abbreviations: St = starch; Gel = gelatin; G = glucose; Gal = galactose; L = lactose; M = maltose; S = sucrose.

Table 32–3. ACTINOMYCOTIC MYCETOMA*

Species	Grain	Histology (H and E)	Colonial and Microscopic Characteristics	Physiologic Profile†						
				C	T	X	ST	GEL	U	AX
Nocardia asteroides	Rare; white, soft, irregular, 1 mm	Homogeneous loose clumps of filaments; rare clubs	Rapid growth (37° C; 98.6° F); glabrous, folded, heaped; orange-yellow, tan, or other. Short rods and cocci; rare branched filaments; acid-fast	–	–	–	–‡	–	+	–
Nocardia brasiliensis	White to yellow, soft, lobed, 1 mm	Same as above; clubs common	Rapid growth (30° C; 86° F); colonial and microscopic same as above; acid-fast	+	+	–	–‡	+	+	–
Nocardia caviae	Same as above	Same as above	Same as above; acid-fast	–	–	+	–‡	–	+	–
Actinomadura madurae	White, rarely pink, soft, oval to lobed, large, 5 mm	Center empty, amorphous; dense mantle peripherally; basophilic wide pink border; loose fringe; clubs	Rapid growth (37° C; 98.6° F); cream white, rarely clot red; wrinkled, glabrous. Delicate nonfragmenting branched filaments; arthrospores; non-acid-fast	+	+	–	+	+	–	+
Actinomadura pelletierii	Red, hard, oval to lobed, small, 1 mm	Round homogeneous dark staining; light peripheral band; hard – fractures easily; no clubs	Slow growth (37° C; 98.6° F); small, dry, glabrous; light to garnet red. Delicate nonfragmenting branched filaments; non-acid-fast	+	+	–	–‡	+	–	–
Streptomyces somaliensis	Yellow, hard, round to oval, large, 2 mm	Variable size; amorphous center; light purple with pink patches; dark filaments at edge, entire; no clubs	Slow growth (30° C; 86° F); cream to brown; wrinkled, glabrous. Delicate nonfragmenting branched filaments; arthrospores; non-acid-fast	+	+	–	±	+	–	–

Actinomyces israelii is also a cause of light-grained mycetoma

*From J. W. Rippon. 1973. *In* Burrows, W.: Textbook of Microbiology. 20th ed. W. B. Saunders Co., Philadelphia. p. 695.
†Abbreviations: C = casein; T = tyrosine; X = xanthine; St = starch (amylolytic); Gel = gelatin (proteolytic); U = urea; AX = acid from arabinose and xylose.
‡Some strains are positive.

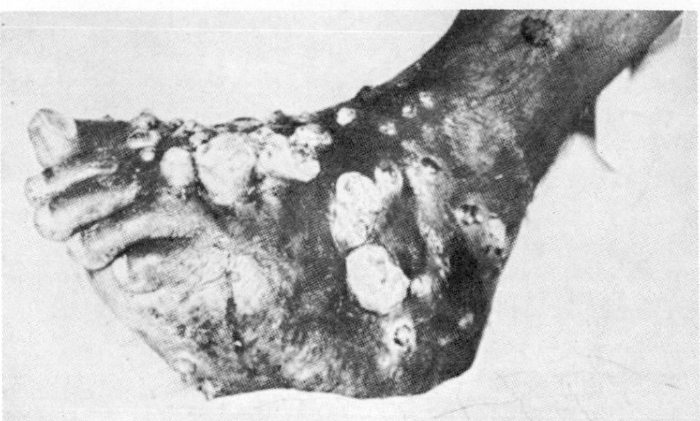

Figure 32–4. Mycetoma.

mali coast); *Nocardia brasiliensis* in Mexico and Central America; *Actinomadura madurae* in India and Southwest Asia; and *Allescheria boydii* in the United States and other temperate areas.

Etiology. The clinical entity of mycetoma is caused by a variety of soil bacteria (actinomycetes) and fungi (Tables 32–2 and 32–3).

Pathology. There is extensive invasion by the fungus or actinomycete. The early lesion is granulomatous in character, with the granules or colonies in edematous granulation tissue infiltrated with mononuclear cells and polymorphonuclear leukocytes. As the lesion progresses it is surrounded by a dense fibrous capsule and often intersected by fibrous trabeculae. There are extensive necrosis of tissue and thrombosis of vessels. In advanced cases the foot becomes a mass of cystlike areas with intercommunicating sinus tracts and multiple externally draining sinuses. In these instances there is complete destruction of muscles, bones and tendons. Bone involvement is more common in actinomycotic than mycotic mycetoma.

Clinical Characteristics. The initial lesion usually appears on the sole of the foot as a superficial or deep cutaneous nodule. The overlying skin becomes discolored and

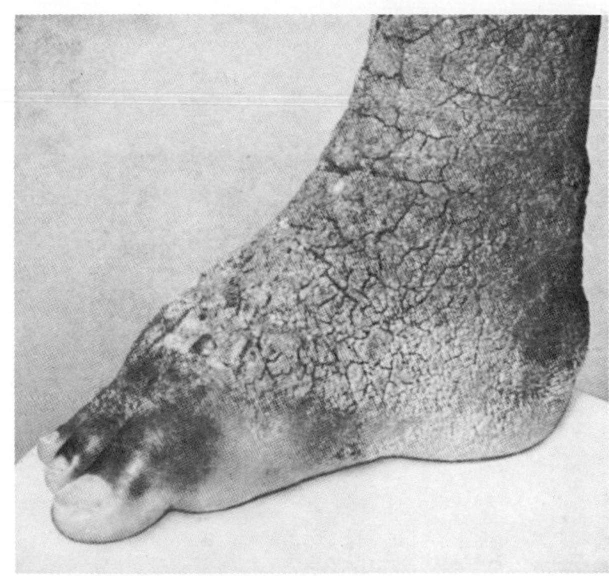

Figure 32–5. Mossy foot: a superficial verrucous dermatitis of varied bacterial etiology. (Courtesy of Dr. Alan Fisher for the Office of the Coordinator of Inter-American Affairs.)

breaks down, and a persistent sinus tract develops. In other instances the process may begin as a deep abscess, ultimately opening externally. As extension occurs, the foot becomes enlarged, presenting a convex sole and swollen dorsum. Nodules appear in uninvolved areas of the skin, breaking down to form new sinuses (Fig. 32–4). Ultimately, the foot may be enlarged to three or four times the normal size. There is little or no systemic reaction and in uncomplicated cases little or no lymphangitis or lymphadenitis.

Diagnosis. The triad of tumefaction, draining sinuses and grains defines the clinical entity mycetoma. The etiologic agents of mycetoma may also cause other clinical diseases as actinomycosis, nocardiosis, chromomycosis or mycotic granuloma. It must be differentiated from mossy foot (Fig. 32–5), chromomycosis and sporotrichosis.

Treatment. Early diagnosis may allow successful treatment by surgical intervention. Actinomycotic mycetoma has been treated with penicillin, streptomycin and especially with the sulfas. Sulfadiazine has largely been replaced by long-acting sulfas, such as sulfadimethoxine and sulfamethoxypyridazine in dosages of 0.1 to 0.5 gm per day for 6 months or more. Eumycotic mycetoma has been consistently resistant to treatment. Amphotericin B has been tried but without much success. Since the treatment and prognosis are so different, it is important to recognize whether the patient has actinomycotic or mycotic mycetoma.

REFERENCES

Actinomycosis

1. Peabody, J. W., and Seabury, J. H. 1960. Actinomycosis and nocardiosis: a review of basic differences in therapy. Am. J. Med. *28*:99–115.
2. Mohr, J., Rhoades, E. R., and Muchmore, H. G. 1970. Actinomycosis treated with lincomycin. J.A.M.A. *212*:2260–2261.

Nocardiosis

3. Kurup, P. V., Randhawa, H. S., and Gupta, N. P. 1970. Nocardiosis: a review. Mycopathologia *40*:194–219.
4. Causey, W. A. 1974. *Nocardia caviae*: a report of 13 new isolations with clinical correlation. Appl. Microbiol. *28*:193–198.
5. Aron, R., and Gordon, W. 1972. Pulmonary nocardiosis. Case report and evaluation of current therapy. S. Afr. Med. J. *46*:29–32.
6. Evans, R. A., and Benson, R. E. 1971. Complicated nocardiosis treated with trimethoprim and sulfamethoxazole. Med. J. Austral. *58*:684–685.

Mycetoma

7. Zaias, N., Taplin, D., and Rebell, G. 1969. Mycetoma. Arch. Dermatol. *99*:215–225.
8. Feiger, J. W. 1963. Mycetoma: review of the literature. Mil. Med. *128*:762–765.

CHAPTER 33

Cutaneous Mycoses

The dermatomycoses are superficial infections of the skin or its appendages caused principally by members of three closely related genera of the Fungi Imperfecti: *Trichophyton* (sexual stage *Arthroderma*), *Microsporum* (sexual stage *Nanizzia*) and *Epidermophyton*.[1] They do not usually invade the deeper tissues of the internal organs. Members of the genus *Trichophyton* attack the hair, the skin and the nails. The fungus may be confined to the cortex of the hair, appearing as chains of spores arranged in parallel rows (endothrix), or it may be on the surface of the hair in chains of small (microspore type) or large (macrospore type) spores (ectothrix). In the skin and the nails these fungi present segmented, branching, mycelial elements, with or without chains of spores, and are indistinguishable from *Microsporum* and *Epidermophyton*.

The genus *Microsporum* attacks the hair and the skin. Infected hairs from the scalp commonly present a characteristic appearance produced by a sheath of small spores surrounding the shaft of the hair and tending to be in a mosaic arrangement rather than in parallel rows as in *Trichophyton* infections. In the skin, species of *Microsporum* form segmented mycelial elements which are identical in appearance with those of *Trichophyton* and *Epidermophyton*.

The genus *Epidermophyton* attacks the skin and nails, forming segmented, branching mycelial elements which are indistinguishable from those of *Microsporum* and *Trichophyton* (Table 33–1).

Diagnosis of Dermatomycoses. A diagnosis of dermatomycosis may be made by direct microscopic examination in potassium hydroxide of an infected hair or of scrapings from the margins of lesions of the skin or nails. Infection of the hair by a few species of the genus *Microsporum* can be detected by a Wood's lamp, which causes the hair to fluoresce. Although a clue to the particular genus may be obtained by such examination in the case of *Trichophyton* or *Microsporum* infections of the hair, definitive diagnosis can be made only by study of the growth characteristics of the fungi in artificial culture media. Since the morphology of all three genera in infected skin and nails is identical, differentiation and species identification must be based entirely upon the cultural characteristics, both macroscopic and microscopic.

Microscopic Examination. For the microscopic examination of scrapings from the skin or nails,[2] or of fragments of hair, the material should be placed in a drop of 10 to 40 per cent potassium hydroxide on a clean microscope slide, covered with a coverglass and heated gently. If clearing is not adequate, additional potassium hydroxide may be run under the coverglass and the preparation reheated. Following such treatment the mycelia and spores are easily distinguished.

Cultures. Similar material should be used for culture. Hair or scrapings should be placed between two slides previously wrapped in paper and sterilized. After rewrapping, the material may be transported to the laboratory for immediate inoculation on Sabouraud's glucose agar to which antibiotics have been added. Such a medium will inhibit bacterial growth. Cycloheximide may also be added (0.5 mg per ml) to the above medium to inhibit saprophytic fungus growth. All cultures should be maintained at room temperature for 2 to 3 weeks. Differentiation of the genera and identification of the species are based upon the gross and microscopic characteristics of the colonies and their elements.

Table 33-1. The Common Dermatophytes and the Diseases That They May Cause*

			Species	Disease in Man	Geographic Distribution
Invading the hair and hair follicles	Small spore varieties		*Microsporum audouinii*†	Prepubertal ringworm of the scalp; suppuration rare	Commonest in Europe, producing about 90 per cent of infections; in the United States, 50 per cent
			Microsporum canis†	Prepubertal ringworm of scalp and glabrous skin; suppuration not infrequent; kerion occasional; from pets	Uncommon in Europe; responsible for about half the infections in the United States
			Microsporum gypseum	Ringworm of the scalp and glabrous skin; suppuration and kerion common; from soil	Relatively rare in the United States; common in South America
			Microsporum fulvum	Ringworm similar to *M. gypseum*	Same as above
			Microsporum ferrugineum†	Similar to *M. audouinii*	Africa, India, China, Japan
	Large spore varieties	Endothrix type	*Trichophyton tonsurans*	Blackdot ringworm of the scalp and smooth skin; sycosis; tinea unguium; suppuration common; the hair follicles are atrophied	Common in Europe, Russia, Near East, Mexico, Puerto Rico and South America, but uncommon in the United States until recently
			Trichophyton violaceum	Blackdot endothrix in both scalp and smooth skin; onychomycosis; suppuration is the rule and kerion frequent	Common in south Europe, the Balkans and the Far East; rare in the United States
			Trichophyton soudanense } *Trichophyton gourvilii* }	Inflammatory scarring; ringworm of scalp	Central and West Africa

		Species	Clinical features	Distribution
		Trichophyton yaoundeii		
	Ectothrix type	*Trichophyton mentagrophytes*	Commonest cause of intertriginous dermatophytosis of the foot ("athlete's foot"); ringworm of the smooth skin, suppurative folliculitis in scalp and beard	Ubiquitous; common in animals
	Ectothrix type	*Trichophyton verrucosum*	Ringworm of the scalp and smooth skin, suppurative folliculitis in scalp and beard; from cattle	Ubiquitous; especially rural, associated with cows
	Ectothrix type	*Trichophyton megninii*	Sycosis is the most common lesion; infection of smooth skin and nails	Sporadic distribution, Portugal, Sardinia
No spores in hair		*Trichophyton schoenleinii*†	Favus in both scalp and smooth skin; scutulum and kerion	Europe, Near East, Mediterranean region; rare in the United States
Not invading the hair and hair follicles		*Epidermophyton floccosum*	Cause of classic eczema marginatum of crural region; causes minority of cases of intertriginous dermatophytosis of foot; not known to infect hair and hair follicles	Ubiquitous, but more common in tropics
Not invading the hair and hair follicles		*Trichophyton rubrum*	Psoriasis-like lesions of smooth skin; tinea unguium, mild suppurative folliculitis in beard; rare invasion of scalp hair; endo- and ectothrix described	Ubiquitous
Not invading the hair and hair follicles		*Trichophyton concentricum*	Commonest cause of tinea imbricata; infection of hair and nails uncertain	Common in South Pacific islands, Far East, India, Ceylon; restricted areas in Central America and South America

*Modified from J. W. Rippon. 1973. *In* Burrows, W.: Textbook of Microbiology. 20th ed. W. B. Saunders Co., Philadelphia. p. 706.

†Infected hairs show fluorescence by Wood's lamp.

Tinea capitis

Synonyms. Tinea tonsurans; herpes tonsurans; ringworm of the scalp.

Definition. A fungal infection of the stratum corneum of the scalp and the hair, most common in children, characterized by scaling, occasionally by dermatitis, and by breaking of infected hairs; it usually disappears spontaneously at puberty or may extend into adult life, dependent upon the fungus responsible for the infection.

Distribution. This infection is widespread, without geographic limitations, and may occur epidemically in schools and among crowded populations in an unsanitary environment.

Etiology. Tinea capitis is produced by several species of *Microsporum* and *Trichophyton.* Of special interest is the recent publication of new species of *Trichophyton* causing scalp infection in several countries of Africa *(T. yaoundeii, T. soudanense, T. gourvilii).*

Pathology. The fungus first invades the stratum corneum of the scalp, producing a minute, rounded, scaling patch or a reddish papule from which a hair projects. Subsequently there is invasion of the hair follicle and then of the deeper or superficial portions of the shaft of the hair. More severe reactions lead to kerion formation and an edematous pustular infection of the scalp.

Clinical Characteristics. The infected hairs become lusterless and brittle and finally break, leaving short stubs projecting from the lesion. Temporary or permanent alopecia may result (Fig. 33–1). The more severe infection or kerion is a painful, weeping, pustular infection with crusting.

Diagnosis. Microscopic examination of a potassium hydroxide preparation of scrapings from the scalp or of the hair is done initially to detect the presence of fungi. Cultures should be made and the etiologic agent specifically identified.

Treatment. Treatment was difficult and often unsatisfactory until griseofulvin was shown to be an antifungal antibiotic. Griseofulvin is an orally administered compound that has been found to be a specific drug for the treatment of infections caused by the dermatophytes *Trichophyton, Microsporum* and *Epidermophyton.* The dose is 500 mg per day (micronized) for adults and 250 mg per day for children in four divided doses after a fatty meal. Treatment may require several months. Tolnaftate (Tinactin) and haloprogin (Halotex) are without benefit in tinea capitis. If secondary bacterial infection is present, warm saline compresses should be used as well as a specific antibiotic chosen after cultural sensitivity studies.

Tinea favosa

Synonym. Favus.

Definition. A fungal infection of the scalp, of the nonhairy skin of the body or of the nails commonly seen in children. It may extend into adult life; it is characterized by the formation of yellowish crusts overlying shallow ulcers called scutula.

Distribution. Classic favus is common in China and central Asia. It is not uncommon in North Africa, the Balkan region, central Europe, Iran, Greenland, the Middle East, and among the Bantu of South Africa (Witkop). The disease is rare in other areas. As is the case with tinea capitis, it may occur epidemically.

Etiology. This condition is usually caused by *Trichophyton schoenleinii* (Fig. 33–2) and rarely by *Trichophyton violaceum* and *Microsporum gypseum.*

Clinical Characteristics. The initial lesions appear as minute, whitish, scaly patches; subsequently sulfur-colored crusts are produced, piling up to form an elevated mass with raised edges. These crusts are very adherent. Removal reveals a superficial ulcer oozing serum or blood-tinged exudate. This infection may cause permanent alopecia.

Diagnosis. This may be obtained by microscopic examination of a potassium hydroxide preparation of scrapings from the early lesions and identification of the fungus by culture.

Treatment. The methods advised for tinea capitis should be used. Griseofulvin has been shown to have excellent curative effects.

Tinea barbae

Synonyms. Tinea sycosis; barber's itch; ringworm of beard.

Definition. A fungal infection of the bearded area and neck of men, involving the skin, hair and hair follicles, usually resulting in a chronic, deep suppurative lesion.

Distribution. This infection is widespread, without geographic limitations, but may occur in small epidemics as a result of contact with infected cattle.

Etiology. *Trichophyton mentagrophytes* and *Trichophyton verrucosum* are the most common etiologic agents. The latter is difficult to isolate on media. *Trichophyton megninii* is an uncommon agent found in Portugal, Sardinia and Africa.

Pathology. Superficial infection of the skin produces scaling circular lesions with a vesiculopustular border. Deep infection of the skin produces suppurative lesions with follicular pustules, kerion formation and extensive abscess formation.

Clinical Characteristics. The superficial lesions resemble those of tinea corporis of the glabrous skin (Fig. 33–9). Progressive infection may lead to a suppurative folliculitis, forming large nodular crusted lesions which extrude pus on slight pressure. The infected hairs are brittle and easily removed; few are seen in older lesions.

Diagnosis. Microscopic examination of potassium hydroxide preparations of skin and hair should reveal fungous elements. Cultures of such material are necessary to determine the etiologic agent of a given case.

Treatment. Treatment of chronic suppurative lesions is difficult. Compresses twice daily for ½ hour, with Burow's solution (1:15), Vleminckx's solution (1:33) or hypertonic saline solution may be helpful. Antibiotics or sulfonamides or both should be used to control secondary bacterial infections, and the antifungal antibiotic griseofulvin should be used for specific treatment.

Tinea pedis and Dermatophytids

Synonyms. Trichophytosis, epidermophytosis, ringworm of hands and feet, Hong Kong foot, athlete's foot.

Definition. Tinea pedis is a chronic, superficial infection of the skin, especially of that between the toes, with maceration and cracking, occasionally extending to involve adjacent skin areas.[3] Less commonly it may affect the hands, groin, axillae and other regions. It is accompanied by intense itching.

Distribution. The infection is widespread and may be particularly troublesome in the moist tropics and subtropics.

Etiology. It is usually due to a species of *Trichophyton,* or less commonly *Epidermophyton floccosum* or *Candida albicans.*

Epidemiology. This infection is extremely common and widespread. The fungi are resistant and persist indefinitely in shoes and other contaminated leather objects. They may be transmitted by towels and clothing unless these are sterilized. They frequently contaminate the floors of baths and washrooms. The infection is acquired directly from contact with an infected individual or indirectly from contaminated floors and articles of clothing. A hot, humid climate and wet feet are predisposing factors.

Pathology. The infection is limited to the cornified layer of the skin, producing acute, chronic and hyperkeratotic lesions. The acute stage is accompanied by erythema, scaling and cracking of the affected

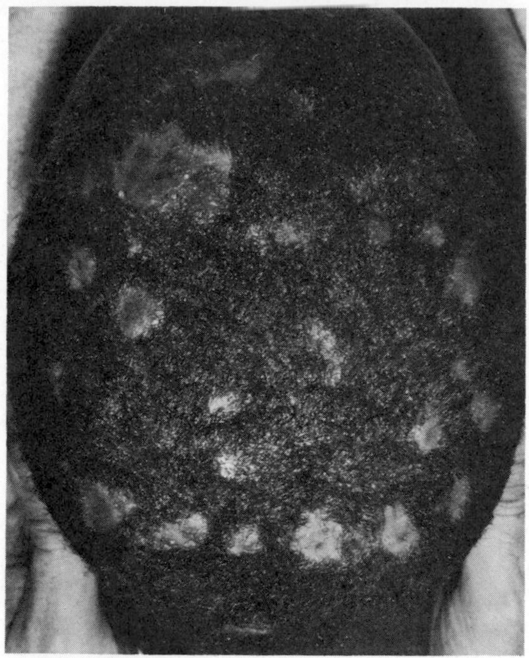

Figure 33–1. Tinea capitis, a triple infection caused by *T. tonsurans, M. audouinii* and *C. albicans.* Note the severe inflammation and areas of alopecia. (From J. W. Rippon. 1974. Medical Mycology. W. B. Saunders Co., Philadelphia. p. 113.)

skin. Secondary infection is common. Invasion of the nails (onychomycosis) is frequent.

Remote skin sensitization may occur and be accompanied by eruptions, dermatophytids, on various parts of the body (Figs. 33–3, 33–4). These do not contain the fungi and subside with control of the active focus.

Clinical Characteristics. The interdigital areas, especially between the third and fourth and fourth and fifth toes, are the usual sites of infection. The lesion may consist of simple erythema with scaling. Fissuring between the toes is common, and the process may be complicated by secondary bacterial infection. In chronic infections the skin is thickened, white and macerated. Not infrequently, deep shotty vesicles appear on the soles of the feet and the palms of the hands. These are accompanied by pruritus and contain clear mucoid material. In severe cases eczematoid lesions may occur involving the foot, ankle, groin, axilla, hand and other areas. These may present an acute inflammatory process with edema and cellulitis due to secondary bacterial invasion (Figs. 33–5, 33–6). Less commonly there may be involvement of the perianal skin with severe pruritus.

Involvement of the nails, especially the toenails, is frequent, and characteristically one or more escape invasion. The affected nail becomes deformed, discolored, opaque and friable (Fig. 33–7). Onychomycosis is resistant to therapy and consequently constitutes an important reservoir for reinfection.

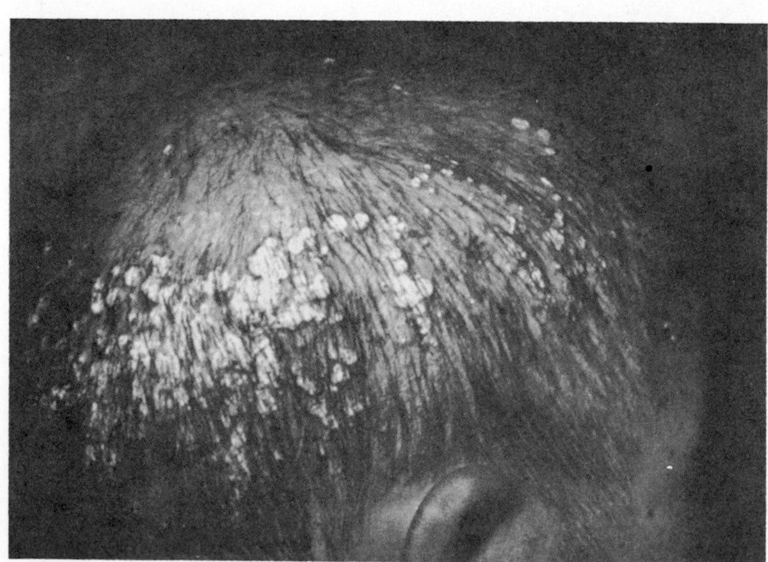

Figure 33–2. Favus showing alopecia and crusted lesions of scalp.

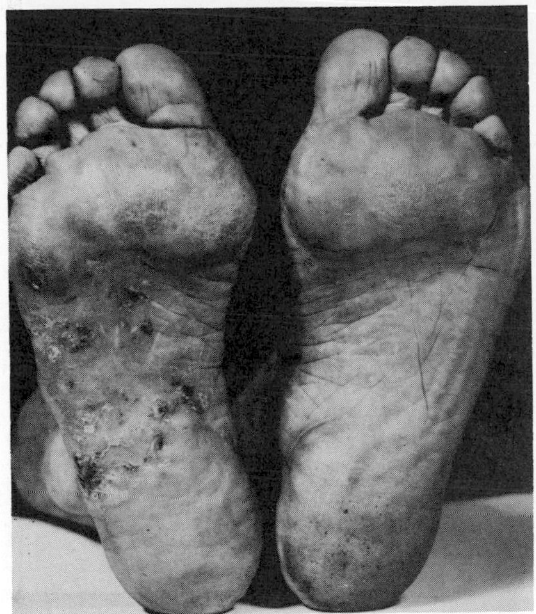

Figure 33-3. Tinea pedis of feet. (From J. W. Rippon. 1974, Medical Mycology. W. B. Saunders Co., Philadelphia. p. 138.)

The remote skin rashes or dermatophytids are considered to be an allergic reaction following cutaneous sensitization to the fungus. The lesions are not distinctive and may be acute, chronic or eczematoid in nature. They usually appear immediately following a flare-up of the infection between the toes (Fig. 33-3).

Diagnosis. It is extremely important to make a careful examination of the skin between and beneath the toes. Scrapings should be made from the margin of the lesion with a sharp scalpel. Microscopic examination of the potassium hydroxide preparation of this material or of the epithelial covering of vesicles will reveal the mycelia of the fungi. Cultures should be made for specific identification of the fungus. (See Chapter 73.)

Treatment. Simple tinea pedis is amenable to topical drugs such as haloprogin (Halotex) or tolnaftate (Tinactin). Severe and chronic infections may require systemic griseofulvin therapy or 10 per cent thiabendazole cream. Infections caused by *Candida* respond to topical nystatin.

Prophylaxis. The prophylaxis of dermatophytosis consists of careful drying of the skin, especially between the toes, the use of slippers in public baths and washrooms, the avoidance of borrowed clothing, and proper sterilization of clothing, including socks and towels. The regular use of a foot powder consisting of calcium propionate, 15 per cent in a talc base, is a highly efficient prophylactic measure. Prophylactic use of griseofulvin has been tried with some success, but appears impractical.[1]

Onychomycosis

Synonyms. Tinea unguium, ringworm of the nail.

Definition. Onychomycosis is a disease of the nail caused by a dermatophyte, *Candida albicans* or some other fungus.[2] True tinea unguium is of two types: (1) leukonychia mycotica (superficial white onychomycosis), where invasion is restricted to patches or pits on the nail surface (Fig. 33-8); and (2) invasive subungual disease, where invasion begins in the lateral or distal edges of the nail (Fig. 33-7). In this latter form the fungus is found on the bottom of and deep within the nail plate.

Distribution. Onychomycosis is of worldwide distribution.

Etiology. Leukonychia mycotica is commonly caused by *Trichophyton mentagrophytes.* Invasive disease is most commonly due to *Trichophyton rubrum* and *C. albicans.* Almost all species of dermatophytes as well as such fungi as *Scopulariopsis, Candida* species, and others have been isolated from infected nails.

Pathology. In leukonychia mycotica the fungus invades the surface of the nail, causing the formation of pits. Distorted mycelia are seen in invasive disease. The myce-

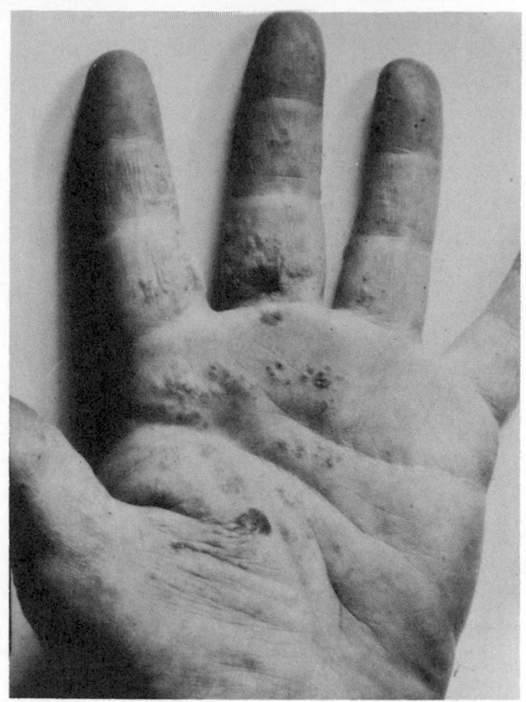

Figure 33–4. Dermatophytid "pomphlox type" of hand. (From J. W. Rippon. 1974, Medical Mycology. W. B. Saunders Co., Philadelphia. p. 138.)

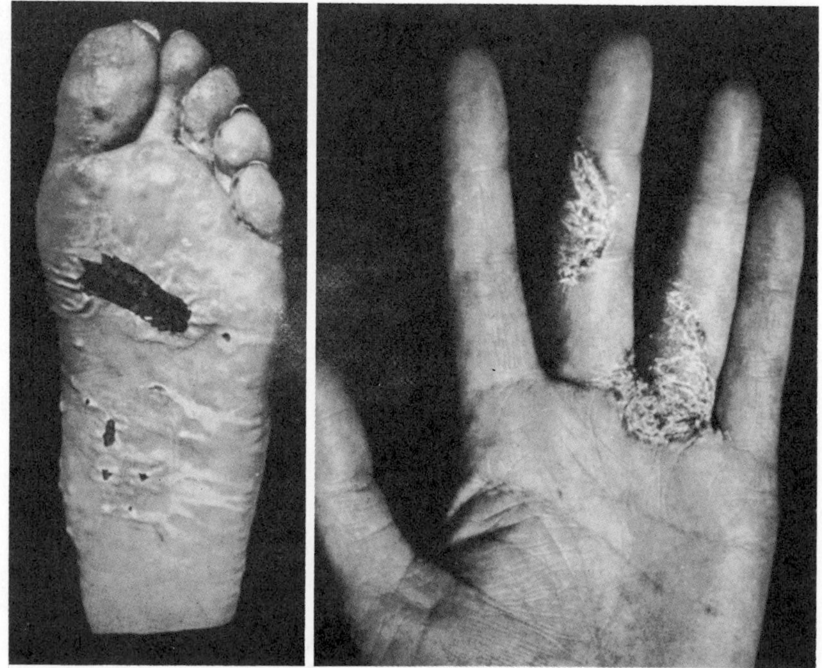

Figure 33–5 **Figure 33–6**

Figure 33–5. Dermatophytosis of foot: advanced lesions showing undermining, bullous response with vesicles and pustules. (Courtesy of Dr. Ray O. Noojin, Duke University.)

Figure 33–6. Dermatophytosis of hand. (Courtesy of Dr. J. Lamar Callaway, Duke University.)

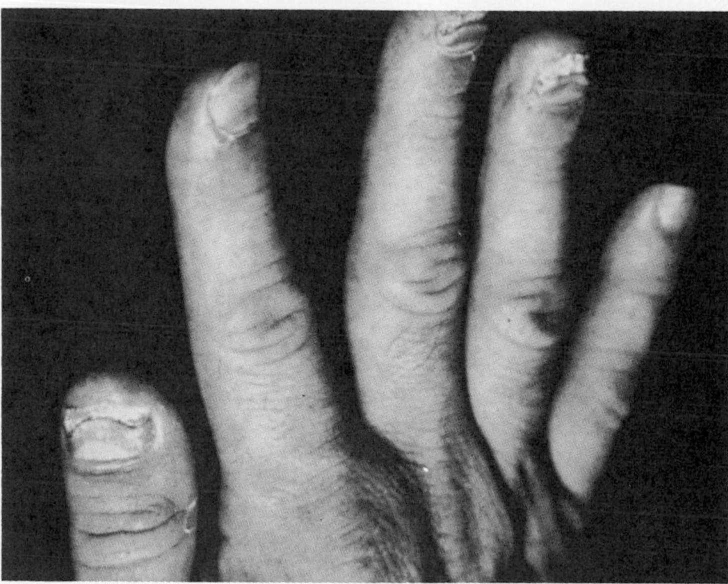

Figure 33-7. Onychomycosis invasion of the nails. (Courtesy of Dr. J. Lamar Callaway, Duke University.)

lium grows along the bottom of the nail plate.

Clinical Characteristics. White spot of the nail is easily recognized as one or more white patches on one or several toenails. There is no other symptomatology. Invasive disease is characterized by grossly distorted nails due to the accumulation of soft friable keratin, produced by the nail bed (usually inactive) and stimulated by the fungus. Nails invaded by *Candida* lack the gross distortion and accumulated detritus.

Diagnosis. Culture and direct examination of white spot are fairly easy. In invasive disease, however, the fungus is deeply buried in the debris along with a large flora of saprophytic bacteria and fungi. Repeated cultures may be necessary.

Treatment. White spot is easily treated by topical antidermatophyte drugs. Invasive disease very rarely responds even to griseofulvin given for a year or more. Infected fingernails respond to treatment more often than do toenails. Onychomycosis represents a constant source of reinfection for other forms of dermatophytosis.

Tinea corporis

Synonyms. Tinea circinata, tinea glabrosa, trichophytosis, "ringworm" of the body.

Definition. Ringworm of the body is a superficial fungous infection that is eczematoid or, if chronic, granulomatous with generalized encrusted lesions. It is often pruritic.

Distribution. This infection has a widespread distribution but is more common in the tropics and subtropics than in the temperate zones.

Etiology. It is due to infection of the skin by species of *Microsporum* and *Trichophyton.* A similar disease is produced by *Candida albicans.*

Clinical Characteristics. The early lesions of tinea corporis appear as flattened, reddish papules having a marked tendency to peripheral spread and central healing. The margins of the lesion are sharply defined and scaly or vesicular. The infection may be accompanied by a varying degree of inflammatory response or an eczematoid reaction, as well as other variations (Fig. 33-9).

Diagnosis. Examination of potassium

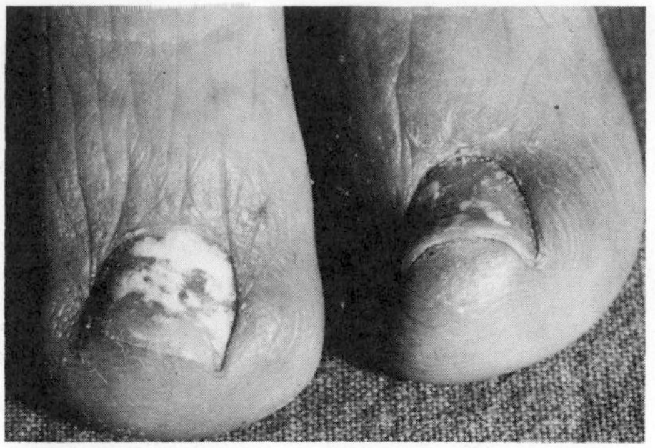

Figure 33-8. Leukonychia mycotica caused by *T. mentagrophytes.* (Courtesy of Dr. N. Zaias, Mt. Sinai Hospital, Miami, Florida.)

hydroxide preparations of scrapings from the lesions reveals the fungal etiology. (See Chapter 73.) Cultures should be made for specific identification.

Pathology. The stratum corneum is invaded by the fungus. Fungal enzymes and metabolic products cause a toxic or allergic dermatitis or both to develop in the epidermis underneath. Lanugo hair may be invaded and acts as a reservoir for reinfection.

Treatment. Uncomplicated tinea corporis usually resolves spontaneously in a few months. It is amenable to several topical drugs, such as tolnaftate and haloprogin. Severe cases are treated with thiabendazole (10 per cent cream) or griseofulvin.

Tinea cruris

Synonyms. Dhobie itch, eczema marginatum, ringworm of the groin, crotch itch, jock itch.

Definition. Tinea cruris is a superficial fungous infection of the skin, primarily of the upper and inner aspects of the thighs. In

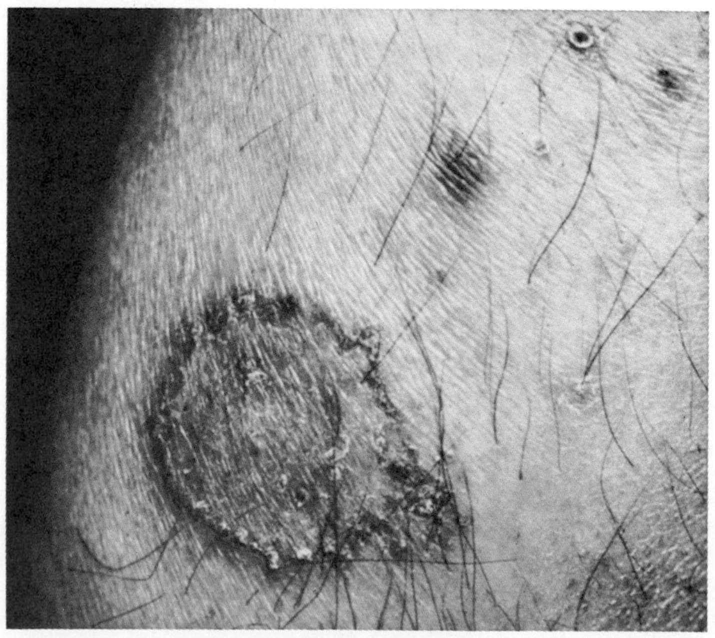

Figure 33-9. Tinea corporis: active vesicular border and scaling of center of lesion. (Courtesy of Dr. J. Lamar Callaway, Duke University.)

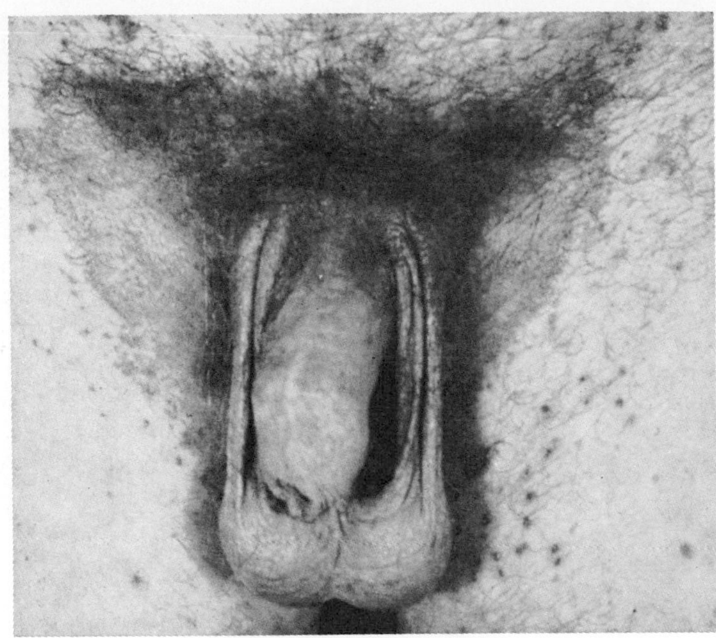

Figure 33–10. Tinea cruris, showing margination and scattered active foci which may later coalesce. (Courtesy of Dr. J. Lamar Callaway, Duke University.)

severe cases it may extend to involve adjacent skin areas and the axillae.

Distribution. The infection is widespread without particular geographic limitation. It is particularly a problem in tropical and subtropical environments.

Etiology. It is commonly due to infection by *Epidermophyton floccosum, T. rubrum* and other species of *Trichophyton. Candida albicans* is a very common agent in the tropics (dermatocandidosis).

Epidemiology. Heat, humidity, excessive perspiration and friction from clothing are predisposing causes. Indirect transmission occurs through the use of unsterilized towels and borrowed clothing.

Clinical Characteristics. Tinea cruris is characterized by brownish or reddish lesions having a scaly surface and presenting a papular or finely vesicular border. These spread peripherally and tend to clear in the center. Small satellite lesions are not infrequent. The infection may extend to adjacent areas, particularly the scrotum, perineum and lower abdomen, and in severe cases the axillae may be involved (Fig. 33–10).

Diagnosis. The diagnosis of tinea cruris is based in part upon the appearance and distribution of the lesions and in part upon the microscopic examination of potassium hydroxide preparations of scrapings from the margin of an active lesion. Such examination will reveal the mycelia of the fungus. Specific identification requires examination of cultures. (See Chapter 73.)

Treatment. The treatment is the same as for tinea corporis. Infections with *Candida* respond to topical nystatin and haloprogin.

Tinea imbricata

Synonyms. Tokelau, Burmese ringworm, Malabar itch.

Distribution. Tinea imbricata is restricted to the tropics, chiefly the islands of the South Pacific and the Malay Archipelago. It also occurs in southern China, southern

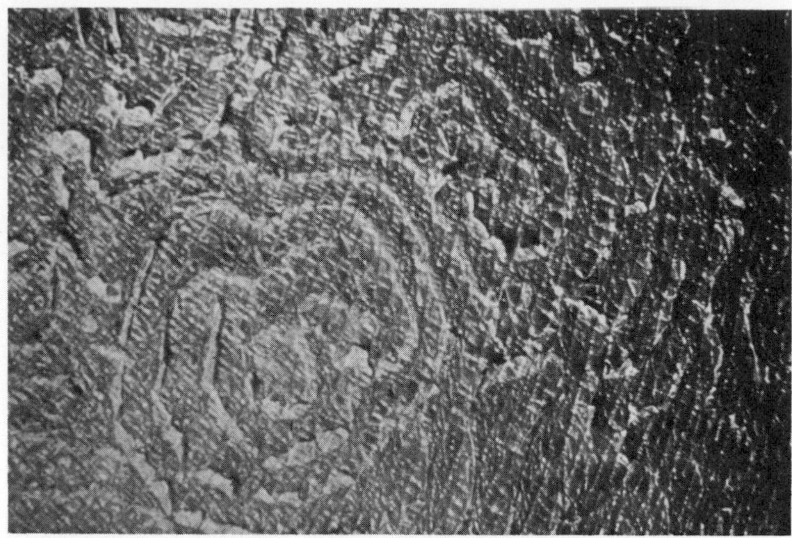

Figure 33–11. Tinea imbricata: typical concentric scales. (Courtesy of Dr. R. Mayorga, Universidad de San Carlos, Guatemala.)

India, Ceylon and central Africa. It has been reported from Colombia, Panama, Brazil and Guatemala.

Etiology. It is due to infection of the skin by *Trichophyton concentricum.*

Clinical Characteristics. The early lesion of tinea imbricata appears as a raised brownish or reddish plaque which gradually extends peripherally. The superficial epithelium desquamates, producing a scaling margin with the free inner edges of the scales turned up and directed toward the center of the lesion. Peripheral extension of the process leaves a smooth central area in which a new and similar lesion appears, producing a further circle of scales within the peripheral circle. These scaled circles following one another may be 1/8 to 1/2 inch apart, producing rosette-like lesions (Fig. 33–11). There is no accompanying inflammatory reaction. The axillae, groin, face, palms of the hands and soles of the feet are much less often affected than in the other cutaneous mycoses. The scalp is not involved. Itching is frequently intense.

Diagnosis. The clinical appearance of the lesions is characteristic, and microscopic examination of a potassium hydroxide preparation of scrapings from the margin will reveal the mycelia of the fungus. (See Chapter 73.) Cultures should be made and identified. (See Chapter 73.)

Treatment. Since extensive skin areas are usually involved, the antibiotic griseofulvin is used. Treatment is unwarranted unless the disease is causing distress to the patient.

Publications dealing with this subject should be used for more extensive information concerning the cutaneous mycoses (dermatomycoses).[1-4]

Pityriasis versicolor

Synonym. Tinea versicolor.

Distribution. This is a very common though unimportant mycotic infection of the skin.

Etiology. It is due to overgrowth of *Pityrosporum orbiculare,* a lipophilic yeast which is part of the normal flora. The high frequency of this disease in the tropics is thought to be due to slower epidermal turnover.[5]

Clinical Characteristics. Pityriasis versicolor is characterized by yellowish or

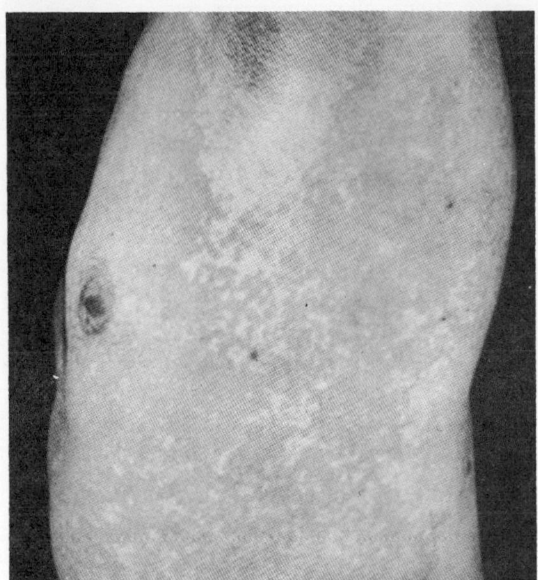

Figure 33–12. Pityriasis versicolor: brownish pigmented eruption. (Courtesy of Dr. J. Lamar Callaway, Duke University.)

brownish irregular macular patches which occur especially on the skin over the shoulders, chest, upper back, axillae and upper abdomen. The individual lesions show fine scaling. Healing is frequently followed by partial depigmentation (achromia parasitica) which may persist for a number of weeks or months (Fig. 33–12).

Diagnosis. Potassium hydroxide preparations of scrapings from the lesion will reveal the characteristic clumping of round bodies, and mycelial fragments and lesions will have a yellow fluorescence under a Wood's lamp.

Treatment. The following preparations are recommended:

1. Fifteen per cent solution of sodium hyposulfite should be sponged on twice daily, or:
2. Pragmatar ointment may be applied to the lesions twice daily, or:
3. Three per cent sulfur and 3 per cent salicylic acid in petrolatum ointment may be applied each night, or:
4. Selenium sulfide (1 per cent solution) ointment may be applied each night.
5. Daily baths with removal of all scales are necessary and are rendered somewhat more efficacious by the use of vinegar, which tends to loosen the scales.

Otomycosis

Synonyms. Singapore ear, myringomycosis.

Distribution. It is common in the moist tropics and likewise is frequently observed in regions of high wind and dust.

Etiology. Many different saprophytic fungi have been isolated from this infection but the disease is primarily one of bacterial etiology.[6]

Clinical Characteristics. Otomycosis is a rare mycotic infection of the skin of the external auditory canal and may present variable clinical phenomena. In mild cases the skin of the canal is reddened and scaly, producing an appearance often confused with seborrhea. In other instances the canal may be packed with a grayish mass of mycelia, having an appearance of wet, grayish blotting paper. Complications involving deeper structures are exceedingly rare. Infection of the canal by bacteria may result in mild symptoms or in pustule formation, cellulitis, edema and occasionally intense pain.

Diagnosis. Microscopic examination of a potassium hydroxide preparation of scrapings from the lesion or of a portion of the mycelial mass reveals the mycelia and spores of *Candida* or the mycelia and so-called fruitheads of *Aspergillus* or *Penicillium*. The bacterial flora should be cultured and identified (Chapter 73). With few exceptions the fungi isolated exist on the detritus caused by a primary bacterial infection (*Pseudomonas* sp., *Proteus* sp., *Staphylococcus* sp., *Streptococcus* sp. or others).

Treatment. If cellulitis with bacterial infection is present, the condition must be treated with compresses of saline or boric acid solution for 1 hour 3 times daily. This should be followed by local application of chemotherapeutic agents selected by sensitivity tests against the cultured bacteria.

If there is no bacterial infection, as much as possible of the mycelial mass, cerumen and other debris should be removed with a curette, after thorough soaking with hydrogen peroxide. After this, one of the following regimens is recommended.

1. The external canal is packed for 12 hours with a pledget of wool saturated with 1 per cent thymol in Cresatin. The patient should be instructed to remove this if it produces severe burning. Thereafter 1 per cent thymol in Cresatin drops is placed in the ear night and morning.

2. Three per cent salicylic acid in 70 per cent alcohol may be swabbed in the external auditory canal and on the affected part of the ear twice daily.

3. After being cleaned and dried with warm air, the canal is packed for 12 hours with wool saturated with Cresatin. Thereafter for 8 days the canal is packed daily for 9 minutes, using a 1 per cent solution of thymol in alcohol. For 3 days thereafter thymol iodide is dusted into the canal 3 times daily. Concurrently the patient should take potassium iodide 1.8 gm by mouth daily for 3 days.

4. After being cleansed with hydrogen peroxide solution, the canal should be swabbed out with 12 per cent silver nitrate. Alcohol drops should be introduced 3 times daily.

5. Soap and water should be avoided locally, and the patient should not be allowed to go swimming.

Prophylaxis. The prophylaxis of this infection is not satisfactory. The use of plugs in the canal does not confer protection. Precautions should be taken to keep the canal dry and protected against trauma with the finger or objects small enough to enter the canal.

REFERENCES

Cutaneous Mycoses

1. Hildick-Smith, G., Blank, H., and Sarkany, I. 1964. Fungus Diseases and Their Treatment. Little, Brown, & Co., Boston. 494 pp.
2. Zaias, N. 1972. Onychomycosis. Arch. Dermatol. *105*:263–274.
3. Blank, H., Taplin, D., and Zaias, N. 1969. Cutaneous *Trichophyton mentagrophytes* infection in Viet Nam. Arch. Dermatol. *99*:135–144.
4. Allen, A. M., Reinhardt, J. M., and Akers, W. A. 1973. Griseofulvin in the prevention of experimental human dermatophytosis. Arch. Dermatol. *108*:233–236.
5. Roberts, S. O. B. 1969. Pityriasis: a clinical and mycological investigation. Br. J. Dermatol. *81*:315–326.
6. Beaney, G. P. E., and Broughton, A. 1967. Tropical otomycosis. J. Laryngol. Otol. *81*:987–997.

CHAPTER 34

Subcutaneous Mycoses

This is a group of mycoses in which the subcutaneous tissues are invaded. The infections are long chronic diseases and systemic invasion is rare. The portal of entry is usually by traumatic implantation of soil fungi into the cutaneous and subcutaneous tissue.

Sporotrichosis

Definition. A subacute or chronic granulomatous fungous infection caused by *Sporothrix schenckii* producing gumma-like nodules, ulcers and abscesses, usually confined to the skin and superficial lymph nodes.[1]

Distribution. Worldwide.

Etiology. Sporotrichosis is produced by infection with *Sporothrix schenckii,* which is widely distributed in nature. In infected experimental animals this organism produces gram-positive, yeastlike forms which may be seen in polymorphonuclear leukocytes. They are rarely seen in materials from man. At 25°C (77°F) it grows as a spore-producing blackish mycelial mat.

Pathology. The gumma-like nodules usually show a central necrotic area surrounded by granulation tissue, epithelioid cells and giant cells with a peripheral zone of connective tissue. Unless the periodic acid–Schiff or methenamine silver stains are used, organisms will not be seen in smears or tissue sections.

Clinical Characteristics. The initial lesion usually appears as a hard, movable, elastic nodule beneath the skin. This enlarges and becomes attached to the skin, which becomes red, inflamed and then necrotic, with the formation of a chronic ulcer (sporotrichotic chancre). Similar nodules develop along the superficial lymphatics draining the

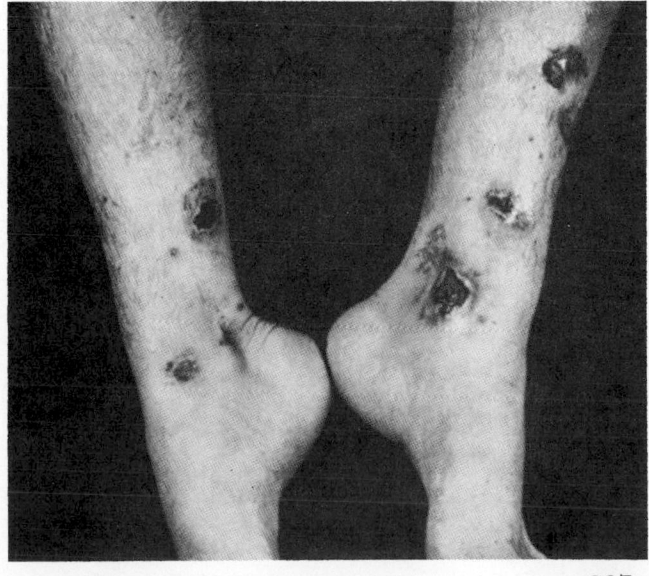

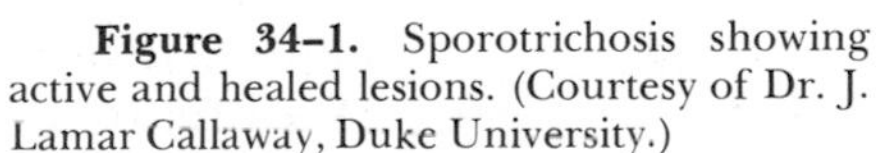
Figure 34–1. Sporotrichosis showing active and healed lesions. (Courtesy of Dr. J. Lamar Callaway, Duke University.)

area, resulting in the formation of secondary ulcers. The lymphatic channels between the lesions are frequently palpable, thickened and cordlike (Fig. 34–1).

Other structures, including mucous membranes, muscles, the skeletal system and the viscera, are involved in systemic infection. Pulmonary sporotrichosis is not a common form of the disease but should be considered in infections of unknown etiology.[2] This form is produced from inhalation of the spores.

Diagnosis. *Sporothrix schenckii* is rarely demonstrable in material from the lesions in man. Diagnosis is based upon the cultural characteristics after inoculation of infected material on Sabouraud's medium. (See Chapter 73.)

Treatment. Potassium iodide is a specific for this infection and should be administered for cutaneous and localized lymphangitic infections from the outset in massive dosage. The treatment begins with 10 drops of a saturated solution of potassium iodide 3 times daily and increases 5 drops with each of the daily doses until as much as 30 to 40 drops are being given 3 times a day. The drug may be given in water or milk. In order to avoid recurrences the treatment should be continued for 4 to 6 weeks.

Systemic sporotrichosis may not respond to oral potassium iodide, in which case amphotericin B should be administered.

Chromomycosis

Synonyms. Chromoblastomycosis, cladosporiosis, phaeosporotrichosis.

Definition. A fungous infection of the skin, producing verrucous, wartlike nodules or papillomas which may or may not ulcerate.

Distribution. This disease occurs sporadically in many areas of the world but is particularly prevalent in tropical areas.

Etiology. Chromomycosis is produced by trauma to the skin and the introduction of one of a variety of fungi—*Phialophora verrucosa, Fonsecaea pedrosoi, Fonsecaea compactum* or *Cladosporium carrionii.* All of these present an identical appearance in pus or in sections of tissue from the lesions. They appear as clusters of large, spherical, dark brown sclerotic cells which reproduce by equatorial splitting and not by budding. Specific identification is based upon the characteristics in culture on Sabouraud's medium at room temperature.[3]

Pathology. The pathology is essentially that of an infectious granuloma with numerous giant cells, mononuclears, phagocytes, epithelioid cells and plasma cells. The organisms may be seen lying free within dermal abscesses or within giant cells.

Clinical Characteristics. Chromomycosis is a very chronic infection, usually occurring on the extremities. It appears first as pustules, which subsequently develop into elevated, scaling, warty nodules or papillomas; the infected extremities gradually become covered with these lesions (Fig. 34–2). When infection occurs on the face, neck or buttocks the lesions are often atypical. Rarely, fatal metastases to the central nervous system occur.

Diagnosis. Diagnosis is based upon demonstration of the characteristic sclerotic cells in smears of exudate or in potassium hydroxide preparations of scrapings from the lesions.

Treatment. When the infection is superficial and not too extensive, surgical excision is recommended. Iodides have no effect. Local administration of amphotericin B has been used with reported successful treatment.[4] Clinical trials with 5-fluorocytosine are under way.

Rarely the agents of chromomycosis and another species, *Cladosporium trichoides,* may disseminate to the brain and cause a fatal abscess. The lesion is seen to contain dark brown mycelial elements.

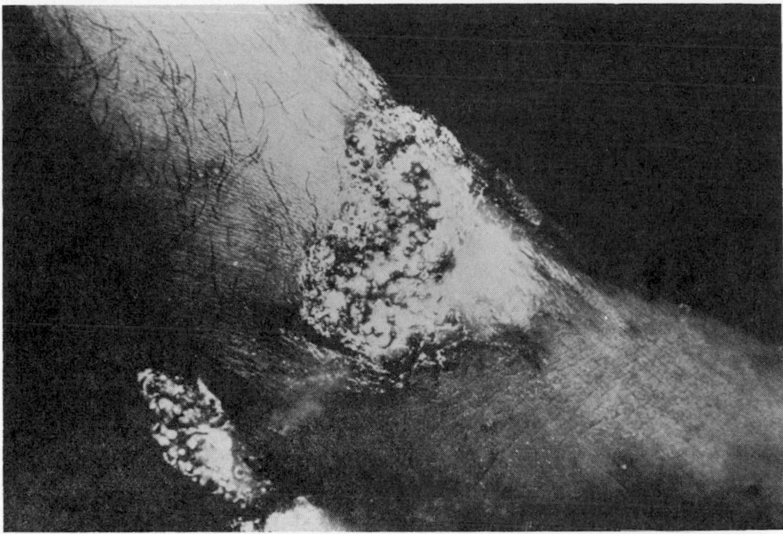

Figure 34–2. Chromomycosis caused by *Fonsecaea pedrosoi.* (Courtesy of Dr. E. Macotela Ruiz, Instituto Mexicano del Seguro Social.)

Entomophthoromycosis

Definition. This entity consists of two distinct diseases that have closely related etiologic agents. The first, subcutaneous phycomycosis, is caused by *Basidiobolus haptosporus*. The disease consists of hard movable subcutaneous swellings on the neck, trunk, back or legs. They respond to potassium iodide therapy. Infections have been recorded in Indonesia, India, Southeast Asia and several African countries. Tissue sections show broad nonseptate hyphae 20 μm in diameter, surrounded by an eosinophilic halo. The lesions are granulomas. The second disease is rhinoentomophthoromycosis. It is a rare disease of tropical climates involving the nose. Palpable hard swellings occur across the nasal bridge. The histology is identical to subcutaneous phycomycosis. The etiologic agent is the insect pathogen *Entomophthora coronata*.[5]

Rhinosporidiosis

Definition. An infection of the mucous membrane of the nose, mouth and pharynx, occasionally of other parts of the body, caused by *Rhinosporidium seeberii* and characterized by the development of pedunculated multiple polypoid masses.

Distribution. The disease is endemic in India and Sri Lanka and sporadic in other parts of the world.[6]

Etiology. The causative organism, *R. seeberii*, has never been cultured but is presumed to be a fungus.

Pathology. The soft nodular tumors are covered by a squamous cell epithelium beneath the surface of which are imbedded numerous sporangia in various stages of maturity up to 300 μm in size containing innumerable spores. When liberated into the tissues, they incite a chronic inflammatory reaction with conspicuous plasma cell and lymphocyte infiltration. Giant cells may be seen in proximity to empty sporangial cells.

Clinical Characteristics. The nose is the common site of infection, with the devel-

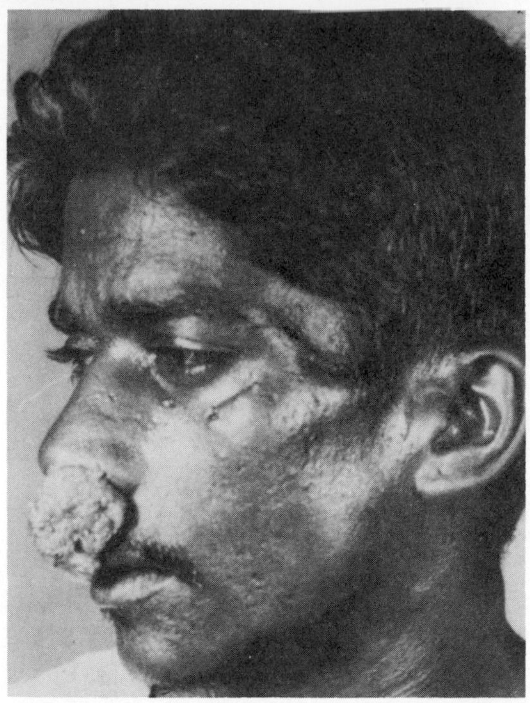

Figure 34–3. Rhinosporidiosis. Pedunculated mass hanging from nose. (Courtesy of Dr. C. Satyanarayana, Madras Medical College, Madras, India. From J. W. Rippon. 1974. Medical Mycology. W. B. Saunders Co., Philadelphia. p. 287.)

opment of tumor masses which become pedunculate, hang free and bleed readily when traumatized (Fig. 34–3). Infection of the nasopharynx and the development of large papillomatous tumors may cause obstruction leading to dyspnea and dysphagia. Tracheobronchial infection may cause death by obstruction.

Conjunctival infection may cause no symptoms when the lesion is small, but continued growth resulting in a large strawberry-like mass may cause eversion of the lid, photophobia and lacrimation.

Rare disseminated rhinosporidiosis has been reported.

Diagnosis. Direct examination of the material expressed from the polypoid mass reveals sporangia, and spores or the occurrence of sporangia in tissue sections allows definitive diagnosis. The organism cannot be cultured.

Treatment. Superficial lesions should be removed by careful surgical dissection. In advanced cases, intensive surgery will be necessary. There is no specific drug for this disease.

REFERENCES

Sporotrichosis

1. Manhart, J. W., Wilson, J. A., and Kobitz, B. C. 1970. Articular and cutaneous sporotrichosis. J.A.M.A. *214*:365–367.
2. Mohr, J. A. 1972. Primary pulmonary sporotrichosis. Am. Rev. Respir. Dis. *106*:260–264.

Chromomycosis

3. Al-Doory, Y. 1972. Chromomycosis. Mountain Press, Missoula. 203 pp.
4. Hughes, W. R. 1967. Chromoblastomycosis: successful treatment with topical amphotericin B. J. Pediat. *71*:351–356.

Entomophthoromycosis

5. Williams, A. O. 1969. Pathology of phycomycosis due to *Entomophthora* and *Basidiobolus* species. Arch. Pathol. *87*:13–20.

Rhinosporidiosis

6. Karunuratre, W. A. E. 1964. Rhinosporidiosis in Man. The Athlone Press, University of London. 146 pp.

CHAPTER 35
Systemic Mycoses

DIMORPHIC PATHOGENIC FUNGI

These infections result from the inhalation of spores. Initially they produce a primary pulmonary disease. Most such infections are subclinical and resolve spontaneously. People living in highly endemic areas usually have residual lesions in the lung representing resolved focal infections. Only rarely do the diseases become clinically apparent and serious. The fungi grow in soil as spore-producing hyphae but convert to budding yeasts (histoplasmosis, blastomycosis, paracoccidioidomycosis) or endospore-containing spherules (coccidioidomycosis) in tissue (Table 35–1).

Table 35–1. Dimorphic Pathogenic Fungi*

Disease and Organism	***Saprophytic Phase*** (25° C; 77° F)	***Parasitic Phase*** (37° C; 98.6° F)
Histoplasmosis *Histoplasma capsulatum* *Histoplasma capsulatum* var. *duboisii*	Septate mycelium, microaleuriospores, tuberculate, macroaleuriospores. Colonies white-beige and fluffy	Budding small yeast 1 to 5 μm Large yeast (5 to 12 μm) in African histoplasmosis *(duboisii)*
Blastomycosis *Blastomyces dermatitidis*	Septate mycelium, microaleuriospores pyriform, globose, or double. Colonies white-buff and fluffy or glabrous	Thick refractile wall, budding yeast 8 to 20 μm. Broad-based bud
Paracoccidioidomycosis *Paracoccidioides brasiliensis*	Similar to *B. dermatitidis*	Large, multiple, budding yeast cells 20 to 60 μm
Sporotrichosis *Sporothrix schenckii*	Pyriform conidia on delicate conidiophores. Delicate septate hyphae. Colonies verrucous white with black underside	Fusiform, oval, budding cells in culture 5 to 8 μm. Asteroid cigar-shaped bodies only in tissue
Coccidioidomycosis *Coccidioides immitis*	Branched, vegetative mycelium which fragments into barrel-shaped arthrospores. Colonies moist and wooly, "moth-eaten"	Spherules 10 to 60 μm with endospores. Up to 200 μm in mice
Rhinosporidiosis *Rhinosporidium seeberii*	Not known in culture	Spherules 100 to 300 μm with endospores
Adiospiromycosis *Emmonsia parva* *Emmonsia crescens*	Dense, dry, flattish, tan colony, aleuriospores on pedicis, 3 to 4 μm	Spherules 40 μm *(E. parva)*, 500 μm *(E. crescens)* also induced at high temperature (40° C; 104° F). No endospores

*From J. W. Rippon. 1973. *In* Burrows, W.: Textbook of Microbiology. 20th ed. W. B. Saunders Co., Philadelphia. p. 722.

Histoplasmosis

Synonyms. Darling's disease, reticuloendothelial cytomycosis, cave disease.

Definition. A self-limited primary pulmonary infection which heals by calcification, or a progressive systemic disease of the reticuloendothelial system caused by *Histoplasma capsulatum*.[1]

Distribution. The majority of reported cases have been from the Mississippi and Ohio valleys and the Appalachian Mountains in the United States. There are isolated reports of cases from the Panama Canal Zone, Philippine Islands, Honduras, Guatemala, Costa Rica, Argentina, Brazil, Java, Japan and England. A disease referred to as African histoplasmosis differs from the classic type in the appearance of large yeast forms of the fungus *H. capsulatum* var. *duboisii* in the tissues.[2]

Etiology. *Histoplasma capsulatum* appears as a small budding yeast, 1 to 5 μm in diameter, in mononuclear cells in the blood and in the reticuloendothelial cells of the internal organs and bone marrow.

Cultivation on blood agar at 37° C (98.6° F) produces a yeastlike growth of small, oval, budding cells. On Sabouraud's medium at room temperature growth is moldlike, at first cottony and white, later becoming brown. The sexual stage is an ascomycete *Emmonsiella capsulata.*

Epidemiology. *Histoplasma capsulatum* has been isolated from the soil and from numerous animals. Infection in man occurs

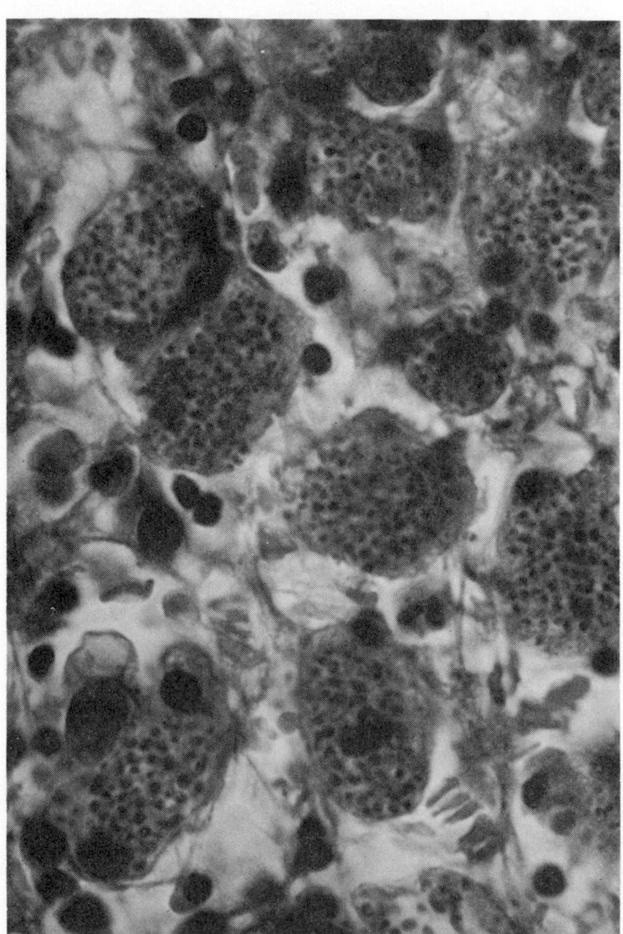

Figure 35–1. Histoplasmosis. Numerous budding yeasts within a macrophage. Note the clear area "capsule" around the cytoplasm. This is the unstained cell wall. The yeast does not have a capsule. (From J. W. Rippon. 1974. Medical Mycology. W. B. Saunders Co., Philadelphia, p. 334.)

by inhalation of infectious particles from soil. There is no evidence of animal to man transmission.

Pathology. Systemic histoplasmosis is a disease essentially of the reticuloendothelial system. Grayish or white nodules, or more or less extensive areas of necrosis surrounded by granulomatous tissue, are produced. The organisms multiply in the reticuloendothelial cells and may be seen in phagocytic cells in the lesions (Fig. 35–1).

Clinical Characteristics. Primary pulmonary infection may be asymptomatic or simulate a mild cold, bronchitis, influenza or tuberculosis. Such an infection results in sensitivity to histoplasmin and spontaneous recovery usually results in miliary calcification which may be detected years later by routine x-ray. In many areas of the United States large population groups have been found to have nontuberculous pulmonary calcifications with a positive histoplasmin skin test and a negative tuberculin skin test. Such individuals are thought to have had primary histoplasmosis as described above.

Systemic progressive infection may result in nasopharyngeal ulcerations resembling carcinoma, pulmonary infection with diffuse or localized consolidation, abscess or cavitation resembling tuberculosis or visceral infection resembling leishmaniasis. Not infrequently lymphadenopathy suggests lymphosarcoma, Hodgkin's disease or leukemia. The solitary pulmonary residual lesion, histoplasmoma, resembles the tuberculoma.

Diagnosis. The organisms stain well with Wright's stain in blood or bone marrow smears in systemic infections, and in infected cells they may be confused with Leishman-Donovan bodies or *Toxoplasma.* Tissues should be stained with methenamine silver for best results. (See Chapter 73 for procedure.) Final identification is based on cultures which demonstrate typical colonies and tuberculate spores of *H. capsulatum.*

Treatment. Amphotericin B provides prompt and complete clinical response with resulting remission in acute disseminated histoplasmosis. In chronic progressive histoplasmosis, amphotericin B therapy is associated with resolution of lesions and clinical improvement; however, organisms may persist in areas of cavitation or caseation. The usual course of treatment consists of 1 mg per kg of body weight to a total of 1 to 3 gm. The drug is very nephrotoxic.

Blastomycosis

Synonyms. North American blastomycosis, Gilchrist's disease.

Definition. A primary pulmonary infection due to *Blastomyces dermatitidis* that frequently disseminates to the skin and other organs. The secondary cutaneous type is characterized by granulomatous ulcerating lesions; the systemic type by a close resemblance to tuberculosis, with involvement of the lungs and less often the abdominal viscera, the skeletal system and the central nervous system.

Distribution. Blastomycosis, until recently, was recognized as present only in the United States and Canada. However, recent publications have confirmed the diagnosis of this disease in Africa.[3] Unlike the situation seen in histoplasmosis and coccidioidomycosis, there does not appear to be a large population with resolved primary infections. It is probable that a progressive disease generally develops following primary infection. The organism appears to be rare in nature; it has not been recovered with regularity from soil.[3]

Etiology. *Blastomyces dermatitidis* appears in tissue and pus as single-budding, round or ovoid yeastlike cells 8 to 15 μm in diameter. They have a thick refractile outer wall, often giving a double-contoured appearance. Mycelia are not present (Fig. 35–2).

Growth in culture at 37° C (98.6° F) is yeastlike, and at room temperature moldlike, with cottony growth of branched aerial mycelia-bearing characteristic spores. The sexual stage is an ascomycete *Ajellomyces dermatitidis.*

Pathology. The visceral type closely

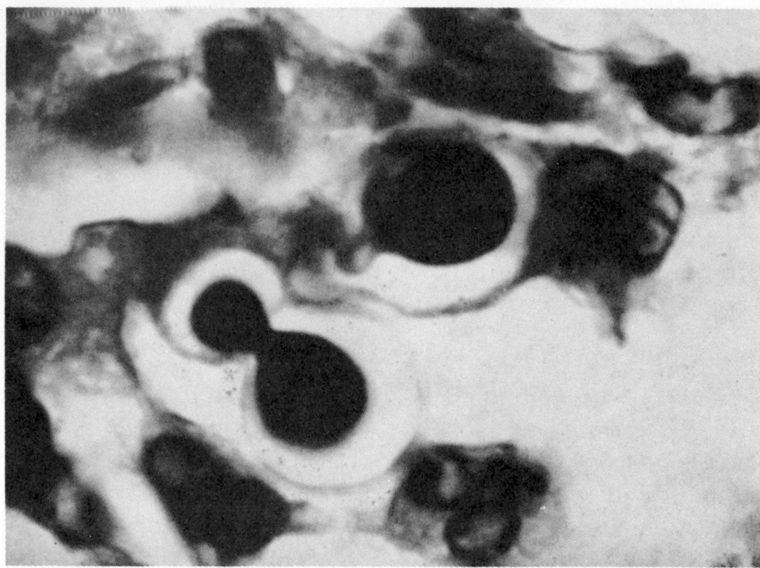

Figure 35–2. *Blastomyces dermatitidis.* Budding yeastlike cells in tissue section.

simulates tuberculosis, but numerous small abscesses with polymorphonuclear leukocytic infiltration are produced.

The primary infection is in the lung, which results in a mixed granulomatous-pyogenic tissue reaction. Secondary involvement of the skin is characterized by pseudoepitheliomatous hyperplasia and micro abscesses containing yeast cells (Fig. 35–3).

Clinical Characteristics. The cutaneous lesions of blastomycosis usually occur on the face, neck, hands, wrists, arms, feet or legs, appearing first as papules or pustules and extending to form the chronic ulcers. There is usually little pain, tenderness or systemic reaction and commonly no lymphadenitis. Such lesions evolve as metastases to the subcutaneous tissues from an established systemic infection (Figs. 35–4, 35–5).

Systemic infections resulting from a primary disease in the lungs frequently produce a clinical picture that is confused with tuberculosis or malignant neoplasms.

Diagnosis. The characteristic budding organisms are found within giant cells in granulation tissue and in necrotic material from the lesion. They may be demonstrated in the sputum in cases of pulmonary infection.

Treatment. Dihydroxystilbamidine or amphotericin B or both can be used for specific treatment of blastomycosis. These drugs are toxic, however, and the patient should be closely watched for signs that may contraindicate their continued use.[4]

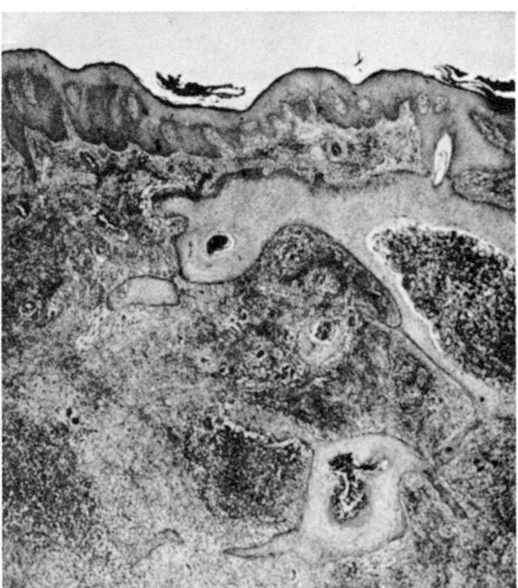

Figure 35–3. Blastomycosis. Granulomatous lesion in subcutaneous tissues.

Coccidioidomycosis

Synonyms. Coccidioidal granuloma, San Joaquin fever, valley fever, Posada-Wernicke disease.

Definition. An acute, benign, self-limited, primary, pulmonary infection; and a chronic, malignant, disseminated infection caused by inhalation of infectious particles of *Coccidioides immitis.*[5]

Distribution. The disease is endemic in the arid southwestern United States, the northern states of Mexico, Honduras, Guatemala, Venezuela and the Chaco region of Bolivia, Paraguay and Argentina. Sporadic cases outside of known endemic areas result from contact with contaminated materials exported from such areas.

Etiology. *Coccidioides immitis* appears in tissue and exudates as round, nonbudding, thick-walled spherules measuring 20 to 60 μm in diameter and containing numerous endospores. Culture on Sabouraud's medium at room temperature produces a cottony white growth, becoming brownish in color, with branching septate filamentous hyphae which subsequently break up with the formation of arthrospores.

Epidemiology. *Coccidioides immitis* has been recovered from the soil and from pulmonary lesions in various wild rodents and other animals, such as cattle, sheep and dogs, in the endemic areas in the southwestern United States. Infection of man occurs by inhalation of dust containing the highly infectious arthrospores. There is no evidence of direct animal to man or man to man transmission. Primary infections have a definite seasonal incidence, occurring predominantly in the hot dusty autumn months.

Pathology. The fundamental pathology is that of a granulomatous process, acute, subacute or chronic in nature, accompanied by varying degrees of fibrosis, with or without central necrosis of the lesion.

In chronic lesions of the lung, cavity formation or pleurisy with effusion may occur. The organisms are surrounded by giant cells, epithelioid cells, lymphocytes and plasma cells.

Occasional granulomatous masses may reach considerable size without necrosis. Abscess formation, however, is more frequent than in tuberculosis. A residual arrested pulmonary lesion, coccidioidoma, as seen by x-ray, may be mistaken for a tuberculoma or carcinoma.

Clinical Characteristics. Primary pulmonary infection produces the clinical picture of pneumonia or acute bronchitis with or without sputum and is occasionally accompanied by pleurisy with effusion. Physical signs may be absent. In the majority of cases recovery occurs in 2 to 3 weeks without sequelae. Sensitivity to the organism frequently develops and may be manifested by erythema multiforme or erythema nodosum. This form of the disease is known as "San Joaquin fever" or "valley fever." These infections are accompanied by an initial leukocytosis with a normal differential count. Later, there is lymphocytosis with an increase in large mononuclear cells and eosinophilia.

The secondary or chronic phase of the disease, coccidioidal granuloma, develops by dissemination of the infection from the primary focus, either in the course of the acute attack or subsequently. Lesions may occur

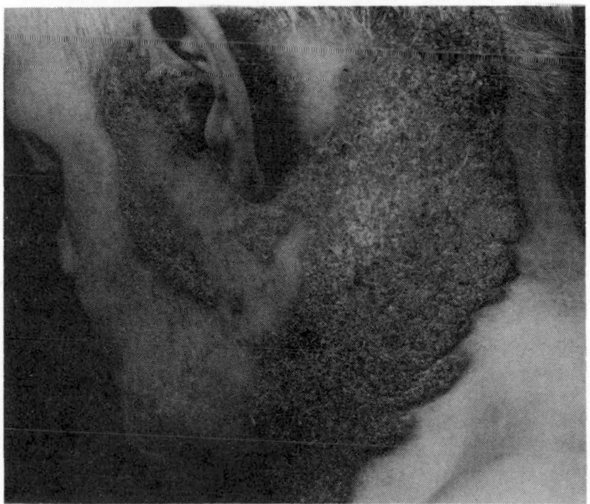

Figure 35–4. Blastomycosis. Secondary cutaneous lesions in a case of long duration. The fungus is found in the advancing border in the verrucous vegetations. The central areas clear with the formation of scar tissue. (Courtesy of Dr. A. Lorincz, University of Chicago, From J. W. Rippon. 1974. Medical Mycology. W. B. Saunders Co., Philadelphia. p. 305.)

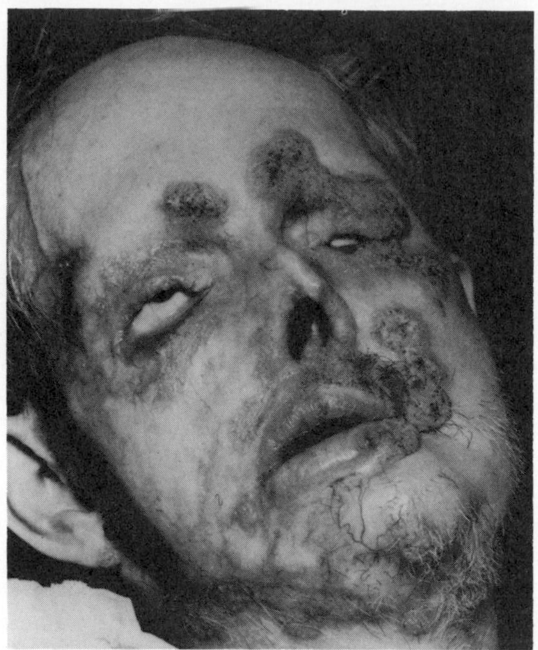

Figure 35–5. Blastomycosis. Same patient as in Figure 35–4. Note the destruction of facial features and the telangiectasia in the areas of scar tissue. Yeasts could be seen in aspirates from vesicles on the advancing border but were absent in the central areas of the lesions. (Courtesy of Dr. A. Lorincz, University of Chicago. From J. W. Rippon. 1974. Medical Mycology. W. B. Saunders Co., Philadelphia, p. 305.)

anywhere in the body, producing a variety of signs and symptoms.

Diagnosis. Diagnosis is based upon demonstration of the large, nonbudding, thick-walled spherules containing numerous endospores in clinical materials (Fig. 35–6) and the development of a cottony culture with typical arthrospores on Sabouraud's glucose agar. Intratesticular injection of infected material or culture fragments into guinea pigs produces lesions containing the typical endospore-filled spherules.

A positive skin test to coccidioidin has the same significance as the tuberculin test in tuberculosis—past or present infection.

Precipitins are present only in recent infections, and complement-fixing antibodies in chronic infection. There is increase in titer of the latter as the disease disseminates.

Differential Diagnosis. This entails differentiation from tuberculosis, syphilis, bacterial osteomyelitis, malignant neoplasms, and other mycotic infections.

Treatment. Most primary infections heal without specific treatment. Amphotericin B offers specific treatment in chronic infections.[5, 6]

Paracoccidioidomycosis

Synonyms. South American blastomycosis, Lutz-Splendore-Almeida disease.

Definition. A primary pulmonary infection by *Paracoccidioides brasiliensis* which has a predilection for lymphatic tissue. The secondary disease appears in two forms: a cutaneous type usually starting about the mouth, and a lymphaticovisceral type with involvement of the lymphatics, liver and spleen. The disease may remain limited to the lungs or become generalized.[7]

Distribution. South America, principally Brazil, but it also occurs in Central America and Mexico. Among the population in the endemic areas, the extent of subclinical resolved infections is unknown. Recent epidemiologic studies indicate that such infections are numerous, a picture similar to that seen in histoplasmosis and coccidioidomycosis. The organism has been recovered from soil.

Etiology. *Paracoccidioides brasiliensis* appears in the lesions as thick-walled round or ovoid yeast cells reaching diameters of 60 μm. Multiple-budding forms are the characteristic structures which allow identification of *P. brasiliensis.* In culture at 25°C (77°F) the colony and spores resemble those of *Blastomyces dermatitidis.*

Clinical Characteristics. The portal of entry is the lungs with secondary involvement of the buccal cavity. A slowly extending ulcer is produced. This has a granular base presenting numerous pinpoint yellowish white areas in which the fungus is particularly abundant. The infection may extend to

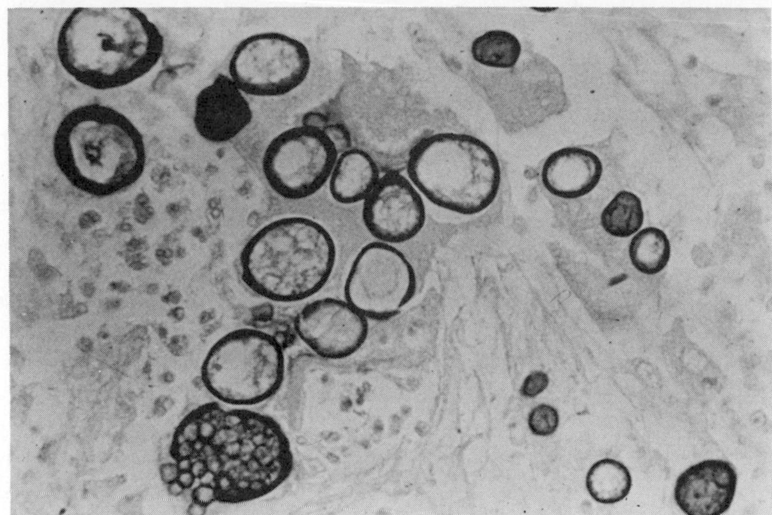

Figure 35–6. Coccidioidomycosis. Tissue section showing developing and mature spherules, some containing endospores. (From J. W. Rippon. 1973. *In* Burrows, W.: Textbook of Microbiology. W. B. Saunders Co., Philadelphia. p. 726.)

adjacent skin areas, producing lesions similar to those of blastomycosis, mucocutaneous leishmaniasis and yaws. The lesion may extend directly to the tonsils and secondarily to lymphoid follicles in the gastrointestinal tract, producing nodules and follicular ulceration. This may be followed by involvement of the regional lymphatics and invasion of the spleen and the liver (Fig. 35–7). The primary pulmonary lesions are often inapparent.

Diagnosis. Diagnosis is based upon demonstration of the large, multiple-budding, yeastlike forms and isolation and identification of the fungus.

Treatment. Amphotericin B has been reported to be curative.

Opportunistic Fungi

These are organisms of very low inherent virulence that are ubiquitous. They are unable to initiate a disease in a normal healthy host but have the potential to invade if the host's defenses are abrogated. The debilitation may be only transient and relatively minor, but colonization may occur very rapidly.[8]

Candidosis

Synonyms. Candidiasis, moniliasis.

Definition. An infection of the skin or mucous membranes (dermatocandidosis) or deeper tissues, particularly lungs, kidneys and meninges, by the yeastlike fungus *Candida albicans* or related species.

Distribution. *Candida albicans* is found in the normal mouth, throat, vagina and intestinal tract of many healthy individuals all over the world as well as in those suffering from candidosis.

Etiology. *Candida albicans* is an ubiquitous fungus of the intestinal tracts of birds and mammals for which there are over a hundred synonyms. It produces small, round, budding forms in the lesions with occasional

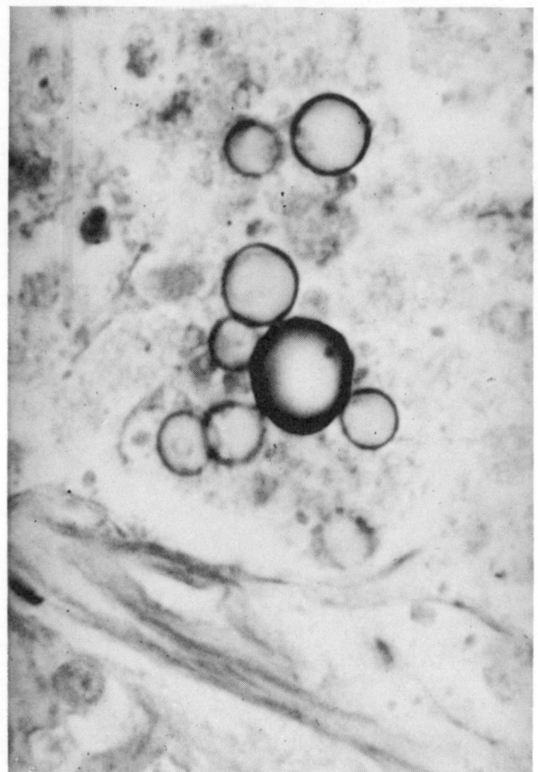

Figure 35-7. Paracoccidioidomycosis. Multiple budding yeast in tissue section. (Courtesy of Dr. P. Graff, University of Chicago. From J. W. Rippon. 1973. *In* Burrows, W.: Textbook of Microbiology. W. B. Saunders Co., Philadelphia. p. 730.)

pseudomycelia. On Sabouraud's medium, white, yeastlike colonies that have a yeasty odor are formed. Many factors may predispose *C. albicans* to invade the body from its endogenous habitat.[9]

Clinical Characteristics. *Candida albicans* is commonly present in the sputum of normal patients as well as of those with pulmonary tuberculosis or carcinoma of the lung. It is likewise frequently present in the stools of normal patients as well as of those with pernicious anemia, sprue and various other gastrointestinal diseases. It is usually difficult to ascribe definite etiologic significance to the presence of this fungus.

Candida albicans has been shown to be capable occasionally of producing a primary bronchitis, infections of the skin and systemic infections. The most common conditions attributed to it are thrush, onychia, paronychia and dermatitis in moist skin areas, particularly the axillae, beneath the breasts and in the intergluteal folds (dermatocandidosis). The rare systemic infections, which are often fatal, include abscess formation and meningitis (Fig. 35-8).

Secondary or opportunistic infection with *C. albicans* may follow extensive therapy with wide spectrum antibiotics (tetracyclines) and corticosteroids, cytotoxins and radiation. During prolonged treatment with such drugs, therefore, the patient must be observed constantly to avoid secondary infections which may prove serious.

Other predisposing factors leading to serious infection by *C. albicans* include debilitating diseases such as lymphoblastoma and leukemia; operative procedures such as thoracic or cardiac surgery; and the necessity for the use of indwelling intravenous catheters.[10] *Candida albicans* is one of the most notorious "opportunistic" fungi.

Diagnosis. The ubiquity of this fungus necessitates extreme caution in etiologic diagnosis. Examination of scrapings from the skin or nails, or of sputum or other material, in 10 per cent potassium hydroxide preparations demonstrates the round, single or budding yeast forms and, occasionally, mycelia.

Treatment. Cutaneous infections by *C. albicans* may be treated as follows:

1. Soaking twice daily for 30 minutes with 1:1500 potassium permanganate solution.

2. Daily application of 1 per cent solution of gentian violet.

3. Topical application of nystatin or haloprogin.

Oral lesions should be treated with nystatin solutions used as a mouthwash and retained in the mouth for a few minutes before swallowing. For vaginitis, douches of potassium permanganate 1:1500 or gentian violet 1:10,000; propionate and nystatin vaginal jelly are also recommended.

Esophageal and gastrointestinal candidosis can be treated with oral nystatin. Systemic infections require intravenous amphotericin B therapy.

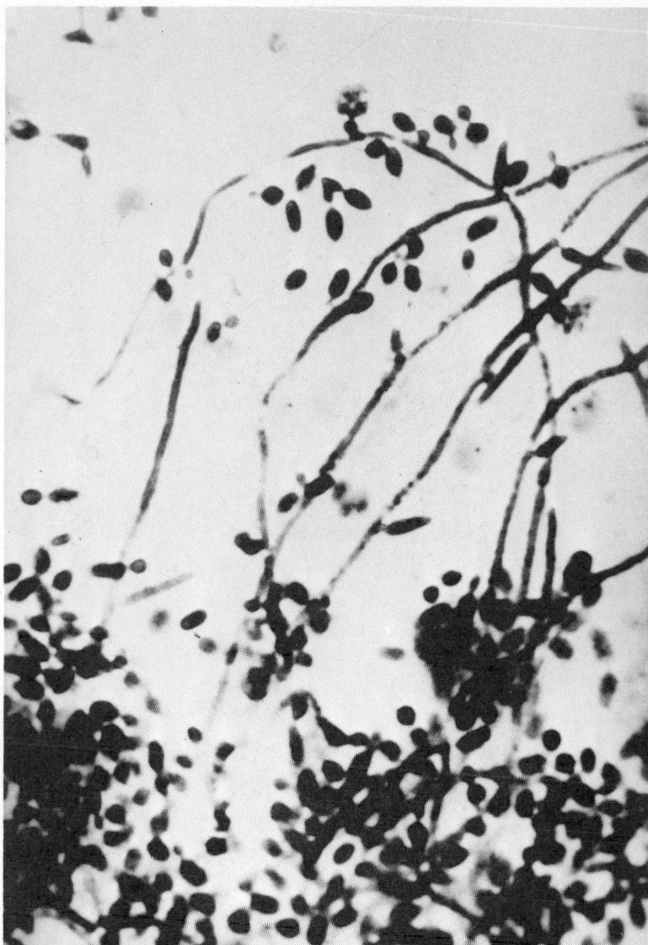

Figure 35–8. Candidosis. Gram stain of a sputum specimen from a patient with invasive pulmonary disease. The presence of the yeast form mixed with mycelium indicates the fungus has colonized and is invading tissue. In normal sputum only the yeast form is seen. (From J. W. Rippon. 1974. Medical Mycology. W. B. Saunders Co., Philadelphia. p. 197.)

Cryptococcosis

Synonyms. European blastomycosis, Busse-Buschke disease, torula meningitis.

Definition. A subacute or chronic infection by a yeastlike fungus, *Cryptococcus neoformans,* in which a primary pulmonary infection is followed by invasion of the body, especially the central nervous system.[11]

Distribution. The fungus is widely distributed in nature throughout the world and has been isolated from the soil and from bird excreta (especially that of pigeons).

Etiology. Cryptococcosis is produced by *C. neoformans,* a budding yeastlike organism. In tissue and in exudates it appears as an ovoid or spherical body measuring 5 to 20 μm in diameter; it has a single bud and is surrounded by a characteristic wide, refractile, gelatinous capsule. In culture it presents a brownish, mucoid, yeastlike growth, with the budding cells exhibiting the characteristic capsule, which is readily seen in India ink preparations (Fig. 35–9). It is the only encapsulated yeast of medical importance.

Pathology. The cutaneous form may produce acneform lesions, granulomatous ulcers and deep nodules or tumor-like masses which are filled with gelatinous material. There is usually little acute inflammatory reaction, but there may be infiltration with giant cells, "foam" cells, plasma cells and lymphocytes, together with fibroblasts and newly formed connective tissue. At times typical tubercles are produced.

In the central nervous system a variety

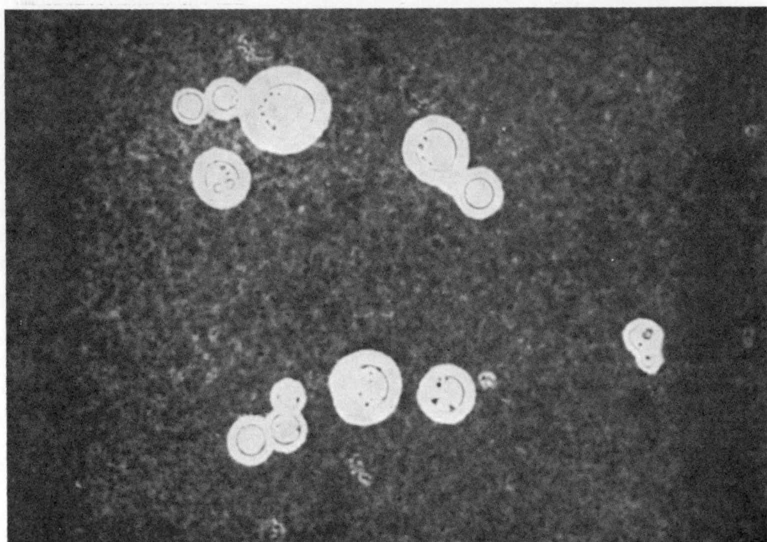

Figure 35-9. *Cryptococcus neoformans* in pus. (Courtesy of Dr. Donald S. Martin, Center for Disease Control, U.S.P.H.S.)

of pathologic changes may be seen, including diffuse meningitis, granulomas in the meninges, endarteritis, infarcts, areas of softening, increase in neuroglia, and extensive destruction of nerve tissue. Tissues should be stained with mucicarmine or alcian blue for best demonstration of the organism and capsule.

Clinical Characteristics. It is often difficult to assess the factors predisposing to infection by *Cryptococcus*. The *cutaneous type* is an expression of systemic infection. It is characterized by pustule formation, granulomatous ulcers of the skin or subcutaneous tumors.

The *generalized type* is usually characterized by symptoms and signs of extensive and progressive involvement of the central nervous system. In this form the onset is ordinarily insidious, although occasionally sudden, with fever, headache and vomiting. Death usually occurs after the onset of coma with signs of increased intracranial pressure. The spinal fluid is often under increased pressure and the cell count increased to 200 to 800 per cu mm; the cells are chiefly mononuclear. The organisms may be present in small numbers and may be mistaken for erythrocytes or small lymphocytes. This form of the disease is often mistaken for tuberculous meningitis since the dynamics, histology and chemistry of the spinal fluid are identical in both diseases.

Involvement of the lungs is accompanied by cough and signs of chronic bronchitis with peribronchial involvement, which may be confused with pulmonary tuberculosis. A low-grade intermittent fever may be present.

Rarely, invasion of the liver, spleen and joints occurs. Among the latter, the knees are most commonly affected.

The prognosis is grave in both the cutaneous and generalized forms. Untreated central nervous system infections are invariably fatal.

Diagnosis. The fungi appear in infected tissue, spinal fluid, sputum, or the gelatinous content of subcutaneous nodules as characteristic round or ovoid, single-budding, yeastlike bodies with heavy capsules. Satisfactory demonstration of the capsule requires smears in India ink of the sediment from centrifuged spinal fluid or of pus (Fig. 35-9).

Treatment. Amphotericin B treatment is required. The usual dosage schedule is used but the cumulative dose necessary is often 3 to 5 gm. Relapses occur.[12] 5-Fluorocytosine alone has been disappointing but used together with amphotericin B may be beneficial in cryptococcosis and systemic candidosis.

Aspergillosis

Definition. Broadly defined, aspergillosis is a group of diseases in which members of the genus *Aspergillus* are involved. (1) Allergic bronchopulmonary aspergillosis is characterized by aspergilli growing in the lumen of the bronchioles, mucus plugging and eosinophilia.[13] There is no invasion of tissue. *Aspergillus* is a common cause of asthma also. (2) Colonizing aspergillosis. Fungal balls or aspergillomas[14] develop within preformed cavities within the lung as a sequela of tuberculosis and sarcoidosis. Patients often have severe hemoptysis. (3) Invasive aspergillosis. This is the rare opportunistic infection of the debilitated patient. It is usually fulminant and rapidly fatal.[15]

Distribution. Since species of *Aspergillus* are ubiquitous in nature, they are a constant threat as infectious agents which can be isolated from diverse clinical syndromes. Their constant occurrence in moist environments as typical "molds" makes their spores readily available as aerosolized infectious particles.

Etiology. *Aspergillus fumigatus* is a primary pathogen for animals and birds and is often associated with human pulmonary and systemic disease. Other species, *Aspergillus terreus* and *Aspergillus flavus,* may be associated with pulmonary lesions, tuberculosis and cancer when they grow in the necrotic tissue. Many species may grow in the bronchial mucus without involving the bronchial wall. Also, species of *Aspergillus* may be found in infected nails, otitis externa, mycotic keratitis, mycetoma and subcutaneous granulomas.

Pathology. Saprophytic growth of an *Aspergillus* in the mucus on a bronchial wall causes little or no reaction (bronchitis), does not penetrate the tissue, but may be coughed up and repeatedly cultured.

Occasionally, such a growth in the presence of a pre-existing pathologic condition (tuberculosis, carcinoma, bacterial bronchitis) will penetrate the bronchial wall and invade the lungs (Fig. 35–10).

Bronchiectatic cysts may become in-

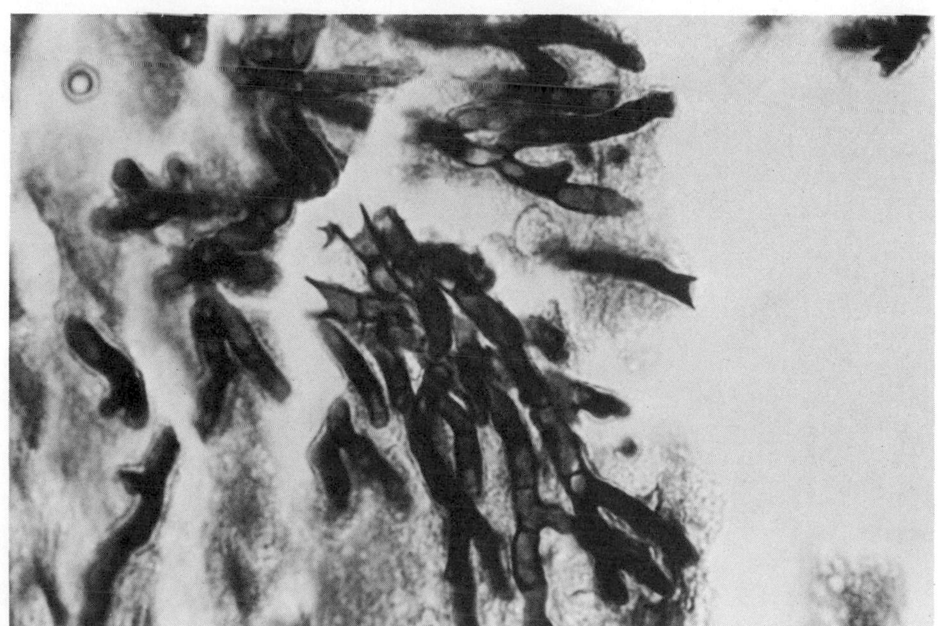

Figure 35–10. Aspergillosis. Septate, dichotomously branched hyphae in a case of fatal invasive disease. The patient was on cytotoxins as treatment for lymphoma.

vaded with *Aspergillus,* which forms a fungus ball or aspergilloma. Ordinarily, the fungus does not penetrate the epithelialized cyst wall.

Bronchopulmonary aspergillosis may result in consolidation and collapse in different areas of the lung. Secretions of mucus and cellular exudate form plugs which block the bronchi (Fig. 35–11), causing shifting shadows seen by serial radiographs.

Invasive aspergillosis is notable for the lack of cellular response. Necrosis and a pyogenic and sometimes a granulomatous reaction may be present and vary in relation to the degree of debilitation of the host.

Clinical Characteristics. Bronchial aspergillosis simulates infection by any infectious agent. Chronic bronchitis may result from prolonged ineffective antibacterial therapy, causing a harassing cough, occasionally blood-tinged expectorate and asthmatic symptoms.

Bronchiectasis of bacterial etiology may be complicated by invasion of the cysts by *Aspergillus* species. Repeated hemoptysis may ensue.

Bronchopulmonary disease is characterized by periods of pyrexia, severe cough and purulent sputum containing fungus "plugs." Expectoration of these plugs relieves bronchial blockage and symptoms.

The debilitated patient with primary disease (Hodgkin's, leukemia, lymphoma) may become secondarily infected with *Aspergillus fumigatus* and manifest the signs and symptoms of widespread systemic infection.

Diagnosis. The repeated isolation of *A. fumigatus* from the sputum, mucous plugs and other exudates from the pulmonary tree must be regarded with suspicion until a definitive diagnosis of pulmonary disease is obtained. However, the occurrence of *Aspergillus* species in known bronchiectatic lesions, tuberculosis and carcinoma may indicate serious complications.

A high eosinophilia in bronchopulmonary disease demands a differential diagnosis of pulmonary eosinophilia and bronchopulmonary aspergillosis. Fungus plugs found in the sputum in the latter disease should establish the diagnosis. Serology is also helpful.

Treatment. Allergic bronchopulmo-

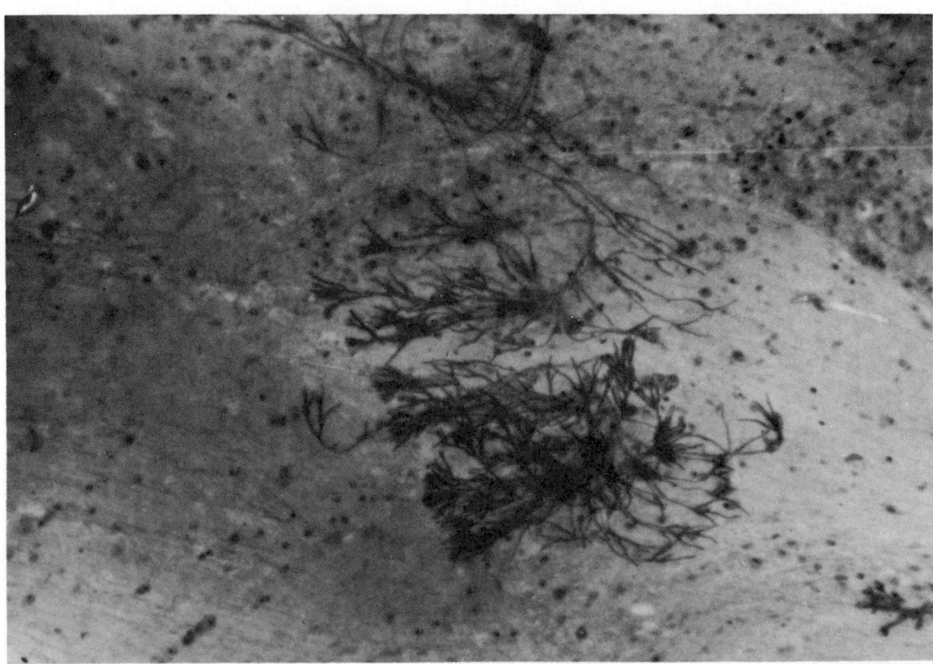

Figure 35–11. Allergic bronchopulmonary aspergillosis. *Aspergillus* growing in a mucous plug within the lumen of a bronchiole. (From J. W. Rippon. 1973. *In* Burrows, W.: Textbook of Microbiology. W. B. Saunders Co., Philadelphia. p. 737.)

nary disease is treated with steroids and good respiratory toilet. Aspergillomas require surgical intervention to prevent exsanguinating hemoptysis. Systemic disease is treated with amphotericin B but is rarely successful. No other drugs are available.

Mucormycosis

Synonyms. Phycomycosis, hyphomycosis, zygomycosis.

Definition. Mucormycosis is an infection of the sinuses, orbital tissue, central nervous system, lungs, skin or other tissue by members of the *Mucorales* order of the Zygomycetes.

Distribution. The zygomycetes are ubiquitous in nature. Members of the order *Entomophthorales* are common in leaf detritus and may cause human infection. (See Chapter 34.) A second order of the Zygomycetes, the *Mucorales,* contains some thermophilic species involved in opportunistic human infections: *Mucor, Rhizopus* and *Absidia.* All are common "molds" of warm, damp places and are found on bread, fruit and starch- and sugar-containing foods.

Etiology. *Rhizopus oryzae* and *Rhizopus arrhizus* account for most cases of rhinocerebral disease found in the acidotic diabetic.[16] Mucormycosis of the lung is associated with leukemia and malignant lymphoma. The species involved are in the genera *Rhizopus* and *Mucor.*[17] Mucormycosis of the gastrointestinal tract is associated with malnutrition particularly of children in tropical countries. It may be a sequela of kwashiorkor or marasmus.[18] Several species and genera have been isolated from such infections. The presence of wide, nonseptate hyphae in tissues (Fig. 35–12) has indicated, in the absence of cultures, infection with a member of the *Mucorales* in patients having extensive burns, leukemia and severe malnutrition.

Pathology. Cerebral mucormycosis is initiated in the uncontrolled diabetic by germination of spores contaminating the nares. Hyphal growth penetrates the tissues and extends rapidly along the walls and in the lumen of blood vessels, producing thrombi and infarction with resulting necrosis and a polymorphonuclear and lymphocytic response. The broad, nonseptate, branching hyphae stain deeply and are readily seen in H-E sections.

Invasion of the wall and lumen of the pulmonary artery and veins produces

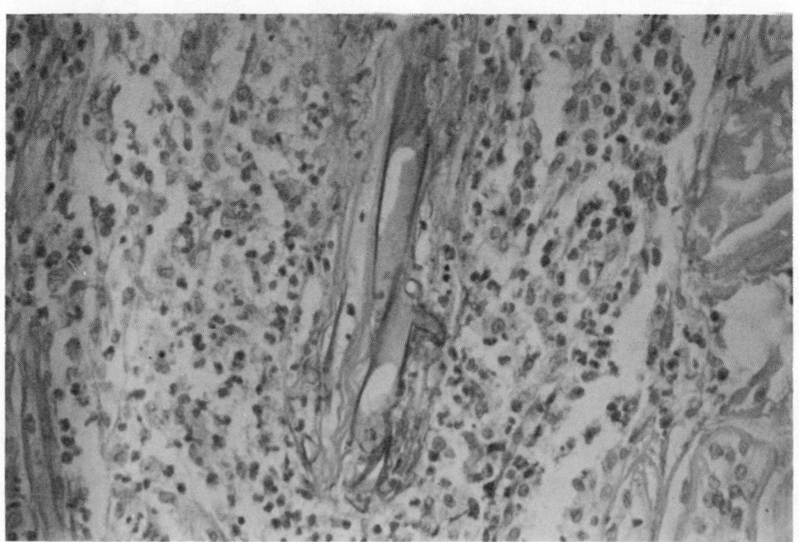

Figure 35–12. Mucormycosis. Broad nonseptate hyphae in necrotic nasal tissue from a case of rhinocerebral mucormycosis. The etiologic agent was *Rhizopus oryzae.*

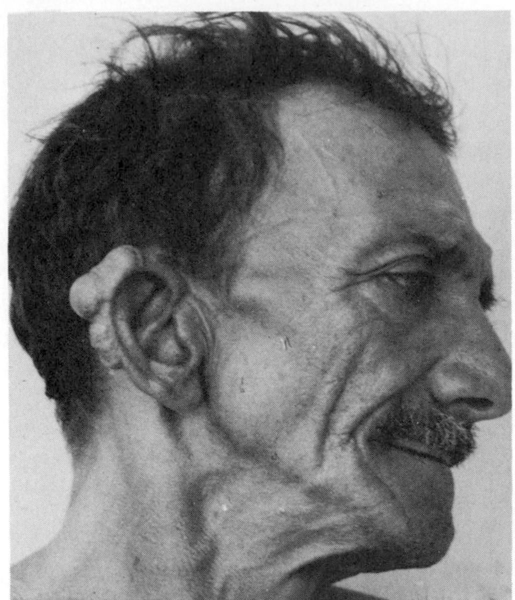

Figure 35-13. Lobomycosis. Typical keloid-like lesions on the ear. (Courtesy of Dr. F. Battistini, Universidad de Oriente, Ciudad Bolivar, Venezuela.)

thrombi and infarction. This leads to massive necrosis of the involved tissues in pulmonary infections.

Clinical Characteristics. Cerebral mucormycosis in the uncontrolled diabetic simulates a cavernous sinus thrombosis of bacterial origin. The rapidity of the infection usually precludes successful management of the patient, who presents a classic triad of acidotic diabetes mellitus, intraorbital infection and meningoencephalitis.

Pulmonary mucormycosis in the diabetic or leukemic patient usually develops rapidly as a nonspecific bronchitis and pneumonia. Signs and symptoms of thrombosis and infarction manifested by severe chest pain, pleural friction rub and bloody sputum appear.

Gastrointestinal mucormycosis presents with vague signs of gastrointestinal distress accompanied by bleeding and extensive tissue necrosis. Multiple thrombi containing fungi are seen in the major vessels at autopsy.

Diagnosis. The demonstration of wide, nonseptate hyphae in the walls and lumen of blood vessels and in the adjacent tissues allows a diagnosis of mucormycosis. Cultures of infected tissues and identification of the resulting fungus growth establish specific etiology of a given infection—*Rhizopus, Mucor, Absidia* and others.

Treatment. The primary disease, such

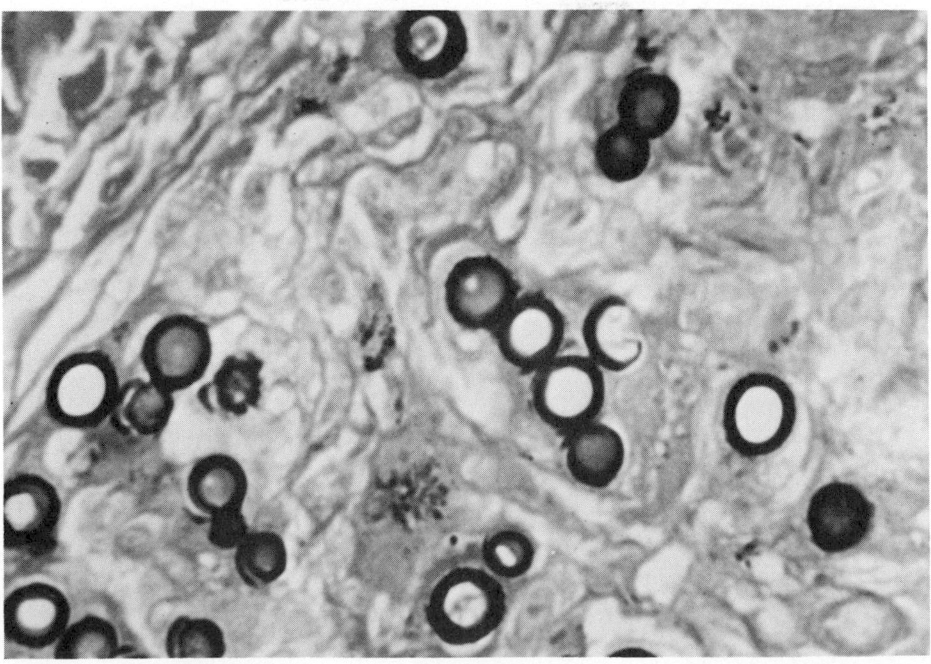

Figure 35-14. Lobomycosis. Numerous yeasts in chains of *Loboa loboi.* (From J. W. Rippon. 1973. *In* Burrows, W.: Textbook of Microbiology. W. B. Saunders Co., Philadelphia. p. 720.)

as diabetes mellitus, leukemia, lymphoma and others, should be rapidly controlled. Previous treatment with antibiotics, adrenocorticotropic hormone (ACTH), corticosteroids, antitumor drugs, and radiation therapy should be re-evaluated in the presence of suspected or proven mucormycosis.

Medical treatment with amphotericin B has proved effective in some cases when used in conjunction with surgical debridement.[17]

Miscellaneous Mycoses

There are a number of minor mycoses found in the tropics and subtropics. Among these are the superficial infections: **piedra,** a lump on the hair either black (caused by *Piedraia hortae*) or white (caused by *Trichosporon cutaneum*); and **tinea nigra,** an infection of the stratum corneum of the palm or sole, characterized by dark serpiginous blotches and caused by *Cladosporium werneckii* in Central and South America and *Cladosporium mansonii* in India, tropical Asia and Africa. **Lobomycosis** is a nodular granulomatous infection of the subcutaneous tissue caused by the as yet uncultivated fungus *Loboa loboi* (Figs. 35–13, 35–14). In tissue stains of yeasts (av. 10 μm) a keloid-like reaction is seen. It is found in northern South America in man and in dolphins in the Caribbean.

REFERENCES

Histoplasmosis

1. Ajello, L., Chick, E. W., and Furcolow, M. L. (eds.). 1971. Histoplasmosis. Proceedings of Second National Conference. Charles C Thomas, Springfield, Illinois. 516 pp.
2. Cockshott, W. P., and Lucas, A. O. 1964. Histoplasmosis duboisii. Q. J. Med. *33*:223–238.

Blastomycosis

3. Furcolow, M. L., and Smith, C. D. 1973. A new interpretation of the epidemiology, pathologenesis and ecology of *Blastomyces dermatitidis* with some additional data. Trans. N.Y. Acad. Sci. Ser. 2, *35*:421–430.
4. Lockwood, W. R., Allison, F., Jr., Batsan, B. E., and Busey, J. F. 1969. The treatment of North American blastomycosis. Ten years experience. Am. Rev. Respir. Dis. *100*:314–320.

Coccidioidomycosis

5. Ajello, L. (ed.). 1967. Coccidioidomycosis. Proceedings of Second Coccidioidomycosis Symposium. University of Arizona Press, Tucson. 434 pp.
6. Winn, W. A. 1964. The treatment of coccidioidal meningitis. The use of amphotericin B in a group of 25 patients. Calif. Med. *101*:78–89.

Paracoccidioidomycosis

7. Paracoccidioidomycosis. 1972. Proceedings of the First Pan American Symposium. P.A.H.O. Sci. Publ. No. 254, Washington, D.C. 325 pp.

Opportunistic Infections

8. Mirsky, H. S., and Cuttner, J. 1972. Fungal infections in acute leukemia. Cancer *30*:348–352.

Candidosis

9. Winner, H. I., and Hurley, R. 1964. Candida albicans. Little, Brown & Co., Boston. 300 pp.
10. Curry, C. R., and Quie, P. G. 1971. Fungal septicemia in patients receiving parenteral hyperalimentation. N. Engl. J. Med. *285*:1221–1225.

Cryptococcosis

11. Littman, M. L., and Zimmerman, L. E. 1956. Cryptococcosis. Grune & Stratton, New York. 205 pp.
12. Littman, M. L., and Walker, J. E. 1968. Cryptococcosis: current issues. Am. J. Med. *45*:922–933.

Aspergillosis

13. Golbert, T. M., and Patterson, R. 1970. Pulmonary allergic aspergillosis. Ann. Intern. Med. *72*:395–403.
14. Ikemoto, H., Watanake, K., and Mari, T. 1971. Pulmonary aspergilloma. Sabouraudia *9*:30–35.
15. Meyer, R. D., Young, L. S., Armstrong, D., and Yu, B. 1973. Aspergillosis complicating neoplastic disease. Am. J. Med. *54*:6–15.

Mucormycosis

16. Fleckner, R. A., and Goldstein, J. H. 1969. Mucormycosis. Br. J. Ophthalmol. *53*:542–548.
17. Medoff, G., and Kobayashi, S. 1972. Pulmonary mucormycosis. N. Engl. J. Med. *286*:86–87.
18. Neame, P., and Rayner, D. 1960. Mucormycosis - a report of twenty-two cases. Arch. Pathol. *70*:261–268.

SECTION VI
Protozoal Diseases

CHAPTER 36
The Intestinal Protozoa

Infection of the human intestine by certain members of the Protozoa is common in many parts of the world. This chapter deals with the morphology of several species of amebae, flagellates and sporozoa of medical importance. Of these, the ameba *Entamoeba histolytica* and the ciliate *Balantidium coli* are recognized pathogens for man. The ameba *Dientamoeba fragilis,* the flagellate *Giardia lamblia,* and the sporozoa *Isospora hominis* and *I. belli* also may cause symptomatic infections. The remaining organisms are of importance partly because of diagnostic problems which they may present and partly for the evidence they furnish as to the environment in which their host has previously lived. Those organisms whose modes of transmission are known are spread from one individual to another by contamination of food or drink with human feces. In the case of *B. coli* it is probable that infection of man originates from the pig as well as from infected humans.

The flagellate *Trichomonas vaginalis* is included in this section because of its morphologic resemblance to *T. hominis,* a resident of the human intestinal tract. A yeast, *Blastocystis hominis,* is likewise described because of its common occurrence in stools and the frequency with which it may be confused with encysted forms of certain of the intestinal protozoa.

Most of the intestinal protozoa of man pass through two stages, an active trophozoite stage and a resting nonmotile or encysted stage. The trophozoites are motile; they feed actively and undergo multiplication by binary fission. Subsequently, certain of the trophozoites cease feeding, lose their motility and secrete a cyst wall. These encysted forms, or cysts, are much less susceptible to changes of environment than are the trophozoites, and they are primarily responsible for transmission of the infection. Trophozoites do not long survive in nature, outside the favorable environment of the intestinal tract.

Identification of the individual protozoan is based upon certain specific characteristics of the trophozoite and of the cyst. These distinguishing features include the type of motility of the trophozoite, food inclusions, the number and structure of the nuclei and other morphologic details. Similarly, the encysted forms may be distinguished by differences in size and shape, by the number and structure of the nuclei, by the characteristics of chromatoidal bodies when these are present, by the amount and distribution of contained glycogen, and by other details of the internal morphology (Figs. 36–1 to 36–8). To demonstrate all of these features it is frequently necessary to examine not only unstained fresh preparations but also films stained by iodine and fixed smears stained by Heidenhain's or other iron-hematoxylin methods. The latter techniques are essential for demonstration of the finer morphologic details upon which specific identification is based.[1] These methods are described on pages 817 to 828.

Certain of the intestinal protozoa may be isolated and maintained in artificial culture media (p. 829).

The important differential features of the trophozoites and the cysts are indicated in Tables 36–2, 36–3 and 36–4.

Table 36–1. Some Important Intestinal Protozoa of Man

Organism	*Potential Pathogen*	*Always Non-Pathogenic*	*Stages of Organism*	
			Trophozoite	*Cyst*
Amebae:				
Entamoeba histolytica	+	–	+	+
E. hartmanni	–	+	+	+
E. coli	–	+	+	+
E. polecki	–	+	+	+
Iodamoeba bütschlii	–	+	+	+
Endolimax nana	–	+	+	+
Dientamoeba fragilis	?	?	+	–
Flagellates:				
Chilomastix mesnili	–	+	+	+
Trichomonas hominis	–	+	+	–
T. vaginalis	+	–	+	–
Giardia lamblia	+	–	+	+
Retortamonas intestinalis	–	+	+	+
Enteromonas hominis	–	+	+	+
Ciliate:				
Balantidium coli	+	–	+	+
Sporozoa:				
Isospora hominis	+	–	*	*
Isospora belli	+	–	*	*

*See pp. 321–322 for stages of intestinal sporozoa.

ENTAMOEBA HISTOLYTICA

Entamoeba histolytica Schaudinn, 1903 is an important pathogenic parasite of man. It localizes principally in the colon and only rarely invades the terminal ileum. Metastatic lesions, particularly of the liver, may follow invasion of the blood stream. The life cycle includes both trophozoite and encysted stages. (See p. 312 and Tables 36–1, 36–2 and 36–3 for *Entamoeba hartmanni.*)

The Trophozoite. Iron-hematoxylin–stained specimens are usually 15 to 25 μm in diameter. There is a single spherical nucleus with a delicate nuclear membrane, the inner surface of which is lightly encrusted with a layer of minute chromatin granules. Within the nucleus there is a small punctiform karyosome. Ingested erythrocytes may be present in the cytoplasm.

The living unstained organism exhibits active progressive motility, which is characteristic of this species. The ameba usually assumes a sluglike form and moves across the microscope field by continuous flowing of cytoplasm into the leading element (Fig. 36–1). This "anterior" portion or pseudopod of ectoplasm is clear and glasslike, often contrasting sharply with the less hyaline or finely granular endoplasm of the ameba. The nucleus is usually not visible. Motility is rapidly lost as the trophozoite is cooled below the temperature of the human body, at which time the distinction between the glasslike pseudopodia and the more granular endoplasm becomes more marked.

The Cyst. The cysts are spherical bodies varying from 10 to 20 μm in diameter. Young cysts are uninucleate, possessing a large ringlike nucleus which may be one-third the diameter of the cyst. As nuclear division occurs, binucleate as well as the fully developed quadrinucleate forms are produced, the size of the individual nuclei decreasing as they increase in number.

In iron-hematoxylin–stained preparations the hyaline single wall of the mature cyst is unstained and the cytoplasm appears grayish white. The delicately beaded nuclear membranes and the small, fine karyosomes

Table 36–2. SALIENT FEATURES OF VIABLE TROPHOZOITES OF SOME INTESTINAL PROTOZOA OF MAN

*Parasite**	*Size (μm) Living*	*Normal Motility*	*Pseudopodia*	*Stained Nucleus*	*Other Characteristics*
Entamoeba histolytica	10–25 (Rounded forms)	Active, progressive, streaming; cytoplasm flows into pseudopod	Tonguelike, explosively formed	Round; minute karyosome; fine chromatic lining of membrane; ringlike	Living nucleus not visible
E. coli	20–30 (Rounded forms)	Sluggish, not progressive	Blunt, hemispheric, semilunar	Round; coarse karyosome; coarse chromatic lining of membrane; ringlike	Living nucleus visible
E. polecki	16–18 (Rounded forms)	Usually sluggish	Rounded, extruded slowly, occasionally two or more	Round; karyosome usually small; nuclear membrane thin; ringlike	Living nucleus occasionally seen
Iodamoeba bütschlii	9–13 (Rounded forms)	Like *E. coli*	Like *E. coli*	Round; large round karyosome	
Endolimax nana	8–12 (Rounded forms)	Usually nonmotile; occasionally slightly progressive	Round, budlike	Round; large, irregular karyosome	
Dientamoeba fragilis	5–20 (Rounded forms)	Usually sluggish or nonmotile	Triangular (tentlike), rectangular, veil-like, cloverleaf	2 (or 1) nuclei, with mass of chromatin granules embedded in clear matrix	
Chilomastix mesnili	13–24 × 6–11	Flagellate; spiral; body rigid	– – –	Round; small eccentric or central karyosome	Body pear-shaped; buccal structures prominent; spiral twist in body
Trichomonas hominis	10–15 × 5–8	Flagellate; continuous, jerky, wobbly; body plastic	– – –	Round or oval; karyosome more or less central	3–5 anterior flagella; undulating membrane and axostyle present
T. vaginalis	10–30 × 5–15	Similar to *T. hominis*	– – –	Elongate oval; chromatin granules small and uniformly distributed	4 anterior flagella; undulating membrane short
Giardia lamblia	11–18 × 6–9	Active; tumbling and turning like falling leaves; spinning	– – –	Right and left nuclei; ovoid with prominent irregular karyosomes	Has sucking disk, 8 flagella
Retortamonas intestinalis	4–9 × 3–4	Flagellate; jerky and progressive	– – –	Round; membrane delicate; karyosome eccentric	2 anterior flagella and 2 blepharoplasts near nucleus
Enteromonas hominis	4–10 × 3–6	Similar to *R. intestinalis*	– – –	Ovoid; membrane delicate; karyosome large	Body pear-shaped; 3 anterior flagella and 1 along flattened surface and extending free posteriorly
Balantidium coli	50–70 × 30–60	Ciliate; strong progressive swimmer; rapid, gliding	– – –	Macronucleus sausage-shaped; micronucleus ovoid or round	**V**-shaped peristome; anus at posterior end

*See page 312 and Table 36–1 for information on *Entamoeba hartmanni;* similar in morphology to *E. histolytica,* but smaller and nonpathogenic.

Table 36–3. Salient Features of Cysts of Some Intestinal Protozoa of Man

*Parasite**	*Usual Shape*	*Usual Size (μm)*	*Number Nuclei*	*Nuclear Karyosome*	*Glycogen Mass (In Iodine)*	*Chromatoidal Bodies*	*Other Characteristics*
Entamoeba histolytica	Round	10–15	1–4	Small granule	Diffuse, brown. In young cysts	Rod-shaped or thick bars	In fresh unstained cyst: nuclei not visible; chromatoids conspicuous when present
E. coli	Round	15–20	1–8	Coarser than in *E. histolytica*	Large, deep brown. In young cysts	Splinterlike, or filamentous	Nuclei usually visible in unstained cyst; cyst wall heavy
E. polecki	Round	12–14	1; rarely 2	Large, massed	– –	Rod-shaped or spherical; ends angular, pointed or round	Spherical, ovoid or irregular inclusion body may be present
Iodamoeba bütschlii	Ovoid; round	6–15	1–2	Bulky, round	Large or small, sharply delimited, deep brown	None	Usually granular mass next to karyosome
Endolimax nana	Ovoid; round	7–10 × 6–7	1–4	Eccentric mass	Occasionally present in young cysts	None	Often cytoplasmic volutin granules confused with karyosomes
Chilomastix mesnili	Lemon-shaped	7–9 × 4.5–6	1	Mass at one pole	Sometimes present	None	Oral apparatus beside nucleus
Giardia lamblia	Ovoid	8–12 × 6–10	4	Punctiform, central	None	None	Nuclei at anterior pole; fibrils in cytoplasm
Retortamonas intestinalis	Pear-shaped	4–7 × 3–5	1	Slightly eccentric	None	None	Cyst wall appears double in fresh preparations; margin of cytostome may show when stained
Enteromonas hominis	Elongate; ovoid	6–8 × 4–6	1–4	Small; central	None	None	1 or 2 nuclei at each end; well defined cyst wall
Balantidium coli	Round	50–65	1 macronucleus 1 micronucleus	– –	None	None	Macronucleus kidney-shaped, large, conspicuous; contractile vacuole present
Isospora hominis	Ovoid	Sporocyst 10 × 15	– –	– –	None	None	Oocyst wall usually absent; sporocysts single or paired
I. belli	Ovoid	Oocyst 12 × 30	– –	– –	None	None	Oocyst wall present; 2 sporocysts 9 × 11μm each within oocyst wall
Blastocystis hominis (A yeast, not a protozoan)	Round	10–15	1–8	– –	None	None	Nuclei marginal, between inner and outer wall

*See page 312 for information on *Entamoeba hartmanni;* morphologically similar to *E. histolytica*, but cysts are less than 10 μm in size.

Table 36–4. Differentiation of Common Intestinal Amebae in Direct Fecal Smears of Unpreserved Fresh Stools

Trophozoites

Unstained Saline Smear (Fig. 36–7)

1 (4) Trophozoites usually large (except for "small races," i.e. *E. hartmanni**) 2
2 (3) Progressive motility with cytoplasm flowing into pseudopod; motile forms have sluglike shape; may contain ingested red cells; nucleus usually not visible without stain (Fig. 36–1) .... *E. histolytica*
3 (2) No progressive motility; cytoplasm does not flow into pseudopod; blunt pseudopodia extended and retracted; a ringlike nucleus frequently visible unstained .... *E. coli*
4 (1) Trophozoites usually small or medium sized; ordinarily motility is sluggish 5
5 (6, 7) Pseudopodia often blunt or round, resembling a yeast budding .... *E. nana*
6 (5, 7) Pseudopodia angular (triangular or tentlike), rectangular or lobulated; outline of nonmotile trophozoites perfectly round or cystlike .... *D. fragilis*
7 (5, 6) Pseudopodia blunt; resemble small *E. coli* trophozoites .... *I. bütschlii*

Iodine-Stained Smear

1 (2) Ringlike nucleus present .... *E. histolytica* or *E. coli*
2 (1) Ringlike nucleus absent .... *E. nana, I. bütschlii* or *D. fragilis*
(Differentiation of trophozoites of the above species must be made from saline or iron-hematoxylin–stained smears.)

Cysts

Unstained Saline Smears (Fig. 36–7)

1 (3) Chromatoidal bars (rodlike or sausage-shaped) if present (Fig. 36–2) 2
2 Present in *some* infections .... *E. histolytica**
3 (1) Chromatoidal bars always absent .... Other amebae

Iodine-Stained Smear (Fig. 36–8)

1 (4) Ringlike nuclei present 2
2 (3) Medium sized (10–15 μm) or small cysts with 1 to 4 nuclei .... *E. histolytica**
3 (2) Large cysts with 5 or more nuclei .... *E. coli*
(Immature cysts of *E. coli*—with less than 5 nuclei—may be identified by the similarity of their size and cytoplasm to mature cysts in same smear.)
4 (1) Ringlike nuclei absent 5
5 (6) Small, round or oval cyst with nuclei appearing as vacuole-like areas .... *E. nana*
6 (5) Medium sized cyst with dark brown mass sharply delimited from the cytoplasm... *I. bütschlii*

*Small trophozoites and cysts (less than 10 μm in diameter) probably represent *Entamoeba hartmanni*, which are similar in morphology to *E. histolytica*, but nonpathogenic. (See p. 312 and Table 36–1.)

are deep black, and blunt-ended black-stained chromatoidal bodies are occasionally present in the cytoplasm.

In unstained fresh smears the colorless cytoplasm has a finely granular appearance, and the nuclei can only rarely be seen as delicate rings of fine refractile granules. In young or immature cysts chromatoidal bars are commonly but not invariably observed. These appear as blunt-ended rods or rounded bodies which are more refractive than the cytoplasm of the cyst. They are distinctive (Fig. 36–2). The chromatoidal bodies of *E. histolytica* contain RNA particles arranged in a crystalline lattice which accounts for its different refractive index.

In iodine-stained preparations the cysts of *E. histolytica* can usually be differentiated from the cysts of the other intestinal protozoa. The cytoplasm appears yellowish in color and occasionally contains a diffuse mass of glycogen staining mahogany brown. The nuclei, which resemble gold wedding rings, are readily seen. Although the chromatoidal bodies may be visible, they are more easily seen in the unstained or hematoxylin-stained smears or in iodine-stained preparations of formalin-ether concentrates.

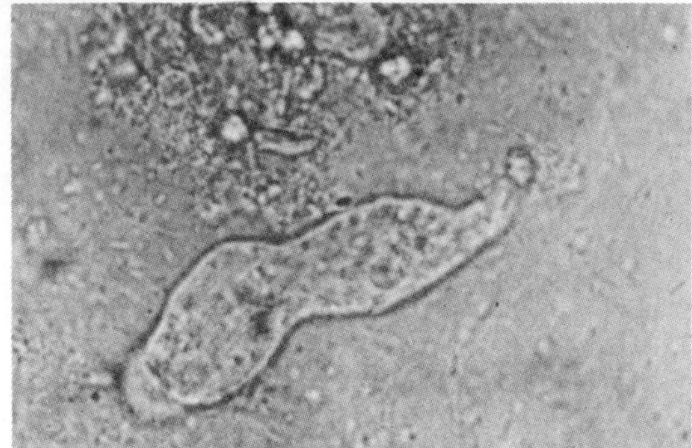

Figure 36-1. Trophozoite of *Entamoeba histolytica* with a sluglike form. (Photomicrograph from Army Medical Museum Collection.)

As indicated in Tables 36-1, 36-2 and 36-3, small races of *E. histolytica* occur. Frequently the term "small race" is applied when the average cyst diameter is less than 10 μm. However, the name *Entamoeba hartmanni* is widely accepted for the "small race of *E. histolytica*" based upon the size difference and the assumption that these forms are nonpathogenic. There is evidence that the size of strains of *E. histolytica* may change.[2] Further, at times some strains of small size may invade tissue. There is, however, evidence of antigenic difference between larger strains of *E. histolytica* and the so-called "small race of *E. histolytica*" as measured by microfluorimetric techniques.[3] Another proposal to the effect that morphologic differentiation can be made between a true small race of *E. histolytica* and *E. hartmanni* has added complexity to the specific identity of the small forms.[4] No doubt there are noninvasive luminal forms of *E. histolytica*. Parasitism by strains of *E. histolytica* may occur in humans without production of lesions, and a state of commensalism may exist.[5] However, whether intestinal infection will remain confined to the lumen of the intestine or will be followed by tissue invasion and produce clinical disease is unpredictable.[6] Factors may change and, as a result, conditions in the intestine may supervene which permit invasion of the wall. From the practical standpoint, the interest of the patient should be borne in mind when amebae with typical characteristics of *E. histolytica* are encountered.

ENTAMOEBA COLI

Entamoeba coli (Grassi, 1879) Casagrandi and Barbagallo, 1895 is a common nonpathogenic ameba of the human colon. Its importance lies in possible confusion with *E. histolytica.* Its presence in the stool provides evidence concerning the sanitary environment to which the host has been exposed. The life cycle includes both trophozoite and encysted stages. The average prepatent period in human experimental infections was 10 days.[7]

The Trophozoite. The motile ameba averages 20 to 30 μm in diameter. In iron-hematoxylin-stained smears the single nucleus is relatively large and coarse. The nuclear membrane is thicker and the chromatin granules larger than in *E. histolytica,* whereas the karyosome is coarser. The cytoplasm is coarsely granular and typically contains many food inclusions, such as bacteria, yeasts and detritus.

The living unstained organism is sluggishly motile, extending and withdrawing pseudopodia with little progressive motion. The pseudopodia are shorter and more blunt than those of *E. histolytica.* The nucleus is frequently visible, appearing as a large refractile ring containing a small hyaline

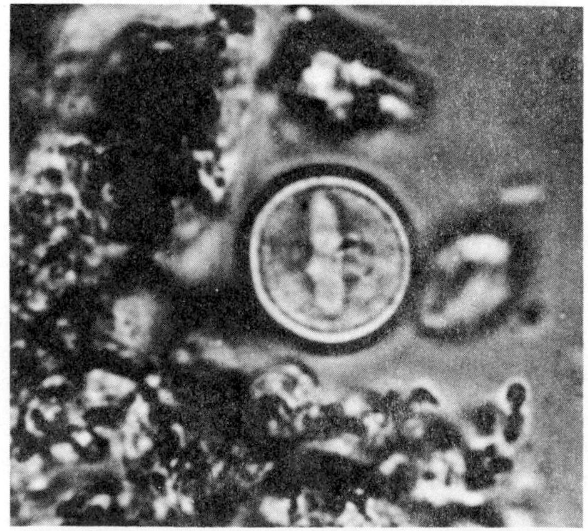

Figure 36-2. Cyst of *E. histolytica* in unstained portion of a direct fecal smear. A chromatoidal body with typical rodlike shape and blunt ends is visible. (Courtesy of the Louisiana State University School of Medicine, New Orleans.)

mass representing the karyosome (Fig. 36–7). This ameba rarely ingests red blood cells.

The Cyst. The cysts of *E. coli* are spherical or ovoid bodies, usually ranging between 15 and 20 μm in diameter. The younger forms are uninucleate or binucleate. Successive nuclear divisions occur to produce the characteristic eight nuclei of the mature cyst; rarely, there may be 16 to 32. The individual nucleus decreases in size and becomes more delicate with each division.

In iron-hematoxylin–stained smears the cyst wall is unstained. The nuclear membrane is heavier than that of *E. histolytica,* and the chromatin granules are coarser. The karyosome is relatively large. Chromatoidals are occasionally observed in immature cysts and characteristically appear as black-staining splinterlike bodies or as masses with jagged ends (Fig. 36–3).

In unstained fresh smears some of the nuclei are often visible. The chromatoidal bodies likewise may be seen when present. The contour of the latter and the visibility of the nuclei in unstained preparations have diagnostic significance (Fig. 36–7).

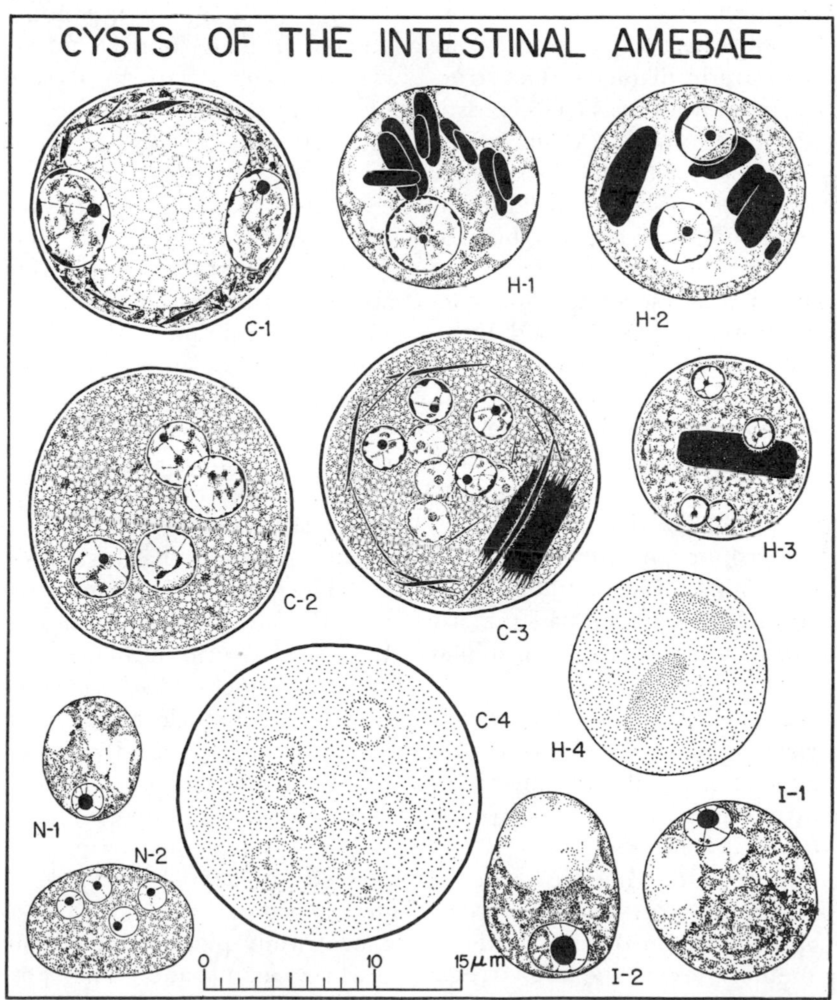

Figure 36–3. *C-1,* Iron-hematoxylin–stained binucleate cyst of *Entamoeba coli. C-2,* Iron-hematoxylin–stained quadrinucleate cyst of *E. coli. C-3,* Iron-hematoxylin–stained mature cyst of *E. coli. C-4,* Unstained mature cyst of *E. coli. H-1,* Iron-hematoxylin–stained uninucleate cyst of *Entamoeba histolytica. H-2,* Iron-hematoxylin–stained binucleate cyst of *E. histolytica. H-3,* Iron-hematoxylin–stained mature cyst of *E. histolytica. H-4,* Unstained cyst of *E. histolytica* showing chromatoidal bars. *N-1,* Iron-hematoxylin–stained uninucleate cyst of *Endolimax nana. N-2,* Iron-hematoxylin–stained mature cysts of *E. nana. I-1, I-2,* Iron-hematoxylin-stained mature cysts of *Iodamoeba bütschlii.*

The ringlike nuclei are clearly visible in iodine-stained smears and, when present, the glycogen mass stains a deep mahogany brown (Fig. 36–8). The splinterlike chromatoidal bodies usually do not appear.

ENDOLIMAX NANA

Endolimax nana (Wenyon and O'Connor, 1917) Brug, 1918 is a small nonpathogenic ameba of man. Both trophozoite and encysted stages are known. The bionomics of infections with *E. nana* have been studied in human volunteers. The average prepatent period was 12 days.[8]

The Trophozoite. The trophozoite averages 8 to 10 μm in diameter. The structure of the spherical nucleus is characteristic and diagnostic in iron-hematoxylin–stained smears. The nuclear membrane lacks chromatin beading. The karyosome is large, irregular or lobulated in shape and may be central or eccentric in position. The cytoplasm is granular and vacuolated and contains bacteria, yeasts and other food inclusions. Red blood cells are not ingested.

In fresh unstained preparations the trophozoite is sluggishly motile, extruding and withdrawing short blunt hyaline pseudopodia but exhibiting little progressive motion. Often, round pseudopodia are present. These give the trophozoite the appearance of budding (Fig. 36–7). The trophozoites of *E. nana* are approximately one-half the size of those of *E. histolytica* and *E. coli,* but similar in size to *E. hartmanni.*

The Cyst. The cysts are thin-walled, oval or spherical bodies varying from 7 to 10 μm in diameter. The single nucleus of the young form undergoes division to produce the mature four-nucleate cyst.

The structure of the nucleus is clearly shown in iron-hematoxylin–stained preparations. The absence of chromatin beads on the nuclear membrane and the large irregular eccentric karyosome are characteristic (Fig. 36–3).

The nuclei are usually not visible in fresh unstained preparations, and chromatoidal bars are absent (Fig. 36–7). In iodine-stained smears the nuclei appear as punched-out holes, resembling small vacuoles. A small dot, representing the karyosome, sometimes may be detected on the periphery of the vacuolelike nuclear outline. In contrast to *E. histolytica* and *E. coli,* the nuclei do not appear ringlike in iodine-stained smears (Fig. 36–8). The absence of ringlike nuclei in *E. nana* is of importance in differentiating it from *E. hartmanni.*

IODAMOEBA BÜTSCHLII

Iodamoeba bütschlii (v. Prowazek, 1911) Dobell, 1919 is a nonpathogenic intestinal ameba of man. Both trophozoite and encysted stages occur in its life cycle. The prepatent period in human volunteers who received cysts of *I. bütschlii* averaged about 7 days.[8]

The Trophozoite. In iron-hematoxylin–stained preparations the trophozoite averages 9 to 13 μm in diameter. The large spherical nucleus consists of an achromatic nuclear membrane and a very large, deeply stained round karyosome. The cytoplasm contains bacteria, yeasts and other inclusions. This ameba does not ingest red blood cells. In unstained warm smears from freshly passed stools, the ameba exhibits sluggish progressive motility and protruding, broad hyaline pseudopodia (Fig. 36–7).

The Cyst. The cysts are very irregular in shape, a distinctive characteristic, and vary from 6 to 15 μm in diameter. The cysts are relatively thick-walled, usually uninucleate, occasionally binucleate, and characteristically contain a large round or oval, sharply demarcated glycogen mass.

In iron-hematoxylin–stained preparations the single nucleus presents a thin unbeaded nuclear membrane. The large, deeply stained, round karyosome is often eccentrically placed and in contact with the nuclear membrane. The position of the glycogen mass is indicated by a large vacuole (Fig. 36–3).

In unstained smears the nucleus is usually not visible, and the glycogen mass appears as a vacuole (Fig. 36–7).

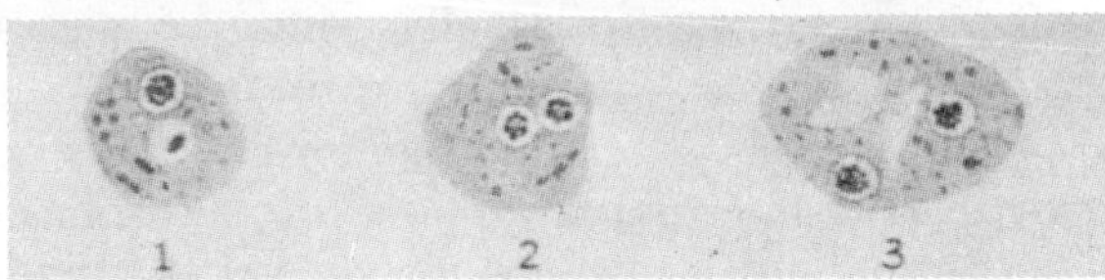

Figure 36–4. *Dientamoeba fragilis. 1,* Uninucleate ameba; *2, 3,* Binucleate amebae. (After Dobell and O'Connor. *In* Craig, C. F.: Amebiasis and Amebic Dysentery. Charles C Thomas, Springfield, Illinois.)

In iodine-stained preparations the large, sharply defined, deep mahogany colored glycogen body is the most striking feature of the cyst (Fig. 36–8). The single nucleus usually does not appear ringlike. Occasionally, a small yellow mass representing the karyosome may be visible if not obscured by the glycogen mass.

DIENTAMOEBA FRAGILIS

Dientamoeba fragilis Jepps and Dobell, 1918 is known only in the trophozoite stage. An encysted stage has not been identified, and the exact means of transmission are in doubt.

The Trophozoite. This ameba varies from 5 to 20 μm in diameter. A majority of the specimens seen are binucleate. The structure is characteristic in iron-hematoxylin–stained preparations. The nuclear membranes of the two nuclei are very delicate and often invisible. The centrally placed, coarse, lobulated karyosome is composed of a group of chromatin granules (Fig. 36–4). The cytoplasm is granular and contains a variety of food inclusions. Red blood cells are not ingested.

In warm smears from freshly passed stools, these amebae at first appear as immobile spherical bodies. After a variable period sluggish, usually nonprogressive motility begins.

The pseudopodia are clear, glasslike, sharply differentiated from the endoplasm and characteristically triangular, rectangular or clover-leaf in outline (Fig. 36–7). The nuclei are rarely visible. Motility ceases promptly on cooling, and the ameba rounds up into a spherical body.

OTHER AMEBAE

ENTAMOEBA POLECKI

Entamoeba polecki von Prowazek, 1912 is an apparently rare intestinal parasite of man. Originally it was described from pigs and later from monkeys, sheep and cattle. The life cycle includes both trophozoite and cyst stages.

The Trophozoite. This ameba measures between 10 and 25 μm, with an average of 16 to 18 μm. Its motility in normally passed stools is sluggish, like *Entamoeba coli.* Pseudopodia are generally rounded, extruded slowly and, occasionally, two or more may be extended at the same time from different sides of the ameba. In warm, liquid stools, progression may resemble *E. histoly-*

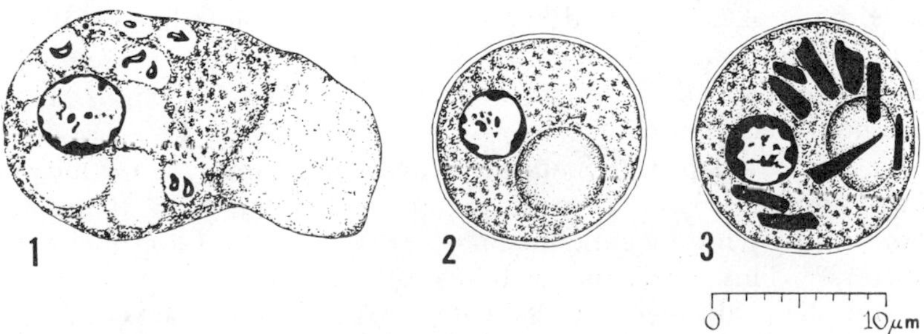

Figure 36–5. *1,* Trophozoite of *Entamoeba polecki.* Note coarse vacuoles. *2,* Cyst of *E. polecki* showing inclusion mass, but without chromatoidal bodies. *3,* Cyst of *E. polecki* with oval inclusion mass and chromatoidal masses, which are rod-shaped, some with rounded ends but most with angular ends. Adapted from Kessel and Johnstone. (Courtesy of the Louisiana State University School of Medicine, New Orleans.)

tica. The trophozoites of *E. polecki* are coarsely vacuolated and usually contain ingested bacteria, yeasts and other protozoa. A distinct line of demarcation generally exists between the endoplasm and the ectoplasm. The nucleus is occasionally seen in the living organism. It is generally round or slightly oval. The karyosome usually is small, consisting of a single granule or cluster of granules, but variations occur. The nuclear membrane is thin.[9, 10] (See Fig. 36–5.)

The Cyst. The cysts contain a single nucleus, rarely two. The chromatoidal masses are rod-shaped or spherical. The rods possess angular or rounded ends, the angular ends at times being pointed. The karyosome is usually massed and large, occasionally being small and at times dispersed. A spherical, ovoid or irregular inclusion body may be visible in the cyst (Fig. 36–5). This structure differentiates it from *E. histolytica* or *E. coli.*

Entamoeba polecki is apparently nonpathogenic for man and appears also to be a commensal in its other known hosts.

This ameba is less easy to culture and responds less readily to amebicidal therapy than *E. histolytica.*[9]

ENTAMOEBA MOSHKOVSKII

Entamoeba moshkovskii Tshalaia, 1941 was discovered in sewage. It resembles *E. histolytica* closely in both its trophozoite and cyst stages. This apparently free-living ameba has a wide geographic distribution as it has been reported from Russia, England, Italy, Singapore, parts of Central and South America, the United States and Canada. *Entamoeba moshkovskii* probably does not parasitize man and is not infective for rats.[11] However, it may be able to adapt to a parasitic existence, since abscesses have been produced experimentally by intrahepatic inoculation of hamsters.[12] This ameba is an anaerobe and can be cultivated at 24° C (75.2° F) as well as at 37° C (98.6° F).[11] Antigenically it is different from most strains of *E. histolytica* with which it has been compared by means of fluorescent antibody techniques.[13]

GIARDIA LAMBLIA

The flagellate *Giardia lamblia* Stiles, 1915 inhabits the duodenum, the upper jejunum and occasionally the gallbladder of man. The life cycle comprises both trophozoite and encysted stages.

The Trophozoite. This flagellate resembles a longitudinally cut pear in shape and measures 11 to 18 μm in length by 6 to 9 μm in width. It is convex dorsally and concave ventrally, with an ovoid sucking disk occupying the anterior ventral surface. There are eight flagella. It has been shown by electron microscopy that the ovoid disk is a rigid structure connected to the exterior by a canal containing flagella. The beating of the flagella is believed to produce a negative pressure in the concavity for attachment to the mucosa. Multiplication occurs by longitudinal fission.

The detailed structure is visible only in iron-hematoxylin preparations (Fig. 36–6). A pair of axostyles, originating anteriorly from a pair of blepharoplasts, are continued backward to extend posteriorly as flagella. The two anteriorly situated nuclei lie on either side of the axostyles. Three additional pairs of flagella, an anterolateral, a posterolateral and a ventral, originate from the blepharoplasts. The cytoplasm does not contain food inclusions or red blood cells.

In fresh unstained preparations the trophozoite is actively motile, combining irregular progression, rotation and rocking movements. The eight flagella become visible only as motility almost ceases. The cytoplasm is hyaline or finely granular in appearance.

The Cyst. The cysts of *G. lamblia* are ovoid in contour. They measure 8 to 12 μm in length and 6 to 10 μm in width. They contain two to four nuclei, usually situated near one pole.

In iron-hematoxylin–stained preparations the individual nucleus is seen to consist of a delicate nuclear membrane and a small central or eccentrically placed karyosome.

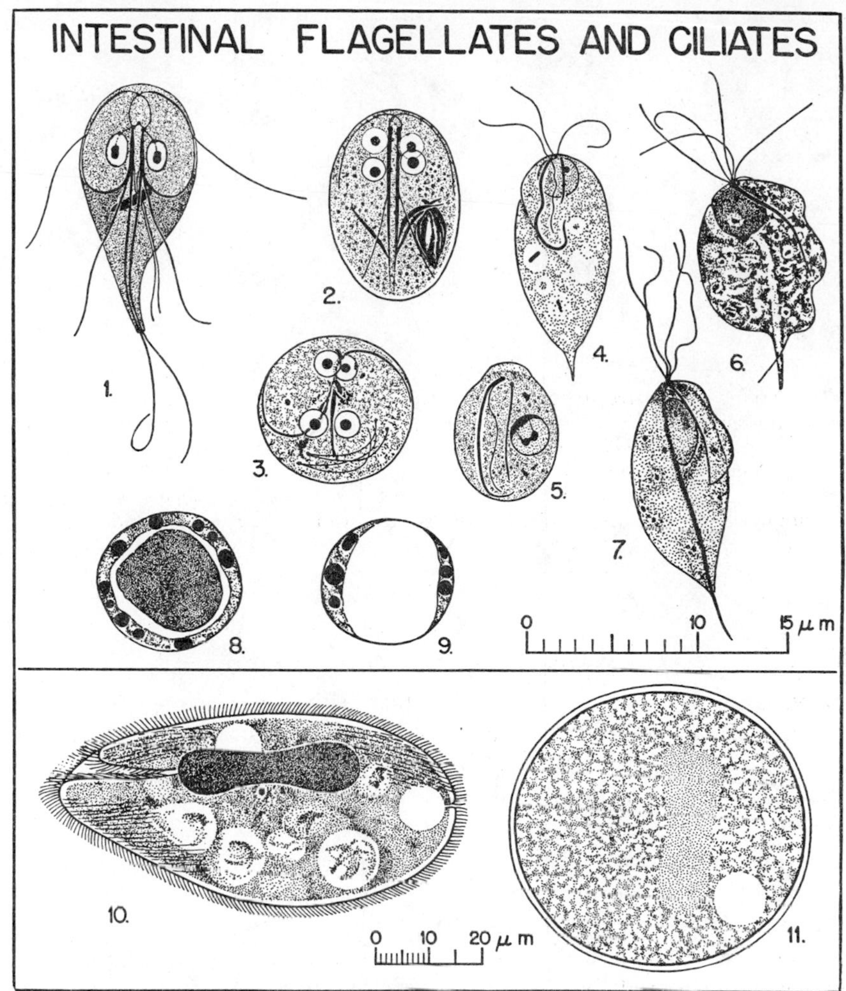

Figure 36–6. *1,* Iron-hematoxylin–stained trophozoite of *Giardia lamblia. 2,* Iron-hematoxylin–stained cyst of *G. lamblia. 3,* Iron-hematoxylin–stained cyst of *G. lamblia* end-view. *4,* Iron-hematoxylin–stained trophozoite of *Chilomastix mesnili. 5,* Iron-hematoxylin–stained cyst of *C. mesnili. 6,* Iron hematoxylin–stained trophozoite of *Trichomonas hominis. 7,* Iron-hematoxylin–stained trophozoite of *Trichomonas vaginalis. 8,* Iron-hematoxylin–stained *Blastocystis hominis. 9,* Unstained *B. hominis. 10,* Trophozoite of *Balantidium coli. 11,* Unstained cyst of *B. coli.*

The axostyles appear as two longitudinally placed curved rods, and the flagella as groups of stained fibrils (Fig. 36–6).

In unstained smears the cysts appear as ovoid, colorless, hyaline bodies with a thick cyst wall in which refractile structures, representing the axostyles and flagella, may sometimes be seen.

In iodine-stained smears the longitudinal axostyles and fibrils representing the flagella may be seen; usually the nuclei are indistinct (Fig. 36–8). The cytoplasm stains a brownish color and may contain diffuse glycogen.

CHILOMASTIX MESNILI

Chilomastix mesnili (Wenyon, 1910) Alexeiff, 1912 is a nonpathogenic flagellate inhabiting the large intestine of man. It is frequently found in normal individuals in many parts of the world. Both trophozoite and encysted stages occur in its life cycle.

The Trophozoite. This flagellate is 13 to 24 μm in length and 6 to 11 μm in breadth. Occasionally, minute, almost spherical forms less than 5 μm in length are observed. The typical specimen has a rigid pear-shaped body with a spiral groove and is

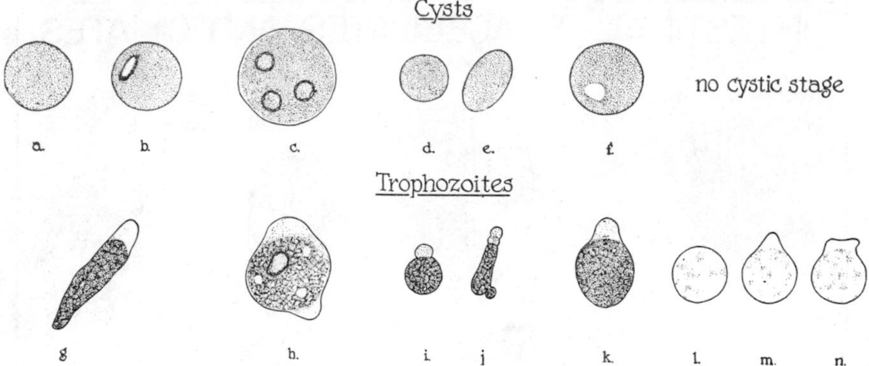

Figure 36–7. Cysts (a–f) and trophozoites (g–n) of common intestinal amebae in direct saline fecal smears, fresh, unpreserved, unstained. *a, Entamoeba histolytica,* no nuclei visible. *b, E. histolytica* with refractile chromatoidal bar. *c, Entamoeba coli* with a few ringlike nuclei visible. *d, e, Endolimax nana,* small and round or elongate-oval. *f, Iodamoeba bütschlii,* glycogen vacuole slightly refractile. *g,* Sluglike trophozoite of *E. histolytica,* nucleus not visible. *h, E. coli,* nucleus visible. *i, j,* Budlike pseudopodia of *E. nana. k, I. bütschlii. l, Dientamoeba fragilis,* spherical shape. *m, n, D. fragilis,* triangular and rectangular pseudopodia. (Courtesy of Dr. J. C. Swartzwelder in Am. J. Clin. Pathol., *22*:379–395, 1952.)

pointed at the posterior end. Multiplication occurs by binary fission.

In iron-hematoxylin–stained preparations the spiral groove is clearly visible. The cytoplasm is finely granular. A mouthlike cytostome, appearing as a cleft, originates anteriorly and extends posteriorly for nearly one-half the length of the body. The nucleus, situated anteriorly near the point of origin of the cytostome, has a well defined nuclear membrane and a small, round, centrally or eccentrically placed karyosome. Three free anterior flagella and one oral flagellum originate from a blepharoplast complex in the anterior portion of the organism (Fig. 36–6).

In warm smears from freshly passed stools the trophozoites are actively motile, progressing in a jerky, spiral fashion. The cytoplasm is colorless or faintly greenish. In sluggishly motile specimens the three anterior flagella, the cytostome and the spiral groove may be visible.

The Cyst. The cysts of *C. mesnili* are ovoid in shape, averaging 7 to 9 μm in length by 4.5 to 6 μm in breadth. A blunt protuberance at one pole gives them a lemon-shaped appearance. There is a single spherical nucleus.

In iron-hematoxylin–stained smears the nuclear membrane is distinct, and the karyosome may be central or eccentric and in contact with the nuclear membrane. The condensed cytostome is longitudinally placed in close proximity to the nucleus. The flagella may appear as dark-stained fibrils (Fig. 36–6).

In unstained preparations the cysts are colorless, and the internal structures are not visible.

In iodine preparations they are stained yellowish brown, and the nucleus and cytostome may sometimes be faintly seen (Fig. 36–8). One or more small glycogen masses may rarely be demonstrated.

TRICHOMONAS HOMINIS

The flagellate *Trichomonas hominis* (Davaine, 1860) Leuckart, 1879 is an inhabitant of the large intestine of man. It is widely distributed throughout the world. Only the trophozoite stage is known. *Trichomonas hominis* is nonpathogenic. When diarrhea of nonparasitic etiology occurs, the flagellate may flourish and become the predominant organism in the stool. It is possible that, under such conditions, *T. hominis* may prolong a diarrhea initially of other etiology. Symptomatic treatment to control the diarrhea results in reduction in the numbers of the trophozoites.

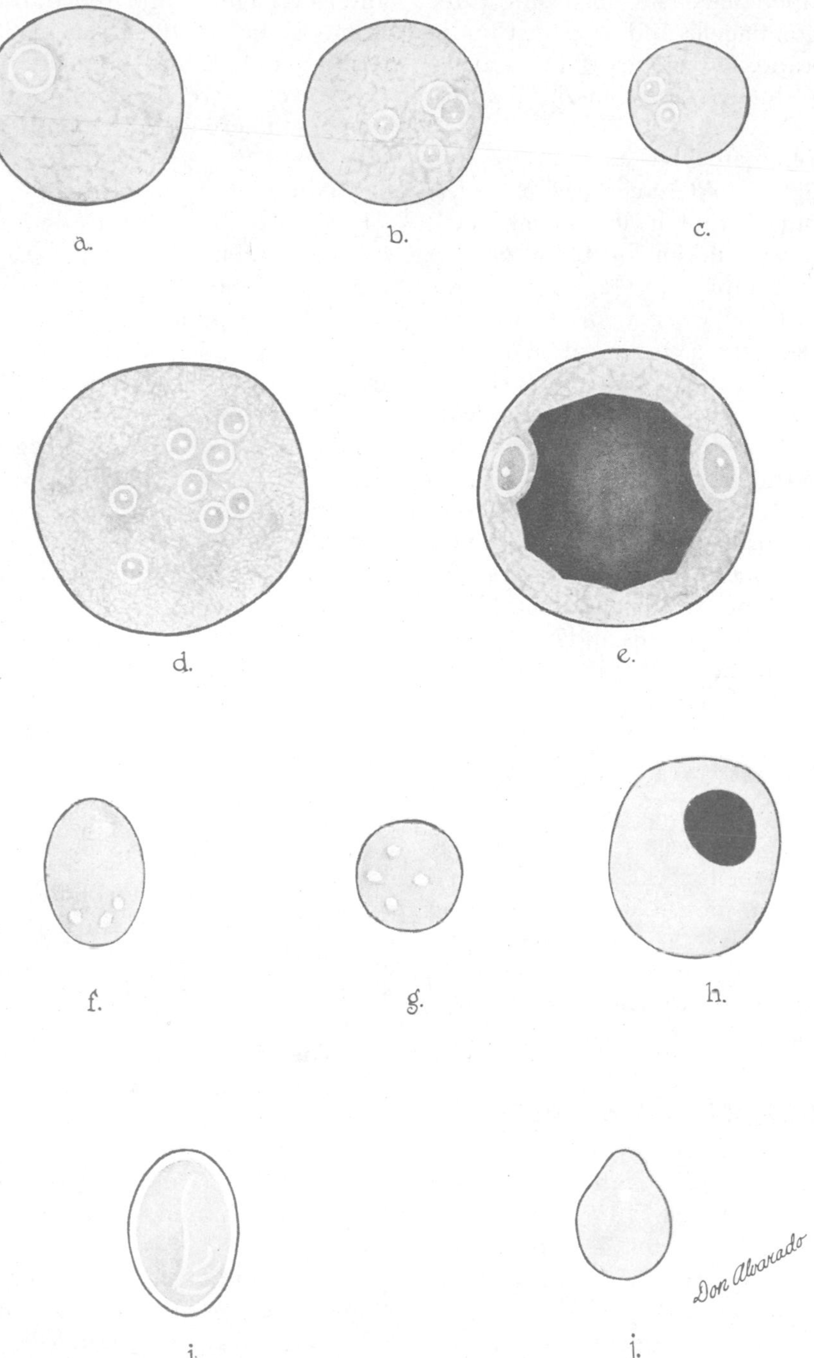

Figure 36–8. Cysts of some intestinal protozoa in direct fecal smears, fresh, unpreserved, iodine-stained. *a,* Uninucleate cyst of *Entamoeba histolytica. b,* Quadrinucleate cyst of *E. histolytica. c, Entamoeba hartmanni* ("small race" of *E. histolytica*). *d,* Mature cyst of *Entamoeba coli. e,* Immature cyst of *E. coli. f, g, Endolimax nana. h, Iodamoeba bütschlii. i, Giardia lamblia. j, Chilomastix mesnili.* (Courtesy of the Louisiana State University School of Medicine, New Orleans.)

The Trophozoite. *Trichomonas hominis* is a pear-shaped flagellate possessing three to five anterior flagella and a distinct undulating membrane. It averages 10 to 14 μm in length. Reproduction is by longitudinal fission.

In iron-hematoxylin–stained preparations the single ovoid nucleus with central karyosome and delicate nuclear membrane is visible near the anterior or blunt end. A blepharoplast complex just anterior to the nucleus provides the origin of: (1) the anterior flagella; (2) a marginal flagellum, which shortly leaves the body to form the edge of the undulating membrane; and (3) an axostyle, which is continued longitudinally through the body and protrudes posteriorly for a variable distance (Fig. 36–6).

In fresh unstained preparations it exhibits active, wobbly progressive motion due to the activity of the flagella and the undulating membrane. The nucleus and other internal structures are not visible in the colorless finely granular cytoplasm.

TRICHOMONAS TENAX

One other species, *T. tenax* (O. F. Müller, 1773) Dobell, 1939, has been found only in the human mouth, where it occurs in dental cavities, in alveolar pus pockets and in the tartar of the teeth. It is the only flagellate known to inhabit the human mouth and is nonpathogenic.

TRICHOMONAS VAGINALIS

Although it does not inhabit the intestine, *T. vaginalis* Donné, 1837 is discussed here with related flagellates. The usual habitats of *T. vaginalis* are the vagina, urethra and the prostate gland. This flagellate is observed much more frequently in women than in men. It is pathogenic and may be associated particularly with a form of vaginitis. It is widely distributed throughout the world. Multiplication occurs by longitudinal fission. This organism is known only in the trophozoite stage.

The Trophozoite. *Trichomonas vaginalis* closely resembles *T. hominis.* It is larger, measuring 10 to 30 μm in length; there are four anterior flagella, and the undulating membrane is shorter than that of *T. hominis,* extending only about one-half the length of the body, where its marginal flagellum terminates. There is no free posterior flagellum (Fig. 36–6).

Although the three species of *Trichomonas* have distinct morphologic and biologic differences, all possess an undulating membrane. When the motility of trichomonads is sufficiently slow, the rippling wavelike motion of the undulating membrane may be observed. For practical purposes, the presence of an undulating membrane on a flagellate in (1) vaginal secretion, urine or prostatic fluid, (2) stool and (3) material from the oral cavity is sufficient to identify it as to species by its source: *T. vaginalis, T. hominis* and *T. tenax,* respectively.

BALANTIDIUM COLI

Balantidium coli (Malmsten, 1857) Stein, 1862 is the only ciliate pathogenic for man. It inhabits the large intestine and less commonly the lower portion of the ileum. *Balantidium coli* is widely distributed throughout the world. Forms morphologically indistinguishable from *B. coli* in man parasitize the pig, various species of monkeys, and rats. Both trophozoite and encysted stages occur in its life cycle.

The Trophozoite. *Balantidium coli* is the largest of the protozoan parasites of man, 50 to 70 μm in length by 30 to 60 μm in breadth. It is ovoid in shape and actively motile. Multiplication occurs by transverse binary fission and by conjugation of two trophozoites.

In iron-hematoxylin–stained preparations the external surface is seen to be covered with cilia arranged in longitudinal rows. The oral apparatus or peristome is a V-shaped groove or depression at the anterior end lined by somewhat larger cilia. The mouth lies at the base of this structure, opening into the gullet. A large kidney-shaped macronucleus and a smaller micronucleus, usually in apposition to the concave surface of the former, are situated in ap-

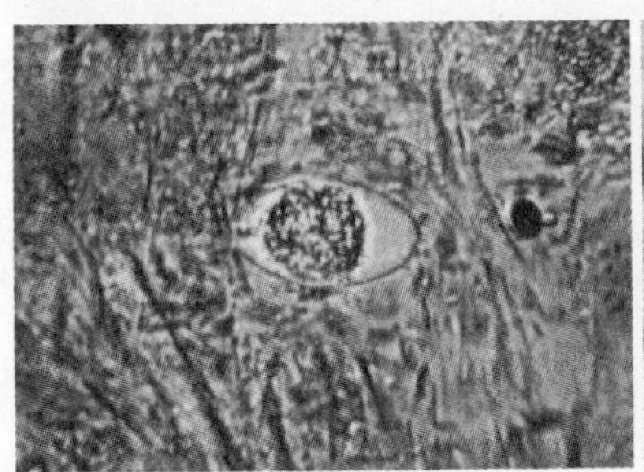

Figure 36–9

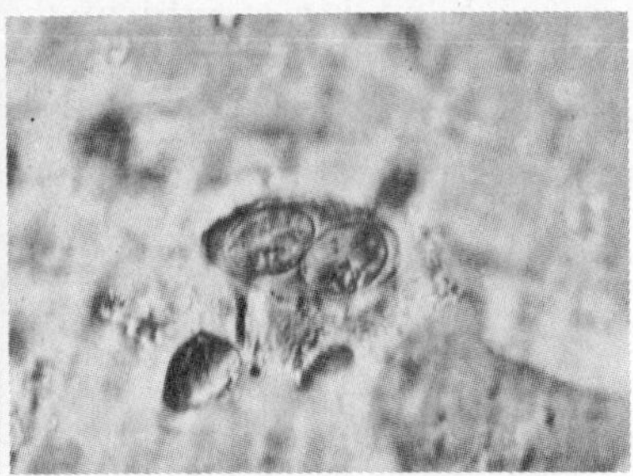

Figure 36–10

Figure 36–9. Immature oocyst of *Isospora belli* from freshly passed feces (1000 ×). (Courtesy of Dr. T. B. Magath, Mayo Clinic.)

Figure 36–10. Older oocyst of *Isospora belli* showing two sporoblasts (1000 ×). (Courtesy of Dr. T. B. Magath, Mayo Clinic.)

proximately the central portion of the body. There are two contractile vacuoles, one anterior and one posterior. The cytoplasm contains a variety of food inclusions, including red blood cells, leukocytes, starch granules and bacteria (Fig. 36–6).

In unstained fresh smears the trophozoite moves actively with a smooth gliding motion. The rapidly beating cilia cannot be seen. The macronucleus often is visible, but the micronucleus is not readily discerned.

The Cyst. The cysts of *B. coli* are oval, measuring 50 to 65 μm in greatest diameter, and the cyst wall appears to have a double outline. They stain poorly with either iodine or hematoxylin although the nuclei and the unstained contractile vacuoles are easily seen (Fig. 36–6).

In unstained preparations the organism may show motility within the cyst wall. The cytoplasm has a faintly greenish tinge. The macronucleus and the contractile vacuoles may be faintly visible.

ISOSPORA BELLI

Isospora belli Wenyon, 1923 is a relatively uncommon sporozoan parasite of man. Although *I. belli* is believed to inhabit the ileum, the finding of oocysts in duodenal drainage fluid suggests that the sites of infection may include the duodenum and possibly the biliary tract. Although details of the development of *Isospora* species in man are unknown, they are presumed to resemble those of coccidia of the dog and cat. Schizogonic development presumably occurs in the epithelial or subepithelial levels of the intestinal mucosa. In the sexual cycle gametocytes are formed. Fertilization of the macrogametes by microgametes, either within or outside of the host cell, results in the zygote. With the

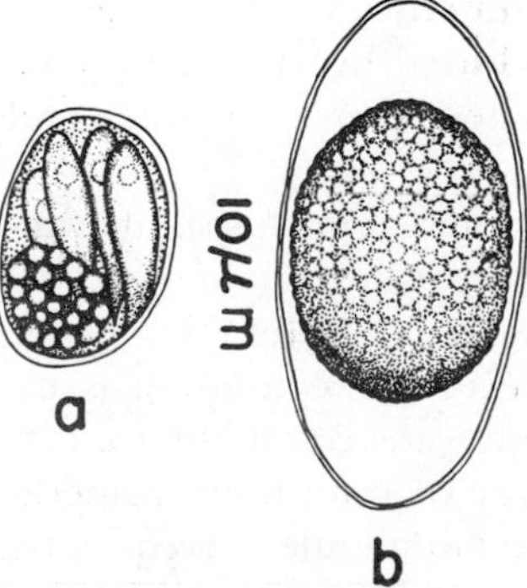

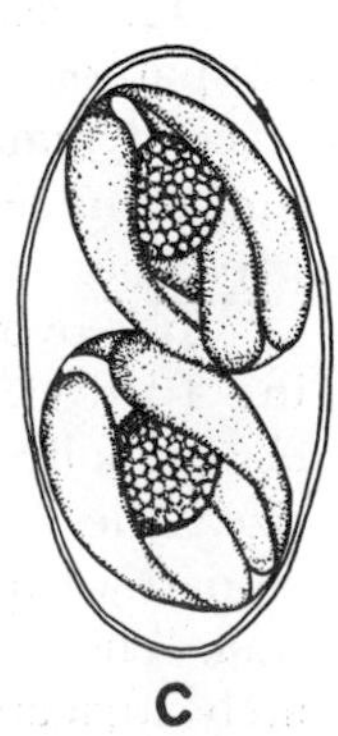

Figure 36–11. *a,* Single sporocyst of *Isospora hominis. b,* Immature oocyst of *I. belli. c,* Mature *I. belli* oocyst. (Courtesy of Dr. R. Elsdon-Dew.)

secretion of a cyst wall, an oocyst is formed. Maturation of the oocyst outside of the intestine occurs as the inner granular nuclear mass divides to form two sporoblasts. Each of these, in turn, secretes a wall and becomes a sporocyst. The nuclear material within each sporocyst divides twice to produce four crescentic sporozoites. Upon ingestion of the infective oocysts, the sporozoites escape and invade the mucosal cells where schizogony and sporogony occur.

The Oocysts. These are ovoid and somewhat elongated and measure 30 by 12 μm. They may be passed at all stages of development; immature forms mature in up to 5 days. The contained sporocysts measure 11 by 9 μm. Typically there is no oocystic residual body. The sporocystic residual body is finely granular, with a limiting membrane that is compact and centrally located between the four sporozoites (Figs. 36–9 to 36–11).[14]

ISOSPORA HOMINIS

In contrast to *I. belli,* the oocysts of *I. hominis* (Rivolta, 1878) Dobell, 1919 ordinarily are passed fully developed and the oocyst wall is usually absent. The sporocysts may be single or coupled in pairs, each being 15 by 10 μm. The sporocystic residual body is composed of coarse, loosely aggregated granules that appear polar in position and separate from the four sporozoites (Fig. 36–11).[14]

BLASTOCYSTIS HOMINIS

The yeast *Blastocystis hominis,* although a nonpathogenic commensal in the digestive tract of man, is included because it may be mistaken for encysted forms of intestinal protozoa.

It is ovoid or spherical in shape, averaging 10 to 15 μm in greatest diameter, and occasionally reaches a considerably larger size. The hyaline refractive cytoplasm is included within a membrane resembling a cyst wall. The outer layer of cytoplasm immediately adjacent to the membrane is frequently differentiated, creating the appearance of a double-walled cyst. This outer layer contains refractile granules and one or more nuclei which are visible in unstained preparations. The central portion is structureless and resembles a large vacuole. Dividing forms are common and exhibit marked variation in size and shape.

In iron-hematoxylin–stained preparations the central cytoplasmic mass appears grayish in color; the peripheral band is unstained except for the nuclei and their large centrally placed karyosomes (Fig. 36–6). Iodine also stains the nuclei, and the central cytoplasm may appear clear or brownish in color.

REFERENCES

1. Brooke, M. M. 1974. Intestinal and urogenital protozoa. *In* Lennette, E. H., Spaulding, E. H., and Truant, J. P. (eds.): Manual of Clinical Microbiology. 2nd ed. American Society for Microbiology, Washington, D.C. pp. 582–601.
2. Ahmad, H., and Ball, G. B. 1963. Increase in size of *Entamoeba hartmanni* trophozoites cultured on an enriched medium. Am. J. Trop. Med. Hyg. *12*:709–718.
3. Goldman, M. 1959. Microfluorimetric evidence of antigenic difference between *Entamoeba histolytica* and *Entamoeba hartmanni.* Proc. Soc. Exp. Biol. Med. *102*:189–191.
4. Burrows, R. W. 1957. *Endamoeba hartmanni.* Am. J. Hyg. *65*:172–188.
5. Elsdon-Dew, R. 1971. Amebiasis as a world problem. Bull. N.Y. Acad. Med. Ser. 2, *47*:438–447.
6. Stamm, W. P. 1970. Amoebic aphorisms. Lancet *2*:1355–1356.
7. Rendtorff, R. C. 1954. The experimental transmission of human intestinal protozoan parasites. I. *Endamoeba coli* cysts given in capsules. Am. J. Hyg. *59*:196–208.
8. Rendtorff, R. C., and Holt, C. J. 1955. The experimental transmission of human intestinal protozoan parasites. V. Multiple infections produced with three species of amebae. Am. J. Hyg. *61*:321–325.
9. Kessel, J. F., and Johnstone, H. G. 1949. The occurrence of *Endamoeba polecki* Prowazek, 1912, in *Macaca mulatta* and in man. Am. J. Trop. Med. *29*:311–317.
10. Burrows, R. B., and Klink, G. E. 1955. *Endamoeba polecki* infections in man. Am. J. Hyg. *62*:156–167.
11. Neal, P. A. 1953. Studies on the morphology and biology of *Entamoeba moshkovskii* Tshalaia. Parasitology *43*:253–268.
12. Artigas, J. 1958. Investigaciones protozoológicas. *Entamoeba moshkovskii* Bol. Chil. Parasit. *13*:36.
13. Goldman, M., Gleason, N. N., and Carver, R. K. 1962. Antigenic analysis of *Entamoeba histolytica* by means of fluorescent antibody. Am. J. Trop. Med. Hyg. *11*:341–346.
14. Elsdon-Dew, R. 1953. Coccidiosis in man: experiences in Natal. Tr. Roy. Soc. Trop. Med. Hyg. *47*:209–214.

CHAPTER 37

Amebiasis and Related Infections

Amebiasis

Synonyms. Amebic dysentery, amebic enteritis, amebic colitis.

Definition. Amebiasis is an infection by the pathogenic ameba *Entamoeba histolytica.* Intestinal amebiasis is characterized by acute or chronic phases, or both, and by a variable clinical picture. The so-called chronic cyst-passer may exhibit few or no significant symptoms. In other instances, infection may be characterized by intermittent episodes of constipation and diarrhea; in still others, the diarrhea may be relatively severe and the stools contain varying amounts of blood and mucus. Acute amebic dysentery is frequent in some areas of the tropics but is less common in the temperate zone. Any of the clinical types of this infection may be followed promptly or after prolonged periods by serious complications, such as amebic abscess of the liver; less frequently metastatic abscesses occur in other organs.

Distribution. Amebiasis has a cosmopolitan distribution and is not restricted to the tropics. Epidemics of amebiasis have occurred in temperate areas, such as the United States, Japan and Korea.

Etiology. *Entamoeba histolytica* Schaudinn, 1903 is the most important of the intestinal protozoa of man. Its life cycle has three distinct stages. The cyst is the infective stage and is ingested in food and drink. Both the mature four-nucleate cysts and the immature cysts are infective. As the cysts pass through the intestine they are acted upon by the digestive secretions. They excyst in the small intestine, and the trophozoites that emerge usually are four-nucleate amebae, which soon divide into uninucleate trophozoites. The uninucleate trophozoite is the actively growing and multiplying stage. Multiplication is by binary fission and two uninucleate trophozoites form from the parent ameba. These actively growing trophozoites may invade the tissue of the large intestine, producing colonies in the intestinal wall and ulcerative lesions.

Cysts are formed as the trophozoites are carried in the lumen contents toward the rectum where the fecal material is dehydrated, but the exact stimulus that produces cyst formation is not known. The mature trophozoite first eliminates food vacuoles and other cytoplasmic inclusions and becomes a precystic ameba. The precystic form then secretes a cyst wall, forming a uninucleate immature cyst, which continues to develop, as a rule, to the typical four-nucleate cyst. This entire cycle takes place within the intestinal tract of man and a few other animals. Cysts of some strains of *E. histolytica* develop in suitable culture media. Cysts do not develop in the tissues, nor from trophozoites after passage from the body. Immature cysts may mature outside the body under favorable conditions.

Epidemiology. The actively motile trophozoites present in the freshly passed feces of patients suffering from amebic diarrhea or dysentery are short-lived outside of the body. It is unlikely that they can survive exposure to the hydrochloric acid and digestive enzymes of the stomach and upper intestinal tract. They are therefore of little, if any, importance in the transmission of the disease.

The encysted forms, however, are resistant to marked changes in their environment and are responsible for transmission. The infection is acquired by the ingestion of these encysted forms in food or drink contaminated by the feces of infected individuals.

The cysts of *E. histolytica* are readily destroyed by drying; they are also killed rapidly at 55° C (131° F). They will survive as long as 1 month in water at about 10° C (50° F). The cysts are relatively resistant to chlorine and are not destroyed by concentrations customarily used for water purification. If dependence is to be placed upon chlorination alone, the concentration and contact time must be adjusted in accordance with the temperature and hydrogen ion concentration of the water.

Dilute disinfectants as ordinarily used are not markedly effective in destroying the encysted forms. In moist feces survival time is reduced to approximately 12 days and is controlled by the rate of putrefaction and the temperature. At 4° C (39.2° F) cysts remain viable for at least 60 days in both sewage and natural surface waters.

Man is the principal reservoir of infection. However, amebae that are morpho-

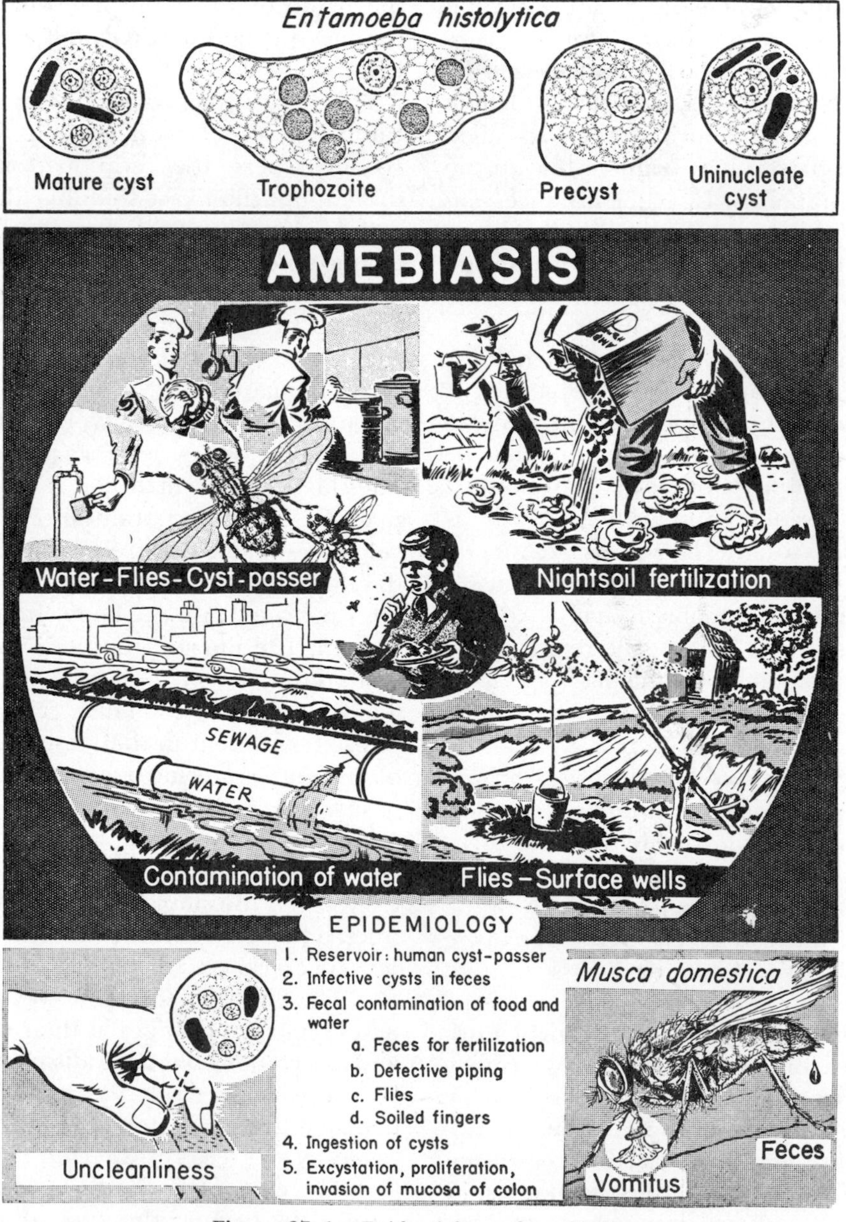

Figure 37–1. Epidemiology of amebiasis.

logically similar to *E. histolytica* have been recovered from the dog, cat, rat, pig and various species of primates.

Transmission of the infection from one individual to another may be accomplished by a variety of mechanisms (Fig. 37–1). The infected individual passing large numbers of cysts in his stools is an important potential source of infection, especially if engaged in the preparation and handling of food. There are numerous instances, especially in family outbreaks, that indicate the hazard of such employment of the cyst-passer.

The housefly and the cockroach feed upon human feces when available, and cysts of *E. histolytica* have been recovered from the intestinal tracts of these insects, apparently undamaged, after periods as long as 48 hours. In some areas flies probably are important in the epidemiology of amebiasis (Fig. 37–1).

Polluted water may likewise be an important vehicle of infection. Fecal contamination of water commonly occurs by surface run-off into springs, unprotected shallow wells and streams, or by discharge of crude sewage into streams and rivers. Less frequently cross seepage between water and sewer pipes laid in the same ditch, or direct cross connections with siphonage of sewage into the water supply system are responsible for outbreaks of infection. The freshening of vegetables with contaminated water or even with crude sewage before sale is widely practiced in many parts of the world. In many regions human excreta, night soil, is widely used as garden fertilizer. This practice may be responsible for heavy contamination of root and leafy vegetables which customarily are eaten raw.

Epidemic outbreaks of amebiasis are uncommon, and all reported instances have been traced to a heavily contaminated water supply or to fly transmission.[1] The disease occurs characteristically in endemic form. The infection rate is low in young children, but in the school age group the incidence reaches that of the general population of the area in which they live.

Pathology. The fundamental pathology of amebiasis is characterized by penetration of the host's tissues by *E. histolytica*, necrosis of tissue cells, and absence of inflammatory reaction. Only the trophozoite stage is found in tissue. Under ordinary circumstances *E. histolytica* is dependent for its survival in culture upon bacterial associates, which provide metabolites essential for the continued multiplication of this ameba. Studies in germ-free animals indicate that, in the absence of microbial associates, *E. histolytica* is not capable of independent survival in the intestine and fails to produce lesions. In contrast, acute ulcerative amebiasis developed in animals which harbored bacteria, e.g. *Escherichia coli* or *Enterobacter aerogenes*, as monocontaminants that were similarly inoculated with *E. histolytica*. Axenic culture of *E. histolytica* with supporting requisite nutritional factors is possible. However, under these conditions pathogenesis of the amebae appears to be reduced. Although *E. histolytica* is unquestionably the causative organism of intestinal amebiasis, the responsibility for the disease must be shared with other microorganisms.[2,3]

Lesions are most commonly found in the cecum, ascending colon, sigmoid and rectum. In the early stage lysis of the epithelium and the underlying stroma produces superficial erosions of the mucosa. Macroscopically these appear as shallow ulcers having a necrotic base and a narrow surrounding zone of hyperemia with normal mucosa intervening. Extension occurs peripherally and downward into the submucosa (Figs. 37–2 to 37–4). In other instances small amebic abscesses are found in the submucosa, eventually opening through the surface to produce the characteristic flask or bottleneck ulcer (Fig. 37–5). Both the superficial and the deeper lesions may form the "sea anemone" ulcer with a deep crater and partly necrotic undermined edges which are raised above the level of the surrounding mucosa.

Initially, there is little edema and no leukocytic response. Secondary bacterial infection of the ulcers occurs rapidly, however, producing a varying, severe inflammatory reaction. Occasionally, shigellosis is superimposed; rarely, secondary infection by *Clostri-*

Figure 37–2

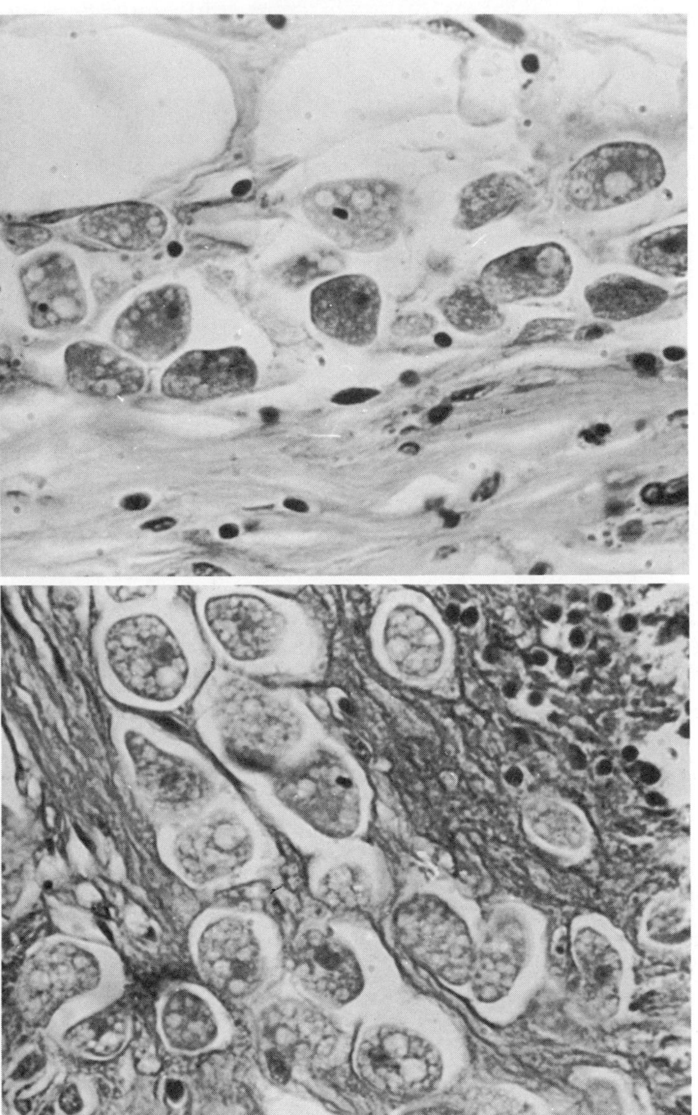

Figure 37–3

Figure 37–2. Trophozoites of *E. histolytica* in submucosa of the colon. (Courtesy of the Louisiana State University School of Medicine, New Orleans; photomicrography by Dr. Mark R. Feldman.)

Figure 37–3. Numerous trophozoites of *E. histolytica* in wall of appendix. (Courtesy of the Louisiana State University School of Medicine, New Orleans; photomicrography by Dr. Mark R. Feldman.)

dium perfringens may produce a rapidly spreading and fatal gangrene of the colon. In some instances, extensive and rapid invasion of the colonic wall by the amebae may lead to severe or fatal hemorrhage or perforation (Fig. 37–6). The resulting ulcer, the so-called "Dyak hair" ulcer, is sharply circumscribed, and the base is formed by fringelike projections of the more resistant supporting tissues.

On microscopic examination of the particles of mucus, the cellular exudate is characteristic. Leukocytes are considerably less numerous than in shigellosis, while bacteria are much more numerous (Figs. 20–1 and 20–2, p. 175). Erythrocytes are often found clumped. Eosinophils, pyknotic bodies and Charcot-Leyden crystals may be present in the dysenteric exudate.[4] Conversely, peripheral eosinophilia of the blood is not characteristic of amebiasis. Macrophages are not common, except after arsenical therapy.

Invasion of the submucosa may be followed by entry of *E. histolytica* into radicles of

Figure 37–4

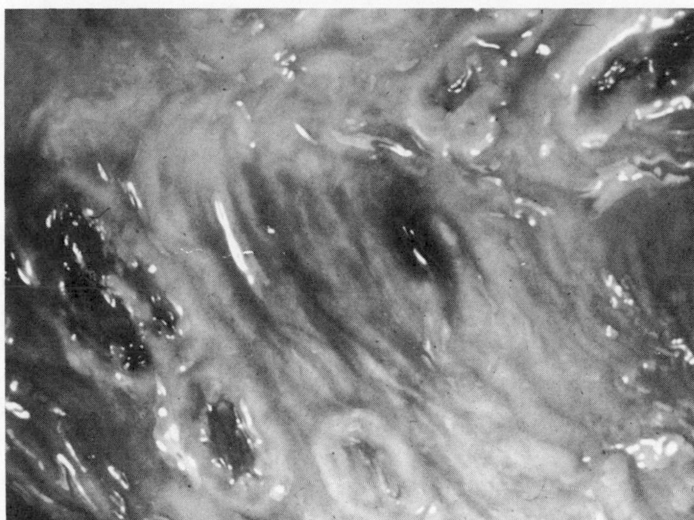

Figure 37–4. Amebic ulcers of the large intestine. Note raised margins of ulcers. (Courtesy of the Louisiana State University School of Medicine, New Orleans.)

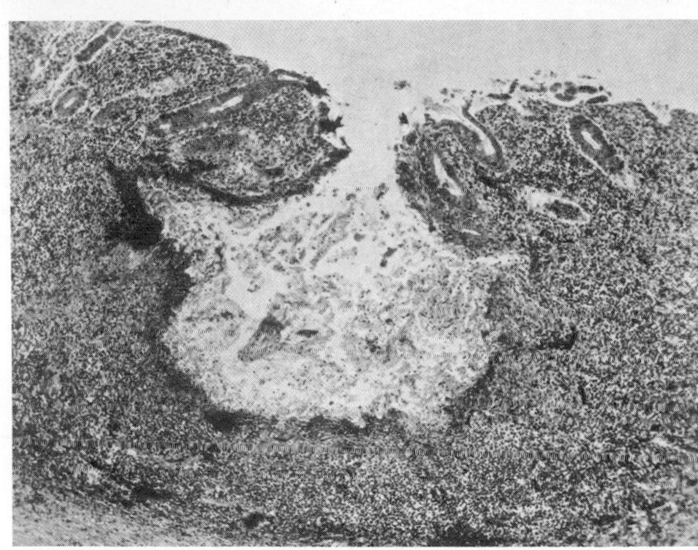

Figure 37–5

Figure 37–5. Section of colon showing flask-shaped chronic amebic ulcer involving the mucosa and submucosa. The neutrophilic infiltration of the border of the lesion suggests secondary bacterial invasion. (From Medical Museum Collection, Armed Forces Institute of Pathology. *In* Craig's Amebiasis and Amebic Dysentery. Charles C Thomas, Springfield, Illinois.)

the portal vein and metastasis of the infection to the liver (Fig. 37–7). This is followed by amebic abscess of the liver. Such abscesses may be single or multiple, acute or chronic (Figs. 37–8, 37–9). Multiple foci of necrosis may coalesce to form a single large abscess. Leukocytic infiltration of the wall occurs even in the absence of secondary bacterial infection. Right lobe abscesses of the liver commonly extend upward and may penetrate the diaphragm and rupture into the lungs (Fig. 37–10). Amebic abscess of the brain and other organs occurs rarely (Figs. 37–7, 37–11, 37–12). Secondary amebic infections of the skin and subcutaneous tissues, the bladder, uterus and vagina have been reported. (See Figs. 37–7, 37–13, 37–14.)

Clinical Characteristics. The clinical response to infection by *E. histolytica* is extremely variable and depends upon the localization of the amebae, the intensity of the infection, possibly differences in virulence of strains, bacterial flora, diet and other factors. The ratios of amebic abscess of the liver, acute dysentery and diarrhea to the known prevalence of amebic infection in the popu-

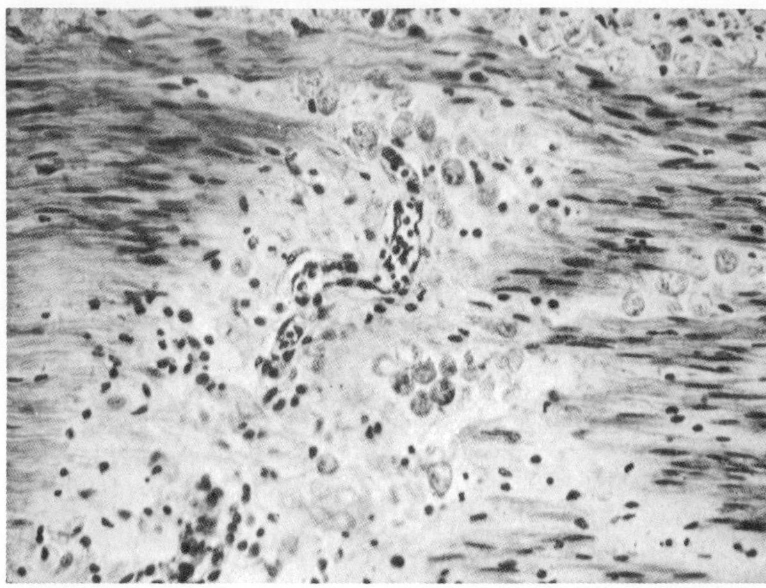

Figure 37-6. Invasion of muscularis along penetrating vessel. (Collection of Dr. W. M. James and Dr. Lawrence Getz.)

lation are low. It is generally recognized that frank amebic dysentery is more common in the tropics and subtropics than elsewhere and that in the temperate zones it is more prevalent in the warmer months of the year.

Large and "small races" of *E. histolytica* have been identified. Those with cysts less than 10 μm in diameter are generally accepted as *Entamoeba hartmanni,* which is considered to be nonpathogenic. (See p. 312 and Tables 36-1 to 36-4.) Some large strains of *E. histolytica* apparently exist as commensals in the large intestine. However, invasion and severe clinical disease may result with changes in diet or in bacterial flora, and in the presence of superimposed debili-

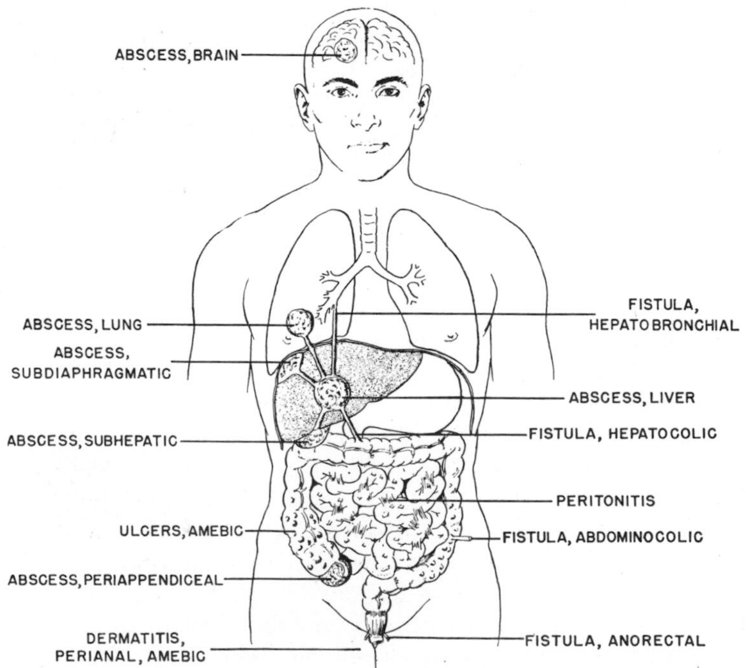

Figure 37-7. Complications of amebiasis. (Courtesy of Ash and Spitz, Pathology of Tropical Diseases. 1945. W. B. Saunders Co., Philadelphia.)

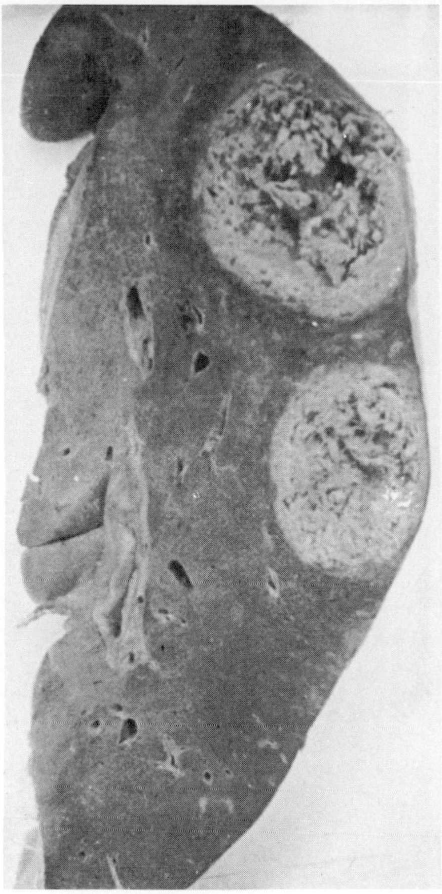

Figure 37–8

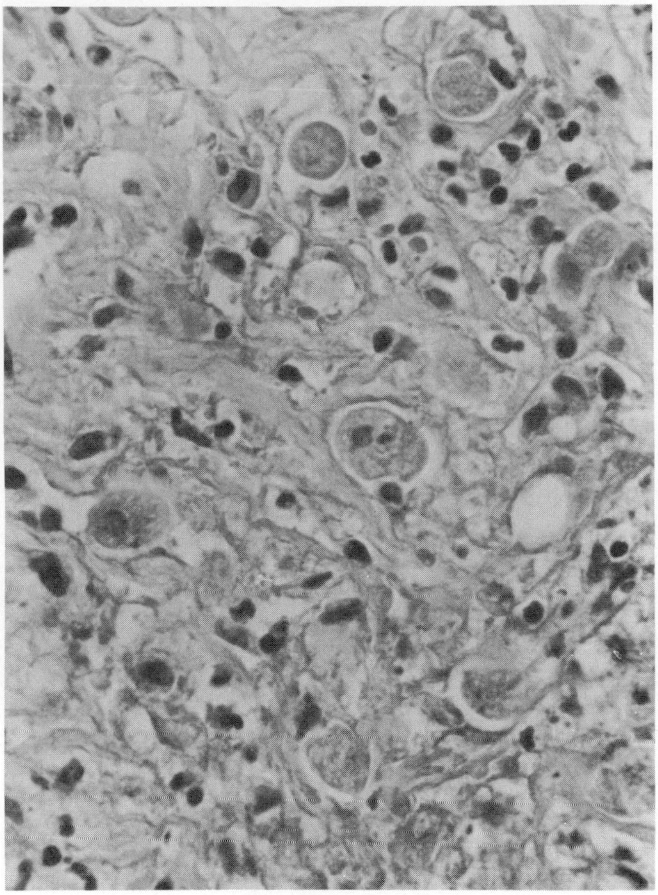

Figure 37–9

Figure 37–8. Multiple amebic abscesses of the liver. (Courtesy of the Louisiana State University School of Medicine, New Orleans; photomicrography by Dr. Mark R. Feldman.)

Figure 37–9. Trophozoites of *E. histolytica* in the liver. (Courtesy of the Louisiana State University School of Medicine, New Orleans; photomicrography by Dr. Mark R. Feldman.)

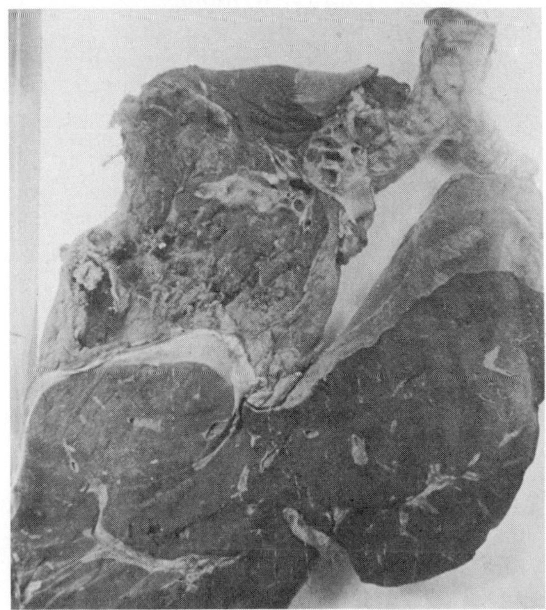

Figure 37–10. Extensive amebic lesion of the lung. Usually lung involvement results from extension of amebic liver abscess. In this case the lesion followed perforation of the hepatic flexure of the colon and penetration of the diaphragm by the trophozoites of *E. histolytica.* (Courtesy of the Louisiana State University School of Medicine, New Orleans.)

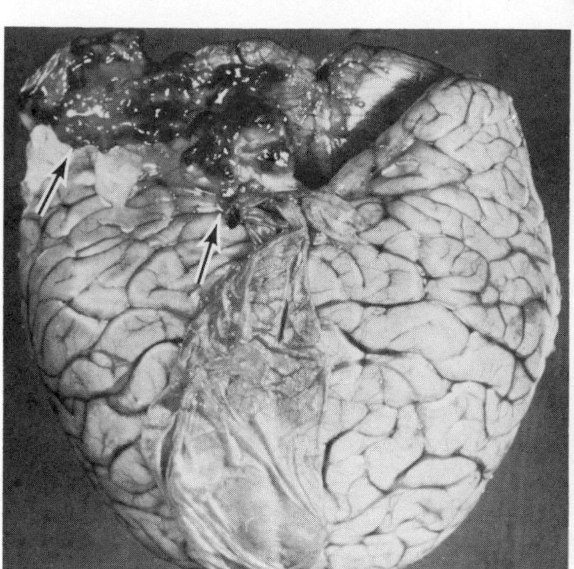

Figure 37–11

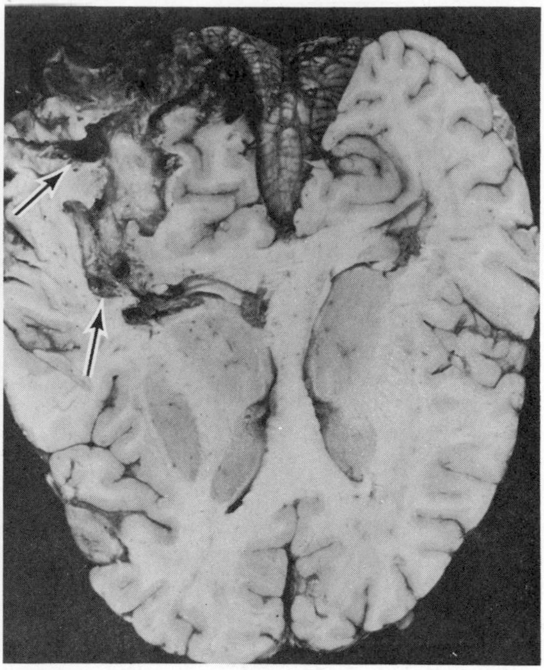

Figure 37–12

Figure 37–11. External view of a brain with an amebic abscess. (Courtesy of the Louisiana State University School of Medicine, New Orleans.)

Figure 37–12. Coronal section of the brain showing extent of the amebic lesion. (Courtesy of the Louisiana State University School of Medicine, New Orleans.)

tating diseases, malnutrition associated with alcoholism, or other factors. From the practical standpoint of the clinician and in the interest of the patient, it should be borne in mind that one cannot predict whether or not a strain of *E. histolytica* will remain in the lumen or later invade tissue. Therefore, treatment is advised.

Infection by this parasite may persist for many years, running a protracted course that is frequently characterized by periodic exacerbation of intestinal symptoms, and by remissions during which the patient may be largely or even entirely free of symptoms.

THE CYST-PASSER. The cyst-passer is the commonest clinical type. Two classes are recognized: those who have acquired the infection but have not experienced active clinical disease; and convalescents who, following acute dysentery or amebic diarrhea, retain a chronic infection and more or less continuously show encysted forms in their stools.

The relationship between the asymptomatic carrier state and active disease is controversial. Some authorities state that not more than 10 per cent of cyst-passers have clinical manifestations from the infection. Others hold that at least 50 per cent exhibit symptoms attributable to *E. histolytica* at some time during the infection. The problem is complicated by the fact that many of the symptoms present cannot be considered as specific responses to the amebic infection. Obviously, in many tropical, subtropical and temperate areas amebiasis is overdiagnosed clinically.[5] Response to therapy cannot be used as sound evidence of a causal relationship between infection and symptoms.[6] As antibodies arise only as a result of invasion and persist after treatment, their prevalence in a community is an index of the frequency of invasion.[5] Thus serology provides a parameter, of at least partial value, in determining relationship of symptoms. On the other hand, it is known that infected individuals may be essentially symptom-free for periods of years only to develop without warning acute involvement of the liver with actual abscess formation. Therefore, the infected individual not only is a source for potential spread to others but also, if tissue invasion occurs, may subsequently develop acute symptoms and serious disease.

The clinical picture of the chronic cyst-passer characteristically lacks specificity. Abdominal distention and flatulence accompanied by constipation are common complaints. Although the constipation may be interrupted by occasional brief periods of loose stools, these ordinarily do not attract attention, especially since gross blood and mucus are not present in the feces. These symptoms are commonly accompanied by vague abdominal discomfort and a sense of abnormal fullness of the abdomen, particularly on the right side. Many infected individuals exhibit the lassitude and other phenomena associated with neurasthenia; however, these complaints appear to have no relationship to amebic infection.

AMEBIC DIARRHEA. When the host-parasite balance is less exact, periodic bouts of diarrhea occur with several loose or liquid stools a day. Abdominal discomfort and cramps may be present; tenesmus does not occur, and fever is usually absent. There is usually little change in the white blood count, although there may be a slight leukocytosis. Careful examination of the stools commonly may reveal small flecks of blood-tinged mucus in which there are large numbers of trophozoites. The spontaneous cessation of diarrhea is usually followed by a variable period of constipation during which the vague symptoms of the cyst-passer may dominate the clinical picture.

AMEBIC DYSENTERY. Acute amebic dysentery occurs in a small percentage of persons with intestinal amebiasis. The incubation period may be as short as 8 to 10 days, and in approximately 50 per cent of cases the onset is sudden. This is especially true of

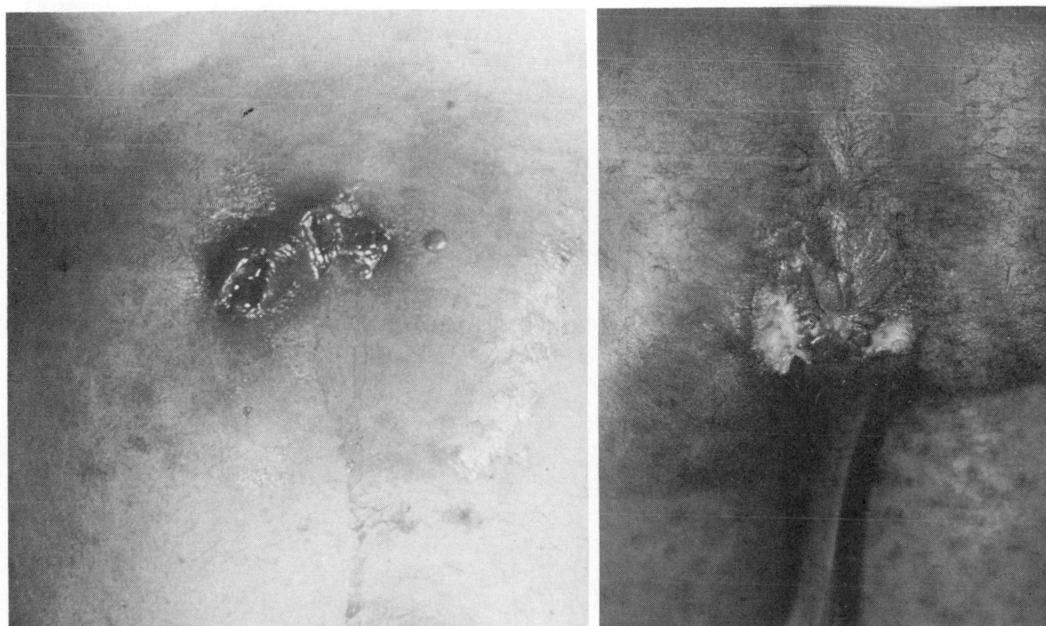

Figure 37–13 **Figure 37–14**

Figure 37–13. Amebiasis cutis. Lesions of anterior abdominal wall resulting from extension of an amebic liver abscess. (Courtesy of the Louisiana State University School of Medicine, New Orleans.)

Figure 37–14. Amebiasis cutis. Two lesions lateral to the anus which communicated by sinus tracts with the rectum. (Courtesy of the Louisiana State University School of Medicine, New Orleans.)

mixed infections with *Shigella.* In other instances acute dysentery may occur in the previously asymptomatic cyst-passer who has carried his infection for long periods.

When the onset is acute it may be accompanied by headache, nausea, chills, fever, severe abdominal cramps and, if there are lesions of the descending colon, by tenesmus. The stools consist of liquid fecal matter containing flecks of bloody mucus, the so-called "sago-grain stools." The white blood count may vary from 5000 to 15,000 with a polymorphonuclear leukocytosis as high as 85 per cent. The presence of a moderate leukocytosis suggests the concurrent existence of an amebic liver abscess; this possibility should be thoroughly explored.

In very severe cases extensive involvement of the colon may lead to massive destruction of the mucosa and the formation of a pseudodiphtheritic membrane which may be passed intact, or actual gangrene of large portions of the colonic wall may occur. In severe cases the deeply penetrating ulceration may produce serious or even fatal hemorrhage. However, death, when it occurs, usually is the result of cardiac failure and exhaustion, or of perforation of the colon and peritonitis.

Repeated and inadequately treated attacks of acute dysentery or of amebic diarrhea may be followed by chronic dysentery. This is the result of long continued mixed infection of the colonic wall by *E. histolytica* and by bacteria. It is associated with progressive scarring and deformity of the colon, and differs little clinically from chronic bacillary dysentery or so-called idiopathic ulcerative colitis. It is characterized by recurrent acute attacks of fever and by diarrhea with blood and pus in the stools. In the intervals between acute attacks the stools are generally loose, increased in number and mixed with variable amounts of blood, mucus and pus. Chronic dysentery is commonly accompanied by malnutrition and cachexia.

Ulcerative colitis, carcinoma of the large intestine and colonic dysfunction of other etiology may simulate chronic amebic dysentery, and cells in the exudate in these conditions may be confused with amebae.[7, 8]

Amebic Appendicitis. Infection of the appendix by *E. histolytica* may occur, and with secondary bacterial invasion the clinical picture of subacute appendicitis may be encountered. In instances when the appendix occupies a retrocecal position, the clinical picture may be exceedingly confusing. Demonstration of *E. histolytica* in the patient's stools, however, should be regarded as potentially significant evidence, and in the absence of imperative indications for operation, antiamebic therapy should be given before laparotomy is decided upon.

Amebic Granuloma (Ameboma). In certain instances intestinal amebiasis is accompanied by the formation of granulomatous lesions of the colon which are commonly misdiagnosed as carcinoma (Fig. 37–15). They may occur in any area from the cecum to the rectum. Those that can be visualized through the sigmoidoscope, or even better through a colonoscope, may present many of the characteristics of adenocarcinoma. In other instances, roentgen examination following a barium enema may reveal a picture characteristic of an annular carcinoma producing partial or even complete obstruction of the colon. Surgical removal without use of amebicidal drugs may result in fatality, whereas medical treatment usually results in disappearance of the tumor.

Coincidental Amebic Infection. Any infection like amebiasis that is prevalent in a significant proportion of the population at times may be present but coincidental to another infection or disorder in the same patient. Thus, amebiasis may occur in persons with carcinoma, ulcerative colitis, shigellosis, psychoneurosis, colonic dysfunction of psychosomatic origin or other conditions. An intestinal neoplasm may be invaded by amebae. With antiamebic therapy the mass is reduced in size and then remains static. The presence of an underlying neoplasm should be suspected when this occurs.[6] The possibility that the amebiasis may not be the primary cause of any or all of the patient's complaints should be borne in mind. This is particularly true when bleeding or other findings and complaints continue after a reasonable amount of antiamebic therapy has been em-

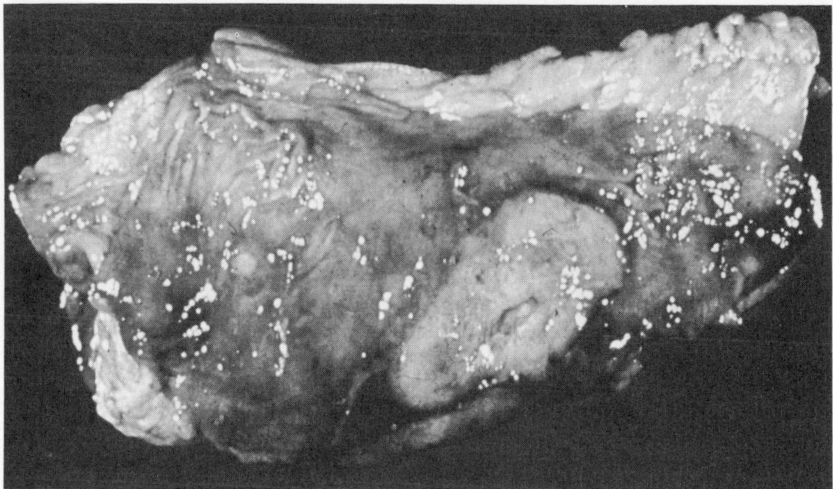

Figure 37–15. Amebic granuloma or ameboma in the cecum. (Courtesy of the Louisiana State University School of Medicine, New Orleans.)

ployed for patients in whom *E. histolytica* initially had been demonstrated.[7, 8]

Diagnosis. The diagnosis of intestinal amebiasis depends upon demonstration of *E. histolytica* in the feces of the infected person. Three normally passed specimens collected over a 7- to 10-day period should be examined. This may be supplemented by examination of a liquid specimen obtained after a saline cathartic, in selected nondiarrheic and nondysenteric cases, which will reveal additional infections. Specimens obtained within 3 days after a barium meal are not suitable for diagnosis. If the individual is passing formed stools, ordinarily only cysts will be found. In the rare instances of active ulceration predominantly confined to the rectum, however, trophozoites may be found in flecks of blood-stained mucus adherent to the surface of the stool. If there is active diarrhea or acute dysentery, on the other hand, only the trophozoites are to be expected. These do not survive long after passage from the body and, especially when exposed to chilling, rapidly lose the motility and normal morphologic characteristics upon which identification must be based (Table 37–1). The detailed morphology is described on page 308. In contrast to the lack of need for haste in examining a formed specimen, a diarrheal stool should be examined at the earliest possible moment unless the PVA or MIF technique is employed. (See pp. 818 and 825.)

Examination of Formed Stool. A small portion of the excreta should be emulsified in saline solution on a glass fecal slide and covered with a coverslip. The prepara-

Table 37–1. Diagnostic Characteristics of *Entamoeba histolytica*

	Form	*Where Found*	*Morphology*
Liquid stools	Trophozoites	Blood-stained mucus or feces	Progressive motion; glasslike pseudopodia; sluglike shape; may contain red blood cells
Formed stools	Cysts	In the fecal mass	Saline preparation: Blunt-ended chromatoidals may be visible; nuclei not visible except after formalin fixation Iodine preparation: 1–4 nuclei at different levels; chromatoidals usually not visible except after formalin fixation
Semiformed stools	Cysts and/or trophozoites	In the fecal mass	Same as above

tion should be of a density that just permits the reading of newsprint through it. A similar fecal emulsion should be made with D'Antoni's iodine solution on the same slide.

In the unstained suspension the cysts of *E. histolytica* appear as pearllike, round refractile bodies in which no nuclei are visible or in which the nuclei can barely be distinguished. When the condenser of the microscope is racked down, the characteristic and diagnostic blunt-ended chromatoidal bar may be seen in some cysts in some, but not all, infections (Fig. 36–2, p. 312).

In the iodine suspension the ringlike nuclei are easily visible (Fig. 36–8). These are four in number in the mature cysts, but it is not unusual to observe younger forms which are uninucleate or binucleate. Chromatoidal bars are usually not visible in iodine suspensions (p. 319).

The major problems in the laboratory diagnosis of amebiasis include *missed diagnoses* and *misdiagnoses* (false diagnoses). Errors result from: (1) failure, because of poor technique or inadequate search, to detect the organism; (2) confusion of various nonparasitic objects in the stool or in sigmoidoscopic aspirate with *E. histolytica;* and (3) confusion of other intestinal protozoa with this pathogen. Erroneous laboratory findings, in turn, lead to incorrect clinical diagnoses. Thus, the laboratory diagnostician should require that objects observed in fecal smears or sigmoidoscopic aspirate meet the accepted morphologic criteria for *E. histolytica.* Otherwise, cells or artefacts present in almost any specimen may be mistaken for this ameba.[7, 8]

In light infections demonstration of the cysts is facilitated by concentration methods. The formalin-ether centrifugal concentration technique is a desirable supplement to direct fecal smears for routine stool examination. These techniques are described in the section on Diagnostic Methods, pp. 817 and 819.

Examination of Diarrheal Stool. The freshly passed stool should be kept at body temperature by immersion of the container in warm water, unless examination can be carried out immediately after evacuation. Refrigeration or incubation at 37° C (98.6° F) of liquid or formed stools usually has a deleterious effect on trophozoites and cysts. A small quantity of liquid feces should be poured into a Petri dish and carefully scrutinized for small flecks of blood-stained mucus. Such a particle of mucus should be placed on a slide, covered with a coverglass and examined immediately. In the presence of an active amebic infection many of the flecks of bloody mucus contain large numbers of motile trophozoites, which appear as elongated sluglike amebae exhibiting progressive motion across the microscopic field (Fig. 36–1). The glasslike pseudopodia and the characteristic progressive motion are diagnostic. *Entamoeba histolytica* trophozoites in dysenteric exudates frequently contain ingested red blood cells. Conversely, trophozoites in diarrheal stools, without gross blood, often contain no red blood cells. It is to be emphasized that the amebae are much more numerous in the flecks of mucus than in the fecal material of the stools. *Entamoeba histolytica* may be isolated in culture (pp. 829–830).

Charcot-Leyden crystals are frequently present in the stools. Although suggestive, they are not pathognomonic of infection by *E. histolytica,* since they occur in association with other parasitic infections and with any chronic ulcerative condition of the colon.

Stools in amebic dysentery usually contain few leukocytes and many bacteria. In contrast, in the exudate of shigellosis, leukocytes are extremely numerous and bacteria are scanty (Figs. 20–1, 20–2, p. 175).

Proctoscopic Examination. Proctoscopic, sigmoidoscopic or colonoscopic examination of the chronic cyst-passer seldom yields information of value. In the more active clinical types of infection, however, lesions may be observed which are characteristic. These are small, discrete, inflamed areas scattered about an otherwise normal mucous membrane (Fig. 37–4). They appear as isolated superficial erosions, pits, small nodules with a petechial ulceration on their surface, or as yellow spots, surrounded by a narrow band of hyperemia. Immediate microscopic examination of the contents expressed with a spatula or aspirated with a glass tube and rubber bulb through the proctoscope will reveal *trophozoites.* Cysts usually are not found in proctoscopic material.

Biopsy scrapings may be obtained from the rectal mucosa by a long-handled Volkmann spoon manipulated through a proctoscope under proper illumination. The material in the bowl of the spoon should be placed on a slide immediately, compressed under a coverglass, and examined for *E. histolytica* trophozoites. Confusion of amebae with the cellular elements in the exudate and mucosal tissue must be avoided.

Trophozoites can also be identified readily in hematoxylin-eosin-stained slides in a high percentage of punch or snip biopsies of amebic ulcers of the rectum. All fragments of tissue and the adherent mucus should be included when preparing the tissue block. Biopsy of rectal ulcers should be employed as a supplement, not a substitute, for examinations of stools and material aspirated during proctoscopy. In selected cases where large ulcers are present, biopsy may be employed effectively for differential diagnosis between amebiasis and lesions of other etiology.

X-RAY EXAMINATION. Roentgen examination of the colon is not a dependable aid in diagnosis, since demonstrable lesions are by no means always present. However, in acute cases, the barium enema may reveal spasm and evidence of ulceration, particularly in the proximal colon, and some degree of deformity of the cecum is not unusual in longstanding chronic infections. In the presence of amebic granuloma a filling defect suggestive of carcinoma may be seen.

CULTURE. Many strains of *E. histolytica* may be cultured on Boeck-Drbohlav or other suitable media (p. 829). However, some strains are difficult or impossible to culture. Culture technique for intestinal amebiasis is a supplemental procedure which may be employed with benefit in selected cases, particularly when large amebic trophozoites are encountered, the identity of which cannot be determined owing to lack of motility. Cultures of stools for *E. histolytica* seldom yield positive results when a thorough microscopic examination has failed to demonstrate the presence of the ameba.

SEROLOGY. The improvement in serologic methods for amebiasis has provided useful epidemiologic tools as well as adjuncts to clinical diagnosis. The indirect hemagglutination test (IHA) is very sensitive for the diagnosis of amebic liver abscess and of invasive amebiasis. Antibodies may persist for over 3 years after termination of an infection. A combination of microimmunoelectrophoresis pattern analysis and IHA titer level provides differentiation between active infection and antibodies persisting after treatment.[9,10] A latex agglutination test kit for invasive amebiasis, commercially available in some areas, has sensitivity and specificity similar to that of the gel diffusion test, but is easier to perform and provides results more rapidly.[11] The complement-fixation test for amebiasis is less sensitive than the IHA for invasive intestinal amebiasis, but is useful for diagnosis of hepatic amebiasis.[3,9]

Treatment. Basic to the problem of therapy in amebiasis are the nature of the pathologic process and the natural habits of the parasite. Some of the trophozoites reside in the intestinal contents, some are found on the surface of the mucosa, and others are found at various depths within the bowel wall or in other organs of the body. The location of the amebae both in the lumen and deep in the tissues makes it necessary to deliver an active amebicide in adequate concentrations to the trophozoites in the intestinal contents and in the tissues. Amebic therapy is directed to the trophozoites, not the cysts. The amebicides now in use vary considerably in their pharmacology and sites of action. A careful selection of drugs is necessary in order to eliminate the amebae from the intestinal contents of the bowel and from the tissues wherever the lesions occur.

DRUGS. The recommended drugs fall into several groups based upon their chemical composition. The arsenicals, such as Carbarsone and Milibis, have largely been supplanted by other intestinal amebicides and are not included. A summary of treatment of amebiasis, including dosages and duration of therapy, is presented in Table 37–2 (p. 339).

Nitroimidazoles. METRONIDAZOLE (Flagyl). This amebicide, 1-2′-hydroxyethyl-2-methyl-5-nitroimidazole, acts directly on the trophozoites of *E. histolytica*. The drug is quickly absorbed, partly metabolized, rapidly excreted, and without cumulative effect. It is useful for treatment of chronic nondysenteric intestinal amebiasis, amebic dysentery, hepatic abscess and possibly other extraintestinal forms of amebiasis. In view of the effectiveness of this amebicidal drug against both clinical intestinal and extraintestinal forms of the disease and the infrequent side effects, the compound has been widely used for this disease.[12, 13]

Patients have developed amebic abscess of the liver 1 to 3 or more months after apparently successful treatment of amebic colitis with metronidazole. This suggests that although metronidazole is a highly effective amebicide, it should not be used as the single agent for therapy of amebic colitis.[14] This would probably apply to other nitroimidazoles.

Mild gastrointestinal symptoms and headache occur infrequently. Vertigo, incoordination, ataxia and paresthesia have been reported on rare occasion; some of the latter may be of doubtful relationship to therapy. A transitory leukopenia can occur. In contrast to emetine, the drug does not produce any alteration of the electrocardiogram or affect the cardiovascular system. Administration is per os. Recently evidence has been presented that metronidazole is carcinogenic in rodents and mutagenic in bacteria. A currently expressed view is that although there are risks associated with the drug, they are probably worth taking in some patients with amebiasis. The latter is particularly true for patients with extraintestinal amebiasis.

TINIDAZOLE (Fasigyn). This nitroimidazole compound, like metronidazole, has shown marked therapeutic effect for clinical intestinal amebiasis and amebic liver abscess.[15–17] Their similar derivation probably also accounts for the therapeutic action of both compounds on human trichomoniasis and giardiasis (p. 348, p. 347). Occasional side effects include mild nausea and dizziness. Tinidazole presently is not widely available geographically or approved for medical use in many areas including the United States.

Halogenated Hydroxyquinolines. DIIODOHYDROXYQUIN (Diodoquin), 5,7-diiodo-8-hydroxyquinoline, contains 63.9 per cent iodine. This drug is relatively insoluble and acts primarily and directly on the lumen-dwelling trophozoites. It is most effective in asymptomatic and carrier patients, but of no therapeutic value per se for amebic liver abscess. It may also be used in conjunction with the treatment of extraintestinal amebiasis for elimination of the primary intestinal source of such complications. This drug is very useful for treatment of either adults or children. Optic atrophy and blindness have been observed after treatment with diiodohydroxyquin (Diodoquin) after prolonged use, usually at greater than recommended doses.[18–20] The recommended dosage for children is 30 to 40 mg per kg per day for 20 days. Other side effects occasionally encountered with this drug are skin eruptions, nausea and diarrhea. Use of this compound for prolonged periods of time or at excessive dosage should be avoided.

Entero-Vioform (iodochlorohydroxyquin) is *not* recommended. The halogenated hydroxyquinolines have been shown to be associated with a gastrointestinal-neurologic syndrome, subacute myelo-optic neuropathy (SMON).[18] In view of the hazard of neurotoxicity from such compounds, other effective and safer intestinal amebicides which are available should be employed.

The halogenated hydroxyquinoline compounds should not be used for the treatment of nonspecific diarrhea.[18] Also, their use as a prophylaxis against amebiasis is not justified in view of the hazard of optic damage. The safety of halogenated hydroxyquinolines for the fetus has not been demonstrated. In view of the similarity of their chemical structure to chloroquine, which can cause deafness in children from prenatal exposure, they should not be prescribed during pregnancy.[18]

Anilines. These are derivatives of 4-

aminophenol. Diloxanide furoate (Furamide) is the 2-furoic acid ester of dichloroacet-4-hydroxy-N-methylanilide. It is rapidly absorbed and appears in the serum mainly as a glucuronide, which is excreted in the urine. Since the drug is active against *E. histolytica* only in the presence of living bacteria, its amebicidal action may be indirect. It is not effective against extraintestinal amebiasis, such as amebic liver abscess. The primary use of diloxanide furoate is for treatment of patients with asymptomatic or nondysenteric mild clinical intestinal amebiasis.[12] Also, it may be employed for elimination of the primary intestinal source of infection as part of the overall treatment for amebic hepatic abscess. This compound is very safe and well tolerated. Side effects occur only occasionally and include mild gastrointestinal complaints and flatulence.

Aminoquinolines. 4-AMINOQUINOLINE, CHLOROQUINE (Aralen, Nivaquine, Avloclor), is supplied as chloroquine diphosphate in tablet form. Each 0.5 gm of the salt is equivalent to 0.3 gm of the base. It is rapidly absorbed from the gastrointestinal tract but slowly excreted. Chloroquine is stored in the liver in high concentration, much less in other tissues of the body. It is highly effective against amebae in the tissues, especially in the liver, and relatively ineffective in intestinal amebiasis. The drug is used in the treatment of amebic liver abscess Chloroquine is usually well tolerated, but in some individuals it may cause mild headache, pruritus, mild gastrointestinal symptoms, blurring of vision, incoordination, epileptiform convulsions, peripheral neuritis, diminution of electrocardiographic T waves and bleaching of the hair. Retinopathy may develop with long-term administration, but not with the usual dosage for amebiasis. Chloroquine can cause deafness in children prenatally exposed to it; thus, it should not be prescribed during pregnancy. The serious hazard of chloroquine to children when taken in excess should be borne in mind.[21]

Alkaloids. EMETINE. EMETINE HYDROCHLORIDE has been a valuable drug for the treatment of amebiasis even though when given alone it will eliminate infection from the intestine in only a small percentage of cases. Emetine affords prompt relief of symptoms in acute amebic dysentery and is a potent therapeutic for hepatic and other forms of extraintestinal amebiasis. The greater concentration and duration of emetine in the liver than in the intestinal wall are consonant with its high efficacy for hepatic amebiasis and its low parasitic cure rate for intestinal amebic infection. Since use of emetine requires hospitalization and bed rest and the drug is somewhat cardiotoxic, other amebicides have largely supplanted it for the treatment of amebic dysentery and as a diagnostic tool when an amebic hepatic abscess is suspected.

Emetine is a general protoplasmic poison that is eliminated from the body slowly, and consequently it may produce cumulative effects. In overdosage it produces focal necrosis of cardiac muscle and may cause cardiac failure and sudden death. Even with a dosage that is generally considered safe, toxic effects on the myocardium are frequently demonstrable during a standard treatment course. The toxic manifestations are elevation of pulse rate, fall of systolic blood pressure and electrocardiographic changes including depression or inversion of the T waves. These changes in the electrocardiogram are reversible.

Emetine should not be used in patients with myocardial disease or marked hypertension. Owing to its toxicity, it should not be used in ambulatory patients; bed rest, with bathroom privileges, during therapy is recommended. Patients receiving emetine should have electrocardiographic monitoring during treatment. The pulse and blood pressure should also be monitored regularly while on medication. The use of emetine in children, except under unusual circumstances, is not advised. It should not be administered during pregnancy unless absolutely necessary. Because of the cumulative action of emetine, when repetition of therapy is indicated, at least 6 weeks should elapse before further administration of the drug.

Emetine is prepared as a hydrochloride

for parenteral injection. It should always be given intramuscularly. When administered subcutaneously it is extremely irritating and produces painful indurations which may persist for considerable periods. It should never be given intravenously.

DEHYDROEMETINE. Dehydroemetine, a synthetic compound (2,3 bisdehydroemetine hydrochloride Δ isomer II) with emetine-like properties, has given results in acute amebic dysentery similar to those obtained with emetine hydrochloride. A high rate of cure of amebic liver abscesses also may be obtained with this drug.[22] Significant toxicity was not encountered. The concentration of dehydroemetine in the heart is less than that of emetine and it is more rapidly excreted from this and other organs. Electrocardiographic changes are less frequent and more transient than with emetine. Dehydroemetine may be administered by intramuscular or deep subcutaneous injection.

Antibiotics. Many of the antibiotics have been studied to determine their potential value in the treatment of amebiasis. A large number have shown some degree of therapeutic value for intestinal amebiasis. The most efficacious are discussed below.

TETRACYCLINES. The broad spectrum antibiotics such as oxytetracycline and chlortetracycline have been found to be effective in the treatment of acute amebic dysentery as well as nondysenteric amebiasis. Further pharmacologic studies of these two antibiotics have proved that the active principle in both is tetracycline. The antibiotics are of no value in the treatment of extraintestinal amebiasis. In acute amebic dysentery and in symptomatic intestinal infections, oxytetracycline (Terramycin), when given alone in adequate dosage, has been found to be better than 90 per cent effective in eliminating amebae from the tissues and contents of the intestine. It produces a similar cure rate of mild or asymptomatic infections. Tetracycline (Tetracyn, Achromycin) should afford equivalent results. The mode of action of tetracyclines in intestinal amebiasis is primarily indirect, since they affect the bacterial associates, the presence or metabolites of which are essential to the amebae. Antibiotics are useful for the treatment of selected cases of intestinal amebiasis, particularly when dysentery is present.[23, 24]

TREATMENT FOR NONDYSENTERIC AMEBIASIS. Symptomless carriers and persons with occasional loose stools or other mild symptoms can be treated satisfactorily as ambulatory patients usually with either diiodohydroxyquin or diloxanide furoate. Frequently, it is desirable to supplement the above luminal amebicides with a course of chloroquine diphosphate as a protective measure in the event that hepatic invasion may have occurred. Although the tetracycline antibiotics are effective against asymptomatic or mild clinical intestinal amebiasis, their use in such cases ordinarily is not justified. In children, a course of diiodohydroxyquin usually eliminates the infection and is tolerated well, but excessive or prolonged dosage must be avoided. Since amebicides are active, directly or indirectly, against the trophozoites, their eradication results in the termination of the passage of cysts in the stool. (See Table 37–2 for dosages.)

Tetracycline antibiotics are effective for the treatment of moderate clinical intestinal amebiasis, as well as for amebic dysentery.[23, 24] Since they are intestinal amebicides, it is often advisable to supplement tetracyclines with chloroquine diphosphate as described. For moderate or chronic intestinal disease, metronidazole may be used.[12] However, it should be supplemented by a course of an intestinal luminal amebicide.[14] (See p. 336 for risks in the use of metronidazole.)

TREATMENT FOR AMEBIC DYSENTERY. The patient suffering from amebic dysentery or severe amebic diarrhea should be confined to bed, although he may be given bathroom privileges. The diet should be high in protein, low in carbohydrate, and supplemented by ample sources of vitamins, especially of the B complex. Although dehydration and toxemia are much less frequent and less severe than in acute bacillary dysentery, adequate fluid balance must be maintained.

There is a wide choice of amebicides for treatment of amebic dysentery. The tetracyclines provide a suitable alternative to

Table 37–2. Summary of Treatment of Amebiasis

Drug	Primary Clinical Usage	Daily Adult Dosage Employed	Duration of Therapy in Days
Nitroimidazole			
Metronidazole (Flagyl) (Note: Before this drug is prescribed, risks associated with its use should be weighed against therapeutic benefits.)	Symptomless carriers to moderate clinical nondysenteric amebiasis	400–800 mg 3 times daily	5
	Amebic dysentery	800 mg 3 times daily	5
		or	
		2.0–2.4 gm every day	3
	Hepatic abscess and other forms of extraintestinal amebiasis	400 mg 3 times daily	5
		or	
		2.0–2.4 gm every day	2–3
Tinidazole (Fasigyn)	Mild clinical to dysenteric amebiasis	2 gm every day*	2–5
	Liver abscess	1.2 gm every day*	7
		or	
		400–800 mg 3 times daily*	1
Halogenated hydroxyquinolines			
Diiodohydroxyquin (Diodoquin)	Symptomless carriers and *mild* clinical nondysenteric intestinal amebiasis	650 mg 3 times daily	20
Anilines			
Diloxanide furoate (Furanimide)	Symptomless carriers and mild and chronic nondysenteric intestinal amebiasis	500 mg 3 times daily	10
Aminoquinolines			
4-aminoquinoline, Chloroquine diphosphate (Aralen, Nivaquine, Avloclor)	Amebic liver abscess	500 mg twice daily followed by 500 mg every day	2 and 12 or 19
Alkaloids			
Emetine hydrochloride	Amebic dysentery; amebic liver abscess; and other forms of extra-intestinal amebiasis	65 mg (1 gr) every day† intramuscularly	Up to 4–10‡
Dehydroemetine	Same as emetine	1–1.5 mg per kg intramuscularly or deep subcutaneous injection	Up to 5–10§
Antibiotics			
Oxytetracycline (Terramycin)	Amebic dysentery; mild to moderate nondysenteric intestinal amebiasis	250–500 mg 4 times daily	Up to 10
Tetracycline (Achromycin, Tetracyn)	Same as oxytetracycline	250–500 mg 4 times daily	Up to 10

*Preliminary dosages; subject to change.

†Daily dosage of emetine hydrochloride is 1 mg per kg; total daily dose not to exceed 65 mg (1 grain).

‡Maximum duration of therapy with emetine hydrochloride is 10 days; total dose for this period not to exceed 10 mg per kg (650 mg or 10 grains). For amebic liver abscess, 10 days; for amebic dysentery, 4 to 6 days as needed to control the dysentery.

§Dehydroemetine, up to 5 days for amebic dysentery; 10 days for liver abscess.

metronidazole, being particularly suitable for children. Dehydroemetine or emetine achieves prompt clinical alleviation of acute dysenteric amebiasis in adults. Since the parasitic cure rate of these two alkaloids is low, their use should be supplemented by effective luminal intestinal amebicides such as diiodohydroxyquin, a tetracycline or diloxanide furoate. Metronidazole is very effective.[12] However, it should be supplemented with a luminal intestinal amebicide. (See p. 336 for hazards.) Tinidazole also appears to be useful for treatment for severe intestinal amebiasis; clinical response to therapy with this nitroimidazole compound is rapid.[16, 17] (See Table 37–2 for dosages.)

As a general rule, if a patient has been treated two or more times for any form of intestinal amebiasis and laboratory reports still indicate *E. histolytica* is present, the validity of the laboratory findings should be questioned. Similarly, if clinical findings or complaints remain or recur after two courses of treatment with amebicides, the diagnosis should be reconsidered and another sought.[7, 8]

Complications. Amebic abscess of the liver is the most common grave complication of intestinal amebiasis. Hepatic involvement results from metastasis of the infection in the wall of the colon to the liver by the portal blood stream.

Other less common extraintestinal complications include abscesses of the lung and brain, cutaneous amebiasis or amebiasis cutis and lesions in other organs. (See Figs. 37–7, 37–10 to 37–14.)

Amebic Abscess of the Liver. Amebic abscess of the liver is commonly a late complication of amebiasis, occurring up to 20 or more years after the probable time of initial infection. However, it may develop within a relatively few months after the initial infection. In some cases there is concurrent dysentery or a history of it. Conversely, many patients with amebic liver abscess give no history of diarrhea or dysentery. The great majority of amebic abscesses of the liver occur in the right lobe; approximately 16 per cent are in the left lobe. The cavity may be large and single, or multiple abscesses, caused by the invasive trophozoites, may be present (Figs. 37–8, 37–9).

Although the clinical picture may be variable, certain salient features should alert the physician to consider amebic liver abscess in the differential diagnosis. These include fever, pain in the right hypochondrium or lower chest, tenderness over the area of the liver, and a moderate leukocytosis. Amebic liver abscess, undiagnosed and untreated, has a very high mortality rate. Conversely, with early diagnosis and prompt institution of specific therapy, the prognosis is excellent and the mortality rate is virtually nil.

In many cases there is a history of weight loss extending over a considerable period of time, with or without periods of low-grade fever. In most cases fever becomes prominent and is usually irregularly remittent, reaching 40° C (104° F). The marked variations in temperature, often accompanied by chills and profuse sweats, may suggest malaria. Variable and irregular pain referred to the right upper quadrant is often present. This is accompanied sometimes by a variety of digestive complaints which may arouse suspicion of chronic cholecystitis or even appendicitis. Jaundice rarely occurs although the levels of alkaline phosphatase and the transaminases often are elevated.

Right lobe abscesses commonly extend upward to involve the diaphragm. In such cases irritation of the basal pleura frequently causes unproductive cough and pain on respiration. Pain referred to the right shoulder is a frequent complaint (Figs. 37–16, 37–17).

With further involvement of the pleura there may be signs of consolidation in the right lower lobe, with or without pleural effusion, leading to an erroneous diagnosis of pneumonia, empyema or tuberculosis. If the process remains unrecognized, spontaneous rupture into the right lower lobe with evacuation of the abscess contents through the bronchial tree may occur. Occasionally the abscess may rupture into the abdominal wall. (Fig. 37–13).

Diagnosis. Careful physical examination of the patient suffering from large single abscess of the liver should immediately arouse suspicion of the true nature of the lesion. Enlargement of the liver is asymmetric. The edge of the right lobe is usually easily palpable, and palpation typically elicits deep pain. If the abscess is in the left lobe, that portion of the liver is similarly affected. When the abscess is on the right, the right hemidiaphragm is commonly elevated and its mobility is impaired; this may be demonstrable on physical examination as well as by roentgen examination and fluoroscopy. An erect posterior-anterior view of the chest may reveal partial or complete obliteration of the costophrenic angle due to the enlarged liver. In some cases "tenting" of the

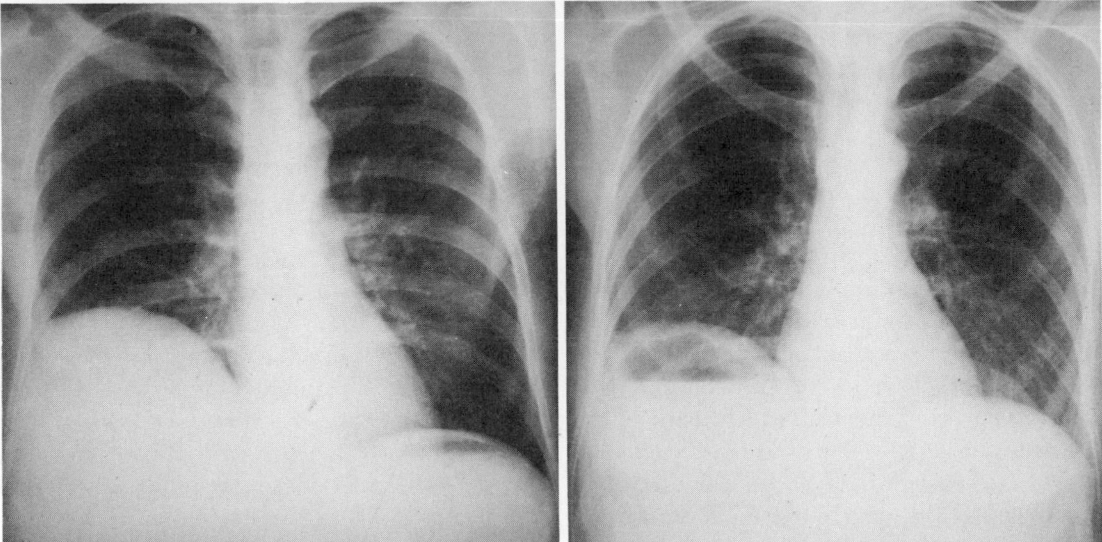

Figure 37-16 Figure 37-17

Figure 37-16. Amebic liver abscess. X-ray film showing marked elevation of the right hemidiaphragm. (Courtesy of Dr. P. A. Muhleisen, Veterans Administration Hospital, New Orleans.)

Figure 37-17. Hepatic amebiasis. X-ray film taken after closed aspiration, showing outline of cavity (air injected) and fluid level under right hemidiaphragm. (Courtesy of Drs. E. Hull and D. Harlee, the Louisiana State University School of Medicine and Charity Hospital, New Orleans.)

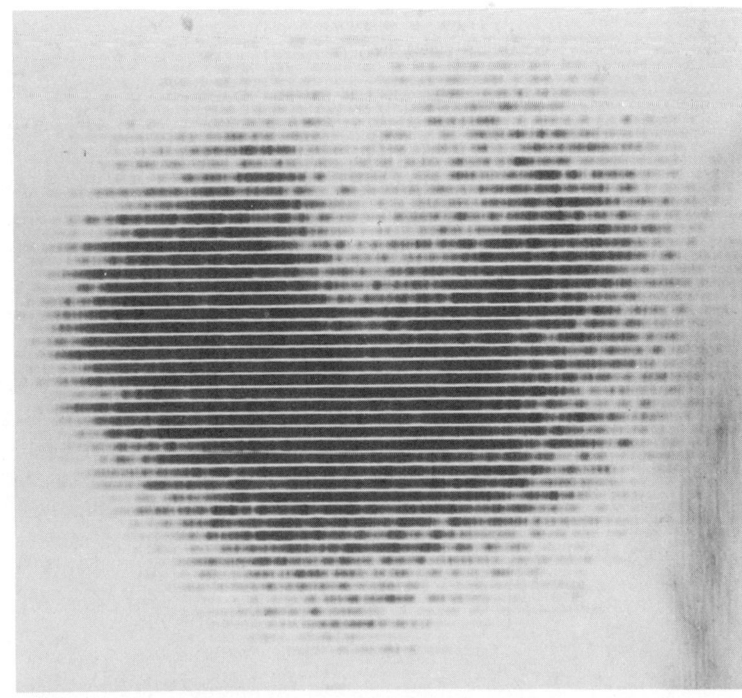

Figure 37-18. Radioisotopic liver scan, lateral view, showing typical "cold area" caused by an amebic abscess. (Courtesy of the Veterans Administration Hospital, New Orleans.)

right hemidiaphragm may be observed. Radioisotopic liver scans reveal "cold areas," indicating the size of the abscess (Fig. 37–18). Heavy percussion of the chest wall in the region of an abscess elicits deep pain. As peripheral extension occurs toward the capsule of the liver, a small area of intercostal tenderness may be noted. When present it is the site of election for aspiration.

The white blood count usually is *elevated moderately,* with an increased percentage of polymorphonuclear leukocytes. Eosinophilia is not characteristic of amebic hepatic abscess, but may be caused by concurrent helminthic infections or other conditions.

Serologic methods are highly sensitive and reliable for confirming the clinical diagnosis of hepatic amebiasis (p. 335). However, initiation of treatment should not be delayed by waiting for results of serologic tests.

A prompt favorable clinical response to specific therapy with extraintestinal amebicides provides a satisfactory means of differential diagnosis and is justified after a careful differential diagnosis has ruled out other possible causes. If secondary bacterial infection complicates an amebic liver abscess, the initial prompt reduction of fever may be followed by return of pyrexia. Also, in large amebic abscesses the reduction in fever may be delayed until therapeutic aspiration of the abscess is instituted. Amebic hepatic abscess is a life-threatening disease. Therefore, a diagnosis of an incurable disease, e.g. hepatoma, in the presence of an unsuspected amebic abscess, can result in fatality from an undiagnosed curable disease. Thus, the obvious cardinal clinical rule relative to diagnosis and prognosis should be kept in mind and amebic hepatic abscess considered in the differential diagnosis when a febrile condition accompanied by subdiaphragmatic involvement on the right side is encountered.[8]

Diagnosis of the presence of an amebic liver abscess is initially based upon clinical evidence. If time permits, the diagnosis can be confirmed or excluded by serologic testing. Although aspiration of an abscess is best reserved for treatment of patients with large abscesses in danger of rupture or when clinical response to specific therapy is delayed or inadequate, it may be desirable or necessary to employ the procedure diagnostically. This is done particularly when serologic testing is not available or when the time required to obtain the results, in the patient's interest, militates against delay of the drainage procedure. Diagnostic aspiration of abscesses in the left lobe should never be attempted.

For aspiration of the right lobe a large caliber needle attached to a syringe should be used and equipped with a stop, so that the point cannot be introduced for a distance greater than 2½ inches from the skin. In the absence of finger-point intercostal tenderness, the site of choice is in the interior axillary line in the ninth interspace. After procaine anesthesia of the skin and deep infiltration, the aspiration needle should be introduced medially and cephalad.

The contents of an amebic abscess of the liver are usually semifluid and chocolate in color. The brown color is pathognomonic for amebic liver abscess, although in old chronic abscesses the aspirate may be yellowish or even white. Amebae may be scanty in the necrotic contents of the cavity and therefore difficult or impossible to demonstrate in the aspirate in many cases. Addition of 10 units of streptodornase per ml of the tenacious pus and incubation at 37° C (98.6° F) with repeated shaking, followed by centrifugation, facilitates detection of the trophozoites. They are, however, more numerous in the advancing border of the abscess wall (Fig. 37–9). The contents of such an abscess are usually bacteriologically sterile. Attempts to culture amebae from the sterile abscess contents invariably fail unless bacteria that will support the growth of *E. histolytica* trophozoites in vitro are used. The addition of *C. welchii* or of other compatible bacteria or bacterial complexes, obtained by separation from stock cultures of *E. histolytica,* to the cultures when they are inoculated with the abscess material frequently results in successful cultivation of amebae from liver abscess aspirates.

Initially, a series of stools should be examined for cysts or trophozoites of *E. histolytica,* depending upon the consistency of the feces. Sigmoidoscopy may be performed. The aspirate should be carefully examined for *trophozoites,* not cysts, of *E. histolytica,* remembering that macrophages are frequently confused with trophozoites.[6, 7]

Differential diagnosis is frequently difficult. An acute abscess may be confused with acute hepatitis, acute cholecystitis, subphrenic abscess or malaria. In the presence of chronic liver abscess the clinical picture may simulate carcinoma of the liver, cirrhosis of the liver, pleurisy with effusion, atypical pulmonary tuberculosis, arthritis of the cervical spine or shoulder, and chronic cholecystitis or appendicitis.

Treatment. The high mortality previously associated with abscess of the liver was in large part due to the universal use of open drainage and the great difficulty in preventing secondary infection. Although open drainage is not recommended for right lobe abscesses, obviously it no longer would result in such a high mortality rate because of the introduction of antibiotics. With the advent of emetine and the use of closed aspiration of the cavity, the mortality was reduced to about 2 per cent.

In cases of right lobe abscess a course of metronidazole should be given. Alternative drugs include dehydroemetine, emetine, chloroquine diphosphate or tinidazole. Luminal amebicides should be used concurrently with any of the above drugs as a supplement to eliminate the primary intestinal infection. (See Table 37–2.) This usually is followed within a few days by reduction of both fever and leukocytosis and by marked diminution in liver pain and tenderness. If there is no prompt clinical response after the institution of therapy, the contents of the abscess cavity should be emptied as completely as possible by closed drainage and treatment with one of the antibiotics instituted at the same time. In patients with large abscesses, fever, pain and leukocytosis may recur or increase a few days after the primary aspiration. This constitutes an imperative indication for further drainage of the cavity. It does not necessarily indicate failure of specific therapy. Such repeated closed drainage should be continued as indications require. Also, occasionally the recurrence of fever following an initial clinical response to specific antiamebic therapy for liver abscess may indicate the presence of a concurrent bacterial infection of the usually sterile amebic liver abscess. Supplementing the amebicidal treatment with an appropriate antibiotic for the secondary bacterial invader usually results in a sustained clinical response and cure of both infections.

Laparotomy is required for drainage of left lobe amebic abscess because of the proximity of the pericardium.

PLEUROPULMONARY AMEBIASIS. These complications usually result from extension or rupture of an amebic liver abscess. Rarely, pulmonary amebiasis may occur either by hematogenous spread of the trophozoites from lesions in the large intestine or by amebic perforation of the hepatic flexure of the colon with penetration of the diaphragm and invasion of the pleural cavity and pulmonary tissue (Fig. 37–10). In the presence of an hepatobronchial fistula, abscess contents with characteristic color, odor, and taste may be coughed up. Frequently there may be scant radiographic evidence of involvement of lung tissue, while in other instances consolidation and cavitation resulting in lung abscess may be present. Dry pleurisy and nonpurulent pleural effusions are common in liver abscess; empyema also may occur.

Demonstration of the existence of the usual underlying liver abscess is basic to the diagnosis of pleuropulmonary amebiasis. Radiographic, serologic and other appropriate procedures for detection of hepatic and intestinal amebiasis are indicated. Sputum with discharged abscess contents should be examined carefully for trophozoites, but ordinarily this is not rewarding. A prompt clinical response to an extraintestinal amebicide, such as emetine or metronidazole, supports a clinical diagnosis. Specific treatment should not be withheld by awaiting results of serology.

Conservative treatment usually suffices. Amebicidal drugs as used for the treatment of hepatic abscess, postural drainage for lung abscess, and, if necessary, drainage of the residual liver abscess are effective. Treatment for the primary intestinal amebic infection should be included (Table 37–2). Prognosis is good if diagnosis and treatment are prompt.

When secondary infection of pulmonary lesions is evident from purulent sputum and culture, appropriate antibiotics should supplement antiamebic treatment. For empyema, regular and thorough aspiration should be employed at 2-day intervals. Continuous drainage may be required, intercostally, if aspiration does not adequately remove the exudate. Again, appropriate antibiotics for secondary infection should supplement specific treatment with extraintestinal amebicides for the underlying abscess in the liver.

Dientamoeba Diarrhea

Synonyms. None.

Distribution. Worldwide.

Clinical Characteristics. *Dientamoeba fragilis* has been considered to be a cause of chronic though mild intestinal symptoms. There is controversy, however, concerning its actual pathogenicity. Its ability to invade the tissues of the host has not been demonstrated.[25, 26] The syndrome commonly ascribed to this organism consists of recurring episodes of lower abdominal discomfort and flatulence associated with the evacuation of two or three loose "mushy" stools each day. There is no mucus, blood or inflammatory exudate in the feces. The symptoms usually cease following treatment with amebicides.

Diagnosis. Microscopic examination of a fresh, loose stool will reveal the trophozoites with characteristic spherical shape and some with extended pseudopodia (p. 315 and Fig. 36–7). Red cells are not ingested, and no encysted stage is known. *Dientamoeba fragilis* may be isolated in culture (p. 829).

Treatment. The infection usually may be eliminated by diiodohydroxyquin (Diodoquin). The adult dosage is 650 mg 3 times daily for 10 days. Also, a tetracycline, 250 mg 4 times daily for 7 days (adult dose), may be employed as an alternative therapeutic.

OTHER PATHOGENIC AMEBIC INFECTIONS

Naegleria and *Hartmannella* (or *Acanthamoeba*) Infections

Clyde G. Culbertson

Synonyms. Infections by "free-living soil-amebae," primary amebic meningitis, hartmannellosis, acanthamebiasis, terramebiasis.

Definition. A disease of humans and animals that affects the respiratory, nervous and, rarely, other systems, which is caused by amebae of the genera *Naegleria* and *Hartmannella* (or *Acanthamoeba*).

Distribution. The distribution of the few cases (fewer than 100 altogether), though worldwide, appears to be confined to the temperate zones.[27–29]

Etiology. These afflictions in the human host are not common. Most of them are caused by *Naegleria,* which enter the nasal cavity and invade the brain via the olfactory nerve or the perineural space through the cribriform plate to the brain. A lesser but definite group of similar infections is caused by *Hartmannella* (or *Acanthamoeba*), i.e. H-A amebae (Fig. 37–19). While the pathogenesis of the *Naegleria* infection, "primary amebic meningitis," has been confirmed by postmortem studies, the preinvasive stage of H-A disease has not been determined in the human.

Epidemiology. The *Naegleria* infec-

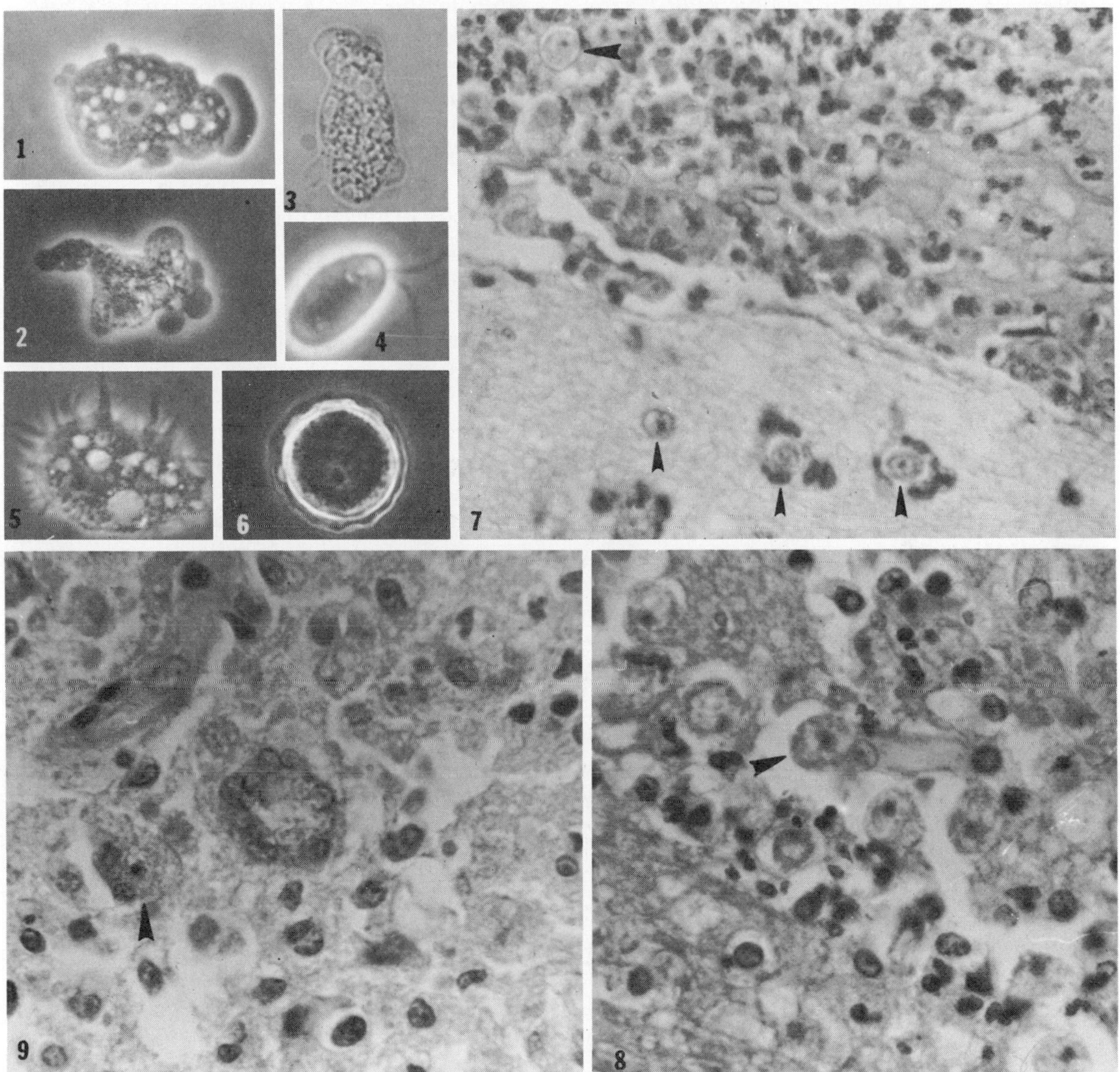

Figure 37–19. Forms of *Naegleria* and *Hartmannella* spp. and lesions produced by these free-living soil-amebae. *1* and *2*, Trophozoites, *Naegleria fowleri* (phase microscopy, 1000×). *3*, Same under light microscopy, 1000×; note lobate pseudopodia in all three. *4*, Biflagellate form appearing after addition of distilled water to culture. *5*, Trophozoite, *Hartmannella culbertsoni* (phase, 1000×); note filiform, spine-like pseudopodia *(Acanthamoeba)*. *6*, Cyst of *Hartmannella rhysodes* (phase, 1000×); note wrinkled outer surface. The cyst of *H. culbertsoni* is similar, but wall is nearly smooth. *7*, Cerebellum, showing meningeal exudate containing amebae. Also, three amebae are invading the brain tissue beneath the exudate (arrows) (H & E × 700). *8*, Hartmannellid amebae in perivascular space in cerebrum (arrow); note amebae are larger than in number 7 (H & E × 700). *9*, Brain. Granulomatous lesion due to amebae resembling soil-amebae (*Hartmannella?*); note mononuclear exudate, giant cell and ameba at arrow. Only the small, round nucleus calls attention to the ameba (H & E × 700). (Composite of illustrations courtesy of Dr. C. G. Culbertson.)

tions are associated with swimming in lakes and pools. There is no known epidemiologic pattern for H-A amebic disease.

Pathology. The pathology of the *Naegleria* infection is that of widespread meningitis with amebic encephalitis involving the entire central nervous system, more intense in the basilar portion of the cerebrum and cerebellum. The H-A infections cause irregularly distributed meningitis, with abscess and granuloma formation in addition to varying degrees of the diffuse invasion more common to the *Naegleria* disease. Thus, the H-A amebae are known to produce acute, subacute and chronic lesions (Fig. 37–19). No chronic or subacute disease due to *Naegleria* has yet been described outside of the experimental infection in mice, where partially effective treatment was given to prolong the life of the animal. Visceral infections are known as experimental lesions in guinea pigs following subcutaneous injection of *Naegleria,* and some spontaneous infections in domestic animals due to H-A amebae, but not in man.[27, 28]

The amebic morphology in tissue sections is quite distinct from that of *E. histolytica.* The soil amebae have large nucleoli, whereas the nucleolus of *E. histolytica* is very small and almost invisible in H and E–stained sections. The H–A amebae are the largest (15 to 30 μm) and may be accompanied by the characteristic double-walled cyst. The *Naegleria* are smaller (8 to 15 μm), and the cyst of *Naegleria* has not been found in central nervous system lesions.[28–30]

Clinical Characteristics. The clinical picture of the *Naegleria* infection is much like that of acute meningococcic meningitis, whereas the H-A amebae have caused disease that resembles chronic virus or mycotic disease of the brain. Thus far *Naegleria* has affected robust young persons, and the H-A amebae have affected those with depressed immune function.[28, 29]

Diagnosis. The key to the antemortem diagnosis is found in examination of cerebrospinal fluid by careful direct microscopy of the fresh sediment, using subdued illumination in the light microscope, or by phase microscopy, which is preferable. Cultures can be made in a number of ways, but most simply by using plates of plain 1.5 per cent agar containing either no sodium chloride or not more than 0.4 per cent, and no nutrient. A loopful of *E. coli* growth from a 24- to 48-hour agar slant culture is spread in a circle in the center of the plate, 1 to 2 cm in diameter, and the suspected amebic inoculum is applied to the middle of the bacterial circle. After incubation the plate is examined for the presence of outgrowing amebic cells. Details of identification are published elsewhere.[30-32]

Treatment. The known cases of *Naegleria* infections have in nearly all instances been fatal, and most of them were diagnosed at autopsy. Amphotericin is effective in experimental mouse infections, but only in a single reported case was there indication of improvement by use of this drug in the human. Sulfadiazine is markedly effective in H-A experimental disease, but has not been tested against this infection in man.[28, 29]

Prophylaxis. Restriction of swimming is advocated unless careful attention is paid to known sanitary measures, such as filtration, chlorination and prevention of soil being carried into the water.[33] Ordinary chlorination does not appear to be lethal to the amebae; periodic hyperchlorination of swimming pools possibly may be of some benefit.

Giardiasis

Synonyms. None.

Distribution. Worldwide.

Etiology. *Giardia lamblia* has been recovered from the duodenum and occasionally from the gallbladder. It has been associated with symptoms referable to the duodenum. This flagellate, which adheres in large numbers to the mucosa, thus coating the proximal portion of the small intestine, has long been considered a noninvasive lumen-dweller. However, there is histologic evidence that *G. lamblia* may invade the mucosa.[34] Further, by electron microscopy, it has been demonstrated that trophozoites of *G. lamblia* can be seen within mucosal cells.[35]

Clinical Characteristics. Frequently,

infections with *G. lamblia* may cause no symptoms. However, in a small percentage of cases of giardiasis, epigastric discomfort, nausea and flatulence may be present. Occasionally, in heavy infections, diarrhea may occur. The stools in some cases are light-colored and contain excessive amounts of fat. The infection is more common in children than in adults. The chronic or subacute stage may mimic gallbladder or ulcer disease; in the acute stage there may be steatorrhea and substantial weight loss.[35a] Symptoms may be related to IgA deficiency.[35b] Giardiasis can also mimic pancreatic steatorrhea by inducing mucosal malabsorption in patients whose pancreatitis alone is not sufficient to cause steatorrhea.[35c] In experimental infections in human volunteers, the prepatent period ranged from 6 to 15 days, with an average of 9 days.[36]

Diagnosis. The cystic stage is observed far more frequently than the trophozoite in stools (Figs. 36–6, 36–8). Actively motile trophozoites occur in some diarrheal stools and may be present in large numbers in duodenal drainage fluid. The detailed morphology is described on page 316. Attempts to culture this flagellate have not been successful.

Treatment. Quinacrine hydrochloride (Atabrine) is a highly effective drug against *G. lamblia.* It should be given by mouth after meals for 5 days. The individual dosage is 50 mg twice daily for children 1 to 4 years of age; 100 mg twice daily for those 4 to 8; and 100 mg 3 times a day for persons over 8 years, including adults. Only occasionally is a second course required to eliminate the infection.

An oral suspension of furazolidine (Furoxone) gave an 81 per cent cure rate in children below 9 years of age. It may be the preferred drug for this age group. The following doses, 4 times a day for 10 days, were employed: less than 1 year, 1/2 to 1 teaspoonful; 1 to 4 years, 1 to 1½ teaspoonsful; 5 or more years, 1 tablespoonful. Reversible hypersensitivity reactions occur rarely.[35a]

Metronidazole (Flagyl) is very effective for treatment of giardiasis. Side reactions are less frequent than with quinacrine hydrochloride and consist of occasional vomiting and abdominal pain. The dose is as follows: less than 2 years, 125 mg; 2 to 4 years, 250 mg; 4 to 8 years, 375 mg; and for youths over 9 years, 500 mg. For children the tablets may be crushed, mixed with sweetened liquids, and taken in divided doses after meals for 5 days.[37] The dosage for adults is 250 mg 3 times daily for 10 days. Metronidazole is considered an investigational drug for giardiasis by the U.S. Food and Drug Administration. Since it has been shown recently that metronidazole is carcinogenic in rodents and mutagenic in bacteria, quinacrine hydrochloride should be employed for treatment of giardiasis in patients in whom side effects are not marked.

Tinidazole (Fasigyn), at a dosage of 150 mg twice daily for 7 days, was curative in all cases in a small series of adult patients with giardiasis. No clinical side effects were observed.[38] This nitroimidazole derivative shows promise as an additional therapeutic for giardiasis if its safety is adequately established. This compound presently is not widely available geographically.

Trichomonas Vaginalis Infection

Synonyms. None.

Distribution. Worldwide.

Etiology. *Trichomonas vaginalis* is a flagellate often associated with a specific vaginitis or urethritis. Infection becomes established when the acidity of the vaginal secretions is reduced. *Trichomonas vaginalis* will not survive at the normal vaginal acidity of pH 3.8 to 4.4 which is maintained by the conversion of glycogen in the epithelium to lactic acid by the normal bacterial flora and, indirectly, by activity of the sex hormones.

Coitus plays an important role in transmission. The possibility of transmission of trichomoniasis by common use of douche equipment, clothing and towels in families or by contaminated instruments used for examination of patients should not be excluded in some cases. Vaginal trichomoniasis is not acquired from the intestine by fecal contamination. *Trichomonas vaginalis* and *T. hominis* are distinct species that are not interchangeable in their location in the body.

Clinical Characteristics. Trichomonas vaginitis is accompanied by vulval pruritus, often intense, and a more or less profuse and irritating vaginal discharge which, in untreated cases, may lead to actual excoriation of the vulva and dermatitis of the adjacent skin of the thighs. The vaginal mucosa is usually diffusely congested and inflamed. A chronic urethritis may be seen in men.

Diagnosis. Although *T. vaginalis* at times may be detected in the urine of both women and men, vaginal and urethral secretion and prostatic fluid are the best diagnostic sources for demonstration of the flagellates. The detailed morphology of *T. vaginalis* is described on page 320 and in Fig. 36–6. It may be isolated in culture (p. 832).

Treatment. Successful treatment of trichomonas vaginitis is difficult and time-consuming and requires persistence and complete cooperation by the patient. The basic principles are cleanliness, restoration of normal vaginal epithelium and secretions, and destruction of the trichomonads by chemotherapeutic agents. Patients who have passed the menopause may require estrogen therapy, and lesions of the cervix must be corrected.

Various chemotherapeutic agents, including arsenicals, sulfonamides, antibiotics, and oxyquinoline derivatives, used locally in the form of powders, vaginal tablets and jellies have been recommended. They are used in conjunction with measures for maintaining vaginal acidity. Treatment of vaginal trichomoniasis is not always successful. Local application of trichomonicides may fail to reach sites of residual infection such as glands and ducts. An infected man may reinfect his coital partner. Oral or systemic drugs for vaginal trichomoniasis such as Tritheon and Flagyl have been employed with some success. Flagyl, Tritheon and Aureomycin have shown significant effectiveness in eliminating trichomoniasis in men.

Metronidazole (Flagyl), 250 mg 3 times daily for 10 days (adult dosage), with insertion of one 500 mg vaginal tablet high in the vagina for the same 10 days, will eliminate most infections with *T. vaginalis* in women. To prevent reinfection, which otherwise is common, the sexual partner may receive the same oral medication over the same period. Since metronidazole (Flagyl) recently has been shown to be carcinogenic in rodents and mutagenic in bacteria, it should not be used for *Trichomonas* infections that can be made asymptomatic by other means. Metronidazole should generally not be used in pregnant women.

Tinidazole (Fasigyn), which has a wide spectrum of antiprotozoal activity (p. 336, p. 347), is also highly effective against *T. vaginalis* infections in females and males. A single dose of 1.4 or 1.8 gm was curative for vaginal trichomoniasis.[39, 40] In males with *T. vaginalis* infection, most of whom had symptoms, the cure rate with a single dose of 2 gm of tinidazole was 97 per cent. Side effects, only mild and transient gastrointestinal complaints, occurred infrequently.[40] Further study of this drug for safety is indicated.

Balantidiasis

Synonyms. Balantidial dysentery.

Distribution. Worldwide.

Etiology. *Balantidium coli* is a pathogenic ciliate which occasionally infects the colon of man and may produce diarrhea and dysentery (Fig. 37–20).

Epidemiology. Presumably the pig is an important animal reservoir of balantidial infection. Man is only an occasional host of the parasite. About 25 per cent of people with reported infection have a history of contact with pigs. The infection may be contracted from human sources under unsanitary institutional conditions.[41] Species of *Balantidium* occur in man, lower primates, pigs, rats and guinea pigs. The *Balantidium coli* of man can be transmitted to the pig, monkey, guinea pig, cat and rat. Limited attempts to infect man with the *Balantidium* of hogs and monkeys have been unsuccessful. However, epidemiologic evidence points strongly to the hog as the chief source of human infection with balantidiasis.

Pathology. *Balantidium coli* penetrates the mucosa, producing necrosis and ulceration. There is no leukocytic infiltration until

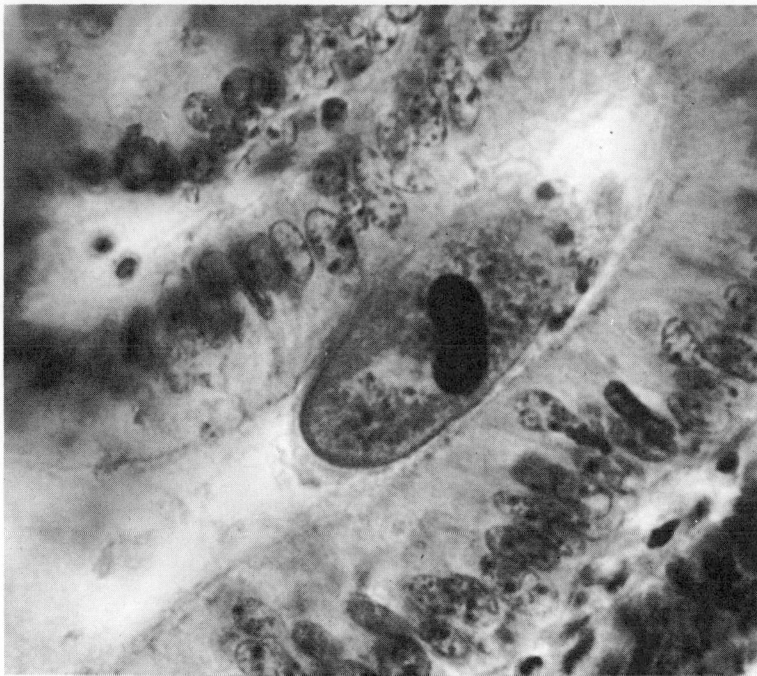

Figure 37–20. *Balantidium coli* trophozoite entering mucosa of large intestine. (Courtesy of the Louisiana State University School of Medicine, New Orleans.)

secondary bacterial infection occurs. Occasionally masses of balantidia are found in the submucosa in a collagenous stroma without an accompanying inflammatory reaction (Fig. 37–21).

As the ciliates invade the mucosa, secondary infection rapidly occurs. Superficial erosions are produced that extend laterally and penetrate into the deeper layers of the intestinal wall. These are often hemorrhagic and in their gross appearance resemble the "Dyak hair" ulcers of amebic dysentery. The lesions are discrete and the intervening mucosa is normal (Fig. 37–22).

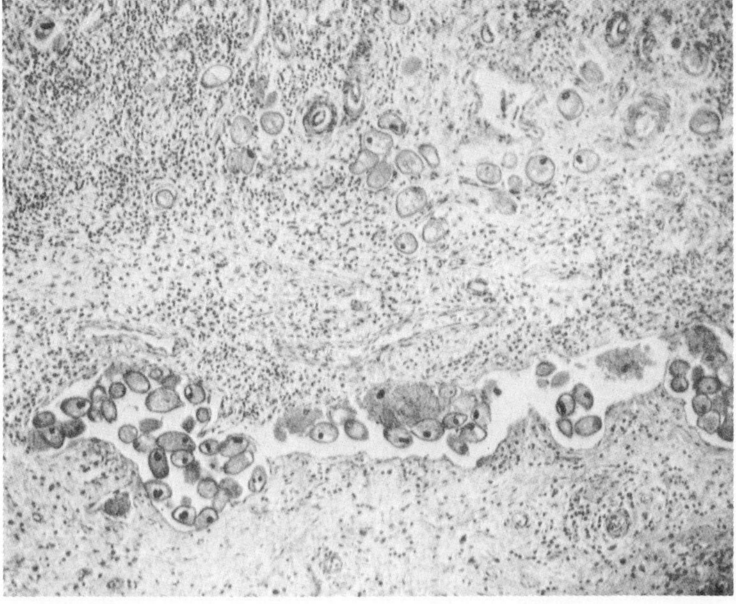

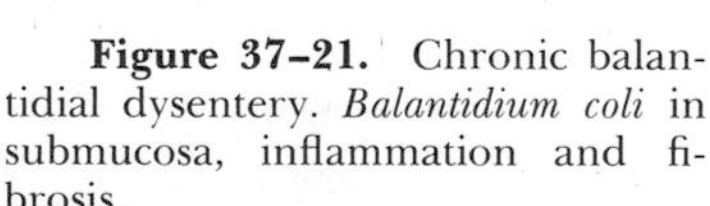

Figure 37–21. Chronic balantidial dysentery. *Balantidium coli* in submucosa, inflammation and fibrosis.

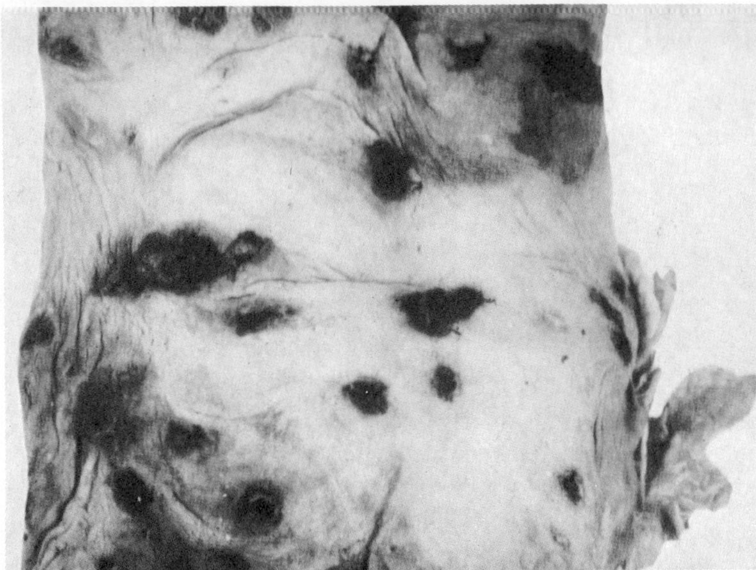

Figure 37-22. Balantidial dysentery. Ulcerations of colon with intervening normal mucosa.

Clinical Characteristics. Balantidiasis may be asymptomatic or may be associated with diarrhea or dysentery.

Diagnosis. Diagnosis depends upon demonstration of *B. coli* in the feces. The motile trophozoites will be found when the stools are liquid or semiliquid; the cysts are seen in semiformed or formed stools. The trophozoite is the more important diagnostic stage, since it is observed in most, perhaps all, of the clinical cases of balantidiasis; the cysts are seen only infrequently.[42] The detailed morphology of the ciliate is described on page 320. (Also see Fig. 36-6, p. 317.)

Treatment. Several of the antiamebic drugs are effective therapeutics for balantidiasis. Favorable results have been obtained with oxytetracycline, 500 mg 4 times daily for 10 days. An alternate method of treatment consists of diiodohydroxyquin (Diodoquin), 650 mg 3 times daily for 20 days. (See Table 37-2.)

Isosporiasis

Synonyms. None.

Distribution. Widely distributed, especially in the southwest Pacific and Philippines. Infection has been reported from man also in southern Europe, the Middle East, Africa, Japan, Vietnam, Manchuria, South, Central and North America and parts of the West Indies.

Etiology. *Isospora belli* and *I. hominis* are mildly pathogenic coccidial parasites of the small intestine of man.

Clinical Characteristics and Pathology. The infection in some instances is asymptomatic However, diarrhea, fever, abdominal pain and tenderness, flatulence, nausea, anorexia and headache may result from infection with these coccidia. Although no lesions have been demonstrated at autopsy, it is believed that transient microscopic lesions must be produced in the epithelial cells. Infections are self-limited. In experimental infections in man symptoms developed in a week, oocysts were recovered 9 to 15 days after ingestion and persisted for less than a month.[43, 44]

Diagnosis. Diagnosis depends upon demonstrating the unstained oocysts in the stool (p. 322 and Figs. 36-9 to 36-11). Oocysts of *I. belli* have been found in duodenal drainage fluid.

Treatment. None, as the infection is self-limited.

PROPHYLAXIS AGAINST INTESTINAL PROTOZOAL INFECTIONS

Infection by the intestinal protozoa does not produce a protective immunity, and artificial immunization has not been accomplished in humans. Prophylaxis, therefore, depends upon avoidance of infection. These organisms reach man through water or food polluted by human feces, and foods contaminated by the droppings and vomitus of flies or by the soiled hands of infected foodhandlers (Fig. 37–1, p. 324). Ice may be a vehicle of infection and should not be used in beverages or placed in contact with food in areas where it may be contaminated. In heavily endemic areas all water for human consumption should be chemically treated or preferably boiled before use. Raw vegetables must be scrupulously avoided, and fruits should be scalded before consumption. The exposure of fresh vegetables to acetic acid or vinegar for a minimum of 15 minutes would provide considerable, but not necessarily complete, protection against any *E. histolytica* cysts present on the foods. Whenever practicable, food handlers should be examined and treated if infected. Latrines should be fly-proofed and kitchens and dining rooms adequately screened.

REFERENCES

1. Le Maistre, C. A , Sappenfield, R., Culbertson, C., Carter, F. R. N., Offutt, A., Black, H., and Brook, M. M. 1956. Studies of a water-borne outbreak of amebiasis, South Bend, Indiana. I. Epidemiological aspects. Am. J. Hyg. *64*:30–45.
2. Phillips, B. P., Wolfe, P. A., Rees, C. W., Gordon, H. A., Wright, W. H., and Reyniers, J. A. 1955. Studies on the ameba-bacteria relationship in amebiasis. Am. J. Trop. Med. Hyg. *4*:675–692.
3. Faust, E. C. 1961. The multiple facets of *Entamoeba histolytica* infection. Internat. Rev. Trop. Med. *1*:43–76.
4. Beaver, P. C. 1958. The exudates in amebic colitis. Proc. 6th Internat. Congr. Trop. Med. Mal. *3*:419–434.
5. Elsdon-Dew, R. 1971. Amebiasis as a world problem. Bull. N.Y. Acad. Med. Ser. 2, *47*:438–447.
6. Stamm, W. P 1970. Amoebic aphorisms. Lancet *2*:1355–1356.
7. Swartzwelder, C. 1952 Laboratory diagnosis of amebiasis. Am. J. Clin. Pathol. *22*:379–395.
8. Swartzwelder, J. C. 1972. Diagnosis of tropical diseases. *In* Chapter VIII, Proc. VIII World Congr. Anat. Clin. Path. Internat. Congr. Series No. 285. Excerpta Medica, Amsterdam. pp. 287–290.
9. Krupp, I. M., and Powell, S. J. 1971. Antibody response to invasive amebiasis in Durban, South Africa. Am. J. Trop. Med. Hyg. *20*:414–420.
10. Krupp, I. M., and Powell, S. J. 1971. Comparative study of the antibody response in amebiasis. Persistence after successful treatment. Am. J. Trop. Med. Hyg *20*:421–424.
11. Morris, M. N., Powell, S. J., and Elsdon-Dew, R. 1970 Latex agglutination test for invasive amoebiasis. Lancet *1*:1362–1363.
12. Powell, S. J. 1971. Therapy of amebiasis. Bull. N.Y. Acad. Med. Ser. 2, *47*:469–477.
13. Antani J., and Srinivas, H. V. 1970. Clinical evaluation of metronidazole in hepatic amebiasis. Am. J. Trop. Med. Hyg. *19*:762–766.
14. Weber, D. M. 1971. Amebic abscess of liver following metronidazole therapy. J.A.M.A *216*:1339–1340.
15. Bunnag, D., and Harinasuta, T. 1974. Clinical trial of tinidazole in amoebic liver abscess using low doses. Proc. 3rd Internat. Congr. Parasit. *3*:1276.
16. De Esesarte, G., Nava, C., and Garcia Reyes, J. A. 1974. Effect of tinidazole in amoebiasis. Proc. 3rd Internat. Congr. Parasit. *3*:1277.
17. Tschl-hyun, J. 1974. Use of tinidazole (Fasigyn) on treatment of intestinal and hepatic amebiasis. Proc. 3rd Internat. Congr. Parasit. *3*:1279.
18. Oakley, G. P. 1973. The neurotoxicity of the halogenated hydroxyquinolines. J.A.M.A. *225*:395–397.
19. Behrens, M. M. 1974. Optic atrophy in children after diiodohydroxyquin therapy. J.A.M.A. *228*:693.
20. Anonymous. 1974. Blindness after Diodoquin (diiodohydroxyquin), United States. C.D.C. Morbidity and Mortality Weekly Report *23*:254.
21. Conn, H. M., and Verhulst, H. L. 1961. Fatal acute chloroquine poisoning in children. Pediatrics *27*:95–102.
22. Powell, S. J., McLeod, I., Wilmot, A. J., and Elsdon-Dew, R. 1962. Dehydroemetine in amebic dysentery and amebic liver abscess. Am. J. Trop. Med. Hyg. *11*:607–609.
23. Sappenfield, R. W., Carter, F. R. N., Culbertson, C., Brooke, M. M., Payne, F. W., and Frye, W. W. 1955. Therapeutic aspects of a water-borne outbreak of amebiasis in South Bend, Indiana. J.A.M.A. *159*:1009–1012.
24. Elsdon-Dew, R., Wilmont, A. J., and Powell, S. J. 1960. The tetracyclines in amebiasis. Antibiotics Annual 1959–1960. pp. 829–833.
25. Knoll, E. W., and Howell, K. M. 1945. Studies on *Dientamoeba fragilis;* its incidence and possible pathology. Am. J. Clin. Med. *15*:178–183.
26. Burrows, R. B., Swerdlow, M. A., Frost, J. K., and Leeper, C. K. 1954. Pathology of *Dientamoeba fragilis* infections of the appendix. Am. J. Trop. Med. Hyg. *3*:1033–1039.
27. Carter, R. F. 1970. Description of a *Naegleria* sp. isolated from two cases of primary amoebic meningoencephalitis, and of the experimental pathological changes induced by it. J. Pathol. *100*:217–244.
28. Culbertson, C. G. 1971. The pathogenicity of soil amebas. Ann. Rev. Microbiol. *25*:231–254.

29. Duma, R. J. 1972. Primary amoebic meningoencephalitis. C. R. C. Crit. Rev. in Clin. Lab. Sci. *3*:163–192.
30. Singh, B. N. 1972. Classification of amoebae belonging to the Order Amoebida with special reference to pathogenic free-living forms. Curr. Sci. *41*:395–403.
31. Page, F. C. 1970. Taxonomic and ecological distribution of potentially pathogenic free-living amoebae. *OR* Taxonomy and morphology of free-living amoebae causing meningoencephalitis in man and other animals. J. Parasit. *56*:257–258.
32. Fulton, C. 1970. Amebo-flagellates as research partners: the laboratory biology of *Naegleria* and *Tetramitis*. *In* Prescott, D. M. (ed.): Methods in Cell Physiology. IV. Academic Press, New York. pp. 341–476.
33. Cerva, L. 1971. Studies of *Limax* amoebae in a swimming pool. Hydrobiologia *38*:141–161.
34. Brandburg, L. L., Tankersley, C. B., Gottlieb, S., Barancik, M., and Sartor, V. E. 1967. Histological demonstration of mucosal invasion by *Giardia lamblia* in man. Gastroenterology *52*:143–150.
35. Morecki, R., and Parker, J. G. 1967. Ultrastructural studies of the human *Giardia lamblia* and subjacent jejunal mucosa in a subject with steatorrhea. Gastroenterology *52*:151–164.
35a. Wolfe, M. S. 1975. Giardiasis. J.A.M.A. *233*:1362–1365.
35b. Zinnemann, H. H., and Kaplan, A. P. 1972. The association of giardiasis with reduced intestinal secretory immunoglobulins. Am. J. Dig. Dis. *17*:793–797.
35c. Sheehy, T. W., and Holley, H. P., Jr. 1975. *Giardia*-induced malabsorption in pancreatitis. J.A.M.A. *233*:1733–1735.
36. Rendtorff, R. C. 1954. The experimental transmission of human intestinal protozoan parasites. II. *Giardia lamblia* cysts given in capsules. Am. J. Hyg. *59*:209–220.
37. Rubio, M., and Cuello, E. 1963. Tratamiento de la giardiosis intestinal con un derivado de nitroimidazol. Bol. Chil. Parasit. *18*:60–63.
38. Pawlowski, Z., Kociecka, W., and Gerwel, M. 1974. Nifuratel and tinidazole as the drugs effective in giardiasis. Proc. 3rd Internat. Congr. Parasit. *3*:1283–1284.
39. Osaki, H., Saito, H., Yagyu, M., and Furuya, M. 1974. Single-dose treatment of *Trichomonas vaginalis* infections with tinidazole. Proc. 3rd Internat. Congr. Parasit. *3*:1290.
40. Chune-Kamrai, W. 1974. The diagnosis of trichomoniasis in the male and its treatment with a single dose of tinidazole (Fasigyn). Proc. Internat. Congr. Parasit. *3*:1291.
41. Young, M. D. 1950. Attempts to transmit human *Balantidium coli*. Am. J. Trop. Med. *30*:70–71.
42. Swartzwelder, J. C. 1950. Balantidiasis. Am. J. Digest. Dis. *17*:173–179.
43. Barksdale, W. L., and Routh, C. F. 1948. *Isospora hominis* infections among American personnel in the southwest Pacific. Am. J. Trop. Med. *28*:639–644.
44. Elsdon-Dew, R., and Freedman, L. 1953. Coccidiosis in man: experiences in Natal. Tr. Roy. Soc. Trop. Med. Hyg. *47*:209–214.

CHAPTER 38

Malaria

Martin D. Young

Synonyms. The synonyms of malaria in general are ague, jungle fever, paludism. Synonyms of malaria due to *Plasmodium vivax:* benign tertian, *vivax* malaria. Synonyms of malaria due to *Plasmodium falciparum:* malignant tertian, subtertian, estivo-autumnal, E-A, *falciparum* malaria. Malaria due to *Plasmodium malariae* is designated quartan malaria or *malariae* malaria. Malaria due to *Plasmodium ovale* is designated *ovale* malaria.

Definition. Malaria is an acute and chronic infection characterized by fever, anemia, splenomegaly and often serious or fatal complications. It is caused by protozoa of the genus *Plasmodium.* Four species occur naturally in man, namely: *P. vivax* (Grassi and Feletti, 1890), Labbé, 1899; *P. falciparum* (Welch, 1897) Schaudinn, 1902; *P. malariae* (Laveran, 1881) Grassi and Feletti, 1890; and *P. ovale* Stephens, 1922. There are many strains in these four species.

Distribution. The normal range of malarial infections is between 45° north and 40° south latitude. In certain areas these limits are wider (Fig. 38–1). Malaria due to *P. vivax* is more widely distributed than the other types. It is the prevalent infection in most areas within the temperate zones but is widespread throughout the tropics as well. *Plasmodium malariae* is comparatively rare; it is observed most commonly in temperate areas and in the subtropics. *Plasmodium falciparum* tends to predominate throughout all tropical regions. *Plasmodium ovale* is relatively uncommon; the majority of cases have been reported from Africa, although some have been found in Asia, Europe and South America.

Etiology. The *life cycle* of the parasites causing malaria in man consists of an exogenous sexual phase, termed sporogony, with multiplication in certain anopheline mosquitoes, and an endogenous asexual phase, termed schizogony, with multiplication in man.

The *exogenous,* or *anopheline, phase* of the cycle begins when a suitable anopheline mosquito ingests blood containing the mature sexual forms, the gametocytes. Within a few minutes after reaching the insect's stomach, the male cell or microgametocyte extends actively motile flagellum-like structures, each of which contains a portion of the nuclear chromatin of the parent cell (Fig. 38–2). These flagella shortly become detached to form microgametes, which migrate to the female cell or macrogametocyte. Meanwhile the latter has undergone maturation in preparation for fertilization. Completion of these changes marks the end of gametogony; subsequent fertilization of the macrogamete by a microgamete initiates the processes of sporogony.

When a microgamete enters the female cell, fusion of the nuclear chromatin from each parent occurs, and shortly thereafter the fertilized cell elongates and becomes motile, forming the ookinete or traveling vermicule. This penetrates the wall of the mosquito's stomach, finally lodging beneath the outer layer.

It then undergoes progressive vacuolization to form a growing oocyst (Fig. 38–3). The nuclear chromatin subdivides repeatedly, its particles becoming arranged along cytoplasmic strands bordering the vacuoles. From each particle of chromatin in the protoplasmic mesh a filamentous structure extends into the lumen of a vacuole. The chromatin particles become incorporated in these filaments to form sporozoites. At maturity the oocyst consists of a spongelike spherical body that projects into the body cavity of the insect. In a suitable infected vector several hundred oocysts may be found on

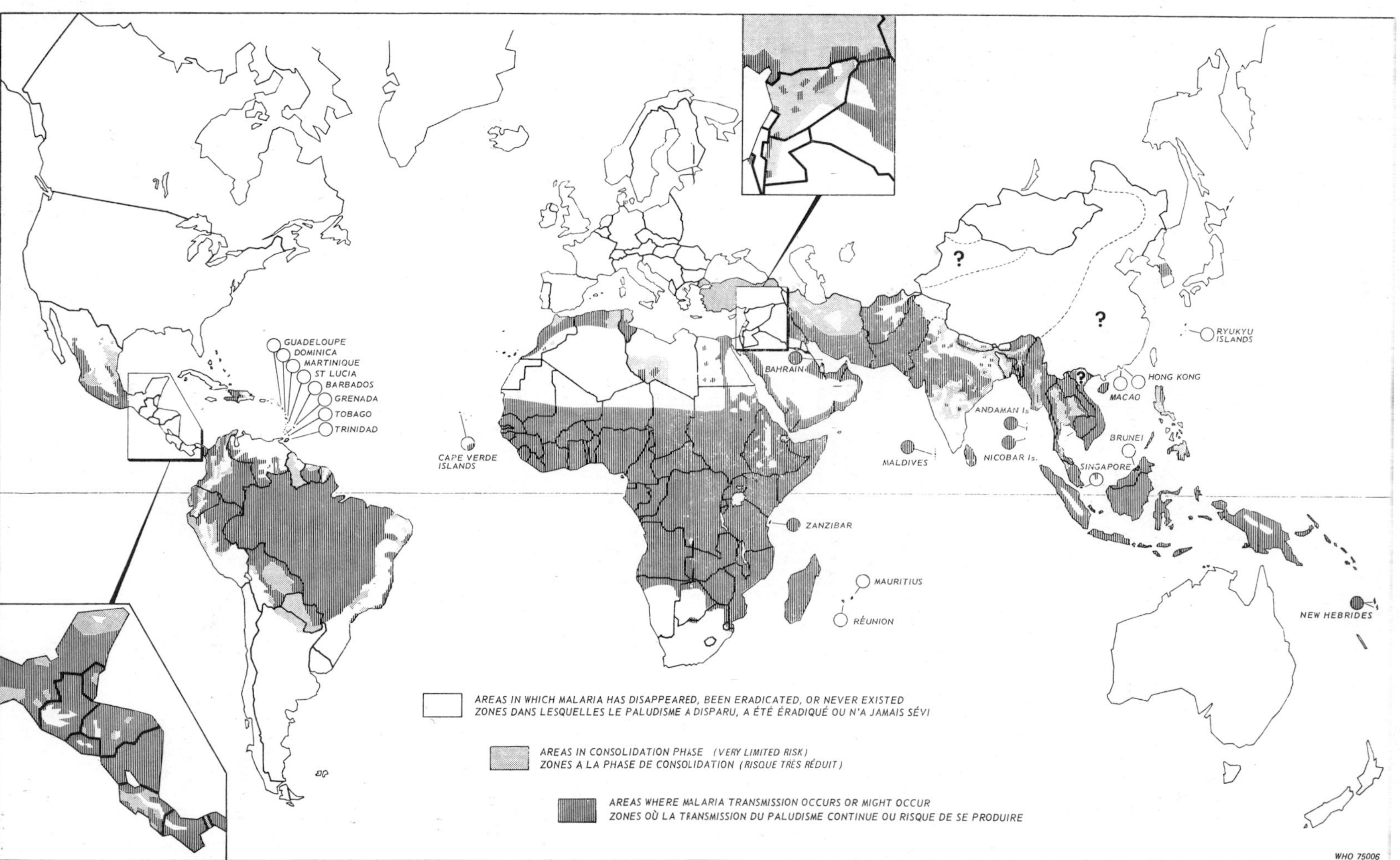

Figure 38–1. Epidemiological assessment of the status of malaria, December 1973. (Courtesy of the World Health Organization, Wkly. Epidem. Rec. No. 6, Feb. 1975.)

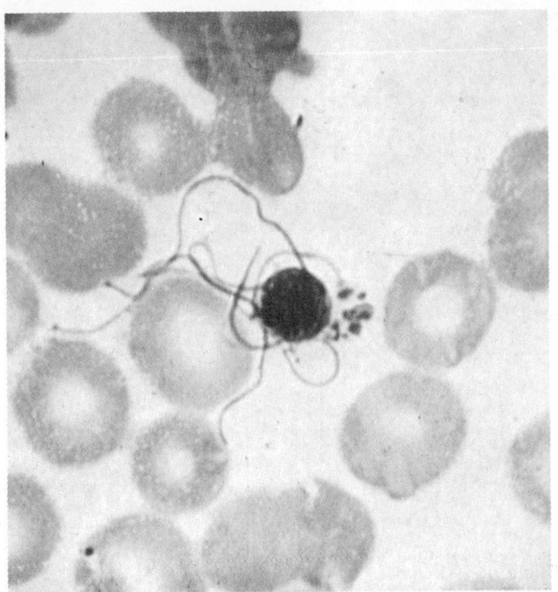

Figure 38–2. Exflagellation of male gametocyte.

the stomach wall, although as a rule they are scarce (Figs. 38–3, 38–4).

Spontaneous rupture of the oocyst finally occurs. Liberated motile sporozoites, which may number several hundred to several hundred thousand, migrate throughout the body cavity of the mosquito, certain ones reaching and entering the salivary glands. Here they remain dormant until injected into man (Figs. 38–5, 38–6).

The duration of the exogenous phase of the cycle, termed the extrinsic incubation period, varies with the species of *Plasmodium,* with the vectors, and with conditions of temperature and humidity. Under favorable conditions, *P. vivax* and *P. falciparum* complete their development in the mosquito within 7 to 14 days; *P. ovale* requires several

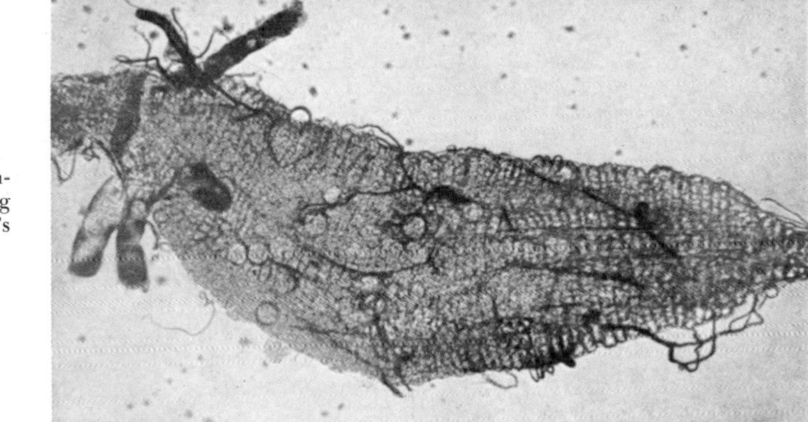

Figure 38–3. Fresh unstained preparation showing oocysts on wall of mosquito's stomach.

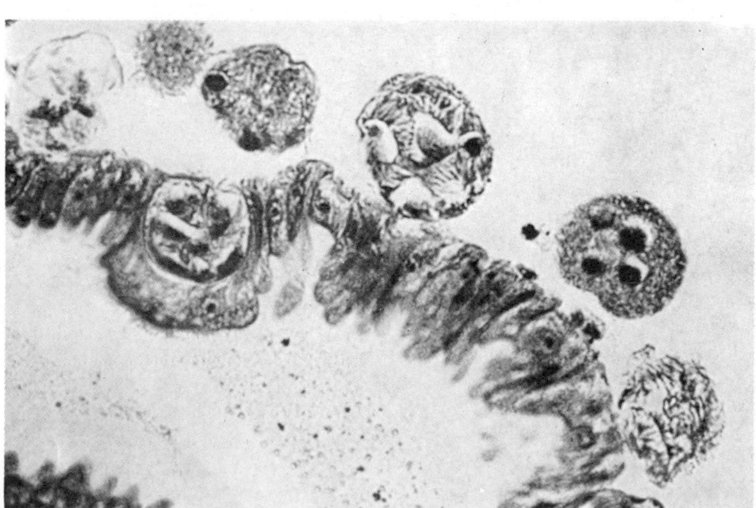

Figure 38–4. Various stages in development of oocysts – showing sporozoite formation and pigment masses. (Courtesy of Mr. P. G. Shute, F.R.E.S., Ministry of Health, Epsom, England.)

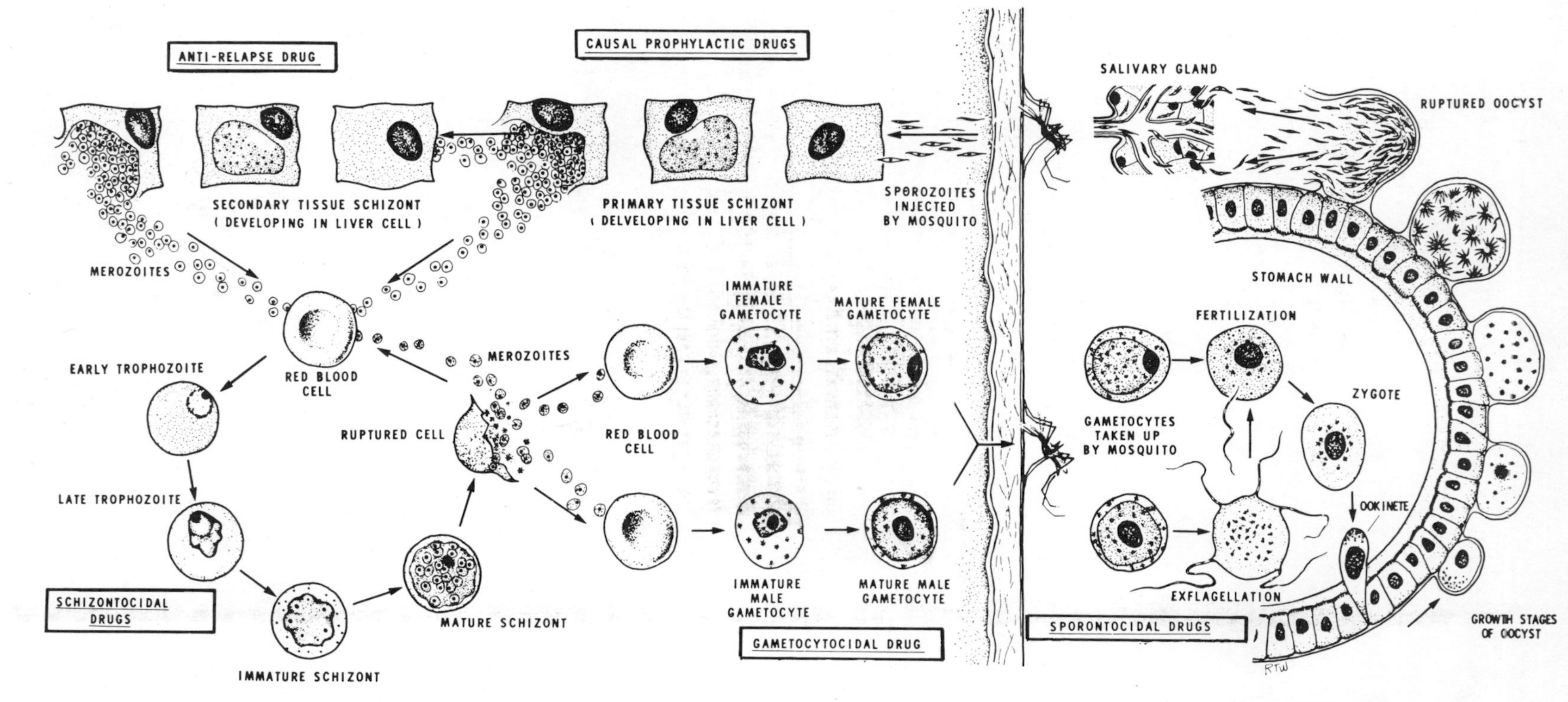

Figure 38–5. Life cycle of *Plasmodium.* (Modified from Bruce-Chwatt and Alvarado. Courtesy of the University of Florida College of Medicine, Gainesville.)

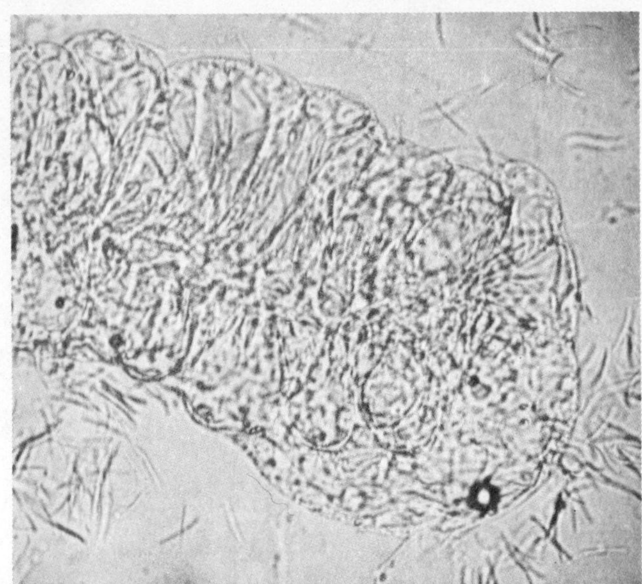

Figure 38–6. Sporozoites in salivary gland of mosquito and in surrounding fluid.

days longer and *P. malariae,* the slowest, may require 3 weeks or more.

The *endogenous* or *human phase* of the cycle begins with the injection of sporozoites by an infected anopheline mosquito. The sporozoites disappear from the peripheral blood after about a half hour, initiating the exo-erythrocytic stage. The parasites next appear in the parenchymal cells of the liver.

The *P. falciparum* parasites in the liver are 15 μm in diameter by the third day after inoculation, contain 40 or more nuclei, and small vacuoles may be present (Fig. 38–7*A*). As the parasite grows, there is a gradual increase in the number of nuclei; cords or islands of cytoplasm appear from which the merozoites are formed. After about 6 days the parasite is mature, is irregular in shape with lobes or projections, is about 60 μm in longest diameter and produces about 40,000 merozoites. The release of the merozoites from the mature schizont coincides with the appearance of ring stages in the erythrocytes of the peripheral blood (Fig. 38–7*B*). This primary development constitutes the pre-erythrocytic stage of the endogenous cycle.

The rate of development and some of the morphologic characteristics of the parasite in the liver vary with the species of parasites: *P. vivax* has a cycle length of 8 days, with a mature schizont that is round, 45 μm in size, and which contains 10,000 merozoites; *P. ovale* requires 9 days for development, has an irregular multilobular mature schizont about 80 × 50 μm, and produces 15,000 merozoites; *P. malariae* requires 15 days, with a mature schizont that is oval, mean diameter of 51 μm, and produces 7500 to 18,600 merozoites.

The pre-erythrocytic parasites do not contain pigment. Except for the destruction of the parasitized parenchymal cells, there is little evidence of injury to the liver.

In relapsing malarias, such as *P. vivax,* the evidence indicates that the exo-erythrocytic parasites persist in the liver parenchymal cells. After a latent period, merozoites are produced which invade the erythrocytes (Fig. 38–7*B*), producing a parasite relapse and, if in sufficient quantities to produce symptoms, a clinical relapse (Fig. 38–5).

MORPHOLOGY. All forms that occur in the blood stain well with Romanowsky stains; the cytoplasm is blue and the chromatin or nuclear substance is bright red. Pigment produced by the parasite in its growth appears as brownish or blackish granules. The earliest form seen in erythrocytes consists of a small ring of blue-stained cytoplasm with one or two dots of chromatin, giving rise to

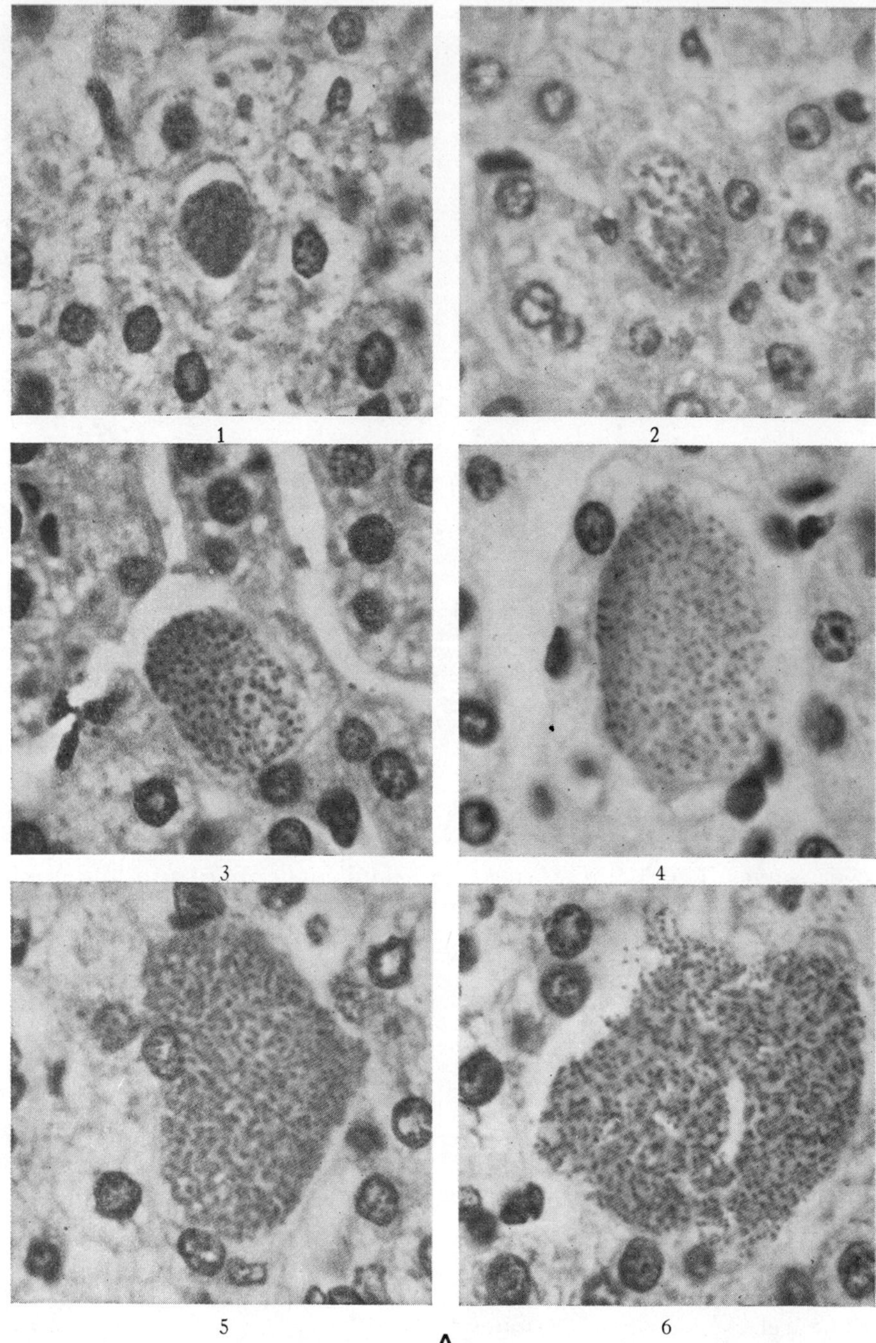

Figure 38–7. *A*, Exo-erythrocytic stages of *Plasmodium falciparum* in liver. *1*, This is one of the smallest parasites seen. Diameter 15 μm. Probably 3 days old. *2*, A larger parasite than that shown in *1*. Sections cut at 2 μm and stained with Delafield's hematoxylin. *3*, A larger stage than that in preceding figures. *4*, A still larger stage with nuclei and cytoplasm more condensed on the left side. Note that although sinusoids may be seen clearly on each side of the parasite, the parasite is not in contact with these spaces. *5*, A parasite approaching maturity with vacuolization cutting the cytoplasm into cords and islands (Shortt's "pseudocytomeres"). Note the growth of the parasite around the unchanged nucleus of the hepatic epithelium. *6*, A mature schizont. Note the cords and islands in the parasite and the formation of merozoites, especially at the top of the parasite. Diameter about 60 μm. (Courtesy of Jeffery, Wolcott, Young, and Williams: Am. J. Trop. Med. Hyg. *1*:917, 1952.)

Illustration continued on the opposite page.

the descriptive term "signet ring." In the course of a few hours the ring develops into an actively motile ameboid form, the trophozoite. This term is applied to all the more mature intermediate stages in which the chromatin still appears as a single mass. Later in development the chromatin undergoes repeated division. Stages that exhibit cleavage of the chromatin without segmentation of the cytoplasm are referred to as presegmenting schizonts. When division of both the chromatin and cytoplasm has been completed, the form is termed a mature schizont, each member of the resulting new generation of parasites being called a merozoite.

Gametocytes are less numerous than asexual forms and therefore do not become readily apparent during the first schizogonic generations of *vivax, ovale* and *malariae* infections. In *falciparum* infections, gametocytes appear about the tenth day of parasite patency. In *vivax, ovale* and *malariae* infections, all forms from the early ring to the mature schizont and gametocyte are found in the peripheral blood. In *falciparum* infections, on the other hand, only rings and gametocytes are usually demonstrable. The intermediate development of this species occurs in the capillaries of the viscera, and the intermediate stages are seen in the peripheral blood only infrequently and are usually associated with heavy infections.

Plasmodium vivax. The young plasmodia appear in Giemsa-stained blood films as delicate rings of blue cytoplasm, each with a red bead of chromatin, the so-called "signet ring." They are approximately one-third the diameter of a normal red blood cell. The chromatin dots are usually but not invariably single, and ordinarily not more than one parasite is observed within a single red cell. The ring undergoes rapid growth and development, the cytoplasm becomes heavier and thicker, and the chromatin mass enlarges. Within 5 or 6 hours yellowish brown pigment granules appear within the substance of the parasite, which now develops into an actively motile trophozoite with bizarre outlines in the stained film. The infected red cell is enlarged; it stains less deeply and may present a diffuse bright red stippling, the Schüffner's dots; this stippling is not present in all cases. When the parasite fills or nearly fills a considerably enlarged and pale red cell, motility ceases, and the chromatin undergoes successive divisions into 12 to 24 fragments, with an average of 16. The cy

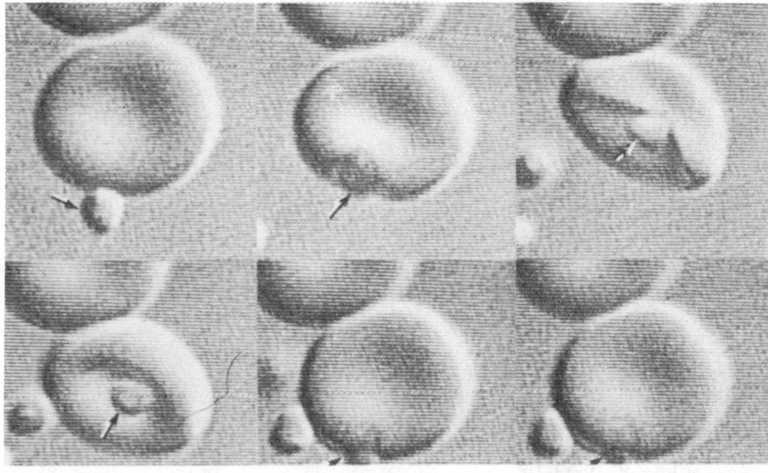

B

Figure 38–7 *Continued*

B, This inverted microscope sequence shows (from upper left to lower right) the invasion of a red blood cell by a malaria parasite (*arrow*). Following attachment of the parasite to the red blood cell, there is a marked distortion of the red blood cell followed by the relatively slow invasion of the red blood cell by the parasite. (Courtesy of B. Plocinik: The NIH Record, March 25, 1975.)

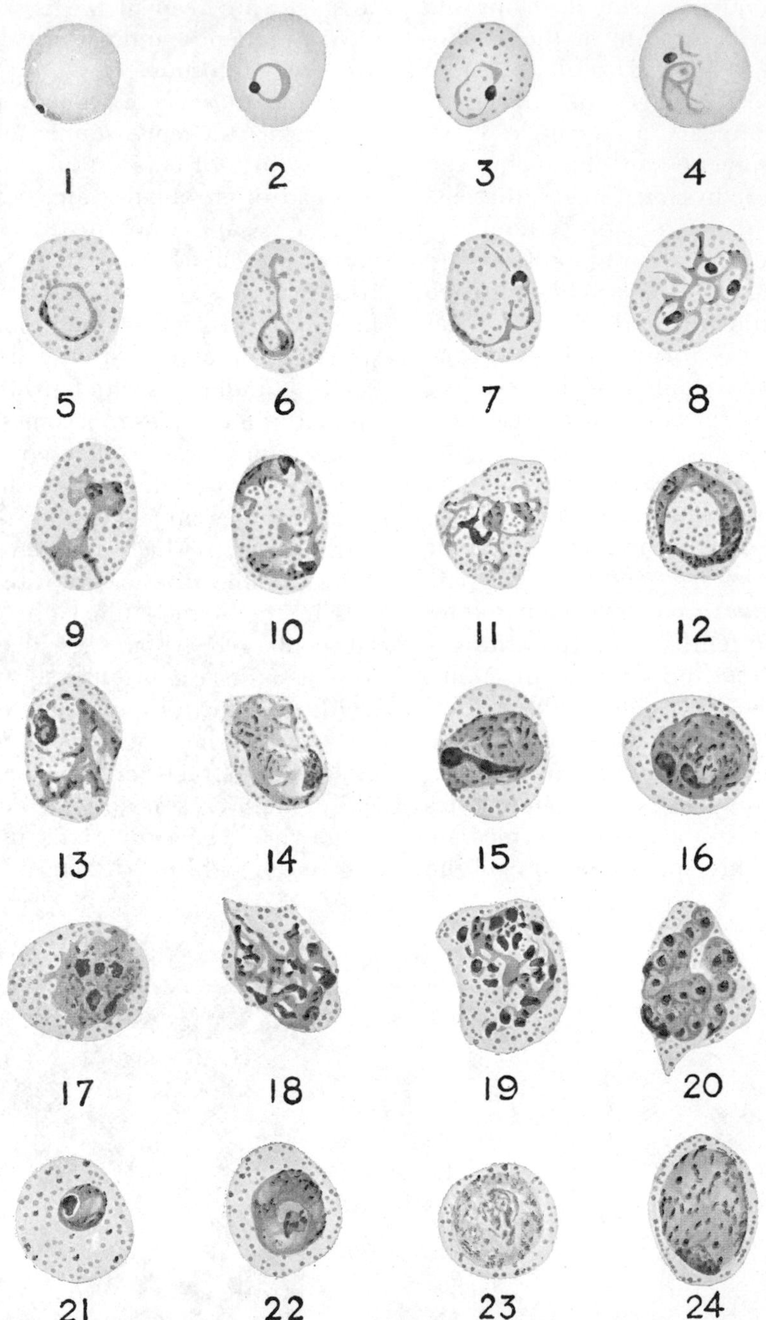

Figure 38–8. *Plasmodium vivax. 1,* Normal sized red cell with marginal ring form trophozoite. *2,* Young signet ring form trophozoite in a macrocyte. *3,* Slightly older ring form trophozoite in red cell showing basophilic stippling. *4,* Polychromatophilic red cell containing young tertian parasite with pseudopodia. *5,* Ring form trophozoite showing pigment in cytoplasm, in an enlarged cell containing Schüffner's stippling. (Schüffner's stippling does not appear in all cells containing the growing and older forms of *P. vivax* as would be indicated by these pictures, but it can be found with any stage from the fairly young ring form onward.) *6, 7,* Very tenuous medium trophozoite forms. *8,* Three ameboid trophozoites with fused cytoplasm. *9, 11, 12, 13,* Older ameboid trophozoites in process of development. *10,* Two ameboid trophozoites in one cell. *14,* Mature trophozoite. *15,* Mature trophozoite with chromatin apparently in process of division. *16, 17, 18, 19,* Schizonts showing progressive steps in division (presegmenting schizonts). *20,* Mature schizont. *21, 22,* Developing gametocytes. *23,* Mature microgametocyte. *24,* Mature macrogametocyte. (Courtesy of the National Institutes of Health, U.S.P.H.S.)

toplasm then undergoes similar subdivision, each portion including one of the chromatin masses. This mature schizont contains the new generation of asexual parasites, called merozoites, and also the pigment formed during the period of growth clumped into one or two loose masses (Figs. 38–8, 38–9). The length of the asexual cycle varies from 42 to 47 hours, depending upon the strain of *P. vivax.*

The mature male gametocyte is often about the size of a normal red cell and lies within an enlarged decolorized erythrocyte; its cytoplasm stains a light grayish or pinkish

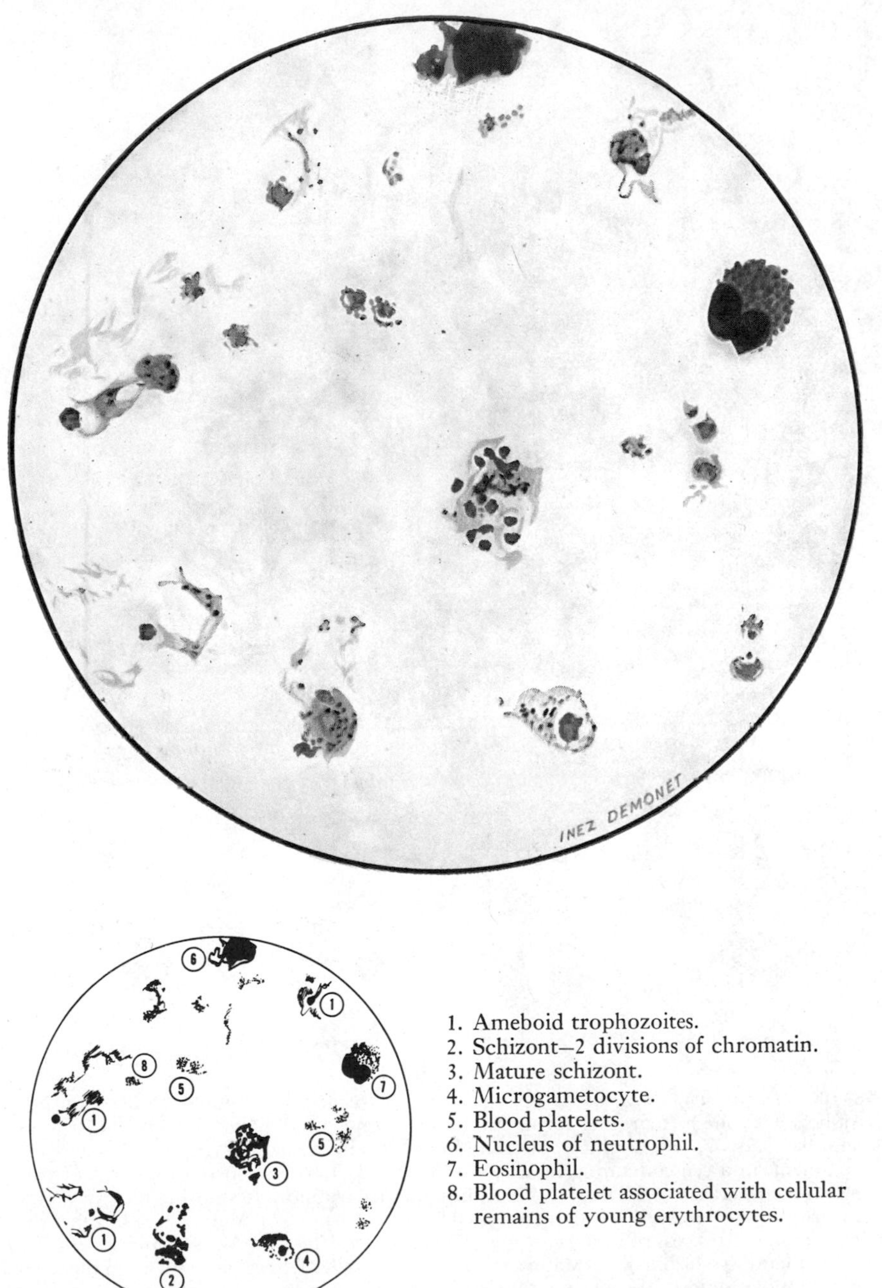

1. Ameboid trophozoites.
2. Schizont–2 divisions of chromatin.
3. Mature schizont.
4. Microgametocyte.
5. Blood platelets.
6. Nucleus of neutrophil.
7. Eosinophil.
8. Blood platelet associated with cellular remains of young erythrocytes.

Figure 38–9. *Plasmodium vivax* in thick smear. (Courtesy of the National Institutes of Health, U.S.P.H.S.)

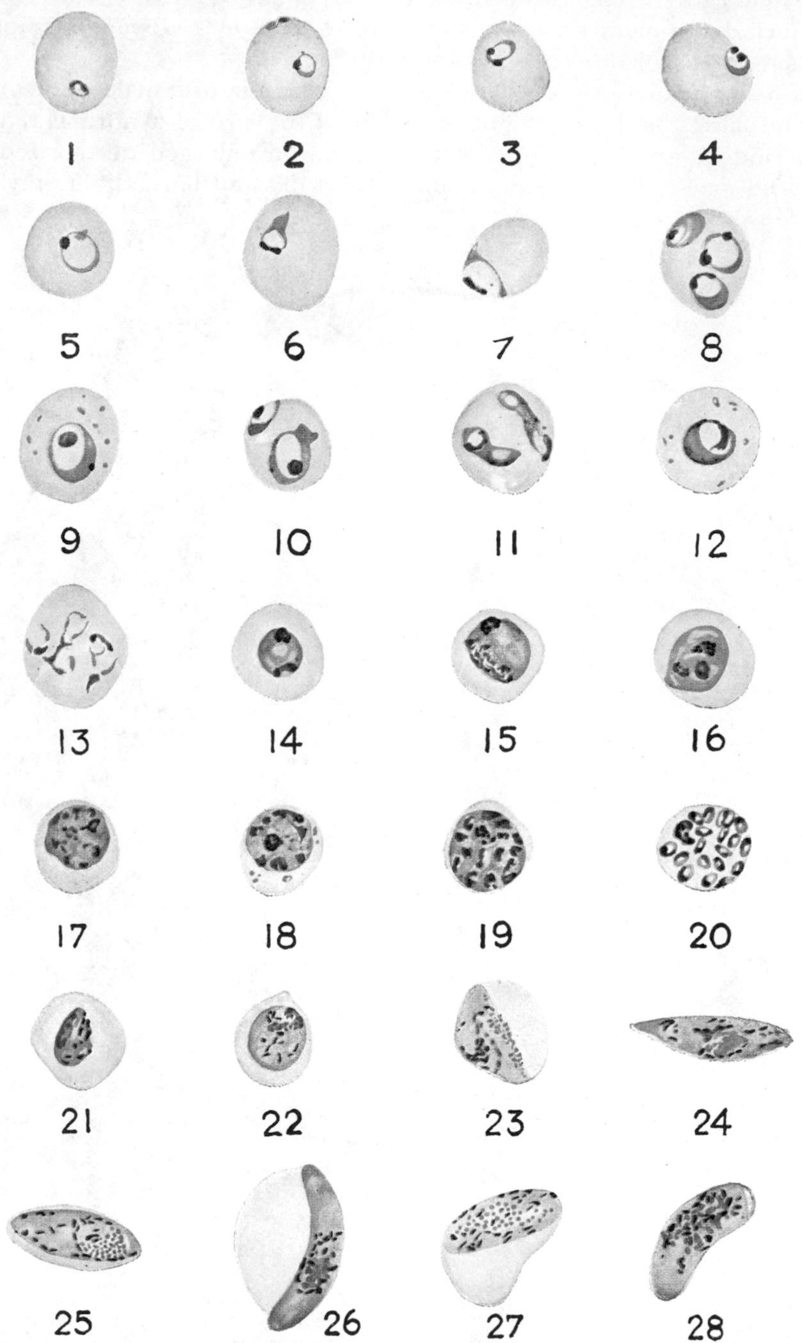

Figure 38–10. *Plasmodium falciparum. 1,* Very young ring form trophozoite. *2,* Double infection of single cell with young trophozoites, one a "marginal form," the other "signet ring" form. *3, 4,* Young trophozoites showing double chromatin dots. *5, 6, 7,* Developing trophozoite forms. *8,* Three medium trophozoites in one cell. *9,* Trophozoite showing pigment, in a cell containing Maurer's dots. *10, 11,* Two trophozoites in each of two cells, showing variation of forms which parasites may assume. *12,* Almost mature trophozoite showing haze of pigment throughout cytoplasm. Maurer's dots in the cell. *13,* Estivo-autumnal "slender forms." *14,* Mature trophozoite, showing clumped pigment. *15,* Parasite in the process of initial chromatin division. *16, 17, 18, 19,* Various phases of the development of the schizont (presegmenting schizonts). *20,* Mature schizont. *21, 22, 23, 24,* Successive forms in the development of the gametocyte—usually not found in the peripheral circulation. *25,* Immature macrogametocyte. *26,* Mature macrogametocyte. *27,* Immature microgametocyte. *28,* Mature microgametocyte. (Courtesy of the National Institutes of Health, U.S.P.H.S.)

blue, and the chromatin appears as granules loosely aggregated in the center or distributed as a transverse band. The pigment is darker than in the schizont and is uniformly distributed. The female gametocyte may be almost twice the size of a normal erythrocyte; its cytoplasm takes a deep blue stain, and the chromatin is compact, usually situated near the periphery.

Plasmodium falciparum. The young rings are smaller and more delicate than those of *P. vivax;* they are often hairlike and may show single or double chromatin dots. Multiple infection of erythrocytes is com-

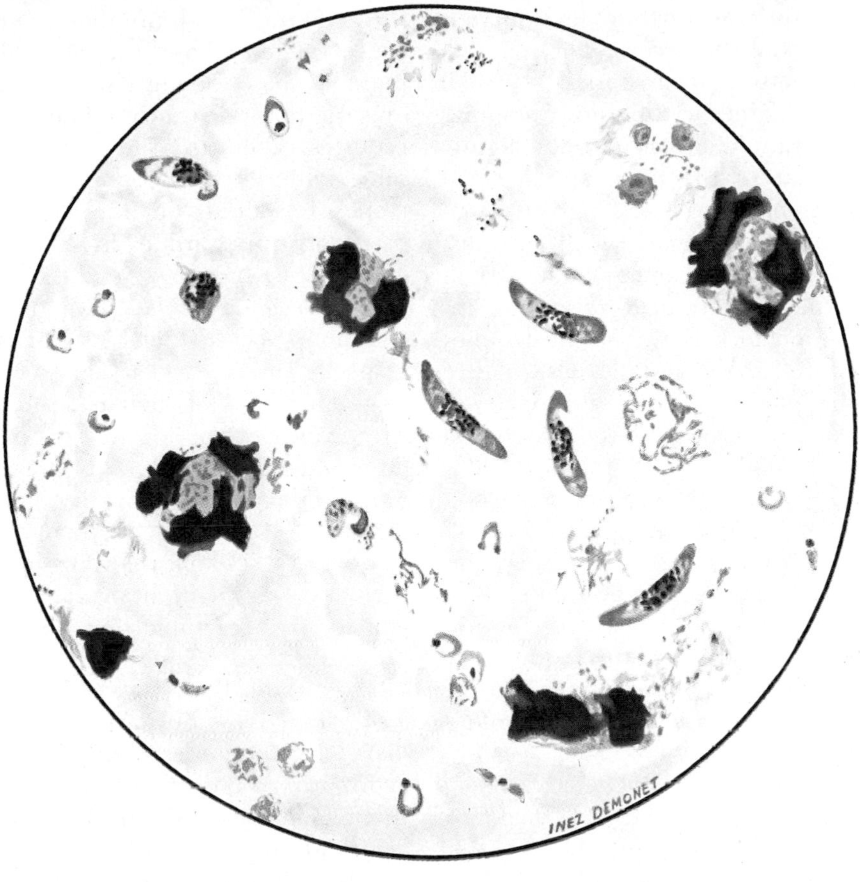

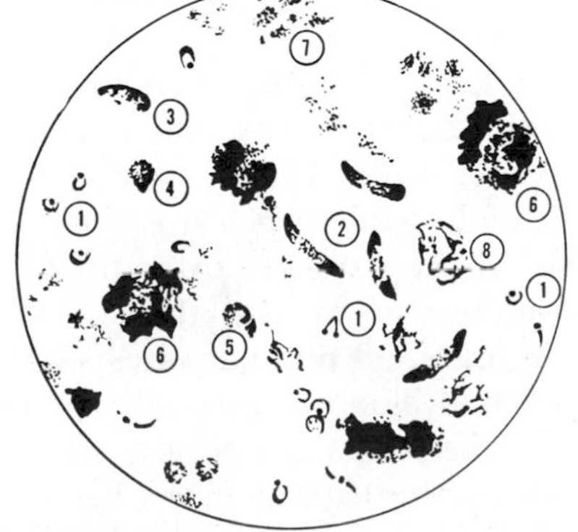

1. Small trophozoites.
2. Gametocytes–normal.
3. Slightly distorted gametocyte.
4. "Rounded-up" gametocyte.
5. Disintegrated gametocyte.
6. Nucleus of leukocyte.
7. Blood platelets.
8. Cellular remains of young erythrocyte.

Figure 38–11. *Plasmodium falciparum*–thick film. (Courtesy of the National Institutes of Health, U.S.P.H.S.)

mon. The frequently seen accolé or appliqué form appears as a fine blue line with a delicate chromatin dot, apparently applied to the margin of a red cell. *Plasmodium falciparum* remains in the ring stage longer than most species of *Plasmodium.* The rings increase only slightly in size and remain smaller and more delicate. After a few hours ring forms disappear from the peripheral circulation to undergo further development in the capillaries of the viscera. There, intermediate and mature forms appear as small masses of light-stained cytoplasm containing a chromatin granule, which is only slightly larger than that of the ring, and a small round mass or block of black pigment. Unlike *P. vivax* and *P. malariae,* which have diffuse pigment that forms an aggregate late in schizogony, the pigment of *P. falciparum* appears as a solid block in the young trophozoite shortly after the ring stage. The mature stages of the parasite are only about two-thirds the size of a normal red blood cell (Figs. 38–10, 38–11).

Parasitized cells of the peripheral blood may show cleftlike or commalike red markings, Maurer's dots. These are larger and less numerous than the Schüffner's dots. The infected red blood cells are not enlarged or decolorized. The time required by *P. falciparum* for completion of one generation of schizogony is about 48 hours. From 8 to 24 merozoites are formed.

The gametocytes are elongated, usually curved, sausage-shaped bodies. The male, or microgametocyte, stains lightly. Its chromatin is loose and scattered, and abundant granular brownish pigment is dispersed through the cytoplasm. The female, or macrogametocyte, is often more slender, longer, and stains more deeply blue. Its chromatin tends to appear as a compact mass in or near the center, and the pigment is usually closely approximated to the chromatin. The gametocytes or "crescents" first appear after several generations of schizogony and subsequently recur in successive waves, usually following waves of trophozoites.

Plasmodium malariae. The ring forms of *P. malariae* are about the size of those of *P. vivax.* Trophozoites are more compact, less ameboid and tend to assume round or ovoid shapes. Band forms are common, the parasite extending as a band across the infected cell. The pigment is darker brown, coarser, and appears in greater quantity and earlier than with *P. vivax.* The mature schizont fills or nearly fills an unenlarged and normally stained red cell. Six to 12 merozoites are formed; the usual number is eight. These are arranged about the centrally collected pigment mass, giving rise to a "daisy head" or rosette appearance. The asexual cycle requires 72 hours. Gametocytes present the same differences between the sexes with respect to staining qualities and arrangement of chromatin granules as in *P. vivax* (Figs. 38–12, 38–13).

Plasmodium ovale. This relatively uncommon species resembles *P. vivax* in many respects. Infected cells very early may show large numbers of coarse Schüffner's dots. The growing trophozoites exhibit relatively little ameboid activity and consequently are more compact and more regular in outline than *P. vivax.* Band forms are noted frequently. The mature schizonts form six to 12 merozoites, with an average of eight. The gametocytes resemble those of *P. vivax* and are difficult to distinguish from them. The infected red cells are less enlarged than in *P. vivax* infections but are decolorized. The margin of the infected cell is often crenated or fimbriated and the cell tends to be oval in shape (Fig. 38–14). The asexual cycle lasts about 50 hours.

Host-Parasite Relationship. Following injection of sporozoites by infected mosquitoes at the end of the extrinsic incubation period, the parasites develop in the liver parenchymal cells. Upon the maturation of these pre-erythrocytic stages, merozoites are released which invade erythrocytes, marking the end of the *prepatent period.* For the detection of the parasites by ordinary microscopic examination of the thick blood smear, a minimum of ten parasites per cubic millimeter of blood is normally required.

The prepatent periods vary according to species, the usual lengths being: *P. vivax,* 12 to 14 days; *P. falciparum,* 10 to 13; *P. ovale,*

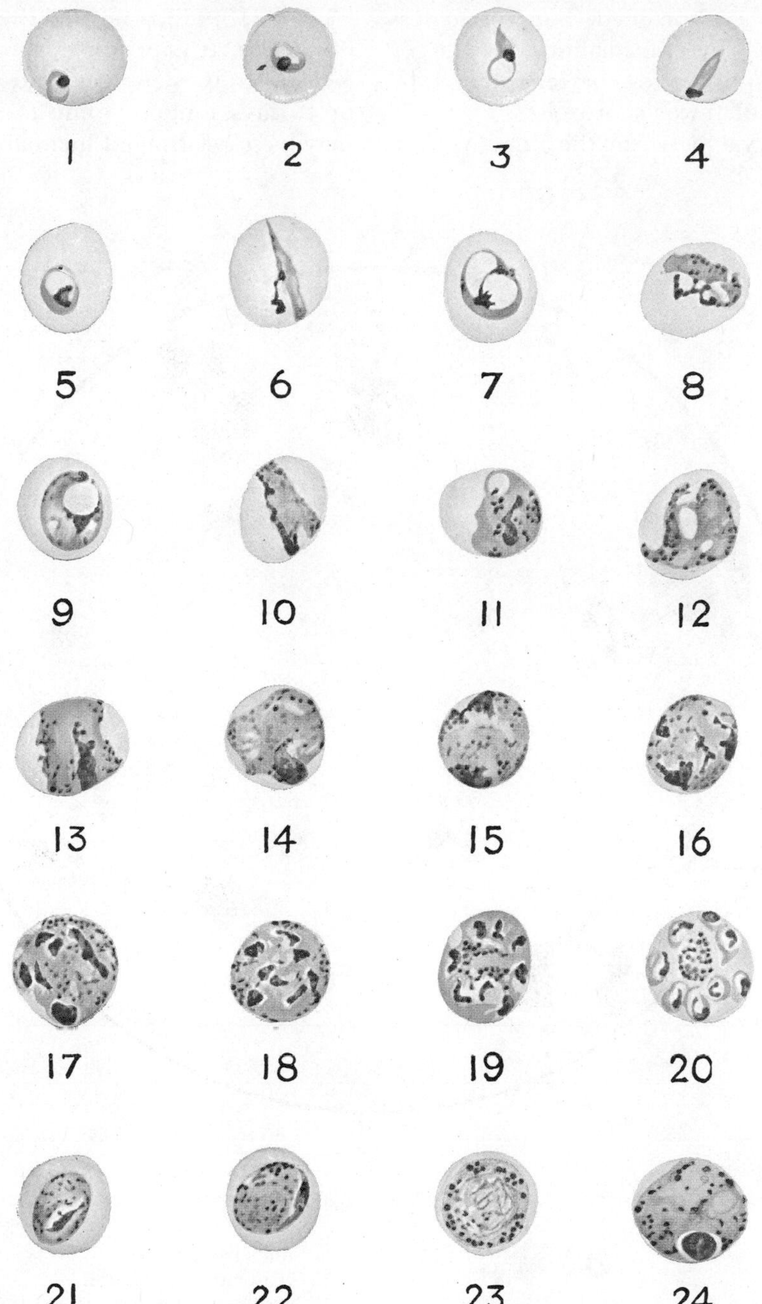

Figure 38-12. *Plasmodium malariae. 1,* Young ring form trophozoite of quartan malaria. *2, 3, 4,* Young trophozoite forms of the parasite showing gradual increase of chromatin and cytoplasm. *5,* Developing ring form trophozoite showing pigment granule. *6,* Early band form trophozoite—elongated chromatin, some pigment apparent. *7, 8, 9, 10, 11, 12,* Some forms which the developing trophozoite of quartan may take. *13, 14,* Mature trophozoites—one a band form. *15, 16, 17, 18, 19,* Phases in the development of the schizont ("presegmenting schizonts"). *20,* Mature schizont. *21,* Immature microgametocyte. *22,* Immature macrogametocyte. *23,* Mature microgametocyte. *24,* Mature macrogametocyte. (Courtesy of the National Institutes of Health, U.S.P.H.S.)

12 to 20; and *P. malariae,* 27 to 37. These periods may be shortened, but not to less than 5 days, by inoculations of larger numbers of sporozoites, or lengthened by the injections of fewer sporozoites.

The interval between the infective bite and the first elevation of temperature to 37.8° C (100° F) is termed the *intrinsic incubation period.* It may coincide with the *prepatent period,* rarely is shorter, and more often is 1 or 2 days longer. Some *P. vivax* infections may have protracted incubation periods of 9

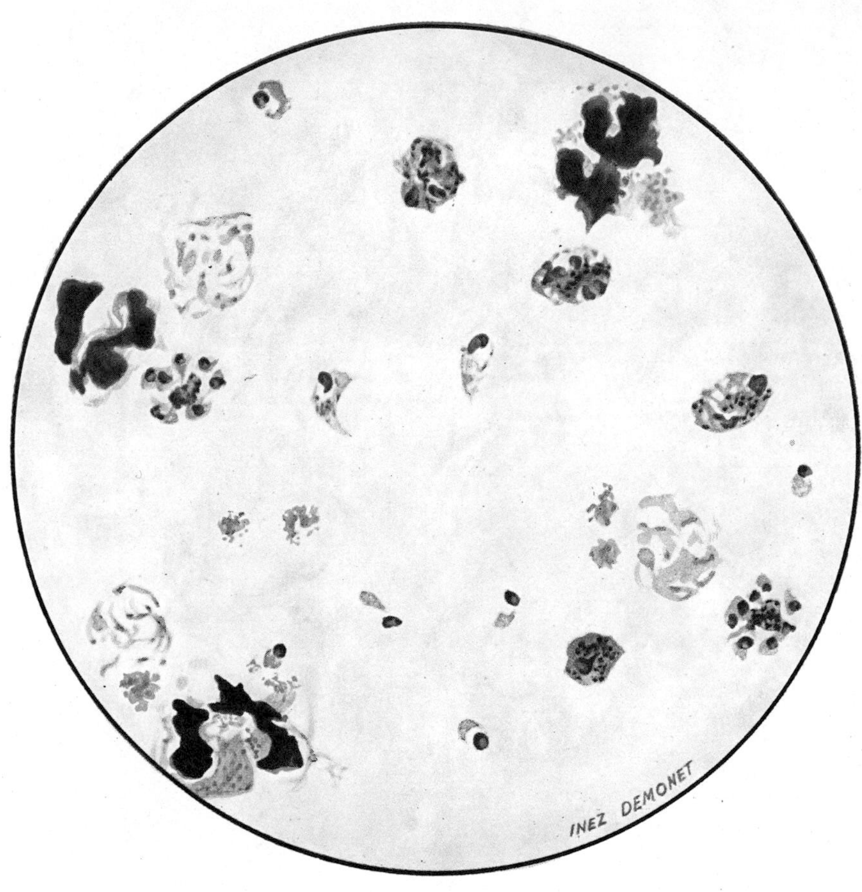

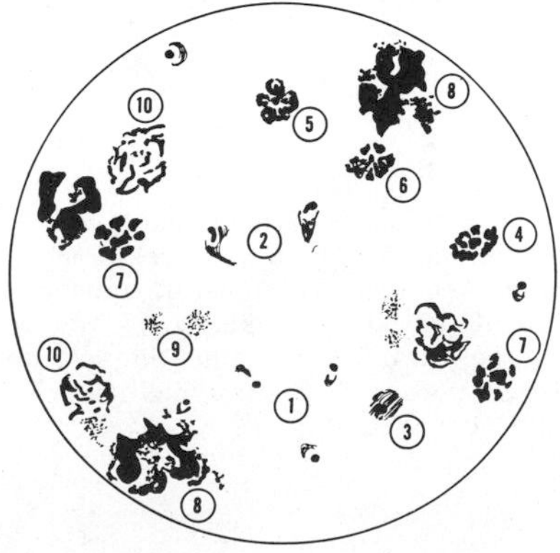

1. Small trophozoites.
2. Growing trophozoites.
3. Mature trophozoites.
4, 5, 6, Schizonts (presegmenting) with varying numbers of divisions of the chromatin.
7. Mature schizonts.
8. Nucleus of leukocyte.
9. Blood platelets.
10. Cellular remains of young erythrocytes.

Figure 38–13. *Plasmodium malariae* in thick smear. (Courtesy of the National Institutes of Health, U.S.P.H.S.)

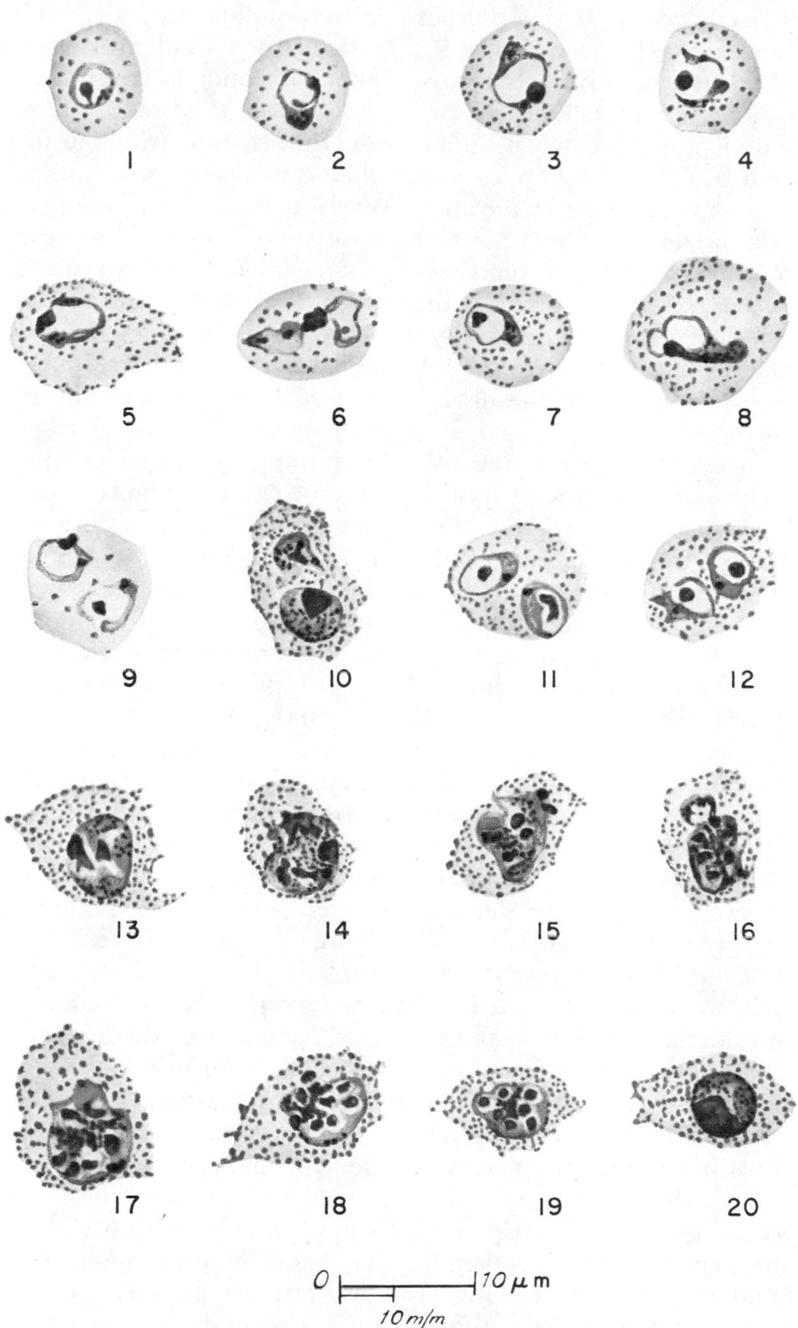

Figure 38–14. *Plasmodium ovale. 1,* Young ring-shaped trophozoite. *2, 3, 4, 5,* Older ring-shaped trophozoites. *6, 7, 8,* Older ameboid trophozoites. *9, 11, 12,* Doubly infected cells, trophozoites. *10,* Doubly infected cell, young gametocytes. *13,* First stage of the schizont. *14 15, 16, 17, 18, 19,* Schizonts, progressive stages. *20,* Mature gametocyte.

Free translation of legend accompanying original plate in "Guide pratique d'examen microscopique du sang appliqué au diagnostic du paludisme" by Georges Villain. Reproduced with permission from "Biologie Medicale" supplement, 1935.

(Courtesy of Aimee Wilcox, National Institutes of Health Bulletin No. 180, U.S.P.H.S.)

months or more, and *P. ovale* of several years. The febrile reaction is related to the sporulation of parasites. The densities of the parasites at the first fever in a nonimmune person usually are between 10 and 100 per cu mm, but they may be below densities (10 per cu mm) detectable by ordinary microscopic examination or, especially in persons with high immunity, may be in the thousands per cu mm. In general, *P. falciparum* has greater densities in all stages of the asexual cycle than do the other species.

There are fundamental differences in the invasive characteristics of these three species of *Plasmodium*. These differences are to a considerable extent responsible for the marked variations in severity of the disease produced by them.

Plasmodium vivax attacks the reticulocytes almost exclusively and appears incapable of invading mature erythrocytes. This imposes a limit on the magnitude of the parasitemia, which usually ranges from 8000 to 20,000 per cu mm and only rarely exceeds 50,000 per cu mm.

Plasmodium falciparum, however, invades all the red cells irrespective of age. There is consequently no limiting factor to prevent progressively increasing parasitemia. Very high densities may therefore be encountered in *falciparum* infections. A parasitemia of 500,000 parasites per cu mm carries a grave prognosis, and even low parasite densities should be considered dangerous. Unlike *P. vivax* and *P. malariae, P. falciparum* induces physical changes in the infected red blood cells which contribute importantly to the pathology of the infection. The infected cells agglutinate and adhere to the capillary endothelium. These effects produce capillary obstruction and ischemia in many tissues of the body.

Plasmodium malariae attacks predominantly the mature erythrocytes. Parasitemias exceeding 20,000 per cu mm are uncommon. After the acute primary attack, the infection tends to become chronic, often persisting for years in a patent or subpatent condition.

CHARACTERISTICS OF P. VIVAX INFECTIONS. In the early stages of infection by *P. vivax,* usually two groups of parasites undergo schizogony concurrently, maturing on alternate days. This results in the release of a new generation of merozoites each day and a corresponding quotidian febrile reaction. Gradually or suddenly one group may drop out. Maturation of the single group or brood of parasites then occurs in 42 to 47 hours, and the accompanying febrile curve becomes characteristically tertian, appearing progressively earlier every other day. In an untreated case a second group ultimately may reappear, its members gradually increasing in numbers as the others decrease, and the fever again becomes quotidian. The naturally evolving *vivax* infection, therefore, consists of a series of such alternating and overlapping groups with corresponding periods of tertian and quotidian fever. The latter type of curve depends upon this phenomenon and not, as has been said in the past, upon double infection acquired on different days. Gametocytes infective to mosquitoes appear in the peripheral blood within a few days after the end of the prepatent period.

CHARACTERISTICS OF P. FALCIPARUM INFECTIONS. Infections by *P. falciparum* differ in certain important respects from those by *P. vivax.* The period required for maturation of the parasites is approximately 48 hours, and schizogony is less synchronized. Release of the new generation of parasites is continued over a longer period. As a result, the febrile episodes are less regular and more prolonged in duration. In severe infections the fever frequently is continuous.

Gametocytes do not appear in the peripheral blood until about 10 days after the onset of the primary parasitemia. They become infective for mosquitoes about 4 days later. In naturally evolving infections, as the gametocyte count rises, the trophozoite count diminishes, and clinical improvement or remission of symptoms frequently occurs. The primary parasitemia is characterized by such a series of successive trophozoite-gametocyte waves. Parasite counts in *falciparum* malaria characteristically fluctuate much more markedly than do those of *vivax,* often showing alternating high and low densities on successive days.

CHARACTERISTICS OF P. MALARIAE INFECTIONS. In the early stages of infections by *P. malariae,* there is usually only one group of parasites undergoing schizogony. The febrile episodes, therefore, recur at intervals of approximately 72 hours. Subsequently one or two additional groups may appear, producing a double quartan fever or even quotidian fever. Gametocytes usually are scanty.

CHARACTERISTICS OF MIXED INFECTIONS. When two species of malaria are present in the human host simultaneously, there appears to be an antagonism between them. If *P. falciparum* and *P. vivax* are both present, the former predominates initially, after which the *vivax* runs its course. When *P. vivax* and *P. malariae* are together, the *P. vivax* is the dominant species initially, sometimes to the complete expulsion of the *P. malariae. Plasmodium vivax* is even more dominant over *P. ovale* when the two are together than over *P. malariae.*

THE PRIMARY ATTACK AND RELAPSES. Study of naturally induced mosquito-transmitted *vivax* infection indicates that in wholly susceptible persons the patent primary parasitemia may persist for as long as 3 months. In the course of this period, however, there may be transitory intervals when the parasite densities are depressed. Such depressions are accompanied frequently by clinical remissions. The duration of clinical symptoms is considerably shorter than the total period of primary parasitemia, and it may be continuous or interrupted by one or more remissions. Any clinical activity occurring within this period is considered part of the primary attack of malaria.

Disappearance of the asexual parasites for several weeks, either naturally or because of treatment, marks the end of the primary attack. The exo-erythrocytic parasites persist in the parenchymal cells of the liver; and it is believed that, after a latent period, these produce parasites which again invade the erythrocytes, causing relapses. The intervals to relapse after noncurative treatment vary. In some *vivax* strains, this interval may be 9 to 10 months, in others several weeks. In contrast to *vivax* infections, the exo-erythrocytic forms of *falciparum* are short-lived and do not persist in the liver.

The natural duration of malaria infections varies. Experimentally induced infections of a single *vivax* strain may persist for 12 or 18 months. Some of the *vivax* strains acquired in the Pacific during World War II persisted for as long as 4 years. *Plasmodium falciparum* experimental infections endure an average of 7 to 9 months, with a small proportion lasting 17 months. *Plasmodium malariae* may persist for many years, most of the time without a demonstrable parasitemia or clinical symptoms. *Plasmodium ovale* apparently relapses only infrequently and only rarely persists longer than 1 year.

Immunity. Experimental studies have indicated that infections by *P. vivax* and *P. falciparum* produce a partial homologous immunity. This is strictly strain-specific, the individual becoming partially or totally refractory to subsequent reinfection by the strain previously used. He is not immune, however, to other strains of the same species, although the severity of the infection produced by them may be modified. There is no cross-immunity between species; thus, infection by *P. vivax* confers no immunity against *P. falciparum,* and the clinical disease produced by the latter is unmitigated in severity. The Negro race has an immunity against *P. vivax.*[1]

The development of immunity is characterized initially by the acquisition of *tolerance* to the infection. This is expressed by cessation of clinical phenomena despite persistence of a parasitemia considerably in excess of that which accompanied the onset of the initial clinical activity. It apparently represents a form of immunity depending upon a persisting latent infection. The defense mechanism, however, is probably largely cellular in nature. This immunity, expressed as tolerance and premunition, is of great importance in the epidemiology of malaria. Agglutinins, precipitins, complement-fixing and fluorescent antibodies are produced. There is a marked increase in immunoglobulins IgM, IgA and IgG shortly after parasite patency with a decrease in the albumin-globulin ratio. The rise in titers of the immunoglobulins generally parallels the increase in parasite density until the parasitemia peak. At that time IgM and IgA decline; IgG may remain elevated for long periods.

Fluorescent antibodies contribute to the increase of total immunoglobulins but tend to persist long after the percentages of the latter have returned to preinfection levels. The IgG fluorescent antibodies persist longer than the IgM or IgA so that the former may be used epidemiologically to measure past infections. Since IgM disappears more rapidly, a high response to it and to IgG indicates a current infection or an infection within the past 1 to 3 months.

Persons with elevated immunoglobulin levels may develop parasitemias owing to relapses or reinfections.

A small fraction of the IgG and IgM antibodies may exert a protective effect against infections. When given to malarious children, parasitemias were suppressed and symptoms were alleviated temporarily.

Attempts to produce vaccines in the past met with little success. Recently, however, a merozoite vaccine of *P. knowlesi*, a monkey malaria, gave partial or complete protection against challenges of the same or variant strains in rhesus monkeys. Also, the first active immunization of man against sporozoites has been achieved.[2] Several volunteers who received large numbers of X-irradiated *P. falciparum* or *P. vivax* sporozoites were protected against later exposure to homologous and heterologous strain sporozoites of the same species. The duration of this immunity does not appear to exceed 6 months and it was ineffective against blood-induced infections.

Congenital malaria appears to be relatively common in babies born to nonimmune but infected mothers. However, congenital malaria is very rare in African babies of immune mothers, although the placentas are frequently infected, sometimes heavily, with *P. falciparum* (Fig. 38–15). The birth weight of these babies is often subnormal. The reason for the rare occurrence of congenital malaria in highly endemic areas is not known.[3]

It has been suggested that sickle-cell trait or glucose-6-phosphate dehydrogenase deficiency confers some protection against malaria. This would be mainly by increasing survival rates.

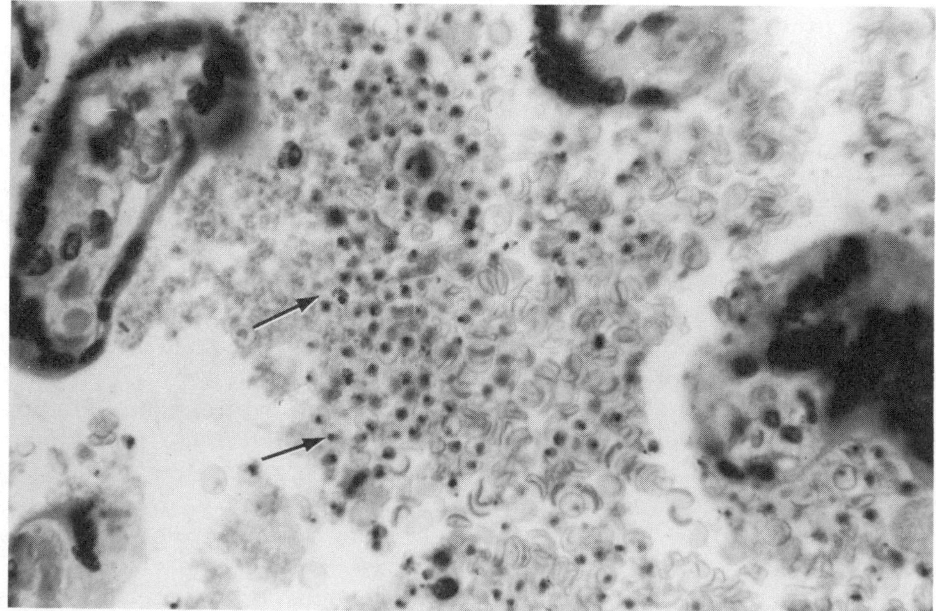

Figure 38–15. Section of placenta from a patient with *P. falciparum* infection. Numerous red blood corpuscles in the intervillous space (maternal side) are parasitized (*arrows*); the corpuscles in the chorionic villus (fetal side) are not parasitized. (Courtesy of the Louisiana State University School of Medicine, New Orleans.)

Epidemiology. Malaria has a high morbidity rate and until recently was responsible for more deaths per year than any other transmissible disease. As recently as 1955, it was estimated that there were 250 million cases of malaria with 2.5 million deaths annually. Eradication programs in many parts of the world have greatly reduced the prevalence of malaria. At the end of 1972, it was estimated that of the 1840 million people then living in the originally malarious areas of the world for which information is available, 73 per cent were in areas where malaria has been eradicated or where eradication programs were in progress. The remainder, approximately 494 million, were in areas where eradication programs were not yet in operation, although control measures were in effect in some places. Malaria is the major health problem in many countries,

Text continued on page 376

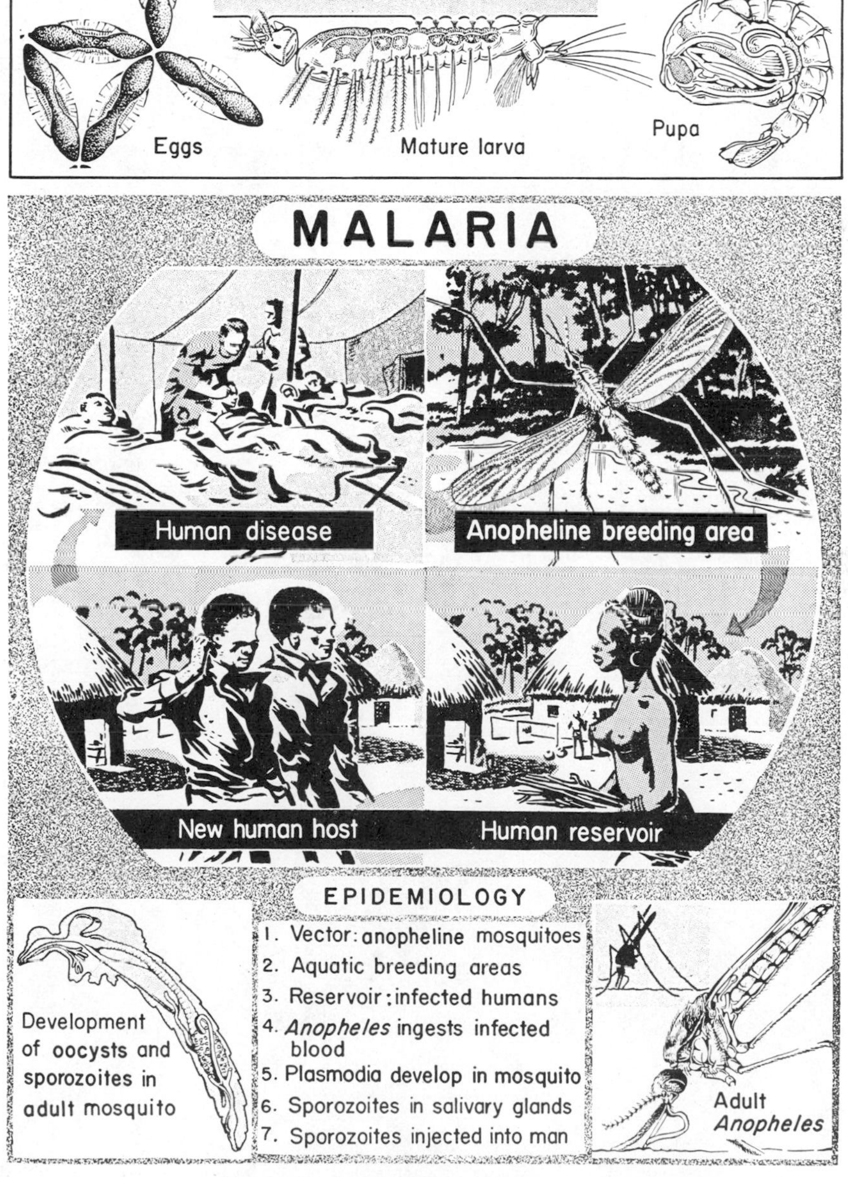

Figure 38–16. Epidemiology of malaria.

Table 38–1. Principal Vectors of Human Malaria*

Region	Area	Species	Type of Breeding Place: Light Requirements	Type of Breeding Place: Water, Vegetation, etc.	Adult Behavior	Efficiency as Vector
Nearctic	United States (and bordering areas):					
	Drier portions of Rocky Mountain and Pacific area and N.W. Mexico	*Anopheles freeborni*	Sun	Fresh, clear seepage from ditches, rice fields, edges of slow streams; irrigation water	Enters houses; feeds readily on man	Was dangerous in interior valleys of west coast of U.S.
	Coastal Mexico to New Hampshire and Ontario west to Minnesota	*A. quadrimaculatus*	Sun usually, sometimes in partial shade	Fresh pools, ponds, lakes, lagoons, swamps, slow flowing rivers, in dense aquatic vegetation	Active at night; feeds on human or animal blood; may remain in houses all day	Was most important carrier in the eastern U.S.
Neotropical (Largely)	Mexico, Central America (and bordering areas):					
	S.E. Texas, through Mexico and West Indies, south to Colombia and Ecuador; east through northern Venezuela	*A. albimanus*	Sun or partial shade	Fresh or brackish fairly pure, stagnant water; matted vegetation favorable in large lakes; swamps; lagoons; hoof prints	Nocturnal; prefers man, but also bites animals; enters houses, usually leaves at dawn after feeding	Most important vector in Central America and Caribbean, especially in rainy season
	Mexico	*A. aztecus*	Sun	Ground water, canals and pools of clear water with emergent or submerged vegetation	Enters and rests in houses	Sole important vector in some areas
	See South America, etc. for:	*A. darlingi*	....	....	....	....
	South Central U.S., south to Chile and Argentina; Grenada	*A. pseudopunctipennis pseudopunctipennis*	Sun	Clear pools, streams and springs rich in algae, in dry season	Enters houses and feeds readily on man in certain areas only	Important in mountain valleys of South America, Central America and Mexico
	Mexico, through Central America and Trinidad to Peru, Brazil	*A. punctimaculata*	Shade preferred	Shaded pools, swamps, sluggish streams	Abundant in undrained jungle; strong flier; enters dwellings; feeds on man	Vector in parts of Panama; proved vector in parts of W. Colombia
	Caribbean area;					
	See Mexico, Central America for:	*A. albimanus*	....	....	....	....
	Panama, Trinidad, Lesser Antilles, south to Brazil	*A. aquasalis* (*tarsimaculatus* of certain authors)	Sun or shade	Brackish tidal swamps; rarely in fresh water of rice fields (inland Trinidad)	May fly 3 miles; enters houses, feeds on man (less true in Panama?)	Important in many localities: Trinidad, coastal Brazil
	Trinidad and Venezuela to Brazil	*A. bellator*	Partial shade	Leaf bases of bromeliads (epiphytic on *Erythrina* and other trees)	Prefers man; bites at night or in shade (daytime); enters dwellings occasionally, returns to forest	Important in cocoa-growing areas of Trinidad, and in coastal states of Brazil
	South America (and bordering areas):					
	See Mexico, C.A. for:	*A. albimanus*	....	....	....	....
	S. Brazil	*A. cruzii*	Partial shade	Leaf bases of bromeliads	Bites man readily; enters houses	Important in coastal states of S. Brazil
	Guatemala to N.E. Argentina and Paraguay; Trinidad	*A. albitarsis*	Some shade (not extreme)	Among mats of aquatic vegetation in large ponds, marshes, overflows near rivers; hoof prints; artificial containers	Enters houses and shows preference for human blood in some areas	Important in Brazil and probably N.E. Argentina
	Colombia, Venezuela	*A. nuneztovari*	Sun to partial shade	Muddy pools and lagoons	Bites and rests outdoors	Important in some areas
	Central America (Belize and Guatemala); South America (Venezuela to Argentina)	*A. darlingi*	Shade	Clear, fresh lagoons, overflows, etc., among debris, surface vegetation; avoids brackish water	Invades houses; prefers human blood. A domestic species	Most dangerous vector in tropical S. America from Venezuela, the Guianas to S. Brazil
	See Mexico, C.A. for:	*A. pseudopunctipennis pseudopunctipennis*	....	....	....	....

Palearctic	Europe: S. Palearctic North of Mediterranean; from England to Japan; from Sweden and Siberia to Portugal, Spain, Italy, Mongolia	*A. labranchiae atroparvus*	Sun	Brackish water along coast; fresh water inland	Frequents houses; feeds readily on man, also stabled animals	Formerly carried "house malaria" of winter months, especially in Netherlands
	N.W. Africa, Spain, Sicily, Sardinia, Corsica, Italy, Dalmatian Coast, islands of central Mediterranean	*A. labranchiae labranchiae*	Sun to partial shade	Brackish, coastal marshes; fresh water of rice fields, upland streams; other situations	Prefers human blood; enters houses in large numbers	Important vector
	Norway and Sweden to Italy; England to Black Sea; eastern Mediterranean	*A. messeae*	Sun	Cool, fresh standing water; lakes, marshes	Prefers animal to human blood; hibernates in barns, houses	Vector in Hungary and Albania
	N.E. and central Italy, Sardinia, Balkans; U.S.S.R. to W. China	*A. sacharovi* (= *elutus*)	Sun	Open inland marshes and coastal marshes even if brackish	Feeds without preference on man, animals; enters houses (bedrooms); hibernates in cold weather, but feeds on cattle in lowlands during winter	Important in Balkans, Israel; preference for cattle reduces its importance as vector in other areas
	See Persian Gulf, etc. for:	*A. superpictus*	....	....	....	....
	North Africa, Middle East: Europe, N. Africa, Asia Minor, Turkestan	*A. claviger* (= *bifurcatus*)	Sun or shade	Marshes, rock pools, wells, cisterns	Domestic in Palestine; enters houses, bites man freely (wild in some regions)	Was most important urban vector in Israel, Syria and Lebanon
			....	....	....	....
	See Central and South Africa for: See Europe for: Canaries, Algeria, Tunisia, Egypt, Israel, Syria, N.W. India	*A. pharoensis* *A. sacharovi* *A. sergenti*	Sun to partial shade	Rice fields, borrow pits, slow irrigation flows (dense vegetation); seepage, neglected drains	Enters houses readily; bites mostly after dark; may migrate 2 miles	Vector in Egypt and Israel
			....	....	....	....
	Persian Gulf and Caucasian area		Relative shade	Wells, cisterns, flower pots, cans, roof-gutters	Feeds readily on man; rests in barracks, houses, cowsheds	Important in urban areas
	See Europe for: E. Arabia, S. Iraq; Iran, India, Burma	*A. sacharovi* *A. stephensi stephensi*	Sun	Freshwater pools, streams, drains, seepages, especially in hill districts	Prefers human blood; readily enters houses, tents, barracks; strong fliers	Important in Europe, Middle East, Pakistan
	Spain, Italy, Balkans to southeast Asia	*A. superpictus*				
	Japan, North and Northeast China, Korea, South Ukraine See Burma, etc. for: China (not south of 30° N. lat.)	*A. sinensis* *A. pattoni*	.... Sun	.... Among algae along stream margins; rain pools, small pools of stream beds in hills	.... Bites man	.... Important vector
Ethiopian	Central and South Africa: Tropical Africa, north to Ethiopia	*A. funestus funestus*	Partial shade	Clear water of swamps, weedy banks of streams, rivers, ditches; margins of lakes, ponds; underground seepages	Enters houses in large numbers; feeds freely on human blood; a few migrate up to 4½ miles	Always important (also carries filariasis)
	Tropical Africa, Arabia, Malagasy Rep., Reunion, Mauritania, Liberia; other points	*A. gambiae*	Sun or light shade	Puddles, shallow ponds, borrow pits, hoof prints, ditches, overflows; rarely rain barrels, cisterns	Prefers human blood; abundant in huts and houses; a few migrate up to 3½ miles	Always important (also carries filariasis)
	Sierra Leone, Liberia, Cameroon, Uganda, Zaire	*A. hancocki*	Sun to slight shade	Clear water in grassy holes, native wells, streams, swamps	Found commonly in human dwellings	Important where prevalent
	Sierra Leone, Liberia, S. Nigeria, Gabon, Zaire	*A. hargreavesi*	More or less shade	Among *Pistia* in open jungle; swamps, stream margins (vegetation)	Abundant in huts in Nigeria; bites at midnight or later	Important where common
	Zaire, Uganda, Cameroon	*A. moucheti moucheti*	Sun to slight shade	Among vegetation on margins of pools, streams, permanent swamps	Often found indoors	Rather important where common
	Southern Nigeria	*A. moucheti nigeriensis*	Sun, largely	Clear water, in swamps (*Pistia* and other vegetation)	Found in native huts	Rather important where common

Table continued on the following page

Table 38–1. Principal Vectors of Human Malaria *(Continued)*

Region	Area	Species	Type of Breeding Place: Light Requirements	Type of Breeding Place: Water, Vegetation, etc.	Adult Behavior	Efficiency as Vector
	Sierra Leone, Liberia, Ghana, Nigeria, Cameroon – eastward to Mozambique	*A. nili*	Heavy shade	Among vegetation along sides of running streams	Common in huts and camps, but rare in houses	Possibly important where prevalent
	Coastal West Africa	*A. melas*	Shade	Breeding associated with black mangrove trees (*Avicennia* sp.) in brackish water, coastal streams and tidal swamps	Feeds more on dark nights; most remain in huts after feeding	Important in some coastal areas of West Africa
	Many parts of Africa; Malagasy Rep., Israel	*A. pharoensis*	Sun to partial shade	Swamps and rice fields; vegetation essential	Enters houses in large numbers; bites man readily but prefers animal blood	Important in upper Nile Province, Sudan, Mali
	E. Central and S. Africa, Zambia, Rhodesia, Sudan	*A. rufipes*	Sun	Pools, marshes, hoofmarks, artificial containers	Rests in crevices and outdoor haunts near breeding places; occasionally found in large numbers indoors	Rhodesia, Former Fr. W. Africa, Sudan; usually of secondary importance
Oriental	Afghanistan, Pakistan, India, Burma, Sri Lanka (Ceylon)					
	India, S. China, Taiwan, entire Malay region and Philippines	*A. annularis* (= *fuliginosus*)	Sun to partial shade	Large tanks or freshwater ponds, slowly moving streams, lake margins (with aquatic vegetation)	Prefers cattle to man; flies great distances; occurs up to 2100 m.	Of secondary importance
	W. Pakistan to Burma; Sri Lanka, Thailand, Tonkin Prov., S. Arabia	*A. culicifacies*	Sun to partial shade	Wide variety of places; prefers fresh, clean water in pools but can survive in brackish	Prefers cattle but bites man freely; rests in cow sheds and houses during day	Most important vector in India; only vector in Sri Lanka
	In foothills from W. Pakistan to Burma; S. India, Turkestan, Thailand, Tonkin Prov.	*A. fluviatilis* (= *listoni*)	Sun	Stream edges, stream pools, springs, irrigation channels; more rarely swamps, lakes	Prefers human to animal blood; found in houses, cow sheds	Important vector in rural foothills (300–1500 meters)
	E. and S. India, Burma, Thailand, Vietnam, S. China, Taiwan	*A. minimus*	Sun	Slow-running streams, springs, with grassy margins, irrigation ditches, rice fields, seepage areas	Remains in houses and cow sheds after feeding	Always important; especially so in India, Burma, Thailand, S. China up to 1700 meters
	India, Burma, Malaya, Thailand, Vietnam, Indonesia, Philippine Islands	*A. philippinensis*	Sun to partial shade	Pools, drains, ditches, tanks, swamps, borrow pits, rice fields; grass-covered stagnant waters	Found in houses, stables, cattle sheds	Important in Bengal; probably *not* vector in Philippine Islands
	See Persian Gulf, etc. for:	*A. stephensi*	....	....	....	....
	India, Burma, Thailand, Malaya, Sumatra, Java, Borneo, Lesser Sunda Islands, S. Celebes	*A. sundaicus*	Sun	Brackish or salt water in lagoons, swamps and behind coastal embankments	Prefers human blood (?); found in large numbers in cow sheds, houses; strong fliers	Important in Bengal, Malaya, Vietnam, Indonesia
	See Persian Gulf, etc. for:	*A. superpictus*	....	....	....	....
	India, Burma	*A. varuna*	Sun or shade	Stagnant water of pools, ditches, wells, slow streams, irrigation ditches	Feeds readily on man; found in houses, cow sheds	Proved vector in some localities
	India, Sri Lanka, Burma, Thailand, S. Vietnam, Malaya, Sumatra, Java, Borneo, Celebes	*A. aconitus*	Sun to partial shade	Irrigation ditches, swamps, ponds, rice fields, pools in creek beds, storm drains; reservoirs with grassy margins	Feeds readily on man, animals; found in houses, cow sheds (350 to 750 m.); strong fliers	Important in Vietnam
	See Afghanistan, N.E. India, etc., for:	*A. culicifacies*	....	....	....	....
	Burma, Vietnam, China, Korea, Japan, Taiwan, Okinawa, Indonesia	*A. sinensis*	Sun	Stagnant water in rice fields, pools, ponds, swamps; rarely stream or lake margins	Not recorded as domestic	Vector in S. Japan, Korea, Okinawa, Indonesia and in China
	India, China, Tonkin Prov., Burma, Taiwan	*A. jeyporiensis candidiensis*	Sun to slight shade	Running water in ditches	Not recorded as domestic	Vector in Tonkin Prov.

	India, Sri Lanka, Burma, S. China, Thailand, Malaya, Indonesia, Vietnam, Taiwan, Philippines	*A. maculatus maculatus*	Sun to very slight shade	Stream and river beds, seepages; also pools, rice fields, lake margins, ditches	Enters houses temporarily; bites humans	Important in Malaya and Indonesia
	See Afghanistan, etc. for:	*A. minimus*	....	....	....	....
	See Afghanistan, etc. for:	*A. sundaicus*	....	....	....	....
	India, Burma, Thailand, Malaya, Laos, Cambodia, Vietnam, Indonesia, Borneo	*A. balabacensis*	Shade	Pools	Feeds in forest canopy and on ground on monkeys and man. Enters houses	Important
	E. India, Tonkin Prov., Malaya, S. Vietnam, Sumatra, Java, Borneo, Celebes	*A. umbrosus*	Shade (can tolerate sunlight)	Stagnant jungle pools and morasses; brackish water in mangrove swamps	Fierce biter, found in dense forests, jungles, also in houses; strong fliers	Important in some areas
	Philippine Islands and south to Java	*A. minimus flavirostris*	Sun and shade	Clear water of shaded streams (bamboo roots); rivers, irrigation ditches, pools, wells	Enters houses to attack man; leaves after feeding, rests under overhanging banks	The important vector in the Philippines
	Indonesia:					
	See Burma, etc. for:	*A. aconitus*	....	....	....	....
	India, Sri Lanka, Burma, Thailand, Vietnam, China, Malaya, Sumatra, Borneo, Java, Lesser Sundas, Celebes, New Guinea, Philippines	*A. barbirostris barbirostris*	Sun and shade	Clear water of shaded streams, rivers, vegetated ponds, pools, flowing ditches, canals; borrow pits, rice fields, salt water swamps; wells	Flies by day (in shade); enters houses rarely; prefers blood of domestic animals	Of little importance (found infected in Malaya, Indonesia)
	Malaya, Indonesia, Sarawak	*A. letifer*	Sun and shade	Stagnant drains, pools, dark brown water of peaty soils; found with varying amounts of vegetation: fresh water areas of coastal plains	Enters house, rests outside during day	Important in Malaya, probably other areas
	India, Sri Lanka, Burma, Thailand, Vietnam, China, Malaya, Sumatra, Java, Celebes, Borneo	*A. nigerrimus*	Sun, largely	Rice fields especially; stagnant vegetated canals, borrow pits, lakes, impounded areas; slow streams	A wild species, invades houses rarely; feeds on man or animals	Of some importance in Malaya and Indonesia
	India, Sri Lanka, Burma, Vietnam, Malaya, Sumatra, Java, Borneo, Philippines	*A. leucosphyrus leucosphyrus*	Heavy shade required	Rock pools; stagnant pools in beds of mountain streams	A wild species; found in dense jungles	Found infected in Indonesia
	See Burma, etc. for:	*A. maculatus*	....	....	....	....
	See Afghanistan, etc. for:	*A. minimus*	....	....	....	....
	India, Malaya, Indonesia, New Guinea	*A. subpictus subpictus*	Sun or shade	Fresh, brackish, or contaminated pools, borrow pits, wallows; roof-gutters, containers	Feeds on man, other animals, but prefers cattle; numerous in cow sheds, houses, barracks	Believed important in Celebes
	See Afghanistan, etc. for:	*A. sundaicus*	....	....	....	....
	See Burma, etc. for:	*A. umbrosus*	....	....	....	....
Australasia	New Guinea, New Britain, Solomons, New Hebrides, Admiralties, N. Australia	*A. farauti*	Sun or slight shade	Fresh or brackish water, natural or artificial, clear or polluted	Bites freely both at night and in daytime shade; exclusively anthropophilic	Dominant carrier in this area
	New Guinea, Bismarck Archipelago and Solomon Islands	*A. punctulatus*	Sun	Small rain pools, stream margins; rarely in larger bodies of water	Frequents houses; bites throughout night; strong flier	Important in New Guinea and in Solomons
	New Guinea, Solomons	*A. koliensis*	Sun	Temporary pools in grasslands at edge of jungle	Enters and rests in houses. Active at night	Important in Solomons
	Australia, New Guinea	*A. bancrofti*	Shade	Swampy areas, vegetation	Nocturnal. Enters and rests in houses and sheds	May be important when present in large numbers

*Some secondary and suspected vectors are not included.

especially in the African region. The great importance of malaria as a military problem was demonstrated in World War I when, in the course of campaigns in Macedonia, the British, French and German armies were immobilized by this disease. In World War II it constituted the major problem of military medicine throughout the tropical and subtropical theaters, particularly in the Mediterranean, India, Burma, China, the Philippines and the south and southwest Pacific. In the latter area malaria had a profound effect upon the development and progress of military operations. In this region also a peculiarly resistant strain of *P. vivax* was encountered which was characterized by repeated relapses over an unusually long period. Experience in Korea demonstrated that malaria may be a problem for armies in the field even in the temperate zone. In the recent Vietnam conflict, malaria was a leading cause of casualties, a problem which was compounded by the presence of drug-resistant strains of *P. falciparum.*

The degree of endemicity or the level of transmission of malaria in any region is determined by a variety of interrelated factors. The most important of these are:

1. The prevalence of infection in man—the reservoir.

2. The species of indigenous anopheline mosquitoes, their relative abundance, their feeding and resting behaviors and their individual suitability as hosts for plasmodia—the vector.

3. The presence of a susceptible human population—the new host.

4. Local climatic conditions.

5. Local geographic and hydrographic conditions which determine anopheline breeding areas (Fig. 38–16, Table 38–1).

It is apparent, however, that there must be other controlling influences, for in areas in which the disease is endemic the prevalence of malaria over long periods exhibits cyclic increases and recessions, the causes of which are not understood.

In many parts of the world there is a definite annual fluctuation and a usual sequence in the times of appearance of the different types of the disease. These are probably dependent upon seasonal variations of temperature, humidity and rainfall affecting both the breeding of anopheline vectors and the development of the exogenous phase of the parasites in them.

The average climatic conditions in the temperate zone permit development and transmission of *P. vivax* and *P. malariae* but are less favorable to *P. falciparum.* These factors, together with relapse characteristics, undoubtedly are important in the seasonal incidence of the types of malaria in cooler parts of the endemic areas. In such regions *P. vivax* infections are the earliest to appear in the spring, whereas *P. falciparum* and *P. malariae* do not reach their peak until late summer and early autumn.

In the true tropics rainfall is the determining factor controlling anopheline breeding. In areas where there are wet and dry seasons each year there are commonly two peaks of incidence. The first follows shortly after the beginning of the rains. The second, and frequently the more important, appears at the end of the rainy season when ample anopheline breeding areas are present and when the destructive action of heavy rainfall upon the larvae is diminished.

In mountainous tropical countries both *P. vivax* and *P. falciparum* are prevalent in the hot, moist lowlands. At higher altitudes as the average temperatures more nearly approach those of temperate zones, *P. falciparum* gradually disappears. *Plasmodium vivax,* however, may be heavily endemic in certain regions at altitudes even in excess of 2400 m.

Evaluation of the malaria problem in any area entails study of all the known factors that contribute to the endemicity and the transmission of the disease.

Malaria reconnaissance provides a rapid, superficial and statistically inexact estimate of the situation. The data provided by such an investigation are insufficient for the preparation of a detailed control program.

A *malaria survey,* on the other hand, is an intensive, detailed, often time-consuming study of all relevant local factors. It should be carried on throughout a year to secure accurate information adequate for planning a control program.

EVALUATION OF INFECTION OF THE HUMAN RESERVOIR. Evaluation of the degree of infection of the human reservoir is based upon the following findings:

Spleen Rate. This is the per cent prevalence of splenomegaly in children of the indigenous population 2 to 9 years of age inclusive. The age group may be varied in certain regions.

Adult Spleen Rate. When the number of children is insufficient, adults may be included in the figures. The prevalence of splenomegaly in the adult population is lower, however, and consequently the qualifying term "adult" must be included to avoid misinterpretation of the data.

Parasite Rate. This is the per cent prevalence of blood films showing malarial parasites. Children of the indigenous population 2 to 9 years of age inclusive are often used for this measurement.

Transmission Index. This is the per cent incidence of blood films showing malarial parasites in infants of the indigenous population under 1 year of age. It provides important information concerning variations in the seasonal transmission rate of malaria in the particular area and is the best indication of the effectiveness of control measures.

Certain arbitrary terms have been accepted to express the *intensity of infection* in a given area. These are rates in children 2 to 9 years of age and are as follows:

Hypoendemic: spleen, 0 to 10 per cent; or parasite, 0 to 10 per cent (may be higher during part of the year).
Mesoendemic: spleen, 11 to 50 per cent; or parasite, 11 to 50 per cent (may be higher during part of the year).
Hyperendemic: spleen, over 50 per cent, adult spleen rate also high; or parasite, constantly over 50 per cent.
Holoendemic: spleen, constantly over 75 per cent, adult spleen rate low, adult tolerance high; or parasite rate in infants (1 year age group) constantly over 75 per cent.

THE INSECT VECTOR. The definitive host of the plasmodia is the anopheline mosquito. There are over 200 known species of anophelines, of which over 60 have been incriminated as vectors of malaria.

Determination of the particular species which are or may be efficient vectors and estimation of their relative abundance in an area are essential functions of the malaria survey. The marked variation in the capacity among different species to transmit the disease depends upon certain fundamental biologic differences. Certain individuals within each species are physiologically unsuitable hosts, and the plasmodia cannot complete their development in them. Some anophelines are domestic, breeding and remaining in the vicinity of human habitations; others are forest dwellers, breeding in and rarely leaving the jungle. Many anophelines feed almost exclusively on animal rather than human blood, whereas others feed with equal frequency on blood from man or animals. Some remain in or close to dwellings after obtaining a blood meal; others immediately leave the human environment. Similarly, there are great variations in flight range. Some anophelines are weak fliers and travel only short distances, but the normal flight range of others may be several miles.

Malaria tends to be a "place" disease, with highest incidence close to important mosquito-breeding areas, and the location and description of such areas are therefore essential functions of the survey. In general, anopheline larvae require clear water, with an adequate content of algae for optimal growth. The typical habitats of different species vary greatly. Some species seek only sunlit water; others flourish in shade. Certain ones cannot utilize water containing even small amounts of salt; others thrive in brackish water containing 40 to 60 per cent sea water. Some species utilize streams or seepage areas, others only swamps and marshes. Such variations in specific habitats form the basis for so-called naturalistic control methods which are designed to alter the natural characteristics of a breeding area, rendering it unsuitable for larval development.

The final evaluation of the importance of a particular anopheline species as a vector of malaria is based upon certain specific procedures.

Epidemiologic Index. This expression

represents the attempt to establish a significant correlation between the prevalence of a particular species of anopheline and the transmission of the disease. It is seldom a practicable procedure and rarely affords dependable evidence.

Experimental Index of Infection. Laboratory-raised female anophelines of a given species are fed upon a human gametocyte carrier. They are subsequently dissected, and the percentage showing oocysts on the stomach wall and sporozoites in the salivary glands is noted. This procedure may give accurate information of the biologic suitability of the particular anopheline to serve as a definitive host for the *Plasmodium.* It does not provide information as to the importance of the species as a *natural* vector. A number of species, of no practical importance in the transmission of malaria, may nevertheless yield a high index of experimental infection.

Natural Index of Infection. Large numbers of captured female anopheline mosquitoes are dissected, and the per cent prevalence of oocyst formation on the stomach wall and of sporozoite infection in the salivary glands is noted. The prevalence of salivary gland infection provides the more important information. A salivary gland index as low as 0.1 per cent or even lower nevertheless indicates an important transmitter when the species is very abundant. Much higher rates may be encountered exceptionally. In the course of epidemic malaria in northeastern Brazil the salivary gland infection rate of *Anopheles gambiae* reached 30.2 per cent. (See p. 788.)

The Precipitin Test. The precipitin test applied to the gut contents of engorged mosquitoes provides a means of distinguishing between anthropophilic and zoophilic species (p. 837).

Pathology. Malaria is accompanied by

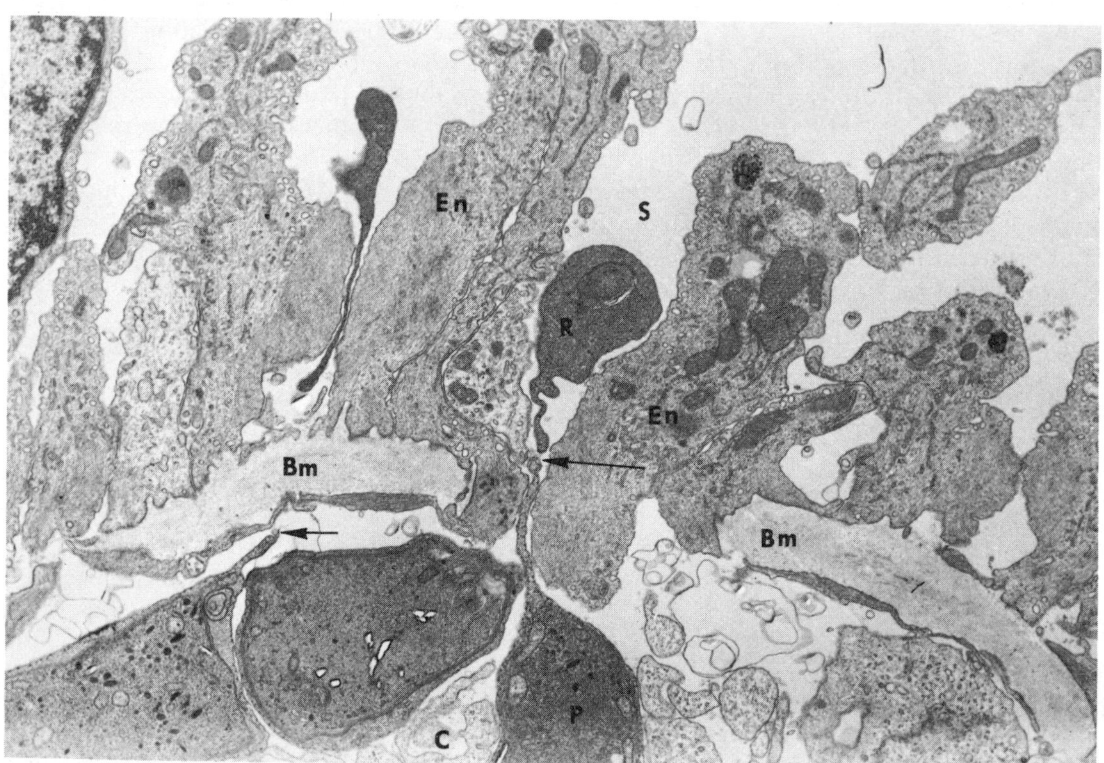

Figure 38–17. An ultrastructural view of the red pulp of the spleen in malaria. Severed (long arrow) red cell (R), one part having passed into sinus (S), with the parasitized (P) part remaining trapped in cord (C). Break has occurred in thin stalk that lies in the fenestration of basement membrane (Bm) and between two endothelial cells (En). Within the cord are two other parasite-containing pitted red cells, one showing a broken red cell stalk (short arrow). × 11,700. (Courtesy of Schnitzer, B., Sodeman, T. M., Mead, M. L., and Contacos, P. G. 1973. Blood *41*:207–218. Used by permission.)

the destruction of enormous numbers of red blood cells, both parasitized and nonparasitized, and by a consequent increase in the bilirubin content of the blood. The hemolysis may be so intense in *P. falciparum* infections as to cause hemoglobinuria and blackwater fever. Sequestration of red cells by the reticuloendothelial system is a major factor in the reduction of erythrocytes. In the spleen, malaria-parasitized erythrocytes are phagocytosed in toto by cordal macrophages, some are pitted of parasites, and others are hemolyzed by splenic microvasculature (Fig. 38–17).[4] Severe grades of anemia may be produced and reticulocyte crisis may follow upon effective therapy. In chronic cases, however, the anemia may be refractory. At least three factors appear to contribute to this: the continued destruction of erythrocytes, the failure of the liver to reconvert liberated iron and, in *P. vivax* infections, the selective parasitization of reticulocytes. Thrombocytopenia accompanies malaria, being most pronounced just preceding the maximum parasitemia. Platelet destruction appears to be caused by sequestration primarily in the spleen.

In chronic malaria there is characteristically a moderate leukopenia with an absolute increase in the number of monocytes.

Malarial pigment (hemozoin) is taken up by circulating polymorphonuclear leukocytes and monocytes and especially by the reticuloendothelial cells of the viscera. One of the striking features of the gross pathologic picture in patients who have died after prolonged infection is a slaty or blackish pigmentation of the organs, especially the spleen, liver and brain (Fig. 38–18).

The spleen varies in size, color and consistency, depending upon the duration and severity of the infection. Usually it is enlarged and dark or slate-colored. After long continued infections it may weigh 1000 gm or more. In acute malaria the spleen is congested and soft; the capsule is distended, and occasionally spontaneous or traumatic rupture may occur. In fatal cases there may be hemorrhagic areas of the pulp, thrombi in the arterioles, and areas of infarction. The majority of cases show distinct diminution in the size of the splenic follicles. In chronic cases fibrosis of the trabeculae is prominent. There is marked hyperplasia of the reticuloendothelial elements.

The presence of malarial pigment in these phagocytic cells is a salient microscopic feature. Both phagocytosed and free pigment are concentrated in the red pulp; however, it is unusual to find phagocytosed pigment in any part of the follicle. From 1 to 50 or more granules of pigment may be present in the cytoplasm of a single cell. The pigment usually appears as single, round, dark

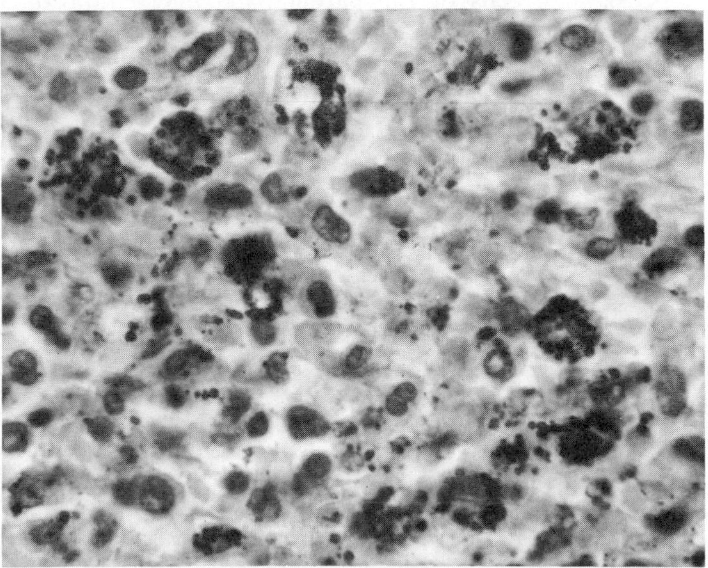

Figure 38–18. Phagocytosed and free malarial pigment in the spleen; numerous individual granules and aggregates of pigment in a single phagocyte. (Courtesy of the Louisiana State University School of Medicine, New Orleans.)

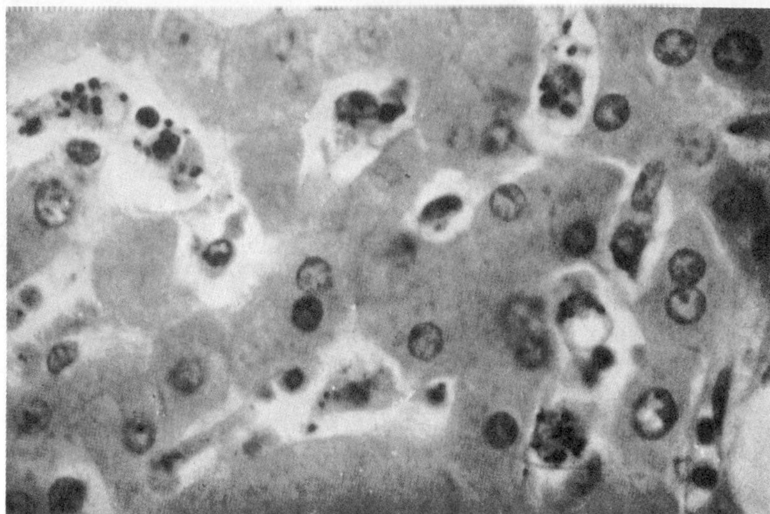

Figure 38–19. Malaria pigment in Kupffer cells of liver.

brown blocks (characteristic of *P. falciparum*) or as small, black conglomerate masses in the phagocyte (Fig. 38–18). Hemozoin must be distinguished from iron pigment, which may be present in the same cell, by the lighter color of the iron, and from formalin pigment by the irregular crystalline shape of the formalin. Dark yellow hemosiderin may be seen in the spleen pulp but not in the malpighian corpuscles.

The liver is usually somewhat enlarged and dark in color. On microscopic examination the endothelial and Kupffer cells are seen to be packed with black pigment (Fig. 38–19). The cells of the parenchyma may contain considerable amounts of hemosiderin and show cloudy swelling and vacuolization. Malarial pigment is not present in the hepatic parenchymal cells. Occasionally, necrotic foci are seen in the portal areas and in the central zones of the liver lobules.

The brain is frequently lead-colored because of the malaria pigment. Engorgement of the cerebral capillaries is a prominent feature; the capillary network of the brain is distended with erythrocytes. There may be extensive capillary plugging by masses of parasitized red cells (Fig. 38–20). In vessels of larger caliber, erythrocytes containing older forms of *P. falciparum,* owing to their adhesive nature, may be seen in contact with the endothelial lining, while the noninfected red cells occupy the lumen. This arrangement of the parasitized corpuscles is referred to as margination (Fig. 38–21*A, B*). In fatal cases hemorrhages are found in the subcortical white matter but not in the gray matter. They are also seen commonly in the pons, medulla and cerebellum. These take the form of ring hemorrhages encircling an area of necrosis in which a central plugged vessel may be discerned. In addition, malarial granulomas (Dürck's nodules) frequently are present. These noninflammatory granulomas resemble the areas of simple hemorrhage, except that with the initiation of a reparative process, a single or multiple layered ring of neuroglial cells is interposed between or mixed with the hemorrhagic belt and the necrotic zone which surrounds the remains of the small, central vessel (Fig. 38–21*C*).

Toxic acute focal or interstitial myocarditis with capillary obstruction in the myocardium also may be present in fatal cases. In the presence of prominent gastrointestinal symptoms, lesions in the stomach and intestines are not uncommon. These are punctate hemorrhages, capillary obstruction by parasitized erythrocytes, necrosis of epithelium and, occasionally, hemorrhage into the lumen. The bone marrow may reveal large numbers of parasitized cells and considerable amounts of malarial pigment.

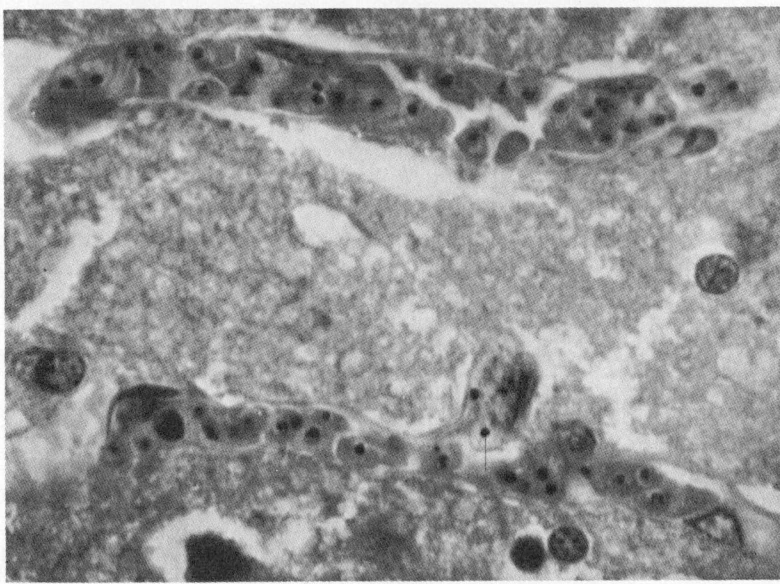

Figure 38–20. Agglutinated parasitized erythrocytes in capillaries of brain—*falciparum* malaria.

Acute malaria may be associated with profound disturbances of body chemistry. There is reduction of the total plasma proteins with reversal of the albumin-globulin ratio but usually not above unity. The serum euglobulin is increased. Cholesterol, lecithin and glucose rise during the chill but usually are slightly decreased during the afebrile period. Plasma potassium is greatly increased by the rupture of erythrocytes. There is a decrease in levulose and galactose tolerance, indicating disturbance of the glycogenetic function of the liver. In heavy infections, bilirubin may be discharged into the blood plasma in considerable quantities, producing an indirect van den Bergh reaction. The blood urea ordinarily does not undergo significant change in malaria; howev-

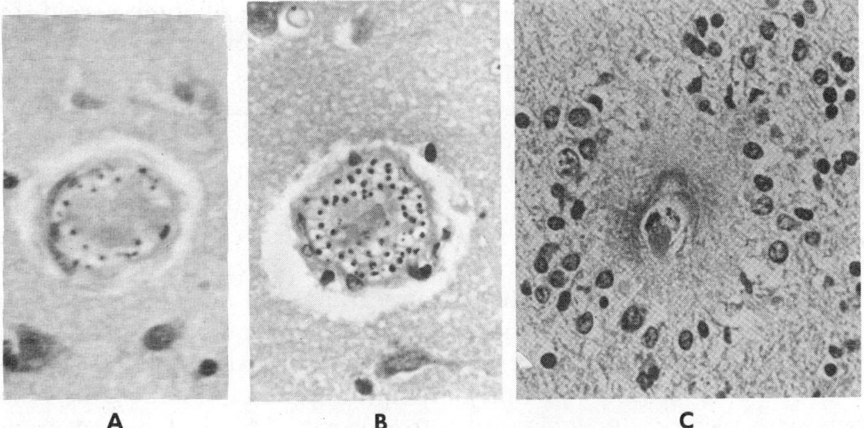

Figure 38–21. *A,* Vessel of brain with parasitized erythrocytes in contact with the endothelial lining (margination) and noninfected red cells occupying the center of the lumen. A pigment granule of *P. falciparum* is prominent in each of the parasitized cells. *B,* Margination with double or multiple rows of adhesive parasitized red corpuscles partially occluding the lumen of the vessel. *C,* Malarial granuloma composed of a central thrombosed vessel, necrotic intermediate zone and peripheral rows of neuroglial cells mixed with erythrocytes (Durck's nodule). (Courtesy of the Louisiana State University School of Medicine, New Orleans.)

er, when there is sufficient damage to the kidneys in malignant *falciparum* or blackwater fever to interfere with renal function, varying degrees of nitrogen retention and uremia may occur.

Clinical Characteristics. Salient features of malaria are periodic fever, splenomegaly, anemia and leukopenia. The characteristic periodicity of the fever (in *vivax* and quartan infections) is associated with the rhythmic maturation of the sporulating forms in the blood and their massive release by rupture of the erythrocytes. The enlargement of the spleen, and to a lesser degree of the liver, is correlated with an increase in reticuloendothelial cells which, as one mechanism of immunity in malaria, phagocytose not only merozoites upon their release but also pigment, parasitized and nonparasitized red corpuscles. Since the malarial organisms live in and at the expense of the erythrocytes, destroying all those attacked, the primary effect of their presence is manifested usually by a normocytic normochromic anemia. Some patients with acute malaria have herpes labialis; others with chronic malaria may have urticaria.

The clinical phenomena accompanying infection by *P. falciparum* differ greatly in their evolution and in the hazard to the infected individual from those accompanying infection by *P. vivax, P. malariae* or *P. ovale. Falciparum* malaria is always dangerous and may be fatal. The other types, although capable of producing severe illness, commonly are free from dangerous complications and grave menace to life. The capacity of *P. falciparum* to invade both mature erythrocytes and reticulocytes is probably directly related to the intense and rapidly increasing parasitemia that accompanies this infection. Furthermore, the infected red blood cells tend to agglutinate and to adhere to capillary endothelium. Large numbers of parasitized red cells distend the visceral capillaries and slow the circulation. This may lead to thrombosis, which produces areas of local anoxemia and ischemia (Fig. 38–21).

The usual intrinsic incubation period for *vivax* malaria is 11 to 15 days; *falciparum,* 11 to 14 days; *ovale,* 14 to 26 days; and quartan from 3 to 4 weeks. Prodromes consisting of malaise, muscle pains, headache, anorexia and slight fever may exist for a few days before the onset of the acute phenomena. In many instances, however, the initial attack comes on abruptly without prodromes.

VIVAX AND QUARTAN MALARIA. The classic clinical picture of malaria with its alternation of "good" and "bad" days is much more the exception than the rule. Even in *P. vivax* infections the initial clinical attack seldom exhibits tertian fever at the outset; usually there are two groups of parasites out of phase with one another and these, maturing on alternate days, produce daily, or quotidian, rather than tertian fever. Later, one group may drop out, and the release of a new generation of parasites will then occur on alternate days, at intervals of 42 to 47 hours. Only then does the fever become tertian (Fig. 38–22).

The typical paroxysms of benign tertian and quartan malaria are similar except for the difference in periodicity. The onset is abrupt and frequently initiated by a rigor which may vary from a slight subjective chilliness to a frank chill accompanied by a sensation of extreme cold, although the temperature meanwhile rises rapidly to 40 to 41° C (104 to 106° F). The pulse is rapid and of small volume. Polyuria, nausea and vomiting are common. After 20 to 60 minutes the hot stage begins, accompanied at first by relief from the sense of intense cold, but shortly followed, however, by an increasing and severe headache and a sensation of intense heat. At this stage the face is flushed and the pulse full. Epigastric discomfort, nausea and vomiting are more prominent. Frequently there is mild delirium, and although the temperature does not remain long at the fastigium, the sweating stage, ushered in by the appearance of moisture on the previously dry skin, increases to a profuse diaphoresis of the entire body. With this change the temperature falls rapidly and the pulse returns to normal. This is followed frequently by sleep, after which the individual awakes somewhat exhausted but otherwise feeling well. The sweating stage lasts 2 to 3 hours and the entire paroxysm averages 10 hours.

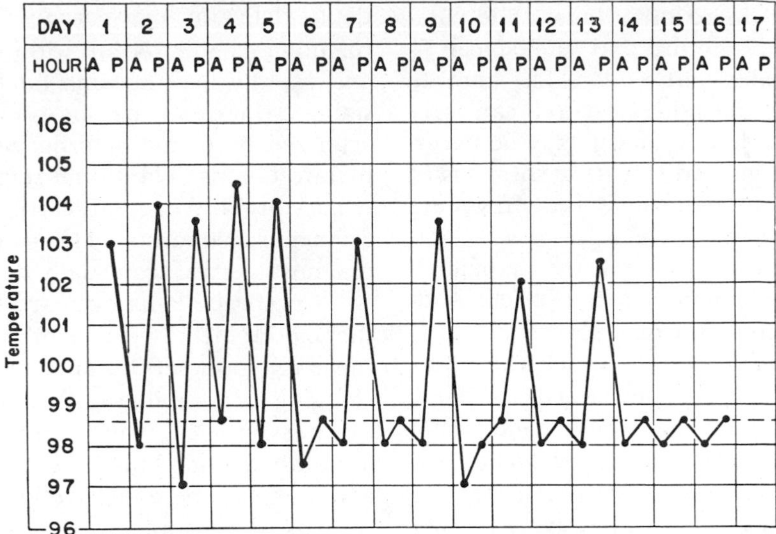

Figure 38–22. Fever chart in a *P. vivax* infection showing an initial quotidian tendency becoming tertian. No specific therapy. A = A.M., P = P.M. (Courtesy of Russell, West, Manwell and Macdonald. 1963. Practical Malariology. 2nd ed. Oxford University Press, London.)

During the paroxysm there is a moderate leukocytosis, whereas in the afebrile period leukopenia with an increase in the number of large mononuclears is usual.

In quartan malaria the attacks occur every 72 hours, if only a single brood of parasites is present. The rise of temperature is less abrupt, and the total duration of the paroxysm averages 11 hours.

Anemia is a common complication of any type of malaria. In addition, rupture of the spleen may occur in *vivax* malaria but is not common. Nephrosis, with large amounts of albumin in the urine, occurs in chronic malaria, chiefly in *P. malariae* infections.

OVALE MALARIA. Infections with this species resemble those due to *P. vivax* but tend to be milder. The untreated primary course is shorter than *P. vivax* and the parasitemia is lower. With a single brood of parasites, the time between clinical attacks averages 49 or 50 hours. Multiple broods cause daily fevers.

FALCIPARUM MALARIA. The onset of malignant tertian malaria is frequently insidious. The individual complains of gradually increasing headache, of gastrointestinal symptoms, or of a clinical complex that is suggestive of influenza and frequently misdiagnosed unless examination of the blood is carried out. In other instances onset is abrupt and dramatic. Characteristically there are: a sensation of chilliness rather than a frank chill; a prolonged and intensified hot stage; and lack of the marked terminal sweating, with its accompanying drop in temperature, characteristically observed in *P. vivax* infections. The fever curve frequently shows prolongation of the fastigium, often with primary fall and secondary rise, before returning to or toward normal. This double-peaked elevation is characteristic when it is observed. Frequently, however, the fever is continuous or remittent instead of intermittent. During the periods of remission there is little or no return of the sense of well-being. Commonly, the tertian periodicity of the infection is indicated by exacerbation of a continuous fever. Defervescence in *falciparum* malaria frequently occurs by lysis rather than by crisis. In those instances in which the fever curve is remittent, the paroxysm often lasts 20 to 36 hours. These variations in the fever curve are to be explained by the phenomena of anticipation and retardation of the events of schizogony as a result of which the new generation of parasites is released over a prolonged period.

Prostration is more marked and the tendency to delirium greater than in *P. vivax* and *P. malariae* infections. Nausea and vomiting frequently occur, and the spleen is generally palpable and tender. The parasite density in the peripheral blood can vary widely in a few hours, and it may be necessary to make repeated smears at intervals of several hours to determine the maximum number of parasites.

PERNICIOUS TYPES. *Falciparum* malaria is notorious for its tendency to produce, suddenly and without warning, severe and dangerous types of disease to which the terms *pernicious* or *malignant* malaria have been applied. These may be rapidly fatal if not recognized promptly and treated adequately. Several clinical types are known. The various types may exist simultaneously, differing only in degree. The tendency of falciparum-infected erythrocytes to clog the small capillaries of the viscera and thus interfere with the blood supply is related to many of the complications associated with this malaria species.

Bilious Remittent Fever. The onset is characterized by marked nausea and profuse, continuous vomiting. Jaundice customarily appears about the second day, earlier than in yellow fever and later than in blackwater fever. The urine frequently contains bile pigment and yields a yellow foam test. Epigastric distress and liver tenderness are marked, and hemorrhage from the stomach may occur, producing coffee-ground vomitus. The temperature tends to be high, and the fever curve is usually remittent rather than continuous. Dehydration and disturbance of the alkali reserve and of mineral balance may develop rapidly.

Cerebral Malaria. The onset of cerebral malaria may be sudden or gradual, and the clinical picture may be varied. The patient may complain of progressively increasing headache with little or no fever and then gradually lapse into coma; or a clinical picture in which there appears little cause for immediate concern may be superseded without warning by a progressive and uncontrollable rise of temperature to levels in excess of 42.2° C (108° F). In addition to hyperpyrexia, convulsive seizures are common. Involvement of the cranial nerves may be evident; delirium may occur. These clinical phenomena may occur within a few hours and rapidly may become fatal. In some instances, the onset may be sudden and characterized by mania or other acute psychotic manifestations. The initial stages of cerebral malaria not infrequently have been mistaken for acute alcoholism. The results of such a diagnostic error are usually disastrous.

Cerebral edema occurs. The viscosity of the blood increases which, combined with the large numbers of infected erythrocytes clogging the capillaries, contributes to the slowing of the circulation and finally to capillary obstruction. This leads to local ischemia and anoxia. The extensive interference with the vascular supply to the central nervous system in cerebral malaria may produce any combination of symptoms and signs indicative of severe and extensive involvement of the brain. In children, convulsions are a frequent presenting symptom. There are no constant or significant changes in the spinal fluid. The spinal fluid pressure, however, may be elevated considerably above normal. In such instances, repeated lumbar drainage is an important therapeutic procedure.

Algid Malaria. The algid forms of *falciparum* malaria accompany extensive vascular involvement of the gastrointestinal tract and other abdominal viscera. Profound prostration, with a tendency to fatal syncope, marked coldness of the skin, subnormal temperature and circulatory collapse occur. Jaundice may be present. Severe grades of anemia may develop rapidly. Acute diarrhea unaccompanied by fever and often ending fatally has long been recognized as an algid form of pernicious malaria.

Other recognized types of pernicious malaria are the gastric, which is characterized by persistent vomiting, and the dysenteric, in which there is a bloody diarrhea due to extensive capillary thrombosis in the intestinal walls. The blood in the stools frequently contains immense numbers of parasites.

Orthostatic hypotension is a prominent clinical feature. Acute renal insufficiency characterized by progressive oliguria may occur in the absence of the rapid hemolysis associated with blackwater fever. Shock, pulmonary edema, and secondary bronchopneumonia are seen in severe *falciparum* malaria.

The general mortality for the pernicious forms of *falciparum* malaria may be as high as 50 per cent.

Diagnosis. The clinical diagnosis of malaria frequently is difficult. It may be confused with many diseases, both cosmopolitan and tropical. This situation is inevitable in view of the pathologic changes, which consist mainly of mechanical interference with the vascular supply in many organs of the body. Among the tropical diseases it may be confused with kala-azar, amebic liver abscess, relapsing fever and yellow fever. Among the cosmopolitan diseases it may frequently simulate typhoid fever, tuberculosis, brucellosis, influenza, pyelitis and other septic conditions, including malignant endocarditis as well as acute or chronic organic disease of the central nervous system. Malaria commonly is associated with positive Wassermann and Kahn reactions.

Definitive diagnosis depends upon demonstration of the parasites. For this purpose the thick blood film is far superior to the thin film technique, since in light infections it may be impossible to find plasmodia in the thin film. The thick film will yield three to four times as many positive findings and will reveal the plasmodia in virtually all active clinical cases. (See Diagnostic Methods, p. 809.) It may be necessary to examine stained thin blood films for positive identification of the particular species present.

Other characteristics of the stained thin blood films may be suggestive. Leukocytes containing ingested malarial pigment may be seen. There is often a leukopenia with a relative increase of monocytes. In chronic cases a sustained submaximal reticulocyte crisis beginning 4 to 7 days after the institution of specific therapy is suggestive.

A history of having been in a malarious area, periodicity of the febrile curve and splenomegaly should arouse suspicion of malaria. In chronic cases, however, there may be little if any significant splenic enlargement. Sternal puncture and examination of the stained marrow smear may be useful in the rare case where parasites cannot be found on a thick blood film.

In view of the marked differences in severity and prognosis between *falciparum* malaria and the other forms of the disease, accurate identification of the species of *Plasmodium* is essential. Table 38–2 presents the significant differential characteristics that may be seen in the stained thin blood film.

Because of the importance of the thick film in the differential diagnosis of human malaria, the characteristics of the three principal species are summarized in Table 38–3. *Plasmodium ovale* usually cannot be identified with certainty in the thick film.

Although immunodiagnosis of malaria has advanced greatly in recent years, the

Table 38–2. Differential Characteristics of the Plasmodia of Man in Stained Thin Film

Characteristics	*P. falciparum*	*P. vivax*	*P. ovale*	*P. malariae*
Infected erythrocyte enlarged	−	+	±	−
Infected erythrocyte, fimbriated and/or oval	Rare	Rare	Frequent	Rare
Infected erythrocyte decolorized	−	+	+	−
Infected erythrocyte, Schüffner's dots*	−	+	+	−
Infected erythrocyte, Maurer's dots*	+	−	−	−
Multiple infections in erythrocytes*	+	Rare	−	−
Parasite, all forms in peripheral blood	Rare	+	+	+
Parasite, large coarse rings	±	+	+	+
Parasite, double chromatin dots*	+	Rare	−	−
Parasite, accolé forms*	+	Rare	−	−
Parasite, band forms*	−	−	+	+
Parasite, sausage-shaped gametocytes	+	−	−	−
Number of merozoites	8–24	12–24	8–12	6–12

*Not invariable but suggestive when seen.

Table 38–3. DIFFERENTIAL DIAGNOSIS OF MALARIAL PARASITIES IN STAINED THICK BLOOD FILMS*

Stage of parasite	*Plasmodium falciparum*	*Plasmodium vivax*	*Plasmodium malariae*	*Comments*
Small trophozoite (early ring)	Small size rings, with small chromatin dot and delicate, scanty cytoplasm. Frequently rings have double chromatin dots. Tendency toward large number of rings. Many ring forms with no older stages—practically certain to be *falciparum* infection. Diagnosis on small number of rings may often be assisted by finding distinguishing gametocyte, though this stage is not necessarily present.	Larger, heavier, ring form than in *falciparum*, often with variety of cytoplasmic patterns and irregularities in shape. Usually older stages of parasite can be found also.	Ring is likely to be heavy, with large dot of chromatin and small amount of cytoplasm, which is often "filled in," without a vacuole. Pigment forms early and may appear as haze in cytoplasm of this stage. Rings practically always associated with older forms. The ring phase is brief, so this stage is not found as often as older stages.	Ring forms often not complete circle—may be "swallow" forms, "exclamation mark," "comma" forms, or "interrupted rings." When rings only are present and number is small, it is practically impossible to differentiate species.
Growing trophozoite	Heavy large rings form—resemble young rings of *vivax*. Sometimes show pigment grains or haze rather clearly in cytoplasm.	Stage usually ameboid in appearance, with large variety of shapes. Cytoplasm frequently fragmented and arranged irregularly in cluster of varying sized pieces or streamers, about or close to a large chromatin mass. Small yellowish brown pigment granules scattered through parts of the cytoplasm. This is the most characteristic stage of *vivax*. Frequently other younger or older stages accompany this one.	Small, usually rounded compact forms, "like marbles in a ring." Profuse, heavy, dark, large-grained pigment. Forms frequently so solid that chromatin seems buried in the mass. This stage and the one that follows are the commonest forms of this parasite seen.	In heavily stained films and in films which have been kept for several days before staining, the "ghost" of the enlarged host cell and persistence of Schüffner's stippling or a pinkness remaining from the stippling may assist in diagnosis of *vivax*.
Large trophozoite	Ring vacuole lost or almost lost. Parasite quite small and compact, cytoplasm often quite pale, irregularly circular or oval. One large chromatin dot. Pigment in blurred mass or small, very dark clump or clumps. Stage is usually found only when the infection is intense and usually accompanied by numbers of ring-form trophozoites.	Frequently quite solid and dark staining. More or less irregular in outline, possibly with one or more vacuoles. Fine brown pigment scattered throughout the cytoplasm. May be confused with macrogametocyte.	Compact, dark, larger than "growing" stages. Sometimes in thinner portion of the smear spreads to normal size. Profuse, fairly coarse, dark brown pigment—often masking the chromatin. May be confused with "rounded up" *falciparum* gametocyte or with gametocyte of *malariae*.	On rare occasions Maurer's dots have been observed in thick films of *falciparum*. The infrequently found stages of *falciparum* are, of course, more readily found in thick films. Band forms have tendency to become rounded in thick films of *malariae*—except perhaps in very thin edge of smear
Schizont (presegmenting)	Stage not often seen and is usually accompanied by large numbers of growing trophozoites when present. Parasite is very small. Contains 2 or more divisions of chromatin and very little cytoplasm (often pale) in which there is located one or more small, dense blocks of very dark pigment.	Irregular or compact clusters of chromatin divisions, often dark reddish purple in color. Cytoplasm in irregular broken masses and wisps, containing light brown pigment granules which are clumped in spots. Usually accompanied by other stages. May be confused with same stage of *malariae*.	Much like *vivax* of the same stage except that parasites are often smaller with darker, larger pigment granules. Often so compact that internal structure is difficult to define. Usually accompanied by other stages. May be confused with presegmenting schizonts of *vivax*.	Schizonts are much like thin film forms of same stages—more compact, smaller in thicker portions of smear. This is the most difficult stage (except infrequent ring forms) on which to diagnose species.

Mature schizont	Seldom seen except in severe cases. Always associated with many small trophozoites. Usually contains around 20 or more tiny merozoites clustered around a small, very dark, pigment mass.	Usually contains around 16 merozoites which are individually larger than those of *falciparum.* Usually relatively larger than other species. Nearly always associated with other stages. Not so often found as other stages.	Most distinctive stage of *malariae* in thick film. Often found in large numbers – usually with trophozoites or presegmenting forms or both. About 8 merozoites each with large chromatin dot and small amount of cytoplasm – may be compact or clearly separated. Frequently the chromatin and pigment only are seen, the chromatin dots being bare and well separated. The dark heavy pigment is more often concentrated, though sometimes dispersed.	Usually smaller than same stage in thin film.
Young gametocyte	Sometimes long, slender and pointed, with pigment scattered to the ends. Usually associated with many trophozoites.	When found is a small, compact, usually rounded parasite, with one chromatin mass which is often in the center of cytoplasm and frequently has unstained area around chromatin mass. Sex is almost impossible to determine.	Same as *vivax* except that parasite is even less frequently found and resembles compact trophozoite so closely that differentiation is impossible.	
Mature gametocyte	Differentiation of sex is difficult or impossible. As "crescent" or "sausage" shapes, may be quite diagnostic of species. In thicker portion of smear may take on oval or rounded, somewhat eroded appearance, which may be confused with *malariae* trophozoite or gametocyte. Often may be distinguished by difference in amount and appearance of pigment or by pink or red "flag" protruding from the edge of the parasite. May be accompanied by ring-form trophozoites or appear alone and infrequently. Often appears in "showers."	Macrogametocyte is larger, as a rule, than in other species; pigment is light, delicate, well dispersed through nonvacuolated cytoplasm. Except in thin edge of film cannot be differentiated from some mature trophozoites of same species. Microgametocyte often distinguishable as large blob of chromatin (varying from pink to purplish red) surrounded by halo of pale or colorless cytoplasm in which pigment granules are more or less evenly dispersed. Other stages of the parasite can usually be found.	As a rule, few in number, somewhat smaller than *vivax,* otherwise have the same distinguishing features except that pigment is coarser and darker. May resemble rounded *falciparum* gametocytes.	

*Courtesy of Aimee Wilcox, Laboratory of Tropical Diseases, NIAID, National Institutes of Health, in "Manual for the Microscopical Diagnosis of Malaria in Man." 3rd ed., 1960; and the American Public Health Association, Standard Methods Committee on Diagnostic Procedures and Reagents: "Diagnostic Procedures and Reagents." 4th ed., New York, 1963.

serologic tests must be interpreted with care, since positive reactions may indicate active infection, or a previous infection, or even only the presence of antibodies against substances antigenically related to plasmodia. Cross-reactions may occur among the various species. The tests used most successfully as an aid to diagnosis, or to establish the prevalence of malaria in a population, or to screen potential blood donors are the complement-fixation, the agglutination and the immunofluorescence. Of these, the indirect hemagglutination (IHA) test[5] and the indirect fluorescent antibody (IFA) test[6] are particularly well suited for epidemiologic surveys.

Prognosis. The prognosis for recovery from the primary attack of malaria due to *P. vivax, P malariae* or *P. ovale* is excellent. *Falciparum* malaria carries a good prognosis if treated adequately; untreated, its mortality is sometimes very high. Radical cure of malaria in the great majority of cases is possible with proper use of the new antimalarial drugs.

Treatment. Drugs have several functions in malaria: treatment of clinical attack; curative therapy to prevent relapses; suppressive and prophylactic action to prevent the acquiring or the clinical manifestations of the disease; and sporontocidal effect, which prevents transmission by mosquito vectors. There are several drugs exerting some of these effects but no one exerts all. The chemical groupings of the drugs are: cinchona alkaloids – quinine; 4-aminoquinolines – chloroquine, amodiaquine; 8-aminoquinolines – primaquine, pamaquine; 9-aminoacridines – mepacrine; biguanides – proguanil; diaminopyrimidines – pyrimethamine, trimethoprim; sulfone – dapsone, sulfonamides – sulfadiazine, sulfadimethoxine, sulfisoxazole, sulfadoxine, sulfalene; antibiotics – tetracycline, doxycycline, minocycline.

The 4-aminoquinoline drugs, amodiaquine and chloroquine, are the drugs of choice for the treatment of acute malaria except where the malaria originates in areas of known resistance to these compounds. In the majority of cases, fever is controlled within 24 hours and thick blood films usually become negative for parasites in 48 to 72 hours. *Plasmodium malariae* responds more slowly than the other species. These drugs will terminate infections by sensitive strains of *P. falciparum.* The gametocytes of *P. falciparum* are not removed or sterilized. For the malarias that have persisting stages, such as *P. vivax,* the addition of primaquine to the regimen generally will prevent relapses, but this varies according to the strain of parasite. Amodiaquine and chloroquine are useful as suppressive agents, in the absence of drug resistance. Some strains of *P. falciparum,* probably relatively few, are resistant to these drugs. Amodiaquine has been reported to be more effective than chloroquine against some resistant strains.

Drugs, especially chloroquine and amodiaquine, should be taken after meals with fluid. This reduces the possibility of occasional nausea, vomiting or mild gastrointestinal disturbances.

Chloroquine. Synonyms: Aralen, Nivaquine. The drug is a white crystalline powder with a bitter taste and is freely soluble in water. It is available in tablets for oral administration, each 0.25 gm equivalent to 0.15 gm of base, and in ampules containing 50 mg per ml equivalent to 40 mg of base for intramuscular and intravenous use.

Absorption is relatively complete and rapid when the drug is taken by mouth. It is stored in the tissues, excreted slowly and does not discolor the skin. Chloroquine usually is well tolerated in the dosages employed clinically. In certain individuals it may cause mild transient headache, visual disturbances, pruritus, trivial gastrointestinal complaints, psychic stimulation and, rarely, a lichen planus–like eruption. When given intravenously undiluted, there is a fall of systolic blood pressure with little or no change in the diastolic pressure. When well diluted and given slowly no significant change occurs. Excretion is accelerated by acidification of the urine.

Amodiaquine. Synonyms: Camoquin, Cam-aqi, Basoquin. Most formulations are prepared as the hydrochloride and distributed in tablets containing 200 mg base. Basoquin is prepared as the base, is tasteless, and is distributed as tablets with 150 mg base or as a syrup, each ml containing 30 mg of base.

Amodiaquine is a yellow crystalline powder and has a bitter taste. It forms a 5 per cent solution in water at room temperature and is rapidly absorbed from the gastrointestinal tract. It is virtually free of toxic effects at normal dosages, although long continued administration in amounts considerably above the recommended therapeutic dosage may be accompanied by loss of energy, insomnia, epigastric discomfort and anorexia.

Quinine. Quinine is rapidly absorbed from the gastrointestinal tract; 60 to 70 per cent is oxidized in the body and the remainder rapidly excreted in the urine. Indications of poisoning appear when the blood level rises to about 10 mg per 100 ml.

Quinine destroys the parasites in the red cells less rapidly than the 4-aminoquinolines. For many years it was the standard drug for treating malaria, and it is still used in some countries where the higher costs of the other drugs are a factor or where the quinine industry exists. There is a wide variation in the responses of different strains of *P. falciparum* to quinine. Some strains require larger total amounts of quinine than others.

Quinine, alone or in combination with another compound, is the drug of choice for treating patients with 4-aminoquinoline–resistant strains of malaria. It is advisable to use quinine initially for acute cases of *P. falciparum* from South America or Southeast Asia.

In therapeutic doses it has little effect on the circulatory system. In excessive dosage it produces an initial rise in pulse rate and blood pressure followed by a depression of both. When given intravenously in too large a dose or too quickly, rapid progressive fall of blood pressure occurs, with the appearance of circulatory collapse due to cardiac depression and vasodilatation.

Cinchonism is the expression of the toxic action of quinine upon the central nervous system. It is characterized by mental depression, giddiness, headache, sense of fullness in the head, tinnitus, deafness, amblyopia and occasional blindness. There may be mental confusion and somnolence as well. True idiosyncrasy to quinine results in the symptoms of cinchonism after small doses that are well within the normal therapeutic range.

Primaquine Diphosphate. This drug is chemically related to pamaquine but is less toxic. It is an orange crystalline solid with a bitter taste and is slightly soluble in water. It is supplied in tablets, 26.5 mg of the salt being equivalent to 15 mg of the base.

The drug may cause severe hemolytic reactions. Dark-skinned races and certain Caucasian groups in the Mediterranean area are particularly susceptible. This reaction is linked with a defect of the glucose-6-phosphate dehydrogenase in the erythrocytes of susceptible persons. Acute intravascular hemolysis may occur in such people after the single administration of 60 mg or the daily administration of 30 mg of the drug. As only the older red blood cells are destroyed, the hemolysis is self-limited. If the usual adult dose of 15 mg base is not exceeded, hemolysis is not of clinical significance. Primaquine administration should be discontinued if severe cyanosis or passage of dark urine occurs.

Primaquine should not be given to subjects receiving at the same time drugs capable of depressing the myeloid elements of the marrow. Quinacrine enhances the toxic effects of primaquine by preventing its metabolic degradation.

Primaquine is relatively ineffective against the erythrocytic forms of malaria. It quickly sterilizes the gametocytes. It is active against the exo-erythrocytic forms and therefore is useful in preventing relapses.

Pamaquine is more toxic than primaquine and has been displaced by the latter.

Dihydrofolate Reductase Inhibitors. This group includes proguanil, pyrimethamine and trimethoprim. They are slow-acting schizontocides and are not drugs of choice to be used alone for the treatment of the clinical attacks. They are normally used in combination with other drugs. The principal use of the first two is for prophylaxis. They are sporontocidal and thus prevent the development of the infection in mosquitoes. Resistance is easily acquired by both the asexual and sexual parasites. Cross-resistance occurs among these drugs.

Proguanil. Synonyms: Chlorguanide, Guanatol, Paludrine. Proguanil hydrochloride is a colorless, bitter pyrimidine compound that is rapidly absorbed from the gastrointestinal tract and is excreted in the feces and urine. There are no significant toxic effects at therapeutic dosage levels.

Pyrimethamine. Synonyms: Daraprim, Malocide. Pyrimethamine is chemically related to chlorguanide. It is a tasteless, odorless, freely soluble white powder. The drug is concentrated in the liver, spleen, brain and bone marrow. It is free from toxic or unpleasant side effects at recommended dosage levels. When administered in amounts far exceeding therapeutic levels it produces megaloblastic changes in the marrow, inhibition of leukopoiesis, marked reduction of erythrocyte, leukocyte and platelet counts, atrophy of lymphatic tissue and degenerative changes in the intestinal epithelium.

Trimethoprim. This diaminopyrimidine is closely related to pyrimethamine. Its principal use has been in the treatment of clinical attacks in combination with other drugs, especially the sulfonamides, with which it has a synergistic effect.

Sulfonamides and Sulfones. Several of the sulfonamides in combination with other drugs have been used to treat clinical attacks, e.g. sulfadiazine, sulfafurazole, sulfadimethoxine, sulfadoxine, and sulfalene. The last two are long-acting. These drugs are often combined with pyrimethamine or trimethoprim.

The sulfones diaphenylsulfone (dapsone) and sulfadiamine (DADDS) are useful as suppressive agents mainly after treatment with some of the more active schizontocidal compounds, such as the 4-aminoquinolines. They are not recommended alone for the treatment of clinical malaria. Resistance occurs easily.

Tetracyclines. Tetracycline hydrochloride, minocycline and doxycycline tend to be curative, but their action is so slow that it is necessary to add a faster acting drug, such as quinine, during the first several days of treatment.

The following 7-day regimens gave good results in limited trials: tetracycline hydrochloride, 1 or 2 gm daily; or doxycycline, 0.2 gm daily; or minocycline, 0.1 to 0.4 gm daily.

The World Health Organization warns against the widespread use of the tetracyclines, sulfonamides, sulfones and trimethoprim because of the danger of inducing concomitant resistance in bacteria. The Organization recommends that the use of the last three compounds be restricted to drug prophylaxis in areas with chloroquine-resistant *P. falciparum.*

Mepacrine Hydrochloride. Synonyms: Atabrine, quinacrine. Mepacrine is a yellow acridine dye with a bitter taste. It is soluble in water; it is absorbed rapidly, deposited in the tissues, especially the liver and gallbladder, and causes a yellow discoloration of the skin. Excretion is slow. The drug is present in the breast milk of nursing mothers.

Mepacrine (quinacrine) usually is well tolerated, although in certain individuals it acts as a gastrointestinal irritant, causing epigastric pain, nausea, vomiting and diarrhea. These symptoms usually are transient phenomena that may be controlled by giving the drug with food or sweetened fluids. With rare exceptions mepacrine may be taken over long periods without ill effect. Rarely, dermatitis occurs. This may take the form of atypical lichen planus, eczematoid or exfoliative lesions. There may be leukoplakia or pigmentation of the mucous membrane of the mouth. Mepacrine should not be administered in conjunction with pamaquine or primaquine because of the danger of acute hemolytic crises.

The drug is active against the erythrocytic forms of the plasmodia. Although a single course of therapy commonly will terminate infections by *P. falciparum,* it is not so effective as the 4-aminoquinolines. It does not affect the relapse rate of *vivax* or *malariae* malaria. When taken as a suppressive, it will prevent *falciparum* malaria. It is an

Table 38–4. CHEMOTHERAPY OF MALARIA

Treatment Schedules

The doses suggested in this summary are for adults of approximately 70 kg (154 lb) body weight. In general they should be adjusted according to the usual rules for weight and age. The doses recommended for prophylaxis and suppression in children are reduced according to weight.

Treatment of the Uncomplicated Attack in Nonimmune Subjects

1. *Amodiaquine dihydrochloride* or *chloroquine phosphate* or *sulfate:* 600 mg of base; 300 mg 6 hours later; 300 mg daily for the next 2 days.

OR

2. *Amodiaquine dihydrochloride:* 600 mg of base first day; 400 mg daily for next 2 days.

OR

3. *Quinine sulfate:* 650 mg of the salt (10 grains) 3 times daily for 7, 10, or 14 days.

Emergency Treatment

4. *Chloroquine dihydrochloride:* 200 mg base intramuscularly repeated in 6 hours if necessary. Transfer to oral therapy as soon as possible. Do not use for *P. falciparum* infections originating from areas where 4-aminoquinoline resistance is present.

OR

5. *Quinine dihydrochloride:* 650 mg salt in normal saline, glucose saline, or plasma injected *very slowly,* repeated in 6 hours if necessary; not more than 3 injections in 24 hours. Or the drug may be administered by intravenous drip at the rate of 2 gm (30 grains) in 24 hours. Transfer to oral therapy as soon as possible. (See text.)

Treatment of Drug-Resistant P. Falciparum

6. Quinine as No. 3 above, if strains do not originate from Southeast Asia.

7. If strains are from Southeast Asia:

Quinine 650 mg 3 times daily for 10 to 14 days

PLUS

Pyrimethamine 25 mg twice daily for 3 days.

To reduce the rate of relapses, the following may be added:

Sulfadiazine 500 mg 4 times daily for 5 days.

OR

Dapsone 25 mg daily for 28 days, beginning on treatment day 7 or 11.

In the rare event that quinine resistance is suspected, regimens combining a sulfonamide and an antifol, such as pyrimethamine or trimethoprim, are often effective against the clinical attacks (one example follows). Relapses may occur.

8. 50 mg pyrimethamine as single or divided dose

PLUS EITHER

1.0 gm sulfadoxine, single dose.

OR

1.0 gm sulfadimethoxine, single dose.

Treatment of Clinical Attack in Semi-Immune Subjects

9. *Chloroquine diphosphate or sulfate:* 600 mg of base, single dose.

OR

10. *Amodiaquine dihydrochloride:* 600 mg of base, single dose.

OR

11. *Quinine sulfate:* 1.0 to 1.5 gm salt (15 to 23 grains) daily for 2 to 5 days.

Radical Cure of Vivax, Ovale and Malariae Infections

12. *Primaquine diphosphate:* 15 mg of base daily, in single or divided doses, for 14 days; reinforced by standard treatment with a schizontocidal drug if given during an acute attack.

Prophylaxis and Suppression

13. *Chloroquine diphosphate or sulfate*:* 300 mg of base plus 30 to 45 mg primaquine once weekly.

OR

14. *Amodiaquine dihydrochloride*:* 300 mg of base plus 30 to 45 mg primaquine once weekly; for partially immunes, 400 to 600 mg every 2 weeks.

OR

15. *Pyrimethamine:* 50 mg and primaquine 40 mg weekly.

OR

16. *Proguanil:* 100 to 200 mg daily.

*Begin taking drugs 1 week before entering and 4 to 8, preferably 8, weeks after leaving malarious area. These regimens may not be completely effective against some strains of *P. falciparum,* especially if resistance is present. Despite prophylaxis, infections of clinical attacks of *P. vivax* and *P. malariae,* and even the rare *P. ovale,* may occur several months or years after leaving the malarious area.

efficient suppressive agent when taken in dosage of 0.1 gm daily. Clinical attacks begin to appear about 2 weeks after discontinuing the medication.

Mepacrine is not used widely.

TREATMENT OF CLINICAL MALARIA. Most simple acute cases respond rapidly to the standard regimens of 1.5 gm of amodiaquine or chloroquine base or 1.4 gm amodiaquine base. *Falciparum* malaria in the nonimmune individual is a highly dangerous infection that requires immediate and effective therapy. The grave complications presented by the pernicious forms of the disease may develop with great rapidity and commonly are accompanied by high mortality rates. Acute *falciparum* malaria and the paroxysms of *vivax* malaria frequently are accompanied by profuse nausea and vomiting. Particularly in the former, it may be necessary to initiate treatment by parenteral therapy. This, however, should be superseded as early as is practicable by oral medication. The drug regimens are shown in Table 38–4. New drugs and combinations are being tested. One of the most effective both curatively and prophylactically is the 4-quinolinemethanol compound WR 142,490 (proposed generic name, mefloquine).

In patients with *falciparum* malaria who have not responded to the chloroquine or amodiaquine treatment, or who have a parasite relapse after a previous response to these drugs, or who are gravely ill with infections which could be resistant to these drugs, the drugs of choice are quinine, 650 mg 3 times daily for 10 to 14 days accompanied by pyrimethamine, 25 mg twice daily for 3 days.

When the patient is unable to retain quinine because of vomiting, or when coma, presumed due to *falciparum* malaria, is present, the drug may be given intravenously. This treatment carries a serious hazard and should be resorted to only when the patient's condition clearly warrants the risk and no other form of treatment is possible. Quinine is administered intravenously as the dihydrochloride, 600 mg in 200 to 600 ml of normal saline, by *very slow* intravenous drip over a period of at least 30 minutes with constant monitoring of the blood pressure and of the pulse to detect hypotension or arrhythmia. The same intravenous dose may be repeated at intervals of 6 to 8 hours if the patient's condition requires. Oral therapy, by stomach tube if necessary, should be utilized as soon as possible.

TREATMENT OF COMPLICATIONS OF MALARIA. Most of the complications are due to high levels of *P. falciparum* parasitemia. The complications must be treated promptly and concurrently with the administration of antimalarial drugs. Dexamethasone, 4 to 6 mg every 4 to 6 hours, has proved useful in the treatment of cerebral and pulmonary symptoms and in blackwater fever. Convulsions should be controlled by a suitable anticonvulsant drug. When the erythrocyte count has fallen to 2 million or fewer cells, transfusion of blood is indicated. Prednisolone phosphate will help control hemolysis. Hemolysis due to primaquine in persons with glucose-6-phosphate dehydrogenase deficiency is self-limited. Shock requires fluid replacement. Corticosteroids may be helpful. In renal failure, careful fluid management is necessary, drug dosage is reduced and either peritoneal or hemodialysis may be required. Hyperpyrexia is reduced by evaporation of water from the body surface, such as by covering with a wet sheet and fanning vigorously. Acute dehydration, dysentery and diarrhea require fluid replacement.

Prevention of Relapses of Vivax Malaria. Relapses of *vivax* malaria may be prevented in the great majority of cases by the standard course of treatment of the acute attack using chloroquine or amodiaquine and concurrent administration of primaquine diphosphate 26.5 mg (15 mg base) daily for 14 consecutive days. An alternate regimen is 600 mg of chloroquine base and 45 mg primaquine base weekly for 8 weeks. Patients receiving this treatment should be under observation for evidence of hemolytic anemia, an indication for discontinuing medication. Particular caution is required in the case of Negro patients (Table 38–4).

SUPPRESSIVE TREATMENT. Although prevention of infection is not possible, clinical attacks of *vivax* and *malariae* malaria can be held in abeyance for prolonged periods by the administration of various antimalarial drugs. However, following cessation of medication, clinical attacks due to infection by *P. vivax* and *P. malariae* may begin to occur after 10 or more days. In the case of infections of *P. falciparum,* suppressive regimens with certain of the available drugs will eradicate the infection without the development of clinical malaria. The routines for suppressive treatment are shown in Table 38–4. If pyrimethamine is used for suppression or prophylaxis, it should be used only in combination with other drugs. The British and Australians continue to use proguanil, 100 to 200 mg daily, as prophylaxis.

To be effective, suppressive treatment must be taken regularly. A breakthrough of clinical activity will occur when drug administration is irregular or insufficient. It may occur likewise in the presence of excessive fatigue, acute infections, trauma and hemorrhage or exposure to high altitudes, since these conditions tend to activate latent malaria. Resistance may appear when pyrimethamine and proguanil are used.

Drug Resistance. Resistance to proguanil and pyrimethamine has occurred widely. Strains of *P. falciparum* resistant to the 4-aminoquinoline drugs, chloroquine and amodiaquine, occur in Colombia, Brazil, Venezuela, Guyana, Surinam and Panama in the Western Hemisphere, and in Assam, Burma, Malaysia, Cambodia, Laos, Thailand, Vietnam, Sabah, Sarawak, Kalimantan and Philippine Islands in the Eastern Hemisphere.[7] Some of these strains also are resistant to the other synthetic schizontocidal drugs, making it necessary to resort to quinine to control and cure the infections. The manifestations of resistance vary according to the strain, ranging from no apparent response to the drug to a temporary response. Failure to reduce drastically the parasitemia at 48 hours after the initiation of treatment or to eliminate fevers 72 hours thereafter probably signifies resistance and indicates the necessity for use of another drug, preferably quinine.

Induced Malaria in Man. For many years, malaria was induced in man for the therapy of neurosyphilis. Many thousands of patients benefited from this treatment. By the study of these controlled infections, much knowledge has been gained in all phases of the biology of malaria, and the development of new drugs has been aided greatly. All four species of the human malarias are transmitted successfully both by infected blood and by sporozoites from the mosquitoes, although a large proportion of the Negro race shows partial or full immunity to *P. vivax. Plasmodium knowlesi,* a monkey malaria, also has been used for malaria therapy of neurosyphilis.

Malaria of Nonhuman Primates. Species of *Plasmodium* found in nonhuman primates include: in the prosimians (lemurs), *P. girardi* and *P. lemuris;* in the monkeys, *P. brasilianum, P. coatneyi, P. cynomolgi. P. fieldi, P. fragile, P. simiovale, P. gonderi, P. inui, P. knowlesi* and *P. simium;* in the apes, *P. eylesi, P. hylobati, P. pitheci, P. reichenowi, P. jefferyi, P. silvaticum, P. rodhani. P. schwetzi* and *P. youngi.* Some subspecies of the above have been proposed.[8]

Some of the simian malarias have been induced experimentally in humans by infected blood (*P. knowlesi, P. inui, P. cynomolgi* and *P. schwetzi*). In general, the infections tend to be much milder and shorter than those caused by the usual malaria parasites of man. Because of these characteristics, *P. knowlesi* was used for many years for the treatment of neurosyphilis. Recent work demonstrating that several of the simian malarias (*P. cynomolgi, P. brasilianum, P. eylesi, P. knowlesi, P. schwetzi*) can be experimentally transmitted to man by the bites of infected mosquitoes suggests the possibility of zoonoses. At present, there is no evidence that such transmissions actually occur in nature to any significant degree, although a recent natural infection in man of *P. knowlesi* and of *P. simium* confirms the zoonotic potential of simian malarias.

Human malaria will grow in splenectomized apes. Recently it was shown that *P. vivax, P. falciparum* and *P. malariae* of human origin will grow well in certain of the small monkeys of the Western Hemisphere. The *Aotus* monkey is the most receptive host, but after adaptation to this host, *P. vivax* will grow in some other species. These models are useful for the study of the biology of malaria and especially for drug development.

Blackwater Fever

Blackwater fever (hemoglobinuric fever) is one of the most dangerous complications of malaria. It is characterized by prostrating chills, profuse vomiting, early jaundice, the passage of dark red to black urine, and a rapidly developing anemia. It is essentially an acute intravascular hemolysis with hemoglobinemia, hemoglobinuria and renal insufficiency.

Etiology and Epidemiology. Blackwater fever ordinarily occurs only in individuals who live or have lived in malarious regions. It was once common in highly malarious areas, but is now greatly reduced and at a low level. Plasmodia may be found in the peripheral blood, and the history generally reveals a succession of malarial attacks. *Plasmodium falciparum* usually is the species involved.

The pathogenesis of the hemolysis in blackwater fever is obscure. Drugs, especially quinine, have been suggested as important factors, as have immune reactions and sensitization to the malaria parasite.

Pathology. Sudden destruction of red blood cells occurs and large amounts of hemoglobin are released. The mechanism for the disposal of blood pigment is overloaded. Hemoglobin, methemalbumin and hemobilirubin accumulate in the plasma. When the renal threshold is reached, hemoglobinuria appears and methemoglobin and bile pigments are present in the urine. Renal anoxia and ischemia are probably of great importance in reducing glomerular filtration and tubular reabsorption. Dehydration increases the hazard of renal failure.

The pathologic changes in the viscera are predominantly those of chronic malaria. In addition, the liver may show either cloudy swelling or necrosis of parenchymal cells, particularly in the regions of the central veins. It is yellowish brown due to hemosiderin.

The kidneys are large and black. Renal tubules are blocked with debris and hemoglobin casts. Cloudy swelling and degeneration of the tubular epithelium and hemoglobin casts, indicative of hemoglobinuric nephrosis, may be present. Glomerular alteration, consisting principally of generalized ischemia, enlargement and increased cellularity of the glomeruli, and hyperchromatism and swelling of the endothelium have been reported in patients with clinical evidence of azotemia. Granular eosinophilic

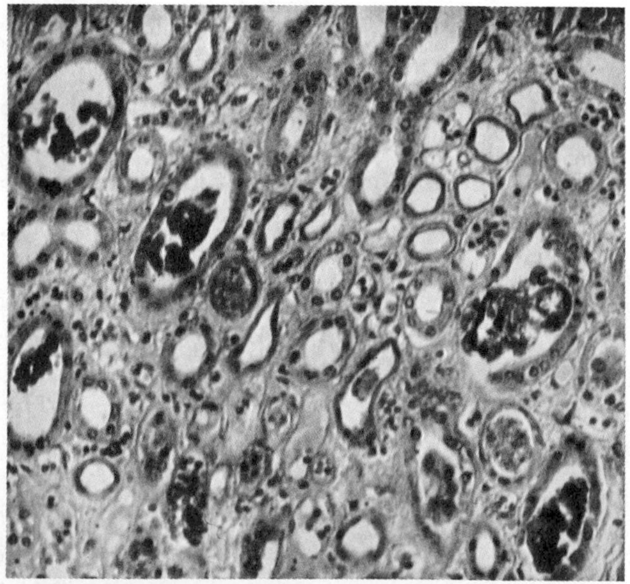

Figure 38–23. Kidney in blackwater fever, showing hemoglobin casts in distal convoluted tubules and degeneration and regeneration of tubular epithelium.

material may be observed within the collecting tubules (Fig. 38–23). Coarse pigmented casts frequently are present in the distal convoluted tubules.

Symptomatology. Blackwater fever presents three cardinal symptoms—hemoglobinuria, fever and jaundice. The onset is usually sudden, with very severe chill, marked prostration, pain over the region of the kidneys and a rapid rise of temperature to 40 or 40.6° C (104 or 105° F). The fever may be continuous or remittent, and rather profuse sweating is apt to accompany drops of temperature. Severe nausea and vomiting accompanied by epigastric distress usually appear early and may be continuous and serious. Jaundice appears within a few hours after the onset and may become intense if the hemolysis is extensive or long continued. Not infrequently the onset of symptoms is accompanied by the desire to void, and the urine specimen presents the color characteristic of the disease. The pulse is usually rapid, feeble and of low tension. Pallor proportionate to the degree of anemia rapidly becomes apparent. The red blood count may fall by as much as 2 million within a period of 24 hours.

The clinical course may terminate after one such abbreviated episode, there may be recurring hemolytic crises, or the process may be continuous, extending over several days in the course of which the fever, hemolysis and hemoglobinuria continue.

Prognosis. The general mortality rate is 25 to 50 per cent. In approximately half the fatal cases death results from renal failure. Marked and persistent vomiting and hiccough are unfavorable signs, as are a rising curve of the blood urea and a falling urinary output. One attack of blackwater fever seems to predispose to subsequent attacks.

Diagnosis. The occurrence of hemoglobinuria, fever and jaundice in an individual known to have had malaria is strong presumptive evidence of blackwater fever. Other causes of hemoglobinuria, however, must be considered.

Parasites are found in only 50 to 70 per cent of cases. When present they may be difficult to find after the first 24 hours.

In addition to the characteristic color of the urine, microscopic examination reveals the presence of much amorphous sediment, occasional red blood cells and casts of various types. Albumin is present in considerable amounts.

Treatment. The principles governing the treatment are essentially those for acute hemolytic transfusion reactions: Mannitol and hydration to institute and maintain diuresis, alkalinization to minimize the formation of hemoglobin casts in the kidney, and the use of peritoneal or hemodialysis if renal failure occurs. An intravenous infusion should be administered and 20 gm of mannitol (110 ml of a 20 per cent solution) given over 5 to 10 minutes after the patient has been sufficiently hydrated. If urine flow in the next 2 hours is under 60 ml per hour, fluids should be restricted and the patient treated as for acute renal failure. If urine flow exceeds 60 ml per hour, then hydration should be continued and 100 ml of 20 per cent mannitol administered often enough to maintain a urine flow of 100 ml or more per hour. The patient must be carefully monitored during prolonged mannitol therapy for sodium loss and possible resultant hyponatremia. Packed red blood cells should be given, if necessary, to combat severe anemia. Corticosteroids are recommended as in other lytic anemias.

Antimalarial Therapy. When malaria parasites are present in the peripheral blood, immediate intensive treatment with a rapidly acting plasmodicidal drug is essential. The drugs of choice are chloroquine and amodiaquine, in the absence of resistance. Otherwise a combination of pyrimethamine and one of the sulfonamides may be tried. Mepacrine and the 8-aminoquinolines are contraindicated. Opinion is divided on the use of quinine and it is not indicated if there is a history of repeated attacks treated with quinine. In the presence of disturbed renal function and fluid and electrolyte imbalance, the administration of quinine entails a serious hazard and requires alert and constant supervision of the patient.

Prophylaxis. In the prevention of blackwater fever, malaria prophylaxis and adequate treatment of clinical malaria, especially when due to *P. falciparum,* are essential. Recognition of the so-called *preblackwater state* is important. This is characterized by toxemia, slight jaundice, enlargement and tenderness of the liver and abnormally dark-colored urine. In the presence of this condition, hospitalization and careful antimalarial therapy are essential. The prevention and control of malaria form the basis of prophylaxis.

REFERENCES

1. Young, M. D., Eyles, D. E., Burgess, R. W., and Jeffery, G. M. 1955. Experimental testing of the immunity of Negroes to *Plasmodium vivax.* J. Parasitol. *41*:315–318.
2. Clyde, D. F., Most, H., McCarthy, V. C., and Vanderberg, J. P. 1973. Immunization of man against sporozoite-induced malaria. Am. J. Med. Sci. *266*:169–177.
3. Anonymous. 1968. Immunology of malaria. W.H.O. Tech. Rep. Ser. No. 396, Geneva. 50 pp.
4. Schnitzer, B., Sodeman, T. M., Mead, M. L., and Contacos, P. G. 1973. An ultrastructural study of the red pulp of the spleen in malaria. Blood *41*:207–218.
5. Kagan, I. G. 1972. Evaluation of the indirect hemagglutination test as an epidemiologic technique for malaria. Am. J. Trop. Med. Hyg. *21*:683–689.
6. Collins, W. E., and Skinner, J. C. 1972. The indirect fluorescent antibody test for malaria. Am. J. Trop. Med. Hyg. *21*:690–695.
7. Anonymous. 1973. Chemotherapy of malaria and resistance to antimalarials. W.H.O. Tech. Rep. Ser. No. 529, Geneva. 121 pp.
8. Coatney, G. R., Collins, W. E., Warren, M., and Contacos, P. G. 1971. The Primate Malarias. U.S. Government Printing Office, Washington, D.C. 366 pp. 54 plates.

CHAPTER 39
Toxoplasmosis

HERBERT E. KAUFMAN
ROBERT ABEL, JR.
JOSEPH H. MILLER

Synonyms. None.

Definition. Toxoplasmosis is a protean disease of man and animals produced by the organism *Toxoplasma gondii.* It varies in severity from a clinically inapparent infection to a severe systemic disease that may terminate in encephalitis and death.

Distribution. Infection of man and animals occurs worldwide.

Etiology. *Toxoplasma gondii* (Nicolle and Manceaux, 1908) is an obligate intracellular parasite with coccidian affinities. Felines have been observed as definitive hosts. Both the classic enteric sexual cycle with oocysts shed in the feces and the extraintestinal asexual forms are seen in these hosts. Animals, including man, as intermediate hosts, harbor only the extraintestinal asexual forms: tachyzoites (proliferative forms) and bradyzoites (encysted forms).[1]

The tachyzoites, rapidly multiplying forms of the acute systemic infection in man, are crescentic in shape, 2 to 4 μm in width and 6 to 7 μm in length (Fig. 39–1). They develop intracellularly in many cell types and multiply by endodyogeny, the formation of two daughter cells within the pellicle of the parent. The host cell degenerates when

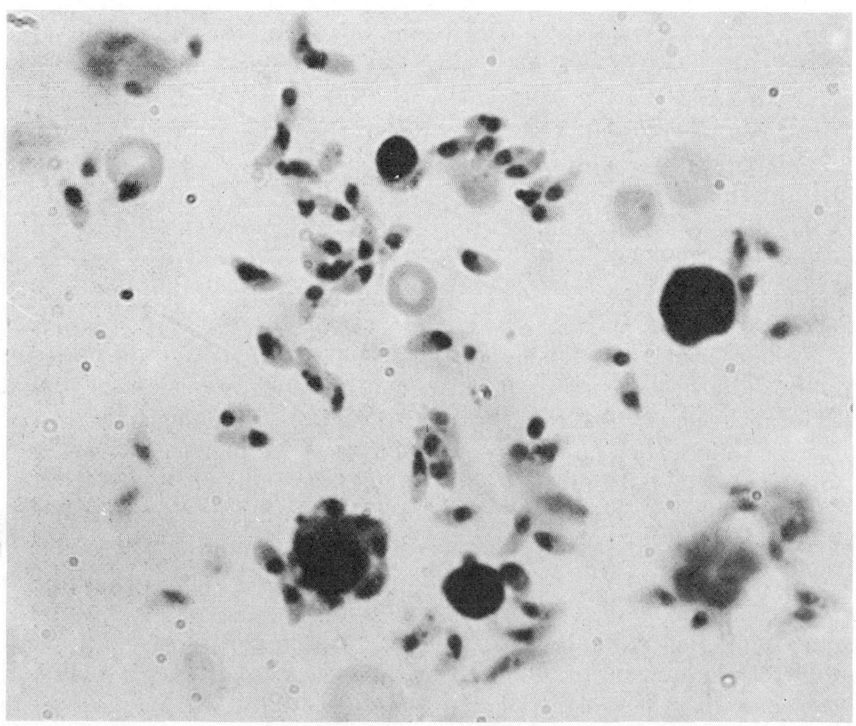

Figure 39–1. Mouse peritoneal fluid demonstrating tachyzoites freed from cells (1000 ×). (Courtesy of the Louisiana State University School of Medicine, New Orleans; photomicrography by Dr. Mark R. Feldman.)

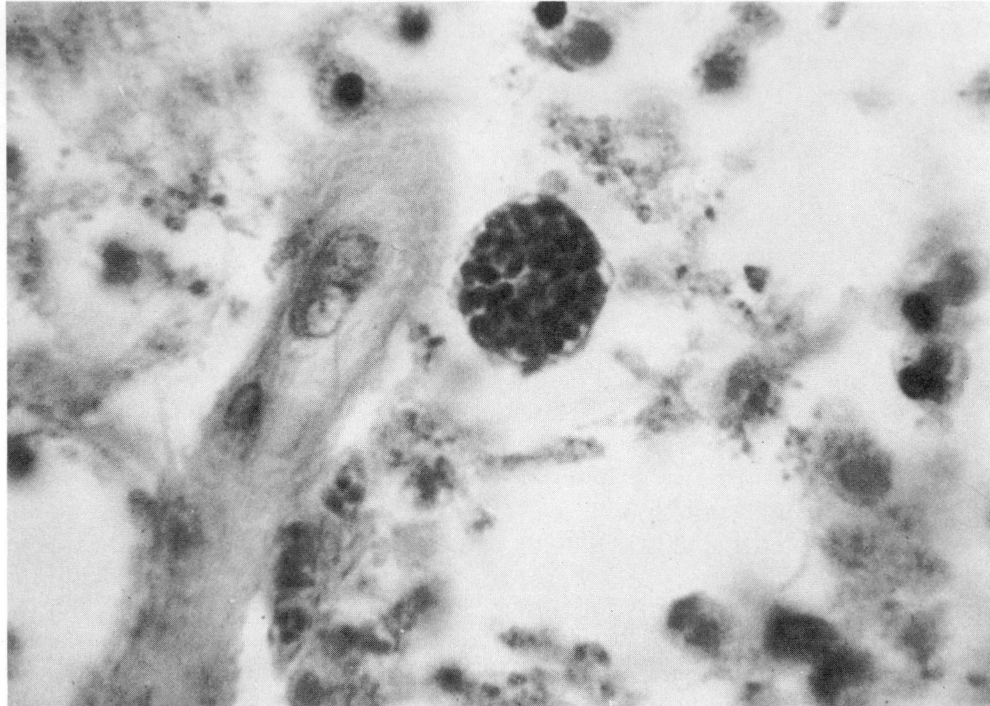

Figure 39-2. Cyst of *Toxoplasma gondii* containing bradyzoites in brain. (Courtesy of Dr. Paul A. McGarry, Louisiana State University School of Medicine, New Orleans.)

from 8 to 16 organisms accumulate and new cells are infected. By the Giemsa method, the cytoplasm stains blue and the nucleus, located near the round end of the parasite, stains red to purple. In chronic infections, 200 to 1000 μm cysts containing numerous bradyzoites, the slowly multiplying resting stages, are characteristic mainly in brain, heart and skeletal muscle (Figs. 39-2, 39-3). When cysts are seen in tissue sections, the organisms may appear similar to leishmanial bodies except for the absence of a rodlike kinetoplast. The tachyzoites in section, however, resemble cellular debris and may be difficult or impossible to recognize in conventional histologic sections, even in tissues that are heavily infected. Cysts may persist for the life of the host, and the release of bradyzoites from cysts by natural causes or traumatic injury maintains immunity. A localized or general relapse may occur when immunity is lowered by natural or artificial conditions. Serologically and immunologically, *T. gondii*, recovered in nature from a variety of hosts, appears to belong to a single species. Strains, however, vary in virulence.

The infection in man may be obtained by ingestion of oocysts containing sporozoites from cat feces, or of cysts containing bradyzoites in inadequately cooked or raw meat.[2] Organisms enter intestinal cells, multiply rapidly, and are disseminated by the lymphatics to lymph nodes and the blood stream. The liver and lungs seem to be the primary sites of multiplication, although many tissues are sites for subsequent multiplication (tachyzoites) or encystment (bradyzoites). A parasitemia occurs during the acute stage that may persist for 2 weeks or longer. Parasites may occasionally persist for weeks or months in the blood stream in macrophages, presumably protected from antibody.[3]

Antibodies begin to appear during the first 4 weeks of infection, during which time there is a diminution and gradual, though variable, cessation of the parasitemia. With this decrease in parasitemia, cysts containing bradyzoites form in most tissues (Figs. 39–2, 39–3). In addition to the cysts, tachyzoites may persist in the brain and eye, in spite of the presence of systemic antibodies. This is probably due to the failure of sufficient levels of antibody to penetrate the blood-brain or blood-ocular barrier.

Epidemiology. Cats become infected by eating mice, rats, birds, or meat containing *T. gondii* cysts. The sexual portion of the life cycle takes place in the intestinal cells of the cat. Immature oocysts are shed in the feces 3 to 5 days after the ingestion of cysts. Oocysts are infective 1 to 5 or more days later after sporulation takes place and are viable for long periods if not subjected to dry or cold climatic conditions. If ingested, oocysts may also infect cats, but shedding of oocysts from this type of infection takes 20 to 34 days. During primary infection, oocysts are shed in 1 to 2 weeks (Fig. 39–4).

Man probably becomes infected primarily by ingestion of poorly cooked or raw meat containing toxoplasma cysts, although accidental ingestion of oocysts from cat feces may play a role. Oocysts seem to be the key to the epidemiology, since they can be dispersed widely in cat feces and produce infections in all animals and birds that have been tested to date.[1] In man, in the United States, approximately 50 per cent in the age group over 20 have antibodies to this organism, with variation from area to area and with age.

Toxoplasmosis may also be acquired congenitally by transplacental transmission after acute maternal infection that is usually asymptomatic or unrecognized (Fig. 39–4). Of 2768 seronegative obstetric patients, six became dye-test positive and two transmitted toxoplasmosis to their infants, supporting the view that the mother must contract the infection during pregnancy in order to transmit the disease to the immunodeficient fetus.[4, 5] There is an association between toxoplasma antibodies and sporadic abortion, but no causal relationship has yet been defined.[6] The evidence of previous infection in man is so common and congenital infection so rare that the presence of stigmata of previous infection, such as retinochoroiditis, in a pregnant woman cannot be considered a cause for alarm. A mother of one infected child can be reassured that her chances of having another infected offspring are extremely remote, and fetal infection from a mother with eye disease does not occur.[4]

Pathology. Congenital toxoplasmosis in its complete form presents a characteristic syndrome of hydrocephalus, sometimes microcephaly with cerebral calcification, hepatosplenomegaly with jaundice, and bilateral

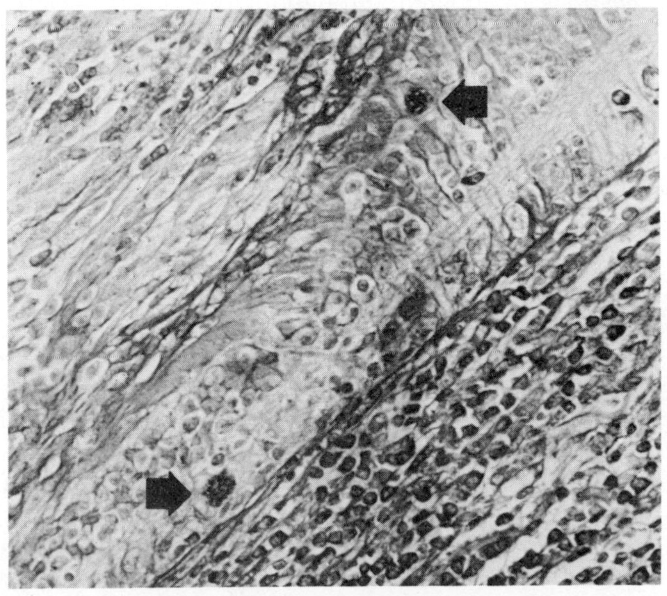

Figure 39–3. Toxoplasma cysts in guinea pig retina. (Courtesy of the University of Florida College of Medicine, Gainesville.)

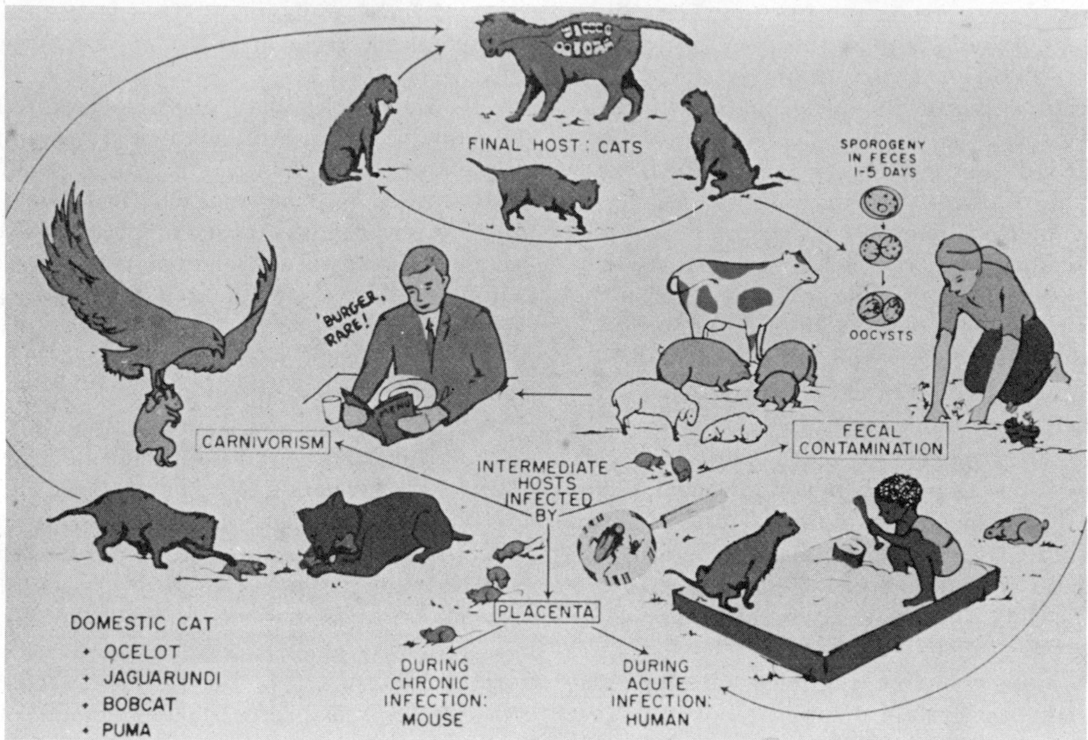

Figure 39–4. Postulated life cycle and transmission of *Toxoplasma.* Cats and certain other felines are shown as final hosts, and other animals and humans as intermediate hosts. Flies and cockroaches can serve as transport hosts. At right, infection with oocysts is shown. At left, transmission by carnivorism is indicated. Below, the transplacental route of transmission is indicated. (Modified slightly from Frenkel, J. K. 1971. Toxoplasmosis. *In* Marcial-Rojas, R. A. (ed.): Pathology of Protozoal and Helminthic Diseases. Williams & Wilkins, Baltimore, p. 260.)

retinochoroiditis. The organism multiplies rapidly in every cell of the body. Roentgenograms of the skull often indicate thin calcifications distributed throughout the cerebral cortex as a result of a multifocal encephalitis which leaves necrotic tissue that later calcifies. The hydrocephalus results from an abnormal proliferation of tissue in the area of the aqueduct of Sylvius, resulting in a stenosis and obstruction. It has been suggested that this tissue, which contains few if any organisms, is a hypersensitivity response on the part of the fetus; but little is known of the pathogenesis. Retinochoroiditis, as seen in children or adults, begins typically as a retinitis, with destruction of the retina and then of the choroid with accumulation of inflammatory debris in the vitreous of the eye. In the inactive stage, a white depressed scar surrounded by pigment is seen (Fig. 39–5).

Retinochoroiditis primarily occurs as a result of the rupture of a cyst with cell death due to invasion and multiplication of tachyzoites in ocular tissue. On the other hand, a severe hypersensitivity response of the host to liberated organisms may also cause eye disease. Although the tachyzoites are exceedingly difficult to see in regular histologic sections, they are easily demonstrated in body fluids or impression smears of lesions. If a histologic diagnosis is sought, a search for cysts under low power magnification is more frequently rewarding, especially in tissues in which the periodic acid–Schiff (PAS) stain can be used, since it reacts with the glycogen content of organisms. Cyst walls are argyrophilic.

Clinical Characteristics. Toxoplasmosis appears in congenital and acquired forms, although the distinction between the two may sometimes be difficult. Congenital toxoplasmosis is readily recognized in its complete form, which usually results in a fatal termination. The finding of hydrocephalus, sometimes microcephaly, encephalitis, sometimes with diffuse cerebral calcifications and psychomotor disturbance, bilateral retinochoroiditis, hepatosplenomegaly and jaundice in a newborn makes the diagnosis most probable. It has become apparent that mild forms of the disease are common in which retinochoroiditis may be the only manifestation. The disease may be inactive at birth and recrudesce later in life. In such children, an esotropia or strabismus is the most frequent finding, since toxoplasmosis typically destroys the macula of the eye. A white reflex, microphthalmia, cataracts, or colobomas may be present.

In adults, the infection is most commonly subclinical although a high proportion of the world's population is infected. When systemic clinical manifestations occur in acquired toxoplasmosis, the most common are (1) retinochoroiditis, or (2) lymphadenopathy, often with fever, and sometimes a maculopapular rash that spares the palms of the hands and the soles of the feet, and hepatosplenomegaly. Since any tissue of the body may be involved, other clinical manifestations of systemic toxoplasmosis are seen. These include a pneumonitis suggestive of primary atypical pneumonia, myocarditis that may result in heart failure without other obvious signs of systemic disease, and encephalitis.

Ocular complications may occur in adult cases and primarily when the central nervous system is affected. The evidence seems to indicate that cases of focal chorioretinitis with positive serologic reactions indicate congenital infection unless there is a recent history of signs and symptoms of toxoplasmosis.[4]

Aside from retinochoroiditis, the most common adult disease is a mononucleosis-like syndrome. There may be prolonged low-grade fever, a feeling of malaise, and enlargement of multiple lymph nodes with reticulum cell hyperplasia which is destructive and diagnostic.

Toxoplasmosis may also recrudesce in a patient with chronic infection whose immunocompetence has been naturally altered by a disease such as leukemia or a lymphoma, or

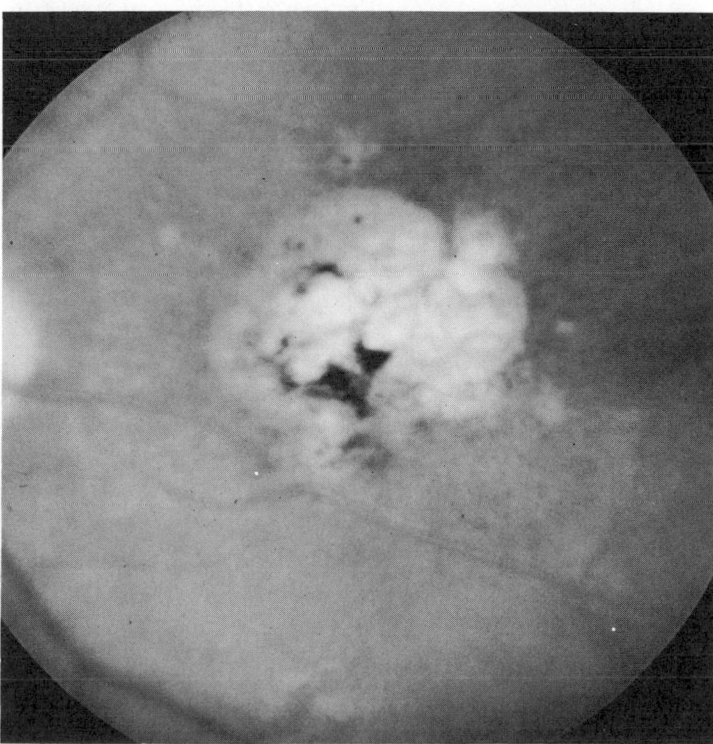

Figure 39–5. Chorioretinal lesion in a suspected case of ocular toxoplasmosis. (Courtesy of the University of Florida College of Medicine, Gainesville.)

artificially by immunosuppressive therapy. In addition, primary toxoplasmosis may occur in both types of patients. Either situation may prove fatal and physicians caring for the chronically ill should be aware of this disease possibility.[1, 7]

Diagnosis. The diagnosis of toxoplasmosis is difficult. Histologic preparations from biopsy specimens that demonstrate cysts do not establish a causal relationship for clinical illness, since they can be found in both acute and chronic infections. Isolation of the organism by passage in mice of tissue from suspect cases is not often successful. The strains that infect humans usually do not kill mice; therefore, they must be tested serologically, sacrificed, and their tissues examined for organisms.

In congenital toxoplasmosis, however, the finding of tachyzoite forms in impression smears of brain lesions at necropsy with the presence of the clinical syndrome establishes the diagnosis.

Since direct demonstration of the organism and the establishment of a causal relationship is difficult, serologic procedures are used to diagnose toxoplasmosis.[8] There are four tests currently in use: the Sabin-Feldman dye test, complement-fixation (CF), indirect fluorescent antibody (IFA), and indirect hemagglutination (IHA). The IFA test is the most widely used serologic procedure for diagnosis. It is as sensitive as the Sabin-Feldman dye test, does not use live organisms, and is therefore safer. It is also more economical and easier to perform. The IHA test is now used almost entirely for adult screening. The IFA and IHA antibodies rise from 10 days to 3 to 4 weeks after infection and are elevated 20 to 30 years, which is identical with the dye test. The CF antibodies rise in about 2 weeks and disappear in a few years. In the interpretation of these tests, low positive titers (1:64 for IFA, IHA and dye test; 1:4 for CF) usually signify previous exposure with immunity. Significant antibody titer (1:256 for IFA, IHA and dye test; 1:8 for CF) usually indicates recent infection, especially with increased titers in repeat specimens. High titers (1:4096 for IFA, IHA and dye test; 1:32 for CF) strongly suggest acute infection.

In congenital toxoplasmosis, an increase of fetal antibody titer to a level higher than the maternal titer indicates congenital toxoplasmosis, but a titer equal to the maternal level in a child less than 6 months of age may be due to passive transfer of maternal antibody. However, more specific of acute disease is the finding of IgM antibody in the fetus, since maternal IgM does not cross the placenta.

Serologic tests for toxoplasmosis, including tests for IgM, are available at the Center for Disease Control, Atlanta, Georgia, and in many state laboratories. A number of commercial kits for IFA testing are available.

Treatment. The present treatment of choice for toxoplasmosis consists of the synergistic combination of sulfadiazine in full therapeutic dosage and pyrimethamine (Daraprim). Pyrimethamine is generally given in a dose of 100 mg initially and 25 mg each day thereafter; in the case of ocular infection, it is continued for about 5 weeks.[9] Since this drug is a folic acid antagonist, a reversible bone marrow suppression may occur.[10] Folinic acid (Leucovorin) does not reduce the efficacy of pyrimethamine, but does reduce the incidence of bone marrow depression and may be given orally 3 times weekly while patients receive the drug. Its use, however, does not obviate the necessity for periodic hematologic study. In the treatment of ocular disease, in which even modest amounts of inflammation can produce sufficient damage to destroy vision, the use of anti-inflammatory corticosteroid therapy may be combined with the pyrimethamine. Treatment with pyrimethamine is to be avoided in females during the first trimester of pregnancy.

Daraprim is effective in killing the tachyzoite forms of the organism but is of limited value against the slowly multiplying encysted bradyzoites. Its effect on chronic or relapsing ocular disease requires further study. Spiramycin (Rovamycin), at this time not available in the United States, is used widely in Europe because of its toxostatic effect. Clindamycin also has toxoplasmacidal properties in rodents and is under investigation in man.

Prophylaxis. Congenital toxoplasmosis of newborns is the primary medical threat of this infection. Therefore, based on the present knowledge of the epidemiology, certain recommendations concerning pregnant women are in order.[8] Pregnant women should not eat raw or poorly cooked meat, since it is well established that *T. gondii* is transmitted in this manner. The role of the cat in the natural transmission of the disease is established, but its role in human transmission, though highly suspect, has not been conclusively elaborated. However, certain precautions are indicated. Cat litter boxes should be emptied daily by other than a pregnant woman to dispose of possible oocysts before they become infective. House cats should be kept indoors and should not be fed raw meat, and outdoor cats or strays should not be allowed into the immediate environment of pregnant women. Present facilities do not permit examination of the large number of follow-up serologic specimens necessary to detect acute infections during all pregnancies. These studies should be employed primarily when, in the opinion of the physician, the patient is thought to be at increased risk and when results of these tests might change the course of clinical management.

REFERENCES

1. Frenkel, J. K. 1973. Toxoplasmosis: parasite life cycle, pathology and immunology of toxoplasmosis. *In* Hammond, D. M., and Long, P. (eds.): The Coccidia: *Eimeria, Toxoplasma, Isospora,* and related genera. University Park Press, Baltimore. pp. 343–410.
2. Frenkel, J. K., and Dubey, J. P. 1972. Toxoplasmosis and its prevention in cats and man. J. Infect. Dis. *126*:664–673.
3. Remington, J. S., Jacobs, L., and Kaufman, H. E. 1960. Toxoplasmosis in the adult. N. Engl. J. Med. *262*:180–186; 237–241.
4. Perkins, E. S. 1973. Ocular toxoplasmosis. Br. J. Ophthalmol. *57*:1–17.
5. Kimball, A. C., Kean, B. H., and Fuchs, F. 1971. Congenital toxoplasmosis: a prospective study of 4,048 obstetric patients. Am. J. Obstet. Gynecol. *111*:211–218.
6. Kimball, A. C., Kean, B. H., and Fuchs, F. 1971. The role of toxoplasmosis in abortion. Am. J. Obstet. Gynecol. *111*:219–226.
7. Levine, A. S., Graw, R. G., Jr., and Young, R. C. 1972. Management of infections in patients with leukemia and lymphoma: current concepts and experimental approaches. Semin. Hematol. *9*:141–179.
8. Krogstad, D. J., Juranek, D. D., and Walls, K. W. 1972. Toxoplasmosis: with comments on risk of infection from cats. Ann. Intern. Med. *77*:773–778.
9. Kaufman, H. E., and Caldwell, L. A. 1959. Pharmacological studies of pyrimethamine (Daraprim) in man. Arch. Ophthalmol. *61*:885–890.
10. Kaufman, H. E., and Geissler, P. 1960. The hematologic toxicity of Daraprim in man. Arch. Ophthalmol. *64*:140–146.

CHAPTER 40
Pneumocystis Pneumonia

JOSEPH H. MILLER

Synonyms. Interstitial plasma cell pneumonia, pulmonary pneumocystosis, parasitic pneumonia.

Definition. This is an opportunistic infection in which *Pneumocystis carinii* produces a diffuse interstitial pneumonia in infants and children with altered host resistance due to prematurity or debilitating disease. Infection also occurs in individuals with congenital or acquired immunodeficiency disease and, in increasing numbers, in patients receiving adrenocorticosteroid and immunosuppressive therapy.

Distribution. The disease was first reported in epidemic form from Europe. However, familiarization with the clinical manifestations and radiologic findings, and an awareness on the part of physicians concerned with the care of patients with chronic disease, especially those receiving immunosuppressive drugs, have resulted in case reports of a sporadic form of the disease from almost every country. It is now accepted as worldwide in distribution.

Etiology and Epidemiology. The taxonomic position of *Pneumocystis carinii* Delanoë and Delanoë, 1912 has not been determined. Most workers believe that *P. carinii* is a protozoan to be classified with *Toxoplasma*,[1] but some maintain that it is a fungus mainly on the basis of its staining reaction. The most easily recognizable stage of the organism is a cystic structure 5 to 12 μm in diameter containing eight small crescent-shaped or ovoid parasites (sporozoites) with eccentric nuclei.[2] Cysts are usually found in a honeycombed exudate in the alveolar sacs (Fig. 40–1). With Giemsa stain the cyst wall is colorless or pale blue, the cytoplasm of the individual parasites is blue, and the nucleus is stained dark purple. Thin-walled pleomorphic trophozoite forms have been described, and it has been suggested that this stage undergoes multiplication by binary fission. Electron microscopy reveals a cyst wall 0.10 μm to 0.30 μm in thickness composed of at least six layers. The sporozoites within measure 1.0 μm to 1.5 μm and their membranes are connected to the cyst wall. Each cyst appears to be surrounded by an anastomosing mass of membranes from its own wall and the membranes from the walls of adjacent cysts. This structural feature probably accounts for the cohesion of cysts and their appearance in clumps in lung imprint preparations.[3]

Although *P. carinii* is widespread in nature (mice, rats, rabbits, guinea pigs, monkeys, sheep, goats, pigs, horses and humans), there seems to be a high degree of host specificity, and transmission from animals to man seems unlikely.[3] Animals given cortisone for prolonged periods develop the disease spontaneously with a clinical and histologic picture identical with human infections. In some of the epidemics that took place among debilitated infants in foundling homes in Europe from 1940 to 1960, healthy adult nursing personnel were carriers and probably spread the infection by aerosol dispersion of respiratory tract secretions. *Pneumocystis carinii* pneumonia was prevalent in South Vietnamese orphans evacuated to the United States in 1975. There is one confirmed instance[4] and five probable cases of transplacental infection, but this seems to be a minor mode of transmission since the organism is rarely found in stillborn infants or infants in the immediate neonatal period.

The sporadic disease that occurs principally in the immunodeficient host may represent a different epidemiologic situation. With modern antibiotic therapy, congenitally immunodeficient infants and children can now live long enough to develop nonbacterial infections. On the other hand, the de-

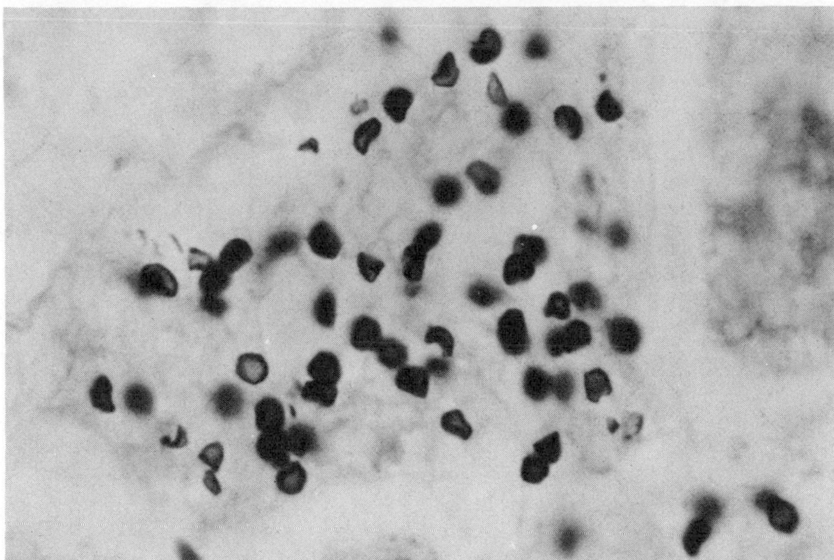

Figure 40–1. Cysts of *Pneumocystis carinii* in alveolar exudate. Note round, crescentic, and other-shaped cysts with collapsed walls; silver methenamine-fast green stain, 1000 ×. (Courtesy of the Louisiana State University School of Medicine, New Orleans; photomicrography by Dr. Mark R. Feldman.)

velopment of sophisticated immunosuppressive therapy has either enhanced the development of disease from latent infections or rendered the host more susceptible to infection from his environment.[3] The definitive method of transmission will remain unknown until the life cycle of this organism is elucidated. However, increasing evidence favors the concept of activation of latent infection as the primary mode of development of the disease in patients undergoing immunosuppressive therapy.[5]

Pathology. In the epidemic or sporadic form there is usually a diffuse panlobular involvement of the lungs; they are enlarged, usually gray, of a firm rubbery consistency, and do not collapse when the chest is opened. Cut surfaces show diffuse consolidation without suppuration and are mucinous. A focal form of the disease has been described displaying similar gross features with less extensive areas of pneumonic consolidation. However, this form may be masked by other pathogens such as cytomegalic inclusion virus and bacterial and fungal organisms. Pleural effusion is usually absent in children with immunodeficiency disease, but may be present in adults with therapeutically induced immunodeficiency. Similarly, mediastinal lymphadenitis may be encountered in the latter group at necropsy.

Histologically, the characteristic finding is the abundant honeycombed material, filling the air spaces, alveoli and respiratory bronchioles (Fig. 40–2). The material is intensely acidophilic and contains occasional desquamated epithelial cells, alveolar macrophages and, rarely, inflammatory cells. The honeycombed appearance results from the cohesion of masses of cysts. The alveolar epithelial cells are hyperplastic, and hyaline membranes may be prominent where there is a concomitant decrease in the amount of honeycombed material. The alveolar septa are broadened by epithelial hyperplasia and inflammatory cell infiltration. These are predominantly plasma cells in the epidemic form of the disease, and lymphocytes, macrophages and eosinophils in the immunodeficient patient.

Interstitial fibrosis and emphysema may be complications where the disease is of long duration.[6] Calcification of the honeycombed material and adjacent lung tissue is a rare occurrence. Cor pulmonale has been reported in some cases of prolonged diffuse pneumocystic pneumonia. Extrapulmonary sites of infection in lymph nodes, liver, spleen and

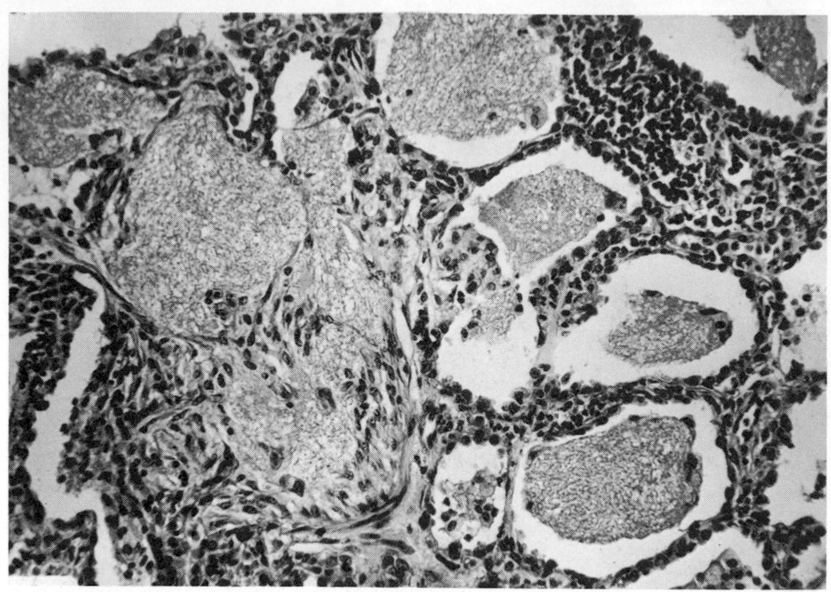

Figure 40–2. Section of lung obtained at thoracotomy showing dilatation of alveolar spaces by foamy material which on one side has been partially replaced by fibroblasts. There is a dense septal infiltrate and hyperplasia of alveolar lining cells. (Hematoxylin-eosin stain × 170.) (Courtesy of the University of Florida College of Medicine, Gainesville.)

bone marrow have been reported infrequently. Pathologic alterations in other organs are secondary to oxygen desaturation resulting from the alveolar capillary block.

Clinical Features. The clinical features of *Pneumocystis* pneumonia are not unique in that they share characteristics with interstitial pneumonias of other causes. The disease begins in an insidious manner with anorexia and weight loss, followed shortly by progressive dyspnea with bluish discoloration around the mouth and nostrils. Within 1 to 3 weeks after the onset of symptoms, respiratory involvement becomes pronounced, with marked tachypnea (90 to 130 respirations per minute), cyanosis, and spells of nonproductive cough without pleurisy or upper respiratory complaints. Despite the severity of the pulmonary involvement, percussion is negative and rales are rare or scanty and chiefly confined to the bases. Fever is prominent in adults but may be conspicuously absent in infants. The course of the disease may be a fulminating or slowly advancing pneumonia. Radiologic examination early in the course of the disease may show localization of interstitial infiltration in one lobe or one lung. Within 24 to 48 hours diffuse interstitial and alveolar infiltrates resembling pulmonary edema develop. In children pneumothorax, subcutaneous and interstitial emphysema, and pneumomediastinum may occur.

The disease usually follows a progressive course, with death in 2 to 6 weeks although deaths have been reported after 2 or 3 days of illness. Mortality has varied from 20 to 60 per cent. However, awareness of the disease and proper early treatment have decreased mortality to less than 3 per cent.

Diagnosis. The demonstration of *P. carinii* in sputum, hypopharyngeal material, and tracheal smears has not been routinely successful. Histologic preparation of open lung biopsy material has been used successfully in children. Hematoxylin and eosin-stained paraffin sections, methenamine-silver nitrate–stained frozen sections, and Giemsa-stained impression smears have all been productive techniques.[3] With the silver stain ovoid and crescent-shaped (collapsed) cyst walls, located in the alveolar exudate, stain black (Fig. 40–1). Needle biopsy has proved successful in some patients, but there are reported lethal complications.

Complement-fixation tests, using an antigen prepared from lung material of patients suffering from the infection, have been used as an epidemiologic tool for the assessment of *Pneumocystis* pneumonia. Recently, direct and indirect immunofluorescent techniques have been developed but are not presently reliable in most areas. Thus, a high index of suspicion based on signs, symptoms, and radiologic and epidemiologic findings is important. The diagnosis may be confirmed by biopsy, but the clinical risks of this procedure should be weighed carefully against the ease of a therapeutic trial.[8, 9]

Treatment. Pentamidine, an aromatic diamidine (available in the United States only from the Parasitic Disease Service, Center for Disease Control), given intramuscularly for 12 to 14 days, gives excellent results. However, early diagnosis and institution of therapy are mandatory if a cure is to be expected. Almost all patients show signs of drug toxicity such as transient nephrotoxicity, oliguria or azotemia, sloughing of injection sites, fasting hypoglycemia, and transient loss of taste. A combination therapy of pyrimethamine, sulfadiazine and folinic acid has given parasitic cures in a few cases. Further trials are necessary to establish the efficacy of this regimen as a safer but more slowly acting therapeutic measure.[3] Supportive measures include high oxygen therapy with volume respirator assistance, antibiotics if indicated, and temporary discontinuance of immunosuppressive drugs. Extracorporeal membrane oxygenation has been used and will be a feasible adjunct in the treatment of certain individuals with further refinements of the technique.[10]

REFERENCES

1. Le Clair, R. A. 1967. *Pneumocystis carinii* and interstitial plasma cell pneumonia: a review. Am. Rev. Respir. Dis. *96*:1131–1136.
2. Kim, H. K., Hughes, W. T., and Feldman, S. 1972. Studies of morphology and immunofluorescence of *Pneumocystis carinii.* Proc. Soc. Exp. Biol. Med. *141*:304–309.
3. Burke, B. A., and Good, R. A. 1973. *Pneumocystis carinii* infection. Medicine *52*:23–51.
4. Pavlica, F. 1962. The first observation of congenital *Pneumocystis* pneumonia in a fully developed stillborn child. Ann. Pediatr. *198*:177–184.
5. Perera, D. R., Western, K. A., Johnson, H. D., Johnson, W. W., Schultz, M. G., and Akers, P. V. 1970. *Pneumocystis carinii* pneumonia in a hospital for children. J.A.M.A. *214*:1074–1078.
6. Nowak, J. 1966. Late pulmonary changes in the course of infection with *Pneumocystis carinii.* Acta Med. Pol. 7:23–41.
7. Meuwissen, J. H., and Leeuwenberg, A. D. 1972. A micro-complement fixation test applied to infection with *Pneumocystis carinii.* Trop. Geogr. Med. *24*:282–291.
8. Robbins, J. B., and DeVita, V. T. 1972. An increasing awareness of *Pneumocystis carinii* pneumonitis. Ann. Thorac. Surg. *14*:445–446.
9. Charles, M. A., and Schwarz, M. I. 1973. *Pneumocystis carinii* pneumonia. Postgrad. Med. *53*:86–92.
10. Geelhoed, G. W., Levine, B. J., Adkins, P. C., and Joseph, W. L. 1972. The diagnosis and management of *Pneumocystis carinii* pneumonia. Ann. Thorac. Surg. *14*:335–346.

CHAPTER 41

The Trypanosomidae

FRANK HAWKING

Introduction. The genera *Leishmania* and *Trypanosoma* are the only members of the family TRYPANOSOMIDAE that are pathogenic for man or animals. There are several important diseases of man caused by these flagellates. Some are produced by species of the genus *Leishmania,* and others are caused by members of the genus *Trypanosoma* (Table 41–1).

All species listed in Table 41–1 have both vertebrate and invertebrate hosts. Their life cycles are carried on partly in certain insects and partly in man or other mammals, the parasites living alternately in the blood or other tissues of the vertebrate and in the gut of the insect. The leishmanial parasites all occur as intracellular organisms, principally in cells of the reticuloendothelial system. The trypanosomes, on the other hand, are extracellular parasites occurring in the blood, lymph or cerebrospinal fluid. *Trypanosoma cruzi* is the only member of the family producing both trypanosomal forms in the blood and leishmanial stages in the tissue cells of man (Table 41–2).

Developmental Stages. In the course of the life cycle in the invertebrate and the vertebrate hosts, multiplication occurs and certain members of the family pass through developmental stages in which they resemble other genera within the family (Fig. 41–1). The nomenclature of these stages has been completely revised.[1]

In the *amastigote (leishmanial) stage* the parasite is an intracellular organism that occurs only in the mammal. It is a nonflagellated round or ovoid body measuring 1.5 to 5 μm in greatest diameter and containing a spherical vesicular nucleus and a smaller kinetoplast complex. Occasionally a fibril, the rhizoplast, may be seen extending from the kinetoplast to the periphery of the parasite (Fig. 41–1).

The *promastigote (leptomonad) stage* occurs in the life cycle of members of the genus *Leishmania* in the insect host and in culture. It has not been found in man. The promastigote form is slender and elongate with a centrally placed vesicular nucleus. A single anterior flagellum arises from a well-developed kinetoplast near the anterior extremity of the body. There is no undulating membrane.

The *epimastigote (crithidial) stage* occurs in the course of the life cycle of members of the genus *Trypanosoma.* Epimastigotes usually occur in the insect vector where multiplication occurs. The typically slender epimastigote form resembles the promastigote in general contour. The vesicular nucleus is centrally placed. The kinetoplast is situated near and anterior to the nucleus. The single

Table 41–1. DISEASES OF MAN CAUSED BY THE TRYPANOSOMIDAE

Disease	***Etiologic Agent***
Kala-azar	*Leishmania donovani*
Oriental sore	*L. tropica*
Mucocutaneous leishmaniasis	*L. braziliensis*
Chiclero ulcer	*L. mexicana*
Trypanosomiasis, West African, Gambian	*Trypanosoma gambiense*
Trypanosomiasis, East African, Rhodesian	*T. rhodesiense*
Chagas' disease	*T. cruzi*

Table 41–2. Stages in Life Cycles of the Trypanosomidae of Man*

Species of Parasite	*Stage in Man*	*Stage in Insect*	*Station*
Leishmania donovani	†Amastigote (leishmanial)	Promastigote (leptomonad)	A††
L. tropica	†Amastigote (leishmanial)	Promastigote (leptomonad)	A
L. braziliensis	†Amastigote (leishmanial)	Promastigote (leptomonad)	A
L. mexicana	†Amastigote (leishmanial)	Promastigote (leptomonad)	A
Trypanosoma gambiense	†Trypomastigote (trypanosomal)	Epimastigote, trypomastigote	A
T. rhodesiense	†Trypomastigote (trypanosomal)	Epimastigote, trypomastigote	A
T. cruzi	†Amastigote, epimastigote (?) trypomastigote (leishmanial, crithidial (?), trypanosomal)	Epimastigote, trypomastigote	P§

*See page 449 for discussion of *T. rangeli.*
† = the multiplicative stage in man.
††A = anterior station.
§P = posterior station.

flagellum continues as the free border of a short undulating membrane that extends to the anterior extremity of the parasite. At this point the flagellum becomes free.

The *trypomastigote (trypanosomal) stage* occurs only among members of the genus *Trypanosoma.* It is represented by a metacyclic phase and a mature phase. The metacyclic form or metatrypanosome is the young infective trypanosome, which develops only in the insect vector. It represents the culmination of the reproductive epimastigote stage, which is not infective to the mammal. When the metacyclic trypanosome is found in the salivary glands of the insect it is said to have an anterior station. When it is developed in

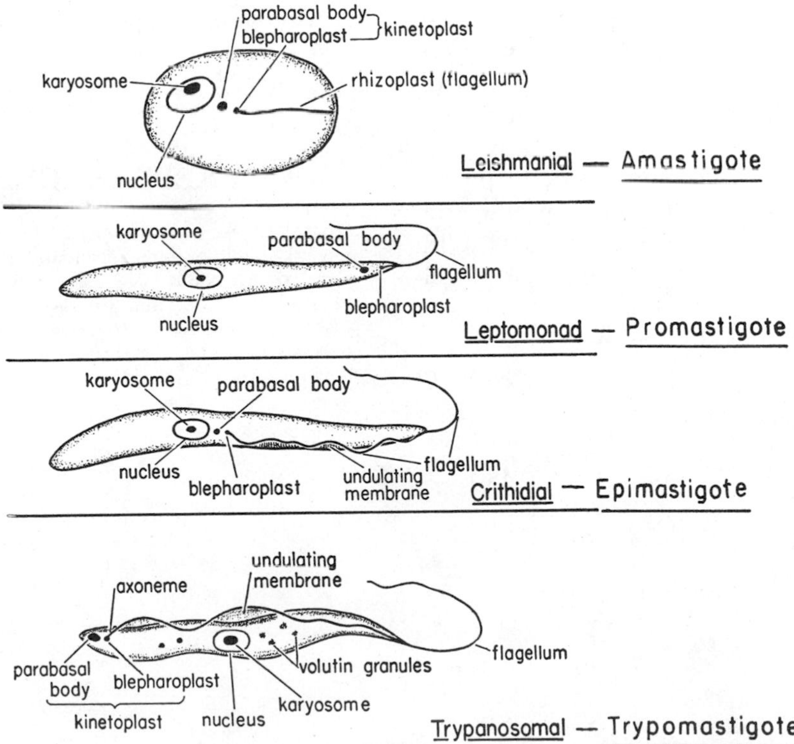

Figure 41–1. Amastigote (leishmanial), promastigote (leptomonad), epimastigote (crithidial) and trypomastigote (trypanosomal) forms of the Trypanosomidae.

the hind gut and is passed in the feces, the term posterior station is used. The metacyclic trypanosome has a relatively short stumpy body with a centrally placed nucleus. The kinetoplast is situated posterior to the nucleus. The single flagellum forms the border of an undulating membrane which extends along the greater portion of the body of the parasite, becoming free at the anterior extremity. The mature trypanosome is longer and more slender. The nucleus is usually centrally placed. The kinetoplast is situated near the posterior extremity. Volutin granules are scattered through the cytoplasm. Two forms of mature trypanosomes may be encountered. In the monomorphic type all individuals are morphologically similar, each possessing a central nucleus, a posteriorly placed kinetoplast, a long undulating membrane and a long anterior flagellum. Those of the polymorphic type, on the other hand, exhibit morphologic differences, particularly with respect to variation in size, position of the nucleus and length of the flagellum. Locomotion of the trypanosome is usually in the direction of the free flagellum.

Multiplication of the parasites in these genera occurs by longitudinal fission. Division of the blepharoplast, the parabasal body and the nucleus precedes division of the cytoplasm. The flagellum when present does not divide, but as division of the blepharoplast occurs a new flagellum rapidly develops while the old flagellum persists. With fission of the cytoplasm two separate flagellated organisms are produced.

The diagnosis of leishmanial and trypanosomal infections in man is based upon demonstration of the parasites in stained smears of blood, spinal fluid, material aspirated from cutaneous lesions, lymph nodes, bone marrow or spleen, or in fixed and stained tissue sections. When stained with the Romanowsky or common tissue stains the cytoplasm of these parasites appears blue, the nucleus pink and the kinetoplast a deep red. The species of *Leishmania and T. cruzi* may be isolated in culture (p. 831). African trypanosomes have been grown on special media with limited success. Xenodiagnosis also is useful in the identification of *T. cruzi* infections; an uninfected reduviid bug is allowed to feed upon the infected individual, and subsequently the trypanosomes may be demonstrated in its feces.

Dogs, cats, monkeys, mice, rats, guinea pigs, Chinese and European hamsters, the gerbil and certain species of squirrels have all been shown to be susceptible in varying degree to infection by species of *Leishmania.* The hamster is one of the best experimental animals. Some species of *Trypanosoma* produce serious disease in domestic animals. particularly cattle in Africa. Human infection with unusual species has been reported occasionally, for instance, recently in India involving *T. lewisi,* a parasite of rats.[2]

REFERENCES

1. Hoare, C. A., and Wallace, F. G. 1966. Developmental stages of trypanosomatid flagellates: a new terminology. Nature *212*:1385–1386.
2. Shrivastava, K. K., and Shrivastava, G. P. 1974. Two cases of *Trypanosoma (Herpetosoma)* species infection of man in India. Tr. Roy. Soc. Trop. Med. Hyg. *68*:143–144.

CHAPTER 42

Leishmaniasis—Introduction

FRANCISCO BIAGI

The term leishmaniasis includes a variety of conditions that may be conveniently subdivided into visceral and tegumentary infections. The geographic distribution of some of these infections is shown in Figure 42-1. These diseases are produced by protozoal parasites belonging to the family TRYPANOSOMIDAE and genus *Leishmania.* The different organisms are morphologically identical but can be distinguished by the anatomo-clinical picture in man, by serology and by metabolic features. *Leishmania donovani* (Laveran and Mesnil, 1903) Ross, 1903; *Leishmania tropica* (Wright, 1903) Luhe, 1906; *Leishmania braziliensis* Vianna, 1911; and *Leishmania mexicana* (Biagi, 1953), Garnham, 1962, are classified as different species within the genus (Table 42-1).

Some subspecies and other species are now under study. A revised classification has recently been proposed for the leishmanias of the Western Hemisphere.[1] Parasites of the *L. mexicana* complex are differentiated from those of *L. braziliensis* by several principal characteristics. Distinguishing characteristics of the *L. mexicana* complex include:

1. transmission by phlebotomines of the *intermediate* group; the parasites do not proliferate in the posterior intestinal triangle of the vector;

Table 42-1. DIFFERENT FORMS OF HUMAN LEISHMANIASIS

		Natural History of Infection in Man				
Name of Disease	***Leishmania spp.***	VISCERAL LESIONS	ULCEROUS CUTANEOUS LESIONS	HEMATOGENOUS METASTASIS TO NASO-ORAL MUCOUS MEMBRANES	SPONTANEOUS CURE	MONTENEGRO INTRADERMAL TEST
Cutaneous leishmaniasis (1)	*L. tropica*	No	Primary	No (3)	Usually in a few months	Positive
Chiclero ulcer	*L. mexicana*	No	Primary	No (3)	Usually in a few months, except in ears (4)	Positive
Mucocutaneous leishmaniasis	*L. braziliensis*	No	Primary	Large, destructive and common in cases infected more than 2 years	Rare	Positive
Visceral leishmaniasis (2)	*L. donovani*	Typical, always in spleen; frequently in other organs	Secondary (if they appear)	Parasites may be found, but usually there are no lesions	Rare	Negative (5)

(1) Cutaneous leishmaniasis has been subdivided into (a) "humid" (*L.t. major*) and (b) "dry" (*L.t. minor*); the former is an acute form, quick healing, strongly immunogenic and zoonotic. In Peruvian valleys of the Andes, another form of cutaneous leishmaniasis called "uta" has been described.

(2) Visceral leishmaniasis has been subdivided according to clinical, geographic and ecologic characteristics into (a) Indian, (b) Mediterranean (*L. infantum*) and (c) African.

(3) In a small percentage of cases, spreading of lesions to mucous membranes by contiguity has been observed.

(4) More than 80 per cent of cases with lesions in the ears, when not treated, remain ulcerated for several years (but they do not originate hematogenous dissemination into mucous membranes).

(5) In some cases, especially in Africa, a positive reaction has been found after cure.

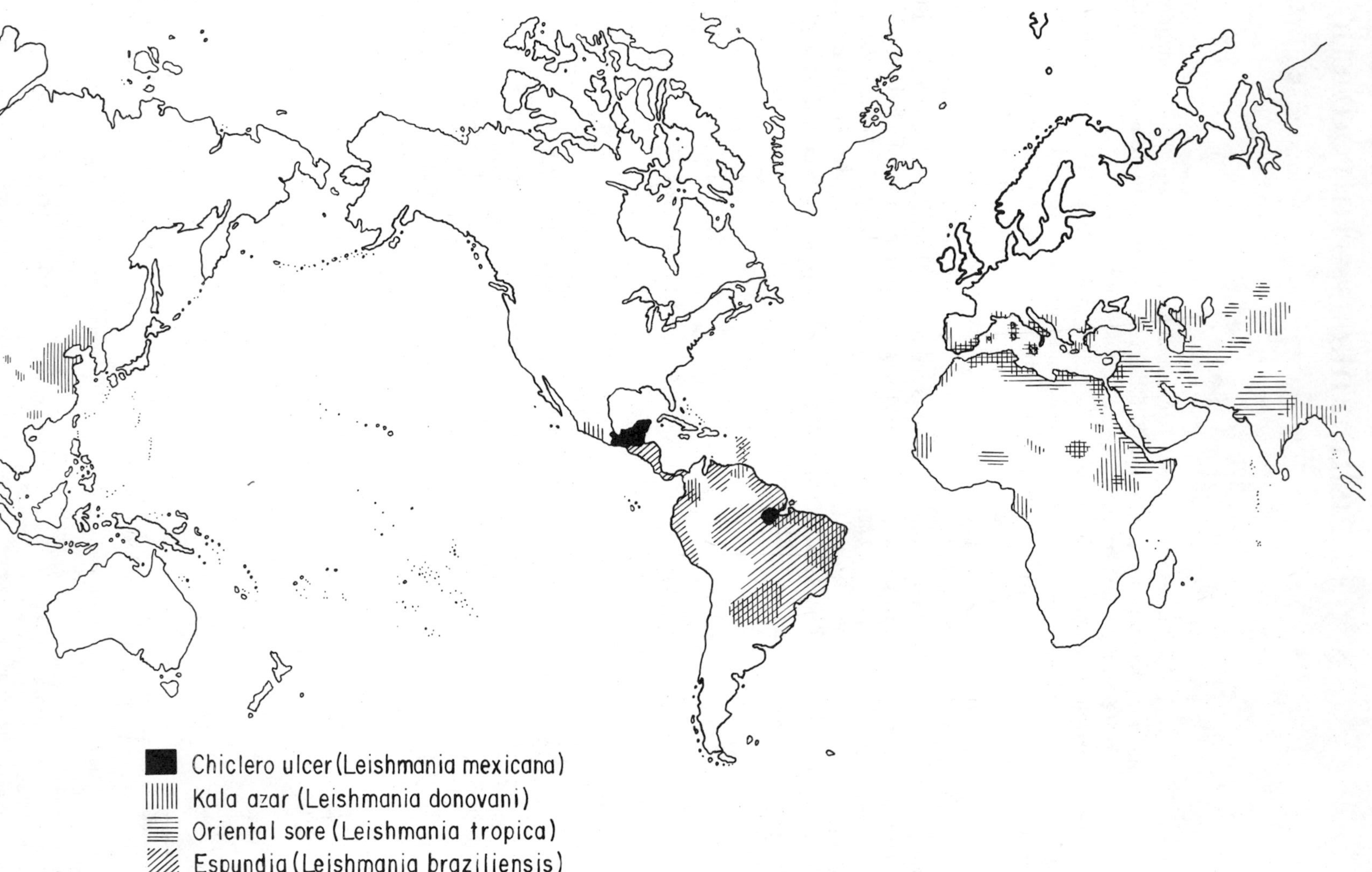

Figure 42–1. Geographic distribution of leishmaniasis.

2. rapid formation of histiocytomas in the skin with abundant amastigotes; propagation by metastases;

3. abundant growth in NNN medium ("fast" growing); and

4. differentiation by DNA buoyant density.

In contrast, parasites of the *L. braziliensis* complex are characterized by:

1. vectoring by phlebotomines of *Psychodopygus* and *intermediate* groups; proliferation occurs in the posterior triangle;

2. slow formation of small nodules or ulcers with sparse amastigotes; no spread by metastases;

3. scanty or moderate growth in NNN medium ("slow" growing); and

4. differentiation by density flotation with DNA.[1]

The proposed classification includes, among the forms now known to produce human disease, the following subspecies of the two complexes: (1) *L. mexicana mexicana, L. mexicana amazonensis, L. mexicana pifanoi* and a *L. mexicana* subspecies from Panama; and (2) *L. braziliensis braziliensis, L. braziliensis guyanensis, L. braziliensis panamensis* and *L. peruviana*.[1]

The amastigotes (leishmania) localize in the reticuloendothelial cells of the viscera or the skin. Thus, in kala-azar a skin inoculation is followed by parasitization and pathologic changes in the spleen, liver and bone marrow. In Oriental sore the lesion, which undergoes spontaneous cure in a few months, is restricted to the skin at the site of the sandfly bite. The chiclero ulcer is also restricted to the site of the sandfly bite, but when located in the ears usually remains active for up to 45 years. In espundia a primary skin lesion also forms at the site of the bite. A few cases show lymphatic spread to the regional lymph glands, and about 2 years later the majority of the patients develop metastatic spread to the mucous membranes of the nose, mouth and pharynx.

In cutaneous leishmaniasis of the Old World, a solid lifelong immunity against other infections with an homologous strain of *L. tropica* develops after the lesion has been allowed to run its full course. Whereas *L. tropica major* protects against a subsequent infection with *L. tropica minor*, the reverse is not true. There is no cross-immunity between *L. tropica* and *L. donovani*, although as a rule the

Table 42–2. KNOWN AND PROBABLE VECTORS OF LEISHMANIASIS

Leishmania donovani – kala-azar	
India, China	*Phlebotomus argentipes* *P. chinensis* *P. sergenti* var. *mongolensis*
Mediterranean, Middle East, Soviet Asia, North Africa (=*L. infantum*)	*P. perniciosus* *P. major* *P. papatasi* *P. caucasicus*
Africa South of the Sahara, Sudan, East Africa	*P. orientalis* *P. martini*
South America (=*L. chagasi*)	*Lutzomyia longipalpis* *L. intermedius*
Cutaneous Leishmaniasis of the Old World Leishmania tropica	
Soviet Asia, Middle East, Mediterranean	*P. papatasi* *P. caucasicus* *Sergentomyia arpaklensis* *P. perfiliewi*
North Africa	*P. sergenti*
Cutaneous Leishmaniasis of the New World	
Chiclero ulcer *L. mexicana*	*Lutzomyia flaviscutellata**
Espundia *L. braziliensis*	*L. migonei* *L. intermedius* *L. gomezi* *L. squamiventris* *L. paraensis* *L. whitmani* *L. pessoai*
Uta (=*L. peruviana*) *L. braziliensis*	*L. peruensis* *L. verrucarum*
Leishmaniasis tegumentaria diffusa (in New and Old World)	Phlebotomine flies

*Under experimental conditions *Leishmania mexicana* has also been artificially transmitted by *Lutzomyia renei, L. longipalpis, L. cruciatus* and *L. paraensis*.

( ) = synonyms

Table 42–3. HUMAN LEISHMANIASIS

Type	*Name*	*Geographic Area*	*Etiologic Agent*	*Main Reservoir*
Visceral	Kala-azar	India	*Leishmania donovani*	Man
		Mediterranean	*L. donovani* (=*L. infantum*)	Dog, fox
		Middle East North Africa Middle Asia Sudan, East Africa	*L. donovani*	Jackal Man Rodent (?)
		South America	*L. donovani* (=*L. chagasi*)	Dog Fox Man
Old World cutaneous	Oriental sore	Rural – moist Urban – dry	*L. tropica* var. *major* *L. tropica* var. *minor*	Gerbil Dog Man
New World cutaneous	Chiclero ulcer	Mexico Belize (Br. Honduras) Amazon basin	*L. mexicana*	Forest rodent
	Espundia	Central and South America	*L. braziliensis*	Forest rodent
	Uta	Peru	*L. braziliensis* (=*L. peruviana*)	Dog
Venezuela, Brazil, Mexico, Ethiopia	Leishmaniasis tegumentaria diffusa		Anergy of the host	

two infections have a different distribution geographically. In cutaneous leishmaniasis of the New World, immunity against reinfection develops with *L. mexicana*, but there is little cross-immunity between the different strains of leishmania in South and Central America.[2] Recent findings suggest that abortive infections followed by solid immunity against *L. braziliensis* may be artificially produced by injection of a small number of parasites in culture.[3] After an attack of kala-azar there is immunity against a second attack. With the exception of Indian kala-azar, the various leishmaniases are zoonoses and have a reservoir in canines or rodents.

Several species of phlebotomine flies are responsible for transmission of the parasites (Table 42–2). These flies are delicate, small and hairy. They are comparatively weak fliers and breed in rodent burrows, tree holes, cracks in masonry, and in rubbish (p. 757). Phlebotomine flies acquire the protozoan by direct ingestion of blood and of tissue debris from the infected skin of men, canines or rodents (Table 42–3). After the amastigotes enter the gut of the insect, they develop into promastigotes. In suitable vector species they occupy an anterior station in the pharynx of the insect and subsequently are introduced to the host by bite.

REFERENCES

1. Lainson, R., and Shaw, J. J. 1974. Las leishmanias y la leishmaniasis del Nuevo Mundo, con particular referencia al Brasil. Bol. Of. San. Panam. *76*:93–114.
2. Heyneman, D. 1971. Immunology of leishmaniasis. Bull. W.H.O. *44*:499–514.
3. Zeledón, R., and Alfaro, M. 1973. Isolation of *Leishmania braziliensis* from a Costa Rican sandfly and its possible use as a human vaccine. Tr. Roy. Soc. Trop. Med. Hyg. *67*:416–417.

CHAPTER 43

Kala-azar

FRANCISCO BIAGI

Synonyms. Visceral leishmaniasis, dumdum fever, tropical splenomegaly, black sickness, splenic anemia of infants, ponos.

Definition. Kala-azar is a disease produced by *Leishmania donovani.* It is characterized by irregular fever of long duration, enlargement of the spleen and often of the liver, emaciation, anemia, leukopenia and hypergammaglobulinemia.

Distribution. Kala-azar is widely distributed; it has geographic types that differ in their epidemiology, clinical features and response to treatment.

Indian kala-azar is endemic in the eastern portion of India in Assam, Bengal, Bihar, Madras and Sikkim, where extensive epidemics with high mortality rates have occurred in the past.

Mediterranean kala-azar, often referred to as infantile kala-azar, is present in the Mediterranean littoral, including southern Italy, France, Spain, Portugal, North Africa, the Mediterranean islands, southern Russia, Transcaucasia, Uzbekistan, North China, Manchuria and Central Asia.

African kala-azar is found in East Africa, Fung and Upper Nile areas of the Sudan, and in isolated areas across Africa to the west coast south of the Sahara. It has recently been reported again from Ethiopia.[1]

American kala-azar occurs chiefly in the northeastern part of Brazil, but also in Argentina, Paraguay, Colombia, El Salvador, Guatemala and Mexico.

Etiology. Kala-azar is caused by *L. donovani* (Laveran and Mesnil, 1903) Ross, 1903. Formerly infantile kala-azar was considered to be due to *L. infantum,* and American kala-azar to *L. chagasi.* Recent studies suggest the possible revalidation of the latter species, but for the present it is considered synonymous.

Leishmania donovani is a round or ovoid organism measuring 2 to 5 μm in diameter and containing a relatively large and peripherally placed vesicular nucleus. A rod-shaped or oval parabasal body and a dotlike blepharoplast in close proximity to it together form the kinetoplast. Occasionally, a short fibril, the rhizoplast, may be seen arising from the blepharoplast and extending to the periphery.

When stained with a Romanowsky stain the cytoplasm appears faintly blue, and the nucleus and kinetoplast are red or reddish purple.

The amastigotes are found within cells of the reticuloendothelial system, monocytes, polymorphonuclear neutrophils and other phagocytic cells.

Epidemiology. Kala-azar is a rural disease. Three factors are essential for transmission of the disease to man: a reservoir of infection, a suitable vector, and a susceptible population. Kala-azar varies from being a complete zoonosis with man involved only accidentally as in Tadzhikistan, through a domestic zoonosis with a reservoir in the dog as in the Mediterranean and South America, to a completely human disease as in India (Fig. 43–1).

When kala-azar appears in new areas, epidemics may occur with a high mortality rate.

The dog is the main reservoir of infection in the Mediterranean and South America. Wild jackals in Tadzhikistan share the infection with domestic dogs, and in Brazil wild foxes with domestic dogs.[2] *Phlebotomus sergenti* and *P. chinensis* in China, and *Lutzomyia longipalpis* in Brazil have been shown to acquire the infection from dogs. Rodents may form a reservoir of infection in the Sudan and East Africa, but their true role has not yet been determined since the *Leishmania* isolated from rodents has not yet been proved pathogenic to man.[3]

Man is the only reservoir in India and is

Amastigote
(Leishmanial) stage
Leishmania
in R-E cell
Promastigote
(Leptomonad)
stage
LEISHMANIASIS
HUMAN DISEASE
Visceral: Kala-azar
Indian & Oriental-L. donovani
Mediterranean-L. donovani
Dermal: Post-kala-azar
Cutaneous:
Oriental Sore-L. tropica
Naso-Oral:
Mucocutaneous-L. braziliensis
Phlebotomus breeding area
rodent
Reservoir
New host
EPIDEMIOLOGY
Leptomonads develop in pharynx of fly.
1. Vector: species of phlebotomines
2. Breeding in cracks & rubble
3. Flies remain in vicinity
4. Reservoir: man, dog, rodent
5. Fly bites infected host
6. Flagellates in insects gut
7. Promastigotes injected into man by bite of fly
8. Amastigotes in reticuloendothelial cells
Phlebotomus

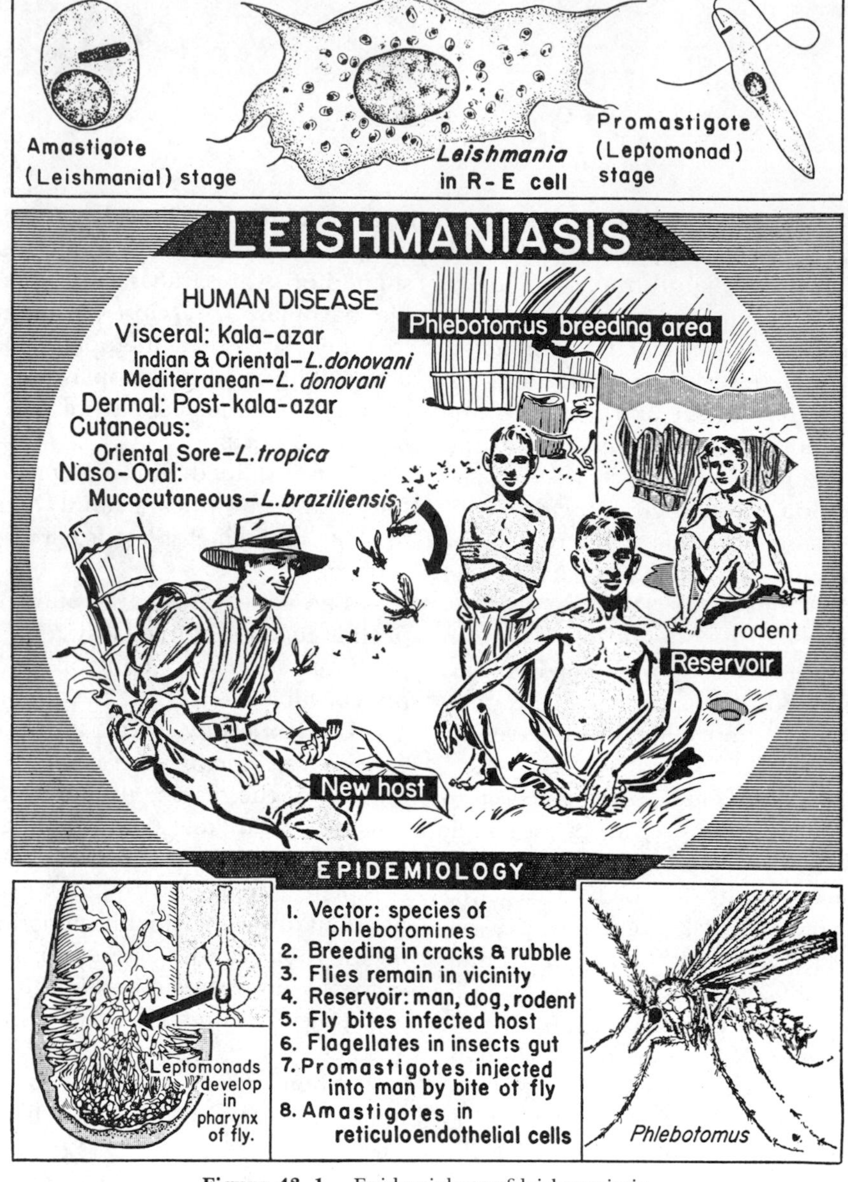

Figure 43–1. Epidemiology of leishmaniasis.

also a considerable source of infection in Brazil, the Sudan and East Africa, where sandflies can easily be infected from his blood. Man plays no part in the spread of the disease in the Mediterranean.

The *sandfly vectors* are most numerous in the immediate proximity of the breeding places. For the most part they remain close to the ground and, consequently, are much less numerous above the first floor in houses. The average life of the sandfly is estimated to be 14 to 16 days. The domestic *Phlebotomus* species are the main vectors of the disease in India *(P. argentipes),* China *(P. chinensis),* and the Mediterranean *(P. perniciosus).* Phlebotomines that live outside houses are the main vectors in the Sudan *(P. orientalis),* East Africa *(P. martini)* and Brazil (*Lutzomyia longipalpis*) (Table 42–2, p. 413).

Amastigotes present in the peripheral blood and the skin in the course of the active disease are ingested by the vector, Promastigotes may be observed in the gut of the insect by the third day after the infective blood meal. They move forward to occupy an anterior station in the pharynx and mouthparts by the fourth or fifth day. From the seventh to the ninth day the flagellates often invade the proboscis, and the flies are then infective. The organisms enter the new host during subsequent biting. Successful transmission by the sandfly to hamsters and to man has been accomplished.

Kala-azar has been transmitted to man by blood transfusion, bite of an infected hamster, and even venereal contact. Amastigotes have been demonstrated in the urine, feces, nasal mucosa and tonsils of infected humans. However, these probably play little or no role in the spread of the infection in view of the sharp geographic limits, the failure of the disease to extend outside these regions, and its absence at altitudes above 600 meters within the endemic areas.

Animals have been shown to acquire leishmaniasis by eating infected carcasses. It is possible that this may be a factor in maintaining the animal reservoir.

Pathology. The essential pathology of kala-azar starts with a primary skin lesion resembling an Oriental sore that does not ulcerate and is so small in nature that it is very seldom observed. After a period of about 4 to 6 months the parasites spread via the blood stream to the viscera, with parasitization and hyperplasia of the cells of the reticuloendothelial system in the spleen, liver, bone marrow and lymph glands. The leishmania multiply within these cells, which ultimately rupture, releasing the parasites which are then taken up by other reticuloendothelial cells. They are ingested to a lesser extent by leukocytes and monocytes, which occasionally may be found containing leishmania in films of the peripheral blood.

The spleen may be greatly enlarged, owing principally to the enormous increase of reticuloendothelial cells, many of which are parasitized. There is replacement of splenic pulp by these parasitized cells and often pressure atrophy of the malpighian bodies. There may be some fibrosis in advanced chronic cases (Fig. 43–2).

The liver is usually, but not always, enlarged in kala-azar. There is marked proliferation of the Kupffer cells, which contain large numbers of amastigotes. Pressure atrophy of the liver cells occurs, and both cloudy swelling and fatty degeneration may be observed. In advanced chronic cases there may be some fibrosis of the parenchyma (Fig. 43–3).

The villi of the small intestine, especially the duodenum and jejunum, may be crowded with parasitized reticuloendothelial cells, and ulceration of the overlying mucosa

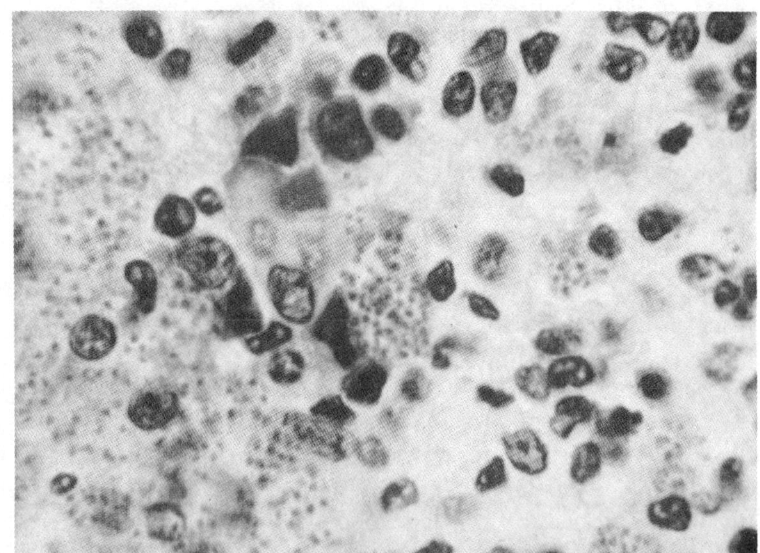

Figure 43–2. Parasitized reticuloendothelial cells in splenic pulp in *Leishmania donovani* infection. (Courtesy of the Louisiana State University School of Medicine, New Orleans.)

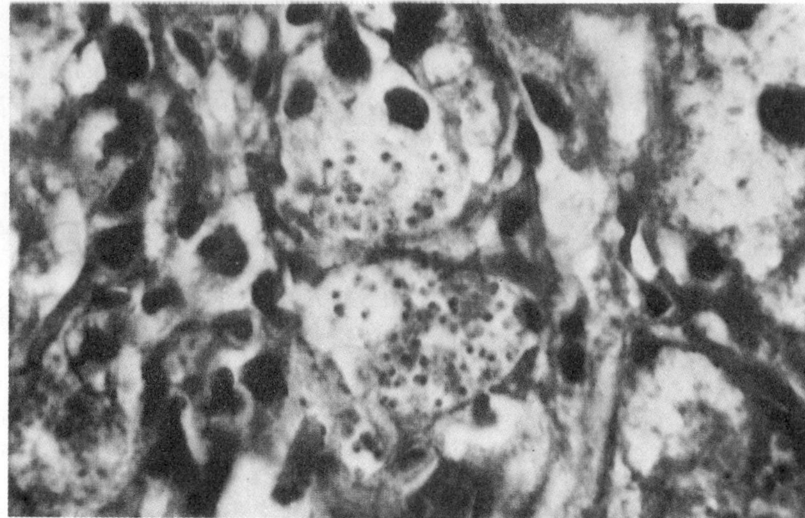

Figure 43-3. Kala-azar: biopsy of liver showing *L. donovani.* (Tissue section courtesy of Dr. J. Rodrigues da Silva, Rio de Janeiro; photomicrograph courtesy of the Louisiana State University School of Medicine, New Orleans.)

occasionally occurs. Less often similar lesions are reported in the colon, and, rarely, cells containing parasites may be observed in the mucous membrane of the stomach.

In the bone marrow there is a progressive replacement of the hematopoietic tissue and the fatty marrow by masses of heavily parasitized reticuloendothelial cells. In experimental infections of animals amyloid disease of the kidneys may be found, and it is probable that similar changes occur in human infections.

There are no characteristic lesions of other organs. Scattered infected phagocytic cells may be observed. The lymph nodes are often enlarged, owing to obstruction of the lymph sinuses by parasitized reticuloendothelial cells. In a number of cases of kala-azar, parasites occur in normal-appearing skin.

Post-kala-azar dermal leishmaniasis usually does not appear until some 2 years after the acute stage of the disease in India. In the Sudan it commonly appears as the visceral disease subsides. The early lesions are depigmented areas that may be ½ inch in diameter, occurring particularly on the face, neck, the extensor surface of the forearms and the inner aspect of the thighs. There is little change in the epidermis, but the pigment in the basal layer is diminished. The subpapillary layer is edematous, the vessels are dilated, and there is infiltration by macrophage cells. Parasites are scanty.

A second type of skin lesion, nodular in character, likewise occurs in post-kala-azar dermal leishmaniasis. In this type there is a thinning of the epidermis over a nodular granulomatous mass of reticuloendothelial cells, some of which contain amastigotes. This condition sometimes develops after inadequate therapy of visceral leishmaniasis with antimony.

Less commonly, xanthomatous lesions of the skin are observed. In these there is a marked increase of connective tissue. Parasites are rare.

Clinical Characteristics. The incubation period of both experimentally and naturally acquired kala-azar is usually from 4 to 6 months but has been as short as 10 to 14 days and as long as 2 years. The primary skin lesion is hardly ever noticed. The onset of the visceral stage may be sudden or gradual. In some instances, it is acute, accompanied by chills, high fever and vomiting. In others, it resembles typhoid and is characterized by general malaise and rising fever, which may reach 40° C (104° F) in about a week. In still others, it is insidious, slow and unaccompanied by any significant febrile reaction.

During the acute stage the fever is

frequently intermittent, with two daily remissions, and each drop in temperature is often accompanied by profuse sweating. Characteristically, the patient's temperature rises in the early afternoon, subsides toward evening and rises again usually before midnight. This may be observed in only 5 to 10 per cent of the early cases. The initial fever may last 2 to 6 weeks. Thereafter, if the disease becomes chronic, it is characterized by recurring febrile waves resembling those observed in brucellosis.

The first noticeable enlargement of the spleen may occur as late as 5 months after the onset, although it is usually at or below the costal margin by the end of the first month. In the early stages of the disease it has a doughy consistency. Each wave of fever is accompanied by further enlargement, followed by some reduction in size during the apyrexial periods. In chronic cases the spleen is often hard and greatly enlarged, extending to the umbilicus or even to the anterior superior spine of the ilium (Fig. 43–4). Soft enlargement of the liver is usually evident after the first month.

Diarrhea and at times even dysentery are not uncommon during the acute stage. Respiratory symptoms also may cause the patient to seek medical attention. As the disease progresses there is marked emaciation, most noticeable in the limbs and chest wall. Drenching night sweats are common. Despite these symptoms and the height of the fever curve, toxemia is inconspicuous. The appetite usually remains good and the tongue clean.

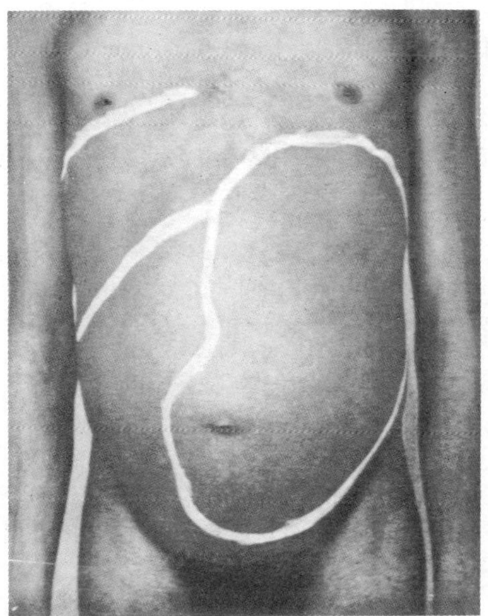

Figure 43–4. Chronic kala-azar: extreme splenomegaly and hepatomegaly.

Atypical forms without splenomegaly resembling acute hemorrhagic fevers, a nephrotic syndrome, or a symptomless generalized lymphadenopathy occur rarely. Mucocutaneous lesions resembling those of South American cutaneous leishmaniasis are found in the African form of the disease. Necrotic lesions of the mouth and nose, such as noma, may occur. Cirrhosis of the liver may be a sequela, and pulmonary tuberculosis often develops.

As the disease advances a characteristic grayish color of the skin develops from which the synonym "black disease" is derived. This pigmentation is most noticeable on the hands, the nails, the forehead and the central line of the abdomen.

The characteristic changes in the blood are produced by hypersplenism. There is a leukopenia with relative increase in the lymphocytes, which may be so severe that agranulocytosis results. There is a moderate normochromic, normocytic anemia, and the platelets may be reduced.

Progressive alteration of the plasma proteins occurs early in the disease. The serum gamma globulin is markedly elevated and may constitute 30 to 63 per cent of the total serum globulins. There is an absolute decrease in the serum albumin. In the late stages of the disease these changes in the plasma proteins commonly lead to ascites and edema.

Purpura, gingivitis, stomatitis and trophic changes of the hair are common. It is probable that they are to be attributed, at least in part, to nutritional deficiencies. Pneumonia, cancrum oris or intercurrent disease are frequent terminal phenomena.

Diagnosis. In endemic areas the diagnosis of kala-azar may be made with reasonable assurance on clinical grounds by about the fourth month, when the characteristic

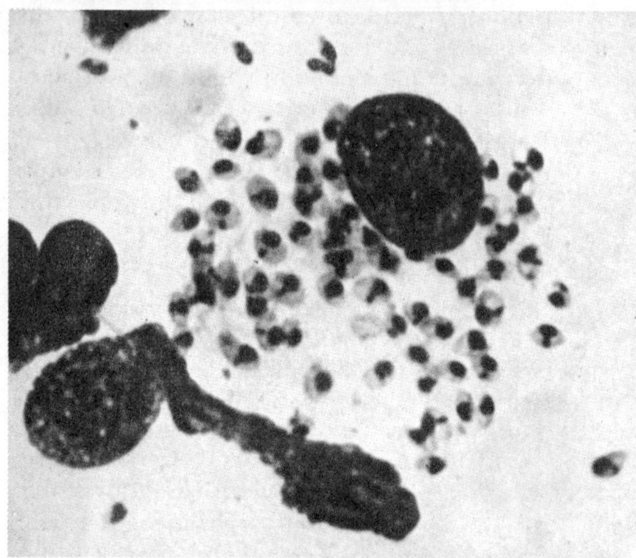

Figure 43-5. *Leishmania donovani* in stained smear from spleen puncture.

features (fever, splenomegaly, hepatomegaly and leukopenia usually below 4000 per cu mm) are ordinarily well established. The serum tests (e.g. formol gel) provide additional but not conclusive evidence. In early cases the characteristic fever curve may be the only significant clinical finding.

DEFINITIVE DIAGNOSIS. This depends upon the demonstration of *L. donovani* in stained smears of spleen, bone marrow, or lymphatic gland juice, and by cultures of the blood and other tissues, or by inoculation into the hamster.

Splenic Puncture. Provided a needle not larger than size 20 is used, splenic puncture in areas where the disease is endemic has not proved hazardous and *L. donovani* bodies are found in over 90 per cent of untreated cases. (Fig. 43-5). In infants and in early cases in which the spleen is soft and not greatly enlarged, some hazard exists from splenic puncture; sternal puncture is preferable.

Sternal Puncture. Leishmania may be demonstrated in 80 per cent of the cases and, although parasites are less numerous than in splenic smears, culture of the material will usually yield positive results.

Liver Puncture. Needle biopsy of the liver is more hazardous in this disease than splenic puncture and will show fewer parasites. However, it is positive in nearly 60 per cent of cases.

Blood Culture. Inoculation of 0.25 ml of blood directly into NNN medium and cultivation at 20 to 24° C (68 to 75° F) will yield promastigotes in from 1 to 4 weeks. With proper technique, positive culture should be obtained in a majority of cases. Cultures should not be discarded for at least 1 month.

Blood Smears. Especially in the Indian form, examination of the buffy coat in stained blood films will reveal leishmania in macrophage cells in almost all cases. In most other endemic areas leishmania are hardly ever seen in films of the peripheral blood.

Formol Gel Test. Positive reactions occur in kala-azar and other rare hypergammaglobulinemias such as macroglobulinemia, multiple myeloma, and schistosomiasis. (See p. 837.)

Complement-Fixation Test. A complement-fixation test has been developed using an antigen prepared from Kedrowsky's acid-fast bacillus. In the great majority of cases of active kala-azar, the test is positive. It reverts to negative after treatment.

Leishmanin Skin Test (Montenegro Reaction). An intradermal test of the delayed sensitivity type using formalinized promastigotes as antigen becomes positive after recovery from the disease. It is negative in active kala-azar. In endemic areas many persons who have not had clinical kala-azar may show a positive skin test.

Differential Diagnosis. The clinical picture of kala-azar frequently may resemble that produced by other diseases that occur in the endemic areas. The early acute stage may be confused with malaria, and in the early weeks it may also resemble typhoid fever. In the chronic stage it may be confused with tuberculosis, brucellosis, infectious mononucleosis, leukemia or other hematologic disorders. Infantile kala-azar has been confused with Banti's disease. The onset of kala-azar in children is frequently insidious. The clinical course is associated with splenomegaly, anemia and general lymphadenitis. The lesions of post-kala-azar dermal leishmaniasis may suggest leprosy.

Treatment. Malnutrition is frequently serious. Patients with severe disease should be hospitalized whenever it is possible.

A diet high in protein and vitamin content is essential. Oral hygiene is of great importance because of the frequency of the highly fatal complication, cancrum oris. Likewise, respiratory infections must be guarded against because of the susceptibility of kala-azar patients to pneumonia. The presence or absence of pulmonary tuberculosis must be determined.

Specific Treatment. The susceptibility of kala-azar to specific drug treatment varies considerably between different geographic areas. The disease in India seems to be most easily cured. The Chinese and Mediterranean forms occupy intermediate positions, and visceral leishmaniasis of the Sudan is notoriously resistant. Prior to the introduction of the currently used drugs the mortality was 95 per cent; it is now 2 to 5 per cent.

Two groups of compounds are recommended: pentavalent organic antimonials and certain aromatic diamidines. One or more of these will meet the requirements of almost all cases.

Pentavalent Organic Antimonials. SODIUM ANTIMONY GLUCONATE. Synonyms: Pentostam, Bayer 561, Solustibosan, Glucantamine. This drug has been widely used and found to be effective in resistant forms of the disease. Toxic effects are rare. A preparation of sodium antimony gluconate is issued under the name of Pentostam and is distributed in a form suitable for immediate injection. It contains 0.1 gm of drug per ml. The dosage is 6 ml (0.6 gm) daily intravenously or intramuscularly. The adult dose may be used for children weighing more than 30 kg, and not less than 0.2 gm should be given to any patient. The dosage for Indian kala-azar is 6 ml daily for 6 days, while the African form of kala-azar requires at least 6 ml daily for 30 days; this may have to be repeated.

NEOSTIBOSAN. Synonym: Bayer 693. Neostibosan is a phenylstibonic acid derivative. The methods of administration and dosage are the same as for sodium antimony gluconate except that this preparation should not be given intramuscularly.

UREA STIBAMINE. The drug is a mixture of compounds of phenylstibonic acid. It has been widely used in India where it has proved effective. It has greater toxicity than Neostibosan and should be administered by the intravenous route only. It should be given on alternate days or every third day in 5 to 10 ml of sterile distilled water. It must not be heated.

The initial recommended dose for an adult is 0.05 gm, the second 0.1 gm, the third 0.15 gm, and the fourth and subsequent doses 0.2 gm.

The mode of action of antimony on the leishmania is not known. The parasites may continue to be present and viable on culture during at least part of the course of treatment, and even for a short period after completion of therapy.

Aromatic Diamidines. The aromatic diamidines are the most powerful known drugs for the treatment of kala-azar. Particularly when given intravenously, reactions of some degree occur in a considerable proportion of patients. These include headache, flushing, faintness, epigastric pain and vomiting, collapse and unconsciousness. There is an associated fall in blood pressure and, at times, lowering of the blood sugar. These reactions can be prevented largely or controlled by intramuscular injection of 0.25 ml of 1/1000 epinephrine or an antihistaminic immediately prior to administration of the drug.

HYDROXYSTILBAMIDINE. This must be given intravenously in doses not larger than

0.25 gm daily for 10 days. In African kala azar three such courses may be necessary. Stilbamidine should not be used.

PENTAMIDINE ISETHIONATE. Synonyms: M & B 800, Lomidine. This is not nearly so effective a drug as hydroxystilbamidine but can be given intramuscularly. The dosage is 4 mg per kg of body weight in 3 ml water.

Amophotericin B and its more soluble form, Fungizone, have been used with success in the treatment of both kala-azar and post-kala-azar dermal leishmaniasis. However, its toxicity is high and creatinine and urea levels should be determined frequently.

TREATMENT OF RESISTANT CASES. A case of kala-azar should not be considered resistant to antimony treatment until repeated and adequate doses of the drug have been given. Hydroxystilbamidine should then be given in adequate dosage for a period. Very large doses of antimony and of hydroxystilbamidine may be necessary. In a truly resistant case, splenectomy may be useful. A postoperative course of antimony should be given.

TREATMENT OF COMPLICATIONS. Antibiotics and blood transfusions are necessary to treat concurrent pneumonia and cancrum oris.

Post-kala-azar dermal leishmaniasis usually responds better to pentavalent antimony compounds than to the aromatic diamidines. The dosage recommended for the visceral infections should be used, but the injections should be spaced 2 or more days apart.

Relapses in kala-azar are not uncommon if insufficient treatment has been given. The relapse is usually accompanied by fever and progressive enlargement of the spleen.

Prognosis. Response to treatment consists of cessation of the fever and a subjective improvement, with rise of the white cell count to at least 6000 per cu mm. The spleen becomes reduced in size after about 2 weeks, and leishmania disappear from the spleen and bone marrow during the first course of treatment. A patient should not be regarded as cured until no parasites can be found or cultured, the spleen can no longer be felt, and the serum globulin has returned to normal. This takes about 6 months. Persistent splenomegaly is due to cirrhosis of the liver and portal hypertension, which occur in about 10 per cent of cases in some areas.

Prophylaxis. There are no specific prophylactic measures for kala-azar. The basic problem centers around the control of the *Phlebotomus* species that act as vectors. Insect repellents furnish temporary protection for the individual. However, DDT and other residual insecticides applied around the doors and windows and to the interior of homes have given remarkable results. Since phlebotomines are weak fliers, some communities can be protected by residual spraying of potential resting and breeding places for about 200 meters beyond the outskirts.

REFERENCES

1. Fuller, G. K., Lemma, A., and Gemetchu, T. 1974. Kala-azar in southwest Ethiopia. Tr. Roy. Soc. Trop. Med. Hyg. *68*:166.
2. Deane, M. D., and Deane, M. P. 1962. Visceral leishmaniasis in Brazil. Geographical distribution and transmission. Rev. Inst. Med. Trop. São Paulo *4*: 149–212.
3. Manson-Bahr, P. E. C., and Southgate, B. A. 1964. Recent research on kala-azar in East Africa. J. Trop. Med. Hyg. *67*:79–84.

CHAPTER 44

Cutaneous and Mucocutaneous Leishmaniasis

FRANCISCO BIAGI

Oriental Sore

Synonyms. Oriental sore; Aleppo, Baghdad, or Delhi boil; bouton d'Orient; bouton de Biskra.

Distribution. Oriental sore is prevalent in many tropical and subtropical regions. Its distribution, however, does not coincide with that of visceral leishmaniasis (kala-azar).

ASIA. Prevalent in parts of China. In Asia Minor, especially prevalent in Syria, Arabia, Iran, Israel, Iraq, the Caucasus, southeast U.S.S.R., Turkmenistan, Pakistan.

EUROPE. In the Mediterranean littoral, in the Mediterranean islands, southern Italy, Spain, the south of France and Greece.

AFRICA. Morocco, Tunisia, Algeria, Ethiopia, the Sudan, Zaire, Lake Chad area, Nigeria and on the west coast south as far as Angola.

Etiology. The etiologic agent of Oriental sore or cutaneous leishmaniasis is *Leishmania tropica* (Wright, 1903) Lühe, 1906. It is morphologically identical with *L. donovani.* There are two subspecies of *Leishmania tropica: L. tropica major,* which causes "moist" or rural leishmaniasis, and *L. tropica minor,* the cause of "dry" or urban leishmaniasis.

Epidemiology. The epidemiology of each of the two forms of cutaneous leishmaniasis is distinct. There are several mammalian reservoir hosts and sandfly vectors.[1] *Leishmania tropica major* produces an infection of gerbils in which lesions occur on the ears and tail. The infection is transmitted from rodent to rodent in their burrows by a sandfly, *Sergentomyia arpaklensis.* Man is only occasionally affected when the infection is transmitted to him by *Phlebotomus papatasi.* Where contact with gerbils is close, as in some Asiatic villages, the infection can be epidemic. *Leishmania tropica minor* causes an infection of dogs, in which lesions occur on the nose and face. The infection is transmitted from dog to dog and occasionally to man by *P. papatasi* and *P. sergenti.* In some areas, such as Baghdad, almost every individual was infected as a child previous to the introduction of DDT. West African cutaneous leishmaniasis may also have canine and rodent reservoirs and be transmitted by *P. duboscgi* and *P. bergeroti.*[2] The affinities of the diffuse cutaneous leishmaniasis which occurs in Ethiopia are as yet uncertain. It is probably more closely affiliated with Oriental sore than with other forms of leishmaniasis. Recent studies indicate that it may be caused by a distinct species named *L. aethiopica.*[1]

Children are more commonly affected than adults. There is no distinctive sex incidence. A fairly solid immunity follows infection in man. This has long been the basis for deliberate inoculation of children in endemic areas, the inhabitants knowing that the induced attack confers protection against naturally acquired infection. Sites are chosen where the resultant scar will be least disfiguring. Vaccination using cultural forms also has been used.

Pathology. Following inoculation of the skin, either through the bite of an infected sandfly or by some other means, a nodule develops that is produced by infiltration of the corium with plasma cells, lymphocytes and large endothelial macrophages. Thinning and atrophy of the overlying epidermis often occur. Perivascular infiltration then becomes prominent and polymorpho-

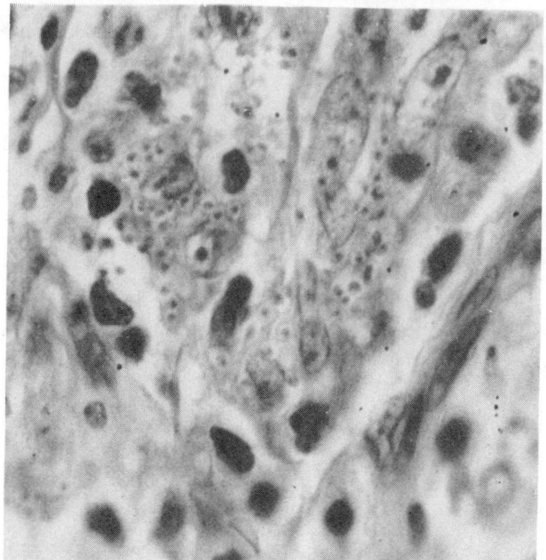

Figure 44-1. Section through the indurated edge of Oriental sore showing cellular infiltration, including heavily parasitized reticuloendothelial cells. (Courtesy of Dr. H. Most, New York University School of Medicine.)

nuclear leukocytes more numerous. Focal accumulations of endothelial phagocytes filled with leishmania are seen (Fig. 44-1).

With further progression, an ulcer develops that has a granulation tissue base and a surrounding zone of inflammation. Infiltration extends into the subcutaneous connective tissue in which reticuloendothelial cells, plasma cells and lymphocytes are prominent. Occasional giant cells are present.

The amastigotes are often difficult to demonstrate in the fully developed ulcer and may be found only at the margin of the lesion or in scrapings from its floor. There is no general dissemination of the parasites. Ultimately, the amastigotes disappear, granulation tissue becomes more abundant and healing occurs, leaving a depressed fibrous scar (Fig. 44-2).

Clinical Characteristics. The incubation period in the case of the moist form is a few weeks to a few months; however, in the dry form it is much longer, extending from many months to over a year. In the moist form ulceration is rapid and the duration of the lesions is short, up to 6 months. In the dry form the lesions last for many months. They appear first as slowly growing papules on an exposed skin area. As ulceration develops they become covered with a crust which exudes a sticky secretion. On removal

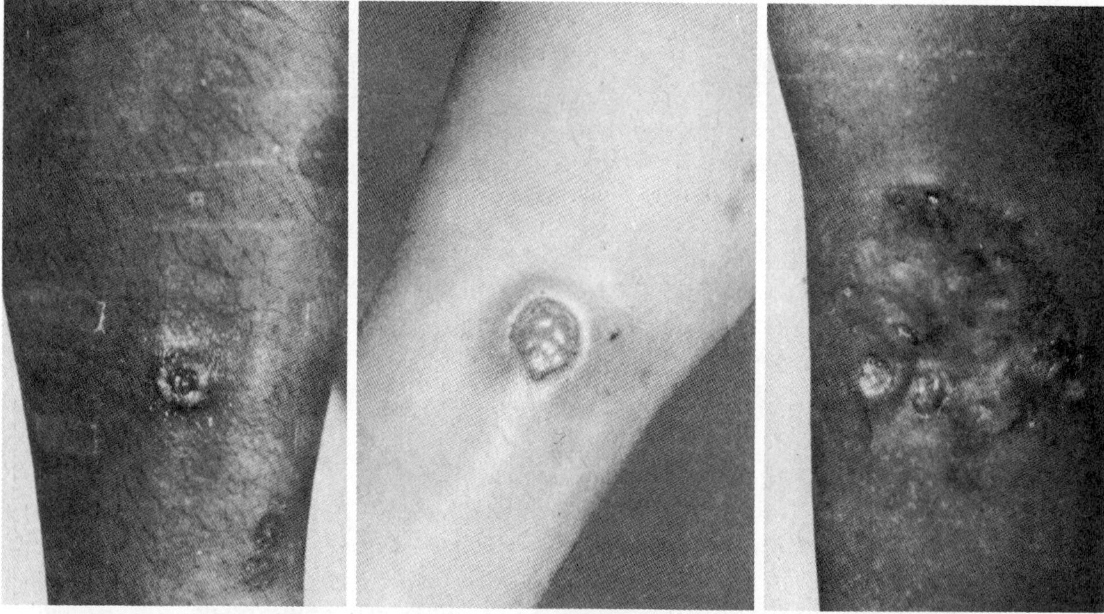

Figure 44-2. The extremities are favorite sites for Oriental sores. Beginning as a small papule, the lesion becomes a plaque (*A*); later, the ulceration extends, showing rolled indurated edges (*B*). Complete healing with scarring usually occurs, but satellite lesions may be formed (*C*) with central scarred areas and secondary ulcerated nodules. (Courtesy of Ash and Spitz: Pathology of Tropical Diseases.)

of the crusts, moist, freely bleeding ulcers are revealed. These ulcers are usually not deep and ordinarily vary from 1 to 3 cm in diameter. Secondary infection is usual and, when severe, greater tissue destruction may result. After effective treatment, or after a number of months if no treatment is given, healing occurs by granulation and a lasting immunity is produced.

In rare cases, spread to contiguous mucous membranes may take place, but it does not occur by metastatic spread through the blood stream.

Diagnosis. The development of one or more cutaneous ulcers on exposed skin areas of the body in a region where Oriental sore is known to be endemic and where sandflies are present should arouse suspicion of this condition. Definitive diagnosis depends upon the demonstration of *L. tropica* obtained from the lesion. Examination of the exudate will seldom be successful. Smears made from curettings of the base or the sides of the ulcer should be used, or a fine hypodermic needle introduced through normal skin may be inserted into the indurated margin of the lesion and material aspirated for preparation of a stained smear. Under sterile conditions, material aspirated from the margin of the lesion may be inoculated into NNN medium and leptomonad forms recovered after incubation at 22° C (72.6° F). Bacterial contamination of cultures for leishmania may be prevented or controlled by the addition of penicillin and other suitable antibiotics. Histologic sections show a granulomatous chronic inflammatory reaction which facilitates the search for parasites within the macrophages.

The leishmanial skin test becomes positive early in the infection and remains positive for life.

The differential diagnosis of cutaneous leishmaniasis must include blastomycosis, sporotrichosis, yaws, tertiary syphilis, cutaneous tuberculosis and lupus.

Treatment. The best results in all cases are obtained following the use of parenterally administered Neostibosan. In general, local injection of mepacrine (Atabrine) or antimony into the edges of the ulcer may enhance the systemic treatment. A total of 10 or 12 injections of Neostibosan intravenously given on alternate days will cure most patients. Antibiotics may be applied to the lesion to combat bacterial infection and to promote healing.

Prophylaxis. In view of the immunity which follows infection in humans with Oriental sore, deliberate inoculation and vaccination have been employed (p. 423). The measures for control of the phlebotomine vectors and insect repellents are discussed on page 800.

Mucocutaneous Leishmaniasis

Synonyms. Espundia, American leishmaniasis.

Distribution. This infection is widely distributed throughout Central and South America with the exception of Chile and Argentina.

Etiology. The etiologic agent is *Leishmania braziliensis* Vianna, 1911.

Epidemiology. This is a zoonotic forest disease especially affecting workers opening new land.[3,4] Epidemics have occurred among soldiers fighting in the forest, as in Paraguay in the Gran Chaco war. Amastigote forms of this species have been found in some wild rodents that are the natural reservoirs.

Clinical Characteristics. A primary cutaneous lesion similar to an Oriental sore appears on uncovered areas of the body. Local spread to the mucous membranes of the nose, mouth and pharynx takes place later in 2 to 50 per cent of cases, particularly after 1 or 2 years of evolution. In some cases, infections have remained occult for as long as 24 years.[5] Ulceration then occurs with widespread destruction of tissue producing marked deformity, especially in the nose and pharynx (Figs. 44–3 and 44–4 *A, B*).

Diagnosis. During the early months of the infection the parasites are very abundant in scrapings or histologic sections of the margin of lesions. Years later, finding of the

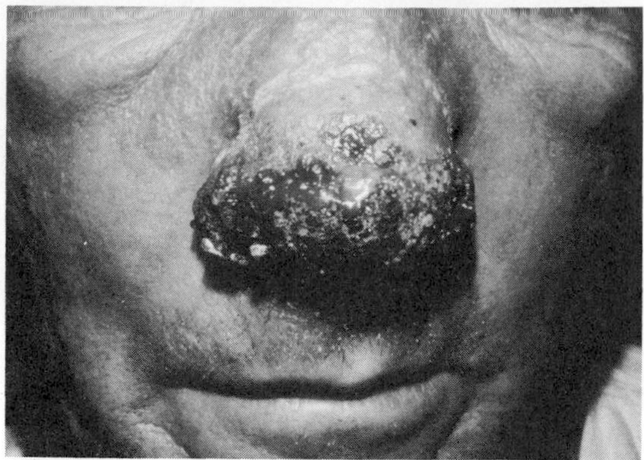

Figure 44-3. Mucocutaneous leishmaniasis. (Courtesy of Dr. Mark R. Feldman, Louisiana State University School of Medicine, New Orleans.)

parasites is very difficult. In certain circumstances culture on NNN medium may be successful.

The Montenegro skin test is very specific and sensitive. It becomes positive 1 or 2 months after infection, and remains positive for life, even after cure.

Differential diagnosis should include syphilis, yaws, leprosy, South American blastomycosis, tuberculosis and malignant tumors.

Treatment. Pentavalent antimonial drugs are used in treatment as in kala-azar (p. 421). More than one course may be necessary. The prognosis of all forms is very good unless metastasis has occurred.

Regression of lesions of dermal leishmaniasis has been observed following treatment with cycloguanil pamoate.[6] The drug was supplied in a suspension of 40 per cent benzyl benzoate and 60 per cent castor oil containing 140 mg of the base in 1 ml of the suspension. It was injected intramuscularly in the following doses: adults, 2.5 ml, containing 350 mg of the base; children, 1 to 5 years, 2.0 ml, containing 280 mg of the base; and infants under 1 year, 1 ml, containing 140 mg of the base. It was helpful to warm the preparation to body temperature and shake the ampule vigorously in order to obtain an even suspension of the drug.

Preliminary studies with an experimental compound (Hoffman-LaRoche No. 7–1051) given orally for 20 days to patients with cutaneous lesions have shown very promising therapeutic results, without side effects. The drug is *N*-benzyl-2-nitro-1-imidazolacetamide. The potential value of an effective and safe oral therapeutic for this disease which occurs in rural areas is obvious.[7]

Bayer 2502 (Lampit), a nitrofurfurylidene derivative, in preliminary studies, was curative in a series of cases of cutaneous and mucocutaneous leishmaniasis in Colombia. In this clinical trial, a dose of 8 to 10 mg per kg daily was employed for 3 to 5 weeks in most of the cases. Tolerance was good, with only mild side effects in a few patients.[8]

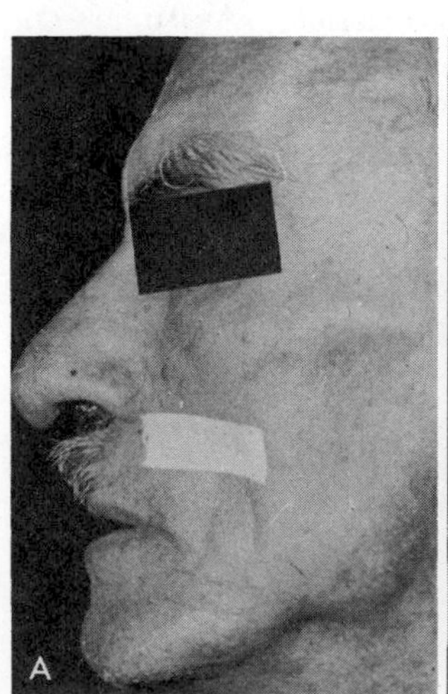

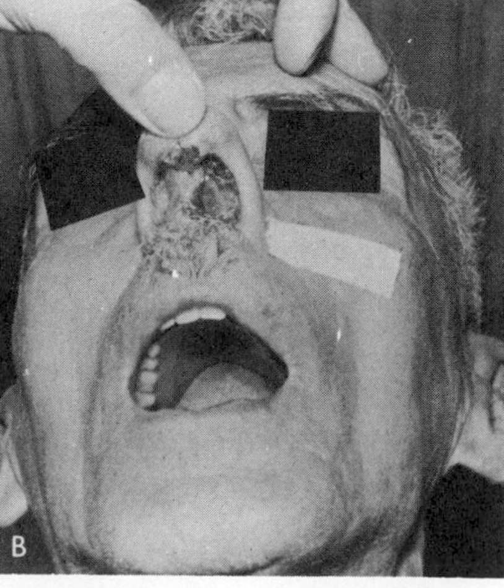

Figure 44-4. Mucocutaneous leishmaniasis in a patient with the disease for more than 15 years (Costa Rica). *A*, Lateral view of the face showing the tapir nose. *B*, Destruction of the nasal septum. (Courtesy of Dr. A. Peña Chavarría, Louisiana State University School of Medicine, New Orleans.)

Chiclero Ulcer

Synonyms. Mexican cutaneous leishmaniasis.

Distribution. The original endemic areas are found in Mexico, southward from the state of Veracruz, in Belize (formerly British Honduras) and northern Guatemala.[9, 10]

Recently, *Leishmania mexicana* has been found in the Amazon basin.[11] It is believed that the parasite is present through the tropical forests of Central America and northern South America.

Etiology. The etiologic agent is *Leishmania mexicana* (Biagi, 1953) Garnham, 1962.[9, 10] (See p. 413 for proposed subspecies of the *L. mexicana* complex.)

Epidemiology. This is a forest zoonosis maintained in nature in *Ototylomys* and other wild rodents.

Man is infected when he enters active foci of transmission that have a spotty distribution along the tropical forests. Not all of the factors influencing the dynamics of transmission are known, but the vector *Lutzomyia flaviscutellata* (called by some authors *L. olmeca*) is more abundant during the long rainy season. This sandfly is also the vector of *Leishmania mexicana amazonensis* in Brazil.[12] It flies and bites predominantly from 5 to 11 P.M. The flight range is very short, so transmission does not take place in towns or even in small villages, but only in the forests. Chicleros working in the jungle during the rainy season acquire the infection much more commonly than other human groups.

Clinical Characteristics. The lesion starts as a pruriginous papule which becomes an ulcer after 1 or 2 months (Fig. 44–5). The ulcer resembles closely that of Oriental sore. Cures occur in almost all cases in less than 6 months, with the exception of the ulcers located in ears. Eighty per cent of the ear lesions remain active for many years and are mutilating (Fig. 44–6). In a few cases regional lymph nodes may be invaded, but this invasion is self-limited. Very rarely a

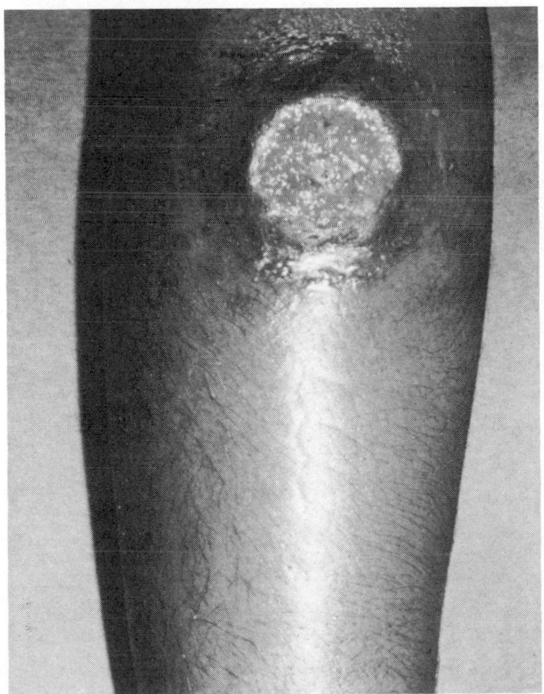

Figure 44–5. Lesion of New World cutaneous leishmaniasis on forearm. (Courtesy of Dr. Mark R. Feldman, Louisiana State University School of Medicine, New Orleans.)

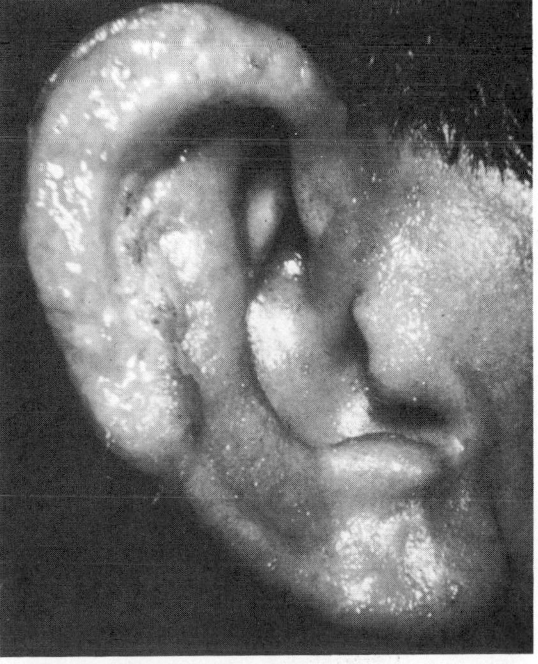

Figure 44–6. Chiclero ulcer. (Courtesy of Dr. Mark R. Feldman, Louisiana State University School of Medicine, New Orleans.)

skin lesion can spread to a contiguous mucous membrane, but metastasis to the naso-oral or other mucous membranes is not observed even in cases with a long-standing infection.

Diagnosis. Parasites are easy to demonstrate in early lesions, but after 2 months of evolution of the infection they are very difficult to find or isolate. The Montenegro intradermal test is very useful for diagnosis and as an epidemiologic survey tool. A recently modified refined antigen for intradermal testing for leishmaniasis has elicited immediately positive reactions.[13] This is in contrast to the delayed hypersensitivity reaction typical of the Montenegro test. Differential diagnosis should be made from cutaneous tuberculosis, sporotrichosis and epithelioma.

Treatment. Treatment is made with antimonials. Metronidazole and cycloguanil pamoate are also useful. Local injection of chloroquine can be useful but painful. Water steam applied daily over the ulcer can be successful. Some of the newer drugs under clinical trial for other forms of leishmaniasis, e.g. RO 7–1051 and Lampit, may prove useful (p. 426).

Prophylaxis. There are no specific measures for most forms of cutaneous or mucocutaneous leishmaniasis, except for deliberate inoculation or vaccination for Oriental sore. Epidemiologically most forms are zoonoses, which renders control unsatisfactory or impracticable. Control measures for phlebotomine vectors and insect repellents are discussed on page 800. However, for laborers in sylvan areas, use of insect repellents is often impracticable. Fine mesh bednets likewise have value, but limited acceptability.

Anergic Cutaneous Leishmaniasis

Synonyms. Leishmaniasis tegumentaria diffusa.

Distribution. This particular type of leishmaniasis has been found in Venezuela, Brazil and Mexico (Fig. 44–7). An Ethiopian form of diffuse cutaneous leishmaniasis with various dermatologic manifestations also occurs[14-18] (Fig. 44–8). In the Sudan, unusual types of leishmanial cutaneous lesions occur, e.g. nodular or nodulo-ulcerative, ulcerative, and nonulcerated diffuse infiltration of skin patches up to 5 cm in diameter.[17]

Etiology. Initially, the name *Leishmania pifanoi* was given to the parasite found in this disease as it occurs in Venezuela. However, it has been demonstrated recently, by studies of human volunteers, that the same parasite isolated from anergic patients with the "diffusa" type of leishmaniasis produced the typical pathology of the cutaneous infection in normal individuals inoculated with this parasite. It has been postulated that the spread of the lesions is due to an immunologic deficiency of the host.

Epidemiology. Sporadic cases occur in endemic areas of other forms of leishman-

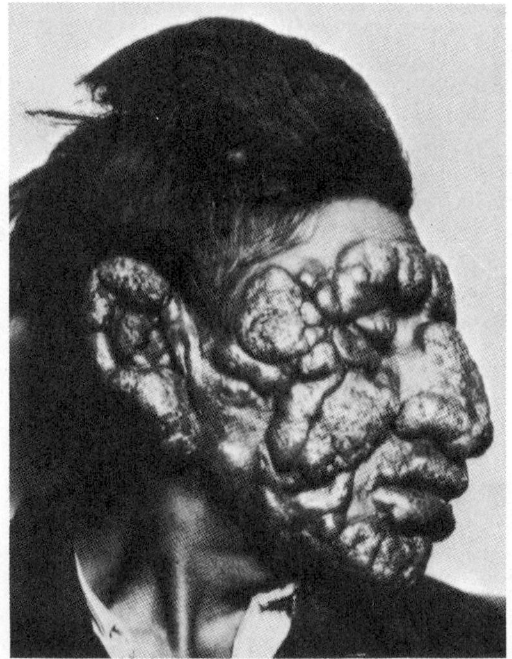

Figure 44–7. Leishmaniasis cutanea diffusa (South America). Diffuse lepromatous lesion. (Courtesy of Dr. P. E. C. Manson-Bahr and Dr. D. J. Winslow. Cutaneous Leishmaniasis. *In* Marcial-Rojas, R. A. (ed.): Pathology of Protozoal and Helminthic Diseases. © 1971, Williams & Wilkins Co., Baltimore.)

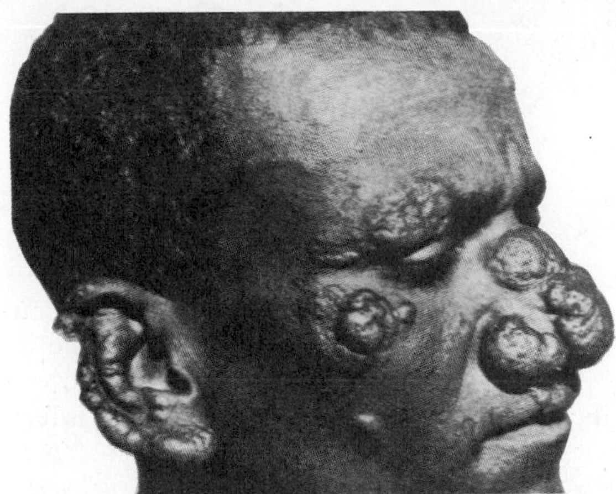

Figure 44–8. Diffuse cutaneous leishmaniasis (Ethiopia) involving nose, cheek, upper lip and ear. (Courtesy of Dr. A. Bryceson. From Dr. P. E. C. Manson-Bahr and Dr. D. J. Winslow. Cutaneous Leishmaniasis. *In* Marcial-Rojas, R. A. (ed.): Pathology of Protozoal and Helminthic Diseases. © 1971, Williams & Wilkins Co., Baltimore.)

iasis. The Ethiopian form of the disease has been studied extensively in recent years, and has a different epidemiology from that of the Sudan. In the latter country, *L. donovani* is thought to be responsible for some of the dermal lesions, as cases occur in areas endemic for kala-azar and dermal lesions may precede visceral; *L. tropica* may be involved in other cases.[17] (See p. 423.) In Ethiopia, the parasite, recently named *L. aethiopica*,[1] is maintained in the reservoir host, the hyrax, and transmitted by *Phlebotomus longipes* and *P. pedifer*.[18]

Clinical Characteristics. After infection, the lesions spread diffusely through the skin, on either the lower areas of the body or the face. There is a broad spectrum of cellular response, from tuberculoid to lepromatous. Usually there is a marked granulomatous reaction producing nonulcerated multiple lepromatoid lesions (Fig. 44–7). The fibrosis of scars is deforming.

Diagnosis. The parasites usually are abundant and easy to find in smears or sections. Isolation of the parasite in culture is readily accomplished. The Montenegro intradermal test is negative.

Treatment. Complete cure is difficult to achieve. Antimonials are useful in some forms; others are antimony-resistant. Relapses are very common.

REFERENCES

1. Bray, R. S., Ashford, R. W., and Bray, M. A. 1973. The parasite causing cutaneous leishmaniasis in Ethiopia. Tr. Roy. Soc. Trop. Med. Hyg. *67*:345–348.
2. Lemma, A., Foster, W. A., Gemetchu, T., Preston, P. M., Bryceson, A. D. M., and Minter, D. M. 1969. Studies on leishmaniasis in Ethiopia. I. Preliminary investigations into the epidemiology of cutaneous leishmaniasis in the highlands. Ann. Trop. Med. Parasit. *63*:455–472.
3. Lainson, R., and Strangways-Dixon, J. 1963. *Leishmania mexicana*. The epidemiology of dermal leishmaniasis in British Honduras. Tr. Roy. Soc. Trop. Med. Hyg. *57*:242–265.
4. Lainson, R., and Strangways-Dixon, J. 1964. Reservoir hosts of *Leishmania mexicana*. Tr. Roy. Soc. Trop. Med. Hyg. *58*:136–153.
5. Walton, B. C., Chinel, L. V., and Eguia y Eguia, O. 1973. Onset of espundia after many years of occult infection with *Leishmania braziliensis*. Am. J. Trop. Med. Hyg. *22*:696–698.
6. Peña-Chavarría, A., Kotcher, E., and Lizano, C. 1965. Preliminary evaluation of cycloguanil pamoate in dermal leishmaniasis. J.A.M.A. *194*:1142–1144.
7. Peña-Chavarría, A. 1974. Personal communication.
8. Restrepo, M., Velasquez, J. P., and Zuluaga, C. B. 1974. Treatment of leishmaniasis with a nitrofurfurylidene derivative (Bay 2502)—Lampit. Proc. 3rd Internat. Congr. Parasit. *3*:1298–1299.
9. Biagi, F. 1953. Síntesis de 70 historias clínicas de leishmaniasis tegumentaria en México (úlcera de los chicleros). Medicina (Méx.) *33*:385–396.
10. Biagi, F., and Velasco. O. 1967. Identidad de *Leishmania mexicana* y su comportamiento en animales de laboratorio. Gac. Méd. Méx. *97*:1412–1417.
11. Ciba Foundation Symposium 20 (new series). 1974. Trypanosomiasis and Leishmaniasis with special reference to Chagas' disease. Associated Scientific Publishers, Amsterdam. 353 pp.
12. Ward, R. D., Lainson, R., and Shaw, J. J. 1973. Further evidence of the rôle of *Lutzomyia flaviscutellata* (Mangabeira) as the vector of *Leishmania mexicana amazonensis* in Brazil. Tr. Roy. Soc. Trop. Med. Hyg. *67*:608–609.
13. Zeledón, R., and Ponce, C. 1974. Parasitological and immunological diagnosis of cutaneous leishmaniasis of the New World. Proc. 3rd Internat. Congr. Parasit. *3*:239–240.
14. Convit, J., Alarcón, C. J., Medina, R., Reyes, O., and Kerdell Vegas, F. 1959. Leishmaniasis tegumentaria diffusa: A new nosological entity. Arch. Venezolanos Patol. Parasit. Med. *3*:218–251.
15. Martínez Ruiz, J. L., Alvarez Fuertes, G., and Biagi, F. 1968. Presencia de la leishmaniasis cutánea generalizada en México. Rev. Invest. Salud Públ. (Méx.) *28*:107–118.
16. Price, E. W., and Fitzherbert, M. 1965. Cutaneous leishmaniasis in Ethiopia. Ethiop. Med. J. *3*:57–83.
17. Abdalla, R. E., Ali, M., Wasfi, A. I., and El Hassan, A. M. 1973. Cutaneous leishmaniasis in the Sudan. Tr. Roy. Soc. Trop. Med. Hyg. *67*:549–559.
18. Ashford, R. W., Bray, M. A., Hutchinson, M. P., and Bray, R. S. 1973. The epidemiology of cutaneous leishmaniasis in Ethiopia. Tr. Roy. Soc. Trop. Med. Hyg. *67*:568–601.

CHAPTER 45

African Trypanosomiasis

FRANK HAWKING

Synonyms. Sleeping sickness; maladie du sommeil (French); Schlafkrankheit (German); Gambian trypanosomiasis or Mid- and West African sleeping sickness; Rhodesian trypanosomiasis or East African sleeping sickness.

Definition. African trypanosomiasis is an acute and chronic protozoal disease produced by hemoflagellates of the genus *Trypanosoma,* family TRYPANOSOMIDAE. It is transmitted by various species of tsetse flies, all of which fall in the genus *Glossina.* The acute disease is distinguished by fever, adenitis, rash and transitory edemas. The chronic form appears when the central nervous system is invaded; it is characterized clinically by meningoencephalitis and meningomyelitis, with wasting and mental and physical apathy which progress into coma and death unless treated.[1]

Distribution. The disease is limited to the tsetse fly areas of Africa. It is endemic throughout most of the tropical area of the continent (Fig. 45–1).

Etiology. *Trypanosoma gambiense* Dutton, 1902, the etiologic agent of Gambian trypanosomiasis, is transmitted by flies of the *Glossina palpalis* group from man to man in whom it produces a chronic disease. *Trypanosoma rhodesiense* Stephens and Fantham, 1910, the causative agent of Rhodesian trypanosomiasis, is transmitted by flies of the *Glossina morsitans* group. *Trypanosoma rhodesiense* is maintained in wild animals, and man is an accidental host; it is more virulent in man than *T. gambiense.* Both *T. gambiense* and *T. rhodesiense* are morphologically identical with *Trypanosoma brucei* Plimmer and Bradford, 1899. The latter trypanosome is maintained in wild animals and usually does not infect man. The taxonomic classification of these three trypanosomes is controversial, and it depends partly on definitions. For practical purposes, *T. gambiense* is a different organism from *T. brucei.* On the other hand, *T. rhodesiense* is merely a name used to indicate strains of *T. brucei* which can infect man.[2,3]

Trypanosoma gambiense and *T. rhodesiense* are slender flagellates tapering to a fine point anteriorly and having a relatively blunt posterior extremity. They vary from about 8 to 30 μm in length. The trypanosomes are polymorphic, some having a free flagellum and some lacking it. When the parasites are present in the blood in considerable numbers, both long and narrow and short and stumpy forms may be seen. The former have a long flagellum, whereas the latter have none, or at most a very short one. At times the nucleus may be situated posteriorly, occasionally close to the kinetoplast. At different stages of the disease trypanosomes may be found in the blood, the lymph and the tissues of the central nervous system.

Epidemiology. RESERVOIR. Man is the reservoir for *T. gambiense;* no important wild animal reservoir has been demonstrated. *Trypanosoma gambiense* probably remains confined to the forest belts because it is unable to produce potent infection in wild animals and because of the behavior of its vector, *Glossina palpalis.*

Trypanosoma rhodesiense is scattered within the savannah fly belts. This species apparently is maintained in wild animals. *Trypanosoma rhodesiense* has been transmitted through sheep, antelope and monkeys. Human volunteers have been infected by a single *G. morsitans* which had fed on experimentally infected sheep, monkeys and several species of wild animals. One strain of polymorphic trypanosomes has been isolated from a naturally infected wild bushbuck (*Tragelaphus scriptus*) and transmitted to man by subinoculation. Several other strains from

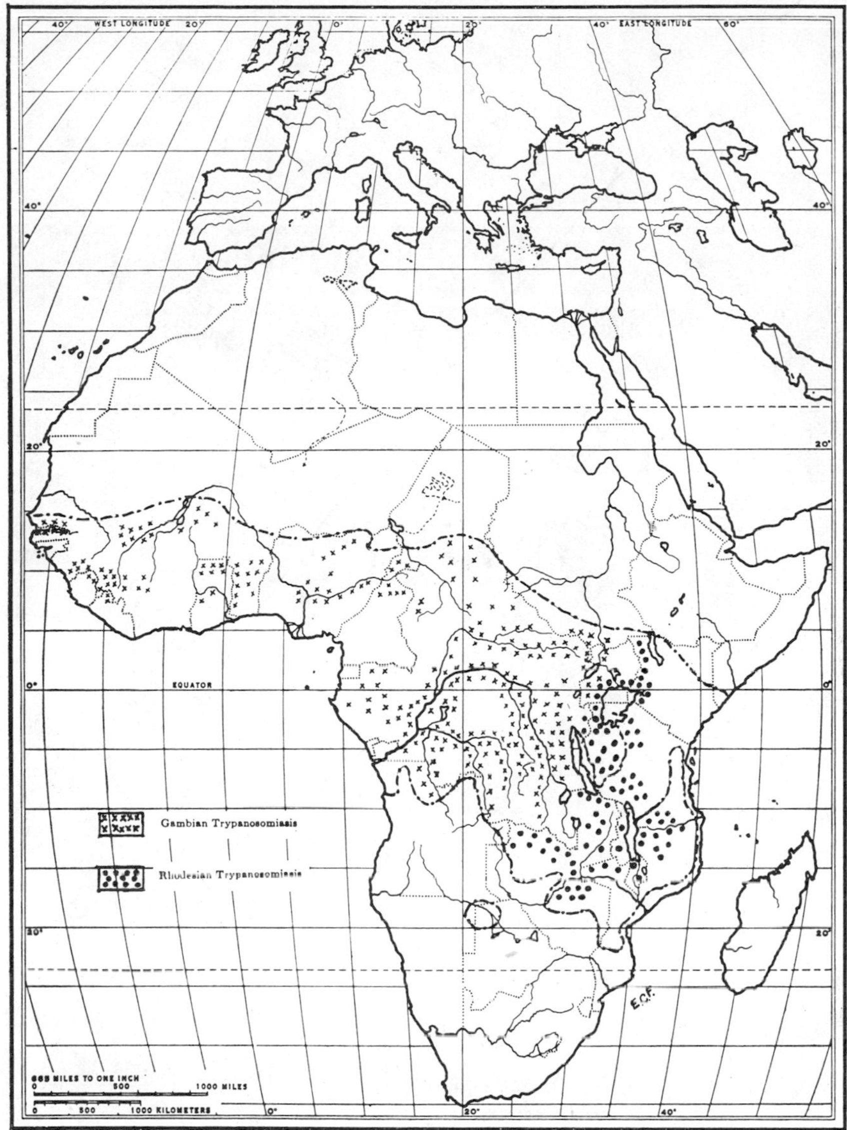

Figure 45–1. Distribution of both Gambian and Rhodesian human trypanosomiasis in Africa. (Slightly modified from Faust, E. C., Russell, P. F., and Jung, R. C. 1970. Clinical Parasitology. 8th ed. Lea & Febiger, Philadelphia.)

game have been found to be resistant to human serum and, therefore, they are probably of the "*T. rhodesiense*" type. It is now clear that "*T. rhodesiense*" can occur in wild game animals and that Rhodesian sleeping sickness is a zoonosis (Fig. 45–2).

VECTOR. These trypomastigotes or trypanosomes undergo cyclical development in various species of *Glossina*, which are the only insect hosts. Endemicity of the infection is therefore limited to tsetse fly–infested areas. The genus *Glossina* contains some 20 species, of which only a limited number have so far been proved to be of importance in the epidemiology of trypanosomiasis (Table 45–1). (See p. 766.)

When these trypanosomes are ingested by the fly they multiply in the midgut. Depending upon conditions of temperature and humidity, long slender forms appear from the eighth to the eighteenth day. These move anteriorly to the proventriculus, then to the salivary glands and ducts where epimastigote or crithidial forms are produced.

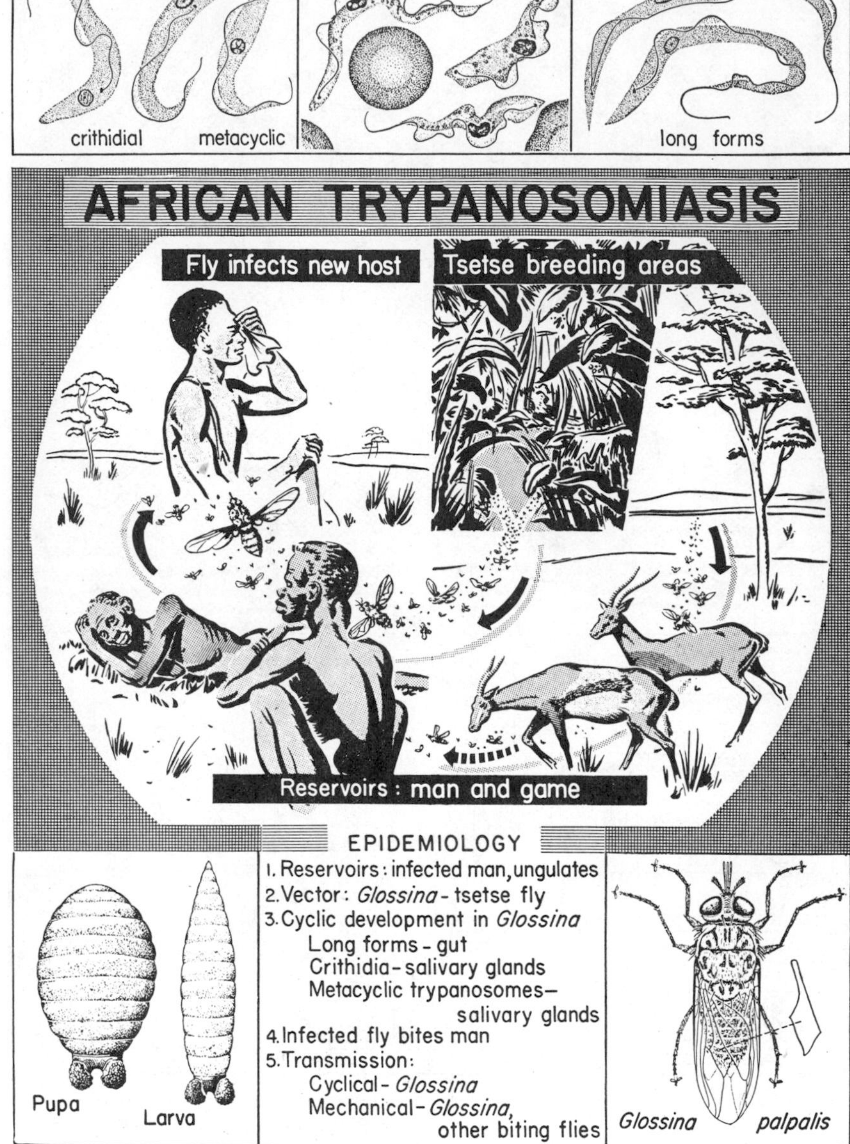

Figure 45–2. Epidemiology of African trypanosomiasis.

Table 45–1. PRINCIPAL VECTORS OF AFRICAN TRYPANOSOMIASIS

Trypanosome Species	*Main Natural* **Glossina** *Vector*
T. gambiense	*G. palpalis* (group); *G. tachinoides*
T. rhodesiense	*G. morsitans; G. pallidipes; G. swynnertoni*
T. brucei	*G. morsitans; G. pallidipes; G. swynnertoni; G. brevipalpis; G. fusca; G. longipennis*

G. palpalis (group) and *G. tachinoides* are mainly riverine-inhabiting tsetse flies.
G. brevipalpis and *G. fusca* are forest-dwelling tsetse flies.
G. pallidipes and *G. longipennis* are associated with thicket vegetation within woodland savannahs.
G. morsitans and *G. swynnertoni* are found in woodland savannahs.

The infective metacyclic trypanosomes, which are similar to the short stumpy trypanosomes observed in the patient's blood in the presence of a heavy infection, are derived from these. They pass down the salivary ducts, entering the bite wound through the channel in the hypopharynx. The fly becomes infective in 18 to 34 days after the infecting meal.

In the presence of epidemic outbreaks of the disease it is possible that mechanical transmission of the trypanosomes from man to man occurs both by the tsetse flies and possibly by the biting fly *Stomoxys* (p. 767). This may occur as the result of interrupted feedings, in the course of which the proboscis has become contaminated with trypanosomes.

INCIDENCE. There is no significant variation in incidence by age, sex and occupation except insofar as these factors may contribute to exposure to the flies. While there is no true racial immunity, it is generally considered that the disease tends to be more acute in the white race than in the colored.

Pathology. The essential pathologic changes of trypanosomiasis are found in the lymph nodes and in the central nervous system.[4] In the early stages there is proliferation of lymphoid tissue. In the chronic stages a productive endarteritis occurs with endothelial proliferation, involving especially the small vessels and accompanied by perivascular infiltration with plasma cells and lymphocytes, giving many of the lesions a histologic appearance similar to those of syphilis. Chronic inflammation of the lymphatic system results in enlargement of the lymph nodes, which in the early stages frequently contain trypanosomes. At this stage, there is usually some enlargement of the spleen. Myocarditis is usually present; there are collections of small round cells between the muscle fibers.

Central nervous system involvement results essentially in a meningoencephalitis and meningomyelitis. These are accompanied by perivascular plasma and round cell infiltration, which is most marked in the pia-arachnoid of the brain and cord, particularly about the vessels of the pons and medulla (Fig. 45–3). The brain and cord are congested; hemorrhages may be present and trypanosomes are frequently scattered through the brain substance. At times, small granulomatous lesions are encountered, especially in the cortex.

Prior to involvement of the nervous system, the cerebrospinal fluid reveals no abnormalities. When lesions are established,

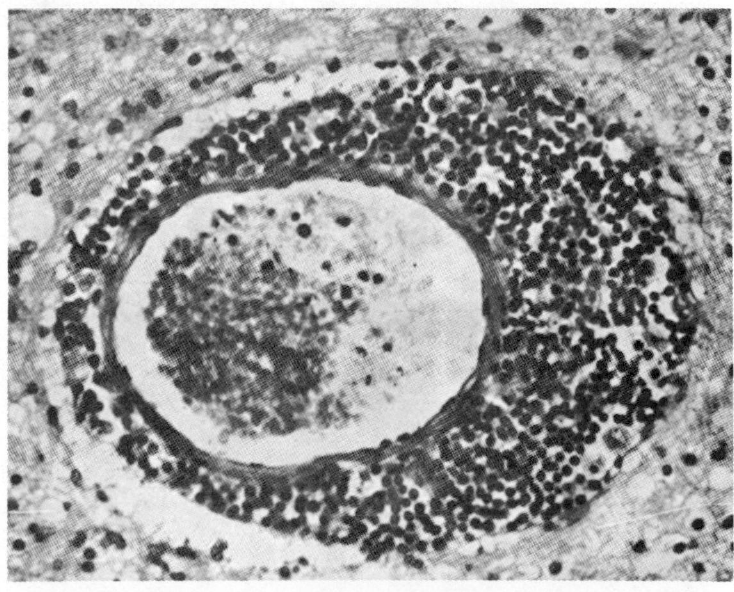

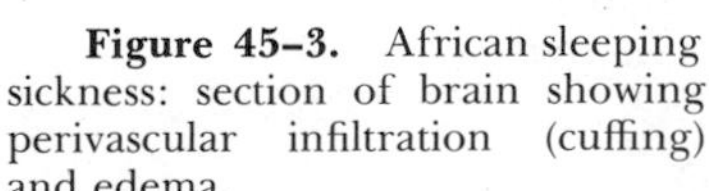

Figure 45–3. African sleeping sickness: section of brain showing perivascular infiltration (cuffing) and edema.

however, the fluid is usually under increased pressure, and the cell count may reach 1000 per cu mm. There is a positive globulin reaction, the total protein is increased, and the centrifuged fluid frequently reveals trypanosomes.

Clinical Characteristics. The clinical manifestations of trypanosomiasis may vary greatly in their intensity and duration. The bite of the infected tsetse fly often is followed by a local inflammatory reaction of the skin that may last 48 to 72 hours or which may develop into a trypanosomal chancre. The incubation period of the disease may show great variation, in occasional instances lasting apparently 2 to 5 years before the appearance of clinical symptoms. Its usual duration, however, is 10 days to 3 weeks.

The disease may be divided into two clinical stages. The first, that of invasion by the trypanosomes, is characterized by fever and lymphadenopathy. The second stage is marked by the onset of central nervous system involvement and is characterized by the symptoms and signs of a meningoencephalitis and meningomyelitis with cachexia and ultimately, in the most severe cases, coma and death.

In the stage of invasion, trypanosomes are present in the peripheral blood but may be more readily demonstrated in fluid aspirated from enlarged lymph nodes (Fig. 45–4). The irregularly remitting fever may be high. Characteristically, the temperature is normal or close to normal in the morning, rising to 39.6 or 40° C (103 or 104° F) at night. The pulse is often faster than would be expected from the height of the temperature. Early in the disease headache, neuralgic pains, insomnia and loss of ability to concentrate are common. In white individuals there is frequently an irregular circinate rash, most commonly observed on the trunk and thighs. This usually appears as irregular oval, pinkish, erythematous areas, having a clear center. Pruritus is common and often severe. Painful local edemas of the hands, the feet, about the eyes and in the vicinity of various joints are frequent and characteristically transitory. All these symptoms and signs, including the febrile reaction, may be irregular and inconstant, disappearing and reappearing after varying intervals.

As the infection becomes established, the superficial lymph nodes become enlarged. This is most evident in the posterior cervical chain where the swelling constitutes one of the most important diagnostic criteria, Winterbottom's sign (Fig. 45–5). This is such a constant accompaniment of African trypanosomiasis that examination for en-

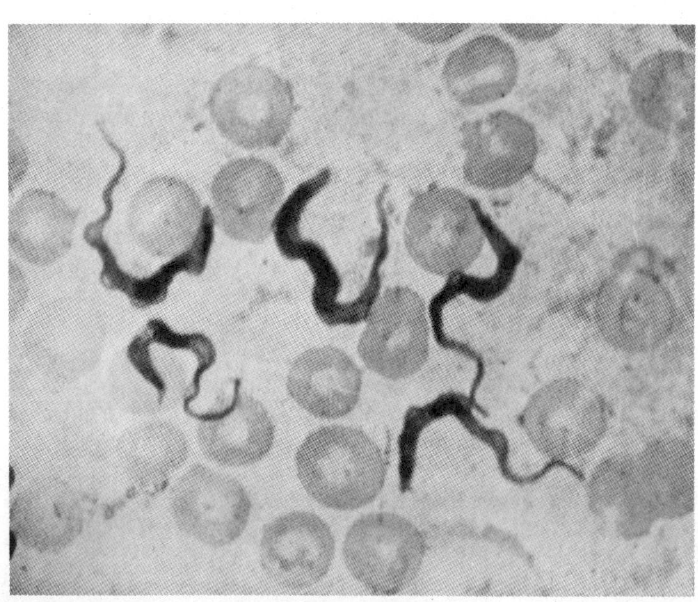

Figure 45–4. *Trypanosoma gambiense* in stained blood film.

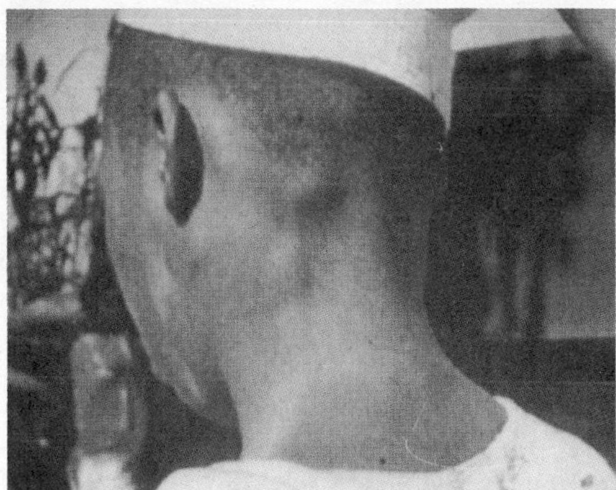

Figure 45-5. Enlargement of posterior cervical lymph nodes—Winterbottom's sign. (Courtesy of Dr. James R. Busvine, London School of Hygiene and Tropical Medicine.)

largement of the posterior cervical nodes is a useful procedure for survey purposes. The individual nodes are discrete, varying from 1.0 to 1.5 cm in diameter. At first they are soft and elastic, later becoming hard as the result of fibrotic changes. The enlargement usually persists from the second to the sixth month of the disease. With the involvement of the lymphatic system there may be some enlargement of the spleen and liver which, with the fever, may be suggestive of a malarial infection.

During this first stage of the disease deep hyperesthesias, especially over the ulna (Kerandel's sign), may occur.

The total leukocyte count is usually normal. There is characteristically a relative mononucleosis, with increased numbers of both large and small mononuclear cells, which may constitute 50 to 70 per cent of the total white blood cells.

The second stage, that of involvement of the central nervous system, may occur early in the clinical course of the infection (Rhodesian type) or may not develop until months or even years later (Gambian type). The onset of this stage is usually insidious. It may be ushered in by tremor of the tongue and fingers, headache, delusions, hysteria, mania and other signs of meningoencephalitis and meningomyelitis. The common presenting symptom is a gradually increasing languor and lassitude. This is followed shortly by the appearance of tremor of the tongue and fingers. With further progression the facial expression is altered; the patient appears apathetic, morose and lethargic; somnolence is common. Speech is slow and mumbling, the gait becomes shuffling, and fine fibrillary tremors of the tongue and of the muscles of the forearms are prominent.

With still further progression the typical sleeping sickness stage is reached. The somnolent state is almost continuous, and it becomes increasingly difficult to arouse the patient. Ultimately, this progresses to true coma. Concurrently, there is progressive

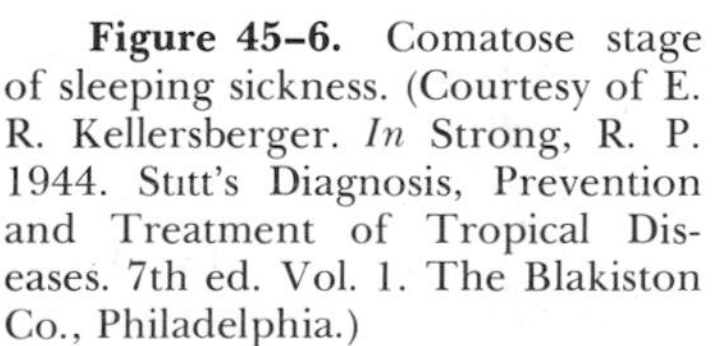

Figure 45-6. Comatose stage of sleeping sickness. (Courtesy of E. R. Kellersberger. *In* Strong, R. P. 1944. Stitt's Diagnosis, Prevention and Treatment of Tropical Diseases. 7th ed. Vol. 1. The Blakiston Co., Philadelphia.)

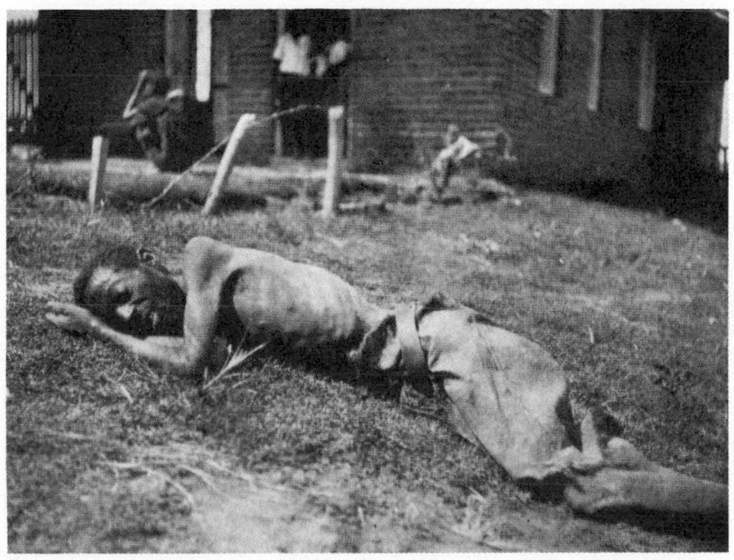

development of marasmus, with wasting, increasing muscular weakness, increasing tremor and dribbling of saliva. Late in the disease epileptiform convulsions may occur. Death ensues as the result of sleeping sickness itself, malnutrition, or intercurrent infection (Fig. 45–6).

Diagnosis. The diagnosis of trypanosomiasis depends upon the demonstration of the trypanosomes in the peripheral blood, in fluid aspirated from enlarged lymph nodes or in the spinal fluid. Frequently trypanosomes are rare or impossible to find in the peripheral blood.

Examination of a stained smear of fluid aspirated from an enlarged elastic lymph node is the most dependable diagnostic procedure in the early stages of the Gambian disease. It is not of value in the later stages when the nodes have become hard and sclerotic. A fine hypodermic needle should be introduced into the substance of a lymph node and the aspirate should be examined under a coverslip with a high dry objective to discover motile trypanosomes. Prolonged search is often necessary. The aspirate can also be used to prepare thick and thin films. These should be stained with Wright's, Giemsa's or Leishman's stains.

Examination of the blood should include the study of both thick and thin smears. It is particularly valuable for Rhodesian trypanosomiasis. The most certain method, however, entails the use of centrifuged citrated blood. The technique is described on page 812.

The cerebrospinal fluid should be examined in all cases. In the stage of early involvement of the central nervous system there may be only a slight increase in the cell count and a positive globulin reaction. Even in this stage trypanosomes may be demonstrable after centrifuging the fluid. As the involvement becomes more extensive, the cell count rises, the pressure is increased and the fluid may have a ground glass appearance or may even be turbid. The cells are predominantly mononuclears.

Examination of the blood of rats, guinea pigs or monkeys after inoculation with blood, lymph node aspirates or spinal fluid from the patient may reveal trypanosomes when other methods fail. Rats are readily infected with *T. rhodesiense*, but *T. gambiense* usually infects only monkeys.

The blood sedimentation rate is markedly increased. An elevated IgM level in the blood, which also occurs in leprosy, kala azar, malaria and syphilis, indicates that prolonged search for trypanosomes should be made. An immunofluorescent test has been described and will probably prove valuable.[5]

Treatment. GENERAL MEASURES. Lumbar puncture should be performed immediately, periodically through the course of treatment, and at least twice at intervals of 6 months after completion of treatment to insure early recognition of central nervous system invasion. It is important to emphasize that the earlier efficient therapy is initiated, the greater are the possibilities of cure.

The drug treatment of trypanosomiasis presents three aspects: the early case; the intermediate and advanced case in which invasion of the central nervous system has occurred; and chemoprophylaxis.[6]

EARLY CASES. Two drugs are recommended for treatment in the stage prior to invasion of the central nervous system.

Suramin (Naphuride, Bayer 205, Antrypol, Moranyl, Fourneau 309, Germanin). The drug is a complex organic chemical that contains no heavy metal. It combines with the plasma proteins and remains in the circulating blood for long periods. It is excreted through the kidneys and frequently acts as a renal irritant, causing albuminuria with yellowish granular casts. More rarely, administration of the drug may be followed by nephritis and uremia. Urinalyses should be performed the day after each treatment, and therapy must be discontinued if there is much albumin and many casts or red cells.

Suramin is still the drug of choice for the early stages of trypanosomiasis and is considered to be particularly useful in cases of infection by *T. rhodesiense.* It is ineffective against infection of the central nervous system. The drug is given intravenously. It must not be given intrathecally because of its irritating effects.

Suramin is administered intravenously

at 5- to 7-day intervals dissolved in 10 ml of distilled water. A preferable schedule is on days 1, 3, 7, 14 and 21. The initial dose should not exceed 0.3 to 0.5 gm because of possible idiosyncrasy. Subsequent doses should be 1.0 gm and should be continued until a total of 7 to 10 gm has been administered. The dosage for children is reduced in accordance with age and weight.

Pentamidine (M&B 800, Lomidine). The drug is an aromatic diamidine available in two forms:

Pentamidine: the isethionate, 1.74 mg equivalent to 1 mg of the base.

Lomidine: the methanesulfonate, 1.56 mg equivalent to 1 mg of the base.

Although it may be administered by mouth, the recommended routes are by intramuscular or intravenous injection. When given too rapidly by vein it may cause a sudden fall of blood pressure. This depressor effect may be prevented by slow administration with the patient in the recumbent position or by intramuscular injection of 0.25 ml of 1/1000 epinephrine or by an antihistaminic given just before the injection of pentamidine. In some instances, blood sugar levels are depressed.

Pentamidine is quite effective in early cases but is less reliable with Rhodesian disease. Solutions of pentamidine must be freshly prepared using sterile distilled water. For intramuscular injection the average dose is 4 mg per kg of body weight dissolved in not more than 3 ml of sterile distilled water; for intravenous administration the dose is 2 to 4 mg per kg of body weight dissolved in 5 to 10 ml of sterile distilled water.

The drug may be given daily or on alternate days for a total of 8 to 10 injections. When administered concurrently with Suramin the depressor effects of pentamidine seem to be reduced.

Another compound, Berenil (diminazene aceturate), has been used very successfully at EATRO, Uganda, for the treatment of early cases. The dosage is 5 mg per kg given intramuscularly, 3 doses at 2-day intervals. This might well become the treatment of choice.

LATER CASES. The onset of the later stages of the disease is marked by the development of central nervous system symptoms and signs and abnormalities of the cerebrospinal fluid. There are two drugs that are useful for the treatment of advanced cases, tryparsamide and Mel B.

Tryparsamide (Tryponarsyl). Tryparsamide contains approximately 25 per cent of pentavalent arsenic, which is reduced in the body to the active trivalent form. It is freely soluble in water. Tryparsamide used to be the main drug used against Gambian sleeping sickness with nervous system involvement but, due to its tendency to produce arsenic resistance in the trypanosomes and to cause optic atrophy, it has now been superseded by melarsoprol and sodium melarsen. It was never effective against *T. rhodesiense.* The drug was given intravenously in doses of 1 gm increasing up to 2 gm in 10 ml of water, weekly for 15 doses. Before each dose, it is important to check visual acuity. This regimen followed a course of Suramin.

Melarsoprol (Mel B, Arsobal). This drug has now replaced tryparsamide wherever medical supervision is available. It is presented as a 3.6 per cent solution in propylene glycol, which is irritant and must be given intravenously. Melarsoprol is effective against *T. rhodesiense* as well as against *T. gambiense,* but it is a dangerous (as well as a very valuable) drug and it should be used with great care. On days 1, 3 and 5, 0.5, 1.0 and 1.5 ml are given respectively; then a rest period of 5 to 7 days; followed by 2.5 ml on each of 3 consecutive days; rest period of 7 days; 3 to 5 ml on 3 consecutive days; rest period of 7 days; 5 ml on 3 consecutive days. A careful watch should be kept on the patient's condition; if side effects appear, the next doses should be postponed.

The important toxic reactions to melarsoprol and other melaminyl compounds concern the nervous system. *Reactive encephalopathy* may occur in up to 13 per cent of Rhodesian cases; from this patients often recover. This occurs more often in late-stage patients, but it may occur in early ones also. It usually develops during or after the first course of injections; if this phase is passed safely, the later courses seldom cause trouble. Apparently the reaction is due to the action of the drug on the diseased brain, the symptoms consisting of increased mental excitement and other signs of cerebral derangement. Treatment is by prompt cessation of chemotherapy at any suggestion of trouble and by sedation if required. A few days after recovery, treatment may be resumed very cautiously. *Hemorrhagic encephalopathy,* which is rare but almost always fatal, seems to be a direct toxic reaction, as occurs with other arsenical compounds. Typically there is sudden loss of consciousness with stertorous breathing and hyperpyrexia.

In spite of these dangers, melarsoprol is a most valuable drug, and will cure many cases of nervous system involvement which would otherwise be incurable and fatal. It should be used with careful supervision, the systemic parasitemia being best removed beforehand by a course of Suramin.

Melarsonyl Potassium (Mel W, Trimelarsan). This is a water soluble analogue of melarsoprol, which may be given by intramuscular or subcutaneous injection. It is similar to melarsoprol in toxicity, but is less effective against Rhodesian disease. The usual dosage is 3 to 4 mg per kg (maximum 200 mg) on 3 to 4 consecutive days, repeated after 2 weeks.

Melarsen (Melarsen sodium). This is the pentavalent form of melarsoprol, analogous to tryparsamide. Its toxicity is little greater than that of tryparsamide, but it has been overshadowed by melarsoprol. Theoretically Melarsen should be more effective in penetrating the nervous system. The dosage is 20 mg per kg intravenously at 5- to 7-day intervals for 8 to 12 injections.

Nitrofurazone (Furacin). This compound acts in some patients but not in others. It should be used in patients who have become resistant to melarsoprol, and who are otherwise incurable. It is given by mouth as 0.5 gm 3 to 4 times per day for 5 to 7 days, repeated once or twice after an interval of 1 week. The toxic symptoms consist of polyneuropathy, and of hemolytic anemia, similar to that caused by primaquine.

In all cases, the success of treatment should be checked by examination of the cerebrospinal fluid at the end of treatment, and 6 and 12 months later.

Prophylaxis. The recognition, isolation and effective therapy of infected persons constitutes one of the most important measures in the prophylaxis of trypanosomiasis.[7] Individuals entering disease-free areas from regions in which the disease is endemic should invariably be examined and subjected to medical control and treatment if infected. This is particularly true of native populations imported for labor purposes.

The second important control measure is directed against the vector.[8, 9] In fly-infested areas individuals should wear suitable clothing, including long sleeves and long trousers. The flies are attracted by moving objects and will frequently follow individuals or automobiles for considerable distances. They bite easily through thin clothing. Motor vehicles passing into a controlled area should be carefully examined for the presence of the tsetse. Insofar as possible, heavily infested areas should be avoided. It has been necessary on occasion in the past to evacuate population groups of considerable size from regions where satisfactory control of *Glossina* was not practicable.

The control of African trypanosomiasis is complicated by the fact that both cattle and man are involved. In the past, therapeutic action for the control of trypanosomiasis has been successful in coping with Gambian sleeping sickness. However, in the *G. morsitans* savannah fly belt it is more feasible to attempt to control the vector. This involves a direct attack against the adult flies by widespread spraying of residual insecticides and also by suitable clearing of the trees and bush. The food supply, i.e. animals, can perhaps be depleted through the use of fences, game control, and opening up the country to agriculture. Other modifications of these basic steps will, of course, be necessary after a detailed study is made of each area where control is attempted.

Two drugs have proved to be effective chemoprophylactic agents: *Suramin* and *pentamidine.* Suramin in dosage of 1 gm every 2 to 3 months exercises a definite protective action. However, pentamidine confers practically complete protection against *T. gambiense* for more than 6 months. The dose is 4 mg per kg (maximum 300 mg) given intramuscularly.

Pentamidine was administered as mass prophylaxis on a large scale in West Africa up to 1961. Since then it has been mostly abandoned because it was unpopular with the local populations.

Chemoprophylaxis is *not* recommended for individuals, owing to the risk of incurring latent infections which might not be detected until too late.

REFERENCES

1. Mulligan, H. W., and Potts, W. H. 1970. The African Trypanosomiases. Geo. Allen & Unwin, London, 950 pp.
2. Rickman, L. R., and Robson, J. 1970. The blood incubation infectivity test: a simple test which may serve to distinguish *Trypanosoma brucei* from *T. rhodesiense.* Bull. W.H.O. *42*:650–651.
3. Hawking, F. 1973. The differentiation of *Trypanosoma rhodesiense* from *T. brucei* by means of human serum. Tr. Roy. Soc. Trop. Med. Hyg. *67*:517–527.
4. Goodwin, L. G. 1970. The pathology of African trypanosomiasis. Tr. Roy. Soc. Trop. Med. Hyg. *64*:797–812.
5. Latif, B. M., and Adam, K. M. G. 1973. Differentiation of *Trypanosoma brucei, T. rhodesiense,* and *T. gambiense* by the indirect fluorescent antibody test. Bull. W.H.O. *48*:401–407.
6. Duggan, A. J. 1973. The treatment of African trypanosomiasis. Trop. Doctor *3*:162–164.
7. W.H.O. Tech. Rep. Ser. No. 434. 1969. African trypanosomiasis. Report of a Joint F.A.O./W.H.O. Expert Committee. Geneva, 25–30 November 1968. 79 pp.
8. Ford, J. 1969. Control of the African trypanosomiases with special reference to land use. Bull. W.H.O. *40*:879–892.
9. Jordan, A. M. 1974. Recent developments in the ecology and methods of control of tsetse flies (*Glossina* spp.) (Dipt., Glossinidae)—a review. Bull. Ent. Res. *63*:361–399.

CHAPTER 46

American Trypanosomiasis

VICTOR M. AREÁN

Chagas' Disease

Synonyms. American trypanosomiasis, schizotrypanosomiasis, opilação, enfermedad de Chagas.

Definition. This is an acute, subacute or chronic disease produced by infection with *Trypanosoma cruzi* which especially affects children and young adults. It is characterized pathologically by the presence of trypanosomes in the blood and leishmanias in the tissues. The acute stage is manifested by fever, facial and general edema, adenitis, anemia and the presence of subcutaneous nodules (paniculitis). The symptoms in the chronic stage depend upon the localization of the parasite in the heart, the central and autonomic nervous systems, liver, spleen and other organs.[1-3]

Distribution. The disease is found chiefly in rural areas. Human infections have been reported from every country in the Western Hemisphere with the exception of Canada, Surinam and Guyana. Patients suffering from diffuse myocarditis have been observed in Trinidad and the United States (Georgia). Serologic tests on these patients suggested that *T. cruzi* was the responsible etiologic agent.[4, 5] Recently, positive serologic tests for Chagas' disease were obtained in Papago native Americans in Arizona.[6] *Trypanosoma cruzi* has been isolated from the insect vectors and from wild rodents in Arizona, California, Georgia, Louisiana, Maryland, New Mexico and Texas.[7] Two authenticated indigenous cases of Chagas' disease have been recorded in the United States, both from Texas.[8] In addition, a patient, originally from Ecuador, was observed in New York with achalasia and a positive Machado-Guerreiro test.[9]

Etiology. *Trypanosoma cruzi* Chagas, 1909 is a pleomorphic trypomastigote or trypanosome having two phases in its life cycle. One occurs in man and other mammals, and one in the transmitting insects. In the infected mammal typical trypanosomes are present in the blood; amastigotes or leishmanias and transformation stages occur in the endothelial and tissue cells.

The trypanosome is approximately 20 μm in length, often spindle-shaped, and

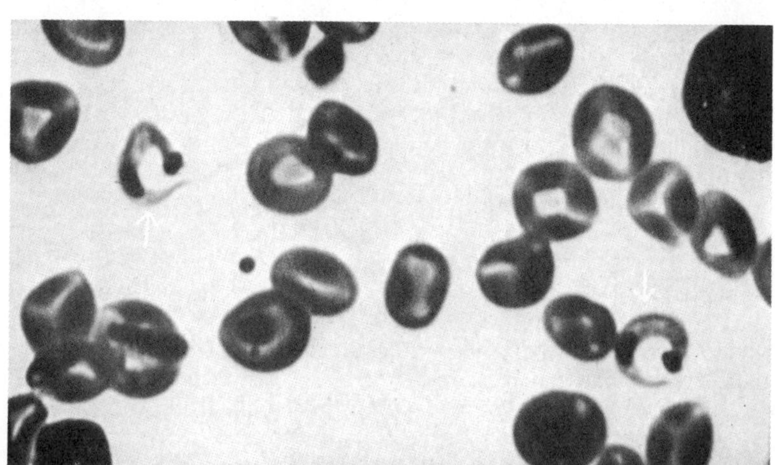

Figure 46-1. *Trypanosoma cruzi* in stained blood film.

presents both long and short forms. The nucleus is centrally placed, and the characteristically large oval kinetoplast is situated posteriorly. An axoneme arises from the dotlike kinetoplast complex and is extended along the margin of a narrow undulating membrane. It presents few folds, becoming a free flagellum anteriorly. Characteristically, this trypanosome presents a sharp wedge-shaped posterior extremity. In stained films the parasites usually appear C- or U-shaped. Dividing forms do not occur in the blood (Fig. 46–1).

The trypanosomes invade tissue cells, lose the flagellum and undulating membrane and assume the leishmanial form; these are round or oval bodies 3 to 5 μm in diameter, presenting both a nucleus and a kinetoplast. *Trypanosoma cruzi* may be grown on artificial culture media. (See p. 831.)

Epidemiology. American trypanosomiasis is primarily a domestic infection in rural areas. The infection is transmitted by species of several genera of reduviid or triatomine bugs (family REDUVIIDAE, subfamily TRIATOMINAE). The reservoirs of *T. cruzi* are man and domestic and wild mammals. Some of the sylvatic reservoir hosts frequent inhabited areas, and triatomine vectors associated with them may enter human dwellings. This establishes a link between wild and domestic cycles of this zoonosis (Figs. 46–2, 46–3). The epidemiology of *T. cruzi* infection is determined, to a large extent, by the triatomine insect vectors involved, the domestic and sylvatic reservoirs and socioeconomic conditions, particularly housing.[10]

Dogs and cats are important domestic animal reservoirs, especially in those areas where *Triatoma infestans,* which has a wide

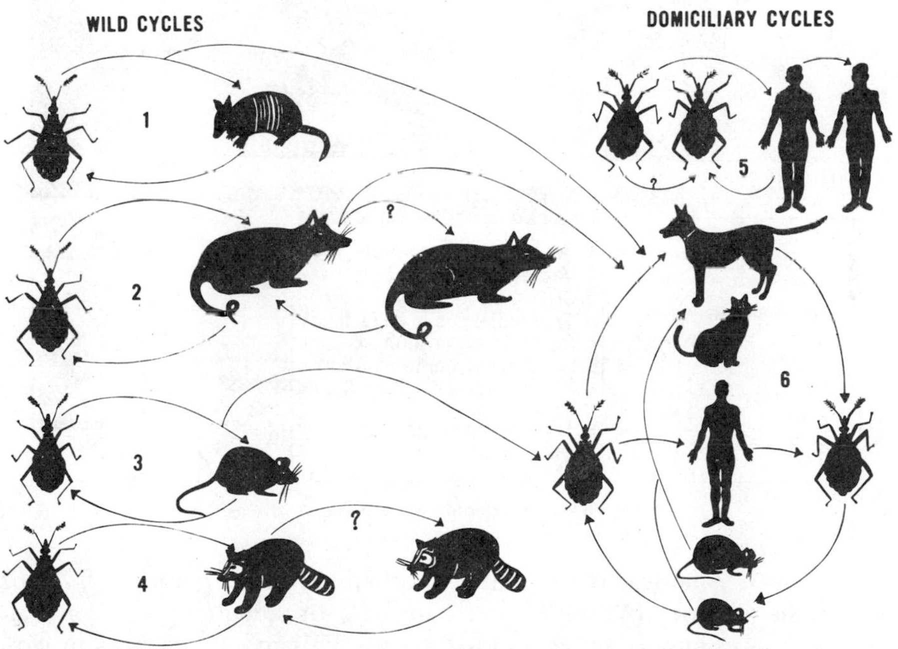

Figure 46–2. Wild and domestic cycles of Chagas' disease – modalities and relationships. *1, Panstrongylus geniculatus* is often associated with armadillos: adults enter houses, attracted by lights. *2,* Opossums (*Didelphis* spp.) are associated with several triatomines and both marsupials and insects visit human dwellings. *3,* Rats and other rodents are associated with insects that also fly to houses. *4,* Raccoons may be associated with triatomines but, as with opossums, they may transmit *T. cruzi* among themselves without participation of the insect. *5,* In the absence of domestic animals there is a cycle between the insect and man. Transmission from one insect to another has been suggested and transmission from man to man is a fact, both transplacentally and transfusionally. *6,* Other domestic animals might participate in the cycle and some of them may become infected by eating small rodents. (From Zeledón, R. *In:* Trypanosomiasis and Leishmaniasis with special reference to Chagas' disease. Ciba Foundation Symposium 20, new series, 1974. Published by Elsevier. Excerpta Medica. North-Holland, Associated Scientific Publishers, Amsterdam. p. 69.)

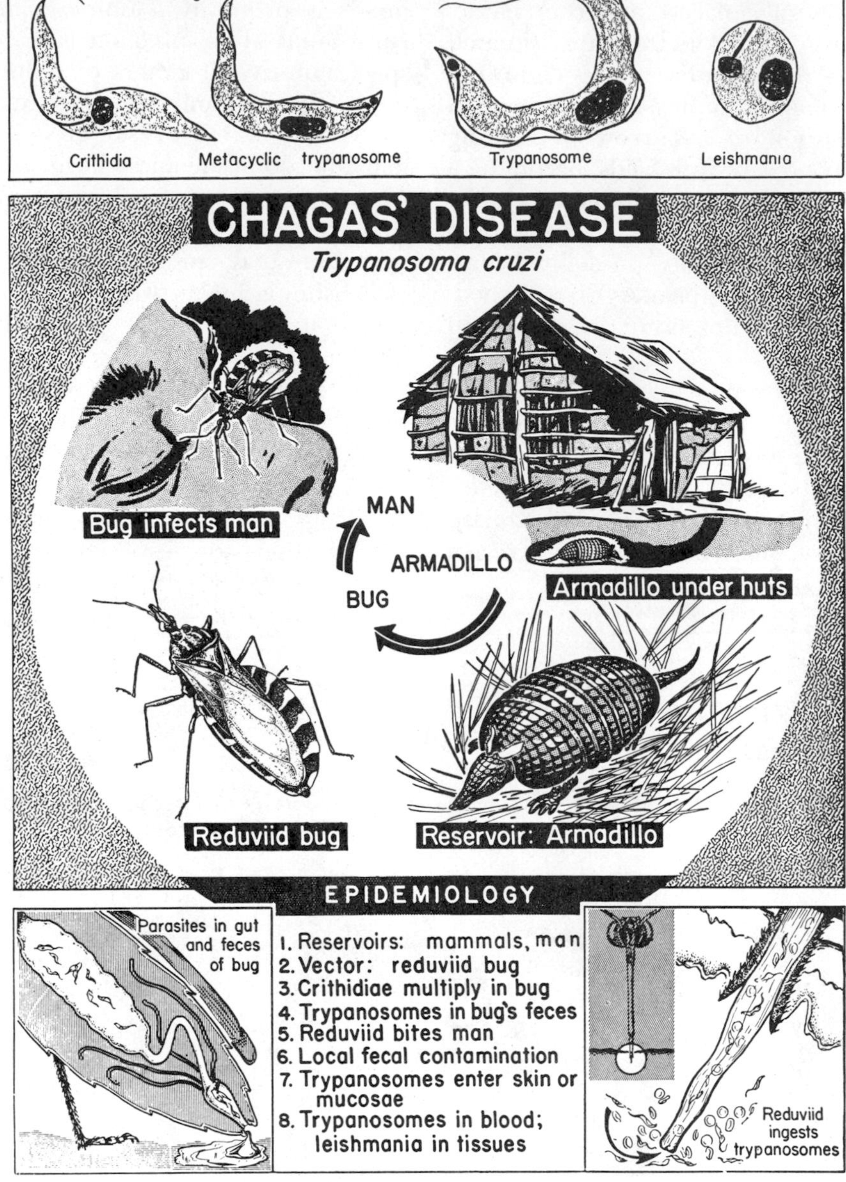

Figure 46–3. Epidemiology of Chagas' disease.

distribution in South America, is the principal vector of the disease. In Bolivia and Peru guinea pigs are important as intradomestic reservoirs. The common rat, *Rattus rattus,* appears to be the main domiciliary reservoir in Panama and Costa Rica. Species of opossum are probably the most important sylvatic reservoirs in the American continent. They have a wide distribution from Argentina to the United States. The common opossum has a long, perhaps lifelong, parasitemia, probably due to lack of adequate immunologic mechanisms. This marsupial lives in close association with several triatomine species, assuring its continued infection. In some areas the armadillo is an important reservoir, with high indices of infection. The raccoon, skunk, domestic pig and a few species of monkeys have been found infected with *T. cruzi.* In all, about 150 species of animals have been incriminated as reservoir hosts of *T. cruzi.*[10]

Triatomine bugs are also called Mexican bedbug, cone-nose bug, wild bedbug, "chinche del monte," assassin bug or kissing bug. The common name of kissing bug is based upon the predilection of the bug to attack the face, particularly of sleeping children. The bugs are avid blood-suckers. Some species have a potent salivary toxin that produces intense local pain. Other species expertly puncture skin and draw blood almost painlessly. Of the approximately 92 known species of triatomines in the New World, about 36 have been found associated with human dwellings; only one-third of these are epidemiologically important as vectors. Species of the genera *Triatoma, Rhodnius, Panstrongylus, Eutriatoma, Eratyrus, Mepraia* and *Psammolestes* reported as vectors of *T. cruzi* in Mexico, Central and South America are listed in Table 70–1 (p. 737). Reduviid bugs naturally infected with *T. cruzi* in the United States are shown in Table 70–2 (p. 737). In North America the most common vector is *Triatoma gerstaeckeri*.[7]

The insect vectors frequently inhabit the nests of opossums and burrows of armadillos (Fig. 46–2) and likewise adapt themselves to living in adobe, mud, cane or poorly constructed rural homes with cracks in walls and dimly lit rooms. They are also found commonly in outbuildings, such as stables and pigsties, and in woodpiles adjacent to or in houses. In Costa Rica, *Triatoma dimidiata* is commonly found with opossums in hollow trees and is passively brought into the house in lumber or firewood. *Panstrongylus geniculatus*, a triatomine frequently associated with armadillos, is readily attracted to human habitations by lights (Fig. 46–3).[10]

The triatomine becomes infective 8 to 10 days after ingestion of *T. cruzi.* It may remain infective for as long as 2 years. After ingestion by the bug the trypanosomes multiply in the midgut by longitudinal fission, with the development of noninfective crithidia, which have a centrally placed nucleus and a kinetoplast toward the anterior end. Subsequently, intermediate forms with a kinetoplast variously situated and metacyclic trypanosomes with the kinetoplast at the posterior extremity are formed. The latter have a well developed undulating membrane and flagellum. The metacyclic trypanosomes are found in the hindgut of the reduviid and are passed in its feces. When the insect feeds, the feces containing metacyclic trypanosomes contaminate the bite wound or an abrasion of the skin, or the organisms may penetrate directly through the mucous membranes of the conjunctiva or lips.

Other means of transmission of Chagas' disease exist. Transmission of *T. cruzi* infection by blood transfusion is rapidly increasing. Another mechanism is via the damaged placenta. Chagasic placentitis can be an important cause of abortion; congenital infection of a child, usually born prematurely, is quite frequent. A microepidemic of Chagas' disease, in the absence of insect vectors nearby, has been attributed to transmission through food contaminated by feces and urine of infected opossums found in the vicinity.[10]

There is no racial or sex distribution of the infection in man. Only 1 per cent of persons infected with *T. cruzi* presents enough clinical symptoms to attract the attention of the physician. The disease is observed at any age, although it predominates in children. The prognosis is less favorable in those under 2 years of age.

Pathology. The parasites multiply rapidly at the site of inoculation, where a severe inflammatory reaction is induced; this is characterized by the presence of neutrophilic leukocytes, round cells, marked interstitial edema and focal lymphangitis (chagoma). The parasites also invade the fat cells of the affected area, where they multiply within the cytoplasm until the host cell disintegrates and a lipogranuloma develops.

During the stage of dissemination the parasites can be found in the blood and in any organ or tissue of the body. However, they show a preference for cells of mesenchymal origin (cardiac and skeletal muscle, reticuloendothelial cells, neuroglia).

In the infected cells the parasite multiplies by binary fission until large numbers of leishmania fill the cytoplasm and distend the cellular membrane, producing a leishmanial pseudocyst (Fig. 46–4). Some amas-

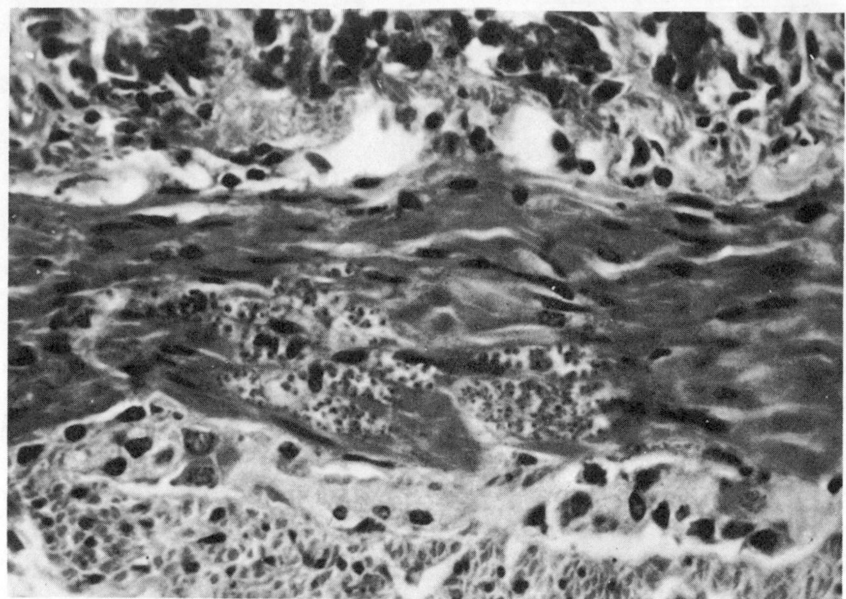

Figure 46-4. Leishmanial pseudocysts in smooth muscle cells of esophagus. (Courtesy of Dr. Fritz Köberle, Ribeirão Preto, São Paulo, Brazil.)

tigotes or leishmania become elongated, produce a flagellum and are transformed into epimastigote or crithidial forms. These in turn undergo binary fission, giving rise to trypanosome forms which may enter the circulation. In humans there is no multiplication of the trypanosomes in the blood stream. The leishmanias that are released into the interstitial spaces by rupture of the pseudocyst must enter a new host cell promptly; otherwise, they quickly lose their capacity to transform into metacyclic forms and soon die. As long as the parasites are intracellular, the inflammatory response is minimal or absent. With disruption of the cell and death of the leishmania, toxic products are liberated that immediately induce an inflammatory reaction, the severity of which is conditioned by the immunologic state of the host.

In early infections the infiltrate is composed mainly of neutrophilic leukocytes, followed later by the appearance of plasma cells, lymphocytes and histiocytes. In older infections the immune state results in the production of granulomatous inflammatory responses of more localized character, with formation of pseudotubercles and presence of giant cells. The adjacent nonparasitized cells may show waxy or hyaline degeneration with partial or complete disappearance of cross striations and necrobiosis. Because the parasite involves cells at random, the inflammatory reaction is at first focal. However, in massive infections or in chronic processes, it adopts a more diffuse character. Healing takes place by fibrosis and results in more or less severe degrees of myocardial insufficiency, depending upon the extensiveness of the inflammation. Involvement of the conduction system of the heart may occur by parasitization of its fibers or secondary to adjacent fibrosis. Similar changes are also detected in skeletal muscle and in subcutaneous fatty tissue. In the spleen, liver, lymph nodes and lungs, there are numerous nodules of hyperplastic reticuloendothelial cells and histiocytic granulomas. The leishmanias can be observed readily in the infected muscle fibers, but are more difficult to see in the reticuloendothelial system or in fat cells.

Meningoencephalitis is an especially severe complication of acute Chagas' disease, fatalities being highest in small children. In the central nervous system the inflammatory reaction is characterized by invasion of

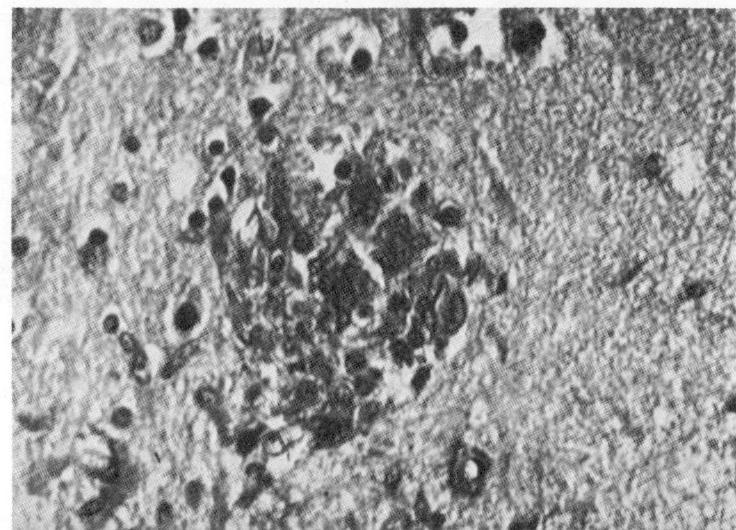

Figure 46-5. Nodules in brain: necrosis, cellular proliferation and infiltration.

neuroglia cells (Fig. 46-5), the presence of numerous glial nodules scattered throughout the white and gray substance, basal ganglia and, more rarely, the cerebellum. Degeneration of neurons, perivascular lymphocytic cuffing, focal endarteritis and leptomeningitis are also encountered.[11]

In recent years attention has been drawn to the frequency of megaesophagus, megacolon and dilatation of other tubular organs in chronic cases of Chagas' disease.[9, 11-17] Pathologic studies have shown that the basic lesion is a degeneration of the intramural autonomic nervous plexuses secondary to the toxic action of *T. cruzi.* In some instances, intramural neurons may be detected, although severe degenerative changes can be recognized in the cytoplasm or nucleus of the affected ganglion cells.[11] Extensive experimental studies have given support to the role played by *T. cruzi* in the genesis of megaesophagus, megacolon and pathologic dilatation of other tubular organs.

Clinical Characteristics. The clinical manifestations of Chagas' disease vary markedly. In general, the younger the individual, the greater the severity of the infection.

Acute Chagas' disease is observed mainly in children under 2 years of age. After an incubation period of 7 to 14 days high continuous fever, which may reach 40° C (104° F), anorexia, vomiting, diarrhea and other systemic symptoms develop, indicating a severe infectious process. Frequently there are unilateral conjunctivitis and edema of the eyelids and face, followed by swelling of the lacrimal glands and of the submax-

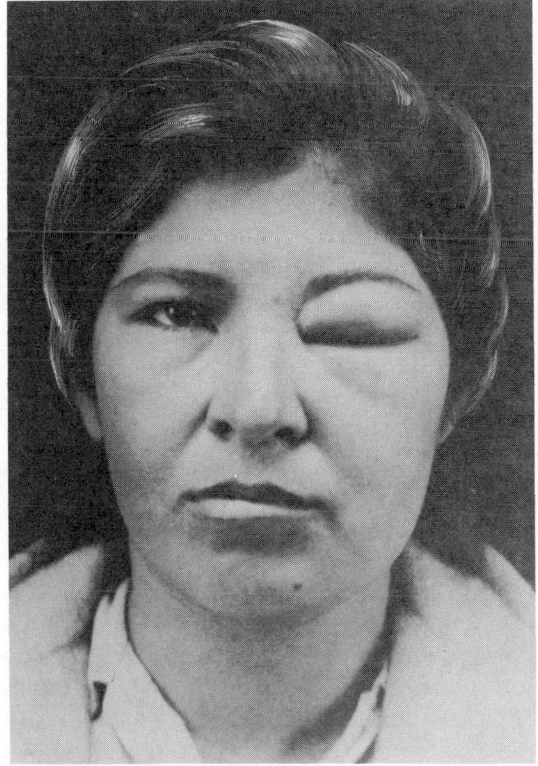

Figure 46-6. Ophthalmoganglionar complex (Romaña's sign) in Chagas' disease. (Courtesy of Dr. Ramon S. Freire, Chaco, Argentina.)

illary lymph nodes (oculoglandular complex, Romaña's sign) (Fig. 46–6). However, Romaña's sign is not always due to the presence of the parasite, but may be related to allergic responses following repeated bites by uninfected reduviid bugs. In severe cases nonpitting edema may spread to other parts of the body. There are generalized enlargement of the lymph nodes, hepatosplenomegaly and meningoencephalic irritation. Cardiac arrhythmias, myocardial insufficiency and collapse are often present and may result in death; sometimes the fatal outcome follows extensive damage to the central nervous system.

Some children develop a milder type of disease characterized by the presence of numerous subcutaneous, painful nodules throughout the body (lipochagomas). There appears to be a peculiar predilection for the involvement of the adipose pad of the cheek (Bichat's pad); because of the extreme tenderness during contraction of the masseteric muscles, the child, after swallowing a few times, refuses to feed and malnutrition develops. In these cases the temperature rises only slightly, but vomiting, diarrhea and signs of tracheobronchitis may be severe and will complicate the picture.

The acute stage may resolve completely in a few weeks or months, or may pass into the subacute or the chronic stage. Parasitemia, which is found consistently during the febrile periods, may also be observed in individuals who no longer show clinical symptoms of the disease. The subacute form is characterized by severe asthenia, mild fever, generalized lymphadenopathy and other symptoms; it may last for months or years. In the chronic stage the clinical manifestations are chiefly secondary to myocardial involvement. In mild cases the cardiac changes may be limited to tachycardia or extrasystoles; some patients show cardiac arrhythmias, atrioventricular or right bundle branch block. In more severe cases there are dilatation of the heart, progressive myocardial insufficiency and, eventually, cardiac failure; in these patients the electrocardiogram shows widening and notching of the QRS complex, and abnormalities in the P and T waves.[12, 13] In young adults the disease may manifest itself in the form of a subacute myocarditis, with death occurring within 1 to 6 months after onset of symptoms.[12–14] Characteristic of this form is the fact that, aside from the symptoms and signs resulting from the massive involvement of the heart, other manifestations of the disease are lacking. It is probable that a number of cases labeled as "idiopathic myocarditis," especially in areas where Chagas' disease is endemic, may actually be due to *T. cruzi* infections. The difficulty in isolating the parasite in these patients, added to the scarcity of leishmanial forms in the tissues, makes it most difficult to establish the correct diagnosis. However, many of these cases give positive serologic tests consistent with a diagnosis of chronic Chagas' disease. In addition there are generalized lymphadenopathy, mild fever, anemia and, occasionally, splenomegaly. In the acute stage a leukocytosis ranging from 18,000 to 30,000 white cells per cu mm of blood and with a predominance of lymphoid elements (70 to 90 per cent) may be seen. A moderate eosinophilia also occurs.[8]

Congenital infections due to transplacental transmission of the parasite seem to be more common than generally suspected.[10, 15, 16] (See p. 443.) As a rule, infants with congenital Chagas' disease are born prematurely and show marked hepatosplenomegaly, abdominal distention and a high susceptibility to bacterial infections, which may lead to death within a short time after birth. Cardiomegaly, megaesophagus and diffuse meningoencephalic lesions testify to the severity and widespread dissemination of the parasite in the newborn. Trypanosomes can be seen in the peripheral blood shortly after birth. The diagnosis has been proved by either xenodiagnosis, serologic tests, or both. Mothers of affected children were also positive upon serologic or xenodiagnostic tests, even when asymptomatic.

A common complication of Chagas' disease is dilatation of tubular organs. In one study, 85.9 per cent of 85 cases with megaesophagus gave a positive complement-fixation test for Chagas' disease. Megaesophagus and megacolon (Fig. 46–7) are frequently

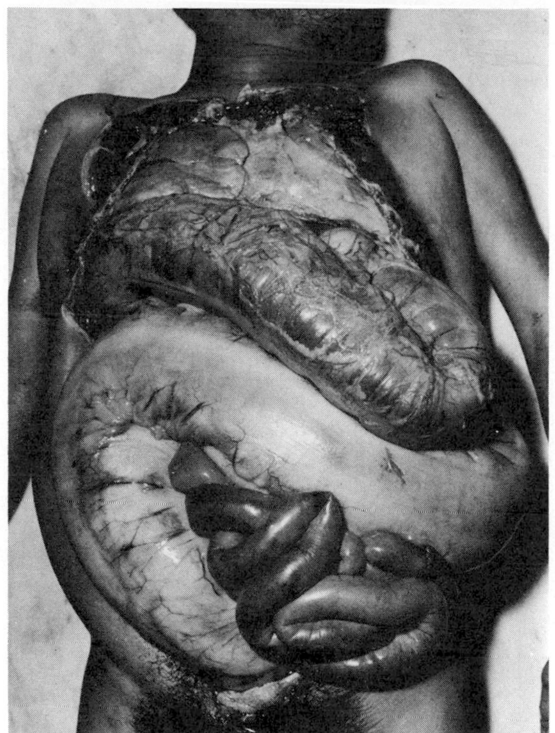

Figure 46–7. Megacolon in chronic Chagas' disease. (Courtesy of Dr. Fritz Köberle, Ribeirão Preto, São Paulo, Brazil. Published in J. Trop. Med. *61*:21–24, 1958.)

observed in endemic areas of trypanosomiasis.[9, 11, 17] Abnormal esophageal function is observed radiologically in 35 per cent of patients with chronic Chagas' disease and the incidence of megacolon is considered to be even higher. Often at autopsy patients will show simultaneous dilatation of both esophagus and colon. Abnormal dilatation of other tubular organs (ureters, urinary bladder, duodenum, stomach) occurs less frequently. Experimental and clinical evidence have proved beyond doubt the causal role of *T. cruzi* in the pathogenesis of neurologic dysfunction leading to these conditions.[11, 17]

On the other hand, the high incidence of hypothyroidism in the same areas, which was once regarded as secondary to chagasic infections, has how been shown to be the result of entirely unrelated causes. Nevertheless, authenticated cases of chagasic thyroiditis are on record.

Diagnosis. The diagnosis of Chagas' disease is based upon identification of the parasite in blood or tissue samples or by serologic procedures. Parasitemia may be demonstrated by the following methods:

1. Examination of fresh blood films.
2. Examination of stained thick and thin blood films.
3. Examination of stained films after centrifuging 5 to 10 ml of citrated blood.
4. Animal inoculations using 5 to 10 ml of the patient's blood. Most laboratory animals are easily infected; the white rat is a suitable test animal. In order to increase the susceptibility of laboratory animals to the infection it is advisable to inject them with 2.5 mg of cortisone at the same time the inoculum is administered.[8] Blood must be checked periodically for 60 days, starting 2 weeks after the inoculation. If no trypanosomes are seen in the blood during this period, the animals should be killed and the heart, liver and spleen studied histologically to determine the presence or absence of leishmanial forms.
5. Culture of blood on NNN medium or culture in blood broth.
6. Xenodiagnosis. Clean uninfected laboratory-bred reduviid bugs are allowed to feed on the suspected patient. Two weeks later the contents of the hindgut are examined for the presence of crithidia and particularly metacyclic trypanosomes. In conducting this test it is essential to use clean insects properly protected, since they can become infected by coprophagy.

It is necessary to keep in mind that xenodiagnosis gives a variable percentage of positivity and that not all reduviids fed on diseased persons become infected. The test gives a higher percentage of positive results when repeated several times.

Positive parasitemia is to be expected only when blood is obtained during the acute febrile stage of the disease or during one of the febrile episodes of the chronic form. When hematologic examinations are negative, an alternative procedure is that of obtaining a biopsy from skeletal muscle for the identification of leishmanial forms in muscle cells. Biopsy of enlarged lymph nodes (mainly those of the retroauricular or submandibular region) may reveal the parasite. Occasionally, needle aspirates from the spleen will render a positive diagnosis, although this is not recommended as a diagnostic procedure. *Trypanosoma cruzi* is seldom encountered in the cephalospinal fluid, and then only in cases showing meningoencephalitic manifestations.

The Machado-Guerreiro test (a complement-fixation test using antigen from *T. cruzi*) is a valuable adjunct in the diagnosis of the disease. Positive results are obtained in over 95 per cent of the cases. Cross-reactions are obtained occasionally in cases of mucocutaneous leishmaniasis. However, the clinical picture and signs of this disease are so strikingly different from those of Chagas' disease that such cross-reactions do not detract from the validity of this test.

Immunoglobulin levels are normal in Chagas' disease, although a slight elevation in IgG may be found in patients with active chronic infections. On the other hand, specific anti-trypanosome antibodies of the IgM class are found in the acute phase and more rarely in the chronic phase. A direct antibody test using epimastigotes as antigen has been employed successfully in the detection of congenitally acquired Chagas' disease. Specific anti-trypanosome antibodies of the IgG and IgA class are found in the acute phase also, but the titers are much higher in the chronic phase of the infection.[18, 19]

An autoimmune mechanism is operative in production of cardiopathy in Chagas' disease. An immune globulin specific for chagasic myocardiopathy, referred to as endothelial-vascular-immunoglobulin (EVI), has been demonstrated.

Intradermal Test. A clear immediate skin reaction can be elicited in chronic Chagas' disease by using soluble protein antigen from parasites grown in culture. The optimum amount of nitrogen in the antigen is about 100 gamma per ml. The reaction can be positive in cutaneous leishmaniasis, but the Montenegro test will differentiate it.[20]

Treatment. At present there is no commercially available curative drug for the treatment of Chagas' disease.[1] A number of nitrofuran compounds have been shown to reduce the number of circulating trypanosomes to the point that they are demonstrable only by xenodiagnosis or by animal inoculation with blood. Furazolidone has been used in chronic infections with encouraging results.[21] Nitrofurazone (5-nitro-2-furaldehyde-semicarbazone), L-furaltadone and Bayer 2502 have been introduced recently in the treatment of this infection. Experimental studies have shown that nitrofurazone will destroy intracytoplasmic leishmanial bodies without damage to normal cells.

Preliminary results with an experimental compound, RO 7–1051, *N*-benzyl-2-nitro-1-imidazolacetamide, indicate that this compound may be useful for the treatment of acute and chronic cases of Chagas' disease.[22] The dosage employed was 8 to 10 mg per kg per day during 30 days in acute and 60 days in chronic cases. A substantial apparent cure rate, based upon xenodiagnosis, was obtained. The serologic tests became negative in a high percentage of the acute cases after treatment, but not in the chronic cases. Skin reactions, in 16 per cent of the cases, were the commonest side effect of the drug. This compound is also being employed experimentally for some forms of cutaneous leishmaniasis (p. 426).

Chlortetracycline and steroids should be avoided since they tend to exacerbate the disease.[8] Otherwise, the treatment is largely symptomatic.

Prophylaxis. Native houses and adobe and thatched huts in the endemic area should not be used for sleeping quarters, since they constitute the normal harborage of the insect vector. Some protection of individuals resident in such structures may be afforded by proper use of bed nets, since the vectors are nocturnal feeders.

Gammexane is highly effective in controlling the reduviid bug population when used as a residual spray inside buildings and huts. It is claimed that entire reduviid bug populations have been eliminated by the use of this chemical. Dieldrin (2.5 per cent emulsion) or lindane (1 per cent in hydrocarbon base) is also effective in killing the reduviids. However, applications of the insecticide must be repeated at 2- to 4-week intervals, as eggs may not be affected by these compounds. (See Table 72–1, p. 796.)

Numerous instances of infection by *T. cruzi* have followed transfusion.[23] Although complement-fixation tests are not dependable for clinical diagnosis, they do provide an important tool for use in screening prospective blood donors. In endemic areas the complement-fixation test should be used routinely, and persons having a positive reaction should be eliminated as potential donors. The addition of 25 ml of a 0.5 per cent solution of gentian violet per each 500 ml of blood 24 hours before transfusing is reported to prevent the transfer of *T. cruzi*.[24]

Trypanosoma Rangeli

Human infections with *Trypanosoma rangeli* (Tejera, 1920) (= *Trypanosoma ariarii* and *Trypanosoma guatemalense*) have been reported from Venezuela, Colombia, Brazil, Panama, El Salvador, Guatemala and Costa Rica. This parasite probably occurs in man in some other Latin American countries where reduviids of the genus *Rhodnius* are common. Natural infections with *T. rangeli* have been found in dogs, monkeys and opossums. Identification was based upon the morphology of the parasite and its evolution in the reduviid vectors. Infection with the organism can be induced in laboratory animals, mainly in rats and mice, by using massive inoculations of cultures, even with those containing only crithidial stages.

Mixed infections of *T. rangeli* and *T. cruzi* are often encountered in man. Evidence of pathogenicity or symptoms have not been observed in persons with natural infections of *T. rangeli* or in human volunteers. Complete knowledge of the development of *T. rangeli* in mammalian hosts is lacking. Dividing forms, which are extremely scanty, have been found in peripheral blood. The organisms may be isolated from the blood, either by xenodiagnosis or by culture, several months after infection. This parasite does not produce intracellular forms as *T. cruzi* does.

The trypanosomal forms in peripheral blood are about 30 μm in length. The nucleus is anterior to the middle of the organism. A small, deeply staining kinetoplast is present.

In the insect vector, the flagellates are found in hemolymph in the body cavity. After a period of active reproduction, they invade the salivary glands where small metacyclic trypanosomes are produced. Promastigote (leptomonad), epimastigote (crithidial) and metacyclic trypanosomes have been found in the reduviid vector *Rhodnius prolixus*, in which the parasite was first observed. The metacyclic trypanosomes have been demonstrated in *R. prolixus* and *R. pallescens*, the latter being the principal vector in Panama.[25] The transmission to man and animals is by the bite of the bug rather than through its excreta, since the metacyclic trypanosome assumes an anterior station.

REFERENCES

1. Ciba Foundation Symposium 20 (new series). 1974. Trypanosomiasis and Leishmaniasis with special reference to Chagas' disease. Elsevier. Excerpta Medica. North-Holland, Associated Scientific Publishers, Amsterdam. 353 pp.
2. Cançado, J. R. (ed.). 1968. Doença de Chagas. Hospital das Clinicas, Belo Horizonte, Brasil. 666 pp.
3. Olivier, M. C., Olivier, L. J., and Segal, D. B. 1972. A Bibliography of Chagas' Disease (1909–1962). U.S.D.A. Index Catalogue of Medical and Veterinary Zoology Special Publication No. 2, Washington. 633 pp.
4. Fistein, B., and Sutton, R. M. P. 1963. Chagas' disease in the West Indies. Lancet *1*:330–331.
5. Farrar, W. E., Kagan, I. G., Everton, F. D., and Sellers, T. F. 1963. Serologic evidence of human infections with *Trypanosoma cruzi* in Georgia. Am. J. Hyg. *78*:166–172.
6. Miller, J. H. 1974. Personal communication.
7. Wood, S. F., and Wood, F. D. 1961. Observations on vectors of Chagas' disease in the United States. III. New Mexico. Am. J. Trop. Med. Hyg. *10*:155–165.
8. Woody, N. C., and Woody, H. B. 1961. American trypanosomiasis. I. Clinical and epidemiologic background of Chagas' disease in the United States. J. Pediatr. *58*:568–580.
9. Scherb, J., and Arias, I. M. 1962. Achalasia of the

esophagus and Chagas' disease. Gastroenterology *43*:212–215.

10. Zeledón, R. 1974. Epidemiology, modes of transmission and reservoir hosts of Chagas' disease. *In:* Trypanosomiasis and Leishmaniasis with special reference to Chagas' disease. Ciba Foundation Symposium 20 (new series). Elsevier. Excerpta Medica. North-Holland, Associated Scientific Publishers, Amsterdam. pp. 51–85.
11. Köberle, F. 1970. The causation and importance of nervous lesions in American trypanosomiasis. Bull. W.H.O. *42*:739–743.
12. Laranja, F. S., Dias, E., Nobrega, G., and Miranda, A. 1956. Chagas' disease: A clinical, epidemiologic and pathologic study. Circulation *14*:1035–1060.
13. Andrade, Z. A., and Andrade, S. G. 1971. Chagas' disease (American Trypanosomiasis). *In* Marcial-Rojas, R. (ed.): Pathology of Protozoal and Helminthic Diseases. The Williams & Wilkins Co., Baltimore. pp. 69–85.
14. Andrade, Z. A., and Andrade, S. G. 1963. Forma subaguda da miocardite chagásica. Rev. Inst. Med. Trop. São Paulo *5*:273–280.
15. Howard, J. E., Rios, C., Ebensperger, I., and Olivos, P. 1957. Enfermedad de Chagas congénita. Bol. Chil. Parasit. *12*:42–45.
16. Rubio, M., Ebensperger, I., Howard, J. E., Knierim, F., and Náquira, F. 1962. Búsqueda de enfermedad de Chagas en 100 madres de prematuros, con hallazgo de un caso de enfermedad de Chagas congénita. Bol. Chil. Parasit. *17*:13–16.
17. Earlam, R. J. 1972. Gastrointestinal aspects of Chagas' disease. Am. J. Dig. Dis. *17*:559–571.
18. Lelchuk, R., Dalmasso, A. P., Inglesini, C. L., Alvarez, M., and Cerisola, J. A. 1970. Immunoglobulin studies in serum of patients with American trypanosomiasis (Chagas' disease). Clin. Exper. Immunol. *6*:547–555.
19. Szarfman, A., Otatti, L., Schmuñis, G. A., and Vilches, A. M. 1973. A simple method for the detection of human congenital Chagas' disease. J. Parasit. *59*:723.
20. Zeledon, R., and Ponce, C. 1974. A skin test for the diagnosis for Chagas' disease. Tr. Roy. Soc. Trop. Med. Hyg. *68*:414–415.
21. Coura, J. F., Ferreira, L. F., and Rodrigues da Silva, J. 1962. Experiencia con a nitrofurazona na fase crónica da doença de Chagas. O. Hospital *62*:957–964.
22. Lugones, H., Rabinovich, B., Cerisola, J. A., Ledesma, O., and Barclay, C. 1974. Preliminary results of the anti-*T. cruzi* activity of Ro 7-1051 in man. Proc. 3rd Internat. Cong. Parasit. *3*:1297–1298.
23. Pereira de Freitas, J. L. 1952. Primeiras verificacoes de transmisão accidental da molestia de Chagas ao homen per transfusão de sangre. Rev. Paulista Med. *40*:36–40.
24. Nussenzweig, V., Amato Nato, V., de Freitas, J. L. P., Nussenzweig, R. S., and Biancalana, A. 1955. Molestia de Chagas em bancos de sangre. Rev. Hosp. das Clinicas *10*:265–283.
25. Sousa, O. E. 1972. Anotaciones sobre la enfermedad de Chagas en Panamá. Frecuencia y distribución de *Trypanosoma cruzi y Trypanosoma rangeli.* Rev. Biol. Trop. *20*:167–179.

SECTION VII
Helminthic Diseases

CHAPTER 47
Introduction

The term "helminth" was originally derived from the Greek and means "worm." As usually interpreted the word connotes several groups of parasitic worms. These are the true roundworms, or Nematoda, and the flatworms, or Platyhelminthes, which include two important groups parasitizing man—the trematodes (Trematoda) or flukes, and the cestodes (Cestoda) or tapeworms. Both roundworms and flatworms are considered as phyla by some authorities. Two smaller phyla, the "hair snakes" or Nematomorpha and the thorny-headed worms or Acanthocephala, are rarely recorded as human parasites. "Hair snakes" or gordiid worms probably reach the intestine of humans by accidental ingestion of free-living stages or by drinking raw water containing the insect hosts in which the worm is developing. Actually, only two species of Acanthocephala have been reported from humans, and infections by these are rare. Therefore, these last two groups will not be considered further in this book.

If one interprets the term "helminth" broadly, one might also include the leeches (Hirudinea, Annelida), which actually are free-living worms except when engorging on the blood of their victim. This group is discussed on page 688.

Parasitic worms infect humans in almost all regions of the world, but there is a particular abundance of them in the tropics—an abundance of both species and infected individuals. This is the result of important climatic and sociologic factors. Many of these parasites require special conditions of temperature and humidity for survival and multiplication. Many others require particular vertebrate or invertebrate hosts such as fish, snails, crustacea or insects for the completion of their life cycles. These hosts, in turn, gain ready access to man in tropical regions owing to the lack of preventive measures by the indigenous populations. Insect vectors, such as various mosquitoes, midges and biting flies, are particularly important among these intermediate hosts.

The distribution of those helminthic parasites whose eggs are passed in human dejecta is affected not only by the climatic conditions of rainfall, temperature and humidity but likewise by the sanitary practices of the population. The custom in many regions of the world of using human excreta (nightsoil) for fertilizer results frequently in widespread pollution of soil, water supplies and certain foods and the transmission of infection.

Moreover, racial food habits often determine the incidence of certain of these parasites in man. The practice of eating raw or partially cooked freshwater fish and shellfish, meat and certain aquatic plants in which, or upon which, encysted larvae of parasitic worms occur permits completion of the biologic cycle and infection of man. Root vegetables pickled in weak concentrations of vinegar or brine are an important potential source of infection, since eggs of *Ascaris lumbricoides, Trichuris trichiura* and even hookworm have been shown to remain viable in such foods for considerable periods.

The parasitic way of life of the helminths has brought about numerous modifications in structure, function and even life cycles. Some of these changes are characteristic of groups while others may be peculiar to given genera or species. For example, the integument or cuticula of helminths, secreted by the underlying cells, forms a hardened, tough and elastic, or delicate covering which is resistant to digestion during the life of the parasite. Often it is specialized to form hooks or cutting plates, such as occur in the buccal cavity of hookworms, the stylets of the microfilariae, or other spines, spicules or hooks. Both the trematodes and tapeworms may possess circular suckers, or acetabula, that serve as holdfast or locomotor organs. However, in some species of tapeworm, such as *Diphyllobothrium latum,* the holdfast device is a poorly developed, although very efficient, pair of sucking grooves. Many helminths possess glands that open near the mouth, and these are believed to secrete enzyme-like substances that cause tissue destruction. Some parasites use this tissue directly as food, whereas for others the destruction merely makes it possible for them to penetrate to a definitive location within the host.

Many organs of locomotion, nutrition and reproduction have undergone marked changes in parasitic organisms. Parasites usually are transported from place to place by the host, and in many instances may be transmitted passively from one host to another. This has been associated with a reduction in the development of locomotor devices. Organs of nutrition have become modified or even lost, as in the case of the tapeworms. On the other hand, the reproductive organs have undergone considerable development and are often larger and more complicated than those found in free-living relatives. Frequently, the production of tremendous quantities of eggs is associated with the slender chance that an egg or larva will succeed in reaching, and establishing itself on or within, another host. These structural or physiologic differences may be characteristics of the large groups, or perhaps only of genera or species.

Helminths almost without exception do not multiply in man as adults, thus differing signally from other disease-producing organisms. The pathologic changes that they induce in the host are the effects of a variety of mechanisms. The hookworm is a voracious feeder upon blood, which it obtains through lacerations of the intestinal mucosa produced by its cutting plates or teeth. Certain of the tapeworms merely rob the host of food, whereas others, utilizing man as an intermediate host for their larval forms, produce single or multiple expanding tumors in many anatomic locations. Other parasites entering the skin cause more or less severe dermatitis, probably the result of toxic secretions, enzymes or metabolites of the larvae after penetration. Certain helminths produce pathologic changes in the subcutaneous tissues, the eye, the lungs and other viscera in the course of the migrations of the larvae or adult worms. Certain of the filarial worms that localize in the vessels of the lymphatic system cause acute and chronic inflammation, which may be followed by lymphatic obstruction. The spined eggs of the schistosomes, deposited in the smaller venous channels of the bowel and vesical walls, produce vascular damage and ulceration into the viscus. Further, the mechanical irritation from the eggs or chemical irritation from products of the contained embryo appears to induce epithelial hyperplasia and metaplasia, which may be followed occasionally by carcinoma.

Thus, the pathologic changes accompanying helminthic infections may be both varied and severe, and the resulting clinical phenomena produce serious and acute or chronic disease. The severity of clinical manifestations is readily enhanced when the frequent combination of malnutrition and parasitism by some species of helminths exists. Infection in the same person with multiple species of helminths, often accompanied by parasitism with various species of protozoa, is a very frequent occurrence. Thus, the physician must think in terms of the possibility of the coexistence of multiple parasitoses in patients, in addition to organic and infectious diseases of nonparasitic etiology which may be obscured by the parasitic infections. A common trinity of intestinal helminthiases includes ascariasis, hookworm infection or disease, and trichuriasis. The spread in the geographic distribution and the increase in prevalence of some species, in an expanded world population with resultant exposure of more people in endemic areas, probably render the classic report of Stoll almost 3 decades ago (p. 489, Reference 29) inadequately reflective of the "wormy world" of the present. The diseases caused by parasitic worms constitute a most important segment of tropical medicine. The practicing physician must be familiar with this group of conditions, their epidemiology, pathology, clinical manifestations, and the life cycles of the parasites in order to practice either therapeutic or preventive medicine successfully.

Endemic areas of worm infections certainly are not limited to the tropics and subtropics. Infections are frequently observed in temperate areas, in migrant population groups or in travelers who acquired their infections in the tropics. Thus, physicians outside the tropics and subtropics also must have adequate knowledge of helminthiases.

CHAPTER 48

Intestinal Nematodes

MORPHOLOGY OF THE NEMATODES IN GENERAL

Introduction. All parasitic nematodes possess certain common characteristics. These will be considered briefly. Other pertinent data dealing with the morphology and biology of the specific subdivisions will be taken up in the subsequent chapters. *Strongyloides stercoralis* is believed by many to be the only heterogenetic nematode infecting man—the only one with both free-living and parasitic generations. All the others are parasitic during part or all of each life cycle.

All nematodes are characterized by their elongate, cylindrical, unsegmented bodies and glistening cuticula. The sexes are separate; the males are smaller than the females and are usually curved ventrally. Nematodes possess a simple, tubular alimentary canal which includes an anterior mouth and a posterior anus (Fig. 48–1).

Intestinal species range in size from those that are essentially microscopic or a few millimeters long *(Trichinella spiralis* and *S. stercoralis* or *Capillaria philippinensis* adults) to 35 cm or more *(Ascaris lumbricoides)*, and some of the nematodes inhabiting blood or other tissues may be nearly a meter long *(Dracunculus medinensis)*.

Nematode Structure. Externally nematodes are covered with a non-nucleated, shiny *cuticula* secreted by underlying subcu-

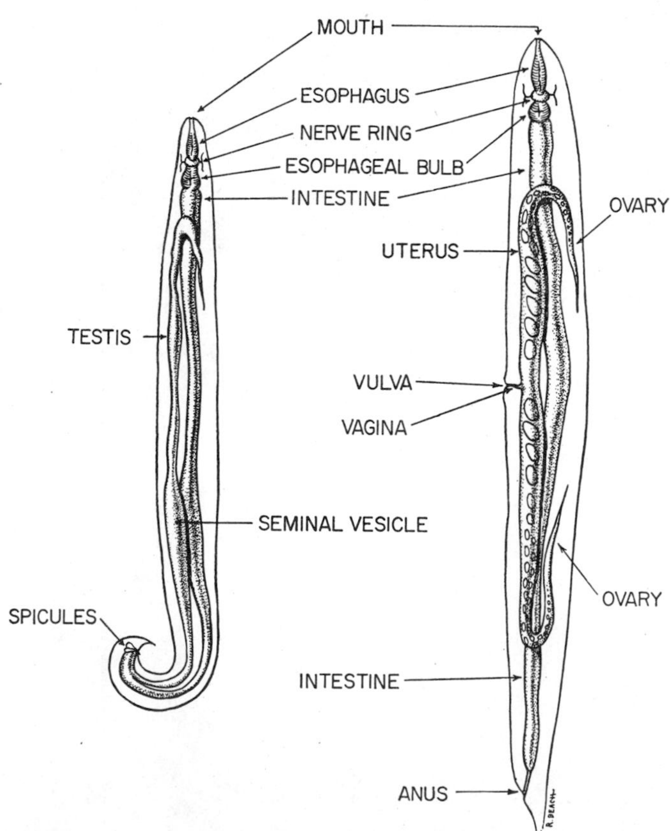

Figure 48–1. Morphology of a typical nematode. (Modified from various authors; courtesy of the University of Florida College of Medicine, Gainesville.)

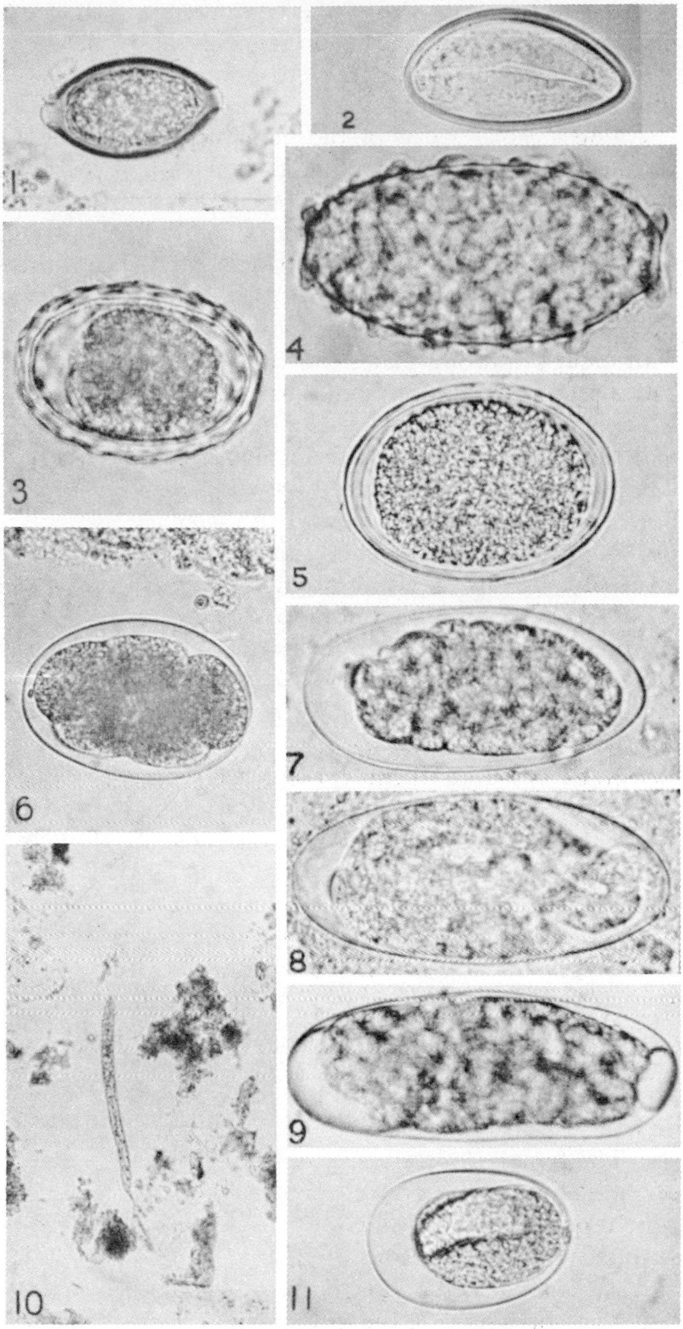

Figure 48–2. Some common nematode eggs: *(1)* whipworm, *Trichuris trichiura; (2)* pinworm, *Enterobius vermicularis; (3)* large roundworm, *Ascaris lumbricoides,* fertilized egg; *(4) A. lumbricoides,* unfertilized egg; *(5) Ascaris,* decorticated egg; *(6)* hookworm egg; *(7)* immature egg of *Trichostrongylus orientalis; (8)* embryonated egg of *T. orientalis; (9)* egg of *Meloidogne javanica,* a plant nematode, which sometimes is found in stools; *(10)* rhabditiform larva of *Strongyloides stercoralis,* the stage usually found in the stool; *(11)* egg of *S. stercoralis,* rarely seen in the stool. All figures 500 × except *(10)* 75 ×. (Nos. *5* and *6* courtesy of the Photographic Laboratory, AMSGS; photos by Milt Cheskis. Nos. *7, 8* and *9* courtesy of Dr. T. B. Magath, Mayo Clinic. All others courtesy of Dr. R. L. Roudabush, Ward's Natural Science Establishment, Rochester, N.Y.; photos by T. Romaniak.)

ticular cells. This integument may be smooth, striated or covered with bosses (elevations) or, occasionally, spines. Some regions contain specialized *sensory papillae* (amphids and phasmids).

Beneath the subcuticula lies a *muscular layer* composed of cells with muscle fibers which constitute the lining of the pseudocoelom or body cavity. The *excretory system* and six longitudinal nerve trunks lie in this layer. In addition, there are a *nerve ring* surrounding the esophagus and sensory devices, previously mentioned, such as *amphids* (papillae), which are located in the cephalic or cervical regions of all nematodes. A minute pair of caudal chemoreceptor organs, *phasmids,* occur in some groups of nematodes. The presence or absence of phasmids is of major taxonomic significance.

The *digestive system* of the nematodes is simple, being composed of a straight tube running from the anteriorly placed mouth to a ventral, posteriorly situated anus. The *buccal* or *pharyngeal cavity* is lined with cuticula and may vary in length; it is surrounded by lips or papillae and is sometimes provided with teeth or cutting plates. Behind the buccal cavity is the typically muscular *esophagus* which, lined with cuticula, varies in structure and shape and functions as a sucking organ. The esophagus is surrounded by well developed valves at its juncture with the *intestine* or "midgut," which is lined with a single layer of cells capable of absorbing food material. Posteriorly, the intestine passes into a rectum and anus, which in males opens into a ventral cloaca. Rectal glands are present in both sexes, except those males (for example, the male hookworm) which have a posterior cloaca modified to form a holdfast device called a *copulatory bursa.* In such cases the rectal glands are modified to serve as cement glands.

The *reproductive system* of the male consists of a single tubule which begins as a testis and passes successively into a vas deferens, seminal vesicle and ejaculatory duct, which opens into the cloaca. Special copulatory devices, such as spicules, a *gubernaculum,* or a posterior extremity modified to form a bursa or holdfast disk, may also occur.

The female reproductive system consists of a delicate, threadlike, tubular ovary, which passes successively into an oviduct, seminal receptacle, uterus, ovijector, vagina and an externally opening vulva. This system may be single, as in the trichina and whipworms; double, as in hookworms and pinworms; or multiple, as in others.

Nematode Eggs. The eggs contain the fertilized cell and yolk granules which are surrounded by a vitelline membrane in a chitinous shell (Fig. 48–2). Sometimes this in turn has an outer protein covering, as in *A. lumbricoides* eggs. Unsegmented, partially developed or embryonated eggs may be discharged, or the larvae may be already hatched. Unsegmented eggs are typical of *A. lumbricoides* and whipworm, whereas the eggs of hookworms usually show signs of development. Pinworm eggs are embryonated when passed, whereas in the case of some microfilariae *(Wuchereria bancrofti)* the original shell is stretched to form the sheath. Larvae or nonsheathed microfilariae are liberated by such parasites as *T. spiralis* and *Onchocerca volvulus,* respectively.

THE GENERALIZED CYCLE OF THE INTESTINAL NEMATODES

The life cycles of the intestinal nematodes fall into one of several categories on the basis of developmental sequences: (1) direct, (2) modified direct and (3) skin-penetrating types.

The Direct Type. No intermediate host is required; the adult worms develop directly from eggs reaching the alimentary canal of man. Whipworm, *Trichuris trichiura,* and pinworm, *Enterobius vermicularis,* are examples of this type. Whipworm eggs passed in the stool require a period for the development of infective larvae within the shell, after which time they become infective for man. Pinworm eggs are embryonated when deposited and become infective for man in a few hours after deposition (Fig. 48–3).

The Modified Direct Type. *Ascaris lumbricoides* eggs are unsegmented when passed in the feces and require a period for embryo-

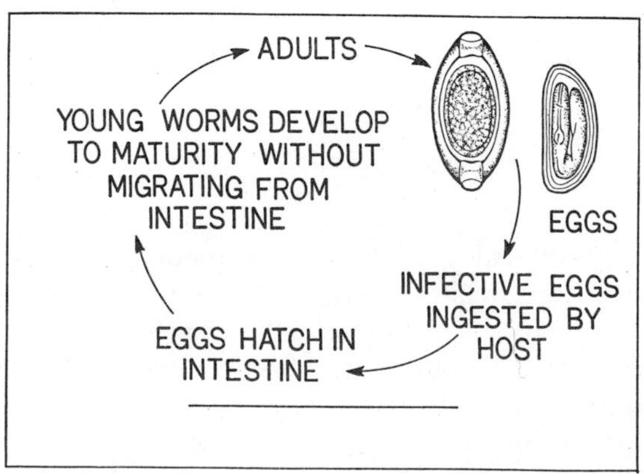

Figure 48–3. Nematode cycle – direct type.

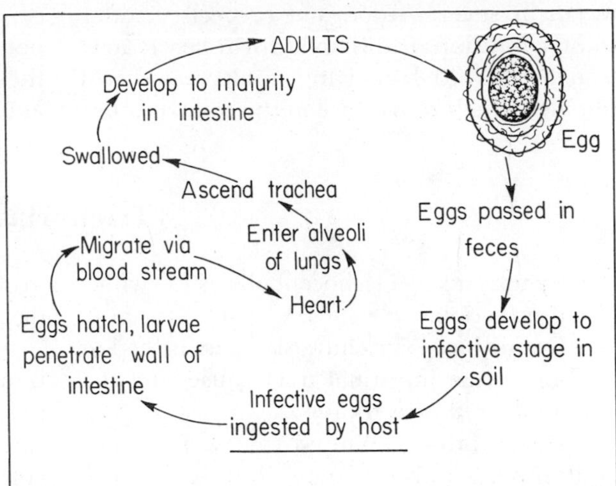

Figure 48–4. Nematode cycle—*Ascaris* type.

nation before becoming infective for man. Ingested embryonated eggs hatch in the intestine of man, and the larvae penetrate the intestinal wall to reach the circulatory system. Surviving larvae leave the capillary beds of the lung and migrate up the respiratory tract to the esophagus and thence down through the stomach to the intestine, where they mature (Fig. 48–4).

The Skin-Penetrating Type. Members of this group pass partially developed eggs or rhabditiform larvae in the stool. The former eventually hatch into noninfective rhabditiform larvae. Such larvae continue to grow, molt several times, and become transformed into infective or filariform larvae capable of penetrating the exposed skin surface of man. Developing eggs are found in the stools of persons infected with hookworms, but larvae are characteristically present in the feces of those infected with *S. stercoralis.*

In both hookworm disease and strongyloidiasis, the filariform larvae which penetrate the skin of man reach the circulatory system and eventually the capillary beds of the lungs. There they leave the capillaries, pass to the alveoli and migrate up the respiratory tract and down the esophagus to the intestine, where maturation takes place (Fig. 48–5).

Strongyloides stercoralis differs from hook-

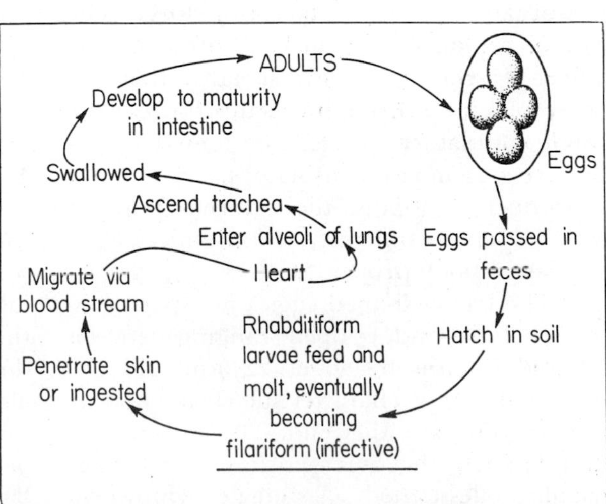

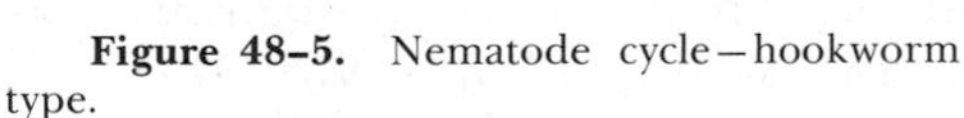
Figure 48–5. Nematode cycle—hookworm type.

worm in several important respects. Under some conditions the rhabditiform larvae may transform into free-living adult males and females which reproduce in the soil. In other cases filariform larvae develop in the intestinal or rectal area. These directly penetrate the bowel or the perianal skin, with resultant autoinfection.

Trichuriasis

Synonyms. Trichocephaliasis, whipworm infection.

Definition. Trichuriasis is an infection of the human intestinal tract caused by the nematode *Trichuris trichiura.*

Distribution. Whipworm is a cosmopolitan parasite but is most abundant in the warm, moist regions of the world. In various areas studied it has been found in 1 to almost 100 per cent of the population.

Etiology. MORPHOLOGY. Adult whipworms, *Trichuris trichiura* (Linnaeus, 1771) Stiles, 1901 [= *Trichocephalus trichiura* (Linnaeus, 1771) Blanchard, 1895], usually are partially imbedded in the mucosa of the large intestine. The parasites have a characteristic whiplike shape. The anterior portion is long and threadlike; the posterior portion is broader and comprises about two-fifths of the worm. The female parasites range between 35 and 50 mm long; the males are slightly smaller, measuring 30 to 45 mm. Anteriorly, the mouth opens into a delicate esophagus, characterized by a narrow lumen surrounded by a single row of cells, which extends through most of the narrow anterior three-fifths of the body. The male reproductive organs open into a posterior cloaca. The caudal region of the male is often coiled. There is a retractile penial sheath with a bulbous spined tip through which protrudes the single copulatory spicule. The female reproductive system also consists of a single set of reproductive organs, the external pore of which opens at the anterior extremity of the thickened body proper.

The barrel-shaped eggs when passed in the stool are undeveloped, ranging between 50 and 54 μm by about 22 μm and are provided with a characteristic clear knob or mucoid plug at either end. The eggs have a double shell, the outer portion of which is usually bile-stained. A female whipworm produces between 3000 and 7000 eggs per day (Fig. 48–2).

DEVELOPMENT. The unsegmented eggs require a minimum of 10 days under optimal conditions of moisture and temperature for development in soil. Under less favorable circumstances embryonation may require several months.

After ingestion the infective eggs hatch in the upper duodenum, and the larvae become attached to the villi of the intestine, where they remain and grow for about a month. At maturity the adult parasites leave their primary site of attachment and pass down the intestine to their final habitat in the cecum and proximal colon. In heavy infections they may also localize in the terminal ileum, appendix and much of the large intestine (Fig. 48–3).

Epidemiology. The distribution of whipworm is largely coextensive with that of *A. lumbricoides,* and the epidemiology of the two species is somewhat similar. (See p. 467.) The former, however, predominates in areas of heavy rainfall, high humidity, dense shade and moist soil. *Ascaris lumbricoides,* on the other hand, is more prevalent in regions of lesser rainfall and shade. The eggs of *T. trichiura* do not withstand exposure to direct sunlight and are destroyed by drying. They are unlikely to develop to the infective stage on cinders, ashes or hardened clay (Fig. 48–15).

Pathology. The anterior portions of the parasites are interlaced through the mucosa of the cecum and appendix. In heavy infections, the nematodes may be found throughout the colon and in the rectum. Ordinarily there is no marked tissue reaction, although liquefaction of the cells and bleeding in proximity to the parasites may occur. Secondary bacterial infection may cause inflammatory lesions (Figs. 48–6, 48–7).

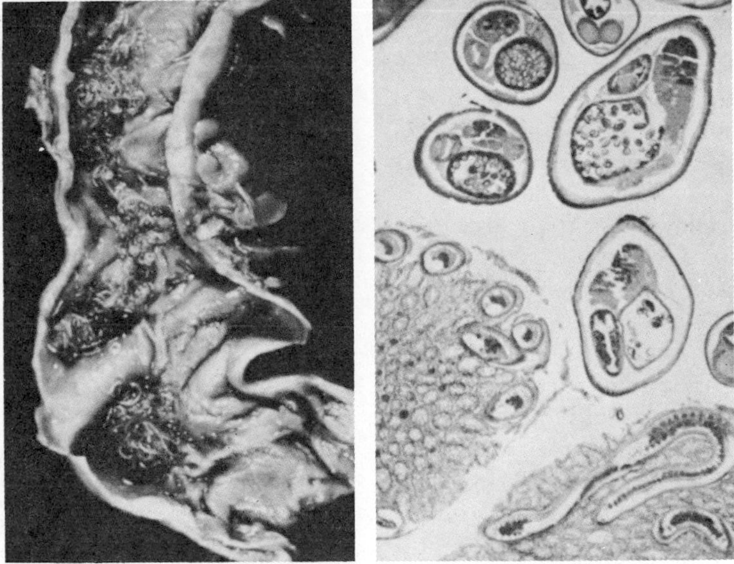

Figure 48-6 Figure 48-7

Figure 48-6. Masses of *Trichuris trichiura* (whipworms) in colon of a child. (Courtesy of the Louisiana State University School of Medicine, New Orleans.)

Figure 48-7. Section of large intestine showing adult whipworms (natural infection of *T. vulpis* in dog). Thin anterior portions of worms are imbedded and threaded in the mucosa; broader posterior parts of worms, containing eggs, are in lumen. (Courtesy of the Louisiana State University School of Medicine, New Orleans.)

Severe infections may be accompanied by a moderate eosinophilia and by anemia; the latter often may be due, in a significant degree, to malnutrition. The dysenteric exudate sometimes contains numerous Charcot-Leyden crystals and eosinophils.[1]

Clinical Characteristics. Light whipworm infections usually produce no symptoms. The presence of a large worm burden may be associated, especially in children, with diarrhea of long duration, dysentery, mucoid stools, abdominal pain and tender-

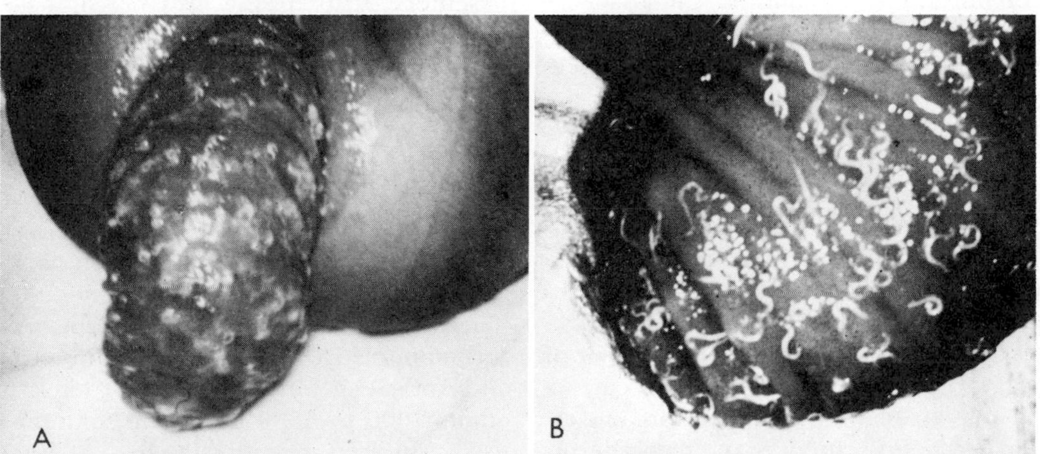

Figure 48-8. *A*, Prolapse of rectum in a heavy infection with *Trichuris trichiura*. *B*, Adult *Trichuris trichiura* attached to prolapsed bowel. (Both figures courtesy of Drs. P. C. Beaver and R. V. Platou, Tulane University School of Medicine, New Orleans, Louisiana.)

ness, dehydration, anemia, weight loss and weakness. Occasionally prolapse of the rectum occurs.[1,2] Adult worms may be observed on the prolapsed bowel (Fig. 48–8 *A*, *B*) or by sigmoidoscopy or colonoscopy (Fig. 48–9). Some patients with heavy infections are acutely ill.

Diagnosis. Diagnosis depends upon the recovery from the feces of the characteristic double-shelled, bile-stained eggs with mucoid plugs. These may be detected in direct smears, by formalin-ether (MGL or AMS III) centrifugal sedimentation methods, or by flotation techniques. (See pp. 819–821.) The intensity of infection should be determined, at least by an egg count per coverslip in a direct smear. This information is necessary for the physician to interpret the clinical significance of the infection. In clinical infections eggs usually are numerous in direct fecal smears. When only a few whipworm eggs are found in a direct smear in patients with diarrhea or dysentery, the helminthic infection probably is coincidental, and other causes of the patient's symptoms should be sought.

Treatment. Mebendazole (Vermox) is an effective therapeutic for trichuriasis. One tablet (containing 100 mg of mebendazole) is administered to children or adults morning and evening for 3 successive days.[3,4,4a,4b] If the patient is not cured 3 weeks after treatment, a second course of the anthelmintic is advised. No special procedures, such as fasting or purging, are required. Until data are adequate to exclude possible adverse effects on the fetus, the drug should not be given to women who are pregnant. Side effects are uncommon. Since mebendazole is also effective against ascariasis, hookworm infection, enterobiasis and certain other helminthiases, it is very useful for treatment of patients with multiple infections. Mebendazole has a highly ovicidal effect on eggs of *T. trichiura* from treated patients. Also, the therapy produces abnormality in size, shape and color of the eggs.[5,6]

Diphetarsone, a pentavalent organic arsenical compound, used as an amebicide for many years, has been shown to have significant therapeutic activity for trichuriasis.[7]

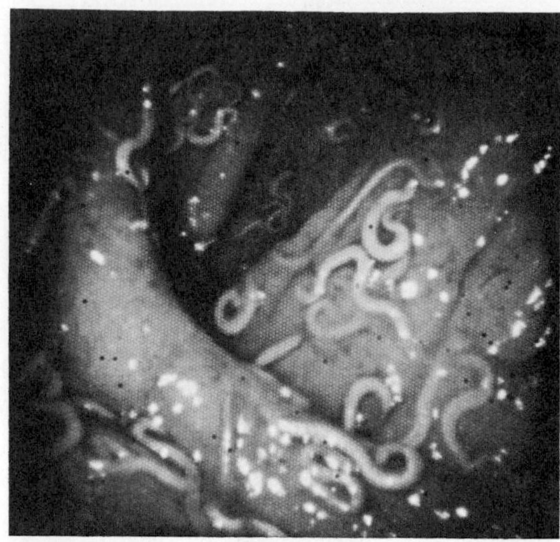

Figure 48–9. Adult *Trichuris trichiura* as observed during colonoscopy. (Courtesy of Dr. Thomas D. McCaffery, Jr., Louisiana State University School of Medicine, New Orleans.)

The dosage employed for adults was 1 gm twice daily with food for 10 days. Children were given a smaller dosage based upon surface area. Occasionally vomiting, diarrhea or a transient erythema occur.

The use of hexylresorcinol retention enemas for clinical trichuriasis no doubt will be supplanted by the new oral trichuricidal drugs. The latter may be employed for either subclinical or clinical trichuriasis. The use of hexylresorcinol enemas has been limited to cases in which either diarrhea or dysentery exists, in the presence of a heavy worm burden. A 2 per cent saline cleansing enema is administered the night before and again 2 hours before treatment is initiated. It is very important that the buttocks, thighs and other areas likely to be exposed to the expelled enemata are coated liberally with Vaseline to protect against the caustic solution. Hexylresorcinol is then given as a retention enema: 3 gm hexylresorcinol, 90 gm mucilage of acacia (and if fluoroscopy is used for monitoring, 90 gm of barium sulfate) and sufficient water to make 1 liter. For adults 1000 to 1500 ml of the solution are used; children receive 100 to 150 ml per year of age. The procedure may be repeated once a week for 2 to 5 weeks, *if necessary,* depending on the severity of the infection, and as indicated by the consistency of the stools.[1]

Prophylaxis. Prophylaxis depends upon sanitary disposal of human feces, washing of the hands before eating, avoiding raw vegetables in areas where human excreta is used for fertilizer and supervision of children to prevent dooryard defecation and coprophagy.

Enterobiasis

Synonyms. Oxyuriasis, pinworm or seatworm infection.

Definition. Enterobiasis is an infection of the human intestinal tract by the pinworm *Enterobius vermicularis.*

Distribution. Enterobiasis is a cosmopolitan infection. Surveys in various parts of the world indicate that *E. vermicularis* is probably the most widely distributed human helminth, its incidence varying from 1 to 100 per cent in the groups studied.

Etiology. MORPHOLOGY. *Enterobius vermicularis* (Linnaeus, 1758) Leach, 1853 [= *Oxyuris vermicularis* (Linnaeus, 1758) Lamarck, 1816] is a spindle-shaped parasite of man. It is usually attached to the mucosa of the lower ileum, cecum or ascending colon. The female is 8 to 13 mm long (Fig. 48–10); the male, 2 to 5 mm. The anterior extremity lacks a true buccal capsule but is characterized by three labia and, laterally, a pair of cephalic, winglike alae. The muscular esophagus terminates in a distinct bulb (Fig. 48–11). The male possesses a strong, ventrally curved tail with caudal alae and a single, large copulatory spicule. The posterior tip of the female is distinctly attenuated, constituting the posterior third of the worm. The paired reproductive system is T-shaped, the vulva opening at the base of the T near the juncture of anterior and middle thirds of the body. The long, clear, pointed posterior end of the female, which is discernible by gross examination, the clear cephalic alae, and the numerous typical eggs within the uteri readily serve to identify this common nematode (Figs. 48–10, 48–11). Adult female pinworms may be recognized in cross sections at appropriate levels by the bilateral crests and by the eggs within the worm (Fig. 48–12).

Females lay embryonated eggs which are flattened on one side, 50 to 60 μm in length and 20 to 30 μm in breadth. The shell consists of three parts: a thick outer albuminous layer, an inner hyaline layer, which is thinner, and the embryonic membrane. An average female produces about 11,000 eggs during the course of her life (Fig. 48–2).

DEVELOPMENT. Pinworm eggs are infective shortly after being deposited. After ingestion the eggs hatch in the upper intestine, liberating the larvae, which migrate to the region of the ileum, moulting twice en route. It is not uncommon for migrating larvae to attach themselves temporarily to the folds and crypts of the jejunum and upper ileum. Copulation of worms takes place in the lower small intestine; the female then migrates into the cecum or lower bowel. As their eggs develop, the worms become detached from the intestinal wall and the parasites pass through the anus. Upon contact with the air they shower their sticky eggs over the perianal skin. Rupture of the worms by scratching to relieve the anal pruritus also serves to liberate the eggs. Development from egg to egg requires a minimum period of about 15 days (Fig. 48–3).

Epidemiology. Pinworm eggs are relatively resistant and withstand desiccation in a humid environment for about 10 days. Infection occurs by ingestion of the eggs, which reach the mouth on soiled hands or in contaminated food or drink. Since the eggs are resistant, dust-borne infections may occur in households. Eggs adhering to the fingers of persons handling contaminated clothing, bedding and bathroom fixtures may cause infection.[8] The intense pruritus ani which is frequently present is an important factor in autoinfection and maintenance of the primary reservoir (Fig. 48–15).

At times retrofection may occur. Eggs

Figure 48–10

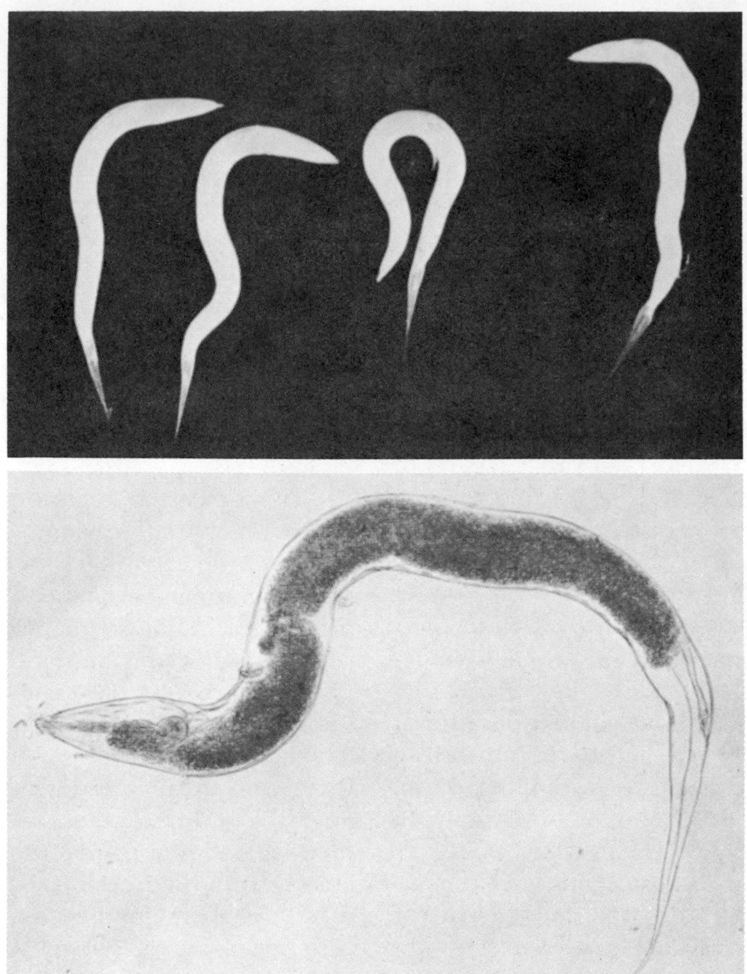

Figure 48–11

Figure 48–10. *Enterobius vermicularis* adult female worms. Note shapes and the clear, attenuated and pointed posterior end. (Courtesy of the Louisiana State University School of Medicine, New Orleans.)

Figure 48–11. Adult female *E. vermicularis* showing cephalic alae, bulb behind esophagus, vulva, egg mass, anus and pointed posterior end. (Courtesy of the Louisiana State University School of Medicine, New Orleans.)

may hatch in the moist anal region. The larvae then enter the large intestine through the anus and mature.

Pinworm infection is commonly a group problem affecting families and others living under crowded conditions. When one individual in a household is infected, it is usual to find several others also harboring *E. vermicularis.*

Pathology. *Enterobius vermicularis* produces no significant intestinal pathologic changes. Minute mucosal erosions may occur in the immediate vicinity of the worms.[9] Pinworms are found occasionally in the wall of the appendix (Fig. 48–13). More rarely pinworms migrate through the genital tract of females to the peritoneal cavity, where nodular or granulomatous formations about the worms result.

The most important effect is the cutaneous irritation in the perianal region produced by the migrating gravid females and the presence of eggs. The intense pruritus causes constant scratching which may lead to dermatitis, eczema and severe secondary bacterial infections of the skin. A vulvovaginitis may occur in young women as a reaction to adult worms which have wandered to these sites.[8] Occasionally eggs of *E. vermicularis* are found coincidentally in Papanicolaou-stained vaginal smears. It has been suggested that a possible relationship exists between enterobiasis and urinary tract infection in young girls.[10] The eosinophil percentage in enterobiasis usually is normal, although a moderate eosinophilia may occur.

Clinical Characteristics. While pinworm infection may be asymptomatic, the most common symptom is the intense pruritus ani already described. Local symptoms during worm migration vary from mild tickling to acute pain. Anorexia, restlessness and insomnia are common in cases of severe involvement. The disturbed sleep results in irritability. There may be changes in behavior attitudes, including inattention and lack of cooperation.[8, 11] Pruritus vulvae and vaginal discharge are not rare. Pinworm infection can be a rare cause of appendicitis. In view of the reportedly high prevalence of pinworms in young females with infection of the urinary tract, it has been recommended that such patients be examined for eggs of *E. vermicularis.*[10]

Diagnosis. Eggs are commonly present in material removed from the perianal skin and, more rarely, are encountered under the fingernails or in the feces. Stool examination is of very little value for the diagnosis of enterobiasis. In heavy infections adult female worms may be found adherent to the surface of the fecal bolus. The most satisfactory method of diagnosing pinworm infections is by the use of a perianal swab. The swab utilizes Scotch tape attached to a slide held sticky side out over the end of a tongue depressor, which is then applied to the perianal region. The tape is placed sticky side down on a clean glass slide and examined for *eggs.* If desired, a drop of toluene or N/10 sodium hydroxide may be added. The swabs should be employed in the morning before the patient bathes or defecates. Since children often are bathed before a visit to a physician's office, the swabs should be collected at home. For practical purposes, three swabs taken on successive mornings may be submitted at one time. For details of the technique, see Figure 48–14 and page 826.

Treatment. There is considerable

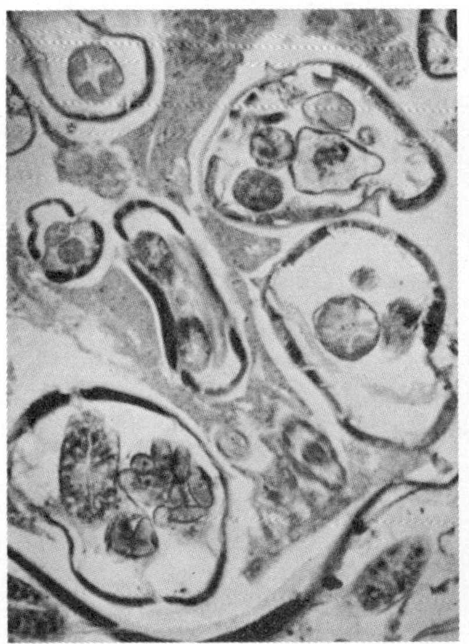

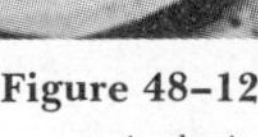

Figure 48–12

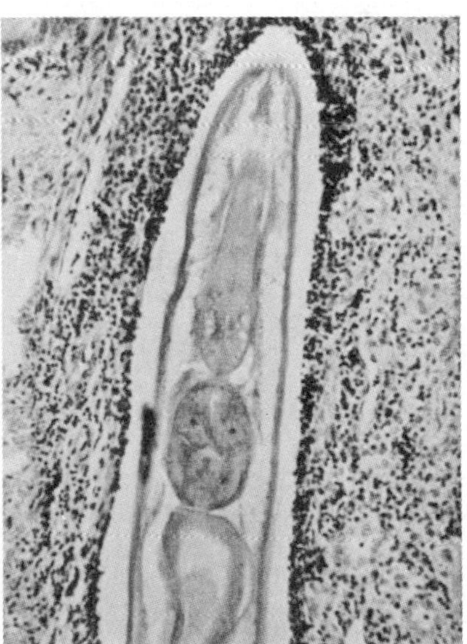

Figure 48–13

Figure 48–12. *Enterobius vermicularis* in lumen of appendix. Cross section of adult pinworms shows bilateral crests; one worm contains eggs. (Courtesy of the Louisiana State University School of Medicine, New Orleans.)

Figure 48–13. *E. vermicularis* in lymphatic nodule of appendix. Longitudinal section shows prominent esophageal bulb. (Courtesy of the Louisiana State University School of Medicine, New Orleans.)

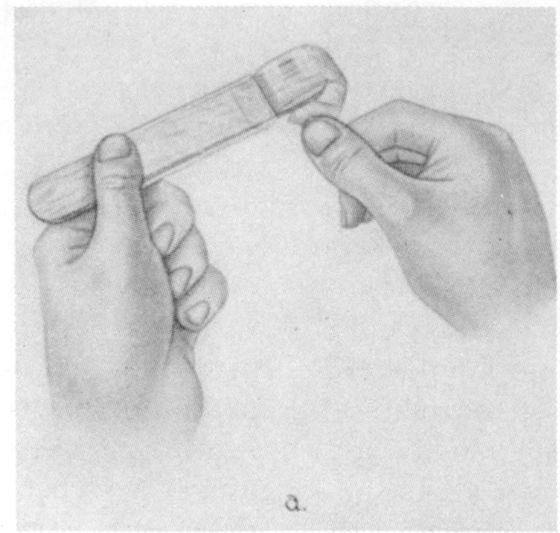

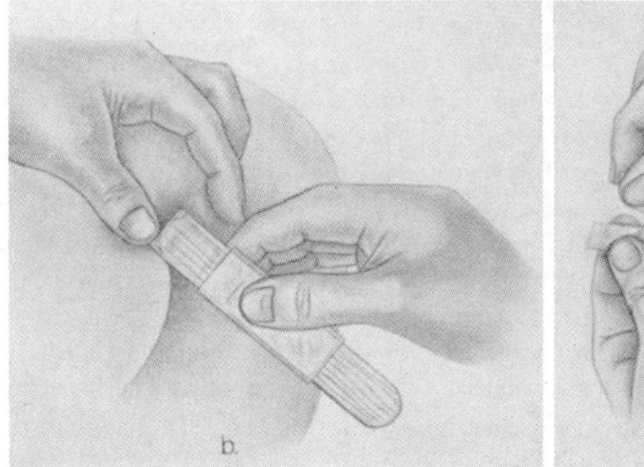

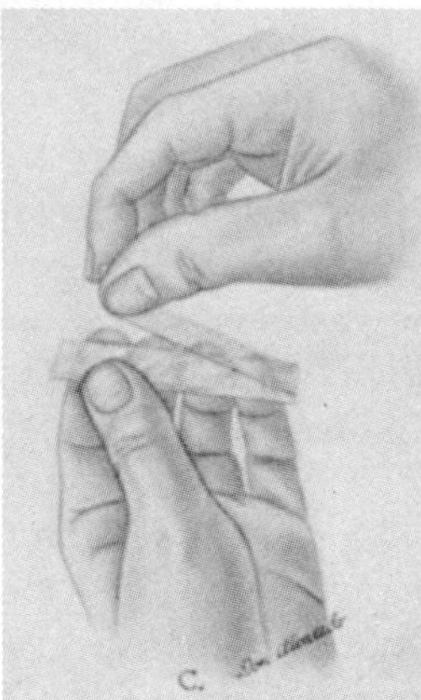

Figure 48–14. Scotch tape slide technique for the diagnosis of enterobiasis. *a,* Tape still partially attached to microscope slide is looped over end of wooden depressor to expose gummed surface. *b,* Gummed surface is pressed against several areas of perianal region. *c,* Tape is replaced on slide preparatory to examination for pinworm eggs. (Adapted from Brooke, Donaldson and Mitchell; Courtesy of the Louisiana State University School of Medicine, New Orleans.)

choice of anthelmintics for treatment for pinworm infection. Among the effective therapeutics for enterobiasis are pyrantel pamoate (Antiminth), mebendazole (Vermox), pyrvinium pamoate (Povan), piperazine citrate (Antepar) and thiabendazole (Mintezol).

Pyrantel pamoate is administered as a single dose of 10 mg per kg of body weight (give 1 ml of suspension per 4.5 kg, maximum quantity 1 gm).[12] Treatment may be repeated after 2 weeks. Occasional side effects reported include nausea, vomiting, diarrhea, cramps, transient elevation of serum glutamic oxaloacetic transaminase (SGOT), headache, dizziness and drowsiness. Many authors consider it suitable for large-scale use.

Mebendazole is given as a single dose of one tablet (100 mg of mebendazole).[4b, 13] The drug appears to be remarkably free from side effects. If the patient is not cured 3 weeks after treatment, a second course is advised.

Pyrvinium pamoate also is an effective single dose therapeutic for enterobiasis.[14] A dosage of 5 mg of pyrvinium base per kg is usually recommended. Nausea, vomiting or cramps occasionally occur. The post-treatment stool is stained by the drug. There are no contraindications to the use of the drug.

Piperazine citrate has been widely used for many years.[15] This anthelmintic is available in syrup, wafer and tablet forms. The recommended dosage is 65 mg per kg of body weight, with a maximum of 2 gm a day for 6 days. It may be repeated in 3 weeks.

Neurotoxicity may occur; the most common signs are due to cerebellar ataxia. Occasionally vomiting, diarrhea, urticaria, tremor, dizziness, visual disturbances and weakness have been observed. Piperazine should not be used in conjunction with phenothiazine compounds.[16]

Thiabendazole is effective against pinworm infection in a dose of 25 mg per kg twice on 1 day, after meals, and repeated 1 or 2 weeks later unless poorly tolerated.[14, 16] The drug is available in a suspension containing 5 mg per 5 ml. Minor side effects are relatively frequent and consist of anorexia, nausea, vomiting, headaches, vertigo and drowsiness. Angioneurotic edema, pruritus, urticaria, chills and fever may occur rarely. A fatal outcome following treatment with thiabendazole for enterobiasis was attributed to hypersensitivity resulting in intrahepatic cholestasis.[16a]

Since pinworm infection frequently is a familial problem, it is often desirable, when practicable, to treat all members of the family simultaneously.[11]

Prophylaxis. Prevention centers around personal hygiene and cleanliness of living quarters. Infestation of the household frequently results in reinfection. Careful washing of the hands and cleaning the fingernails before meals and after each use of the toilet are the most practical measures. Hand restraints to prevent scratching are undesirable and antipruritic anal ointments unnecessary. Usually it is not practical to employ many of the other prophylactic measures described below. Sleeping clothes, sheets, underwear, towels and washcloths, folded without shaking, may be soaked in ammonia water (1 cup of household ammonia in 5 gallons of cold water) for 1 hour or boiled before being laundered. Children may be given a shower bath or stand-up bath daily, preferably in the morning, with thorough washing and rinsing of the perianal area and genitalia. Both of the above measures are of particular value during the first few days of treatment. Bathroom fixtures, floor and toilet seat may be cleansed daily; rugs vacuumed once a day. Fingernails should be kept short; children should keep their fingers away from the mouth and nose. Metal toys may be sterilized in a hot oven; similar plastic articles may be soaked in the dilute ammonia solution.

Ascariasis

Synonym. Large roundworm infection.

Definition. Ascariasis is an infection by *Ascaris lumbricoides*, one of the most common helminthic parasites of man. The adults commonly remain in the small intestine. Passage of the larvae through the lungs is accompanied by pneumonitis of varying intensity.

Distribution. Ascariasis has a worldwide distribution and is particularly common in regions with poor sanitation or no sanitation. The prevalence in some areas is reported to be 90 per cent or more. Endemic regions exist in the United States, especially in southeastern parts of the Appalachian range. It is a common infection, too, in some areas of the southern and Gulf Coast states.

Etiology. MORPHOLOGY. Adult *A. lumbricoides* Linnaeus, 1758 are white, cream or pink in color. They are the largest intestinal nematodes, and their macroscopic appearance is characteristic. The females usually range between 20 and 35 cm in length, whereas the males vary between 15 and 30 cm. The cuticula is finely striated. The anterior extremity is characterized by three lips, one dorsal and two ventrolateral in position. Each lip carries a pair of small papillae on its lateral border. The male possesses a single set of reproductive organs composed of a long, single, tortuously coiled tubule which is sometimes faintly visible through the cuticula. The copulatory spicules are simple and unequal. The posterior end of the male often is coiled slightly or recurved. The vulva of the female is situated midventrally where the anterior and middle thirds of the body meet. The paired female reproductive system is coiled in the posterior two-thirds of the body and, like that of the male, sometimes may be seen through the cuticula. The female produces millions of eggs during her life, laying up to 200,000 per day. Eggs are deposited in an undeveloped stage and may be fertilized or unfertilized. The eggs may be covered with an outer roughened (mammillated) albuminous coat; if this is lacking the egg is said to be decorticated (Fig. 48–2).

DEVELOPMENT. The adults live in the lumen of the small intestine, especially in the jejunum, where they may persist for 6 months or longer. Eggs reach the external environment with the feces. Under conditions of sufficient moisture and oxygenation, and at an optimum temperature of 25° C (77° F) they develop and become infective in about 3 weeks. *Ascaris lumbricoides* eggs develop more rapidly and survive better in

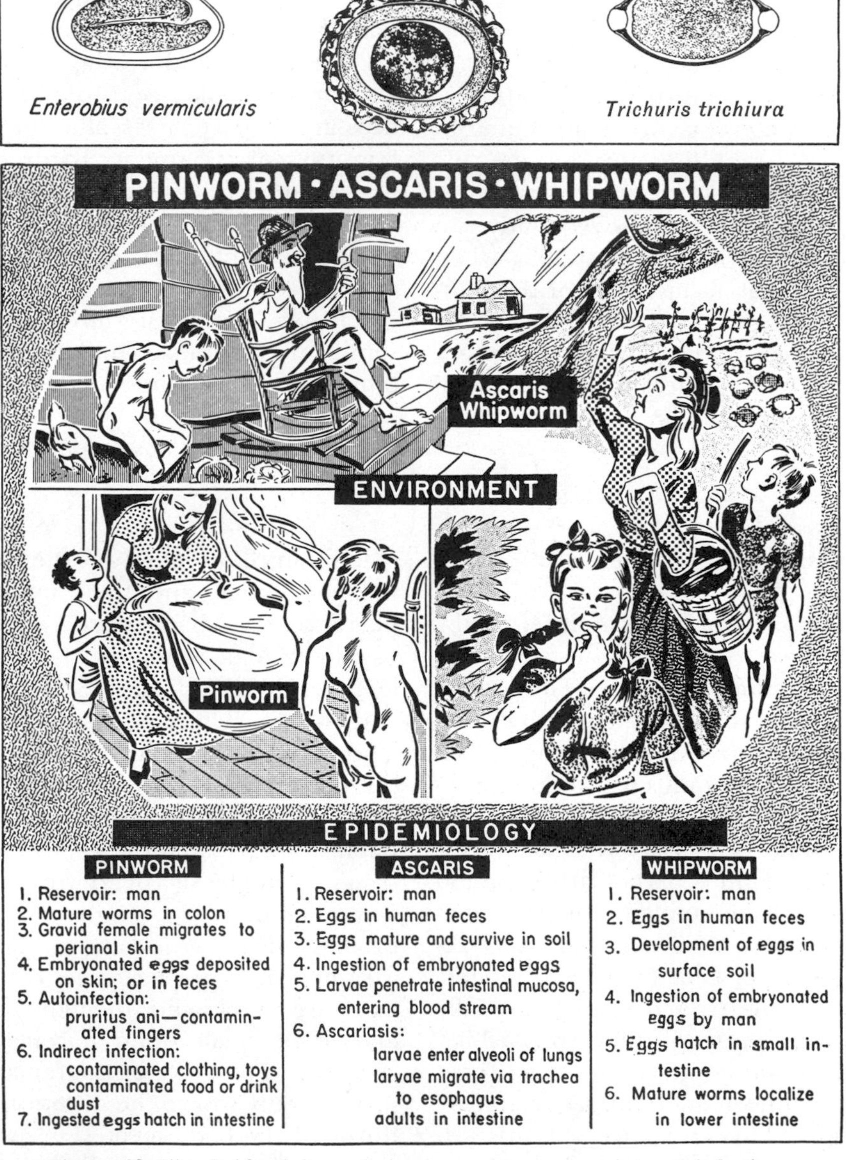

Figure 48–15. Epidemiology of pinworm, whipworm and *Ascaris* infections.

shaded soil containing clay than in shaded sandy soil. Before eggs become infective for man the contained embryo must have undergone one molt within the egg. These eggs hatch in the intestine, liberating minute larvae which promptly penetrate blood or lymph vessels in the intestinal wall. Some larvae thus reach the portal circulation and are carried to the liver; others pass through the thoracic duct. By either route they must finally reach the lungs, where they are filtered out of the blood stream; and, in a few days, many perforate the alveoli. After increasing in size and molting twice, the larvae migrate up the respiratory passages to the epiglottis and then down the esophagus. In this way the parasites again reach the small intestine where maturation and copulation occur. During the migration the larvae increase from about 0.2 to 1.5 mm in length and undergo a total of four molts. A new generation of eggs appears in the feces within approximately 2 months after the ingestion of embryonated eggs (Fig. 48–4).

Epidemiology. Children frequently acquire ascariasis by the ingestion of embryonated eggs which reach the mouth by soiled hands or by geophagia. Ascariasis often is a dooryard infection (Fig. 48–15). Parasitized children who fail to use sanitary facilities contaminate yards with their excrement and thus "seed" the soil with eggs which, upon maturation, provide a source of new infection for others or by reinfection for the original host. Uncooked vegetables from gardens which have been fertilized with human excreta also provide an important source of infection. The eggs are highly resistant to desiccation and to thermal changes under 45° C (113° F); therefore, they may remain infective for a considerable period. Although *A. lumbricoides* usually is more prevalent in children, this helminth is a common parasite of adults in many areas. The magnitude of the global prevalence of ascariasis is such that it probably still represents more than one-fourth of all of man's helminthiases.

Pathology. REACTIONS TO LARVAE. Minute hemorrhages occur at the penetration sites of the larvae through the intestinal wall and into the alveoli of the lungs. In experimental animals exudation of erythrocytes and white blood corpuscles, including many eosinophils, and desquamation of the pulmonary alveolar epithelium occur (Fig. 48–16). Larvae from large numbers of infective eggs, or repeated ingestion of eggs, produce pathologic changes in the lungs characterized by a lobular pneumonitis. This is more often seen in children, since they are usually more heavily infected than are adults.

REACTIONS TO ADULTS. The adult worms cause no specific pathology in the

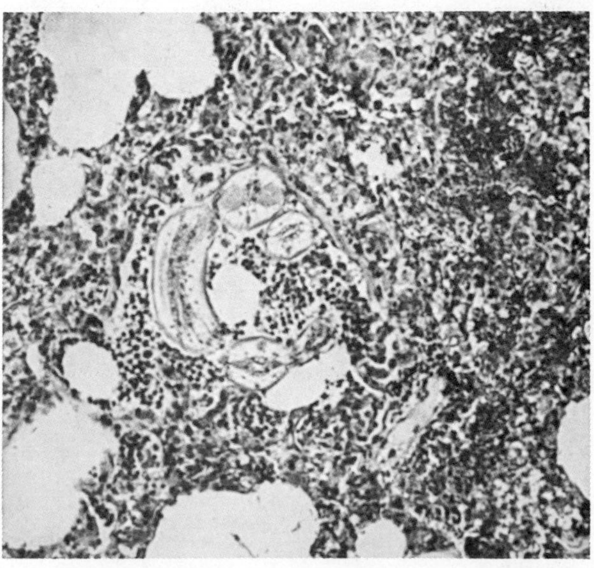

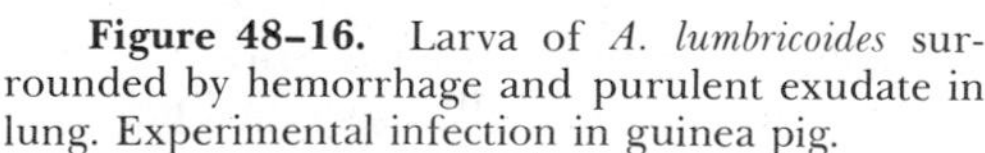

Figure 48–16. Larva of *A. lumbricoides* surrounded by hemorrhage and purulent exudate in lung. Experimental infection in guinea pig.

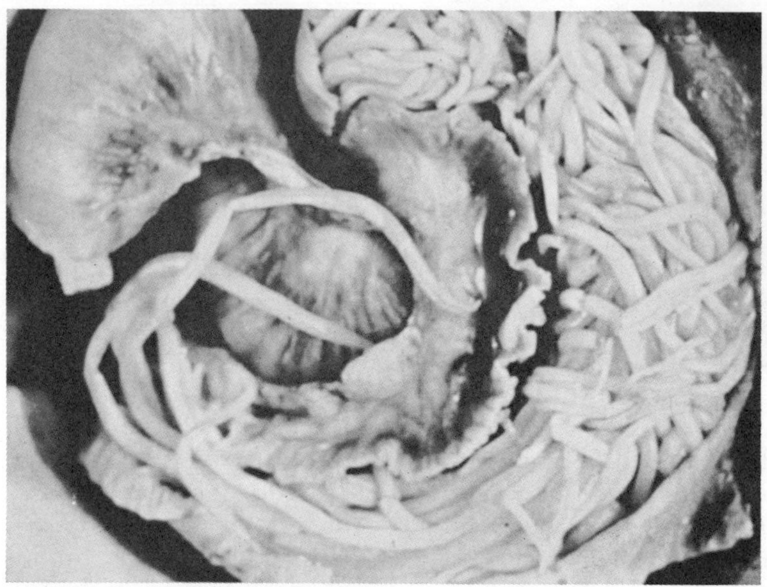

Figure 48-17. Terminal part of ileum opened, showing obstructing bolus of ascarids. (Courtesy of Drs. D. W. Aiken and F. N. Dickman. From J.A.M.A. *164*:1317-1323, 1957.)

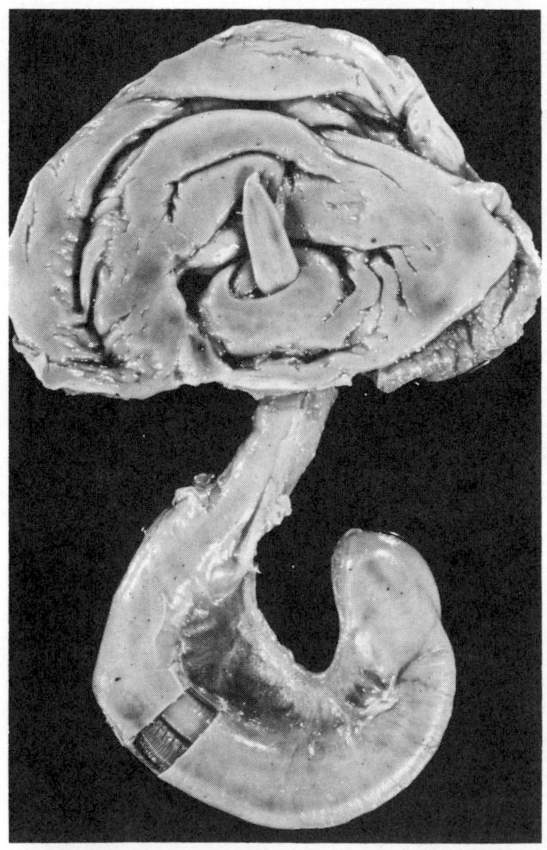

Figure 48-18. Adult *Ascaris lumbricoides* in appendix. (Courtesy of the Louisiana State University School of Medicine, New Orleans; photography by Eugene Wolfe and Eugene Miscenich.)

small intestine. If, however, they are present in sufficient numbers, they occasionally form a bolus which produces partial or complete obstruction (Fig. 48-17). Ascarids infrequently cause appendicitis and rarely perforate the gut wall or invade the bile duct (Fig. 48-18). The presence of *A. lumbricoides* interferes with the digestion and absorption of dietary protein. A moderate eosinophilia is often noted in individuals infected by this worm.

Clinical Characteristics. REACTIONS TO LARVAE. Children are particularly susceptible to ascariasis. If numbers of infective eggs are ingested there may be an elevation of temperature to 39.5 or 40.5° C (103 or 105° F) within a period of 5 days, corresponding to the period of migration of the larvae. This may be associated with frequent spasms of coughing, bronchial rales, evidence of lobular consolidation and hemoptysis. The physical signs often simulate an atypical pneumonia. The presence of the parasites is seldom suspected, and thus a clinical diagnosis of *Ascaris* pneumonitis is rarely made. Since sputum, when obtainable from the children, usually is not examined for migrating larvae, specific diagnosis is seldom achieved. Eosinophilia during this phase is prominent.

Reactions to Adults. Abdominal pain, frequently colicky in nature and located in the epigastrium or umbilical region, is one of the most common complaints of persons with ascariasis. Ascariasis-like symptoms may be provoked in humans by oral administration of *Ascaris* body fluid mixed with barium. Spasm and enhanced peristalsis of the stomach occur initially, followed by stagnation of barium in the stomach.[17] Often a history of passing worms spontaneously is obtained. Abdominal distention and tenderness, vomiting and constipation may be present. Rarely, allergic reactions to the worms, including dyspnea, may occur.[17] *Ascaris* infections often produce no symptoms. It is doubtful that ascarids cause convulsions. The passing of worms in patients with convulsions is probably due to a migration of ascarids induced by fever of another cause. During the intestinal phase of ascariasis, the eosinophil percentage is normal or only slightly elevated, but not a prominent feature.

The most frequent complication of *Ascaris* infection is a partial intestinal obstruction that may proceed to complete obstruction. This complication occurs in a small percentage of persons with ascariasis, more often in those with moderate or heavy rather than light infections. Although intestinal obstruction sometimes occurs after the onset of a febrile infection, or occasionally after use of some anthelmintics, it may develop without any obvious precipitating factor. The usual site of obstruction is the ileocecal region.

Diagnosis. Diagnosis depends upon the demonstration of characteristic eggs in the stool or the recovery of an adult worm. Recognition of both mammillated and decorticated eggs is important. (See Fig. 48–2.) Eggs presenting several different appearances may be encountered in the stool as follows:

Fertilized Eggs. These range from 45 to 75 μm by 35 to 50 μm in diameter. Ordinarily they are covered by a coarsely mammillated, albuminoid, bile-stained outer shell beneath which is a thick, transparent, hyaline inner shell.

Unfertilized Eggs. These are 88 to 94 μm by 39 to 44 μm; they are longer, narrower and have a slightly thinner outer and inner shell than typical fertilized *Ascaris* eggs. Vegetable cells are sometimes erroneously diagnosed as eggs of *A. lumbricoides*, being particularly confused with unfertilized eggs.

Decorticated Eggs. Occasionally, the roughened mammillated outer shell is absent, and only the thick hyaline inner shell remains; these are known as decorticated eggs. They may be fertile or infertile.

Ascariasis can usually be detected by direct smears; however, concentration techniques, such as the MGL or AMS III, insure a diagnosis. (See pp. 819–821.)

Tangled masses of worms are seen from

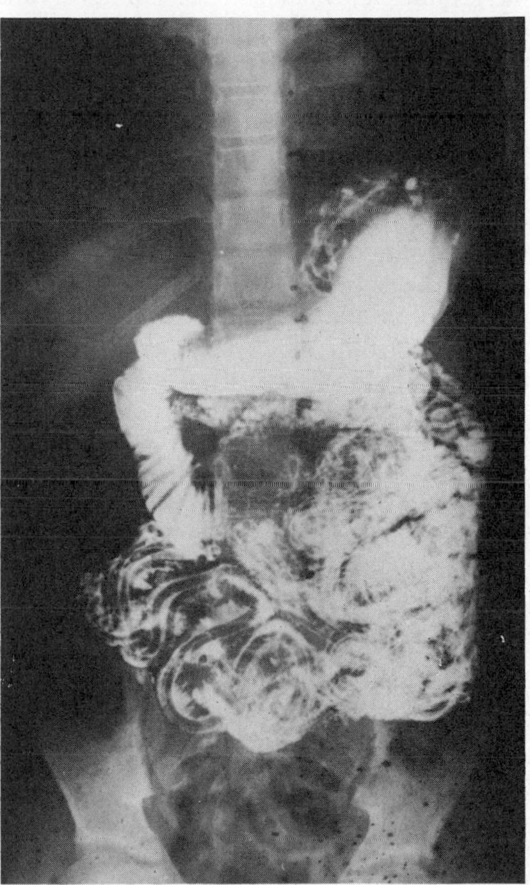

Figure 48–19. Adult *Ascaris lumbricoides* visualized in small intestine by x-ray following barium. Ascarids may be detected at times without barium, by air contrast, but are less distinct. (Courtesy of Dr. David J. Harllee, the Louisiana State University School of Medicine and the Charity Hospital of Louisiana, New Orleans.)

time to time in plain films of the abdomen. This can be of value in patients with obstructive signs; however, obstruction should be attributed to the worms only if a large number are clearly revealed. In the early part of fluoroscopic examination the worms appear as tubular filling defects, often with undulations and coils. As the barium progresses, the worms become more obvious owing to a coating of barium on their surface and, occasionally, thin filamentous streaks in their alimentary canal (Fig. 48–19).[18]

Treatment. Several drugs are now available which are effective therapeutics for ascariasis. Included among these are pyrantel pamoate (Antiminth), mebendazole (Vermox), piperazine citrate (Antepar), tetramisole/levamisole, thiabendazole (Mintezol) and bephenium hydroxynaphthoate (Alcopar, Alcopara). Fasting and post-treatment purgation are not required or indicated. Hexylresorcinol (Crystoids anthelmintic, Caprokol) has been supplanted in many areas by the newer drugs. In view of the hazard of burns of the mouth and pharynx from hexylresorcinol, if the pills are chewed or retained under the tongue or between the teeth and cheeks by children, the present anthelmintic armamentarium offers safer choices. Some of the compounds are effective against other helminths and their range of anthelmintic activity should be considered in selection of drugs for treatment of patients with multiple infections.

Pyrantel Pamoate. This is administered as a single dose of 10 mg per kg of body weight.[16, 19, 20] One ml of the suspension is given for each 4.5 kg. The maximum dose is 1 gm. Pyrantel acts through neuromuscular blockade and subsequent immobilization. (See p. 464 for side effects.)

Mebendazole. This anthelmintic is supplied as tablets containing 100 mg of the drug. The dosage for adults or children is 100 mg morning and evening for 3 days. Reactions are infrequent. Transient symptoms of abdominal pain and diarrhea have occurred in cases of massive infection and the pain was associated with expulsion of worms. The drug exerts its anthelmintic effect by blocking glucose uptake by the susceptible helminths, with resultant glycogen depletion and decreased formation of ATP which is essential for survival and reproduction. Ascariasis and trichuriasis frequently coexist in the same patient and thus, with mebendazole, treatment can be effectively directed at both infections.[3, 4]

Piperazine Citrate. This drug has been employed for many years for the treatment of ascariasis and in the conservative treatment and management of partial intestinal obstruction due to ascarids.[15, 21] An effective regimen is 50 mg per kg of body weight, given in a single dose for 2 days, with a maximum daily dose of 3.5 gm. Piperazine acts by producing neuromuscular block in *A. lumbricoides* through an anticholinergic action at the myoneural junction, in association with decreased succinic acid production by the worms. Both actions are reversible if worms are transferred to a piperazine-free medium where they regain motility. The narcotized worms lose their ability to retain their position against small intestinal peristalsis; they are thus carried down the gastrointestinal tract passively and passed with the feces. (See p. 465 for reactions.)

Levamisole. This levorotatory isomer of tetramisole is an effective anthelmintic for therapy for ascariasis.[22, 23] The dose for individual or mass treatment is 2.5 mg per kg of body weight in a single dose. Treatment may be repeated in a week to cure any failures from the initial dose. Tolerance by patients is very high. Side effects, mild and transient, occur in about 1 per cent of treated patients and may include nausea, vomiting, anorexia, abdominal discomfort, headache or vertigo. Trimestrial administration of levamisole has been used for control of ascariasis.[24] This compound reportedly also has immunostimulating properties. The drug is not advised in early pregnancy or in advanced liver or renal disease. Ascarids are paralyzed by the drug through selective enzyme inhibition; specifically, the inhibition of succinatedehydrogenase activity in the muscle of the worm prevents conversion of fumarate to succinate, with resultant decrease of muscular energy production. The affected worms then are expelled by peristalsis. This anthelmintic is very suitable for mass treatment campaigns.

Thiabendazole. This anthelmintic is administered in a dosage of 25 mg per kg twice a day for 2 days. Single doses should not exceed 1.5 gm with a maximum total daily dose of 3 gm. The precise mechanism of action of this drug on the worms is unknown.[25] (See p. 465 for information on adverse reactions.) While thiabendazole is useful and efficient for ascariasis, it is not the drug of primary choice. It is very useful for other nematode infections such as strongyloidiasis, trichinosis and creeping eruption.

Bephenium. This drug is used primarily for hookworm infections. Since it also is active against ascariasis, bephenium is useful when hookworm infections are complicated by the presence of ascarids. Vomiting is a frequent side effect. It is not a primary choice for treatment for ascariasis.[26] (See p. 480 for dosage.)

INTESTINAL OBSTRUCTION DUE TO ASCARIASIS. *Partial intestinal obstruction* due to *A. lumbricoides* frequently responds to conservative management, and surgical intervention may not be necessary in many instances if this method of therapy is followed.[21] Parenteral fluids are administered as required. If necessary, Wangensteen drainage with a Levin tube is employed for abdominal decompression to relieve distention and vomiting. Saline enemas are given to remove any worms that may have collected in the large intestine owing to decreased peristalsis. After 4 to 6 hours of nasogastric suction, vomiting usually abates, and piperazine citrate syrup is instilled by gravity through the tube. Suction is discontinued for 1 to 2 hours after administration of the drug. The initial dosage of piperazine is 150 mg per kg of body weight, with a maximum of 3 gm (30 ml of the syrup). Subsequently, 65 mg of piperazine per kg, with a maximum of 1 gm (10 ml), is given at 12-hour intervals for 6 doses. If vomiting is not frequent and drainage is unnecessary, the drug should be given by mouth. In such cases, if the initial dose (150 mg per kg) is retained fully, the next dose (65 mg per kg) should be given 24 hours later (instead of 12) and repeated at 12-hour intervals for 6 doses. After the acute illness has subsided, the stools should be examined. If eggs of *A. lumbricoides* are present, the residual infection should be treated as an uncomplicated case of intestinal ascariasis.[21]

Complete intestinal obstruction in ascariasis requires prompt surgical intervention.[27] The prognosis is determined largely by the length of time between onset of the obstruction and the institution of surgical treatment.

Prophylaxis. Effective prophylaxis against ascariasis, as well as trichuriasis, consists especially of sanitary disposal of human excreta, prevention of fecal contamination of top soil, avoidance of eating uncooked vegetables in areas where nightsoil is used as fertilizer, and the institution of proper habits of personal cleanliness. Children's play and hygienic habits should be supervised to prevent defecation in the yards, ingestion of contaminated soil and placing soiled hands in the mouth.

Impressive results in ascariasis eradication have been obtained by repeated mass treatment with piperazine at monthly and trimestrial intervals.[24, 28]

Hookworm Disease

Synonyms. For *Ancylostoma duodenale* infections: uncinariasis, ancylostomiasis, Old World hookworm infection; for *Necator americanus* infections: necatoriasis, New World hookworm infection, American hookworm infection.

Definition. Hookworm disease is an infection of the small intestine by *A. duodenale* or *N. americanus.* Tissue destruction and blood loss attributable to the parasites occur in proportion to the abundance of these invaders. Malnutrition and avitaminosis aggravate the detrimental effects of infection.

Distribution. Hookworm disease is widespread and is one of the most important

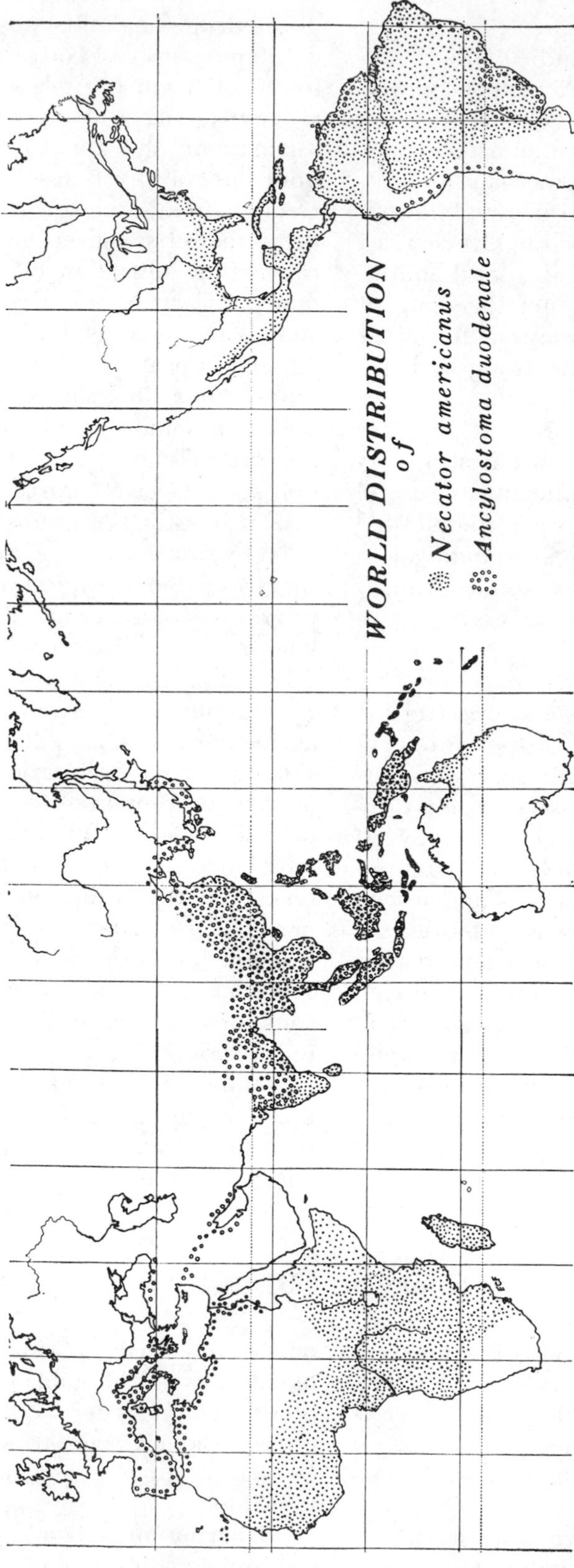

Figure 48–20. World distribution of human hookworm infection. (From Faust, E. C., Russell, P. F., and Jung, R. C. 1970. Craig and Faust's Clinical Parasitology. 8th ed. Lea & Febiger, Philadelphia.)

Table 48–1. DIFFERENTIAL CHARACTERISTICS OF COMMON HOOKWORMS*

	Necator americanus	*Ancylostoma duodenale*	*Ancylostoma braziliense*	*Ancylostoma caninum*
Shape	Head curved opposite to curvature of body, giving a hooked appearance to anterior end	Head continues in same direction as curvature of body	Similar to *A. duodenale*	Similar to *A. duodenale*
Length				
Female	9 to 11 mm × 0.35 mm	10 to 13 mm × 0.60 mm	9 to 10.5 mm × 0.38 mm	14 mm × 0.6 mm
Male	5 to 9 mm × 0.30 mm	8 to 11 mm × 0.45 mm	7.8 to 8.5 mm × 0.35 mm	10 mm × 0.4 mm
Buccal capsule	A pair of dorsal and ventral semilunar cutting plates	Two pairs of curved ventral teeth of nearly the same size, rudimentary inner pair	Two pairs of ventral teeth, inner smaller	Three pairs of ventral teeth, inner smallest
Length of esophagus	0.5 to 0.8 mm in length. Opening small, oval, long axis dorsoventral	1.3 mm in length. Opening oval, long axis transverse	Opening very small, long axis dorsoventral	Opening large, oval, long axis dorsoventral
Bursa of male	Long, wide and rounded, dorsal ray small, bipartite	Broader than long, dorsal ray tripartite	Small, almost as broad as long, with short stubby rays	Large and flaring, with long slender rays
Caudal spine in female	Absent	Present	Present	Present
Vulva	Anterior third to middle of body	Posterior to middle of body	Posterior to middle of body	Posterior to middle of body
Size of eggs (micrometers, μm)	64 to 76 × 35 to 40	56 to 60 × 35 to 40	55 to 60 × 34 to 40	60 to 75 × 38 to 45

*Adapted from D. L. Belding. 1965. Textbook of Parasitology. 3rd ed. New York, Appleton-Century-Crofts. p. 426.

helminthic diseases of man. It occurs in nearly all subtropical and tropical countries. The number of hookworm infections probably is still near the past estimate of nearly 500 million.[29] The ranges of the two species of hookworm infecting man overlap, and both are present in many regions.

Ancylostoma duodenale, the Old World hookworm, is prevalent in southern Europe, northern Africa, northern India, China, and Japan; it is also present in southern India, Indonesia, Burma, the Malay Archipelago, the Philippines, south and central Pacific Islands, Portuguese West Africa, Australia and Paraguay. *Necator americanus* is the predominant human hookworm in southern Asia, Indonesia, the Philippines, Polynesia, Melanesia, Micronesia, central and south Africa, the southern United States, Central and South America and the West Indies. Consult the map in Figure 48–20 for other details. Human infection with *Ancylostoma ceylanicum* Looss, 1911 has been reported in the Philippines and Calcutta.[30]

Etiology. MORPHOLOGY. *Ancylostoma duodenale* (Dubini, 1843) Creplin, 1845, and *Necator americanus* (Stiles, 1902) Stiles, 1903 cause ancylostomiasis and necatoriasis, respectively. Although morphologic differences exist between them, only *A. duodenale* will be described here. Other important diagnostic differential features are presented in Table 48–1.

The adults are pink or creamy white and have a tough cuticula and a pair of prominent cervical papillae that are laterally situated behind the esophageal nerve ring. The oval buccal capsule contains, on the ventral (or apparently upper) side, two pairs of fused teeth. The outer pair is the larger; the inner is provided with a small, inconspicuous accessory median process (Figs. 48–21 to 48–24).

The males are 8 to 11 mm long; the females, between 10 and 13 mm. The posterior tip of the male is expanded to form a typical copulatory bursa supported by fleshy rays, with a pattern that is characteristic of

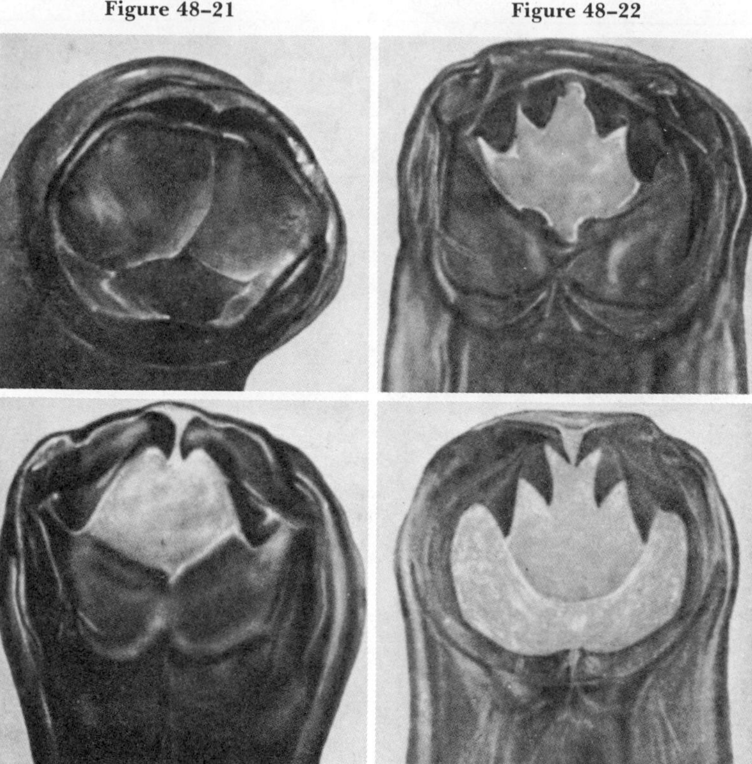

Figure 48–21. Mouthparts of *Necator americanus.* Note two pairs of chitinized cutting plates characteristic of this species. (Courtesy of J. M. Edney through Dr. A. O. Foster.)

Figure 48–22. Mouthparts of *Ancylostoma duodenale.* Note two large pairs of teeth, each of the medial pair bearing a small accessory process. (Courtesy of J. M. Edney through Dr. A. O. Foster.)

Figure 48–23. Mouthparts of *A. braziliense.* Note two pairs of teeth, a large outer pair and a small inner pair without accessory processes. (Courtesy of J. M. Edney through Dr. A. O. Foster.)

Figure 48–24. Mouthparts of *A. caninum.* Note three well developed pairs of teeth. (Courtesy of J. M. Edney through Dr. A. O. Foster.)

the species. The alimentary canal and genital ducts open into this bursa. A pair of long copulatory spicules are regulated by an accessory copulatory device or *gubernaculum.*

The females have a subterminal, ventrally located anus on the conical posterior extremity. The reproductive system is double, the tubules of the ovary being coiled intricately over the alimentary canal and confined to the posterior two-thirds of the body. The vulva is located ventrally at the beginning of the posterior third of the body. During copulation the copulatory bursa of the male surrounds the vulva, thus giving the spermatozoa access to the reproductive system of the female. After mating the male becomes detached. Fertilization takes place in the upper portion of the uterus or in the seminal receptacle.

Differential diagnosis of the various species of hookworms depends upon their length, the number and arrangement of the teeth or cutting plates, the length of the esophagus, the detailed morphology of the bursa of the male, the position of the vulva in the female and the size of the eggs. Table 48–1 summarizes these points in tabular form for the two common hookworms of man and for two closely related species.

DEVELOPMENT. Since the life cycles of

these two species are essentially identical they will be considered together. Adult hookworms live attached to the mucosa of the small intestine. Females liberate eggs into the lumen which are eliminated with the feces in two- to eight-celled stages of cleavage. Eggs vary between 56 and 76 μm in length by 35 to 40 μm in breadth. *Necator* eggs usually are somewhat longer than those of *Ancylostoma.* Eggs that remain in undiluted feces develop slowly. Under optimum conditions of dilution, moisture and temperature, however, they hatch within 24 to 48 hours, each liberating a rhabditiform larva approximately 250 to 300 μm long. Its anterior extremity is bluntly rounded and is characterized by a long narrow buccal cavity. Hookworm larvae in this stage of development may be confused with the rhabditiform larvae of *Strongyloides* (Table 48–2; p. 479). The rhabditiform larvae of the hookworm may migrate several inches beneath the soil, where they feed on bacteria, molt, gradually double in size, and finally undergo a metamorphosis to become infective, or filariform, larvae. During this period of growth a second molt, or ecdysis, occurs, the parasites frequently remaining within their sheaths.

The worms then enter a period during which no food is consumed, but active vertical migration may continue. When these infective larvae come into contact with unprotected human skin, they penetrate the superficial layers, enter the blood stream and are transported to the lungs. There they leave the vascular system, emerge into the alveoli and migrate up the bronchi and trachea and down the esophagus to reach the small intestine where maturity is attained. Eggs appear in the stool 5 or more weeks after invasion of the host by the larvae (Fig. 48–5).

Epidemiology. The infective filariform larvae ordinarily enter the skin. As penetration is difficult, mud caked on the foot or between the toes gives the larvae a purchase for the actual penetration.

In the tropics, coffee and banana groves and sugar cane and sweet potato fields are ideal for the growth and development of the larvae. Conditions most favorable to embryonic development include a loose, moist, shaded, sandy soil, loam or humus, through which the filariform larvae are able to crawl vertically. They cannot, however, climb up rocks or the sides of concrete-lined latrines. Temperatures ranging between 26.7 and 32.2° C (80 and 90° F) are optimal. Because eggs and larvae are readily killed by freezing and desiccation, hookworm disease is endemic only in those tropical and subtropical areas where the rainfall averages 50 or more inches a year (Fig. 48–25).

In many parts of the world special habits or customs of the people are factors in maintaining hookworm infections. In some regions, for example, there are usually certain defecation areas which adults use. These spots often provide the proper environment for the development of infective hookworm larvae. Adults revisit these sites daily, thus exposing themselves to infection and reinfection. Young children often defecate beside the house or in the area in which they play. In other parts of the world, dissemination is furthered by the utilization of untreated nightsoil as fertilizer. Infection results as the fields are worked.

There is a fundamental distinction between hookworm infection and hookworm disease; the two terms are not synonymous and the medical implications are quite different. It is difficult to obtain adequate data on the prevalence and distribution of hookworm disease. The method for routine stool examination merely demonstrates the presence of the parasite; it provides no exact evidence of the magnitude of the hookworm burden. Other methods involving egg count techniques give data on the *intensity* of the infection, thus furnishing a basis for estimating the worm burden of an individual. Persons harboring hookworms may be divided into two groups:

1. The hookworm "carrier"—a person with few worms and no clinical evidence of hookworm disease.
2. The clinical case—a patient carrying many worms who presents clinical evidence of hookworm disease. Clinical cases are severe only when large numbers of the parasites are present.

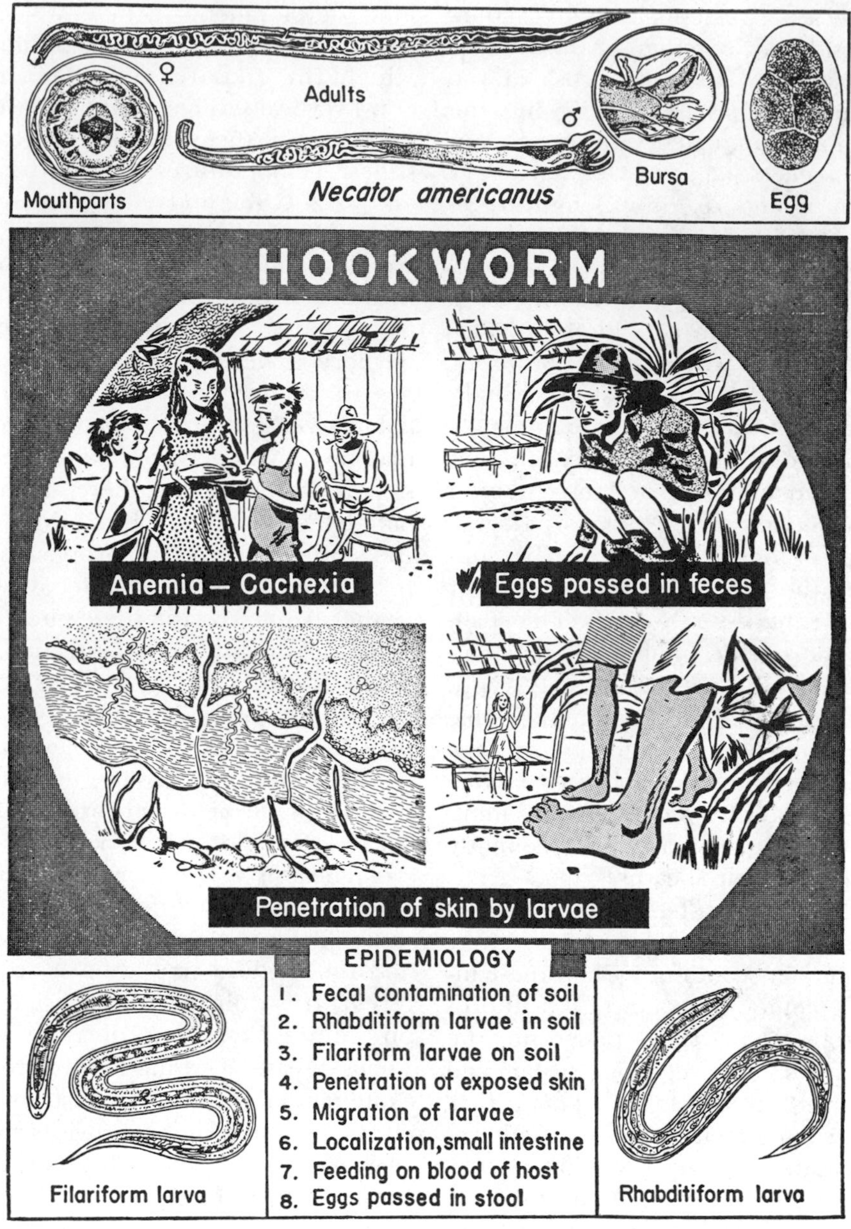

Figure 48–25. Epidemiology of hookworm disease.

It is frequently stated that the highest incidence of hookworm infection occurs in the teen-age group. While this may be true in the United States and certain other areas, it does not conform to the findings in Okinawa, South Korea and Japan, where the incidence increases until old age is reached and the individuals cease working in fields contaminated by nightsoil.[31-33] In many areas men may be more heavily infected than women, but in Okinawa, South Korea and Japan, this is not true; the incidence is approximately the same, but the *worm burden* is higher in women.

It appears probable that some human immunity to hookworm develops; otherwise large numbers of people would die from the disease. However, adequate direct evidence that man develops a firm immunity to hookworm infection is lacking.[34] The prevalence is lower and heavy infections are less often encountered in Negroes than in whites. Knowledge of the development of immunity is based upon experimental studies made with the dog hookworm. It has been found that small repeated infections give almost complete immunity. When such immunity develops, the worms in the gut are eliminated; anemia, however, may prevent the development of immunity. Further experiments demonstrate that pre-existing malnutrition and avitaminosis determine the appearance of hookworm disease after a small inoculum of worms that ordinarily would produce only a subclinical infection. If immunity has been established it can be lost if the diet becomes deficient; it can likewise be restored after an adequate diet has been resumed. This immunity to the invasion of the larvae seems to be a response to their secretions and excretions, the mechanism of which is the formation of precipitates which are deposited around the larvae. Their motion is then slowed and they soon disintegrate and are phagocytosed.

There is also evidence of a gradual and spontaneous reduction in the numbers of hookworms in cases where there is no reinfection. It has been estimated that in *N. americanus* and *A. duodenale* infections there is a 70 or more per cent reduction of the worm burden within 1 or 2 years and a total elimination by the end of 5 to 15 years.

Pathology. The penetration of the skin by the filariform larvae of *N. americanus* often causes a local dermatitis, "ground" or "dew itch," with edema, erythema and a vesicular or papular eruption, which usually subsides spontaneously in about 2 weeks unless secondary bacterial infection occurs. *Ancylostoma duodenale,* however, seems much less prone to produce a cutaneous reaction.

As the migrating larvae leave the capillaries of the lungs and penetrate into the alveoli, minute hemorrhagic lesions are produced. In heavy infections these may be numerous and may be accompanied by round cell infiltration. In general, however, the pulmonary reaction often is not evident clinically or is mild.

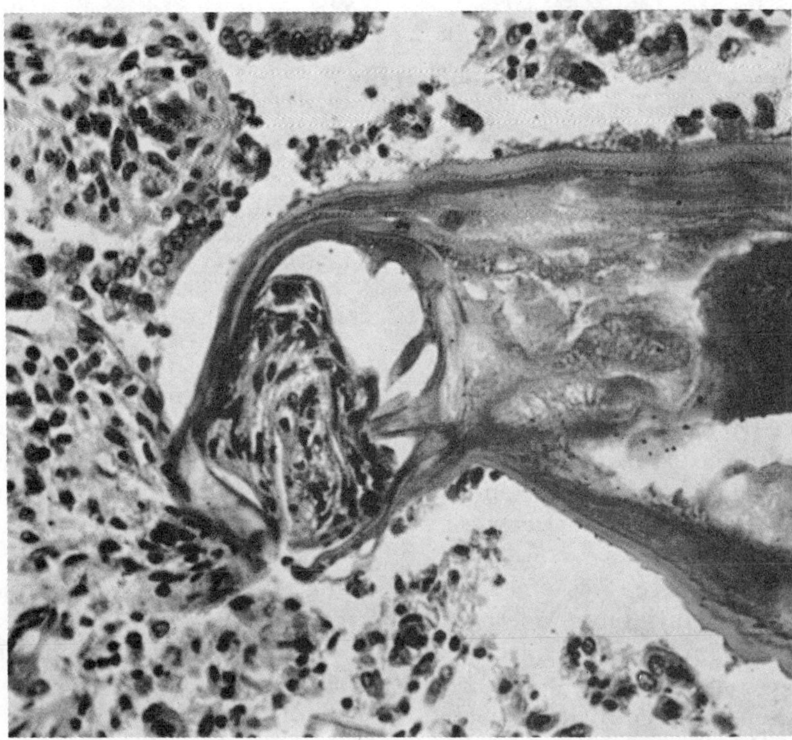

Figure 48–26. Longitudinal section through hookworm attached to intestinal mucosa. (Courtesy of Dr. Pedro Morera, Facultad de Microbiología, Universidad de Costa Rica.)

The adults of both human species inhabit the upper half of the small intestine, where they become attached and suck blood (Fig. 48–26). Of these, *N. americanus* is believed to be the more benign. Injury to the host results from the mechanical and lytic destruction of tissue at the point of attachment. A secondary hemorrhagic anemia is the chief pathologic condition. It has been estimated that a single hookworm may remove as much as 0.03 to 0.06 ml of blood a day.[35] When this figure is multiplied by thousands of worms and repeated day after day for long periods, the resulting anemia is readily understood. Hookworms digest only part of the blood they ingest. Previous points of attachment bleed for some time after the worm moves on to a new site, owing to the anticoagulant secreted by the worm. Study of jejunal biopsies indicates that hookworm infection per se, without the association of other factors such as malnutrition and other parasitic infections, does not as a rule lead to histologic changes in the mucosa that might cause malabsorption of nutrients. No major defects in the various absorption tests could be demonstrated in the majority of cases with heavy hookworm infection.[36]

Clinical Characteristics. The clinical picture of hookworm disease is variable and depends primarily upon the severity of the infection and the diet of the individual. Common symptoms are weakness, fatigue, dyspnea on exertion, cardiac palpitation, pallor, epigastric discomfort and, in heavy infections of long duration, mental and physical retardation. Children harboring this parasite in large numbers are frequently potbellied. Aberrations of appetite, such as a craving for earth (geophagy), wood, charcoal or other abnormal substances, are not unusual. Advanced cases with severe anemia and hypoproteinemia may present extensive edema and cardiac damage.

In many areas where the infection is heavily endemic, malnutrition is widespread in the population.[37] Furthermore, the clinical picture may be complicated by concurrent malaria and other parasitic infections of the intestinal tract. Hookworm disease, therefore, seldom appears as a clear-cut entity.

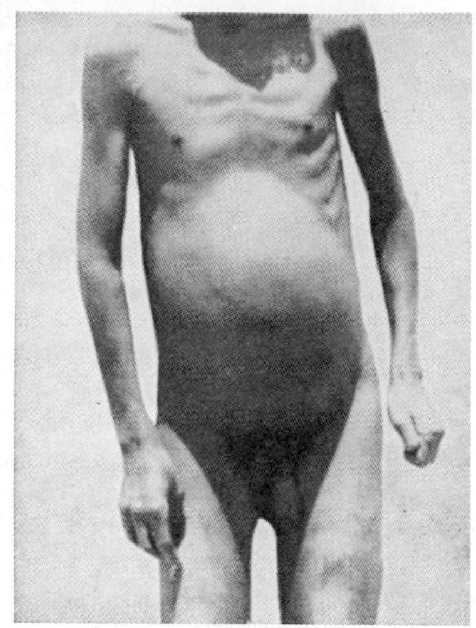

Figure 48–27. Clinical hookworm disease showing emaciation and protuberant abdomen. (Courtesy of Maj. D. S. Glusker, M.C., A.U.S., for the Office of the Coordinator of Inter-American Affairs.)

The most serious effects occur in children (Fig. 48–27); however, blood loss from hookworm infection can influence health and productivity and may even prove fatal in adults.

The anemia of hookworm disease may be severe with hemoglobin values under 15 per cent and erythrocyte counts below 1,000,000 per cu mm. The cells are usually microcytic and hypochromic. However, when the disease is complicated by malnutrition, the anemia may be macrocytic or normocytic in type.[38]

There may be a moderate leukocytosis; more commonly, the total white blood count is within normal limits. A moderate increase in eosinophil percentage may exist. It is less marked, however, in advanced cases.

Penetration of the skin may be associated with a severe pruritus.

Diagnosis. Diagnosis depends upon finding typical eggs in the stool (Fig. 48–2). Differentiation between the eggs of *N. americanus* and *A. duodenale* is not necessary or possible. It is important, however, that the rhabditiform larvae of hookworm, *S. stercoralis*, *Trichostrongylus* spp., and the free-living *Rhabditis* spp. be distinguished from one

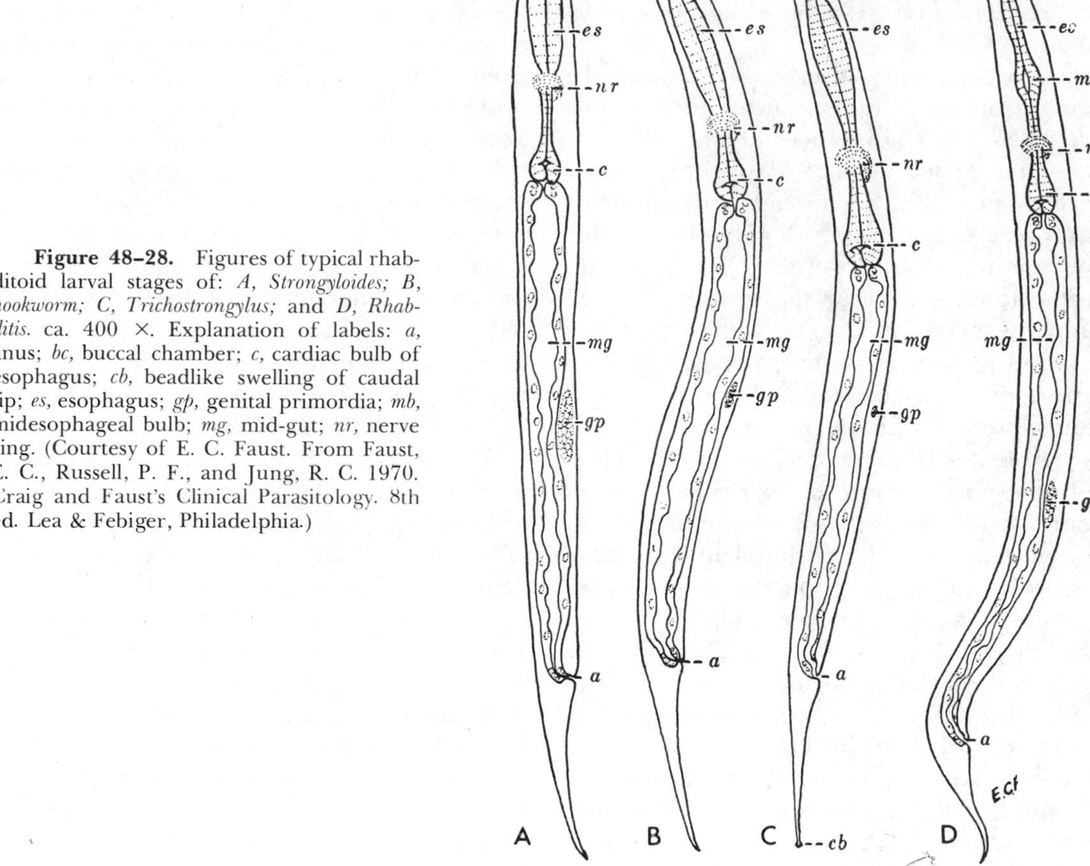

Figure 48–28. Figures of typical rhabditoid larval stages of: *A, Strongyloides; B, hookworm; C, Trichostrongylus;* and *D, Rhabditis.* ca. 400 ×. Explanation of labels: *a,* anus; *bc,* buccal chamber; *c,* cardiac bulb of esophagus; *cb,* beadlike swelling of caudal tip; *es,* esophagus; *gp,* genital primordia; *mb,* midesophageal bulb; *mg,* mid-gut; *nr,* nerve ring. (Courtesy of E. C. Faust. From Faust, E. C., Russell, P. F., and Jung, R. C. 1970. Craig and Faust's Clinical Parasitology. 8th ed. Lea & Febiger, Philadelphia.)

another (Fig. 48–28). In the diagnostic laboratory it is usually a question of differentiating between the larvae of hookworm and *S. stercoralis,* since those of *Trichostrongylus* spp. and *Rhabditis* spp. are rarely encountered. Rhabditiform larvae of hookworm will occasionally be found in stool samples that are held too long before examination. The presence of embryonated eggs and rhabditiform larvae in the stool is suggestive of hookworm infection or mixed infections of hookworm and *S. stercoralis.* If only rhabditiform larvae are present, strongyloidiasis should be suspected. It should be borne in mind that mixed infections are common, especially in the tropics. Rhabditiform larvae of hookworm and *S. stercoralis* may be differentiated by the characteristics listed in Table 48–2.

Stools should be examined by direct smears and by some concentration method such as the MGL, AMS III or zinc sulfate techniques (p. 819). If it is desired to determine the worm burden, the Stoll dilution egg-count technique should be utilized (p. 822). Other useful quantitative egg-count procedures are Beaver's direct egg-count technique (p. 822), McMaster's helminth egg-counting technique (p. 823), and the Kato thick smear technique (p. 821).

DIFFERENTIAL DIAGNOSIS. Hookworm disease may be confused with wet beriberi, malarial cachexia, chronic nephritis and with

Table 48–2. RHABDITIFORM LARVAE

Character	*Strongyloides*	*Hookworm*
Size, average	225 × 16 μm	275 × 17 μm
Posterior tip	Blunter	Sharper
Buccal chamber	Short or absent	Long
Genital primordia	Larger	Smaller

anemias of other etiology. Both beriberi and malaria may coexist with hookworm disease and complicate the diagnostic and the therapeutic problems.

Treatment. *Tetrachloroethylene.* In hookworm infections uncomplicated by ascariasis tetrachloroethylene is an inexpensive therapeutic choice. A dose of 0.10 or 0.12 ml per kg of body weight (maximum of 5 ml in a single dose) is highly effective for the removal of hookworms. The anthelmintic is administered in the morning on an empty stomach, and food is withheld for several hours afterward. No purgative is given before or after treatment. When the drug is administered without purgation, it is tolerated better by anemic patients and is more effective in removal of worms.[39] Two or more treatments at 4-day intervals usually are necessary to achieve complete removal of the worms. If eggs are found only in concentration techniques, either initially or after one or more doses of tetrachloroethylene, treatment or retreatment may not be justified. This regimen has been employed safely and effectively both for mass therapy and for patients with anemia. However, in severely ill young children this drug should be used with caution. Transient vertigo, headache, a burning sensation in the stomach, abdominal cramps, nausea and vomiting sometimes occur following the use of tetrachloroethylene.

Bephenium. Bephenium hydroxynaphthoate (Alcopar, Alcopara) is an effective therapeutic for hookworm infections.[40, 41] It is more active against *A. duodenale* than against *N. americanus.* The mode of action against hookworms is unknown. However, ascarids are excited initially, followed by paralysis associated with loss of muscular reactivity to acetylcholine. The standard dose is 5 gm of the salt (2.5 gm of bephenium base). Usually this dose is given regardless of weight or age; however, for children less than 20 kg of weight, sometimes one-half the above dose is used. The drug, in the form of small dispersible granules, is shaken in one-half glass of water and taken orally on an empty stomach. No food is allowed for at least 2 hours. The bitter taste may be disguised by sweetening. Bephenium is administered as a single daily dose for 3 days. Purgation is not done. Nausea and vomiting may occur with this drug, especially in children. Other side effects, which are mild and transient but not infrequent, include dizziness, cramping abdominal pain and diarrhea. Bephenium is a safe drug, but wide variations in ethnic tolerance exist. In the presence of gastrointestinal ulceration the drug is probably contraindicated. In view of the known side effects, the dosage should be reduced if used in patients during pregnancy. Combined therapy, employing bephenium and tetrachloroethylene, may result in high frequency of side effects.[42]

Mebendazole. Newer drugs, including mebendazole, have added to the choice of therapeutics. A dosage for children or adults of one tablet, 100 mg of mebendazole, twice daily for 3 days, produces a high rate of cure of hookworm infection, based upon studies involving *N. americanus* and *A. duodenale.*[3, 4, 43] Side effects are rare and transient. (See p. 460, under Trichuriasis, for additional information.) This anthelmintic may be used in the presence of coexisting ascariasis against which it is also effective. In view of the limited or lack of availability of tetrachloroethylene for medicinal use for humans in the United States, mebendazole offers a satisfactory alternative. Mebendazole has a highly ovicidal effect on *N. americanus* eggs in treated patients.[5]

Pyrantel pamoate. This compound is highly effective against *A. duodenale* and apparently is of significant potency against *N. americanus.* Single oral doses of 10 or 20 mg per kg have been used for *A. duodenale* infections; however, mild side effects have occurred with marked frequency at the higher dose level.[44] A total daily dose of 10 mg per kg of the drug, given in divided doses 2 or 3 times a day, for 3 days has significant therapeutic effect on *N. americanus* infections.[45] This anthelmintic is used for the treatment of enterobiasis and ascariasis, but has the additional value of being useful for hookworm infections (p. 464).

Other Drugs. Both levamisole and thiabendazole have significant activity against *A.*

duodenale and *N. americanus,* when given for 3 days.[22,25] Neither is, however, a primary drug for intestinal hookworm infections. Phenylene-di-iso-thiocyanate (Jonit) also is active against both species of hookworms. Side effects from the latter compound, though mild to moderate and transient, are of high frequency.[46]

MIXED INTESTINAL HELMINTHIC INFECTIONS. When mixed infections with hookworm, *A. lumbricoides* and *T. trichiura* occur, mebendazole would be a desirable therapeutic choice. Bephenium and pyrantel pamoate are active against both hookworms and ascarids, and could be used when these two parasites coexist. Some of these anthelmintics have a spectrum of activity which also includes *E. vermicularis, Taenia* spp., *Trichostrongylus* spp. and other species of helminths. Thus, in selection of a therapeutic of choice for an individual case or for mass chemotherapy, such additional benefits should be considered.

SUPPORTIVE MEASURES. Anthelmintic treatment may need to be supplemented or preceded by the administration of ferrous sulfate, by the institution of an adequate, balanced diet, and, in some cases with extreme anemia, by transfusion with whole blood or packed red corpuscles. Generally, removal of the worms, an improvement of the diet and administration of iron are sufficient.

Prophylaxis. The prophylaxis of hookworm infection is based upon sanitary disposal of human excreta and the prevention of soil pollution. In heavily endemic areas it is usually necessary to carry out mass treatment of the population to reduce the reservoir of infection; to construct adequate latrine facilities; and, perhaps of even greater importance, to instruct the population concerning the epidemiology of the infection and the necessity for the prevention of soil pollution. The wearing of shoes to prevent contact of exposed skin with infested soil is one of the most important preventive measures. However, in many areas of the tropics, insistence upon this measure would be unrealistic and impracticable for economic, cultural or other reasons. An adequate, balanced diet containing sufficient iron to permit compensation for blood loss will prevent or reduce clinical manifestations.

Tetrachloroethylene was used effectively in an area in Costa Rica to break the chain of transmission of hookworm infection. Mass treatment was given 4 times at 6-week intervals, followed by the usual annual mass therapy. The prevalence and worm burden of hookworm were reduced markedly and remained low for 5 years of observation. Control of hookworm by the regimen employed may be practicable as a public health measure in similar situations common to Latin America and other geographic areas.[47]

Trichostrongyliasis

Synonym. *Trichostrongylus* infection.

Definition. Trichostrongyliasis is an infection caused by any of several species of *Trichostrongylus.* Adult worms lie with their heads embedded in the mucosa of the duodenum and jejunum.

Distribution. Several species of *Trichostrongylus* occur in man. It has been estimated that they parasitize over 5 million humans, principally in Asia and the U.S.S.R.[29] *Trichostrongylus orientalis* has been found as a very common intestinal parasite in some areas. Some of these species normally infect lower animals. The geographic distribution of trichostrongylids reported from humans is shown in Table 48–3.

Etiology. MORPHOLOGY. Adult *Trichostrongylus* spp. are small roundworms, the males measuring 4 to 6 mm in length and the females 5 to 8 mm. The head is unarmed; a distinct buccal capsule is absent, but a definite notch occurs where the excretory pore opens. Males are characterized by a copulatory bursa with rays and spicules that are diagnostic for each species. In the female the paired reproductive system opens through a common vulva. The eggs are elongate, oval, possess a transparent hyaline

Table 48–3. Geographic Distribution of Human Infection with Species of *Trichostrongylus*

T. orientalis Japan, Korea, China (Central and South), Taiwan, Iran, Armenia	*T. probolurus* U.S.S.R. (Siberia), Armenia, Iran, North Africa	*T. axei* Armenia, Mauritius, U.S.S.R. (Siberia), Iran, Japan, Java
T. vitrinus U.S.S.R. (Siberia), Armenia, Iran, Egypt	*T. instabilis* U.S.S.R. (Siberia), Armenia	*T. skrjabini* Armenia, Iran *T. brevis* Japan
T. colubriformis India, Assam (extensive), Japan, Java, Australia (Atherton tableland), Armenia, Egypt, Iran, Israel (possibly Yemen, Syria, Iraq, Turkey, Afghanistan?); U.S.A. (New Orleans, one case)		*Trichostrongylus* spp. (?) Israel, Iraq (Basra), Saudi Arabia (Eastern), Tunisia, Iran (Southern), Zaire, Rhodesia, France, Turkey, Greece (?), Chile, Peru

shell, and resemble those of hookworms except that they are much larger (85 to 115 μm). When found in the feces they are usually in the morula stage (Fig. 48–2).

Development. Under favorable conditions of humidity and temperature the eggs hatch within 24 to 36 hours. However, they are remarkably resistant to long periods of cold or drought. The larvae undergo two ecdyses and reach the infective stage in 60 hours or more. Infection normally occurs when infective larvae are ingested, although adult parasites have been recovered following penetration of the skin. They mature in the small intestine within 25 to 30 days without undergoing a migration through the lungs.

Epidemiology. Man is believed to acquire the infection through contaminated food or drink. The widespread use of nightsoil in the Orient and the resistance of eggs and infective larvae to desiccation often create conditions in farming communities that are ideal for the spread of trichostrongylids. Herbivorous animals are common reservoir hosts.

Pathology and Clinical Characteristics. Little is known concerning the pathology of trichostrongyliasis. In severe infections a mild anemia and general emaciation have been reported. Presumably the worms, with their capillary heads in the mucosa, at times suck blood. Several hundred worms must be present to produce marked clinical manifestations. However, in Japan significant clinical phenomena were not observed even in individuals with high egg counts. A transient eosinophilia (maximum 10 per cent) may occur.

Diagnosis. This depends upon the detection of characteristic eggs or the recovery of adult worms from the stool (Fig. 48–2). Care should be taken to avoid confusion of *Trichostrongylus* eggs with those of hookworm, since tetrachloroethylene is not very active against trichostrongylids.

Treatment. Levamisole effects a high cure rate of trichostrongyliasis, followed by thiabendazole[48] (p. 465) and mebendazole (p. 460).

Prophylaxis. Effective prophylaxis against trichostrongyliasis involves the sanitary disposal of human excreta and the prevention of fecal contamination of the topsoil by infected animals or man.

Strongyloidiasis

Synonyms. Strongyloidosis, *Strongyloides stercoralis* infection, the strongylid threadworm.

Definition. Strongyloidiasis is an infection by the nematode *S. stercoralis,* the female of which usually is embedded in the mucosa of the small intestine of man.

Distribution. Strongyloidiasis occurs primarily in the tropics and subtropics, although it has been reported sporadically from temperate regions.

Etiology. MORPHOLOGY. The parasitic adult female, *S. stercoralis* (Bavay, 1876) Stiles and Hassall, 1902 is minute, about 2 mm long. The cuticula is delicately striated, and the esophagus occupies one-third to two-fifths of the body length. The paired ovaries, oviducts and uteri open through a short vaginal orifice near the beginning of the posterior third of the body. The mature parasitic female lies buried in the mucosa of the duodenum and jejunum where it liberates thin-shelled, ovoid eggs, 50 to 58 μm by 30 to 34 μm that resemble eggs of the hookworm. These are usually embryonated and soon hatch to produce the typical rhabditiform larvae encountered in the stools of individuals with strongyloidiasis. These larvae are 200 to 250 μm long and closely resemble the rhabditiform larvae of hookworm, differing from them chiefly in having a shorter buccal capsule, a larger genital primordium and a more robust posterior extremity (Table 48–2).

The little-known parasitic male is about 0.7 mm long. It possesses two spicules and a gubernaculum but no caudal alae. The tail is pointed and ventrally curved. It is similar morphologically to the free-living adult male observed in strains with an indirect cycle.

Strongyloides fülleborni, which is generally regarded as a parasite of monkeys, has been reported from humans.

DEVELOPMENT. The ecology of *S. stercoralis* is complex. Several cycles are known. The *direct* form of development is most common. In this cycle, rhabditiform larvae are passed in the stool. Under favorable environmental conditions they transform in soil into filariform larvae within 24 hours. These infective larvae are capable of penetrating the intact skin of man.

Less commonly, an *indirect* cycle is observed in which rhabditiform larvae develop into free-living adult males and females. The latter deposit eggs in the soil; the eggs, in turn, develop into rhabditiform larvae. These may transform directly to the filariform stage or into free-living adults. Under suitable conditions, repeated generations of free-living adults may develop, thus continuing the indirect cycle for a limited period. Ultimately, infective filariform larvae are produced.

The infective filariform larvae of *S. stercoralis* resemble hookworm larvae at the corresponding stage of development but are smaller and possess a much longer esophagus and a tail with a minute notch which is diagnostic. The filariform larvae that penetrate the skin eventually reach the lymphatics or capillaries and are carried to the right side of the heart and the pulmonary capillaries. Here the larvae leave the capillary beds and penetrate into the alveoli of the lungs. The parasites then migrate up the respiratory passages, reach the esophagus and pass down into the stomach and intestines. Mating is believed to occur in the duodenum or jejunum. After fertilization the females burrow into the mucosa to oviposit, thus completing the life cycle (Fig. 48–29).

The prepatent period is about 1 month. Since the parasitic adult male *S. stercoralis* has been seen only rarely, it is believed that the parasitic female may be parthenogenetic, like an analogous species, *S. ratti,* in rats.

In certain cases the cycle is completed entirely within the host. Rhabditiform larvae in minute fecal particles that remain in the perianal region after defecation can transform readily into filariform larvae. These penetrate the perianal skin, producing a form of hyperinfection referred to as *external* or *perianal autoinfection.* A fourth developmental cycle is *internal autoinfection.* The rhabditiform larvae that ordinarily would be passed into the stool rapidly metamorphose

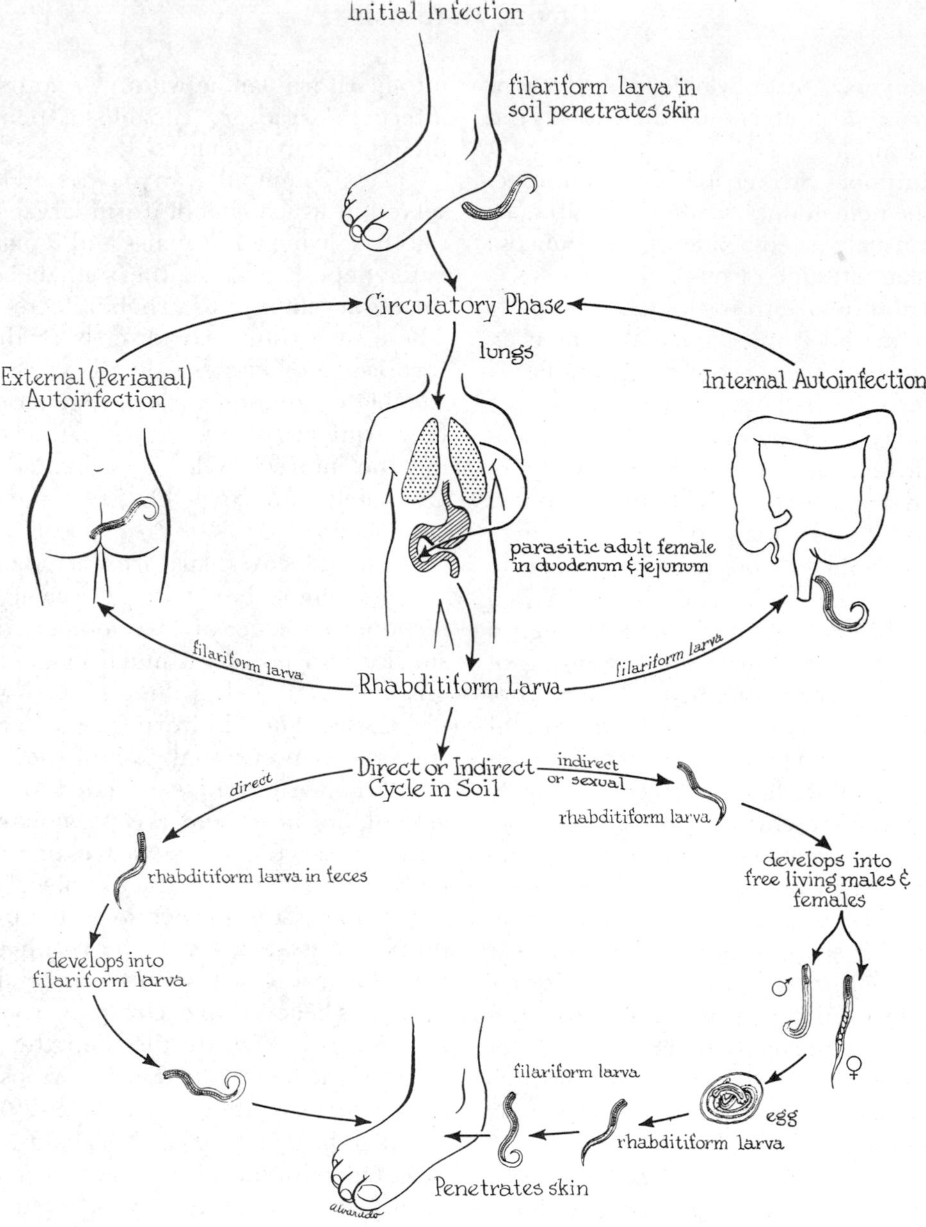

Figure 48–29. The life cycle of *Strongyloides stercoralis.* (Courtesy of the Louisiana State University School of Medicine, New Orleans.)

into dwarf filariform larvae within the bowel These directly penetrate the mucosa of the colon and rectum.

The above two types of hyperinfective cycles provide a built-in mechanism by which the patient's worm burden can be increased or replenished, even though he may never again come in contact with infested soil. It can easily be seen that, once acquired, such an infection can be continued for years—even for life—and that, protected by favorable internal environmental conditions, it can persist in any climate. Repeated autoinfection results in the pyramiding of one generation of adult parasites upon another in the duodenum; this process probably accounts for the frequent recurrences of clinical episodes that characterize this disease.

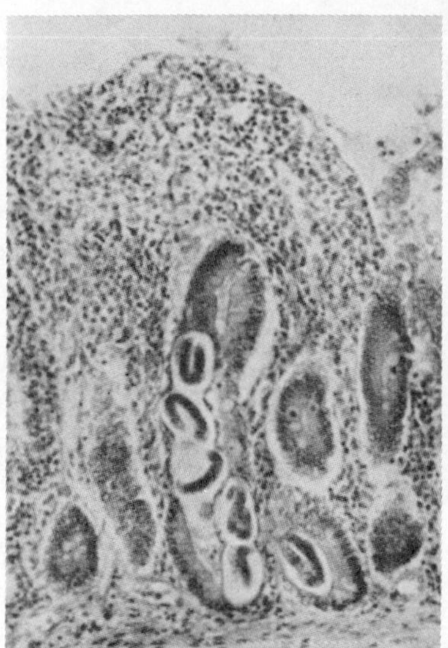

Figure 48-30

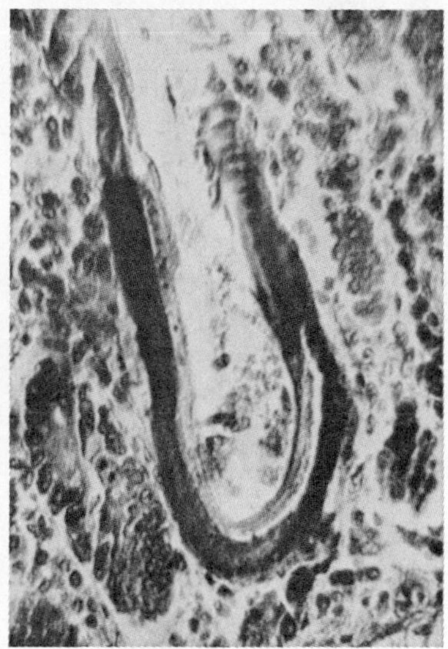

Figure 48-31

Figure 48-30. Embryonated eggs of *Strongyloides stercoralis* in mucosa of duodenum. (Courtesy of the Louisiana State University School of Medicine, New Orleans.)

Figure 48-31. Portion of a parasitic adult female *S. stercoralis* in mucosa of small intestine. (Courtesy of the Louisiana State University School of Medicine, New Orleans.)

Epidemiology. While much remains to be learned concerning the epidemiology of strongyloidiasis, it is known that man usually acquires the infection by skin contact with the infective filariform larvae. Penetration is effected in the same manner as in hookworm infection.

Pathology. Penetration of the skin usually causes no marked reaction. Larvae that reach the blood stream are carried to the lungs, where they migrate into the alveoli. Presumably they cause some bleeding as they erupt from the pulmonary capillaries and excite cellular infiltration. On rare occasions, a scattered patchy kind of infiltration (Loeffler's pneumonia) may occur in this infection. In general, pulmonary pathologic changes in human strongyloidiasis are not marked. The maturation of *S. stercoralis* to the adult stage in the lungs has been demonstrated in an experimental host. This occurs in humans, but is extremely rare. Occasionally, hyperinfective filariform larvae en route to the intestine may be found in sputum. This has been observed principally in patients with pulmonary disorders unrelated to strongyloidiasis, such as emphysema, bronchiectasis and carcinoma.

Normally, the immature females develop rapidly after reaching the duodenum and upper jejunum. There, they invade the mucosa (Figs. 48-30, 48-31) but usually do not go below the muscularis mucosae. Less frequently they may be found in the mucosa of the pyloric region of the stomach or ileum. The females soon produce eggs singly or in nests near the bases of the villi and in the interglandular stroma (Fig. 48-30). Upon hatching, the young larvae gradually work into the lumen of the intestine. In heavy infections the mucosa may be honeycombed by both the adult worms and the hatched larvae. In overwhelming infections, larvae may be found in all layers of the intestinal wall and widely disseminated in the viscera. In some cases, the reaction to the infection results in a duodenitis, which may be detected radiographically. An eosinophilia of about 10 per cent is usual; occasionally, patients are seen with eosinophil percentages in excess of 50 per cent due to strongyloidiasis.

Clinical Characteristics. The symptoms of strongyloidiasis vary. In some patients the parasite produces moderate or severe gastrointestinal disturbances; in others the infection may cause no symptoms. The clinical manifestations relate primarily to the duodenitis. Pain in the midepigastrium is the most common complaint. It is often sharply localized to the right of the midline, does not radiate, and may be described as a burning sensation, a deep dull ache or a cramp. The ingestion of food or alcohol may increase the pain. When the pain is localized, tenderness to deep firm pressure frequently is present. A salient diagnostic combination is the presence of pain in the epigastrium together with eosinophilia.

Nausea and vomiting may begin when the pain appears. A tentative diagnosis of peptic ulcer is often made in patients with strongyloidiasis. Diarrhea, anorexia, weight loss, weakness and generalized urticaria are relatively common complaints. Clinical exacerbations recur at irregular intervals and may be due to hyperinfection. Strongyloidiasis is a chronic disease and may lead to invalidism. Asthma is occasionally associated with strongyloidiasis. Manifestations of pulmonary disease occur when the adults, on rare occasions, parasitize the lungs. Fatalities have been reported in persons with massive hyperinfection but are not common.

Diagnosis. Eosinophilia is the most characteristic feature of the blood picture; polymorphonuclear leukocytosis may be marked or absent.

Examination of several stool specimens may be necessary to demonstrate larvae. The finding of motile rhabditiform larvae in a stool is highly suggestive of strongyloidiasis. Confirmation may be made by carefully checking the morphology of the larvae to distinguish them from those of hookworm. The rhabditiform larvae of *S. stercoralis* possess a short buccal capsule. The formalin-ether (MGL or AMS III) techniques usually reveal larvae if they are in the feces. The Harada-Mori test tuber filter paper method is a simple and efficient procedure to recover larvae of *S. stercoralis.* (See p. 833 for details of the methods.) Eggs of this species are observed in stools only on extremely rare occasions.

In about one-fourth of the cases of strongyloidiasis the larvae will not be found in the stool. If an infection with this parasite is suspected, duodenal fluid may be examined for the presence of larvae (Fig. 48–28) and embryonated eggs after examination of several stools has failed to demonstrate larvae. The method of obtaining duodenal samples devised by Beal and colleagues, consisting of the use of nylon yarn or ribbon coiled inside a weighted pharmaceutical capsule, is simple and effective (p. 816).[49]

Practicable serologic diagnostic techniques for strongyloidiasis are not available. Experimental studies of an indirect fluorescent antibody test show diagnostic value, but cross-reactions with filariasis occur which may be obviated by absorption.[50]

Treatment. Thiabendazole (Mintezol) is the drug of choice for treatment for strongyloidiasis.[25] The recommended dosage is 25 mg per kg twice daily for 2 days. Nausea, vomiting, vertigo, drowsiness, lethargy and headache are not uncommon side effects. Care should be taken in the use of this drug in persons with liver and renal disease.

Pyrvinium pamoate (Povan) also has anthelmintic activity in strongyloidiasis. A dose of 50 mg 3 times daily for 7 days has been employed for adults; an appropriate reduction of the dose is made for children.[51]

Mebendazole apparently has some anthelmintic activity against *S. stercoralis.* However, the cure rate with this drug probably is relatively low.[3]

Prophylaxis. The prophylaxis of strongyloidiasis does not differ from that of hookworm disease. In both, the essential features are prevention of soil pollution by human feces and protection against infection by the wearing of shoes.

Thiabendazole has been used very effectively for community control of strongyloidiasis in Costa Rica, being employed in two single dose treatments of 75 mg per kg of body weight at a 6-week interval.[52] The control program remained effective over a 7-year period of observation.[53]

Capillariasis Philippinensis

Synonyms. Wasting disease, Pudoc mystery disease, intestinal capillariasis.

Definition. Capillariasis philippinensis is a new chronic, wasting disease of man caused by the nematode *Capillaria philippinensis.* The parasite produces a syndrome resembling that of autoinfected, disseminated strongyloidiasis (p. 485) with diarrhea, abdominal pain, muscle wasting, edema and depletion of minerals, often leading to death in 2 to 4 months.[54]

Distribution. The disease was first noted in the Province of Ilocos Norte on the northwest coast of Luzon, the Philippines. It is now known to occur in five adjacent provinces and has recently been reported from southern Thailand.[55]

Etiology. MORPHOLOGY. The adult *Capillaria philippinensis* Chitwood, Valesquez and Salazar, 1968, is a small, slender nematode. The males range from 1.5 to 3.9 mm (average 2.6 mm); the females are larger and measure 2.3 to 5.3 mm (average 3.6 mm). The male spicule has a long sheath without spines. The vulva of the female is proximal to the esophagus; the eggs in utero have flattened bipolar plugs and measure 45 by 21 μm. In feces the eggs are usually unseg-

CAPILLARIA PHILIPPINENSIS		TRICHURIS TRICHIURA
	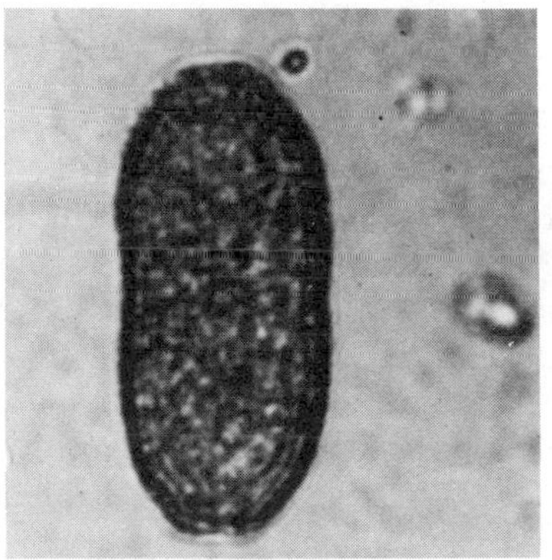	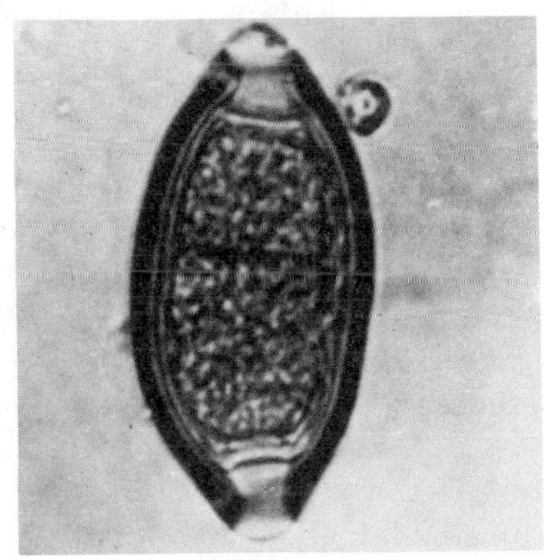
Size:	45 X 21 μm	52 X 26 μm
Shape:	peanut	ellipse
Plugs:	bipolar not protuberant	bipolar protuberant
Shell:	pitted	smooth

Figure 48–32. Comparison of *Capillaria philippinensis* and *Trichuris trichiura* eggs. (Courtesy of U.S. Naval Medical Research Unit No. 2. From G. E. Whalen et al. 1969. Intestinal capillariasis: a new disease in man. Lancet *1*:13–16.)

mented or in the one- or two-cell stage, are peanut-shaped and the outer shell is pitted (Fig. 48–32).[56]

Development. Both oviparous and larviparous females have been found at autopsy, suggesting that autoinfection is a part of the cycle. The presence of both eggs and larvae in the tissues supports this view, as do feeding experiments on gerbils[57] and monkeys.[58, 59]

Epidemiology. The disease has been found in at least 20 municipalities in five provinces along the western coast of Luzon that border on the South China Sea. The majority of cases have occurred in an area 40 by 10 km in the vicinity of Tagudin. Here many families ingest raw freshwater fish known as "birut" *(Eleotris melanosoma),* "bagsang" *(Ambassis miops),* and "bagsit" *(Hypseleotris bipartita).* These have been experimentally infected with *C. philippinensis* and subsequently fed to monkeys who became infected and passed eggs.[59] Currently the disease is known only from this one area of the Philippines and southern Thailand, but it possibly occurs in other regions where small freshwater fish are eaten raw. Possibly of zoonotic origin, the animal habitat of the worm remains uncertain. The disease primarily affects males between the ages of 20 and 50 years, although numerous infections occur in both sexes and in other age groups. During epidemic conditions, prior to the demonstration of effective therapy, the mortality was about 10 per cent.

Pathology. *Capillaria philippinensis* is found in the small intestine, especially the jejunum. The adults are partially imbedded in the mucosa. Small numbers are found free in the larynx, esophagus, stomach and colon, and have been seen rarely near the portal area of the liver.[60] The villi become flattened and the crypts of Lieberkühn atrophied. Histologic sections show a mild inflammatory response with edema of the basement membrane and distention of the mucous glands together with plasma cell and lymphocyte infiltration into the lamina propria. Although parasites have been found principally in the small intestine, pathologic changes also occur in other parts of the body. These are due to reactions to the migration of the parasites into the gut wall and to the effects of malnutrition and electrolyte depletion.

Clinical Characteristics. *Capillaria philippinensis* causes a syndrome suggesting autoinfected, disseminated strongyloidiasis, with initial symptoms of borborygmus, abdominal pain, intermittent and then persistent diarrhea with numerous sprue-like stools a day. Concomitantly there is weight loss, anorexia, malaise, nausea and vomiting. In more advanced cases there is cachexia with general muscle weakness and wasting and hyporeflexia. These are associated with malabsorption of sugars and fats and a marked protein-losing enteropathy resulting in severe peripheral edema. Also there are low levels of carotene, potassium, sodium and calcium.[61] Progressive loss of weight leading to cachexia and death may occur rapidly.

Diagnosis. The diagnosis of capillariasis philippinensis depends upon the detection of the characteristic eggs, which must not be confused with those of *Trichuris trichiura* (Fig. 48–32). Sometimes adult and larval worms are also found in the feces. An intradermal test, using antigen prepared from extracts of adult worms, has proved useful epidemiologically.

Treatment. This involves the replacement of fluids and electrolytes, a high protein diet and anthelmintic therapy. Mebendazole (Vermox) is the drug of choice; the dosage is 400 mg per day for 20 days for the treatment of initial infections and 30 days for those who have relapsed.[62] Thiabendazole (Mintezol) may also be used; the dosage is 25 mg per kg per day for 30 days followed by maintenance doses of 1 gm every other day for 6 months. Levotetramisole, an aminothiazole derivative, gave promising results at 2.5 mg per kg per day for 7 days followed by a similar dosage every other day for 15 days.[63]

REFERENCES

1. Jung, R. C., and Beaver, P. C. 1952. Clinical observations on *Trichocephalus trichiurus* (whipworm) infestation in children. Pediatrics *8*:548–557.

2. Biagi, F., and Gomez Medina, J. R. 1962. Caudro clinico de la trichocephalosis. Bol. Med. del Hosp. Infant. de México *19*:467–470.
3. Peña Chavarría, A., Swartzwelder, J. C., Villarejos, V. M., and Zeledon, R. 1973. Mebendazole, an effective broad-spectrum anthelmintic. Am. J. Trop. Med. Hyg. *22*:592–595.
4. Sargent, R. G., Savory, A. M., Mina, A., and Lee, P. R. 1974. A clinical evaluation of mebendazole in the treatment of trichuriasis. Am. J. Trop. Med. Hyg. *23*:375–377.

4a. Wolfe, M. S., and Wershing, J. M. 1974. Mebendazole. Treatment of trichuriasis in Bahamian children. J.A.M.A. *230*:1408–1411.

4b. Miller, M. J., Krupp, I. M., Little, M. D., and Santos, C. 1974. Mebendazole. An effective anthelmintic for trichuriasis and enterobiasis. J.A.M.A. *230*:1412–1414.

5. Wagner, E. D., and Peña Chavarría, A. 1974. *In vivo* effects of a new anthelmintic, mebendazole (R-17, 635), on the eggs of *Trichuris trichiura* and hookworm. Am. J. Trop. Med. Hyg. *23*:151–153.
6. Wagner, E. D., and Peña Chavarría, A. 1974. Morphologically altered eggs of *Trichuris trichiura* following treatment with mebendazole. Am. J. Trop. Med. Hyg. *23*:154–157.
7. Lynch, D. M., Green, E. A., McFadzean, J. A., and Pugh, I. M. 1972. *Trichuris trichiura* infestations in the United Kingdom and treatment with difetarsone. Br. Med. J. *4*:73–76.
8. Cram, E. B. 1943. Studies on oxyuriasis XXVII. Summary and conclusions. Am. J. Dis. Child. *65*:46–59.
9. Symmers, W. St. C. 1950. Pathology of oxyuriasis, with special reference to granulomas due to presence of *Oxyuris vermicularis (Enterobius vermicularis)* and its ova in tissues. A.M.A. Arch. Pathol. *50*:475–516.
10. Simon, R. D. 1974. Pinworm infestation and urinary tract infection in young girls. Am. J. Dis. Child. *128*:21–22.
11. Royer, A., and Berdknikoff, K. 1962. Pinworm infestation in children; the problem and its treatment. Can. Med. Assoc. J. *86*:60–65.
12. Bumbalo, T. S., Fugazotto, D. J., and Wyczalek, J. V. 1969. Treatment of enterobiasis with pyrantel pamoate. Am. J. Trop. Med. Hyg. *18*:50–52.
13. Brugmans, J. P., Thienpont, D. C., Van Wijngaarden, I., Vanparijs, O. F., Scheurmans, V. L., and Lauwers, H. L. 1971. Mebendazole in enterobiasis. Radiochemical and pilot clinical study in 1278 subjects. J.A.M.A. *217*: 313–316.
14. Mathies, A. W., Jr. 1969. Thiabendazole in the treatment of *Enterobius vermicularis*. Tex. Rep. Biol. Med. *27* (Suppl. 2): 611–614.
15. Brown, H. W., Chan, K. F., and Hussey, K. L. 1956. Treatment of enterobiasis and ascariasis with piperazine. J.A.M.A. *161*:515–520.
16. Most, H. 1973. Office management of common intestinal parasites. Drug Therapy *3*:39–45.

16a. Jalota, R., and Freston, J. W. 1974. Severe intrahepatic cholestasis due to thiabendazole. Am. J. Trop. Med. Hyg. *23*:676–678.

17. Matsumura, T. 1963. Ascaris allergy. Gunma J. Med. Sci. *12*:186–226.
18. Middlemiss, H. 1961. Tropical Radiology. Intercontinental Medical Book Corporation and Pittman Press, Bath, England. 272 pp.
19. Desowitz R. S., Bell, T., Williams, J., Cardines, R., and Tamarua, M. 1970. Anthelmintic activity of pyrantel pamoate. Am. J. Trop. Med. Hyg. *19*:775–778.
20. Villarejos, V. M., Arguedas-Gamboa, J., Eduarte, E., and Swartzwelder, J. C. 1971. Experiences with the anthelmintic pyrantel pamoate. Am. J. Trop. Med. Hyg. *20*:842–845.
21. Swartzwelder, J. C., Miller, J. H., and Sappenfield, R. W. 1957. The use of piperazine for the treatment of human helminthiases. Gastroenterology *33*:87–96.
22. Thienpont, D., Brugmans, J., Abadi, K., and Tanamal, S. 1969. Tetramisole in the treatment of nematode infections of man. Am. J. Trop. Med. Hyg. *18*:520–525.
23. Lionel, N. D. W., Mirando, E. H., Nanayakkara, J. C., and Soysa, P. E. 1969. Levamisole in the treatment of ascariasis in children. Br. Med. J. *4*:340–341.
24. Gatti, F., Krubwa, F., Vandepitte, J., and Thienpont, D. 1972. Control of intestinal nematodes in African schoolchildren by the trimestrial administration of levamisole. Ann. Soc. Belg. Med. Trop. *52*:19–32.
25. Campbell, W. C., and Cuckler, A. C. 1969. Thiabendazole in the treatment and control of parasitic infections in man. Tex. Rep. Biol. Med. *27* (Suppl. 2): 665–692.
26. Jayewardene, L. G., Ismail, M. M., and Wijayaratnam, Y. 1960. Bephenium hydroxynaphthoate in treatment of ascariasis. Br. Med. J. *2*:268–271.
27. Aiken, D. W., and Dickman, F. N. 1957. Surgery in obstruction of small intestine due to ascariasis. J.A.M.A. *164*:1317–1323.
28. Biagi, F., and Rodriguez, O. 1960. A study of ascariasis eradication by repeated mass treatment. Am. J. Trop. Med. Hyg. *9*:274–276.
29. Stoll, N. R. 1947. This wormy world. J. Parasit. *33*:1–18.
30. Chowdhury, A. B., and Schad, G. A. 1972. *Ancylostoma ceylanicum:* a parasite of man in Calcutta and environs. Am. J. Trop. Med. Hyg. *21*: 300–301.
31. Hunter, G. W., III, Ritchie, L. S., Chang, I. C., Kobayashi, H., Rolph, W. D., Jr., Mason, H. C., and Szewczak, J. 1951. Parasitological studies in the Far East. VII. An epidemiologic survey of Southern Korea. Japan Logistical Command. Bull. No. 2. 20 pp.
32. Hunter, G. W., III, Ritchie, L. S., Pan, C., and Lin, S. 1951. Parasitological studies in the Far East. XI. An epidemiologic survey of Okinawa, Ryukyu Islands. Japan Logistical Command. Bull. No. 3. 29 pp.
33. Anonymous. 1951. Parasitological studies in the Far East. XIV. Summary of the common intestinal and blood parasites of the Japanese. Japan Logistical Command. Bull. No. 4. 51 pp.
34. Stoll, N. R. 1962. On endemic hookworm, where do we stand today? Exp. Parasit. *12*:241–252.
35. Roche, M., and Layrisse, M. 1966. The nature and causes of hookworm anemia. Am. J. Trop. Med. Hyg. *15*: 1031–1102.
36. Layrisse, M., Blumenfeld, N., Carbonell, L., Desenne, J., and Roche, M. 1964. Intestinal absorption tests and biopsy of the jejunum in subjects with heavy hookworm infection. Am. J. Trop. Med. Hyg. *13*: 297–305.

37. Scrimshaw, N. W., Taylor, C. E., and Gordon, J. E. 1959. Interaction of nutrition and infection. Am. J. Med. Sci. *237*: 367–403.
38. Borrero, J., Restrepo, A., Botero, D., and Latorre, G. 1961. Clinical and laboratory studies on hookworm disease in Colombia. Am. J. Trop. Med. Hyg. *10*: 735–741.
39. Carr, H. P., Pichardo Sardá, M. E., and Nuñez, N. A. 1954. Anthelmintic treatment of uncinariasis. Am. J. Trop. Med. Hyg. *3*:495–503.
40. Goodwin, L. G., Jayewardene, L. G., and Standen, O. D. 1958. Clinical trials with bephenium hydroxynaphthoate against hookworm in Ceylon. Br. Med. J. *2*: 1572–1577.
41. Rowland, H. A. K. 1966. A comparison of tetrachlorethylene and bephenium hydroxynaphthoate in ancylostomiasis. Tr. Roy. Soc. Trop. Med. Hyg. *60*:313–321.
42. Dutta, J. K., 1970. Treatment of ankylostomiasis with combined therapy of bephenium hydroxynaphthoate and tetrachlorethylene. J. Indian Med. Assoc. *54*:150–152.
43. Banerjee, D., Prakash, O., and Kaliyugaperumal, V. 1972. A clinical trial of mebendazole (R 17,635) in cases of hookworm infection. Indian J. Med. Res. *60*: 562–566.
44. Farahmandian, I., Sahba, G. H., Arfaa, F., and Jalili, H. 1972. A comparative evaluation of the therapeutic effect of pyrantel pamoate and bephenium hydroxynaphthoate on *Ancylostoma duodenale* and other intestinal helminths. J. Trop. Med. Hyg. *75*:205–207.
45. Botero, D., and Castaño, A. 1973. Comparative study of pyrantel pamoate, bephenium hydroxynaphthoate, and tetrachloroethylene in the treatment of *Necator americanus* infections. Am. J. Trop. Med. Hyg. *22*: 45–52.
46. Botero, D., and Perez, A. 1970. Clinical evaluation of a new drug for the treatment of ancylostomiasis. Am. J. Trop. Med. Hyg. *19*: 471–475.
47. Swartzwelder, J. C., Peña Chavarría, A., Kotcher, E., Villarejos, V. M., Arguedas-Gamboa, J., Picado, B., and Esquivel, R. 1972. Control de la infección anquilostomiásica por tratamiento quimioterapéutica masivo en Costa Rica. Rev. Biol. Trop. *20*: 295–307.
48. Markell, E. K. 1968. Pseudohookworm infection—trichostrongyliasis. N. Engl. J. Med. *278*: 831–832.
49. Beal, C. B., Viens, P., Grant, R., and Hughes, J. 1970. Technique for sampling duodenal contents. Am. J. Trop. Med. Hyg. *19*:349–352.
50. DaFalla, A. A. 1972. The indirect fluorescent antibody test for the diagnosis of strongyloidiasis. J. Trop. Med. Hyg. *75*: 109–111.
51. Wang, C. C., and Galli, G. A. 1965. Strongyloidiasis treated with pyrvinium pamoate. J.A.M.A. *193*: 847–848.
52. Kotcher, E., Peña Chavarría, A., Arguedas-Gamboa, J., Guevara, W., and Villarejos, V. M. 1969. Community control of intestinal nematodes by thiabendazole treatment. Tex. Rep. Biol. Med. *27* (Suppl. 2): 629–643.
53. Arguedas-Gamboa, J., Villarejos, V. M., Swartzwelder, J. C., Peña Chavarría, A., Zeledon, R., and Kotcher, E. 1975. Community control of *Strongyloides stercoralis* by thiabendazole. Tex. Rep. Biol. Med. (In press)
54. Whalen, G. E., Rosenberg, E. B., Strickland, G. T., Gutman, R. A., Cross, J. H., Watten, R. H., Uylangco, C. V., and Dizon, J.-J. 1969. Intestinal capillariasis: a new disease in man. Lancet *1*: 13–16.
55. Anond, P., Kampol, P., Chatree, C., and Prasobsri, U. 1973. The first case of intestinal capillariasis in Thailand. S. E. Asian J. Trop. Med. Pub. Hlth. *4*: 131–134.
56. Chitwood, M. B., Valesquez, C., and Salazar, N. G. 1968. *Capillaria philippinensis* sp. n. (Nematoda: Trichinellida) from the intestine of man in the Philippines. J. Parasit. *54*: 368–371.
57. Cross, J. H., Banzon, T. C., Singson, C. N., Basaca-Servilla, V., and Watten, R. H. 1973. Zoonotic aspects of *Capillaria philippinensis*. 9th Internat. Congr. Trop. Med. Mal. Athens, Greece. *1*:154–155.
58. Cross, J. H., Banzon, T., Murrell, K. D., and Watten, R. H. 1970. A new epidemic diarrheal disease caused by the nematode, *Capillaria philippinensis*. Industry Trop. Hlth. 7:124–131.
59. Cross, J. H., Banzon, T., Clarke, M. D., Basaca-Servilla, V., Watten, R. H., and Dizon, J. -J. 1972. Studies on the experimental transmission of *Capillaria philippinensis* in monkeys. Tr. Roy. Soc. Trop. Med. Hyg. *66*:819–827.
60. Fresh, J. W., Cross, J. H., Reyes, V., Whalen, G. E., Uylangco, C. V., and Dizon, J.-J. 1972. Necropsy findings in intestinal capillariasis. Am. J. Trop. Med. Hyg. *21*: 169–173.
61. Watten, R. H., Beckner, W. M., Cross, J. H., Gunning, J.-J., and Jaramillo, J. 1972. Clinical studies of capillariasis philippinensis. Tr. Roy. Soc. Trop. Med. Hyg. *66*: 828–834.
62. Singson, C. N., Banzon, T. C., and Cross, J. H. 1974. Effectiveness of mebendazole in the treatment of intestinal capillariasis. Proc. 3rd Internatl. Congr. Parasit. München. *3*:1361–1362.
63. Singson, C. N., and Banzon, T. C. 1969. A preliminary report on levo-tetramisole: a new drug for intestinal capillariasis. J. Philippine Med. Assoc. *45*:627–632.

CHAPTER 49

Tissue-Inhabiting Nematodes: The Filarioidea

BIOLOGY OF THE FILARIOIDEA

Introduction. Nematodes principally inhabiting the extraintestinal tissues of man include the filarial worms, the guinea worm, the trichina worm and larvae of several other species of nematodes normally parasitic in animals, such as the dog and cat hookworm and ascarids, and the gnathostomes. These belong to the superfamilies FILARIOIDEA, DRACUNCULOIDEA, TRICHUROIDEA, STRONGYLOIDEA, ASCARIDOIDEA and SPIRUROIDEA. Only parasites in the first superfamily will be considered here. Members of the FILARIOIDEA infecting man may be characterized as follows:

1. The threadlike adults inhabit the tissues or body cavities of a vertebrate where the females produce eggs which are partially or completely embryonated.

2. At the time of oviposition, or just prior thereto, the embryos uncoil and are known as microfilariae.

3. The eggshell may persist, accommodating itself to the elongated larva, thus producing a "sheathed" microfilaria. If the shell ruptures, a naked or "unsheathed" microfilaria results.

4. All microfilariae must pass a developmental stage in a bloodsucking insect vector (Fig. 49–1).

Some of the tissue-inhabiting nematodes produce diseases in man. Thus, Bancroft's filariasis is an infection by *Wuchereria bancrofti,* filariasis malayi by *Brugia malayi,* onchocerciasis by *Onchocerca volvulus* and loiasis by *Loa loa.* Two other filariae, *Dipetalonema perstans* and *Mansonella ozzardi,* which are found in man do little if any damage and produce few if any symptoms. In addition to these well recognized parasites, a number of rarer forms also have been re-

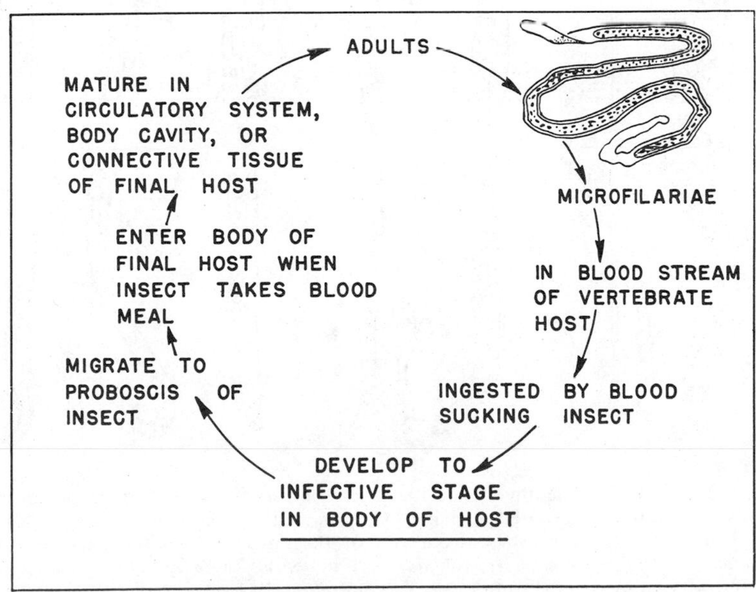

Figure 49–1. Nematode cycle – filarial worm type.

ported in man but will not be considered here.

MORPHOLOGY OF THE FILARIOIDEA

Adults. The adult parasites vary between 19 mm and 60 cm in length, the females often being twice as long as the males. Most are creamy white, filiform worms whose cuticle may be smooth, transversely striated, or covered with annular rings or knoblike bosses. There are species-specific papillae about the head, mouth and usually the tail. In some species the males possess caudal alae, and all have spicules that vary in size and shape. Further details will be found in the discussion of the appropriate species.

Microfilariae. Adult females produce prelarvae known as microfilariae which range from 177 to 300 μm in length. Some of these embryonic forms retain their shells as "sheaths"; others break out and hence are "unsheathed." Sheaths appear as delicate close-fitting membranes that may be de-

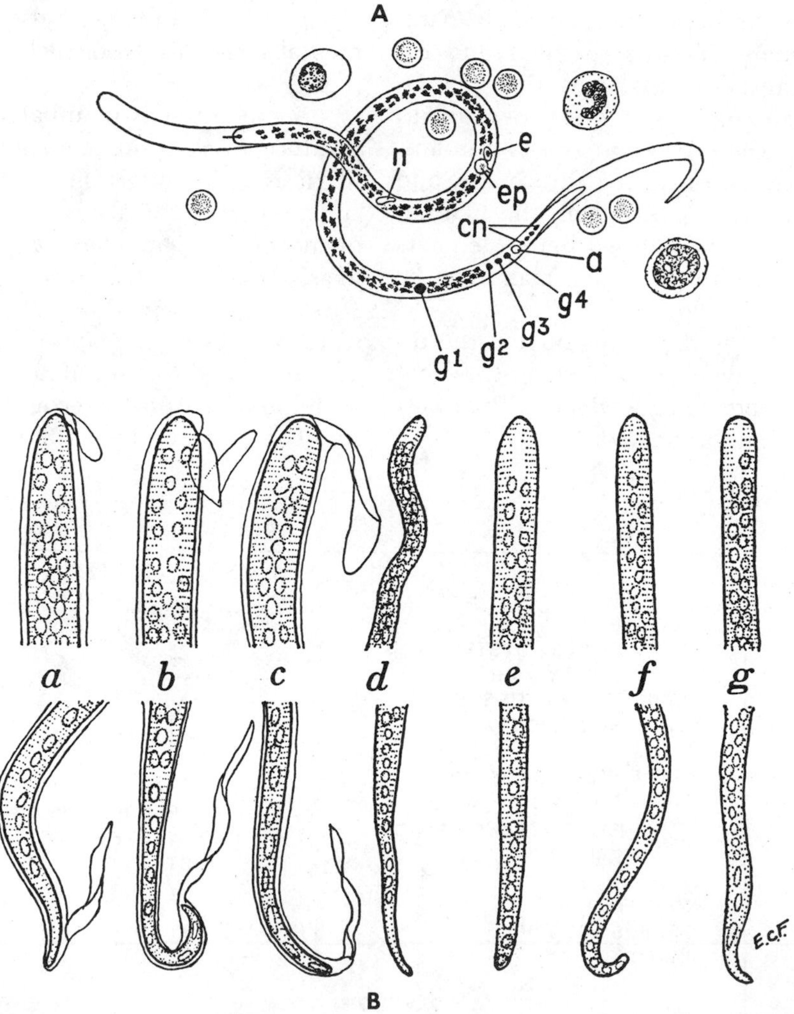

Figure 49–2. *A*, Diagram of a sheathed microfilaria of *Wuchereria bancrofti* from peripheral blood showing characteristic features: *a*, anal pore; *cn*, caudal nuclei; *e*, excretory cell; *ep*, excretory pore; g^{1-4}, genital cells; *n*, nerve ring. (Original.) *B*, Differential characteristics of anterior or posterior ends of the microfilariae of *a. Wuchereria bancrofti; b, Brugia malayi; c, Loa loa; d, Onchocerca volvulus; e, Dipetalonema perstans; f, D. streptocerca* and *g, Mansonella ozzardi.* Greatly enlarged, drawn to scale. (From Faust, E. C., Russell, P. F., and Jung, R. C. 1970. Craig and Faust's Clinical Parasitology. 8th ed. Lea & Febiger, Philadelphia.)

Table 49–1. Vectors of Human Filarioidea

Parasite	*Hosts*
Wuchereria bancrofti and *Brugia malayi*	Many species of mosquitoes belonging to the genera *Culex, Aedes, Mansonia, Anopheles*
Onchocerca volvulus	Black flies: *Simulium damnosum, Simulium neavei, Eusimulium avidum, Eusimulium ochraceum, Eusimulium mooseri,* and probably others
Loa loa	Tabanid flies: *Chrysops dimidiata, Chrysops silacea*
Mansonella ozzardi	Midge: *Culicoides furens*
Dipetalonema perstans	Midge: *Culicoides austeni, Culicoides grahami*
Dipetalonema streptocerca	Probably midge: *Culicoides grahami*

tected only where they project beyond the anterior or posterior ends of the microfilariae. Internally each parasite is seen to consist of columns of nuclei that are believed to represent the anlagen of various sytems and structures. The best means of differentiating various species of microfilariae lie in noting the position of organ precursors of parts of the digestive, excretory and reproductive systems and the position of the caudal nuclei. These stain deeply with hematoxylin and occupy characteristic positions. Certain anatomic landmarks differ in their distances from the anterior tip of the worm. Such structures include the nerve ring, excretory pore, excretory cell in relation to the excretory pore, anal pore, and the four genital cells, g^{1-4} (Fig. 49–2*A*).[1]

A determination of the type of periodicity displayed by the microfilariae is of value in making tentative species identifications, although periodicity can be reversed in some species if the patient works at night and sleeps during the day. For example, the microfilariae of the nocturnally periodic form of *W. bancrofti* occur in greatest numbers in the peripheral blood between 8 P.M. and 2 A.M., while the microfilariae of the diurnal (diurnally subperiodic) strain appear in the peripheral blood at all times but reach a peak between 10 A.M. and 8 P.M.[2, 3] In loiasis the microfilariae are also diurnal. However, the mechanism of microfilarial periodicity is not understood, although many hypotheses have been advanced, including the presence of "animal clocks" built into the 24-hour cycle.[3]

Developmental Stages. All members of the Filarioidea require an insect intermediate host. As this vector feeds on man,

Table 49–2. A Key to the Common Microfilariae Infecting Man

1	(10)	Microfilariae in peripheral blood	2
2	(7)	Microfilariae sheathed	3
3	(4)	Nuclei do not extend to tip of tail; cephalic space equal to diameter of head; nocturnal periodicity (or nonperiodic ?)	*Wuchereria bancrofti*
4	(3)	Nuclei extend to tip of tail in broken or unbroken chain; diurnal or nocturnal periodicity	5
5	(6)	Nuclei extend in solid row to tip of tail; diurnal periodicity	*Loa loa*
6	(5)	Nuclei extend in broken row to tip of tail, resembling *W. bancrofti* except for two small terminal nuclei; cephalic space twice diameter of head; nocturnal periodicity	*Brugia malayi*
7	(2)	Microfilariae unsheathed	8
8	(9)	Nuclei extending to tip of tail, often appearing as a double row; tail straight	*Dipetalonema perstans*
9	(8)	Nuclei not extending to tip of tail	*Mansonella ozzardi*
10	(1)	Microfilariae typically in skin and subcutaneous tissues	11
11	(12)	Nuclei extending to tip of tail, usually as a single row; tail strongly bent in shepherd's crook curve; rarely in blood films	*Dipetalonema streptocerca*
12	(11)	Nuclei not extending to tip of tail	*Onchocerca volvulus*

Table 49–3. The Differentiation of the Microfilariae of the Filarioidea of Man*

Sheathed Microfilariae From Peripheral Blood

Characteristics	Wuchereria bancrofti	Brugia malayi	Loa loa
Periodicity	Usually nocturnal	Nocturnal	Diurnal
Appearance	Graceful sweeping curves	Stiff, secondary kinks	Stiff, secondary kinks
Tail	Tapers to a delicate point, terminal nuclei absent	Slight bulb at tip, 2 terminal nuclei	Gradual tapering, caudal nuclei continuous row into tail
Length	244–296μm (thick films)	177–230μm (thick films)	250–300μm (thick films)
Excretory cell	Small, near excretory pore	Large, far behind excretory pore	Large, far behind excretory pore
G cells	Small, similar in size; g^{2-4} far behind g^1; g^1 – 70.14%‡	Larger; g^1 relatively near and larger than g^{2-4}; g^1 – 68.33%‡	Similar to those of *B. malayi;* g^1 – 68.6%‡
Anal pore	82.48%	82.28%‡	81.9%‡
Intermediate host	Best – *Culex quinquefasciatus* (= *Culex fatigans*), *Anopheles gambiae*	Best – *Mansonia* spp.† *Anopheles* spp.	*Chrysops* spp.
Cephalic space	As long as broad	Twice as long as broad	?
Stylets	1	2	?
Body nuclei	Well defined	Blurred, intermingled	Larger and stain less deeply

Unsheathed Microfilariae From Peripheral Blood

Characteristics	Mansonella ozzardi	Dipetalonema perstans
Stylet	1	0
Tail	5 terminal nuclei not reaching tip of tail	Nuclei extend to tip of tail, often in 2 rows

Microfilariae of Skin and Subcutaneous Tissues

Characteristics	Dipetalonema streptocerca	Onchocerca volvulus
Sheath	Absent	Absent
Stylet	?	None
Tail	Shepherd's crook curve	Slightly curved
Nuclei	?	5–7 near tip

*Modified from Faust's adaptation from Feng, 1933.
†Subgenus *Mansonioides.*
‡Distance from anterior end.

microfilariae are ingested. The parasites soon leave the vector's alimentary canal, undergo a period of development in the thoracic muscles, and finally migrate into the mouthparts, where they are infective for man. When the insect next feeds on man the parasites leave the vector, penetrate the skin surface at or near the bite site and migrate to the definitive location specific for the development of the given species of worm. After maturing and mating, the adult females produce microfilariae (Fig. 49–2). The better known vectors are listed in Table 49–1.

Differentiation of Microfilariae. Microfilariae in onchocerciasis may occur in aspirate of nodules, in thin sections of skin or in tissue fluid obtained by the skin scarification technique. Microfilariae of other species of the Filarioidea are found in films of the peripheral blood, some being diurnal, others nocturnal. Still others display no periodicity. These larvae or prelarvae may be differentiated by the key presented in Table 49–2.

A more detailed summary of the microfilariae infecting man occurs in Table 49–3.

Filariasis Bancrofti

Synonyms. Bancroft's filariasis, *Wuchereria bancrofti* infection.

Definition. Filariasis bancrofti is due to the presence of adult *W. bancrofti* in the lymphatic system or connective tissues of man. The infection may be accompanied by important pathologic conditions related to the lymphatic system, including inflammatory lesions, dilatation and rupture of lymphatics, hypertrophy, hyperplasia and fibrosis. Offspring of the parent worms, known as microfilariae, are characteristically present in the circulating blood; their presence while alive does not contribute to the pathologic changes listed above. Many species of *Anopheles, Culex, Mansonia* and *Aedes* are vectors.

Some workers regard periodic (i.e. nocturnally periodic) filariasis bancrofti as different from the diurnal (diurnally subperiodic) form. Variations in the clinical development of these two entities, their mutual geographic isolation and their different types of periodicity suggest the possibility that two species, or perhaps varieties, of etiologic agent exist.

Distribution. Filariasis bancrofti is widespread throughout much of the tropics and subtropics (Fig. 49–3). In the Western Hemisphere it was formerly established as far north as Charleston, S.C., but no longer occurs there. The disease occurs throughout the West Indies, Colombia (rare), Venezuela and portions of the Guianas and Brazil.

In Europe and the eastern Mediterranean only a single focus of *W. bancrofti* transmission remains, in Alanya in Turkey. Along the North African Coast it occurs spottily from lower Egypt to Morocco. Other areas include a wide belt across the central portion of Africa, Madagascar, the neighboring islands and the east and west coastal regions.

The disease is endemic in the Orient. In many localities its distribution overlaps that of *B. malayi,* which was not described until 1927. The periodic (nocturnal) form has also been reported from coastal Arabia to India and is found with the Malayan form in India, Bangladesh, Southeast Asia, southern China, the Philippines and southern Japan. It occurs in the Pacific area in Micronesia, and in Papua/New Guinea and adjacent islands including the Solomons and New Hebrides; it is transmitted primarily by *Culex* and *Anopheles* mosquitoes.

The diurnal (subperiodic) form of *W. bancrofti* is found only in the South Pacific, in the Polynesian zone, particularly Fiji, and in New Caledonia and the Loyalty Islands. It is transmitted by *Aedes* mosquitoes. A subperiodic form has also been identified in Thailand; since the microfilaremia is mainly nocturnal, it appears to be more closely related to the periodic (nocturnal) form.

The prevalence of filariasis in the Pacific Islands, productive of an epidemic in the American forces in World War II notable for the absence of a detectable microfilaremia,[4] has been considerably reduced in recent years by the use of diethylcarbamazine in mass treatment control projects.

Etiology. MORPHOLOGY. Adult *W. bancrofti* (Cobbold, 1877) Seurat, 1921 localize in the lymphatic vessels and the lymph nodes. The males and females are often closely intertwined. The mature worms are threadlike, cylindrical and creamy white, with a smooth cuticula and bluntly tapering extremities. The slightly swollen cephalic region bears two rings of small papillae. The unarmed mouth opens directly into a cylindrical esophagus which is divided into an anterior muscular and a posterior glandular portion. The male worm can be as long as 40 mm. On the ventrally curved tail may be found a maximum of eight preanal and four postanal pairs of papillae supporting narrow inconspicuous alae; farther caudad there are two pairs of larger papillae and one pair of smaller ones. Copulatory spicules, which vary in size and shape, and a crescent-shaped gubernaculum characterize the male.

The females are longer, ranging between 80 and 100 mm. The vulva opens about 0.8 or 0.9 mm from the anterior tip. The vagina extends to a long, bilateral, coiled uterus which has its origin about 1 mm from the posterior tip.

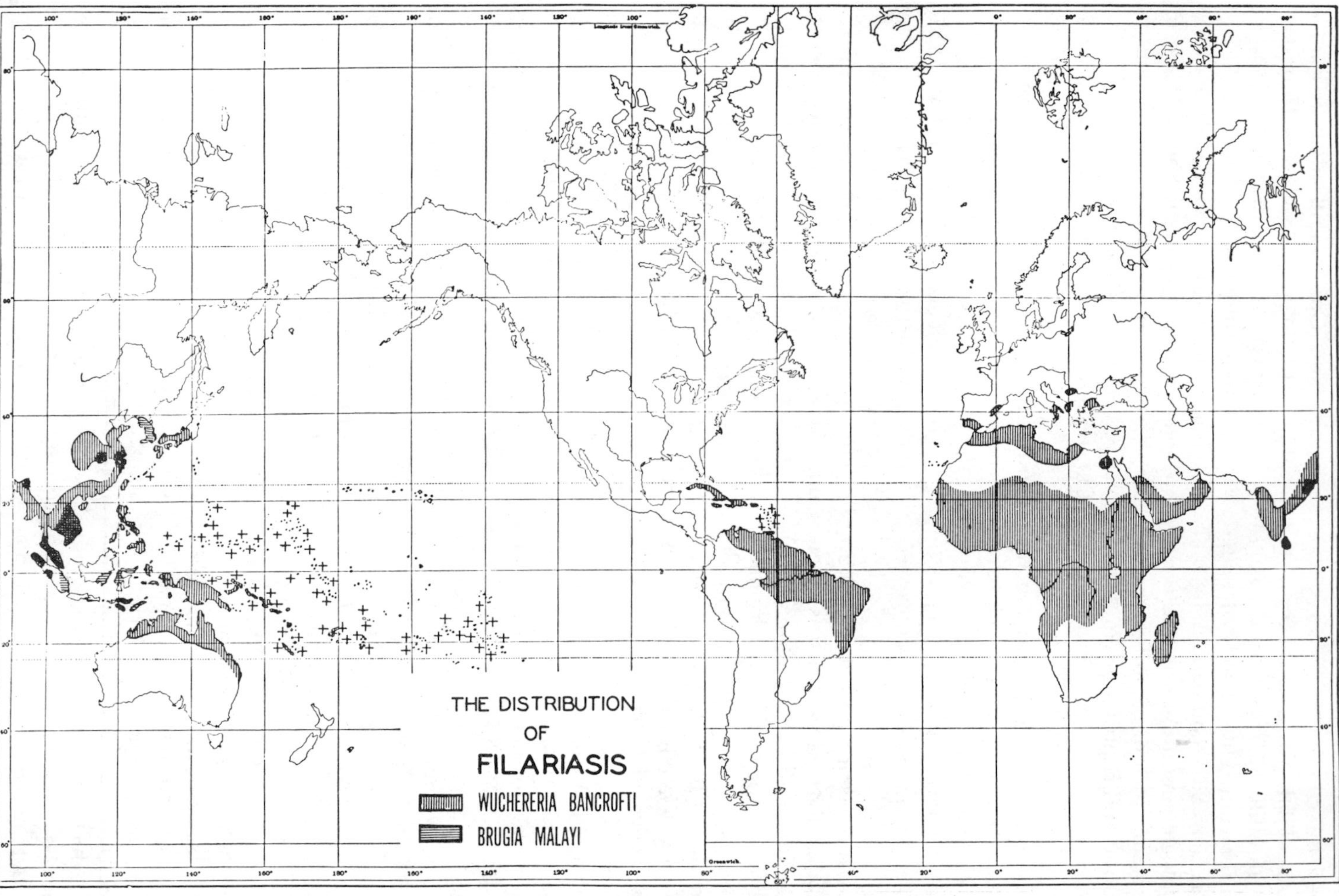

Figure 49–3. Geographic distribution of filariasis due to *Wuchereria bancrofti* and *Brugia malayi*. + indicates presence of one or the other species in Polynesia and the West Indies. (From Faust, E. C., Russell, P. F., and Jung, R. C. 1970. Craig and Faust's Clinical Parasitology. 8th ed. Lea & Febiger, Philadelphia.)

Developing microfilarial embryos are coiled in a membrane or shell averaging about 38 by 25 μm in size. Later this structure elongates to form the microfilarial sheath.

Fully developed, sheathed microfilariae measure 244 to 296 μm in length by 7.5 to 10 μm in breadth. The tip of the head is described as bearing a stylet, and the cephalic space between the column of nuclei and the anterior tip is approximately equal to the diameter of the head. Adequate staining of smears is necessary to determine that the nerve ring is 20 per cent of the body length from the anterior tip; the excretory pore, 29.6 per cent; the excretory cell, 30.6 per cent; the G_1 cell, 70.14 per cent and the anal pore, 82.4 per cent (Fig. 49–2*A*). The last 5 per cent of the body length, the tail, is devoid of nuclei, a point of importance in distinguishing between the microfilariae of this species and *B. malayi* (Table 49–3). Microfilariae of periodic and diurnal (or subperiodic) *W. bancrofti* are morphologically indistinguishable.

DEVELOPMENT. Adult *W. bancrofti* normally inhabit the lymphatics, where they liberate microfilariae. The latter either remain in the lymph or reach the peripheral circulation, where they are ingested by the mosquito vector as it feeds. They complete their intermediate development in the gut and tissues of the insect host.

Within an hour after ingestion, the larvae exsheath and those that are not passed in the mosquito's feces penetrate the stomach wall and migrate within 24 hours to the thoracic muscles. Here the parasites undergo a series of complex morphologic changes, including two molts. During this period the developing larvae pass from a sausage-shaped stage to mature, infective filiform (third stage) larvae between 1.4 and 2 mm in length. Under optimum conditions 10 or 11 days are required for this transformation to occur. The larvae then migrate to the mouthparts of the mosquito, from which point they reach the new host when the mosquito next feeds. Since the larvae usually leave the mosquito by breaking through Dutton's membrane, it is believed they actively penetrate the skin, entering either the puncture site, or possibly even forming their own portal of entry. The filiform larvae that succeed in establishing entrance eventually reach the lymphatic system and are thought to mature within about a year. The details of the migrations and development of these worms within man are not fully known.

Epidemiology. Complete development of the larval forms of *W. bancrofti* has been shown to occur in at least 70 species of mosquitoes included in the genera *Anopheles, Culex, Aedes* and *Mansonia.* However, these mosquitoes are not all necessarily concerned with the transmission of the infection in nature. Some of the most important known vectors are *C. pipiens quinquefasciatus (C. fatigans), C. pipiens, C. pipiens pallens, Anopheles gambiae, A. funestus, A. darlingi, A. punctulatus, A. farauti, Aedes aegypti* and *Aedes polynesiensis.*

The importance of a particular potential mosquito vector depends to a large extent upon whether it feeds on human rather than animal blood and breeds in areas in close proximity to man. The conditions necessary for maintaining filariasis at a high level of endemicity are an adequate human reservoir, a sufficient number of cases having numerous microfilariae in the peripheral blood, and ample breeding of suitable mosquitoes within range of the infected population. This means that where the microfilariae have a diurnal periodicity (diurnally subperiodic) the mosquito vectors basically must be daytime feeders (Fig. 49–4).[3]

The roles of occasional or continuous infection in the development of the syndromes of the disease are not known. It is said that the incidence of demonstrable infection is low in young children and infants and highest after the twentieth year. It is also claimed that the prevalence of clinical disease varies between the sexes in different parts of the world. This may be an expression of differences in occupation of the infected individuals and of variations in the behavior and habitats of the important vectors in different regions. It is probable that persons experiencing asymptomatic infections and the early clinical stages of the disease constitute the important human res-

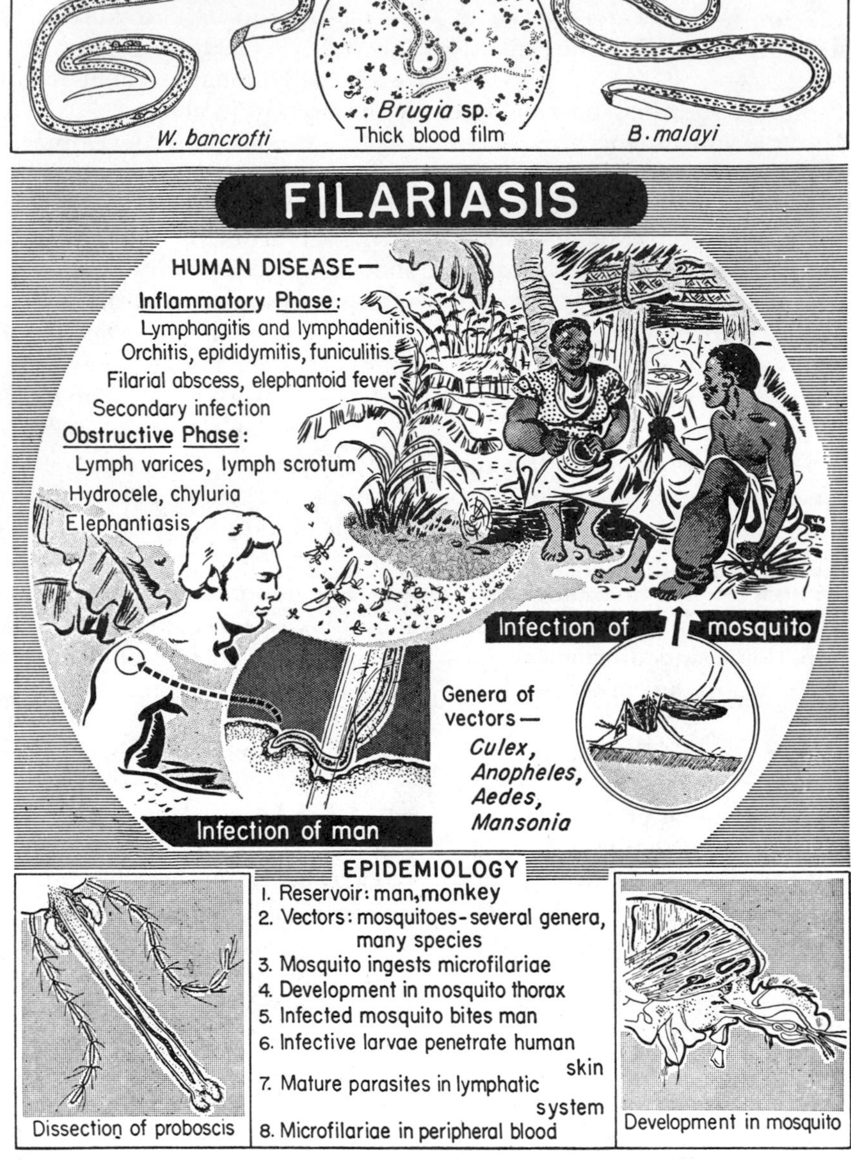

Figure 49–4. Epidemiology of filariasis.

ervoir. In the early or advanced stages, particularly in the presence of elephantiasis, microfilariae may not be present in the peripheral blood.

As previously indicated, periodicity is the alternate increase and decrease in the number of microfilariae present in the peripheral blood. The epidemiologic importance of the phenomenon of periodicity is that it will determine which species of mosquito become infected. Microfilariae with nocturnal periodicity are therefore transmitted almost exclusively by night-biters, while the diurnally subperiodic microfilariae are transmitted primarily by daytime feeders.

There is no natural immunity to human filariasis.

Pathology. The pathology that develops in infections of *W. bancrofti* is the result of several factors, such as: the

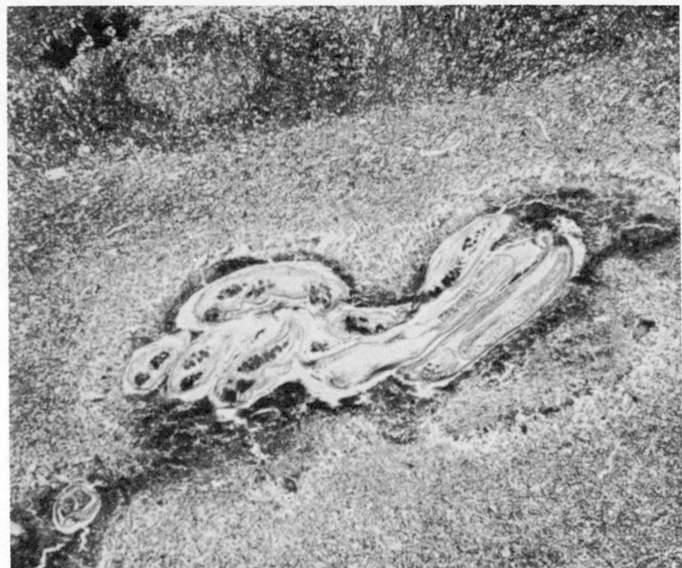

Figure 49-5. Filariasis: acute inflammatory reaction about female worm in a lymph node.

number of microfilariae inoculated into man by the mosquito; the number of infected bites received; whether such bites are received within a short space of time or spread out over years; the location of the sites where the parasites come to rest and develop to maturity; the tolerance of the victim to this foreign protein introduced in the form of a parasite; and, lastly, the possibility of intervening secondary bacterial infections.

The essential pathologic changes in filariasis consist of inflammatory reactions and subsequent progressive obstruction of lymphatic channels by scar tissue (Fig. 49-5). These changes occur especially in the vicinity of adult worms, which are commonly found in the lymphatic vessels, especially those of the abdominal cavity. However, worms may be present in the lymphatics in any part of the body. Common sites are the elephantoid tissues of the external genitalia and the mammary gland, the lymph nodes of the extremities, and the retroperitoneal tissues, particularly about the kidneys. There is no evidence to indicate that circulating microfilariae participate in the production of lesions, although in the lung they may initiate the hypersensitive response characteristic of tropical eosinophilia. (See p. 540.)

Biopsy studies performed on United States troops in the Southwest Pacific infected by the diurnal *W. bancrofti* during World War II have thrown some light on the genesis and the progression of the pathologic changes. The acute stages of filariasis of the lymphatic system may occur as early as 3 months after exposure. Essentially the same lesions were found whether or not adult worms, living or dead, were present. Furthermore, there was no indication that either microfilariae or bacteria participate in the early pathology.

The lesions in the lymph nodes were characterized by granulomatous inflammation, proliferation of the macrophage (reticuloendòthelial) system and eosinophilia of adjacent tissues. The dilated sinuses showed a wide zone of microphages with variable numbers of eosinophils, lymphocytes and foreign body giant cells at the periphery. Necrosis was slight in amount, and there was no increase of collagenous connective tissue.

The lymphatic vessels showed a variety of lesions, including hyperplasia of the lining endothelium and of reticular cells in the walls, acute lymphangitis with or without thrombosis of the vessel and, finally, fibrous obliteration. It would appear that the latter constitutes the basis for the development of lymph blockage and elephantiasis by succes-

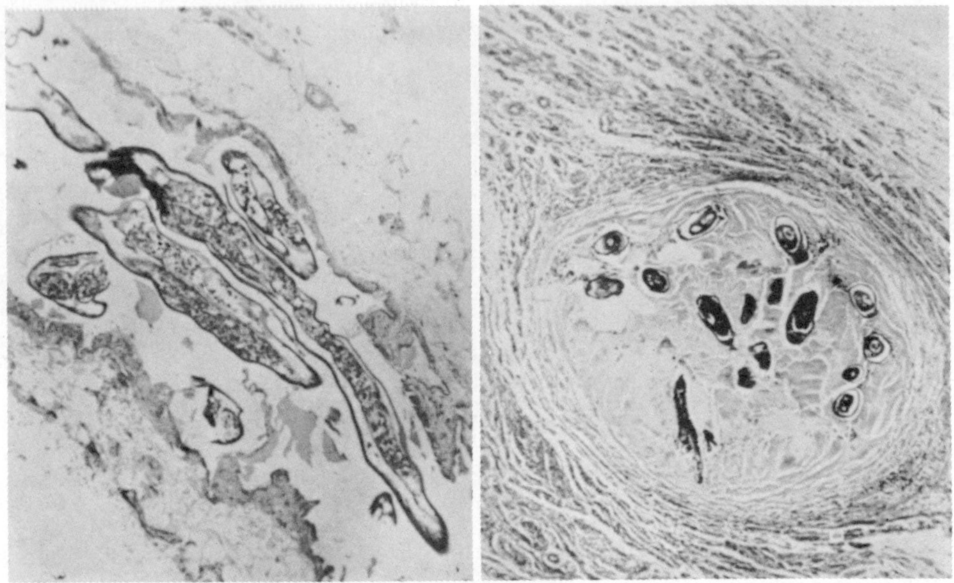

Figure 49–6 Figure 49–7

Figure 49–6. Longitudinal section of intact filarial worm in lymph vessel. (Courtesy of Drs. L. Galindo, F. von Lichtenberg and C. Baldizón and Am. J. Trop. Med. Hyg., vol. 11.)

Figure 49–7. Granuloma containing a partially calcified filarial worm. (Courtesy of Drs. L. Galindo, F. von Lichtenberg and C. Baldizón and Am. J. Trop. Med. Hyg., vol. 11.)

sive thrombosis, organization of the thrombus and fibrosis with obliteration of the lymph channel.

In some infected persons there may be no significant host tissue response to the presence of the adult filariae. In others who are hypersensitive to the filariae, the living or dead worms may cause inflammation or fibrosis. These may be the result of toxic secretions of the parasite, mechanical irritation, or disintegration products left after the death of the worm.

Lymphatic obstruction (Fig. 49–6) is almost invariably followed by acute lymphangitis, which may be accompanied by leukocytosis and eosinophilia. The inflammatory reaction is followed by the deposition of scar tissue about the involved lymphatics and lymph nodes. Degenerated worms ultimately may become calcified (Fig. 49–7).[5, 6]

Following repeated inflammatory episodes, chronic obstruction to the lymphatic circulation occurs and there is progressive fibrosis. The distal lymph channels are distended or thrombosed, and the tissues become edematous and infiltrated with connective tissue. When the thoracic duct is involved, distended lymphatics in the urinary tract may rupture, causing chyluria. When the extremities and superficial structures are involved, the lymphatic obstruction and fibrosis lead to great thickening of the skin and subcutaneous tissues and the development of elephantiasis.

Clinical Characteristics. The infection may produce no symptoms in some persons while in others a variety of manifestations may ensue. The clinical phases of filariasis may be classified as inflammatory or obstructive. The effects of inflammation may include lymphangitis, lymphadenitis, orchitis, epididymitis, funiculitis, filarial abscess, elephantoid fever and secondary bacterial infections, especially by streptococci and staphylococci. The obstructive phase is accompanied by a variety of clinical syndromes. Lymphatic dilatation without rupture produces lymph varices, lymph scrotum and hydrocele. Rupture of the distended lymphatics is responsible for chyluria and chylous ascites. The advanced stages of the obstructive phase are characterized by elephantiasis, which commonly affects the leg, the scrotum, the arm and the mammae.

Clinical filariasis normally has a prolonged incubation period which is seldom of less than 8 to 12 months' duration and may be much longer. However, it is now well established that clinical phenomena may appear within 3 months of exposure. The early stages of the infection are usually accompanied by inflammatory phenomena and fever, which frequently suggest other conditions.

The initial symptoms are largely local and unaccompanied by significant constitutional reaction. They usually consist of pain, swelling or redness of an arm or leg; or pain and swelling in the scrotal region. Stiffness of an involved extremity is common. Local lymphangitis with enlargement of the regional lymph nodes, particularly the epitrochlear, the axillary, the femoral or the inguinal nodes, depending upon the site of infection, frequently accompanies the early symptoms. Fever is usually mild when present. Characteristically, the acute local symptoms are transitory, rarely persisting more than a week or 10 days. Enlargement of lymph nodes, however, tends to persist. Repeated recurrences of these phenomena are usual in the early stages of the disease.

THE INFLAMMATORY PHASE. *Acute lymphangitis* is a common early manifestation, usually involving the lower extremities, accompanied by fever ranging to 40° C (104° F), often with chills, and by more or less severe toxemia. The onset is frequently preceded by a "focal spot" of sharply circumscribed pain and tenderness, often in the region of one of the malleoli, and followed by ascending lymphangitis originating in this area. In other instances, the lymphangitis begins centrally and follows a centrifugal course. The affected part is swollen, often tender and painful, and the involved lymphatics are frequently palpable. The skin may be diffusely reddened or red streaks may be seen over the inflamed lymphatic vessels. When the abdominal lymphatics are involved, the clinical picture may suggest malaria or an acute abdomen. Involvement of the testes and spermatic cord is common. Spontaneous resolution occurs after several days. The skin of the affected part may return to normal, or there may be residual induration. Recurring attacks are usual.

Inguinal lymphadenitis commonly accompanies or may precede filarial lymphangitis. The nodes are usually enlarged, painful and tender during the attack.

Filarial orchitis is a frequent acute manifestation. The onset is usually sudden, with pain in the testicle, fever and, occasionally, rigors. The testicle enlarges rapidly and is extremely tender; this condition is commonly accompanied by hydrocele. Recurrences are frequent.

Funiculitis, a lymphangitis of the spermatic cord, and *epididymitis* are likewise common complications of filariasis (Fig. 49–8).

Filarial abscesses are often deeply seated in intermuscular fascial planes but frequently occur about infected lymph nodes, particularly those of the inguinal, axillary and epitrochlear regions. Dead filarial worms may be present in the abscess cavity. The pathologic process apparently is the combined result of the presence of the parasite and secondary bacterial infection.

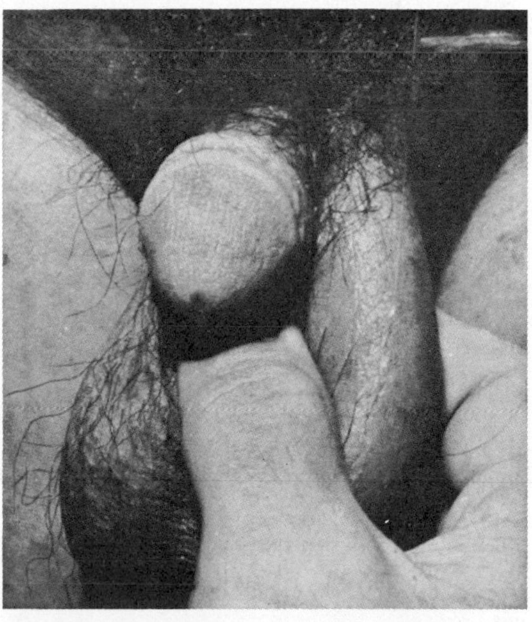

Figure 49–8. Filariasis: thickened spermatic cord.

Elephantoid fever is a recurrent acute febrile condition which may be associated with elephantiasis or lymphangitis. Inflammatory phenomena may be absent; in these instances, it is probable that there is an acute lymphangitis of the visceral lymphatics. The onset is usually sudden, with fever ranging to 40° C (104° F), rigors and sweating. An attack may last from a few hours to several days. Recurrences are common and frequent.

THE OBSTRUCTIVE PHASE. This phase of filariasis is characterized by interference with the lymphatic circulation, edema and accumulations of serous fluid. These manifestations frequently appear in the course of the various phenomena of the inflammatory phase which commonly leave evidence of progressive lymphatic obstruction in their wake. The two phases of the disease, therefore, often exist concurrently, each contributing to the progressive pathologic changes.

Lymph varices, or "varicose glands," commonly affect the inguinal or femoral lymph nodes of one or both sides and, less often, the axillary nodes. These are soft lobulated swellings which usually develop slowly as the result of obstruction and dilatation of the lymphatic vessels. They are not attached to the overlying skin. The dilated lymphatics are palpable and tense, having a soft elastic consistency. The condition is usually painless and insidious. Aspirated fluid may contain microfilariae. Incision may be followed by a persistent lymph sinus (Fig. 49–9).

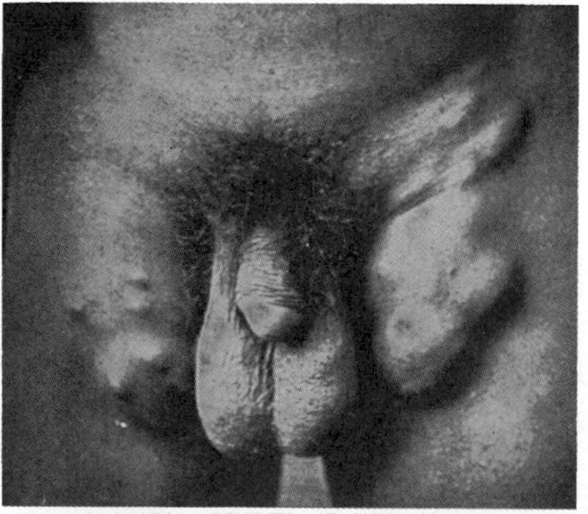

Figure 49–9. Filariasis: varicose inguinal lymph nodes. (After Taniguchi-Kumanoto. From Strong. 1944. Stitt's Diagnosis, Prevention, and Treatment of Tropical Diseases. The Blakiston Company, Philadelphia.)

Lymph scrotum in many instances is associated with inguinal lymph varices and with chyluria. The onset often occurs with fever, swelling of the scrotum, varicose lymphatics and, occasionally, vesicles in the skin, which may rupture and drain for a considerable time. Microfilariae may be present in this fluid. Elephantiasis of the part may follow.

Hydrocele is a frequent accompaniment of filariasis because of the common localization of adult worms in the epididymis. It may develop acutely in the course of filarial orchitis or epididymitis, or more slowly and with relatively few local symptoms. Microfilariae are often demonstrable in the serous fluid.[6]

Chyluria is the result of obstruction and dilatation of the thoracic duct or its chyle-carrying tributaries, followed by rupture of distended lymphatics into the urinary tract and the appearance of chyle in the urine. The urine frequently has the appearance of milk. Blood is often present in varying amounts, giving a pinkish coloration. On standing, the urine separates into an upper fatty layer, a semitransparent gelatinous layer of coagulated lymph, and a pinkish sediment containing lymphocytes, red blood cells and, frequently, microfilariae.

The onset is usually abrupt, often preceded by pain in the back or aching in the lower abdomen and thighs. Fever may be present. The attack commonly lasts only a few days. Recurrences are usual, and there are intermissions of varying duration.

Elephantiasis occurs particularly in the legs and scrotum and less frequently in the arms, mammae or vulva as a late complication of filariasis. It appears in only a small percentage of infected persons. The complication develops gradually in the course of repeated attacks of acute filarial lymphangitis in adults exposed for many years to reinfection of the lymphatics by the parasites. The skin and subcutaneous tissues

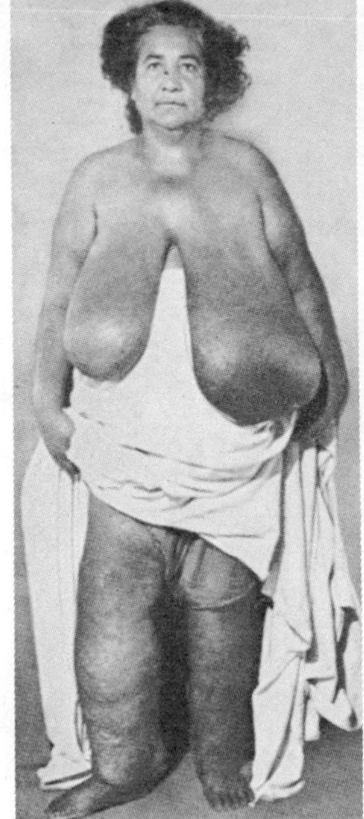

Figure 49–10. Filariasis: elephantiasis of legs and breasts. Cook Islands.

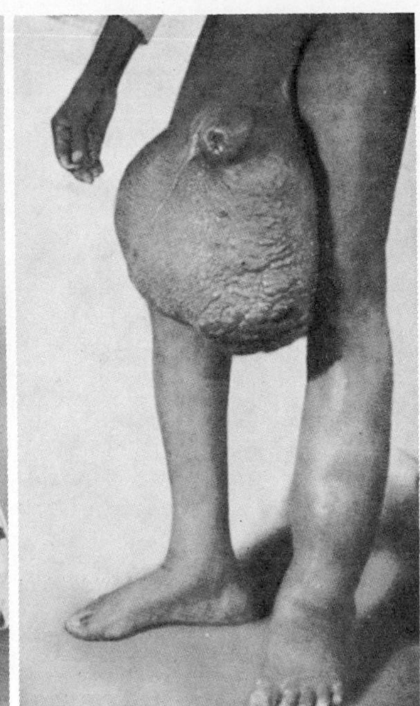

Figure 49–11. Filariasis: elephantiasis of scrotum, lymphedema of leg. (Courtesy of Alan Fisher for the Office of the Coordinator of Inter-American Affairs.)

are greatly thickened and fibrotic, and the regional lymph nodes draining the affected area are usually enlarged. In the majority of cases of elephantiasis, microfilariae are not demonstrable in the blood (Figs. 49–10, 49–11). Some cases may be nonfilarial in origin. (See page 508.)

Diagnosis. In the early stages of filariasis, microfilariae may not be demonstrable in the peripheral blood, and the diagnosis must be based on clinical data alone.[7] A history of exposure in an area of known endemicity, of an incubation period of at least 3 months' duration prior to the appearance of symptoms, and of recurrent inflammatory phenomena is highly suggestive.

Certain objective signs should be carefully sought. Commonest of these is enlargement of the regional lymph nodes draining the affected area, with or without swelling of an extremity or of the scrotal contents. The spermatic cord is frequently thickened, indurated and nodular. Hydrocele of moderate degree is common even in the early stages of the disease and there may be enlargement of the testicle as well.

Lymphangiography is helpful in differentiating filarial lymphedema from lymphostatic verrucosis. In advanced cases of filarial disease there is obliteration of the lymphatic system of the leg.[6]

There is at present no laboratory test that provides dependable diagnostic criteria in the absence of demonstration of the microfilariae. Complement-fixation tests using antigen prepared from related worms *(Dirofilaria immitis)* have not proved to be sufficiently reliable. However, skin tests using antigen from adult *D. immitis* or from microfilariae of *W. bancrofti* have been used widely, with varying effectiveness.[8–10] One of the best of these, a highly purified preparation from *D. immitis*, antigen FST (Sawada antigen),[11] has proved useful although a false positive result may occur with infections of *Schistosoma japonicum*, and up to 25 per cent of microfilaria carriers in some surveys have had a negative test.[12] A soluble antigen fluorescent antibody test has been found valuable by some but not all workers.

Although adult worms may be present in affected lymph nodes, biopsy is emphatically contraindicated, since it further augments lymphatic obstruction. Between acute inflammatory attacks subjection of the individual to heavy physical exertion often initi-

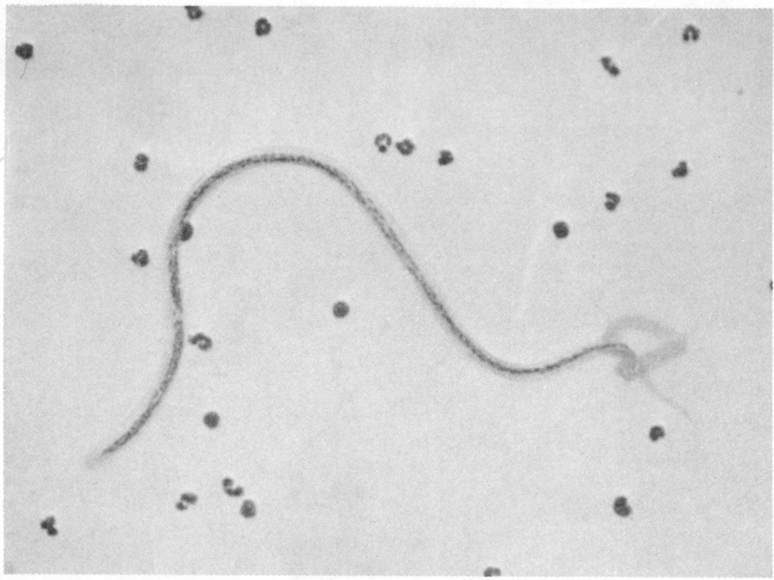

Figure 49-12. Microfilaria of *W. bancrofti* in thick blood film stained with hematoxylin to show sheath and characteristic tail. (Courtesy of National Institutes of Health, U.S.P.H.S.)

ates an acute recurrence accompanied by characteristic clinical phenomena. The acute episodes commonly are accompanied by leukocytosis and eosinophilia.

In the intermediate stages of the disease microfilariae may be demonstrated in the peripheral blood. Frequently, they are absent in the early phases and in the stage of advanced elephantiasis. A thick film of fresh blood is useful in light infections, since the actively motile microfilariae are easily found. Stained thick smears should be used in preference to thin films. Examination of hemolyzed blood in a counting chamber,[13] or concentration on a membrane of the microfilariae filtered from a hemolyzed blood sample,[14] are recently developed methods for making accurate parasite counts. Smears of the sediment from laked centrifuged blood should be used when other methods fail. When infection by nocturnally periodic forms is suspected, blood for examination should be taken at night, preferably after 9 o'clock. Since it is often difficult to obtain cooperation for night blood surveys, a test has been developed that provokes a transitory emergence of these forms into the peripheral circulation during the day—100 mg of diethylcarbamazine are administered, and thick blood films made 1 hour later. The test cannot be used in areas of onchocerciasis or loiasis for fear of provoking severe reactions. Daytime specimens are preferable for the diurnally periodic form. Microfilariae of *W. bancrofti* must be distinguished from such sheathed forms as *B. malayi* and *Loa loa* (Figs. 49-2, 49-12). Airborne spores of saprophytic fungi, such as *Helicosporium lumbricoides,* may contaminate blood films and be mistakenly identified as microfilariae.

Microfilariae may sometimes be demonstrated in fluid aspirated from a hydrocele or enlarged lymph nodes.

Treatment and Prophylaxis. See page 506.

Filariasis Malayi

Synonyms. Brug's filariasis, *Brugia malayi* infection.

Definition. Filariasis malayi is caused by the presence of adult *Brugia malayi* in the lymphatics, lymph nodes or connective tissues of man. A periodic (nocturnal) form of the parasite, with microfilariae appearing in the peripheral blood only at night, predominates in most of the filarial areas of Asia, but a nocturnally subperiodic form showing a secondary daytime microfilaremia occurs in very limited foci in Indonesia, Malaysia, Borneo, Vietnam and islands of the Philippines in the Sulu Sea. *Mansonia* mosquitoes are of particular importance as vectors. In other respects, this disease is fundamentally similar to filariasis bancrofti.

Distribution. Filariasis malayi is found in India, Burma, Malaysia, Thailand, Vietnam, coastal areas of China, Taiwan, South Korea,[15] Japan in a single small focus, Borneo, and Indonesia as far east as Ceram.[12] It has also been found among the Tonkinese in the New Hebrides and the Koreans in Hawaii (Oahu), but without local transmission. In Timor a closely related species predominates as the cause of filariasis. In some parts of Asia the distribution of *B. malayi* and *W. bancrofti* overlaps (Fig. 49–3).

Etiology. MORPHOLOGY. Filariasis malayi is caused by the filarial parasite *B. malayi* (Brug, 1927) Rao and Maplestone, 1940, which bears a close resemblance to *W. bancrofti.* However, the discovery of other *malayi*-like parasites occurring not only in a wide range of animals but also in man resulted in the establishment of the genus *Brugia.*[16] The adults are white, delicate worms that occur coiled and paired in the dilated lymphatics. Two rows of small papillae surround the mouth. The males are smaller, 13 to 23 mm in length, and their posterior extremities undergo about three complete loops. The cloaca is 0.1 to 0.14 mm from the posterior tip. There is a large pair of papillae near the cloaca and one posteriad, and two other smaller pairs are nearby. The copulatory spicules are unequal in length, and a small naviculate gubernaculum is present. The females are about 43 to 55 mm long by 0.13 to 0.17 mm in diameter. The vulva is situated 0.92 mm from the anterior end; the anal pore is 0.94 mm from the posterior tip. Although the measurements made by Dutch and Indian scientists are in essential accord, the descriptions of the papillae differ, indicating the desirability of further morphologic observations.

The sheathed microfilariae of *B. malayi* are 177 to 230 μm in length and 5 to 6 μm in breadth. There is an anterior cephalic space about twice as long as the diameter of the head, the latter bearing double stylets. Staining reveals that an excretory pore is situated 30.09 per cent of the body length from the anterior tip; the large excretory cell, 37.07 per cent; the G_1 cell, 68.33 per cent; and the anal pore, 82.28 per cent. The body tapers from the anal pore, the column of large nuclei terminating some distance before the acuminate tip of the tail is reached. The distal extremity is swollen to accommodate a single distinct nucleus: a second smaller one lies a short distance anteriad. The position of these nuclei and the length of the cephalic space constitute the two characteristic features of this essentially nocturnal microfilaria (Table 49–3).

DEVELOPMENT. The development cycle parallels that of *W. bancrofti* in all essential details. The microfilaria of this species undergoes two molts and completes its development in the mosquito in 6 days under optimum conditions.

Epidemiology. Although the epidemiology is very similar to that of filariasis bancrofti, certain differences exist in the identity and ecology of the vectors and in the periodicity of the microfilariae. The generally accepted mosquito vectors belong to the genera *Mansonia* (subgenus *Mansonioides)* and *Anopheles.* However, *Aedes togoi* (Theobald) is reportedly the vector on Hachijo-Komisha Island in Japan. The vectors may vary geographically as well as ecologically and, consequently, an important transmitter in one region may not be the chief vector in an adjacent area.

The *Mansonia* group constitutes a difficult larval control problem, because these organisms secure their oxygen by attaching themselves to such green aquatic plants as *Pistia* spp. or water lettuce, *Eichhornia crassipes* or *Lemna* sp. In Travancore, India, filariasis malayi was reduced by removing the water plant *Pistia stratiodes,* on which the larvae of the principal vector, *Mansonioides annulifera,* lived. Ordinarily, larviciding measures, such as the use of oil, Paris green or DDT, are ineffective.

The microfilariae of the strain of *B. malayi,* which is responsible for most of the filariasis malayi in man, are essentially nocturnally periodic. This strain is not a natural parasite of other animals, although cats and rhesus monkeys have been infected experimentally. However, the nocturnally subperiodic strain occurring in the swamp-forest regions of Malaya has been found in about 75 per cent of the leaf monkeys *(Presbytis* sp.) examined, as well as in other forest and domestic animals.

Pathology and Clinical Characteristics. The pathologic changes and the clinical syndromes associated with infections by *B. malayi* range from asymptomatic adenitis to periodic attacks of fever and lymphangitis, and to elephantiasis typically involving the feet and legs. Elephantiasis of the upper limbs is seldom seen. Lymph scrotum, chyluria and chylous hydrocele have not been observed, and elephantiasis of the genitalia is rare. Infections in human volunteers were characterized by enlarged lymph glands, a retrograde lymphangitis, a slight eosinophilia and a transient edema of the affected limb. In other cases, pulmonary changes such as bronchial asthma, a high eosinophilia and adenopathy, somewhat suggestive of tropical eosinophilia, were encountered. Treatment as outlined for filariasis in general is indicated.

Diagnosis. The diagnosis rests upon a clinical picture suggestive of filariasis and its confirmation by the demonstration of characteristic microfilariae of *B. malayi* (p. 494). The morphology of the sheathed microfilaria differs from that described for *W. bancrofti* chiefly in the cephalic space, which is twice as long as broad, and the posterior extremity of the worm, which has a slight bulb at the tip with two minute terminal nuclei; the remainder of the tapering posterior extremity is devoid of nuclei (Fig. 49–13). Skin tests, particularly with antigen FST prepared from *Dirofilaria immitis,*[11] may be of value if microfilariae cannot be demonstrated.

Treatment of Filariasis Bancrofti and Malayi. Diethylcarbamazine (Hetrazan, Notezine, Banocide) rapidly decreases the number of microfilariae or eliminates them from circulating blood. Clinical and biopsy evidence indicates that the drug also probably has a direct effect on the adult worms.

Side reactions following the administration of diethylcarbamazine are common, particularly in *B. malayi* infections, but usually are not serious or of sufficient intensity to require termination of therapy. The reactions include fever, malaise, vertigo, ur-

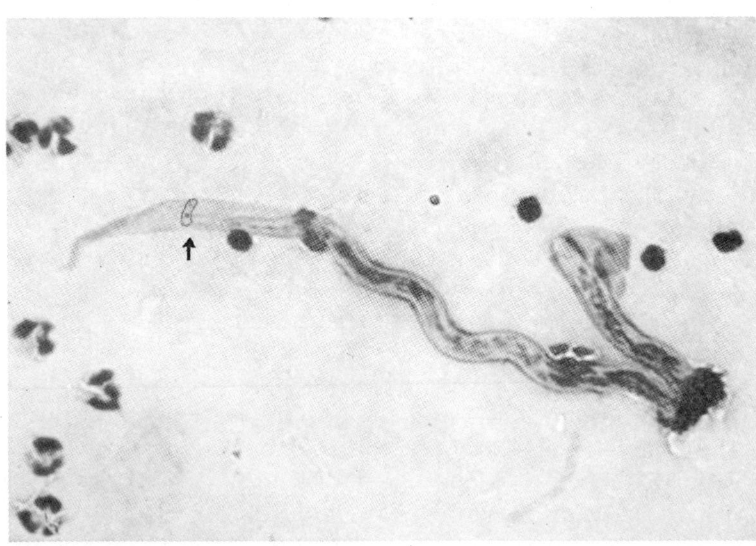

Figure 49–13. Sheathed microfilaria of *B. malayi* in thick blood film (hematoxylin-stained). Note position of characteristic terminal caudal nuclei and cephalic space.

ticaria, headache, nausea, vomiting and inflammatory reactions of the lymph nodes and the scrotal contents. Delayed reactions consisting of bullous eruptions and abscess formation occasionally result. Diethylcarbamazine is nontoxic. The reactions appear to be allergic responses to the products of the parasites following institution of therapy rather than to the drug itself.

The bullous reactions sometimes seen in persons after administration of diethylcarbamazine for filariasis can be arrested promptly by a combination of cortisone and prednisone. *Corticosteroids must be given with extreme caution to patients with secondary bacterial infections.*

For the treatment of individual cases of filariasis bancrofti, a dosage of 4 to 6 mg of diethylcarbamazine citrate (2 to 3 mg of the base drug) per kg of body weight is administered daily for 14 to 21 days. The daily amount may be given either as a single dose or in divided doses, after meals. Permanent elimination of circulating microfilariae and death of adult *W. bancrofti* are dependent upon ingestion by the patient of a total dose of about 72 mg of the drug per kg.[17] Because *B. malayi* infections are susceptible to half this amount, and react more strongly to treatment, they should be treated with a dosage of 2 to 3 mg per kg daily for 14 to 21 days. Concurrent administration of an antihistaminic drug may lessen the incidence and severity of the allergic reactions.

The administration of 100 mg of cortisone daily in divided doses for a month or longer to patients with elephantiasis may be followed by reduction or disappearance of induration, by diuresis and by an increase in the number of circulating microfilariae. The induration reappears after therapy is discontinued through gradually decreased doses, but some degree of improvement may persist for several months. Retreatment with smaller doses of cortisone for short periods as relapses occur seems beneficial.

Treatment of filarial lymphangitis with antibiotics is without direct effect. Antihistaminics are beneficial for symptomatic treatment of this manifestation, but acetylsalicylic acid is more effective in reducing pain and fever.

Hydrocele may be treated satisfactorily by injections of sclerosing agents, such as sodium psylliate and sodium morrhuate.

Chyluria should be treated by complete bed rest; the foot of the bed should be elevated. Cystoscopic treatment and bladder irrigations may be required in severe cases when more conservative measures fail. Marked improvement in an adult patient presenting with chylous ascites requiring paracentesis, and with chyluria, dependent edema and wasting, was recently obtained by administration of metronidazole, 400 mg 3 times a day for 10 days, the use of oral and parenteral diethylcarbamazine having been unsuccessful.[18]

Surgical procedures are contraindicated except for definitive treatment of elephantiasis, especially of the scrotum. Palliative operations directed to improve lymph circulation in elephantiasis of the extremities are seldom successful. Such conditions are best managed by a period of continuous elevation of the affected part. An elastic stocking or elastic bandage must be worn constantly afterward. In cases of early elephantiasis of the lower extremities, elevation and pressure bandages are particularly successful in reducing the swelling. Care must be taken not to bandage too tightly, and the limb must be exercised to prevent venous stasis. In mild cases the leg may assume its original size and the skin a natural texture, remaining normal for a prolonged period without further treatment.

Painful lymph scrotum may be relieved by the use of a suspensory and by keeping the affected parts clean and protected.

Prophylaxis of Filariasis Bancrofti and Malayi. Essential features of prophylaxis against filariasis are mosquito control, individual protection from possibly infected mosquitoes and mass treatment of infected populations. (See Chapter 72.) However, the rapid and unplanned urbanization that is occurring in many countries where Bancroftian filariasis is endemic has exceeded efforts to provide adequate sanitation and disposal of waste water, and a principal vector, *Culex pipiens quinquefasciatus (C. fatigans)*, has prospered accordingly.[17] Drainage of the widespread larval habitats of other vectors of *W. bancrofti, Anopheles* and *Aedes* mosquitoes, and of the *Mansonia* vectors of *B. malayi,* is also extremely difficult. Reliance must continue to be placed on chemical control of these mosquitoes (see Table 72–1), although methods of biological control such as the introduction of larvivorous fish or larval pathogens are applicable to some mosquito breeding sites, and genetic methods are being developed.

Mass treatment of infected populations with diethylcarbamazine citrate, when coordinated with mosquito control measures, is successful against *W. bancrofti* in proportion to the degree of population coverage achieved. A total dose of 72 mg per kg should be given, in divided doses of 5 mg per kg at daily, weekly or monthly intervals. Larger doses should not be given since reactions occur. The mass campaign against *W. bancrofti* may be followed by selective treatment of remaining microfilaria carriers at monthly intervals, the entire community being treated every 3 months. In endemic *B. malayi* areas, unsupervised mass treatment is inadvisable because of the frequency of reactions, and special care should be taken in areas where onchocerciasis and loiasis occur.

NONFILARIAL ELEPHANTIASIS

Elephantiasis of the legs occurs in southwest Ethiopia at an altitude of 1000 to 2000 meters, where *W. bancrofti* (and of course *B. malayi*) are not transmitted. The condition is present in 2.7 per cent of inhabitants aged more than 15 years, the rural peasant population being particularly affected.[19] An important causal factor is believed to be absorption through the skin of the toe clefts of silicon in solution, and less importantly other minerals, particles of which have been identified within macrophages in the inguinal and cubital lymph nodes. Blockage of the sinuses of all nodes develops through proliferation of the littoral cells, and the flow of lymph is progressively impeded.[20]

Onchocerciasis

Synonyms. Onchocercosis, "blinding filarial disease," "river blindness," enfermedad de Robles, volvulosis, erisipela de la costa (Guatemala), mal morado (Mexico), ceguera de los rios (Africa).

Definition. Onchocerciasis is due to the presence of the filarial parasite *Onchocerca volvulus* in the skin, subcutaneous and other tissues of man, where it may produce fibrous nodules. Blindness is a serious complication of this infection. The disease is transmitted by species of buffalo gnats or black flies of the family SIMULIIDAE.

Distribution. In the Western Hemisphere onchocerciasis is largely confined to Mexico and Central America, although foci have been reported in Venezuela, Colombia, Surinam and (in 1973) northwestern Brazil near the Venezuelan border. It is widespread in tropical Africa. In the Americas it occurs principally among persons inhabiting the western slope of the Sierras at altitudes of 600 to 2000 meters. Guatemala and the southern states of Mexico constitute the chief endemic centers. In Africa onchocerciasis is found from Senegal, Sierra Leone and Liberia eastward through Ghana, Dahomey, Nigeria, Chad and Cameroon to the Congo; and in the southern Sudan, Uganda, Kenya, Ethiopia, Tanzania and Malawi. In Arabia, it has been reported in South Yemen and Yemen.

Etiology. MORPHOLOGY. The adult parasite, *Onchocerca volvulus* (Leuckart, 1893) Railliet and Henry, 1910 [= *Onchocerca caecutiens* (Brumpt, 1919)], occurs in tumors in the subcutaneous connective tissue. The living parasites are white or cream colored and transparent, with a cuticula showing distinct striations. Both extremities are blunt. Anteriorly about the mouth are two concentric circles of four papillae each. In addition,

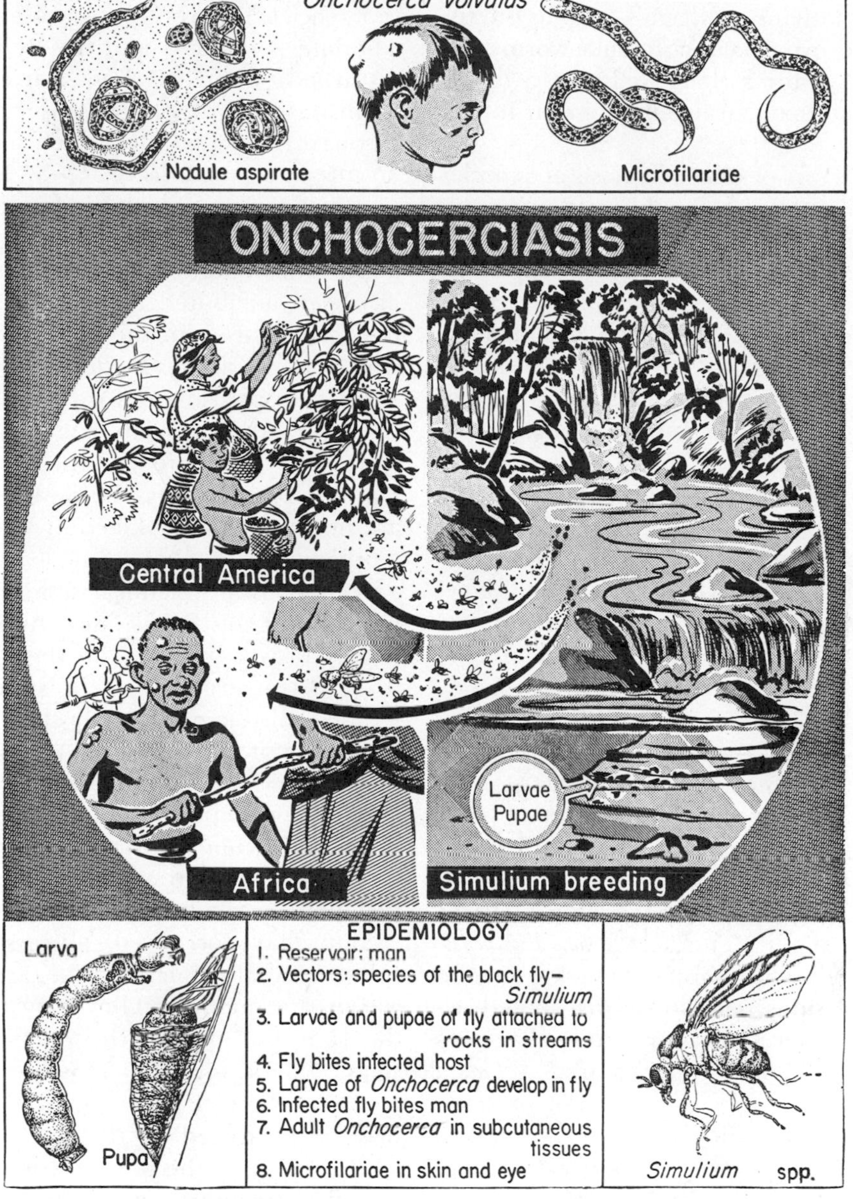

Figure 49–14. Epidemiology of onchocerciasis.

there is a pair of large, oval, lateral papillae situated between these two circles. Posteriorly the tightly coiled males show copulatory spicules and a number of perianal and caudal papillae which, although diagnostic, nevertheless show considerable variation in position. The males are 19 to 42 mm long and the females 33 to 50 cm. The vulva of the female opens posterior to the esophagus. Microfilariae of two sizes, 285 to 368 by 6 to 9 μm and 150 to 287 by 5 to 7 μm, are produced.

Development. The microfilariae of *O. volvulus* probably exsheath soon after leaving the female worm. Both extremities and the excretory pore region of these larvae lack nuclei. The absence of nuclei from the tip of the tail is of diagnostic value. These microfilariae rarely occur in the peripheral blood but are found typically in the subcutaneous nodules near the parent worms, in the stratum germinativum or dermis, and in the tissues of the eye. Fecund female worms are known to live for as long as 15 years, while microfilariae may survive in the skin for 30 months.

The vectors of onchocerciasis are species of black flies of the family SIMULIIDAE (p. 755). These become infected as they suck blood and tissue juices from the skin of an infected host. Ingested microfilariae leave the food reservoir of the fly and, after molting twice, develop to the metacyclic stage. This takes about 6 days. From the time that the infective larvae are introduced to man by the biting fly, 15 to 18 months pass before their microfilarial progeny appear in the skin.[21]

Epidemiology. Man is the reservoir for the filarial worm *O. volvulus.* The following species of the genus *Simulium* are of importance as vectors. (See Chapter 71, p. 757, and Figure 71–2.) In Africa *S. damnosum* Theobald and *S. neavei* Rouband are the chief vectors of onchocerciasis, the latter being the main vector in East Africa assisted by *S. nyasalandicum* and *S. woodi* whose breeding habits are similar. In Guatemala, *S. ochraceum (Eusimulium ochraceum)* is the principal vector, tending to bite on the upper part of the body, while in Venezuela *S. metallicum (E. avidum)* is less efficient and bites low on the body; the lesions tend to be distributed accordingly. Other known or potential vectors in Central and South America are *S. callidum (E. mooseri), S. exiguum, S. veracruzanum, S. hematopotum,* and (in Mexico) *S. gonzalezi.* Most of the species of the SIMULIIDAE transmitting onchocerciasis breed in the riffles of rapidly flowing streams, where the larvae and pupae may be found attached to submerged stones, logs or even vegetation. A few species prefer the more slowly flowing water of roadside ditches (Fig. 49–14). Developing forms of *S. neavei, S. nyasalandicum* and *S. woodi* are found attached to freshwater crabs.

Buffalo gnats, turkey gnats or black flies, as these simuliids are called, are small "hump-backed" flies 1 to 5 mm long. Ordinarily, they are outdoor day biters, but in Guatemala they will bite indoors even at night in the presence of artificial light. African species apparently do not enter houses. The bite is painless and the fly is not easily disturbed when it has started feeding. Transmission of the disease occurs only through the female fly which has fed upon an infected person (Fig. 71–3, p. 756).

Pathology. The primary lesion in onchocerciasis usually follows the initial rash and concomitant pruritus. This reaction has been attributed to: (1) the presence of the microfilariae in the subcutaneous tissue which cannot always be demonstrated; (2) an allergic response; or (3) a deficiency of vitamin A. It has been suggested that the worms may compete with the host for this vitamin. In most cases, the developing worms are not immediately killed by encapsulation, a process which takes a little less than a year, and there is little clinical significance to the infection at this time. These tumors are distributed over regions of the body where there is convergence of the superficial lymphatics. Histologically, they show a relatively low grade of inflammation, a leukocytic infiltration in which eosinophils are conspicuous, and a heavy deposition of collagen fibrils. As a rule, the nodules are solid, though infrequently where the adult parasites die and degenerate, or where secondary bacterial infections have occurred, abscesses have resulted. Usually microfilariae are abundant within the nodules. They may be found in the skin but not in the circulating blood (Figs. 49–15, 49–16). However, a second type of lesion of much greater importance may be produced by the microfilariae that are liberated by the female worms in the encapsulated tumors; these larvae escape into the lymphatics and circulate in these tissue layers. Heavily infected patients may have microfilaruria, associated with lesions in the renal pelvis resembling those of necrotizing papillitis. In many endemic areas in both hemispheres the microfilariae migrate into the eyeball and become associated with lesions that result in a marked impairment of vision or, in some cases, blindness.

The incidence and the severity of the ocular pathologic changes in onchocerciasis bear no relation to the anatomic situation of

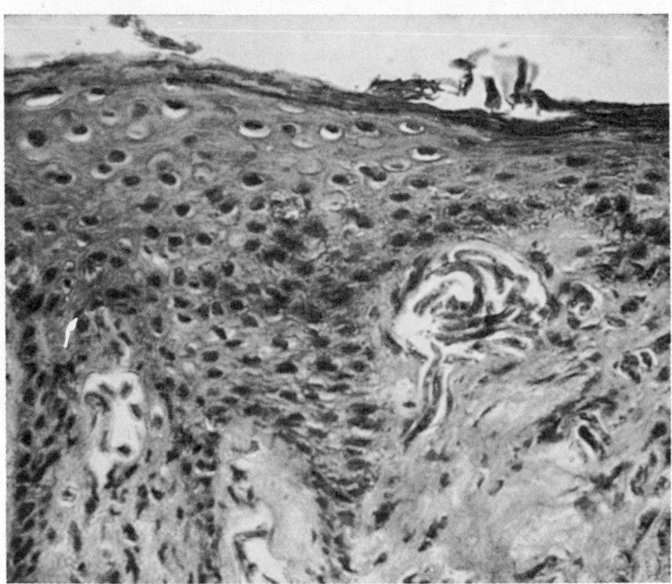

Figure 49-15. Onchocerciasis – microfilariae in skin. (Courtesy of Dr. M. Martínez Baez. Mexico, D.F.)

the nodules, the duration of the infection or the age of the individual. Accumulating evidence indicates that the underlying mechanism is related to the development of sensitivity to antigenic substances of the parasite or its products of metabolism or disintegration.

The essential pathologic process is a low-grade chronic iritis and iridocyclitis, with occasional acute exacerbations that lead to synechia, distorted, contracted, eccentric pupils, pigment deposits and corneal opacities. Superficial punctate keratitis is so common as to be almost pathognomonic. Dead microfilariae have been identified in these minute opacities, and the latter have been observed to increase in number following treatment which kills the microfilariae. Blindness results from pupillary occlusion, corneal opacity or both.

Clinical Characteristics. The subcutaneous nodules are the most characteristic lesions of onchocerciasis.[21] However, these onchocercomas are not always demonstrable.

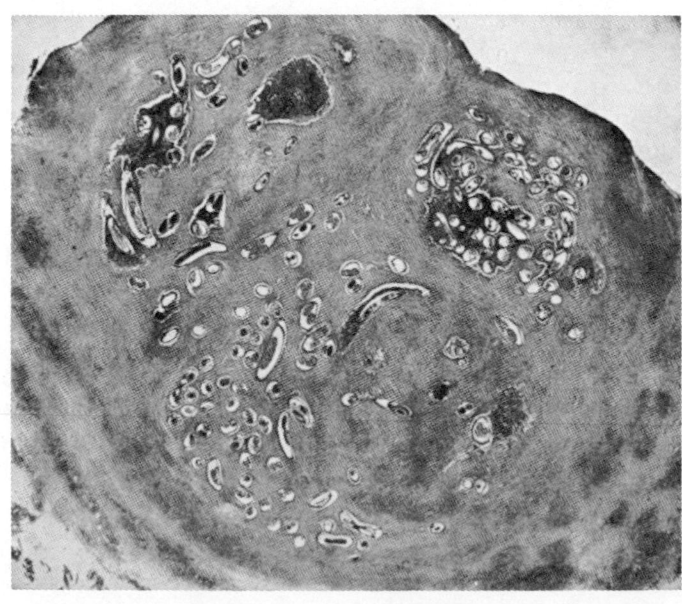

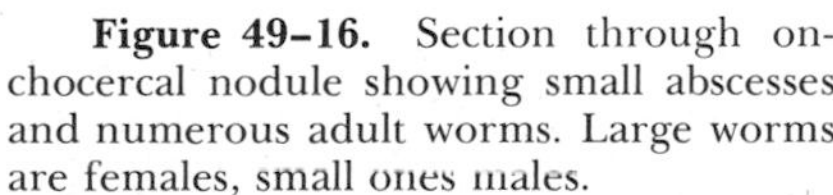

Figure 49-16. Section through onchocercal nodule showing small abscesses and numerous adult worms. Large worms are females, small ones males.

In the Central American form of the disease the nodules are most numerous over the head and thorax; in the African form they are predominantly on the trunk.

In the typical case, following the bite of an infected fly, there is an incubation period of several months before nodules appear. There is little if any systemic reaction. The nodules grow slowly, attaining full size in 3 or 4 years, when they may reach a diameter of 2 to 3 cm. There may be few on one individual and over a hundred on another. Ordinarily, they cause little inconvenience, although in the vicinity of joints they are often painful. Inflammatory reactions may occur in and about certain nodules, occasionally followed by abscess formation. These may be due to secondary bacterial infection or to an allergic reaction. Intensely pruritic skin rashes may be a prominent feature. A facial complication observed in Guatemala, erisipela de la costa, formerly considered to be bacterial in origin, is almost certainly allergic, since it is reproduced exactly in hypersensitive patients following treatment with diethylcarbamazine. This condition is characterized by thickening of the skin over the facial bones with a bluish pigmentation.

Ocular pathologic changes are the most serious feature of onchocerciasis.[21] The incidence of eye lesions has been reported as high as 30 per cent in certain groups in Central America and up to 85 per cent in Africa, particularly in the sub-Sahara savannah areas where in affected communities along streams as many as half the adult male population may be blind.[22] In Guatemala blindness occurs in about 6 per cent of patients with ocular lesions. These complications usually do not appear until some years after the initial infection. The early symptoms include conjunctivitis, lacrimation and photophobia. Serious involvement is indicated by circumcorneal congestion, iritis and punctate keratitis of the cornea.

Two complications of onchocerciasis often seen in the southerly forest areas of West Africa, and in East Africa, are hanging groin and hernia. The hanging groin is a sac of atrophic skin containing sclerosed inguinal or femoral lymph glands. This condition predisposes to hernia. On occasions, microfilariae of *O. volvulus* have been found in the urine; this possibly is the result of the presence of adult worms in the deep tissues of the pelvic region.

Diagnosis. An eosinophilia averaging about 35 per cent is frequently present.

Diagnosis depends upon demonstration of the microfilariae in the skin or nodules (Fig. 49–17).[21] Ordinarily, they are not found in greatest numbers over or adjacent to subcutaneous nodules. In the Central American disease they are most consistently found in the skin of the scapular and neighboring areas, and in the African form in the pelvic girdle and thigh regions.

Skin biopsy, taking a thin section of superficial skin with a razor blade, is the simplest and probably the easiest diagnostic technique. The excised skin should be mounted in saline under a coverglass. A second useful method is by scarification, making several closely approximated superficial linear incisions into the skin and preparing a smear of expressed blood and lymph for staining with hematoxylin or Giemsa's stain. Microfilariae of *O. volvulus* appear to have diurnal periodicity. Maximal density of microfilariae in the skin in Guatemala occurred at 10 A.M. or shortly thereafter; this peak is earlier than reported in Africa.[22a] Aspiration of a subcutaneous nodule and examination of the fluid will frequently reveal large numbers of microfilariae. When microfilariae are too scanty to be revealed by these methods, their presence may be indicated by use of the Mazzotti test: ingestion of 50 mg of diethylcarbamazine should, in positive cases, be followed within 24 hours by a pruritic skin reaction.

Blood smears are of very limited value for the demonstration of microfilariae of *O. volvulus.* However, microfilariae may be found in urine (microfilaruria) in a significant percentage of cases of onchocerciasis in Africa and in the Western Hemisphere. At times the microfilariae may be found in blood and sputum specimens. In some cases, the microfilariae may be detected more readily in these fluids after diethylcarbamazine.[22b, 22c]

While progress is being made in the

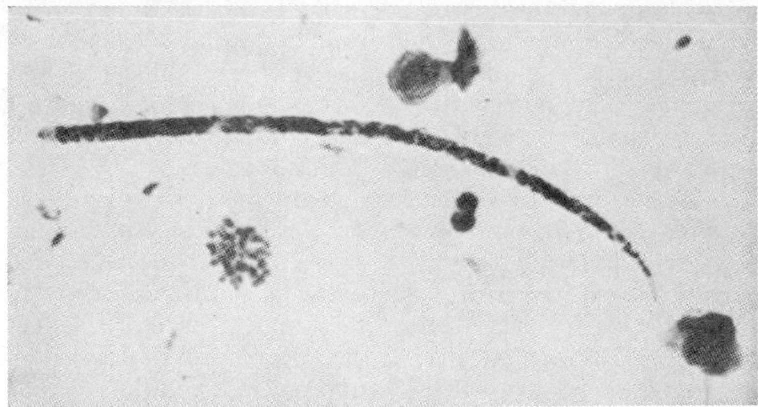

Figure 49–17. Unsheathed microfilaria of *O. volvulus* in aspirate from skin. Caudal nuclei do not reach tip of tail.

provision of specific antigens for diagnostic skin tests, serodiagnostic tests with an acceptable degree of specificity and sensitivity are not yet available.[23]

When the eye is involved, examination of the cornea under oblique illumination will frequently reveal minute superficial opacities—the superficial punctate keratitis which is almost pathognomonic of onchocerciasis.

Treatment. Whenever possible all tumors should be excised, particularly in view of the danger of later ocular complications. This is frequently impracticable, however, when large numbers of the nodules are present. Such treatment is not always followed by disappearance of the microfilariae, probably because other adult worms remain in the host's tissues.

Drug treatment of onchocerciasis must be undertaken with caution in the presence of ocular involvement, since severe reactions may occur in sensitive patients, producing further damage to the eye.

Suramin (Naphuride, Bayer 205, Antrypol, Germanin) is an effective drug. Reported reactions include fever, headache, muscle and joint pains, abdominal pain and nausea. These should be treated symptomatically. Hyperesthesia of the soles of the feet may be troublesome in some individuals. Pruritus and subjective ocular reactions, apparently allergic in nature, may be controlled by antihistamine preparations. Treatment should be discontinued if severe symptoms, peripheral edema or evidence of renal damage occur. Suramin is contraindicated in the presence of renal disease.[24]

Six weekly doses of Suramin should be administered intravenously dissolved in 10 ml of sterile distilled water. For an adult, the initial dose is 0.5 gm and the succeeding doses 1 gm for 5 weeks.

Suramin causes the death of adult worms and the slow disappearance of microfilariae. Whenever possible large subcutaneous nodules should be excised, since abscess formation may follow the death of the adult worms. Not all of the ocular damage in onchocerciasis is reversible, but patients may recover a degree of vision after Suramin therapy.

Diethylcarbamazine is of considerable value in the treatment of onchocerciasis. Although it rapidly kills the microfilariae, severe allergic reactions are not uncommon in sensitized patients, and in the presence of ocular lesions severe damage to the eye may result. It has little or no effect upon the adult worm. The limited effect of diethylcarbamazine on the adult forms of *Onchocerca volvulus* and the severe reactions which frequently follow administration of the drug to persons with this infection constitute serious objections to its use in mass treatment programs. However, administration of corticosteroids, especially betamethasone, minimizes these reactions. Diethylcarbamazine, but not Suramin, tends to mobilize microfilariae, often in large numbers, into the epidermis, cornea, sputum, venous blood and particularly the urine.

Metrifonate (trichlorophone) has recently been used to treat patients in Mexico.[25] The nodules were reduced in size, and adult worms and microfilariae killed. The dermatitis showed marked improvement. Each dose was usually followed by a mild reaction.

Prophylaxis. Satisfactory control measures directed against the breeding places of the vector are difficult and often impractical. In Africa, aerial spraying of DDT and the introduction of DDT into larger streams and rivers has proved effective. A carbamate preparation, Abate, or the dimethyl homolog of Dursban may well replace DDT. In Central America, however, the vectors breed in much smaller, more rapidly flowing streams, and this renders effective control difficult. There is no satisfactory personal prophylaxis other than avoidance of endemic areas. Repellents are of doubtful value.

Onchocerciasis has been shown to persist, with clinical manifestations and progressive ocular disease, over a decade after elimination of transmission by black fly control measures. Therefore, effective control of onchocerciasis requires both the eradication of the vector and the treatment of all heavily infected cases.

Loiasis

Synonyms. Calabar or fugitive swelling disease, eye-worm disease of Africa.

Definition. Loiasis is due to the presence of the parasitic filarial worm *Loa loa* in man, in whom it frequently causes calabar or fugitive swellings. Tabanid flies, *Chrysops* spp., are the intermediate hosts and vectors.

Distribution. Loiasis is transmitted in the West and Central African rain forest and its fringes, being endemic along the Congo River watershed and extending to Angola in the south, the Rift Valley in the east, and Sierra Leone in the west.

Etiology. MORPHOLOGY. The loa or eye-worm, *L. loa* (Cobbold, 1864) Castellani and Chalmers, 1913, produces loiasis or fugitive swellings as the adult migrates about the subcutaneous tissues of man.

The male averages 30 to 34 mm long; the female ranges between 50 and 70 mm. In both sexes the body is filiform, semitransparent and bluntly tapered at both extremities. The head is characterized by two lateral and four small, submedian papillae lying in the same transverse plane a little below the mouth. The latter passes directly into a slender, muscular esophagus. The cuticula of these parasites is covered with small bosses, except for a portion of either extremity of the male.

The posterior end of the male is ventrally curved and possesses narrow lateral alae and eight pairs of perianal papillae (five anterior and three posterior), which are diagnostic. The copulatory spicules are unequal in length and shape, and the cloacal orifice is surrounded by a powerful sphincter.

The broadly rounded posterior tip of the female carries a pair of terminal papillae. The vulva opens about 2.5 mm from the anterior tip in the cervical region and passes into a posteriorly extending vagina which, within 9 mm of its external aperture, bifurcates to form twin uteri and other paired structures of the reproductive system. The uterus contains developing embryos in various embryonic stages. When these are mature, sheathed microfilariae are liberated. These are 250 to 300 μm in length and 6 to 8.5 μm in breadth and are similar in size to corresponding stages of *W. bancrofti.* The percentage distances of the worm's length from the anterior end to various anatomic landmarks are as follows: the widely separated excretory cell and pore, 31.6 and 36.6 per cent, respectively; the G_1 cell, 68.6 per cent; the anal pore, 81.9 per cent. The nuclei extend caudally to the tip of the gradually tapering tail. In many respects the microfilariae of *L. loa* resemble those of *B. malayi* but may be distinguished by the arrangement of the caudal nuclei and the shorter cephalic space.

DEVELOPMENT. The female liberates sheathed microfilariae which enter the blood stream and are diurnal in their periodicity. The intermediate hosts for these worms are certain tabanid or "deer" flies belonging to the genus *Chrysops*. The parasites undergo development in the thoracic muscles and fat body of the fly. About 10 days after infection the mature larvae, about 2 mm in length, migrate to the proboscis and remain infective for about a week. After reaching man by the bite of the fly, the parasites disappear into the subcutaneous tissues and mature slowly.

Epidemiology. Infection is acquired through the bite of infected tabanid flies of the genus *Chrysops*, e.g. *C. dimidiata, C. silacea, C. distinctipennis* and probably other species (p. 764). These flies are diurnal biters, feeding primarily between dawn and 10 A.M. and again between 4 P.M. and dusk. Only the females bite. It has been noted that they prefer darker colors and are found more frequently in wooded areas. Infections develop slowly and are known to persist for at least 15 years. The finding of *Loa loa* in monkeys suggests the existence of a reservoir host.[26]

Pathology. Loiasis is a chronic disease frequently characterized by inflammatory processes and fugitive swellings of the subcutaneous tissues. The adult worms migrate through the subcutaneous tissues at a maximum rate of about a centimeter per minute and have been removed from such locations as the back, axilla, groin, breast, penis, scalp, eyelids, the anterior chamber of the eye and the bulbar conjunctiva. Adult *L. loa* are rarely encapsulated but usually migrate more or less continuously. A marked eosinophilia, sometimes as high as 50 to 70 per cent, may be present. The microfilariae are diurnal and are found in greatest numbers in the peripheral blood during the middle of the day.

Clinical Characteristics. The outstanding clinical feature of the disease is the occurrence of the transient tumors known as fugitive or calabar swellings. These are about the size of a small hen's egg. They appear suddenly, frequently preceded by pain, and in most cases persist for only 2 or 3 days. They may cause inconvenience and disability, such as hampering the use of the hands, and considerable irritability. Fever, urticaria and pruritus may occur.

A number of theories have been advanced in an attempt to explain the occurrence of calabar swellings. It has been suggested that the swellings may be due to : (1) the wanderings of the worm; (2) the liberation of large numbers of microfilariae by the female; (3) toxins secreted by the parasite; and (4) an allergic response on the part of the host. A typical calabar swelling has been produced experimentally in a patient with loiasis by injecting antigen from the dog heartworm *Dirofilaria immitis*, thus supporting the concept of the allergic nature of such responses.

External heat tends to bring the worm close to the surface of the body.

Diagnosis. Diagnostic findings in patients with loiasis include one or more of the following: (1) calabar swellings; (2) worm crossing the eye; (3) edematous outline of the worm under the skin; (4) microfilariae in films of the peripheral blood or in fluid aspirate of the calabar swellings. A marked eosinophilia is usually present.

Microfilariae may be demonstrated in the usual thick smear or by concentration methods (p. 812) (Fig. 49–18).

Differentiation between the microfilariae of *L. loa* and the other sheathed species, *W. bancrofti* and *B. malayi*, is necessary. A detailed comparison is given on page 494. Diurnal periodicity, a tapering tail and the position of the caudal nuclei characterize *L. loa* (Table 49–3).

It has been shown that some filarial worms can be visualized in man by a simple fluorescent method following the administration of tetracycline. The indirect fluorescent antibody test, using *Dipetalonema viteae* from animals as antigen, has been found useful for diagnosis of loiasis.

Treatment. Loiasis responds well to treatment with diethylcarbamazine and, to a lesser extent, to Suramin. In the case of

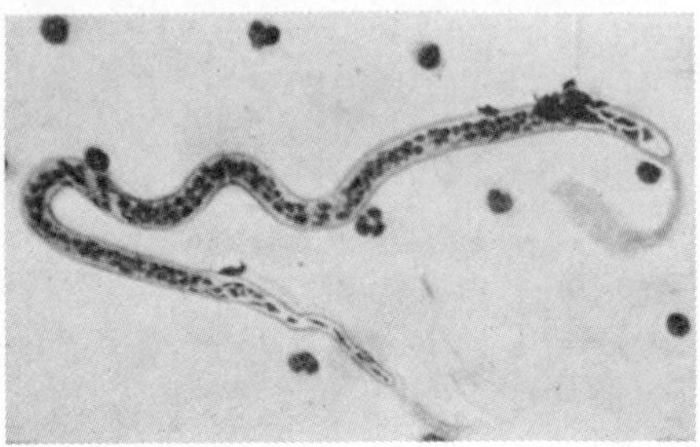

Figure 49–18. Sheathed microfilaria of *Loa loa* in thick blood film. Caudal nuclei extend to tip of tail. (From slide of Liverpool School of Tropical Medicine, loaned by Puerto Rico School of Tropical Medicine. From Bercovitz, Z. T. 1944. Clinical Tropical Medicine. Paul B. Hoeber, Inc., New York.)

diethylcarbamazine, both microfilariae and the adult worms are killed. There may be marked allergic reactions in highly sensitized persons and moderate reactions in others (up to 70 per cent of treated patients). Symptoms include the appearance of calabar swellings, pruritus, fugitive papular erythematous eruptions as well as headache, nausea and arthralgia; more rarely, there may be fever, vomiting and diarrhea. Meningoencephalitic or nephrotic syndromes have been encountered in patients whose cerebral or glomerular capillaries have been blocked by large numbers of moribund microfilariae. These reactions may to some extent be alleviated by antihistamines or corticosteroids, and only in the most marked cases should specific treatment with diethylcarbamazine be temporarily suspended.

In initiating treatment with diethylcarbamazine citrate, in order to reduce allergic reactions a dosage as low as 0.7 mg per kg should be given 3 times a day for 10 days.[27] Mild symptoms of loiasis may reappear a week or two after completion of the course, and additional treatment is often required. For later courses, the dosage may be increased to 2.0 mg per kg and treatment continued for 14 days. A period of at least 2 weeks should intervene between courses. The microfilariae are phagocytosed in the liver and rapidly disappear from the circulating blood. The adult worms tend to appear under the skin, where they are destroyed and small nodules are formed. The initial course of therapy is commonly accompanied by a marked rise of the eosinophil count.

Surgical removal of the migrating adult worms as formerly practiced is not recommended.

Prophylaxis. Protection from bites of *Chrysops* in endemic areas will prevent the disease. Oiling of the surface of the pools over which the flies skim will aid in their elimination as the spiracles or tracheal tubes become occluded by the oil, thus causing suffocation. Repellents such as dimethyl phthalate or indalone are reported to be effective against these flies (Table 72–1, p. 800).

Fly populations are reduced by the clearing of forest, the canopy resting places of adults being eliminated. Also, the resultant exposure and drying out of the forest floor reduce favorable oviposition sites.

Elimination of carriers by mass treatment of village inhabitants with diethylcarbamazine citrate will interrupt transmission, but the hazard of serious reactions in allergic individuals makes it necessary to institute treatment cautiously. For chemoprophylaxis, the drug may be administered in doses of 2.0 mg per kg twice daily for 3 consecutive days each month; some advocate a lesser dosage given for 28 days.

Filariasis Ozzardi

Synonyms. Mansonelliasis ozzardi, Ozzard's filariasis.

Definition. Filariasis ozzardi is due to the presence of *Mansonella ozzardi* in man. The adults inhabit the body cavities; the nonperiodic microfilariae are found in the blood stream. The intermediate host and vector is a midge of the genus *Culicoides.*

Distribution. *Mansonella ozzardi* is confined exclusively to the Western Hemisphere, being native to parts of South America, particularly the Guianas, Colombia, Venezuela and northern Argentina. It is also present in Panama and Mexico (Yucatan), and in such West Indies areas as Puerto Rico, St. Vincent and Dominica; however, there is no indication that it has become established in the Old World.

Etiology. MORPHOLOGY. *Mansonella ozzardi* (Manson, 1897) Faust, 1929, is a nematode, the adults of which are found in the mesenteries, body cavities and visceral fat. A complete male has not been described. The female ranges between 65 and 81 mm in length and possesses an unarmed head, a smooth cuticula and a pair of fleshy lappets or flaps at the caudal extremity. The unsheathed microfilariae are 185 to 200 μm long and about 5 μm broad. Both the cephalic and caudal extremities lack nuclei, the nucleus-free region comprising the anterior 2.2 to 2.5 per cent and the posterior 1.8 to 2.0 per cent of the worm. Other measurements from the anterior tip are as follows: the nerve ring, 21.9 to 22.2 per cent; excretory pore and excretory cell, 30.9 to 31.5 and 35 per cent, respectively; the G_1 cell, 67.9 to 69.3 per cent; the G_4 cell just in front of the anal pore at 79.4 per cent. The outstanding diagnostic characteristics are the lack of a sheath and the absence of nuclei in the posterior tip of the tail. (See Tables 49–2, 49–3.)

DEVELOPMENT. The unsheathed microfilariae are nonperiodic. The larvae require 5 to 7 days for development in the vector, *Culicoides furens*.

It appears possible that the *Microfilaria tucumans* of Argentina is identical with the microfilaria of *M. ozzardi*.

Epidemiology. Even though the epidemiology of Ozzard's filariasis has not been adequately studied, it has been demonstrated that transmission occurs principally through the bite of an infected *C. furens* (Fig. 71–1, p. 754). *Culicoides paraensis* appears to be another vector. In Brazil, the parasite or a closely related species may be carried by *Simulium amazonicum*. The prevalence of this infection is not definitely known for most areas. In endemic areas of the Argentine about 30 per cent of the population are believed to be infected.

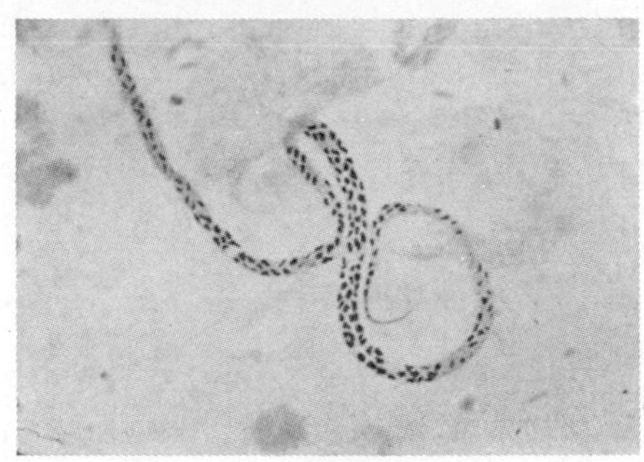

Figure 49–19. Unsheathed microfilaria of *M. ozzardi* in thick blood films. (Courtesy of F. W. O'Connor. From Bercovitz, Z. T. 1944. Clinical Tropical Medicine. Paul B. Hoeber, Inc., New York.)

Pathology and Clinical Characteristics. The adult worms apparently produce few if any pathologic changes or symptoms. An occasional hydrocele or enlarged lymph node has, however, been attributed to *M. ozzardi* infections.

Diagnosis. This is based upon the recovery and the identification of the unsheathed microfilariae from the peripheral blood. The pointed tail and absence of nuclei extending to the posterior tip are important diagnostic characteristics (Fig. 49–19). (See Table 49–3 for additional details.)

Treatment. None recommended. Diethylcarbamazine is not effective against *M. ozzardi*.

Prophylaxis. No effective control measures are known, other than the use of repellents against midges. These insects are so small that screening will not exclude them.

Dipetalonemiasis

Synonyms. Acanthocheilonemiasis, *Dipetalonema perstans* infection.

Definition. Dipetalonemiasis is due to the presence of *Dipetalonema perstans* or closely related species in man. *Dipetalonema perstans* adults inhabit the peritoneal cavity, the pleural cavity, pericardium, mesenteries or retroperitoneal tissues; the nonperiodic microfilariae are found in the blood stream. Adults and microfilariae of *Dipetalonema streptocerca* most commonly inhabit the skin of the trunk. The vectors are various species of *Culicoides.*

Distribution. *Dipetalonema perstans* is common in the tropical regions of South America and Africa. In the Western Hemisphere it has been reported from Panama to northern Argentina as well as in Trinidad. In Africa, where prevalence rates may be high, particularly in banana-growing districts, the parasite occurs in all the tropical countries as far south as Rhodesia, and has been found in Tunisia and Algeria. The infections are often mixed with those of *W. bancrofti.*

Dipetalonema streptocerca has a more restricted range in West Africa and the Congo basin than has *D. perstans,* which it closely resembles (Fig. 49–2, Table 49–2).

Etiology. MORPHOLOGY. Adult *D. perstans* (Manson, 1891) Yorke and Maplestone, 1926 are elongated, cylindrical, creamy white FILARIOIDEA with a smooth cuticle. The anterior tip is unarmed and bluntly rounded, although a shield possessing two large lateral papillae and two pairs of submedian papillae is present. The caudal extremity is somewhat curved ventrally in both males and females and is bifurcated to form a pair of triangular nonmuscular flaps. The female is 70 to 80 mm long; the male averages about 45 mm. The latter possesses four pairs of preanal papillae and one postanal pair with unequal rodlike copulatory spicules.

DEVELOPMENT. The female produces unsheathed microfilariae measuring about 200 by 4.5 μm. These enter the blood stream and are nonperiodic. The intermediate hosts of this parasite include several species of *Culicoides.* Development occurs in the midge which then transmits the infection when it next feeds, allowing the infective stage to reach the skin of man.

Epidemiology. In Africa *C. austeni* Carter, Ingram and Macfie and perhaps *C. grahami* Austen serve as the vectors for this disease (p. 755). The vectors in other areas are unknown.

The incidence of parasitism in man varies markedly. The infection rates in northern Argentina range between 39.1 and 50.6 per cent. In some areas of Africa, such as Uganda, the parasite has been found in about 90 per cent of the population, and in the heavily wooded portion of the Cameroons the infection rate is more than 92 per cent. The parasite is endemic in the Congo River basin.

Pathology and Clinical Characteristics.

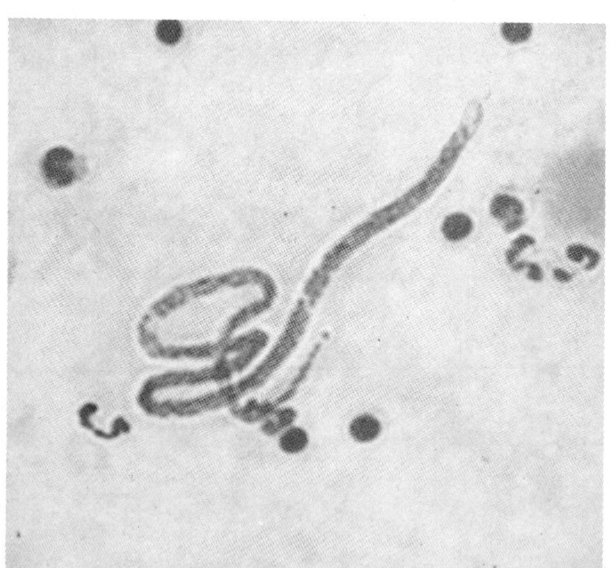

Figure 49–20. Unsheathed microfilaria of *D. perstans* in thick blood film (hematoxylin-stained). Note caudal nuclei extending to tip of tail and other morphologic characteristics. (What appears to be a sheath is merely a halo.)

The consensus of opinion is that *D. perstans* is nonpathogenic. However, vertigo, aching limbs, periodic itching, abdominal and pectoral pain, enlargement of spleen and liver, fever followed by urticaria, edema of lower limbs and scrotum, and marked eosinophilia have been attributed to this filarial infection. *Dipetalonema streptocerca* produces a pruritic rash resembling that of onchocerciasis, from which the condition must be differentiated.

Diagnosis. The detection and identification of the unsheathed microfilariae of *D. perstans* in the peripheral blood are diagnostic. These may be differentiated from the microfilariae of *M. ozzardi* by the position of the caudal nuclei which, in the case of *D. perstans,* extend into the posterior tip of the blunt tail but stop short thereof in the case of *M. ozzardi* (Fig. 49–20).

Treatment. *Dipetalonema perstans* adults and microfilariae are less susceptible to diethylcarbamazine citrate than are *D. streptocerca,* infections of which respond well to dosages of 2.9 mg per kg daily. Because of the unpredictable nature of *D. perstans* infections, however, it appears wise to administer treatment.[28]

Prophylaxis. At present it does not seem feasible to control the breeding of *Culicoides.* Ordinary screening does not exclude these midges. Avoidance of endemic areas and the use of repellents are the only available prophylactic measures.

Other Filariae

Filariae of the genus *Dirofilaria* are occasionally transmitted to man by their arthropod vectors, but in so abnormal a host the parasites die without producing microfilariae. Several species have been identified in man, in the southern United States *D. tenuis* Chandler, 1942, parasitic in the raccoon, being the most common.[29] *Dirofilaria immitis* (Leidy, 1856), the dog heartworm,[30] *Dirofilaria repens* Railliet and Henry 1911, which is normally found in the subcutaneous tissues of dogs in Asia, Europe and South America, and other species of *Dirofilaria* some (such as *D. conjunctivae*) of doubtful validity have been designated as the offending filaria in some cases. At least 30 per cent of the reported cases have occurred in Italy.[31]

The organisms have been found mainly in the subcutaneous tissues, within a nodule or, less commonly, a migratory lesion. However, in several cases they have been located internally in a variety of sites. *Dirofilaria immitis* in particular has been found asymptomatically in the cardiopulmonary system, the granulomas that form around the worms being detected radiologically, reported as "coin lesions," and often mistaken for tumors. The invading worm is usually identified as a female. The worms frequently degenerate at a young age in the human host, apparently because of an unfavorable environment, with a resultant granulomatous reaction. Eosinophils are abundant at the site of the inflammatory reaction about the dead or dying worms. Serologic methods are useful for differential diagnosis.

REFERENCES

1. Nelson, G. S. 1960. The identification of filarial larvae in their vectors. Indian J. Malariol. *14*:585–592.
2. Eyles, D. E., Hunter, G. W., III, and Warren, V. 1947. The periodicity of microfilariae in two patients with filariasis acquired in the South Pacific. Am. J. Trop. Med. *27*:203–209.
3. Mattingly, P. F. 1962. Some considerations relating to the role of *Culex pipiens fatigans* Wiedemann in the transmission of human filariasis. Bull. W.H.O. *27*:569–578.
4. Swartzwelder, J. C. 1964. Filariasis bancrofti. *In* Coates, J. B. (ed.): Preventive Medicine in World War II. Vol. VII. Communicable Diseases. U.S. Government Printing Office, Washington, D.C. pp. 63–71.
5. Galindo, L., von Lichtenberg, F., and Baldizón, C. 1962. Bancroftian filariasis in Puerto Rico: infection pattern and tissue lesions. Am. J. Trop. Med. Hyg. *11*:739–748.
6. Cohen, L. B., Nelson, G., Wood, A. M., Manson-

Bahr, P. E. C., and Bowen, R. 1961. Lymphangiography in filarial lymphoedema and elephantiasis. Am. J. Trop. Med. Hyg. *10*:843–848.

7. Beaver, P. C. 1970. Filariasis without microfilaremia. Am. J. Trop. Med. Hyg. *19*:181–189.
8. Bozicevich, J., and Hutter, A. M. 1944. Intradermal and serological tests with *Dirofilaria immitis* antigen. Pub. Hlth. Rept. *53*:2130–2138.
9. Hunter, G. W., III, Bozicevich, J., and Warren, V. 1945. Studies on filariasis. II. A skin test for filariasis bancrofti utilizing an antigen prepared from microfilariae of *Wuchereria bancrofti*. J. Parasit. *31* (Suppl.):13.
10. Hunter, G. W., III (1958). 1961. Skin testing for filariasis with an homologous antigen. Proc. 6th Internat. Congr. Trop. Med. Mal. *2*:479–483.
11. Sawada, T., Sato, S., Matsuyama, S., Miyagi, H., and Shinzato, J. 1968. Intradermal skin test with antigen FST (FSCD1) on individuals in endemic area. Jap. J. Exp. Med. *38*:405–414.
12. Edeson, J. F. B. 1972. Filariasis. Br. Med. Bull. *28*:60–65.
13. Denham, D. A., Dennis, D. T., Ponnudurai, T., Nelson, G. S., and Guy, F. 1971. Comparison of a counting chamber and thick smear methods of counting microfilariae. Tr. Roy. Soc. Trop. Med. Hyg. *65*:521–526.
14. Bell, D. 1967. Membrane filters and microfilariae: a new diagnostic technique. Ann. Trop. Med. Parasit. *61*:220–223.
15. Hunter, G. W., III, Ritchie, L. S., Chang, I. C., Kobayashi, H., Rolph, W. D., Jr., Mason, H. C., and Szewczak, J. 1951. Parasitological studies in the Far East. VII. An epidemiologic survey of Southern Korea. Japan Logistical Command. Bull. No. 2. 20 pp.
16. Buckley, J. J. C. 1960. On *Brugia* gen. nov. for *Wuchereria* spp. of the '*malayi*' group i.e., *W. malayi* (Brug, 1927), *W. pahangi* Buckley and Edeson, 1956, and *W. patei* Buckley, Nelson and Heisch, 1958. Ann. Trop. Med. Parasit. *54*:75–77.
17. Anonymous. 1974. W.H.O. Expert Committee on Filariasis. Third Report. W.H.O. Tech. Rep. Ser. No. 542, Geneva. 54 pp.
18. Anjaria, P. D., Basantani, G. K., and Mehta, J. K. 1972. Successful treatment of chyluria and chylous ascites. Preliminary communication and case report. J. Assoc. Physicians India *20*:55–56.
19. Oomen, A. P. 1969. Studies on elephantiasis of the legs in Ethiopia. Trop. Geogr. Med. *21*:236–253.
20. Price, E. W. 1972. The pathology of non-filarial elephantiasis of the lower legs. Tr. Roy. Soc. Med. Hyg. *66*:150–159.
21. Buck, A. A. (ed.). 1974. Onchocerciasis. Symptomatology, pathology, diagnosis. W.H.O., Geneva. 80 pp.
22. Duke, B. O. L. 1972. Onchocerciasis. Br. Med. Bull. *28*:66–71.

22a. Anderson, R. I., Fazen, L. E., and Buck, A. A. 1975. Onchocerciasis in Guatemala. III. Daytime periodicity of microfilariae in skin. Am. J. Trop. Med. Hyg. *24*:62–65.

22b. Fazen, L. E., Anderson, R. I., Figueroa Marroquin, H., Arthes, F. G., and Buck, A. A. 1975. Onchocerciasis in Guatemala. I. Epidemiologic studies of microfilaruria. Am. J. Trop. Med. Hyg. *24*:52–57.

22c. Anderson, R. I., Fazen, L. E., and Buck, A. A. 1975. Onchocerciasis in Guatemala. II. Microfilariae in urine, blood, and sputum after diethylcarbamazine. Am. J. Trop. Med. Hyg. *24*:58–61.

23. Mueller, J. C., Mitchell, D. W., Garcia-Monza, G. A., Aguilar, F. J., and Scholtens, R. G. 1973. Evaluation of a skin test for onchocerciasis in Guatemala. Am. J. Trop. Med. Hyg. *22*:337–342.
24. Anonymous. 1966. W.H.O. Expert Committee on Filariasis. Second Report. W.H.O. Tech. Rep. Ser. No. 359, Geneva. 47 pp.
25. Salazar Mallén, M., González Barranco, D., and Jurado Mendoza, J. 1971. Trichlorophone treatment of onchocerciasis. Ann. Trop. Med. Parasit. *65*:393–398.
26. Kershaw, W. E. 1955. The epidemiology of infection with *Loa loa*. Tr. Roy. Soc. Trop. Med. Hyg. *49*:143–150.
27. Hawking, F. 1973. Chemotherapy of tissue nematodes. *In* Cavier, R., and Hawking, F. (eds.): Chemotherapy of Helminthiasis. Vol. I. Pergamon Press, New York. pp. 437–500.
28. Adolph, P. E., Kagan, I. G., and McQuay, R. M. 1962. Diagnosis and treatment of *Acanthocheilonema perstans* filariasis. Am. J. Trop. Med. Hyg. *11*:76–88.
29. Beaver, P. C., and Orihel, T. C. 1965. Human infection with filariae of animals in the United States. Am. J. Trop. Med. Hyg. *14*:1010–1029.
30. Abadie, S. H., Swartzwelder, J. C., and Holman, R. L. 1965. A human case of *Dirofilaria immitis* infection. Am. J. Trop. Med. Hyg. *14*:117–118.
31. Carneri, I. de, Sacchi, S., and Pazzaglia, A. 1973. Subcutaneous dirofilariasis in man—not so rare. Tr. Roy. Soc. Trop. Med. Hyg. *67*:887–888.

CHAPTER 50

Tissue-Inhabiting Nematodes: The Dracunculoidea

The DRACUNCULOIDEA are tissue-inhabiting nematodes of which but a single representative, *Dracunculus medinensis,* infects man. The adults may be distinguished from members of the FILARIOIDEA by their great size and their characteristic larvae, which are 500 μm or more long. Copepods (minute crustacea) serve as intermediate hosts.

Dracunculiasis

Synonyms. Dracontiasis; dracunculosis; medina, serpent, dragon or guinea worm infection.

Definition. Dracunculiasis is due to the presence of the guinea worm, *Dracunculus medinensis,* in the deep connective and subcutaneous tissues of man. Superficial lesions are formed through which the larvae are discharged.

Distribution. The medina, or guinea worm, produces a disease which has been recognized in man for many centuries. It is highly endemic in a number of regions in tropical Africa and over large areas of India. Dracunculiasis occurs also in Arabia (especially along the Red Sea), Iran, Afghanistan and Russian Turkestan. The endemic centers in Africa lie between the equator and the Tropic of Cancer where they are scattered from Mauritania to Gabon, especially in Mauritania, Senegal, Republic of Upper Volta, Ivory Coast Republic, Togo Republic, Ghana, Dahomey, Nigeria and the Cameroons. Endemic centers extend east to Lake Chad and to the southern parts of the Sudan and into Uganda. It is also found in the Nile Valley and in Iraq, Iran, Pakistan and portions of southeastern U.S.S.R.

The western half of India constitutes the next most important endemic center; there is little infection east of Delhi and the central provinces. Dracunculiasis also occurs in limited areas of Indonesia.

Guinea worms morphologically similar to those infecting man have been reported from monkeys, baboons, dogs, leopards, polecats, cattle and horses from the Old World and possibly an identical species from foxes, mink and raccoons in North America. However, many authorities are inclined to consider infections of the latter hosts as due to *Dracunculus insignis.*

Etiology. MORPHOLOGY. *Dracunculus medinensis* (Linnaeus, 1758) Gallandant, 1773 is an elongate, cylindrical, threadlike worm. Males of the species are rare. They range in size from 12 to 40 mm. The female has a smooth cuticula and is much larger than the male, averaging about 1 meter in length.

DEVELOPMENT. As the female becomes gravid she migrates from her location in the body cavity, or retroperitoneal tissues, usually to the subcutaneous tissues of the distal portions of the lower extremities. As she approaches the skin a small papular induration is produced in the dermis which develops into a blister within 24 to 36 hours. Shortly thereafter this blister bursts. If the affected part comes in contact with water, a loop of the uterus of the parasite prolapses through its body wall, ruptures, and liberates large numbers of motile, rhabditiform larvae. These larvae are 500 to 750 μm in length and have a maximum diameter of 15 to 25 μm. Their anterior extremity is bluntly rounded; the caudal extremity is long and attenuated. In order that the life cycle of these parasites be completed, the larvae must be ingested by one of several species of crustaceans (Fig. 50–1). Here they undergo a

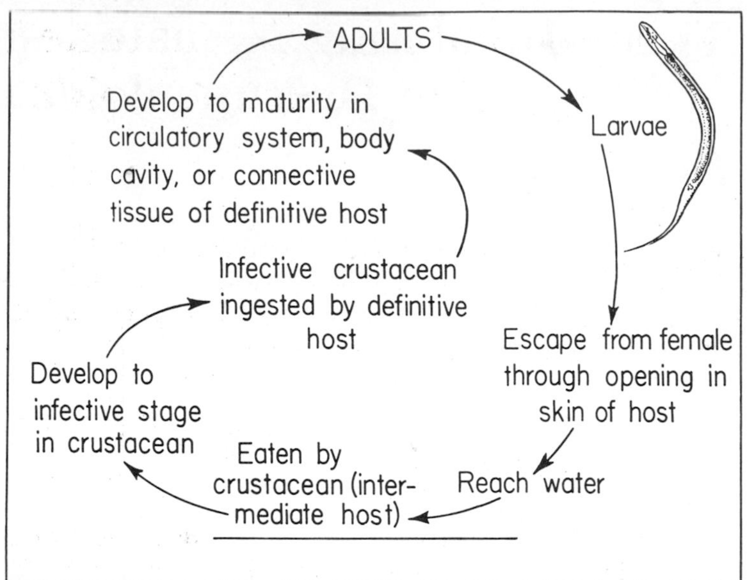

Figure 50–1. Nematode cycle – guinea worm type.

developmental period averaging 10 to 12 days, after which time the copepods become infective. Following ingestion of the intermediate host by man, the parasites probably mate, and the female migrates through the tissues. After 8 months to a year, the fertilized female approaches the skin to liberate her young, thus completing the cycle.

Epidemiology. Man becomes infected from drinking raw water containing infected copepods, many species of which (*Cyclops* spp., *Eucyclops* spp., *Thermocyclops* spp., and others) serve as intermediate hosts. In endemic areas step wells and open wells provide the principal source of infected copepods, the prevalence of infection being much higher in persons using step wells compared with open wells (38 vs. 14.5 per cent) (Fig. 50–2).[1] Lesions in man occur most frequently on the appendages, and larvae are released when an infected person wades in sources of drinking water. In some parts of India religious ablutions include rinsing the mouth, and this custom facilitates infection. The role of reservoir hosts in this disease is unimportant epidemiologically.

Pathology. After an incubation period of 8 to 12 months the female parasite approaches the skin, and in 85 to 90 per cent of the cases migrates to some portion of the lower extremities. Here a reddish papular lesion appears; it has a domelike vesicular center, the margin of which gradually becomes indurated (Fig. 50–3). The entire lesion may be 2 mm to 7 cm in diameter; the size depends upon the amount of exudate underneath the blister and the time elapsing before the blister ruptures. Usually not more than 24 to 48 hours elapse between the first symptoms and the bursting of the lesion. In many instances patients do not present themselves for treatment until after the blister has ruptured; as a result, secondary infection occurs in nearly half the cases. An eosinophilia up to 15 per cent has been recorded in some infected individuals.

Clinical Characteristics. A few hours before the appearance of the worm beneath the skin there are pronounced symptomatic prodromes. These consist essentially of erythema, generalized urticaria, severe pruritus, giddiness, asthma-like symptoms, severe dyspnea and sometimes vomiting and diarrhea. It is believed that these reactions are associated with toxic secretions of the parasite. As the anterior extremity of the worm reaches the skin, intense itching or burning sensations are frequently experienced. The adult worm may migrate to various sites and produce, for example,

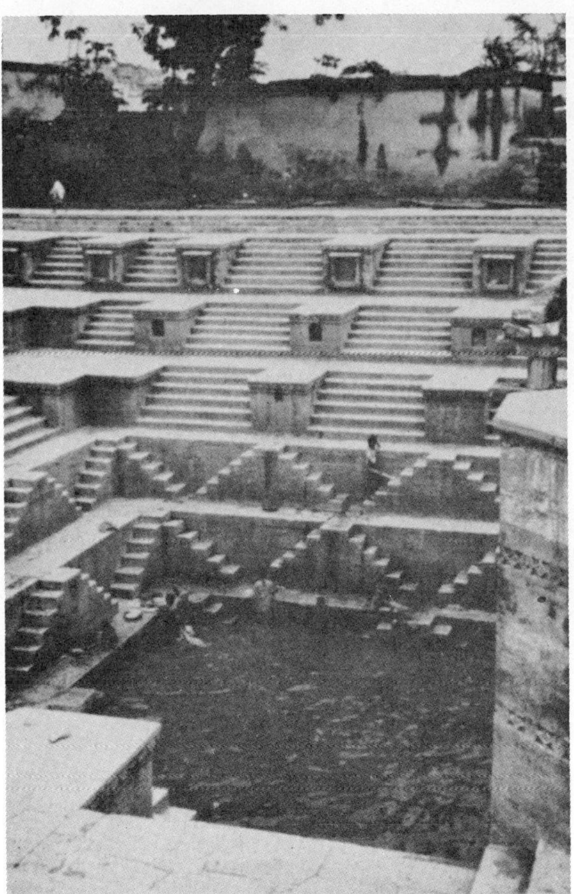

Figure 50-2. Elaborate step well at Rajasthan, India, with water at low level in bottom of basin, where *Dracunculus medinensis* larvae from burst cutaneous lesions of infected persons are discharged while bathing. Other persons contract the infection during bathing by swallowing infected *Cyclops*. (Photograph courtesy of Doctor Paul C. Beaver. From Faust, E. C., Russell, P. F., and Jung, R. C. 1970. Craig and Faust's Clinical Parasitology. 8th ed. Lea & Febiger, Philadelphia.)

spinal extradural abscesses with severe neurologic damage, or intra-articular infection with acute arthritis, particularly of the knee joint.[2]

Diagnosis. Diagnosis cannot be made until the cutaneous lesion has developed or until the adult worm presents itself immediately below the surface of the skin. Intradermal and complement-fixation tests have been used in the past, but the recently developed indirect immunofluorescence (IF) test promises to be more valuable in the diagnosis of prepatent infections. Partially or completely calcified worms may be detected by x-ray. The larvae are found in the washings of the ulcers through which the gravid females discharge their young, or may sometimes be seen in aspirated synovial fluid from joint infections.

Treatment. Diethylcarbamazine (Hetrazan), in large doses taken orally, is lethal to the adult worms. Immature forms of the parasite are destroyed when this drug is employed prophylactically.[3] Single injections of Trimelarsan (Mel W), 5 mg per kg (maximum 200 mg), or oral administration of thiabendazole, 50 to 100 mg per kg daily for 1 to 3 days, or of niridazole, 30 mg per kg daily for 10 days, or of metronidazole, 25 mg per kg daily for 7 to 15 days (or a shorter regimen of metronidazole of 800 mg 3 times daily for 3 to 5 days[4]) have all acted to produce expulsion or lysis of the worm within 3 weeks, with acceleration of healing. Allergic side reactions to these drugs, particularly Trimelarsan and niridazole, may be suppressed by concomitant administration of promethazine. Discoloration of the urine following treatment with niridazole may alarm the patient. Recent studies suggest, however,

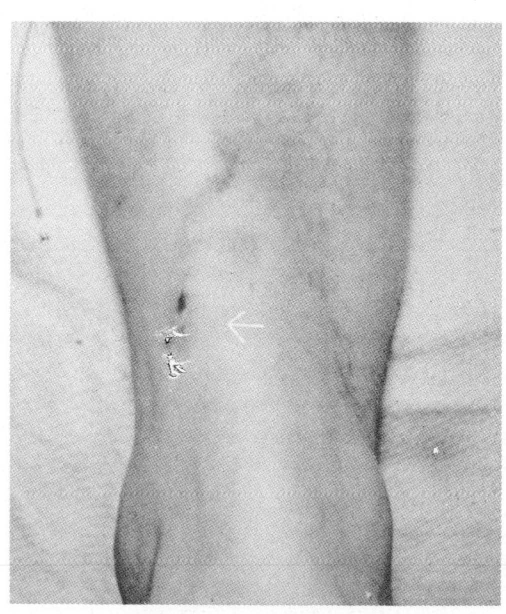

Figure 50-3. Dracunculiasis. Track of part of the worm which became visible in the skin following the appearance of the vesicle. Note that the blister is now crusted and that there is discoloration of the surrounding skin.

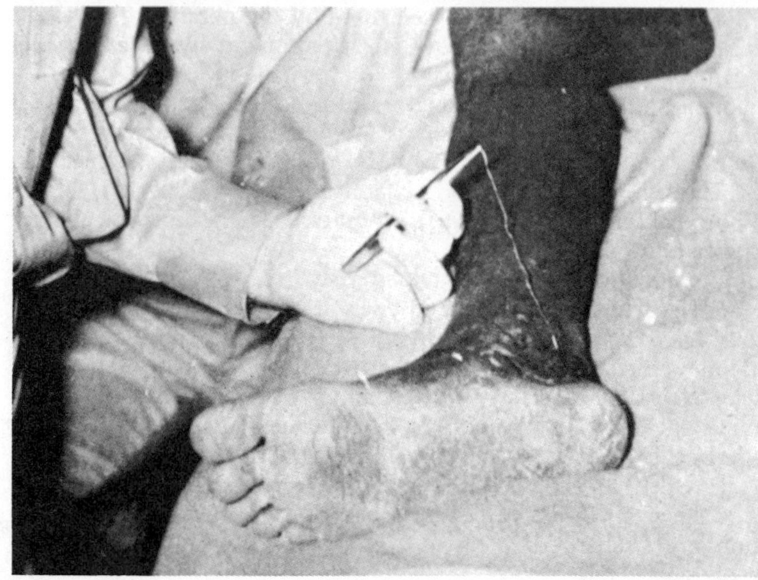

Figure 50–4. *Dracunculus medinensis* partially extracted. (Courtesy of Dr. J. M. Hulsey, Jr., through Dr. Hardy A. Kemp, State Hospital, Larner, Kansas.)

that the efficacy of these drugs may be attributable more to an anti-inflammatory than an antiparasitic action, good results also being obtained by application of 2.5 per cent hydrocortisone cream daily to the blister site.[5] More recently, mebendazole in regimens of 100 mg twice daily for 14 days or 200 mg twice daily for 3, 5 and 10 days have effected cures of dracunculiasis.

The time-honored custom of "forcing" parturition by the use of wet pads and then rolling the worm on a stick is not recommended, as sepsis often results. However, this method will doubtless continue to be used in some areas. Worms localized in deep tissues and producing severe manifestations, such as acute arthritis or extradural abscess, must be removed surgically as soon as possible[2] (Fig. 50–4).

Prophylaxis. As infection comes from swallowing water containing infected copepods, control centers around the destruction of the copepods and the protection of wells so that the water may not be contaminated by infected persons. This may be accomplished as follows:

1. Eliminate the so-called step wells.
2. Construct a cement curb around wells.
3. Treat the water with quicklime in dilution of 1:1000. When used in a strength of 1 ml per liter (80 per cent CaO) this water is potable in 2 days and remains free of copepods for 2 weeks.
4. Copper sulfate in combination with Perchlon is also effective.
5. Introduce DDT, 10 parts per million, in pond water for household use, but not for drinking. Several insecticides, notably the organophosphorus compound Abate in its sand-granule formulation, dichlorvos, fenitrothion and similar compounds are destructive to copepods.[5]
6. Biologic methods of control may be introduced. Almost any small plankton-feeding minnow will keep down the copepods. In Indian step wells *Barbus puckelli* has been found to be a voracious feeder on copepods and their larvae. Actually, each endemic focus must be carefully studied before a practical control method can be developed.

REFERENCES

1. Lindberg, K. 1946. Enquete épidémiologique sur la dracunculose dans un village de Deccan (Inde). Bull. Soc. Path, Exot. *39*:303–318.
2. Reddy, C. R. R. M., and Sivaramappa, M. 1968. Guinea-worm arthritis of knee joint. Br. Med. J. *1*:155–156.
3. Rousett, P. 1952. Essae de prophylaxie et de traitement de la dracunculose par la notézine en Adrar. Bul. méd. Afr. occid. franc. *9*:351–568.
4. Padonu, K. O. 1973. A controlled trial of metronidazole in the treatment of dracontiasis in Nigeria. Am. J. Trop. Med. Hyg. *22*:42–44.
5. Muller, R. 1971. *Dracunculus* and drancunculiasis. *In* Dawes, B. (ed.): Advances in Parasitology. Vol. 9. Academic Press, New York. pp. 73–151.

CHAPTER 51

Other Tissue-Inhabiting Nematodes

Trichinosis

Synonyms. Trichiniasis, trichinelliasis.

Definition. Trichinosis is a disease caused by the parasite *Trichinella spiralis.* It runs an acute and rapid course and is characterized by fever, gastrointestinal symptoms, myalgia and eosinophilia.

Distribution. Trichinosis is widespread through the temperate regions of the world wherever pork or pork products are eaten, with the exceptions of Australasia, the Pacific Islands other than Hawaii, China and Japan. It is endemic in the United States including Alaska and Hawaii, Mexico, Central and South America (Guatemala, Venezuela, Brazil, Uruguay, Chile), East Africa and Nigeria, although African strains are less infective to test animals than are those from the temperate zone. Throughout Africa, including South Africa, trichinosis is enzootic in wildlife, particularly carnivores and bushpig, and man is involved sporadically. The disease is endemic in most European countries. Several hundred cases occur annually in Spain but, inexplicably, virtually none in Portugal. Although prevalent in Sicily, the disease in northern Italy is rare in man (but widespread in foxes); it has been absent from the Netherlands for 20 years, and is extremely rare in Finland where pork has been inspected for more than a century. Endemic foci exist in northern Russia and in parts of Asia including, since 1962, northern Thailand.

Etiology. MORPHOLOGY. The trichina worm, *T. spiralis* (Owen, 1835) Railliet, 1895, is a white roundworm just visible to the naked eye. The adult male ranges from 1.4 to 1.6 mm in length by 40 to 60 μm in diameter; the female is 3 to 4 mm long and about one and one-half times as broad as the male. Both sexes are somewhat attenuate anteriorly and are characterized by a long,

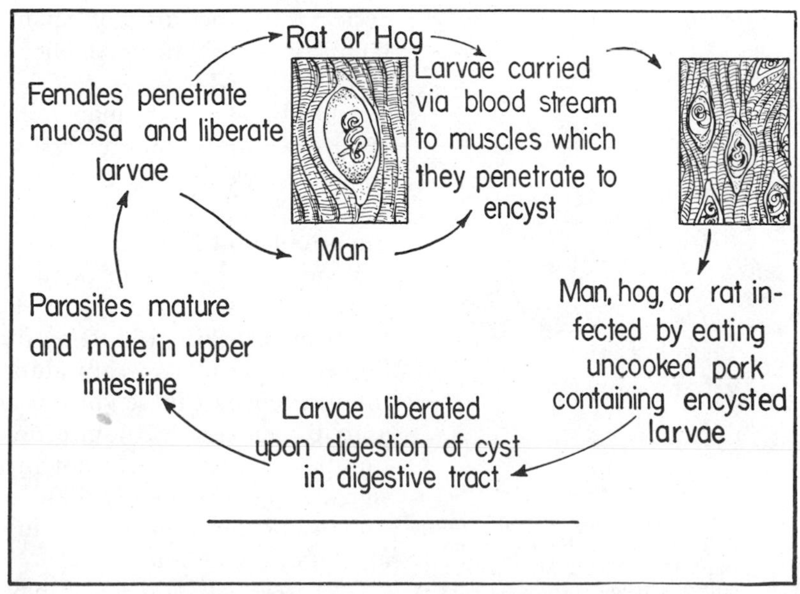

Figure 51–1. Nematode cycle—*Trichinella spiralis.*

slender esophagus extending one-third to one-half the body length surrounded by a single layer of esophageal cells. Posteriorly the eversible cloaca of the male is guarded by two papillae. The vulva of the female lies in the anterior third of the worm, and through this the small infective larvae, measuring only 100 μm in length by 6 μm in cross section, are discharged.

DEVELOPMENT. The worms gain entrance to the digestive tract as larvae encysted in muscle tissue (Fig. 51–1). By the time they reach the small intestine they are freed from their cysts, penetrate the duodenal epithelium and mature within a few days. Within 5 to 7 days the females are fertilized, invade the intestinal mucosa (Fig. 51–2) and produce larvae. It is believed that an adult female discharges between 1000 and 1500 larvae during the 3- to 16-week period she parasitizes man. If many females are present, large numbers of larvae are soon circulating in the blood. The larvae leave the blood stream between the eighth and twenty-third day. They may invade various tissues or cavities of the body, which they may subsequently leave to re-enter the blood stream; those finally reaching skeletal muscles will encyst. Musculature low in glycogen is the site of greatest invasion by the larvae of *T. spiralis*, which usually begins 8 to 9 days following the infecting meal. After reaching this final destination the larvae require a minimum period of 16 days to complete their development and to become infective. Larvae which are filtered out and remain in other organs fail to develop to the infective stage and are destroyed. The encapsulated larvae continue to grow until they reach a size of 0.8 to 1 mm. In man these cysts usually become calcified within 6 months, although some are believed to remain viable for 30 years. Under normal conditions the cycle is completed when viable cysts are ingested by a new host. While both adults and encysted larvae develop in the same animal, two hosts are nevertheless necessary to continue the cycle.

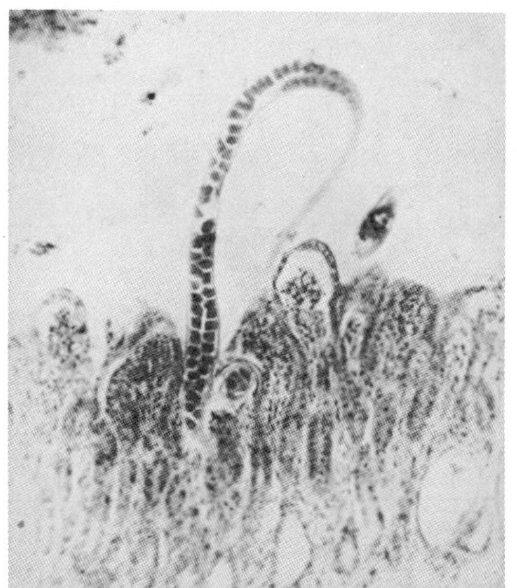

Figure 51–2. Adult female *T. spiralis* penetrating mucosa between villi of experimentally infected mouse. (From Dr. Irving Rappaport. *In* Nauss' Medical Parasitology and Zoology. Paul B. Hoeber, Inc., New York.)

Epidemiology. The most important reservoir of human infection is the hog, although many other flesh-eating mammals occasionally serve as reservoirs. In the United States hogs become infected chiefly from feeding on garbage containing uncooked pork scraps, and thus complete a hog-to-hog cycle. Both hogs and rats having access to the offal remaining after the slaughter of an infected hog may thereby acquire the infection. Other hogs may thus be infected at once, or they may later feed upon infected rats, completing a rat-to-hog cycle. Rats, because of their cannibalistic habits, show a high prevalence of natural infection (Fig. 51–3).

Outbreaks of human trichinosis follow group consumption of fresh, insufficiently cooked pork products containing striated muscle. Sampling of a large proportion of the population 2 and 3 decades ago revealed that nearly 18 per cent of the people in the United States were infected. However, there has been a striking reduction during the past 30 years, the most recent autopsy survey of the incidence of infection revealing a rate of 4 to 6 per cent.[1] An infection by a small number of worms does not produce clinical signs, and consequently these are discovered only by postmortem studies in which the diaphragm is examined.

Occasional outbreaks have also been

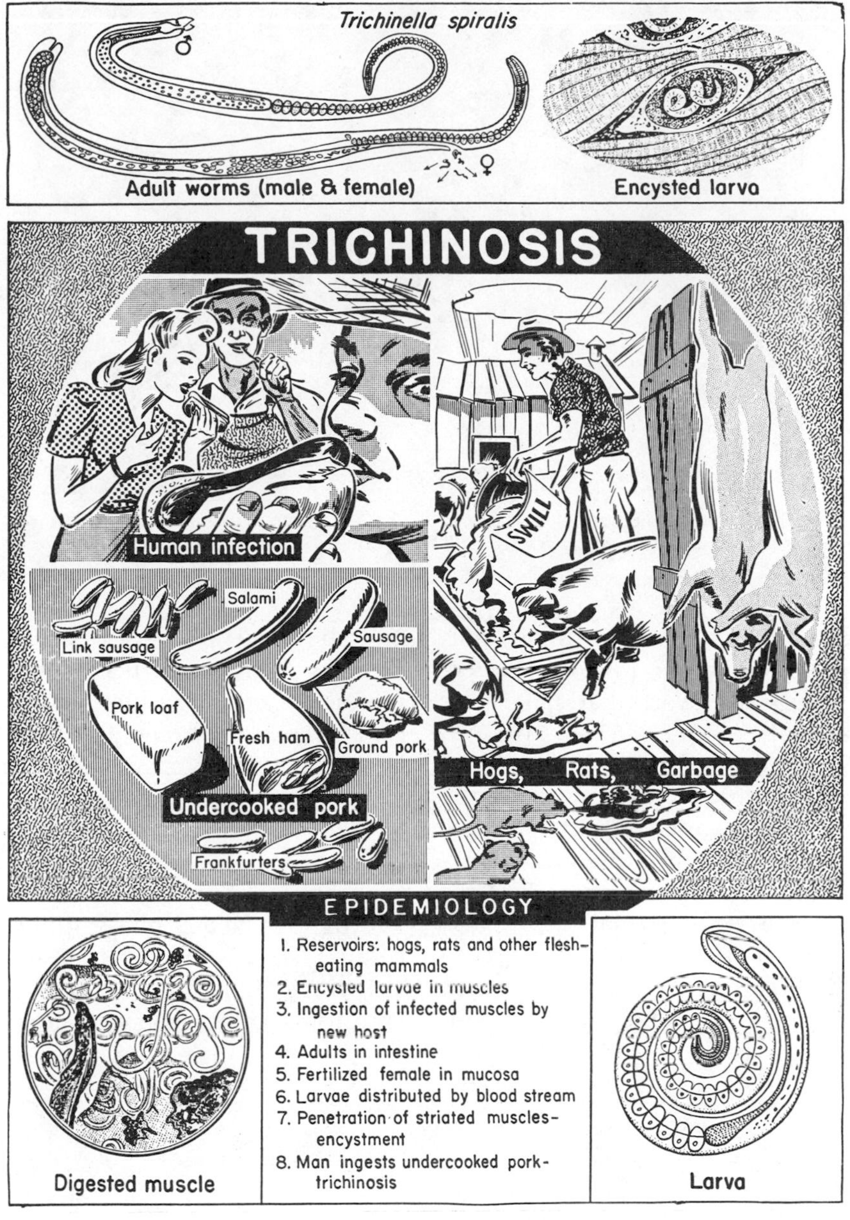

Figure 51-3. Epidemiology of trichinosis.

traced to such unusual sources as jerked infected bear meat.

Pathology. Trichinosis causes localized inflammation and necrosis in muscle tissue. The penetration of striated muscle fibers by the larvae of *T. spiralis* causes the destruction both of the fibers in which the larvae lie and of the adjacent ones. The parasites grow rapidly and, even after encystment, distention of the cysts occurs, causing further damage to adjacent tissues. In severe infections the myocardium may be extensively damaged, presenting cellular infiltration and necrosis and fragmentation of the muscle fibers. Encystment does not usually occur in cardiac muscle. It is believed that the destruction and absorption of host tissue and of many of the larvae cause the generalized toxemia. A high eosinophilia, sometimes reaching 70 per cent, is typical of this disease. In fatal

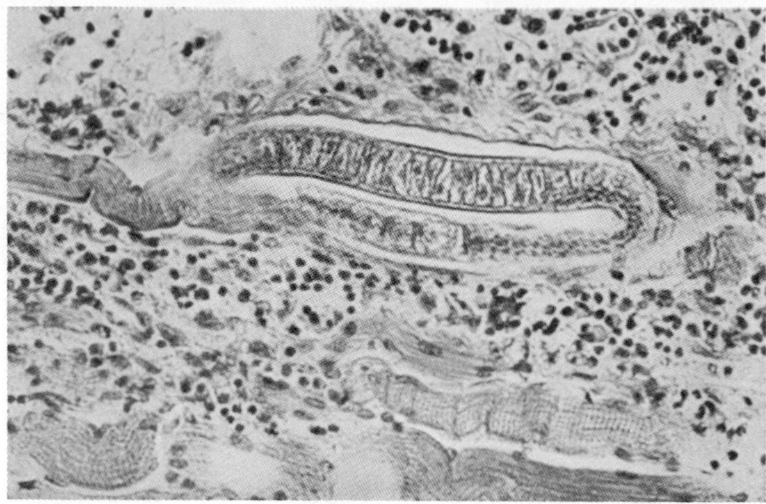

Figure 51–4. Early stage of encystment of larva of *T. spiralis* in man, showing degeneration of muscle fiber and surrounding myositis. (Courtesy of the University of Florida College of Medicine, Gainesville.)

cases death, usually intervening 4 to 8 weeks after the infection, is due to toxemia, secondary pneumonia, myocardial failure or trichinous encephalitis (Figs. 51–4, 51–5).

Clinical Characteristics. The clinical picture may be divided roughly into the stages of intestinal invasion, muscle penetration, and tissue repair (encystment). Twenty-four hours following the ingestion of viable larvae, signs of gastrointestinal disturbance in the form of nausea, vomiting, diarrhea and abdominal pain may become evident. In about a week the females begin to larviposit and the stage of muscle penetration commences. This period is characterized by periorbital edema, which usually occurs between the twelfth and fourteenth day, and irregular but persistent fever lasting 1 or 2 weeks sometimes attaining 40.5° C (105° F). Myositis and "rheumatic pains" are especially noticeable at this time. In severe infections a generalized scarlatiniform rash may occur. During this acute phase differential blood counts reveal a marked eosinophilia. The last stage is characterized by neurotoxic symptoms and possibly myocarditis. In less

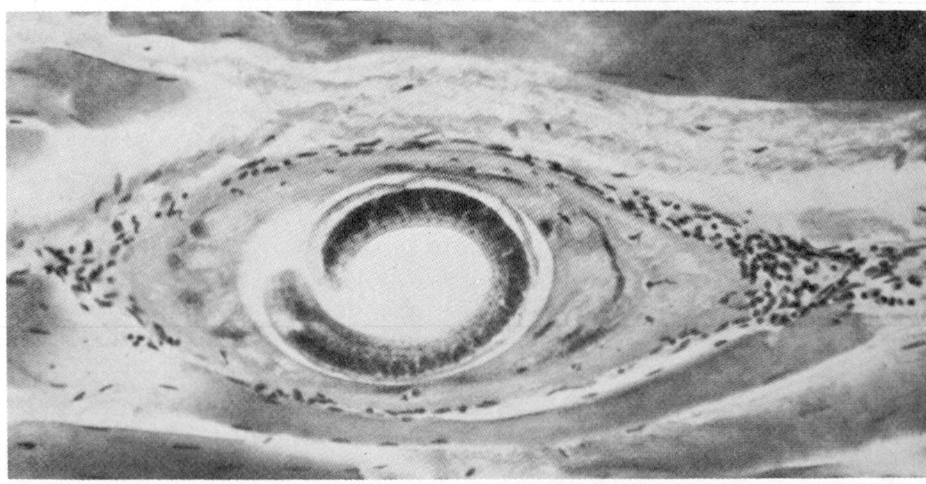

Figure 51–5. Encysted larva of *Trichinella spiralis.* The capsule, cellular infiltration and degeneration of adjacent muscle fiber are evident. (Courtesy of the Louisiana State University School of Medicine, New Orleans.)

severe cases the fever begins to subside and a slow convalescence follows. Loss of weight frequently occurs. Some atypical cases may simulate meningitis or encephalitis.

Diagnosis. An early diagnosis of this disease is difficult or impossible because of the absence of a clear-cut clinical picture. A history of eating raw or undercooked pork is helpful, but as trichinosis is not often suspected, a pertinent history is rarely elicited at the onset. Frequently members of the same family or even several families in one neighborhood will be involved.

Additional presumptive evidence is found in the periorbital edema and fever, coupled with a significant eosinophilia. The intradermal reaction, of the "immediate" type read in 15 minutes, becomes positive 3 weeks after infection occurs and persists for many years after arrest of the condition; however, false negative reactions also appear. Some other diagnostic tests involve flocculation, a saline extract of muscle larvae being coupled to inert carriers such as bentonite (BF test) or latex. (See p. 838.) These tests become positive in a month, and fail in less than 2 years. Although some false positive reactions occur with the flocculation tests, it is felt that the BF test still most nearly meets diagnostic requirements in the acute stage of the disease.[2] Reacting with all classes of immunoglobulin—and so more sensitive than the BF test—is the fluorescent antibody (FA) test, which detects antibodies as early as 7 days after infection. Indirect hemagglutination or complement-fixation procedures give results which vary in different hands. The agar gel diffusion test distinguishes false from true positives, but requires several days for completion. A newly developed test, which may be completed in 1 hour and appears highly reliable compared with the BF test, is counterelectrophoresis using antigens derived from mature muscle larvae.[3]

Direct evidence of the infection rests upon the demonstration of the parasite. Sometimes this may be accomplished by biopsy of the deltoid, biceps or gastrocnemius muscle, part of which should be compressed between glass slides and examined under a microscope, part digested and the remainder sectioned. *Trichinella* larvae may be recovered from the spinal fluid of patients with severe trichinosis.

It is necessary to make a differential diagnosis, especially in the initial stages, to exclude food poisoning and diarrhea or dysentery of other etiology. Later, cardiac, renal, hepatic or central nervous system disease and other causes of fever associated with generalized body pains must be suspected.

The prognosis is good in light infections but becomes grave when heavy parasitization is evident.

Treatment. The treatment of trichinosis is principally supportive, since 95 per cent or more of clinically diagnosed cases recover spontaneously with few sequelae.[4] Symptomatic relief of febrile stages of the disease may be obtained from the use of corticosteroids, but such treatment may permit increase in the numbers of muscle larvae, thus contributing to enhancement of chronic trichinosis. Several drugs are being tested that have specific prophylactic or therapeutic effects or both. Of these, thiabendazole remains the drug of choice although side effects accompany its use in many patients.[5] In a dosage of 50 mg per kg per day for 7 days, muscle stiffness and pain may be rapidly reduced and the general condition improved. Administration in the first week of invasion has prevented the development of clinical symptoms.

Prophylaxis. Infection is due largely to the ingestion of raw or insufficiently cooked pork. The larvae of *T. spiralis* are readily killed by thorough cooking of meat, the thermal death point of trichinae being 60° C (140° F), or by freezing it for 36 hours at −27° C (−16.6° F), for 24 hours at −30° C (−22° F), or for 40 minutes at −35° C (−31° F). It should be remembered that the United States Government *DOES NOT INSPECT MEAT* for the presence of this parasite.

Proper cooking of garbage used for feeding swine is a presently available effective and practicable measure to prevent continued dissemination of trichinosis. Exposure of trichinous pork to gamma radiation from cobalt-60 and atomic waste fission material will prevent the larvae from developing into adult forms when the meat is eaten. Pigs fed a diet containing 0.1 per cent thiabendazole and exposed to larvae of *T. spiralis* developed either no infection or an infection of negligible severity.[6]

Creeping Eruption

Synonyms. Larva migrans, ancylostomiasis braziliensis.

Definition. Creeping eruption results from the presence of the larvae of the dog and cat hookworm, *Ancylostoma braziliense,* in the epidermis of man. A number of other species of skin-penetrating nematode larvae may produce somewhat similar dermatoses (Table 51–1).

Distribution. Ancylostomiasis braziliensis is endemic in the southeastern part of the United States while sporadic cases have been reported as far north as Massachusetts. It is present to a lesser degree along the coastal regions of Texas, Mexico and Central America. Colombia, Venezuela, the Guianas and Brazil are regarded as centers of infection. In Africa, ancylostomiasis braziliensis exists in a band across the tropical portion of the continent with another endemic center on the beaches of Port Elizabeth, Republic of South Africa. It is also reported in Sri Lanka, Malaya, Burma, Thailand, Java, Taiwan, Hong Kong and the Philippines. Adult worms have been reported in scattered instances from the intestine of man in the Philippines, Indonesia, Sri Lanka, India, Thailand, parts of Africa and Brazil, but these probably represent a distinct but closely related species.

Etiology. MORPHOLOGY. The dog and cat hookworm, *A. braziliense* (de Faria, 1910), is the smallest of the "human" hookworms. The males are 7.8 to 8.5 mm long and the females 9 to 10.5 mm. The general morphology of this species is essentially similar to that of *A. duodenale. Ancylostoma braziliense* has two pairs of teeth, a small, curved, inner pair and a larger, outer pair, making the buccal capsule diagnostic of the species. The bursa of the male is smaller than that of other hookworms and is likewise diagnostic; it is almost as broad as it is long and is supported by short stubby rays. The eggs cannot be distinguished readily from those of *A. duodenale.*

DEVELOPMENT. The females produce about 4000 eggs a day. The extrahuman developmental cycle parallels that of the other hookworms. The filariform larvae, however, usually remain localized in the skin of man and do not undergo further development.

Epidemiology. Wild and domestic members of the dog and cat families constitute the normal and reservoir hosts of *A. braziliense.* The eggs are passed in the stools and contaminate the soil where, under adequate conditions of temperature and humidity, infective filariform larvae develop (Fig. 51–6). These, coming in contact with the skin of man, readily penetrate and produce "creeping eruption." Sandy areas of the southeastern states constitute the chief endemic foci in the United States. Beaches, children's sandpiles and areas where dogs and cats defecate are common sources of infection. Less extensive lesions of creeping eruption have been reported for the European dog hookworm, *Uncinaria stenocephala,* and experimentally for the dog hookworm, *Ancylostoma caninum.*[9]

Pathology. The larvae, after penetrating the epidermis, produce serpiginous tunnels in the stratum germinativum of the skin, progressing at a rate of several millimeters or a few centimeters each day. The course of the tunnels is marked by erythema, induration and, at times, overlying vesiculation. Histologic examination reveals local eosinophilic and round cell infiltration. The larvae may remain active in the skin for variable periods up to several months. In some human infections, larvae reach the lungs and may cause transient pulmonary infiltration.

Clinical Characteristics. A reddish pa-

Table 51–1. Differential Diagnostic Chart of Cutaneous Lesions Produced by Some Metazoan Parasites

Parasite	*Character of the Lesions*
Necator americanus "American" hookworm	Penetration of larvae is followed by itching, burning, erythema and edema. Later a papule appears, followed frequently by a vesicle. If secondary infection does not occur, the dermatitis disappears spontaneously in 2 weeks. This is known commonly as "ground itch," or "dew itch."
Ancylostoma duodenale "Old World" hookworm	May cause "ground itch" as above, but not invariably, some cases being asymptomatic.
Ancylostoma braziliense Dog and cat hookworm	The commonest type of "creeping eruption." Lesions serpiginous, extending sinuously through the stratum germinativum from several mm to several cm daily. Erythema, or even purpura, make the "burrows" superficially visible, in addition to elevation of the skin over the tunnels. The chief symptom is intense itching. The worms live for weeks or months. Secondary infection may complicate the disease. Pulmonary involvement develops occasionally.
Ancylostoma caninum The dog hookworm	Penetration is followed by itchy papules; occasionally with linear extension by "burrowing." Symptoms usually disappear in 2 weeks.
Uncinaria stenocephala European dog hookworm	This nematode, the European dog hookworm, produces a condition practically identical with the "creeping eruption" of *Ancylostoma braziliense* but of shorter duration.
Strongyloides stercoralis The strongylid threadworm	On rare occasions infections produce a pruritus at the site of entry within an hour, characterized by an erythematous macule. Generalized urticaria occurs occasionally; serpiginous lesions (larva currens) are seen only rarely.
Strongyloides myopotami (strongylid of nutria)	This parasite of coypu, or nutria, apparently can produce migratory, maculopapular serpiginous or linear lesions in the skin of man.[7]
Capillaria sp.	Migratory, linear, zigzag tract; redness and severe pruritus.[8]
Gnathostoma spinigerum Gnathostomes	This nematode forms boils, abscesses, or deep burrows. Infiltration by white blood cells, especially eosinophils, is seen histologically.
Dermatobia hominis The tropical warble fly	Deeply penetrating, with an open "breathing hole" in skin. No migration. Elevated red itchy painful boil or "bot" or "warble." Duration about 6 weeks (p. 776).
Gasterophilus sp. Horse bot fly	Penetrates to stratum germinativum, then burrows parallel to skin surface, migrating slowly for several months. Looks more like true "creeping eruption" of *A. braziliense* than most other similar lesions and is called larva migrans (p. 775).
Hypoderma sp. Cattle warble fly	Deeply penetrating to subcutaneous tissue. Slow migration occurs during the course of a month. Quite painful. Little itching (p. 778). More serious than *Gasterophilus*.
Schistosoma Species for which man is an abnormal or unfavorable host Blood flukes	Known as schistosome dermatitis or swimmer's itch. Urticarial wheals immediately after penetration of cercariae. Several hours later itching and edema, followed by papules and pustules. Symptoms begin to subside after 3 days (p. 565).

pule, accompanied by pruritus, occurs at the site of invasion within a few hours after the larvae have penetrated the skin. Within 2 or 3 days the parasites begin to migrate, producing an erythematous, serpiginous, linear and elevated tunnel. This migration is accompanied by an intense pruritus. The unoccupied portion of the tunnel soon dries and becomes crusted. Scratching of these lesions frequently leads to secondary infection. The infected person may suffer intolerably, the local symptoms producing insom-

Ancylostoma braziliense
Mouthparts
Bursa
Egg
CREEPING ERUPTION
Lesions Simulating Creeping Eruption:
European dog hookworm– Uncinaria stenocephala Creeping eruption.
Horse botflies– Gasterophilus spp. "larva migrans"
Fecal contamination
EPIDEMIOLOGY
1. Reservoirs and normal hosts: dogs and cats
2. Eggs in feces contaminate soil
3. Development of larvae in soil
4. Contact of hosts with infested soil:
normal hosts — dogs and cats
abnormal host — man
5. Penetration of skin by infective larvae
6. Migration of larvae:
in man — in epidermis — creeping eruption
in natural host — to heart, lungs and gut
— maturation of worms
— reproduction
Early lesion
Infection by larvae

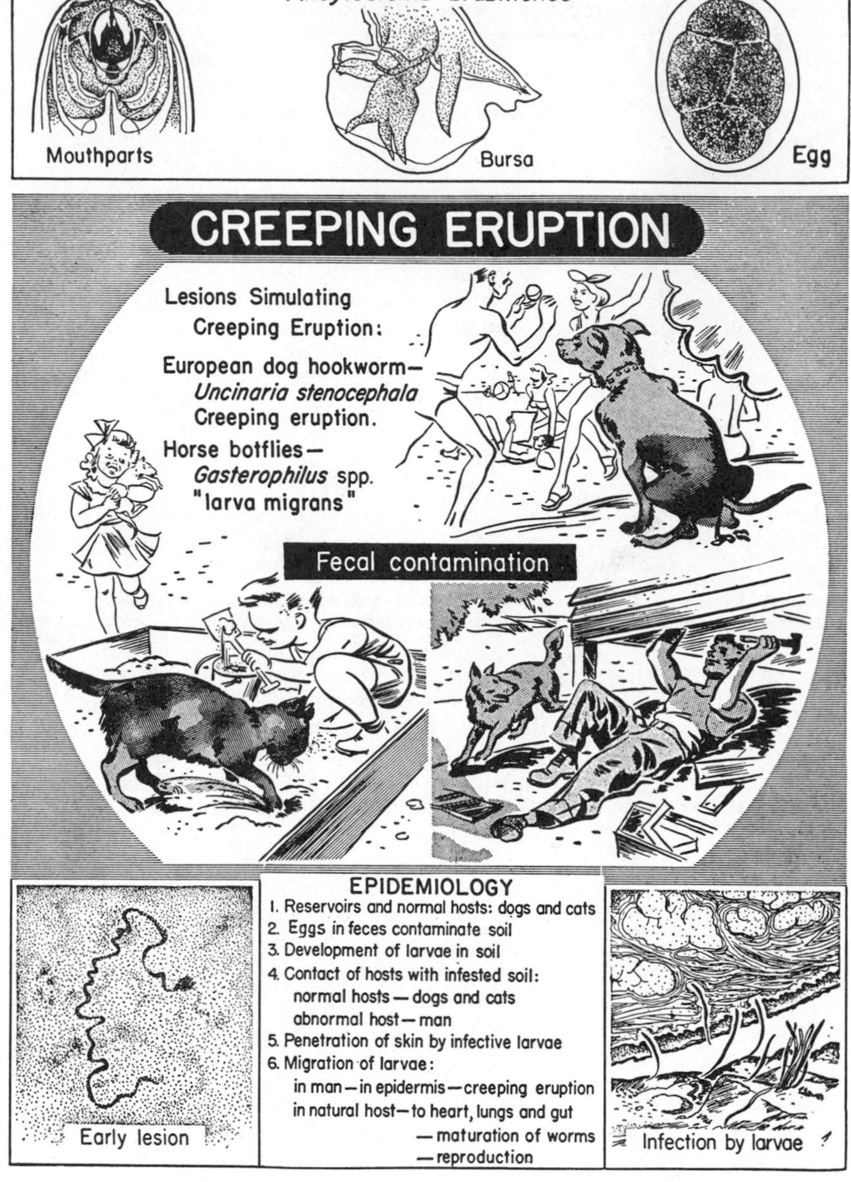

Figure 51–6. Epidemiology of creeping eruption.

nia, anorexia and even loss of weight (Fig. 51–7). Loeffler's syndrome – eosinophilia, cough and x-ray evidence of transient pulmonary infiltrations – occasionally occurs.

Diagnosis. *Ancylostoma braziliense* infection may be diagnosed most readily on the basis of the characteristic serpiginous lesions and a history of exposure in a typical "creeping eruption environment." A differential diagnosis between "creeping eruption" and other types of dermatitis caused by metazoan parasites is sometimes difficult. Considerable confusion is possible, but a careful analysis and reference to the accompanying table should prove helpful (Table 51–1).

Treatment. Permanent relief is obtained by freezing the area just ahead of the lesion with ethyl chloride spray or carbon dioxide snow. This is a commonly employed therapeutic measure but at best is unsatisfactory, especially if numerous lesions are present.

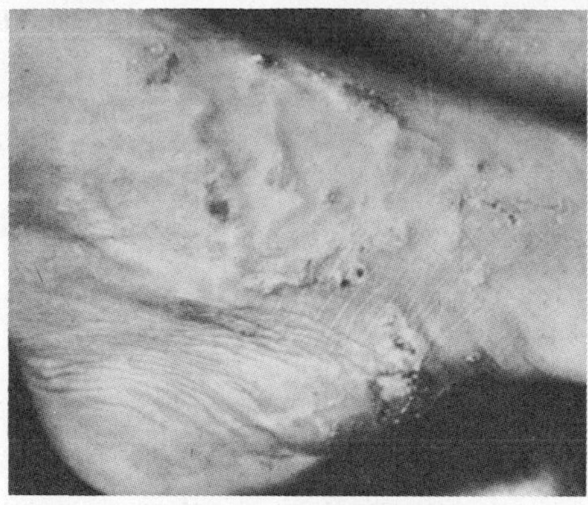
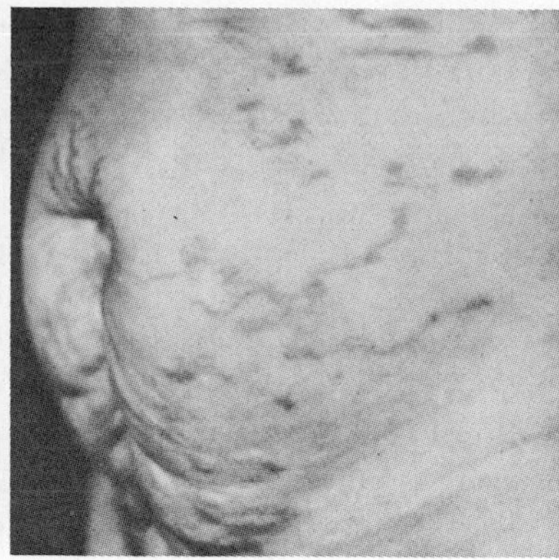

Figure 51–7. Creeping eruption caused by the larvae of *Ancylostoma braziliense.* (Courtesy of the Dermatology Division, University of Miami Medical School.)

The oral administration of promethazine hydrochloride (Phenergan) has been effective, but thiabendazole is now preferred for treatment. The suggested dosage is 25 mg per kg twice a day for 2 successive days, repeated in 3 to 7 days if active lesions remain.[10] Thiabendazole as a topical application was effective in 3 days, being applied locally as a suspension (500 mg per 5 ml) overlaid with 0.1 per cent dexamethasone cream. A polyethylene film was superimposed to occlude the medication.[11] Thiabendazole has been applied topically with dimethyl sulfoxide. It has been administered intracutaneously, using a jet injector.

Prophylaxis. Avoid contact with sandy soil which dogs and cats may leave polluted with feces. Sandboxes and the like should be protected from dogs and especially cats which may select these as defecation sites. Periodic deworming of these domestic animals should be helpful in reducing infection.

Gnathostomiasis

Synonyms. *Gnathostoma spinigerum* infection, larva migrans or creeping eruption.

Definition. Gnathostomiasis is an infection caused primarily by immature *Gnathostoma spinigerum; Gnathostoma dolorosi* and *Gnathostoma nipponicum* also have been incriminated in Japan. The worm may localize in the internal organs but also may occur in the peripheral tissues in nodules or in subcutaneous tunnels in which the worms migrate (hence, larva migrans or creeping eruption). Adult parasites are usually found in wild or domestic cats and more rarely in dogs, hogs or mink.

Distribution. Gnathostomiasis is known from Israel, India, Bangladesh, Java, Malaya, Thailand, China and Japan. In certain areas of Thailand it is highly endemic.

Etiology. MORPHOLOGY. The adult nematode *G. spinigerum* (Owen, 1836) is stout, reddish in color and possesses a globose cephalic bulb or head which is separated from the body proper by a slight constriction and is armed by four to eight transverse rows of recurved spines. The anterior half of the body is spinose also. Males and females range respectively from 11 to 25 mm and 25 to 54 mm in length. The mature female produces ovoid, unsegmented eggs with a greenish tinged, irregularly pitted shell that is marked by a transparent plug at one end; the eggs are 63 to 70 μm long by 37 to 41 μm broad.

DEVELOPMENT. The adult worms lie coiled in tumors along the alimentary canal of cats, dogs and other reservoir hosts. Eggs reach the lumen of the intestine from these lesions and are passed in the feces, where they become embryonated. They hatch upon reaching water, releasing a cylindrical, ensheathed rhabditiform larva which, if ingested by a copepod (*Cyclops*), continues to develop. When the infective copepod is eaten by a fish, frog, snake or bird, a third-stage larva is produced which becomes encapsulated in the flesh of the host. Upon ingestion by the definitive host, the parasite usually becomes localized in the stomach wall, where it matures after about 7 months.

Epidemiology. Man becomes infected with *G. spinigerum* through the ingestion of improperly cooked fish, frogs, birds and snakes containing encapsulated larvae. It appears doubtful that man becomes infected by swallowing infected copepods in water. Prenatal transmission of larvae may occur in humans, as it does in other mammals.

Pathology. Obviously, man is an abnormal host. Only immature worms have been encountered. When the parasites are situated superficially, abscesses or cutaneous nodules may be produced. Subcutaneous tunnels may be formed by the migrating nematodes. Ocular involvement occurs rarely. Two systemic syndromes have been described, the abdominopulmonary believed caused by migration of infective larvae, and the eosinophilic myeloencephalitic caused by migration of immature adult worms. In the latter cases, sometimes fatal, the brain and spinal cord contain tracks of the wandering worm, surrounded by necrotic and hemorrhagic tissue. These tracks are larger than ones made by *Angiostrongylus cantonensis.*[12] The spinal fluid contains many eosinophils, as does the blood.

Clinical Characteristics. Creeping eruption is an obvious form of the infection. The worms, which are situated superficially, usually are encountered between the stratum germinativum and the corium of the skin, producing local inflammation, edema, eosinophilia and leukocytosis. Other symptoms depend upon the location of the parasites, and may be grouped as abdominopleuropulmonary imitating acute appendicitis, pleurisy and other conditions or myeloencephalitis with initial severe trunk and limb pain, followed by ascending paralysis starting in the extremities, early impairment of consciousness, and sometimes death. The first such case was diagnosed in Thailand in 1963,[13] and many more have been reported since then. Infection may persist for long periods—up to 17 years. Human urinary gnathostomiasis, a rarity, has also been reported.[13a]

Diagnosis. Residence in an endemic area is suggestive, but definitive diagnosis depends upon recovery and identification of the parasite. Skin-testing provides a reliable means of diagnosis. The nonmigrating type of infection must be differentiated from abscesses of bacterial origin; the superficial migrating form must be distinguished from cutaneous myiasis (p. 531) or the migrations of larval hookworms, especially *Ancylostoma braziliense* (p. 530). In Thailand, differentiation of eosinophilic myeloencephalitis from eosinophilic meningoencephalitis induced by *Angiostrongylus cantonensis* is based on clinical symptomatology and the intense blood eosinophilia found in the former. The spinal fluid contains many eosinophils in both these syndromes.

Treatment. Diethylcarbamazine (Hetrazan) has some therapeutic value in cutaneous gnathostomiasis. The recommended dosage is 0.5 to 0.7 mg per kg of body weight 3 times daily after meals for 5 to 7 days. Courses of quinine or prednisolone lasting 4 weeks provided temporary relief of edematous swellings in some cases.[14]

Prophylaxis. Since man acquires this helminthiasis by ingestion of infected fish, frogs, birds or snakes, adequate cooking of the flesh of these animals is recommended. Immersion of fish in vinegar for 5½ hours has also been found to be an effective measure.

Visceral Larva Migrans

Synonyms. Human toxocariasis, nonpatent nematodiasis.

Definition. Visceral larva migrans denotes prolonged migration of larvae of animal nematodes in human tissues other than the skin. The syndrome in persons who react significantly to the presence of the larvae is characterized by persistent hypereosinophilia, hepatomegaly and, frequently, by pneumonitis. Larvae of dog and cat ascarids and of other animal nematodes may produce this entity. The infection occurs predominantly in children.

Distribution. Most of the cases have been reported from the United States. The infection probably occurs widely throughout the world.

Etiology. *Toxocara canis* (Werner, 1782), a common ascarid of dogs, probably is the most important etiologic agent.[15] Opportunity for infection of children with eggs of this animal nematode in soil is favored by the close association of dogs with humans and the animal's habit of promiscuous defecation. *Toxocara cati* (Schrank, 1788), an ascarid of cats, is probably of somewhat lesser epidemiologic significance. Some of the other nematodes presently known to be involved in the larva migrans type of infection in man are *Capillaria hepatica* (Bancroft, 1893), a parasite of rodents, certain species of gnathostomes and other spiruroids, species of hookworm including *A. braziliense* and *A. caninum* (Ercolani, 1859) and one or more species of animal filariae of the genus *Dirofilaria*.

Epidemiology. *Toxocara canis* and *T. cati* eggs deposited in yards and scattered by rain may embryonate in soil under favorable environmental conditions. Owing to the habit of toddler-age children of eating dirt, eggs of the ascarids may be ingested. The mode of infection is similar to that of human ascariasis and trichuriasis except that the infective eggs are of animal origin. Adults may acquire the infection from soiled hands and food or water contaminated with *Toxocara* eggs. The larvae emerge from the eggs in the intestine of the human host, penetrate the bowel wall and, by direct migration or through the circulation, reach the various organs of the body. The extensive somatic migration may continue for an undetermined period, probably many months. It is followed by encapsulation of the larvae, which may persist without morphologic change for more than a year. *Toxocara* infections rarely reach maturity in the human intestine since man is not a natural host.

Pathology. Scattered gray nodules up

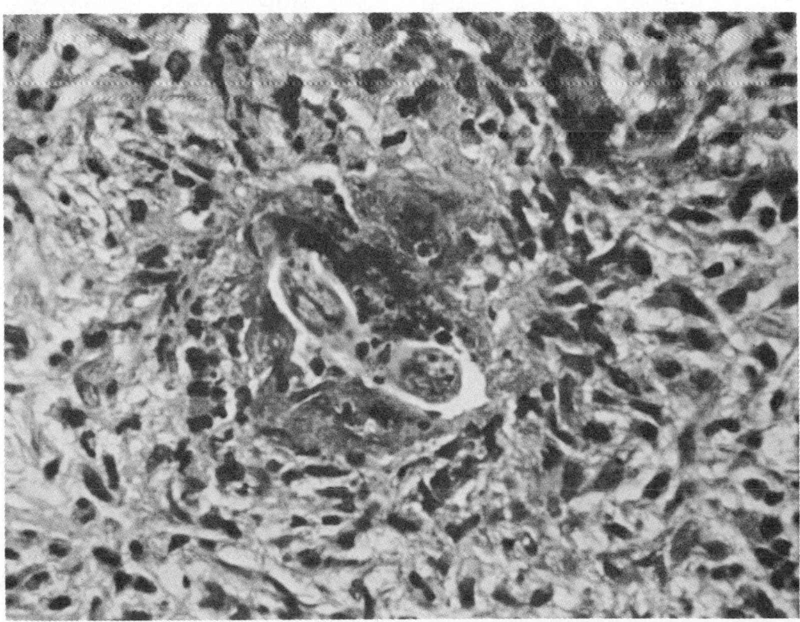

Figure 51–8. Foci of granulomatous inflammation around larva of *Toxocara canis.* Note histiocytic and multinucleated giant cell reaction. The amorphous material around the larva stained bright red. (PAS × 450.) (Courtesy of Dr. V. M. Areán, University of Florida College of Medicine, from material loaned by Dr. Gillermo Carrera, Ochsner Foundation Hospital, New Orleans, Louisiana, in Revista Clínica Española, vol. 94.)

to 0.7 cm in diameter may be seen in the liver, lungs and other organs at autopsy. A granulomatous eosinophilic and neutrophilic inflammatory reaction surrounds the worms and their tracks.[15] Typically the lesion is an eosinophilic granuloma. Charcot-Leyden crystals have been observed in the allergic granulomas. The continuous active movements of the larvae may be responsible for considerable tissue destruction. Meticulous search of many sections usually is necessary to find larvae in biopsy material. Later, they are encapsulated by connective tissue. Larvae are most abundant in the liver, lungs and brain but, to a lesser extent, may invade almost all organs of the body (Fig. 51–8). Irreversible changes in the central nervous system occasionally occur. The bone marrow shows an eosinophilic hyperplasia.

A nematode endophthalmitis represents another form of visceral larva migrans. The most characteristic lesion is an eosinophilic abscess that is frequently located on the underside of the retina, in the retinal folds and in the vitreous membrane.

Clinical Characteristics. Many infections are subclinical, and the only salient finding is a moderate or high sustained eosinophilia. In symptomatic infections a syndrome consisting of hypereosinophilia, hepatomegaly, hyperglobulinemia and frequently a patchy pneumonitis is seen. Intermittent fever, leukocytosis primarily due to the increase in eosinophils, malaise, pallor, anorexia, failure to gain weight, muscle and joint pains, abdominal pain, nausea, vomiting and neurologic disturbances, with convulsions and petit mal attacks, may occur in some cases. An impetiginous pruritic skin rash sometimes appears on the trunk and extremities.

The infection usually runs a chronic benign course, as long as 18 months, and is self-limited in the absence of reinfection. Deaths attributed to this infection have been few. The severity of the infection varies with the number of larvae in the tissues and the immune or allergic state of the infected individual. Before its etiology was known, many cases of visceral larva migrans probably were designated as familial eosinophilia, Weingarten's disease, Frimodt-Möller's syndrome, eosinophilic pseudoleukemia, tropical eosinophilia and Loeffler's syndrome.

A nematode endophthalmitis clinically resembling retinoblastoma may be caused by larvae migrating to the orbit. This entity has been most frequently observed in children.

Diagnosis. A high and persistent eosinophilia in a child should arouse suspicion of visceral larva migrans. The diagnosis is made primarily on clinical grounds. A history of eating dirt or playing on ground frequented by dogs or cats, the presence of these pets at home, and previous or present infection with intestinal helminths which could have been acquired simultaneously help to support a clinical diagnosis. Differential and total leukocyte counts may reveal an eosinophilia of 20 to 80 per cent and 15,000 to 80,000 white blood cells per cu mm. Intradermal tests, using as antigen a solution prepared from a saline extract of desiccated adult *T. canis,* have been increasingly used for epidemiologic purposes.[16] Experimental studies indicate that the indirect immunofluorescence, the hemagglutination or the bentonite flocculation tests may be specific enough to distinguish larval *Toxocara* infections. Since visceral larva migrans frequently is encountered in the same age group in which ascariasis commonly occurs, cross-reactions in serologic tests, resulting from previous or concurrent *A. lumbricoides* infection, may result. In the hemagglutination test for visceral larva migrans, *Ascaris* antibody may be absorbed out, before testing with *Toxocara* antigen, in order to reduce the possibility of cross-reaction.

Since the parasite does not complete its life cycle in man, the patient's stools do not contain *Toxocara* eggs.

Liver biopsy is not recommended. However, the diagnosis of second-stage rhabditoid *Toxocara* larvae in tissue sections can be made from one good cross section at the midgut level; *T. canis* ranges in maximum diameter from 14 to 20 μm and *T. cati* 12 to 16 μm. Both *Toxocara* species have average lengths of 320 μm. Second-stage larvae of *A. lumbricoides* resemble those of *Toxocara,* but the third-stage larvae are much larger and

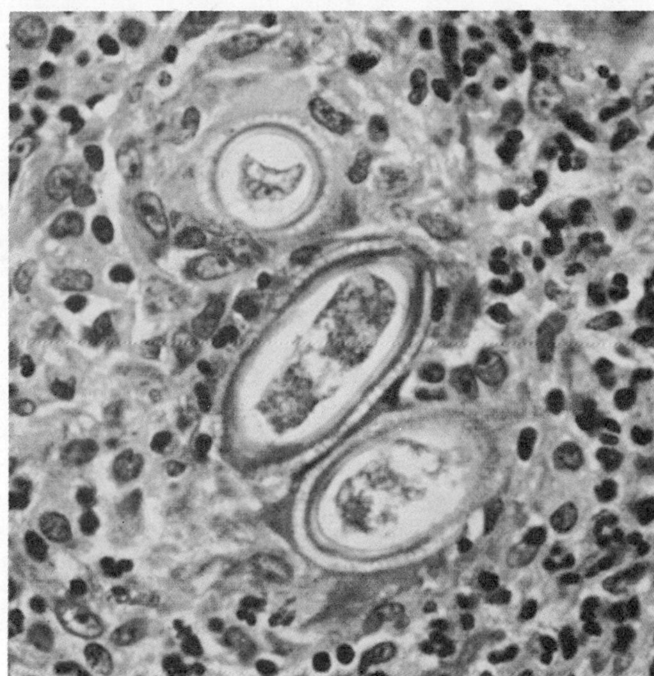

Figure 51–9. Focus of granulomatous reaction around three eggs of *Capillaria* sp. (H and E × 450.) (Courtesy of Dr. V. M. Areán, University of Florida College of Medicine and the Revista Clínica Española, vol. 94.)

measure about 600 μm in length and 24 to 26 μm in diameter.

Differential diagnosis includes pneumonia, miliary tuberculosis, asthma, whooping cough, Loeffler's syndrome, tropical eosinophilia and intestinal helminthiases. Strongyloidiasis, trichinosis and other helminthic infections in which there may be a marked increase in eosinophils may need to be excluded. Larval *A. lumbricoides* occasionally may produce a similar syndrome in some children. Histologically, the lesions may simulate periarteritis nodosa and sarcoidosis, and the blood picture may suggest eosinophilic leukemia. In some instances, retinoblastoma and endophthalmitis of other etiology must be considered. Ocular lesions of visceral larva migrans have been confused with pseudoglioma, Coats' disease and endophthalmitis of unknown origin. Specific diagnosis of nematode endophthalmitis is made only after enucleation of the organ.

Treatment. Opinions differ regarding the value of thiabendazole as a specific for *Toxocara* infections, although it is generally agreed that symptoms may be ameliorated by the use of cortisone. Among recent serologically confirmed cases, a patient with severe respiratory involvement improved rapidly following successive administration of methylprednisolone intravenously and a 3-day course of thiabendazole,[17] and another patient having acute meningoencephalomyelitis with flaccid paraplegia recovered completely following two courses of thiabendazole given for 6 days.[18] Usually no specific treatment is necessary. The prognosis ordinarily is good if the source of infection is removed. Measures to prevent superinfection are extremely important in management of patients with this infection.

Prophylaxis. Dogs and cats should be dewormed at monthly intervals. In some instances, it may be desirable to dispense with these pets. When practicable, play yards should be protected by fences to exclude pets and stray dogs. Paved areas and lawns are preferable to open soil and sandboxes as play sites. Top soil may be turned under to place the eggs out of reach of children. Instruction of children and supervision of their hygienic and play habits to reduce the ingestion of soil and the placing of contaminated hands in the mouth are of great importance.

HEPATIC CAPILLARIASIS

The capillary liver worm is a common parasite of rats, their relatives, as well as a wide variety of other mammals, rarely including man. The adult worms, *Capillaria hepatica* (Bancroft, 1893) Travassos, 1915, inhabit the liver, and the eggs infiltrate into the surrounding parenchyma where a granulomatous reaction occurs (Fig. 51–9).[19] The clinical picture suggests hepatitis with eosinophilia. Diagnosis is by liver biopsy. In a case reported recently from the Transvaal, treatment with diethylcarbamazine was ineffectual, but a slow improvement followed the use of sodium antimonyl gluconate.[20] Prophylactic measures involve the avoidance of consumption of raw livers of the reservoir hosts.

Angiostrongylosis

Synonyms. Eosinophilic meningoencephalitis, angiostrongyliasis.

Definition. A type of meningitis caused by the presence of the rodent lungworm, *Angiostrongylus cantonensis,* and characterized by a pleocytosis with a high percentage of eosinophils (25 to 65 per cent) in the cerebrospinal fluid of infected persons. Parasites have also been reported from the eye and brain of man.

Distribution. *Angiostrongylus cantonensis* has been reported in rodents throughout the Indo-Pacific region, including Madagascar, Mauritius, India, Sri Lanka (Ceylon), West and East Malaysia, Thailand, East Asia and the Western and Central Pacific Islands. It occurs in Australia but not New Zealand. Human angiostrongylosis has been diagnosed in the Pacific Islands and southeast Asia, as far west as Kuala Lumpur.

Etiology. *Angiostrongylus cantonensis* (Chen, 1935) Dougherty, 1946 is a delicate, filiform roundworm ranging between 17 and 25 mm in length, with a maximum diameter of 0.25 to 0.36 mm, a smooth cuticle, and three minute lips at the cephalic extremity. As is the case with other metastrongyles, the male bears a copulatory bursa supported by bursal rays.[21]

The life cycle, described in Australia in 1955,[22] has been further studied. The natural hosts for the parasite are rodents of several genera, including *Rattus rattus,* which acquire the infection by ingesting mollusks containing third-stage larvae. The larvae proceed to the rodent's brain, where they develop in 2 weeks into young adults which migrate to, and establish themselves in, the pulmonary arteries. Eggs are laid and lodge in the lung capillaries, where they hatch. First-stage larvae enter the alveolar spaces, migrate up the trachea and down the alimentary tract, and are excreted with the rodent's feces which attract feeding mollusks. The larvae, which can survive exposure for 2 weeks under humid conditions, are thus ingested by, or penetrate, mollusks. A variety of terrestrial snails, slugs and aquatic snails serve as intermediate hosts of the parasite, which develops principally in the muscular part of the mollusk's foot, molting and becoming infective as third-stage larvae in about 2 weeks. The cycle continues from mollusk to rodent by three routes: infected mollusk tissue is ingested by the rodent; mollusks may contaminate drinking water; or mollusk tissue may be ingested by carrier (paratenic) hosts such as freshwater prawns, land crabs and planarians, the parasite larvae surviving and then gaining access to rodents devouring these carriers. Man is an abnormal mammalian host, the metastrongylid parasite being unable to complete its cycle and dying in his central nervous system.

Epidemiology. A principal method of spread of *A. cantonensis* has been in one of its most effective intermediate hosts, the giant African snail *Achatina fulica.*[23] This snail has spread from Madagascar eastward and its appearance has preceded discovery of infected rodents in countries of the Indo-Pacific region and East Asia; it is still unreported, but the parasite present, only in Australia, New Caledonia and Tahiti. Murine angiostrongylosis probably reached the Pacific early in the present century, but the first human case was not seen until 1944. Incidence in man is correlated with diet, infections being acquired through the ingestion of raw or lightly cooked snails, slugs, crabs, prawns and (on unwashed vegetables) planarians, or in contaminated drinking water.

Pathology. Typical of later reports was the first case of eosinophilic meningitis described.[24] At autopsy there was evidence of encephalomalacia of frontal and temporal lobes and leptomeningitis. Sections of the cerebrum and cerebellum revealed a nematode which in subsequent dissection of brain tissue proved to be *A. cantonensis.* Microscopically, aggregates of eosinophils, monocytes and foreign body giant cells were found about the living worms, while in some cases there was marked necrosis around dead worms. Invariably noted are multiple tortuous tracks in brain and spinal cord, with associated hemorrhages. Vascular lesions with necrosis and aneurysmal dilatation occur. The serum IgG and spinal fluid total protein, albumin, IgG, IgM and IgA are increased.

Clinical Characteristics. Symptoms related to an infecting meal appear 10 to 28 days later, and may include vomiting. Head ache, unremittingly severe and unresponsive to analgesics, and paresthesias and neurologic symptoms are frequently experienced. Signs of meningeal and meningoencephalitic involvement are more specific, and include neck rigidity, impairment of vision sometimes leading to blindness, drowsiness and coma. In most instances meningitis has been of short duration, and complete and spontaneous recovery has occurred.

Diagnosis. Recovery of the parasite by spinal fluid tap or from the anterior chamber of the eye has occasionally been achieved. Patients exhibiting a syndrome of central nervous system involvement, a moderate to high peripheral eosinophilia, and a pleocytosis with an elevated eosinophilic count in the cerebrospinal fluid should be suspect, especially those who reside or have resided in areas where it has been demonstrated that the rodents are infected with *A. cantonensis.* Positive skin or serologic tests are not sufficiently specific to be good diagnostic aids, but negative results rule out the diagnosis. It will also be necessary to exclude infections by other helminths which often induce an eosinophilia, especially those which may involve the central nervous system.

Treatment. Symptoms have been relieved in some cases by administration of prednisone, or thiabendazole, or dehydroemetine, but benefit from these drugs has been inconsistent and occasionally even adverse.

Prophylaxis. Prevention of human infection in areas of endemic murine angiostrongyliasis depends on proper cooking of edible mollusks and thorough washing of salad vegetables, strawberries and other similar sources. It should be remembered that larvae may remain infective in drinking water for 60 hours, and are resistant to standard chlorine or periodide purification methods.

ABDOMINAL ANGIOSTRONGYLIASIS

This condition, present in rodents in Central America, has recently been identified in man in Costa Rica and Honduras.[25] The causative agent, *Angiostrongylus costaricensis* Morera and Céspedes, 1971, is harbored in the mesenteric arteries of various rats (principally *Sigmodon hispidus* and *Rattus rattus*), and has as its intermediate host the slug *Vaginulus (Sarasinula) plebeius* which probably contaminates salad vegetables (p. 684). Clinically, abdominal pain, usually in the right iliac fossa, is associated with anorexia, vomiting, and a fever that may persist for 2 months. The patient's abdomen is distended, and a marked leukocytosis with eosinophilia of 11 to 81 per cent may be present. The worms congregate in the appendiceal area and, in contrast to *A. cantonensis,* may mature in the human host and lay fertile eggs.[26]

Tropical Eosinophilia

Synonyms. Eosinophilic lung, pulmonary eosinophiliosis, tropical pulmonary eosinophilia, Frimodt-Möller and Barton disease, Weingarten's syndrome.

Definition. Tropical eosinophilia is a syndrome often allergic in nature, characterized by hypereosinophilia of 20 to 90 per cent, paroxysms of cough and, frequently, asthmatiform dyspnea. Current evidence suggests that hypersensitivity to nonhuman and sometimes human nematodes results in their destruction in the tissues, especially the lungs, where their remnants stimulate a focal reaction. There are usually radiographic changes.

Distribution. The condition is found in South India, Sri Lanka, northwest and central Africa, Tanzania, China, and the Philippines, Samoa, West and East Malaysia, the West Indies and a few other areas.

Etiology. The syndrome suggests an allergic response and is difficult to distinguish from other instances of hypereosinophilia that result from obscure helminth infections in which the parasites are in intimate contact with host tissue. Among those that may be suspect and are highly eosinophilogenic are *Ascaris lumbricoides* and *Strongyloides stercoralis* larvae during migration, *Trichinella spiralis* before encystation, pulmonary gnathostomiasis, schistosomiasis, *Toxocara* spp. larvae (associated with visceral larva migrans) as well as the larvae of certain spiruroid nematodes. However, there is evidence that at least one type of tropical eosinophilia depends on an occult filarial infection, caused by nonhuman species of *Brugia* or *Dirofilaria,* or human species such as *B. malayi.* Microfilariae, often degenerated, have been identified at autopsy or biopsy in areas of eosinophilic infiltration in the lungs of patients with typical symptoms of tropical eosinophilia but without microfilaremia.[27]

Pathology. The histopathology of this disease is by no means clear, since both biopsy and autopsy material are scarce. The pathology is essentially an eosinophilic bronchitis and bronchiolitis. Serial chest films showed that initially there appears a barely detectable shadow about 1 mm in diameter which enlarges to 3 mm over the next few days and suggests lesions of miliary tuberculosis. However, these do not continue to enlarge or assume the irregular outline typical of tuberculosis and other infectious diseases, but fade after 3 to 4 weeks without leaving signs of calcification. The chest films show diffuse miliary mottling, increased hilar shadows and stranding into the bases.

The most striking lesions are tubercle-like nodules with groups of giant cells in the center and clusters of surrounding monocytes. Liver biopsy specimens show eosinophilic infiltration along the portal tracts and in the sinusoids. There are often areas of focal necrosis with numerous multinucleated giant cells.

Clinical Characteristics. Clinically, the syndrome consists of interstitial inflammation and edema, labored respiration, paroxysmal cough and constitutional debility, including malaise, fatigue, anorexia and loss of weight. In endemic areas the patient presents such a characteristic picture that a tentative diagnosis may be made clinically and confirmed later by the hypereosinophilia and elevated erythrocytic sedimentation rate. The physical signs are those of bronchial asthma. Breathlessness is a major complaint and it varies from shortness of breath with a sense of suffocation following bouts of coughing to expiratory dyspnea. Lymphadenopathy may occur and may be the predominant finding. Patients with tropical eosinophilia that is left untreated usually have frequent remissions.

Diagnosis. As implied previously, the clinical diagnosis is often difficult. The hypereosinophilia is highly suggestive, especially if the total number of eosinophils exceeds 3000 per cu mm and the total leukocyte count is above 10,000 cells per cu mm. In many native populations an eosinophilia of 10 to 12 per cent should be considered as typical due to the high incidence of helminths.

The x-ray picture often superficially resembles chronic bronchitis or bronchiectasis or may be mistaken for Loeffler's syndrome. However, this syndrome has a low total leukocyte count, inflammation of the upper respiratory tract and transitory lung changes. The lung signs may be confused with tuberculosis, but the eosinophilic lesions affect the bases and leave the apices clear. The absence of *Mycobacterium tuberculosis* from the sputum, the blood picture and the response to therapy are all helpful in making a diagnosis. Antigens from various helminths including *Dirofilaria immitis* provide high titers in complement-fixation tests of patients with tropical eosinophilia, but these are too nonspecific to be useful diagnostically.[28]

Treatment. The successful treatment by neoarsphenamine was discovered accidentally when a patient with concurrent syphilis was being treated. Adequate treatment with organic arsenicals has been curative, as has been stibophen, but these drugs have generally been superseded by diethylcarbamazine which has less potentially serious side effects. Piperazine adipate has also proved effective. Levamisole, in a dose of 120 mg administered on alternate days for 6 doses, has been recently tested and provides very rapid clinical improvement with clearing of the chest and fall in eosinophilia, apparently without side effects.[29]

At present, diethylcarbamazine (Hetrazan) is the drug of choice, its efficacy supporting the concept that filarial worms are a main etiologic factor.[30] Various regimens, both oral and parenteral, have been used. Vomiting and other side effects may occur if the dose exceeds 12 mg per kg. Consequently, a course employing 10 mg per kg taken by mouth 3 times a day, for 5 days, has been favored, but lesser amounts may be given for up to 3 weeks. Most patients obtain symptomatic relief in a few days, but radiologic resolution is much more protracted and, in those with sustained erythrocytic sedimentation rates, relapse often occurs.

REFERENCES

Trichinosis

1. Zimmermann, W. J. 1974. The current status of trichinellosis in the United States. *In* Kim, C. W. (ed.): Trichinellosis. Intext Educational Publishers, New York. pp. 603–614.
2. Kagan, I. G., and Norman, L. G. 1970. The serology of trichinosis. *In* Gould, S. E. (ed.): Trichinosis in Man and Animals. Charles C Thomas, Springfield, Illinois. pp. 222–268.
3. Despommier, D., Müller, M., Jenks, B., and Fruitstone, M. 1974. Immunodiagnosis of human trichinosis using counterelectrophoresis and agar gel diffusion techniques. Am. J. Trop. Med. Hyg. *23*:41–44.
4. Zaiman, H. 1970. Drug treatment of trichinosis. *In* Gould, S. E. (ed.): Trichinosis in Man and Animals. Charles C Thomas, Springfield, Illinois. pp. 329–347.
5. Stone, O. J., Stone, C. T., Jr., and Mullins, J. F. 1964. Thiabendazole–probable cure for trichinosis; report of first case. J.A.M.A. *187*:536–537.
6. Campbell, W. C., and Cuckler, A. C. 1962. Effect of thiabendazole upon experimental trichinosis in swine. Proc. Soc. Exp. Biol. Med. *110*:124–128.

Creeping Eruption

7. Burks, J. W., and Jung, R. C. 1960. A new type of water dermatitis in Louisiana. South. Med. J. *53*:716–719.
8. Morishita, K., and Tani, T. 1960. A case of *Capillaria* infection causing cutaneous creeping eruption in man. J. Parasit. *46*:79–83.
9. Hunter, G. W., III, and Worth, C. B. 1945. Variations in response to filariform larvae of *Ancylostoma caninum* in the skin of man. J. Parasit. *31*:366–372.
10. Stone, O. J., and Mullins, J. F. 1964. Thiabendazole therapy for creeping eruption. Arch. Dermatol. *89*:557–559.
11. Eyster, W. H., Jr. 1967. Local thiabendazole in the treatment of creeping eruption. Arch. Dermatol. *95*:620–621.

Gnathostomiasis

12. Nye, S. W., Tanghai, P., Sundarakiti, S., and Punyagupta, S. 1970. Lesions of the brain in eosinophilic meningitis. Arch. Pathol. *89*:9–19.
13. Chitanondh, H., and Rosen, L. 1967. Fatal eosinophilic encephalomyelitis caused by the nematode *Gnathostoma spinigerum*. Am. J. Trop. Med. Hyg. *16*:638–645.
13a. Nitidandhaprabhas, P., Siridana, A., Harnsomburana, K., and Thepsittor, P. 1975. Human urinary gnathostomiasis. A case report from Thailand. Am. J. Trop. Med. Hyg. *24*:49–51.
14. Jaroonvesama, N., and Harinasuta, T. 1973. Comparison of quinine with prednisolone in treatment of gnathostomiasis. J. Med. Assoc. Thai. *56*:312–313.

Visceral Larva Migrans

15. Beaver, P. C. 1956. Larva migrans. Exp. Parasit. *5*:587–621.
16. Wiseman, R. A., and Woodruff, A. W. 1970. Evaluation of a skin sensitivity test for the diagnosis of toxocariasis. Tr. Roy. Soc. Trop. Med. Hyg. *64*:239–245.

17. Beshear, J. R., and Hendley, J. O. 1973. Severe pulmonary involvement in visceral larva migrans. Am. J. Dis. Child. *125*:599–600.
18. Müller-Jensen, A., Schall, J., Weisner, B., and Lamina, J. 1973. Eosinophile Meningo-enzephalomyelitis und viszerales Syndrom durch Askaridenlarven beim Erwachsenen. Dtsch. Med. Wochenschr. *98*:1175–1177.

Capillariasis

19. Areán, V. M. 1964. Los sindromes clinicos de la larva migrante visceral. Rev. Clin. Españ. 94:1–9.
20. Silverman, N. H., Katz, J. S., and Levin, S. E. 1973. *Capillaria hepatica* infestation in a child. S. Afr. Med. J. *47*:219–221.

Angiostrongylosis

21. Chen, H. T. 1935. Un nouveau nématode pulmonaire, *Pulmonema cantonensis* n.g., n.sp., des rats de Canton. Ann. Parasit. *13*:312–317.
22. Mackerras, M. T., and Sandars, D. F. 1955. The life history of the rat lungworm *Angiostrongylus cantonensis* (Chen) (Nematode: Metastrongylidae). Austral. J. Zool. *3*:1–21.
23. Alicata, J. E., and Jindrak, K. 1970. Angiostrongylosis in the Pacific and Southeast Asia. Charles C Thomas, Springfield, Illinois. 105 pp.
24. Rosen, L., Chappell, R., Laqueur, G. L., Wallace, G. D., and Weinstein, P. P. 1962. Eosinophilic meningoencephalitis caused by a metastrongylid lungworm of the rat. J.A.M.A. *179*:620–624.
25. Morera, P., and Céspedes, R. 1971. Angiostrongilosis abdominal. Una nueva parasitosis humana. Acta Méd. Cost. *14*:159–173.
26. Morera, P. 1973. Life history and redescription of *Angiostrongylus costaricensis* Morera and Céspedes, 1971. Am. J. Trop. Med. Hyg. *22*:613–621.

Tropical Eosinophilia

27. Webb, J. K. G., Job, C. K., and Gault, E. W. 1960. Tropical eosinophilia. Demonstration of microfilariae in lung, liver and lymph nodes. Lancet *1*:835–842.
28. Pacheco, G., and Danaraj, T. J. 1963. Ethanol extracts of various helminths in a complement fixation test for eosinophilic lung (tropical eosinophilia). Am. J. Trop. Med. Hyg. *12*:745–747.
29. Zaman, V., and Fung, W. P. 1973. Treatment of eosinophilic lung with levamisole. Tr. Roy. Soc. Trop. Med. Hyg. *67*:144–145.
30. Donohugh, D. L. 1963. Tropical eosinophilia. An etiologic inquiry. N. Engl. J. Med. *269*:1357–1364.

CHAPTER 52

The Schistosomes

Introduction. The schistosomes infecting man, commonly known as blood flukes, are the most important human trematodes. It has been estimated that 180 to 200 million people in 71 countries are infected, and the number is probably increasing. This is especially true where land reclamation projects and associated irrigation projects as well as fish ponds combine to make conditions ideal for the spread of schistosomiasis.

There are three major species that infect man—*Schistosoma haematobium, Schistosoma mansoni* and *Schistosoma japonicum,* each producing its characteristic disease. In addition *Schistosoma intercalatum,* producing an intestinal form of the disease, is important in a limited number of foci in Central Africa. Other species such as *Schistosoma bovis, Schistosoma mattheei* and *Schistosoma spindale,* normally parasites of cattle, have been reported as occasional human parasites. In some areas of Africa the latter occurs in man along with a concurrent infection of *S. haematobium.*

The generic name *Bilharzia,* named for Bilharz who discovered the worms in Egypt in 1852, is sometimes used for *S. haematobium* and *S. mansoni* in Europe and Africa.

Morphology. These parasites differ from other trematodes of man in that they are dioecious (exist as males and females) (Fig. 52–1). They range in length between 6.5 and 26 mm; the females are longer and more slender than the males. They are cylindrical and possess an oral and a ventral sucker or acetabulum, the latter being situated near the anterior end. The most characteristic feature of the males is their ventrally infolded margins, beginning behind the acetabulum and forming a groove or *gynecophoral canal* in which the more slender female is carried during most of its life. The alimentary canal passes from the oral cavity into an *esophagus,* which divides just anterior to the acetabulum forming two *intestinal canals* which fuse near the center of the worm to form a single, serpentine trunk extending to a blind terminus near the posterior end of the worm. The gut frequently appears reddish black owing to the presence of ingested blood. The male reproductive system consists of four to nine *testes,* depending upon the species, located dorsally just posterior to the acetabulum and connected by tubules to the *seminal vesicle* and *genital pore* on the ventral surface. The female system consists of a single *ovary* situated just anterior to the fusion of the two branches of the intestine, a *seminal receptacle* adjacent to it, an *oviduct* leading forward to an *oötype* and *shell gland,* yolk glands *(vitellaria)* occupying the posterior half of the body with ducts leading to the oötype, and a *uterus* passing forward from the oötype to the genital pore

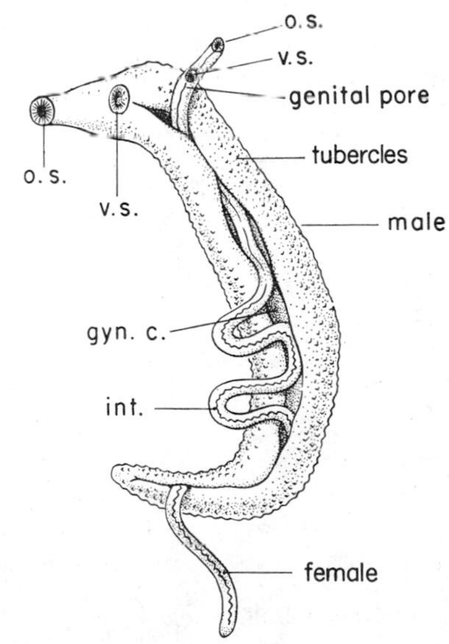

Figure 52–1. Schematic drawing of a male and female *Schistosoma mansoni.* Abbreviations: o.s., oral sucker; v.s., ventral sucker (acetabulum); gyn.c., gynecophoral canal; int., intestine. (Modified from Looss.) (Courtesy of the University of Florida College of Medicine, Gainesville.)

Table 52–1. CHARACTERISTICS OF SCHISTOSOME EGGS

Species	*Length (Micrometers, μm)*	*Breadth (Micrometers, μm)*	*Diagnostic Features*
S. haematobium	112–170 av. 150	40–70 av. 60	Terminal spine
S. mansoni	114–175 av. 150	45–70 av. 60	Lateral spine
S. japonicum	70–100 av. 89	50–70 av. 66	Small spine or knob which often is not seen
S. intercalatum	140–240	50–85	Terminal spine

just posterior to the acetabulum. This location of the genital pore permits the deposition of eggs from the uterus into the smallest venules when the female worm protrudes its head into these vessels. The uterus may contain only a few eggs at one time *(S. mansoni)* or as many as 300 *(S. japonicum).*

Schistosome Eggs. These differ from the eggs of all other trematodes in the absence of an operculum or lid and the presence of a spine or knob on the shell (Fig. 53–2). In addition, schistosome eggs contain a fully developed *miracidium* when they leave the host. Table 52–1 summarizes some of the more important characteristics.

THE LIFE CYCLE OF THE SCHISTOSOMES

The life cycle is outlined in Figure 52–2.

Oviposition. The female worm matures following embracement and fertilization by the male, after which the male carries the female in its gynecophoral canal. The male transports the female against the current of the portal blood stream by means of its suckers into the smaller radicles of the mesenteric veins. In the case of *S. haematobium* the worms migrate through the hemorrhoidal plexus into the systemic veins of the pelvis, especially those of the urinary bladder. Here the female may partially or entirely leave the gynecophoral canal of the male in order to migrate further into the venule. The eggs are deposited in a beadlike row, often in the capillaries of the mucosa, after which the female retreats into a larger venule, allowing the smaller vessels to contract about the eggs. The embryo within the egg rapidly matures and secretes an enzyme which passes through the porous egg shell and causes necrosis of the vessel wall and ad-

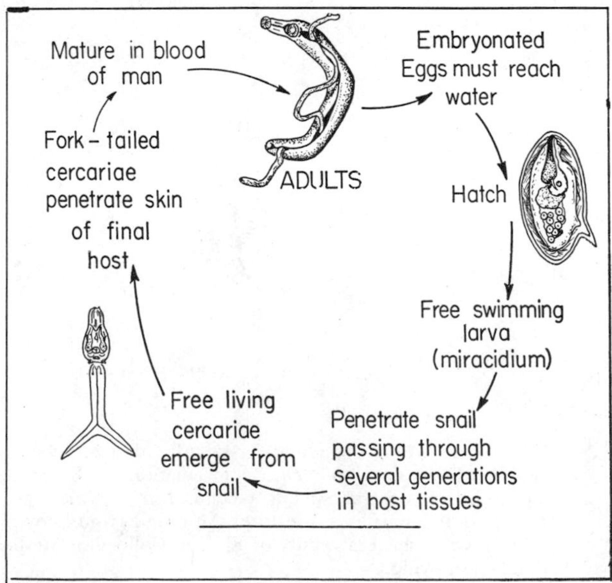

Figure 52–2. Trematode cycle—schistosome type.

jacent tissue. If the egg is very close to the surface epithelium, it quickly breaks into the lumen. If it is deeper in the tissues, it produces a tiny abscess which may rupture into the lumen. The egg reaches water in urine or feces and soon hatches, liberating a free-swimming embryo.

Development in the Snail. The embryo or miracidium is a ciliated, actively swimming organism. It remains infective without feeding for about 6 hours after hatching, during which time it must reach and penetrate a suitable freshwater or amphibious snail if further development is to occur. (See Table 66–1, p. 670 and Fig. 66–4, p. 679 for snail hosts.) It should be noted that the miracidium penetrates several species of these snails, but in an unsuitable host its development is arrested. In a suitable snail the miracidium becomes transformed into a *mother sporocyst* which, in turn, produces many *daughter sporocysts.* These migrate to the gonad and digestive gland of the snail where they, in turn, produce hundreds or thousands of fork-tailed *cercariae,* the infective larvae which escape from the snail. In *S. haematobium* 4 to 8 weeks elapse from the penetration of the miracidium to the liberation of cercariae; in *S. mansoni* under optimum conditions only 4 weeks are necessary; *S. japonicum* requires 5 to 7 weeks. The length of the developmental period in the snail depends upon several environmental factors, one of the most important of which is temperature.

Penetration of the Cercariae. Upon emerging from the snail the cercariae swim about vigorously tail first and, after reaching the surface of the water, gradually sink to the bottom. This behavior is repeated many times, although some cercariae (especially those of *S. japonicum*) remain temporarily attached to the surface film by their suckers until disturbed.

Persons in endemic areas engaged in occupations that necessitate contact with water, e.g. growing rice, washing clothes or vehicles, may acquire schistosomiasis. Drinking infested water or bathing or wading in it can also cause infection. As the water on the skin evaporates, the cercariae penetrate the epidermis by forcing the anterior end of the body through the skin after casting off the tail. Penetration can occur within 5 minutes. It is aided by enzymes from the penetration glands. By the end of 24 hours the larvae have worked their way through the epidermis to the peripheral venules or lymphatics; they are then carried through the blood stream to the right side of the heart and thence to the pulmonary capillaries, where they may be delayed for several days while squeezing through the lumen of the capillaries into the veins. Some apparently leave the lumen of the capillaries and are believed to migrate directly to the portal system and liver. Those working through the capillary bed then journey back through the left side of the heart into the systemic circulation. It is thought that only those survive which pass through the mesenteric arteries and capillaries and reach the portal circulation. Here they develop rapidly, feeding on the nutritious portal blood, and soon crawl back into the larger portal venules. Copulation occurs before the parasites are fully mature. Subsequently, the females mature, and the males carry them into the mesenteric or pelvic venules where they deposit their eggs.

Reservoir Hosts. In many areas man serves as the principal host for both *S. haematobium* and *S. mansoni.* Monkeys and certain rodents can be infected experimentally with both species; the peccary has also been infected in the laboratory with *S. mansoni.* Baboons and monkeys have been found naturally infected with *S. mansoni* and *S. haematobium,* and wild rodents infected with *S. mansoni* have been found in Africa and South America. These animals may prove to be important reservoir hosts in certain areas. In one area of Tanzania baboons have been found to maintain infections of *S. mansoni* among themselves without the intervention of infected humans. *Schistosoma japonicum,* in addition to infecting man, parasitizes water buffalo, horses, cattle, pigs, dogs, cats and field rodents, some of which serve as important reservoir hosts.

Schistosoma intercalatum, which has a terminal spined egg, causes human intestinal schistosomiasis of significance in certain restricted foci in West Central Africa. Several other species of schistosomes have been reported infrequently as parasites of man. One is *S. spindale,* a parasite of cattle, sheep, goats, horses and antelopes of India, South Africa and Sumatra.

HOST RESPONSE

The pathogenesis and clinical manifestations of schistosomiasis are essentially the same for all four species of worms infecting man, differing primarily in the location and egg-laying capacity of the worms. However, certain facts should be borne in mind: the adults do not multiply in man; the immunity that follows the initial exposure is not complete; in most cases man is repeatedly re-exposed; the adult parasites are long-lived and as a result not only does the worm burden increase over the years, but also great numbers of eggs are produced, many of which remain lodged in the tissues; the disease is related to the presence of various stages of the parasite, their excretions and secretions, as well as to the inflammatory response of the host.

SCHISTOSOME DERMATITIS. During the penetration of the skin the cercariae secrete enzymes from their pre- and postacetabular glands that facilitate their passage through the epidermis and dermis. Itching followed by a pruritic papular rash lasting several days results from exposure to large numbers of cercariae, particularly in hypersensitive persons. The term "schistosome dermatitis" is misleading, since this usually refers to "swimmer's itch" which is caused by the penetration of the superficial layers of the skin by cercariae whose normal hosts are birds or other mammals. (See p. 565.)

KATAYAMA FEVER. In the migration of the young worms, or schistosomules, through the lungs and mesenteric vessels, some undoubtedly rupture capillaries causing minute hemorrhages. As the worms mature in the portal and mesenteric veins they serve as antigens. Some 20 to 60 days after exposure, about the time egg-laying starts, a syndrome occurs that has been recognized by the Japanese since the middle of the nineteenth century. It is known as Katayama, Yangtze River, or urticarial fever. It is typically found in persons parasitized by *S. japonicum,* although it also may occur in those exposed to an initially heavy dose of *S. mansoni* cercariae.

The infected person experiences a daily afternoon fever, malaise, chills, sweating, epigastric discomfort, headache, a slight cough and diarrhea. Extensive urticaria often occurs in large patches on various parts of the body. Auscultation of the lungs may reveal localized areas of moist rales along with a generalized lymphadenopathy and frequently hepatosplenomegaly.[1] Katayama fever may persist for several weeks after which it subsides unless death intervenes. The reaction is believed due to the release of large amounts of new antigenic material in the form of eggs; these are added to the cross-reacting antibody produced in response to the presence of the developing worms.[2, 3]

CHRONIC SCHISTOSOMIASIS. In infections caused by *S. mansoni* and *S. japonicum* there appears to be a correlation between the intensity of the infection, i.e. the number of worms present, and the severity of the disease. Patients having a light worm burden have few, if any, symptoms and show little evidence of a pathologic condition. In such cases it may not be necessary to treat the patient.

HEPATOSPLENIC, PULMONARY AND URINARY TRACT SCHISTOSOMIASIS. Heavy worm burdens are a prerequisite for the development of severe disease. It begins with the deposition of eggs in the tissues. The miracidium within the egg matures in 6 days (*S. mansoni*), 9 to 10 days (*S. japonicum*), and probably survives for several weeks in the tissues. During this period it secretes an enzyme that produces a minute abscess containing mainly polymorphonuclear leukocytes, many of which are eosinophils. If a mass of eggs is deposited together, the abscess may be of considerable size and may have an area of necrosis at the center. Abscesses and small ulcers develop in the walls and on the mucosal surfaces of the intestine or bladder, and eggs that are carried by the blood stream as emboli to the liver or lungs produce abscesses where they lodge. The liver becomes enlarged, and the resulting portal obstruction leads to enlargement of the spleen. The eggs add to the foreign protein reaction of the host. The urticaria and pulmonary signs usually persist for only 5 to 7 days, but the fever continues and the eosinophilia increases, often reaching 60 to 80 per cent of the total leukocytes. In severe cases there may be a considerable increase in the blood serum globulin. This acute reaction lasts for about 3 to 10 weeks, the temperature gradually returning to normal. There may be exacerbations, however, and egg deposition will continue during the life of the female worms, which is known to be sometimes as long as 30 years. Recent investigations suggest that these records may be exceptions and that the mean life of the female schistosomes may be as short as 2 years, and is probably not more than 5 years.

The next stage, that of tissue proliferation and repair, begins with the healing of the acute abscess. The polymorphonuclear leukocytes are replaced by epithelioid cells forming a pseudotubercle. Foreign body giant cells appear and surround and invade the dead egg. Ultimately, the egg may become calcified or may disappear entirely, and normal structure returns or a scar is formed. Thickening of the wall of the intestine or bladder occurs, with polyp formation on the mucosal surface and adhesions on the peritoneal surface. In the liver, obliteration of many portal venules leads to a true portal cirrhosis. It is probable that nutritional deficiency adds to the cirrhosis in the late stages of the disease. In the lungs, scarring may lead to obstruction of the pulmonary circulation and result in cor pulmonale. There is no good evidence that toxic substances from the adult worms themselves contribute to the fibrosis which is the end result of the infection.

Other anastomoses besides those of the hemorrhoidal plexus, which is the normal path of migration of *S. haematobium* into the pelvic veins, may permit the migration of adult worms and the deposition of eggs in unusual situations. Anastomoses between portal and hepatic venules in the liver may be large enough to permit the direct passage of eggs to the lungs, and anastomoses between the larger mesenteric veins and the vena cava may permit the passage of both eggs and worms into the vena cava and lungs, especially if portal obstruction causes these anastomoses to enlarge. There are also anastomoses between the lower colonic veins and those of the spinal column through which adult worms can gain access to the central nervous system and deposit eggs in the spinal cord or the brain. Other ectopic locations where worms have been known to deposit eggs are the conjunctiva and skin.

In experimental animals immunity builds up gradually and is mainly stimulated by the presence of adult worms and less by schistosomules, cercariae and eggs in that order. Apparently the same processes occur in man based upon observations in monkeys and man as well as upon epidemiologic grounds in the case of the latter. There is evidence to suggest that schistosomes somehow adsorb host antigens onto their surfaces and so protect themselves against the antibodies of the host.[4] Antibodies to antigens produced from cercariae, adult worms and eggs have been demonstrated in serologic and intradermal reactions, but the relation of these antibodies to immunity is not clear.

DIAGNOSIS

Specific diagnosis of schistosomiasis depends mainly upon the demonstration of the characteristic eggs from the feces or urine. (See pp. 817 and 828 for details.) In cases of schistosomiasis mansoni or japonica, rectal or sigmoidoscopic biopsies or scrapings from the mucosal surface of the rectum are of value if eggs cannot be found in the feces. In schistosomiasis haematobia, biopsied material may be obtained through the cystoscope; sometimes rectal or sigmoidoscopic biopsies may be diagnostic for urinary schistosomiasis. Cervical smears have also revealed the presence of viable eggs of both *S. haematobium* and *S. mansoni,* thus suggesting another possible route for the occasional transmission of eggs.[5] The biopsy specimen or the scrapings should first be pressed between two slides or mounted under a coverslip and examined under low magnification. If eggs are present they should be observed under high power to determine whether they are alive. If alive, the miracidium will be seen to move, or a flaglike motion of its excretory "flame cells" can be observed. In treated cases dead eggs persist for a long time and their presence should not be interpreted as an indication that further treatment is necessary. The biopsy specimen can finally be fixed in formalin for permanent record or for sectioning. Complement-fixation and intradermal tests, preferably with delipidized extracts of adult worms as antigen, give positive reactions for the schistosome group. The cholesterol-lecithin cercarial slide flocculation test and the bentonite flocculation test are useful for serologic diagnosis of schistosomiasis. A delipidized cercarial antigen is employed. The tests may be used in suspected cases when eggs cannot be found, but positive reactions should lead to further search for eggs by concentration or hatching methods, or by rectal biopsy or scraping. These tests often remain positive for several months after completion of curative treatment.

The intradermal test gives an immediate or delayed-type of hypersensitive response.[6, 7] It has been used in surveys of prevalence where fecal or urine specimens are difficult to obtain. An eosinophilia should lead to a suspicion of schistosomiasis in any person who may have been exposed in an endemic area.

Chest radiography in advanced stages of schistosomiasis may reveal granulomas scattered throughout both lung fields, in addition to signs of pulmonary hypertension; a barium swallow may reveal esophageal varices.[7a]

TREATMENT

Even though schistosomiasis has been known for years, there are relatively few drugs that are highly effective. Trivalent compounds of antimony are very useful for the treatment of schistosomiasis. Those most frequently used today are: antimony sodium tartrate (AST), which has generally replaced the potassium salt (the original tartar emetic); sodium antimonyl gluconate (Stibogluconate sodium); and antimony sodium dimercaptosuccinate (Stibocaptate, Astiban). The first two are given intravenously and the third intramuscularly.[8]

Among the nonantimonial compounds, niridazole (Ambilhar) has been found to be effective against all three species of schistosomes in experimental animals. In man it is effective against *S. haematobium*[9] and *S. mansoni* and to a lesser degree against *S. japonicum.* Niridazole is contraindicated for general use when impairment of the liver may be present or when there is a history of psychotic disturbances. Recent experiments using body fluids of man and mice have demonstrated that niridazole is mutagenically active against certain bacteria at low dosages. This suggests the desirability of further studies to evaluate more completely the risks involved, if any, in prescribing this drug.[7b]

Hycanthone, a metabolite of lucanthone, has been found to give cure rates of 65 to 95 per cent for both *S. haematobium* and *S. mansoni.* It may be given orally or intramuscularly. Although still under field trials, it holds considerable promise.[8]

Dosages are given under the appropriate disease.

Patients should be examined at intervals of 1 or 2 months for a year in order to detect relapses. The finding of *living* eggs in the feces or urine is an indication for retreatment with a larger total dose. Reinfection must be considered a possibility in endemic areas and treated patients should be educated to avoid re-exposure.

PROPHYLAXIS

Theoretically, the schistosomes are vulnerable to attack in all stages of their life cycles. The adults can be attacked by chemotherapy. This has been attempted in Egypt and has diminished the severity of the disease in many cases but has not materially reduced the prevalence of infection. The miracidia can be prevented from reaching snails by proper storage or disposal of excreta. The snails can be attacked by chemical molluscicides. Copper sulfate has been used in Egypt for many years with partial success; sodium pentachlorophenate, introduced since World War II, has proved promising in limited endemic areas in Japan and elsewhere (p. 563); Niclosamide (Bayluscide), Frescon (*N*-tritylmorpholine), Organotin compounds[10] as well as soapberry (Endod) have all been found useful under certain field conditions.[11] (See Chapter 66, p. 672.) The advantages of the use of such compounds must be weighed against the temporary elimination of fish, which are important as a source of protein in the diet. The cercariae can be prevented from penetrating man by his avoiding infested water, by protective clothing, by storage and chlorination of water, or by furnishing an adequate, safe water supply.[12] A combination of methods will be necessary in most endemic areas, and education of the people in changing long established habits and methods of working will also be essential. Where animal reservoir hosts are involved, prevention of human infection will be more difficult.

Schistosomiasis Haematobia

Synonyms. Genitourinary bilharziasis, endemic hematuria.

Definition. Schistosomiasis haematobia is due to the presence of the blood fluke *Schistosoma haematobium* in the vesical and pelvic venous plexuses of man.

Distribution. Schistosomiasis haematobia occurs throughout much of Africa and the Middle East. Isolated areas of southern Europe (Portugal and Cyprus) have been under control and there the disease is now virtually extinct. The Nile Valley is one of the chief endemic centers of the disease. The infection also occurs across North Africa to Morocco, and to the south and east (the Sudan, Ethiopia, Somalia, Uganda, Kenya, Tanzania, Mozambique, Malawi, Zambia, Rhodesia, Republic of South Africa and the

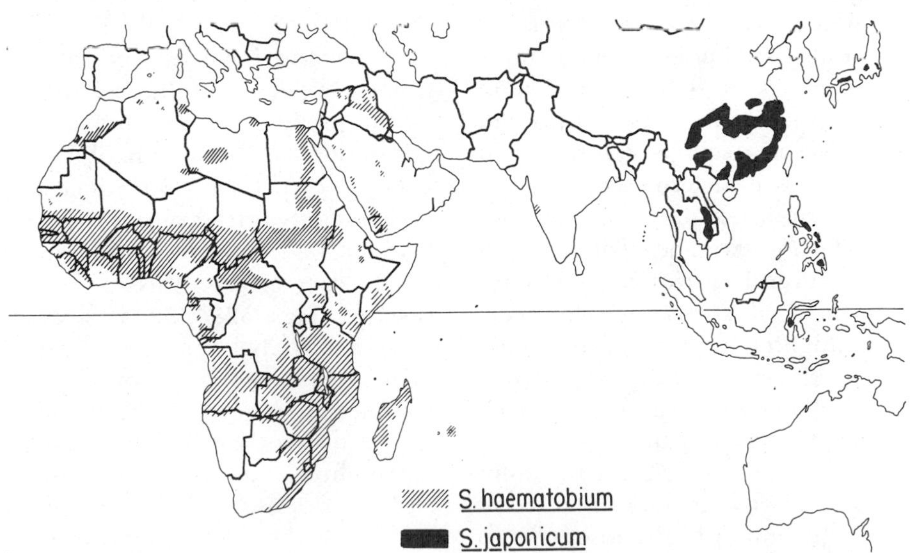

Figure 52-3. World distribution of schistosomiasis due to *S. haematobium* and *S. japonicum.* (Redrawn by Donald M. Alvarado from W. H. Wright: Geographical Distribution of Schistosomes and their Intermediate Hosts. *In* Ansari, N. (ed.): Epidemiology and Control of Schistosomiasis (Bilharziasis). 1973. University Park Press, Baltimore. p. 34.)

islands of Malagasy Republic, Mauritius and Reunion). It occurs extensively in Central Africa and the West Coast of Nigeria to Angola. In the Middle East it is endemic in parts of Aden, Turkey, Israel, Lebanon, Northern Syria, Saudi Arabia, Yemen, Iran and Iraq (mostly along the Tigris and Euphrates valleys). More recently a small endemic focus has been discovered in the Maharashtra State of India, near Bombay (Fig. 52–3).

Etiology. MORPHOLOGY. *Schistosoma haematobium* (Bilharz, 1852) Weinland, 1858 inhabits the vesical and pelvic plexuses of the venous circulation and the veins of the lower colon and rectum. The cuticle of the male is covered with small tubercles; that of the female possesses minute papillae that are limited to the extremities of the worm. In the male four or five testes are located just posterior to the acetabulum. In the female the ovary is located posterior to the middle of the body. There is a correspondingly long uterus, which may contain 50 eggs at one time. The egg is pointed at one end. For other details of schistosomal morphology see page 543.

DEVELOPMENT. The life cycle does not differ markedly from the generalized life history outlined on page 544, except that the worms migrate from the mesenteric to the pelvic veins and the eggs are discharged principally in urine rather than in feces.

Epidemiology. Man is the main reservoir for *S. haematobium.* Baboons and monkeys have been found infected in nature, but their importance as a source of infection in various localities is undetermined. Embryonated eggs hatch when the urine becomes diluted with fresh water. The ciliated miracidia penetrate several species of freshwater snails and in the tissues of susceptible species mother and daughter sporocysts are formed. The latter produce characteristic brevifurcate (short, fork-tailed) cercariae that penetrate the exposed skin of man.

In endemic regions practically the entire population of some communities may be infected. The distribution of the disease is increasing owing to the transfer of snails from infected foci to other areas as new irrigation projects are completed, and owing to the migration of infected people into nonendemic localities where susceptible snail hosts are present. Transmission in certain Mohammedan countries is facilitated by the religious stipulation that the anal and urethral orifices be washed with water after urination or defecation. This custom is usually carried out in a river or canal. Another epidemiologic factor is that the species of snails serving as intermediate hosts for the parasite thrive in sewage.

The chief intermediate hosts for this parasite in North Africa and the Middle East are freshwater snails of the genus *Bulinus.* In Africa south of the Sahara Desert, members of the subgenus *Physopsis* serve as hosts; in Portugal the snail host is a member of the genus *Planorbarius;* and in India it is *Ferrissia tenuis*[13] (Table 66–1, p. 670).

Pathology. The pathologic changes are produced chiefly by the eggs of the worm. The urinary bladder is the principal organ involved. Eggs are deposited in all layers of the bladder wall, and the secretion of the enclosed miracidia produces necrosis and minute abscess formation. Eggs in the mucosa can thus easily break through the epithelium into the lumen, and with them mucus, blood and pus enter the urine, leaving minute ulcers in the mucosa. Eggs which are deposited deeper in the wall may break through later, especially if they are close together and form a larger abscess. Others cannot break through, and the lesion goes on to pseudotubercle and scar formation. Ulceration and irritation of the epithelium lead to polyp formation, which may become malignant. Scarring causes thickening of the bladder wall, with loss of elasticity and ultimate contracture. Masses of eggs become calcified (Figs. 52–4, 52–5), giving the inner surface a sandy appearance, and calculi may form in the lumen. Secondary bacterial infection may occur. Eggs are often deposited in the ureters, causing obstruction and hydronephrosis or pyonephrosis. Eggs may also be deposited in other pelvic organs, such as the seminal vesicles, prostate, urethra, spermatic cord or penis in men, and the uterus, vagina and vulva in women.

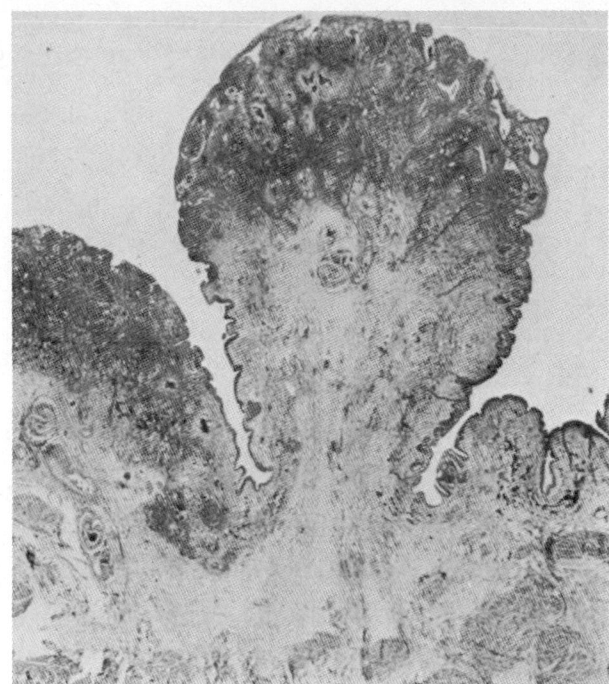

Figure 52–4. Bladder polyp in schistosomiasis haematobia. Note shallow ulceration of surface mucosa, many eggs and minute abscesses in submucosa, cross section of a pair of adult worms in venule of submucosa. (Ash and Spitz. 1945. Atlas of Pathology of Tropical Diseases. W. B. Saunders Company, Philadelphia.)

Even the cutaneous venules may be invaded, with eggs breaking out through the skin. Although some eggs are deposited in the wall of the lower colon and some are carried to the liver, they are rarely numerous enough to produce significant lesions in these locations. The association of bladder carcinoma and *S. haematobium* infections is well known. In Egypt, cancer of the bladder has been reported to occur more frequently in infected than in uninfected groups, and to be associated with increased levels of lactic acid dehydrogenase (LDH), the activity of which can be used as a screening test.[14] Elsewhere in Africa, chronic *S. haematobium* infection is considered an etiologic factor in squamous

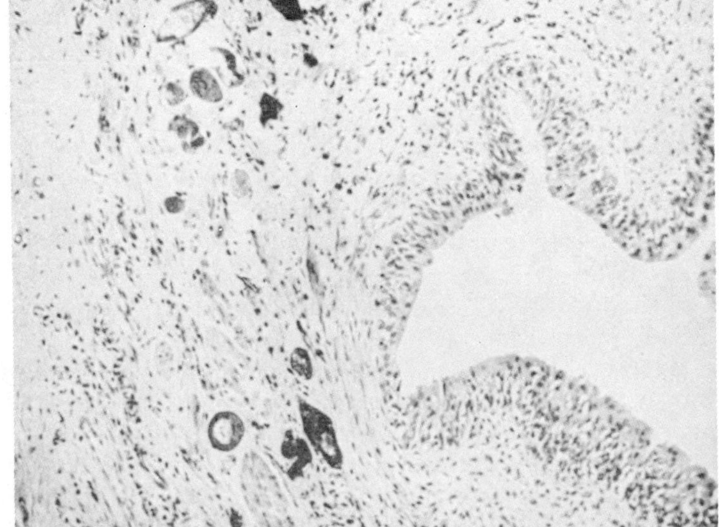

Figure 52–5. Schistosomiasis: fibrosis of bladder wall, eggs of *S. haematobium.*

carcinoma of the bladder.[15] A causal role may be played by β-glucuronidase, which has an increased activity in the urine of people with urinary schistosomiasis, and hydrolyzes inactive glucuronides into potentially carcinogenic substances.[16]

Clinical Characteristics. The incubation period is usually 10 to 12 weeks. The early symptoms of evening fever followed by sweating, lassitude, abdominal discomfort and urticaria vary greatly in individual cases. The fever may last for several weeks and then gradually subside. Urinary frequency is a common early symptom and may be accompanied by a scalding sensation along the course of the urethra during and after voiding. In natives of endemic areas hematuria may be the first symptom noticed. It is frequently gradual in onset, at first microscopic, later becoming gross as frank ulceration of the bladder mucosa develops. At first it is terminal in character, but with extensive ulceration the whole specimen may be bloody, and clots may be present. Pain is variable and is usually referred to the suprapubic region or the perineum. Often it is aggravated by distention of the bladder and is most intense at the end of micturition.[17]

In late cases symptoms of ascending pyogenic renal infection or neoplasia may appear. Urinary obstruction due to scarring or prostatic hypertrophy may occur.

Diagnosis. The finding of terminal-spined eggs in the urine is pathognomonic of this disease (Fig. 53–2, p. 571). These are usually distributed throughout the urinary stream and not concentrated solely in the last few drops of urine at the end of micturition.[18] Viable eggs have been recovered from cervical smears suggesting that occasionally they may be released in this manner.[4] The eggs are easily seen under low power of the microscope.

Cystoscopy will reveal bleeding points, minute ulcers and, in late cases, sandlike excrescences which are usually calcified. Biopsy specimens should reveal eggs. Eggs may also be found in the feces and seminal fluid. Frequently, rectal or sigmoid biopsies reveal eggs.

Treatment. The probable drug of choice is niridazole (Ambilhar), which should be given as 25 mg per kg per day for 7 days, or as 35 mg per kg per day for 5 days. A total of 175 mg per kg of body weight is reported to cure 75 to 95 per cent of *S. haematobium* infections. The drug may be given orally and reaches maximum blood concentrations in 6 hours. (See p. 548 for additional information.) Abdominal pain, anorexia, nausea, vomiting, headache, vertigo and diarrhea have all been reported as side effects. Major side effects involving the central nervous system occur only rarely.[8]

Two other drugs are recommended. The first is antimony sodium dimercaptosuccinate (Stibocaptate, Astiban), which may be given intramuscularly once or twice a week in 5 divided doses for a total dose of 40 mg per kg of body weight. The other is Stibophen (Fuadin), which contains 8.5 mg of antimony per ml. It is given intramuscularly as follows: 1.5 ml followed 2 days later by 3.5 ml and then 5 ml every other day for a total of 80 ml.[9]

Prophylaxis. Methods of breaking the life cycle of the schistosomes have already been outlined (p. 548). There is a special problem in the prevention of *S. haematobium* infection. In Moslem countries, which compose most of the endemic regions, the religious requirement of urination, defecation and ablution before praying or eating is a great source of infection. Water that looks clean may be heavily infested with cercariae. In rice-growing areas such as Egypt, periodic drainage and drying of the irrigation canals have been used, but the snails can burrow into the soil and survive. Clearing vegetation from canals and ponds reduces snail population. However, the extension of irrigated areas and the greater mobility of people tend to increase the extent of endemic areas. Copper sulfate (15 to 50 ppm) has been used in Egypt for many years with only partial success. For other molluscicides see Chapter 66, p. 672.

The improvement of general sanitation, provision of pure water supplies and education of the people can contribute to prevention.

Schistosomiasis Mansoni

Synonyms. Intestinal bilharziasis, Egyptian splenomegaly.

Definition. Schistosomiasis mansoni is an endemic disease with abdominal and dysenteric symptoms and splenomegaly caused by the blood fluke *Schistosoma mansoni.*

Distribution. Schistosomiasis mansoni originally was an African disease but was imported into the West Indies and South America by the slave trade. The total number of human infections has been estimated at 29 million. It occurs commonly in the inhabitants of the Nile Delta, much of the east coast of Africa, parts of West Africa, the Congo River basin, South Africa and the island of Malagasy Republic. It is also present in North Africa (Libya), in Eritrea and in Asia (Saudi Arabia and Yemen and Aden, but no autochthonous cases in Israel, Lebanon, Syria, Turkey, Iran and Iraq where *S. haematobium* occurs). In the Western Hemisphere it is known in parts of Brazil, Venezuela, Surinam and French Guiana, as well as numerous islands in the Caribbean, including a focus in the Hato Mayor area in the Dominican Republic, Puerto Rico, Vieques, Guadeloupe, Martinique, St. Lucia, and probably others (Fig. 52–6).

Etiology. MORPHOLOGY. *Schistosoma mansoni* (Sambon, 1907) superficially resembles *S. haematobium.* The tubercles of the cuticle of the male are more prominent than those of *S. haematobium* (Fig. 52–7). There are six to nine testes. In the female the ovary is located anterior to the middle. The uterus, which is correspondingly short, rarely contains more than one egg. The egg is easily identified by its lateral spine.

DEVELOPMENT. The life cycle of *S. mansoni* conforms to the generalized description on page 544.

Epidemiology. The epidemiology of schistosomiasis mansoni is essentially similar to that of schistosomiasis haematobia, except that (1) different species of snails serve as intermediate host (Table 66–1) and (2) defecation rather than urination by infected persons contaminates the water with schistosome eggs. Untreated sewage emptying into ditches, streams or lakes and the

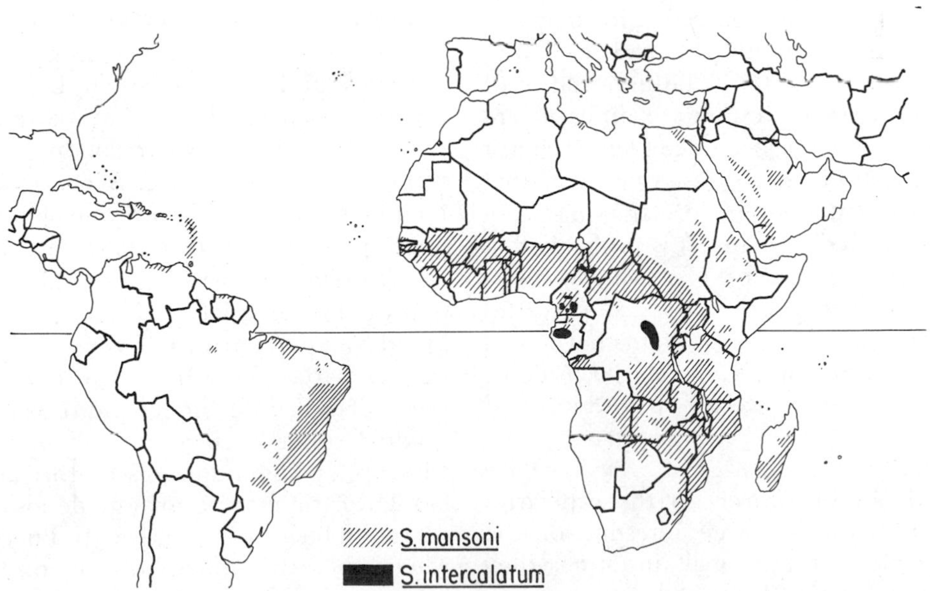

Figure 52–6. World distribution of schistosomiasis due to *S. mansoni* and *S. intercalatum.* (Redrawn by Donald M. Alvarado from W. H. Wright: Geographical Distribution of Schistosomes and their Intermediate Hosts. *In* Ansari, N. (ed.): Epidemiology and Control of Schistosomiasis (Bilharziasis). 1973. University Park Press, Baltimore. p. 35.)

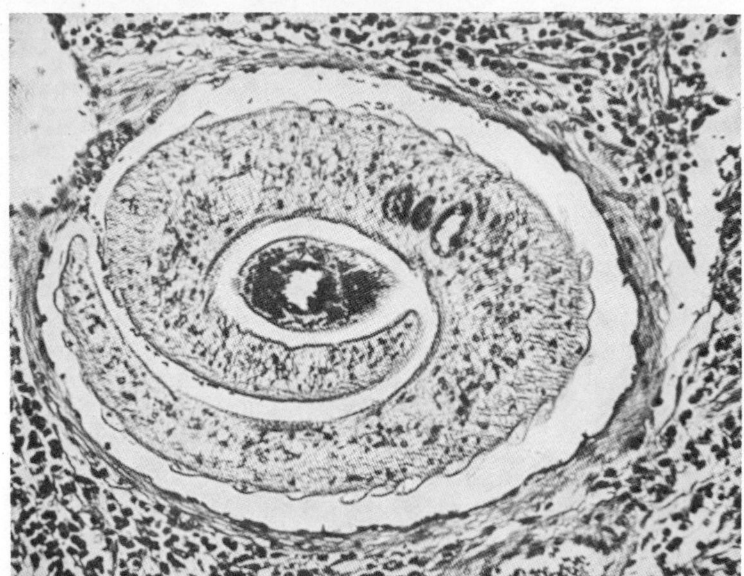

Figure 52–7. Schistosomiasis: male and female *S. mansoni* in lumen of mesenteric vein showing tuberculate cuticula of male.

washing of human excreta by rains into such bodies of fresh water constitute an ever-present menace to the populations in endemic regions (Fig. 52–8).

The known intermediate hosts of *S. mansoni* are all flat freshwater snails of the family PLANORBIDAE. In Africa as well as in South America and the West Indies, they belong to several species of the genus *Biomphalaria.* Within a period of about 4 weeks after penetration by the miracidium, cercariae emerge from the snail and are infective for man.

Baboons and monkeys have been found to be naturally infected. The importance of their role as reservoir hosts in different endemic areas has not been determined, but it has been found, in at least one area, that baboons can maintain the infection in the absence of infected humans. It is probable that some rodents are capable of serving as reservoir hosts, since mice, hamsters, peccaries and several kinds of wild rodents have been infected experimentally, and wild rodents have been found infected in Africa and South America.

Pathology. The eggs of *S. mansoni* are deposited almost entirely in the capillaries and venules of the large intestine or the lower portion of the small intestine; they may also be carried by the blood stream to the liver. In some cases eggs may also be found in the urine.[19, 20] Since there is usually only one egg in the parasite's uterus, eggs are more often deposited singly than in large masses. However, the typical lesion is produced (p. 546), and myriads of eggs produce severe disease. The wall of the intestine becomes thickened (Fig. 52–9), polyps protrude into the lumen, and in heavy infections there may be prolapse of the rectum or perianal masses. In the liver, scarring leads to cirrhosis (Fig. 52–10), and portal obstruction causes splenomegaly and ascites. Anastomoses between the mesenteric-portal veins and the vena cava become enlarged and permit eggs, and even worms, to be carried to the lungs, where fibrosis may cause obstruction to the pulmonary circulation and lead to right ventricular failure. Worms may also migrate to the spinal cord and deposit eggs which produce lesions resulting in paralysis.

Clinical Characteristics. The penetration of the cercariae may cause itching followed by a papular rash in sensitized individuals (p. 546). The worms mature in about 5 weeks. Toward the end of this time there is a gradual onset of fever and malaise, often with upper abdominal discomfort and nausea. Urticaria may occur. Egg deposition and excretion begin a week later. In Puerto Rico, where the early phase of the disease has been studied thoroughly, two clinical types, the dysenteric and the hepatosplenic, have been described. In the dysenteric type, depo-

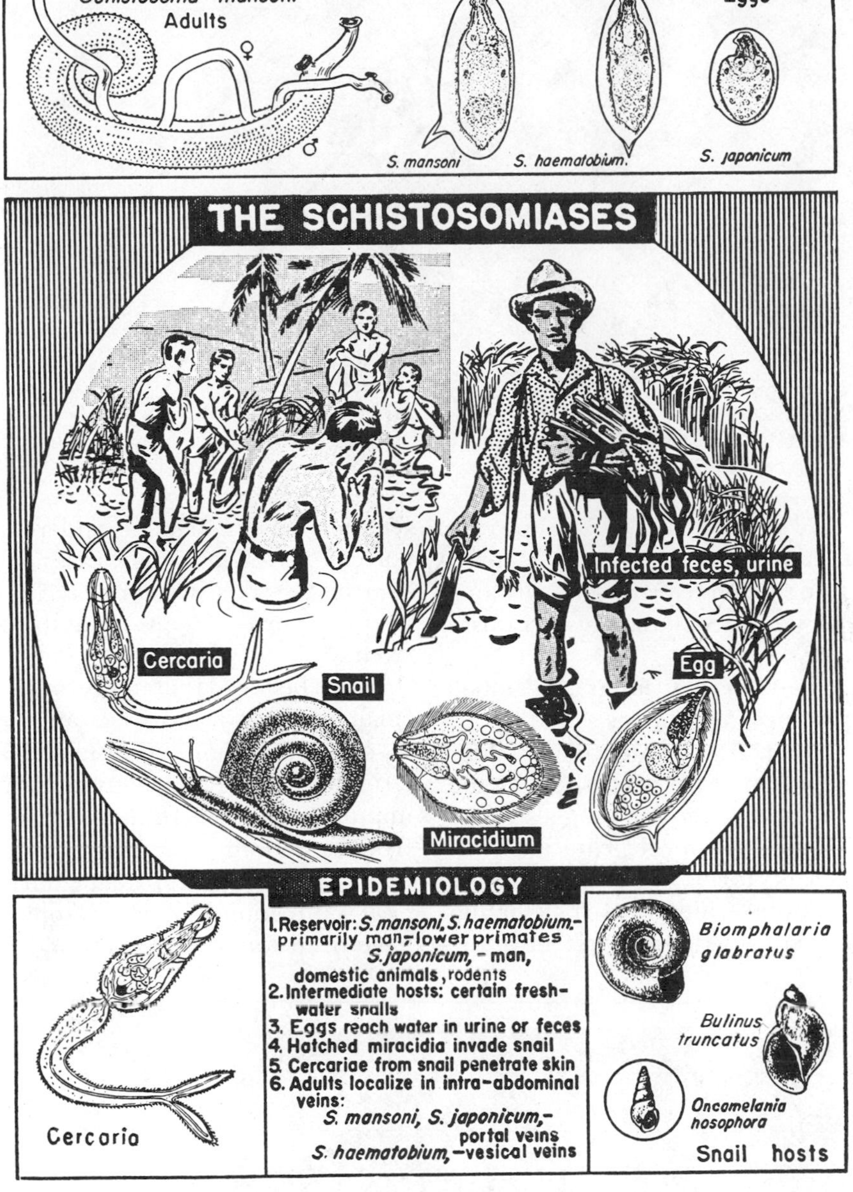

Figure 52–8. Epidemiology of the schistosomiases.

sition of eggs in the wall of the intestine is accompanied by bloody diarrhea, loss of weight, abdominal pain and moderate anemia. Eggs are abundant in the mixture of blood, pus and mucus discharged from the intestine. In the hepatosplenic type there is much less diarrhea, symptoms of upper abdominal discomfort predominate, and there is progressive enlargement of the liver and spleen. In both types the acute symptoms last for several weeks. Recurrence of symptoms is common. Eosinophilia may be as high as 75 per cent.

With the development of fibrosis of the lesions, adhesions and polyp formation may give rise to intestinal obstruction or episodes of abdominal pain. The progressive cirrhosis of the liver may cause esophageal varices with hematemesis. The spleen may become very large. Ascites may require paracentesis;

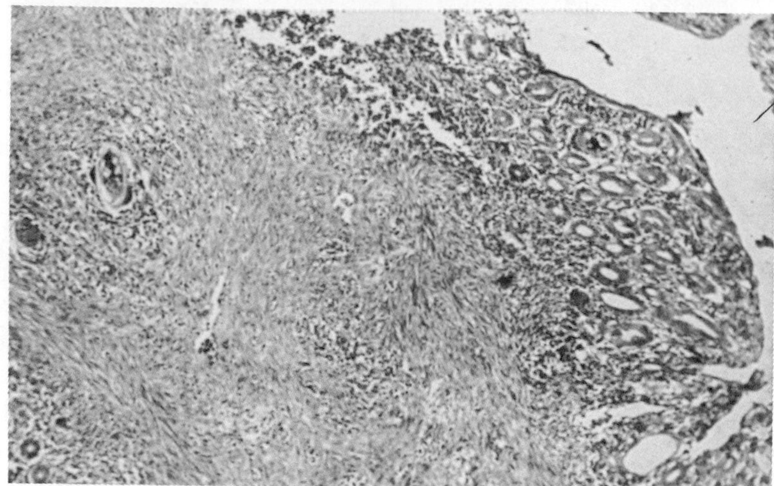

Figure 52–9. Schistosomiasis: ulceration and fibrosis of colon, eggs of *S. mansoni* in submucosa.

leukopenia may develop. The clinical picture of Banti's disease frequently occurs. Hepatic insufficiency may characterize the terminal period. Dietary deficiency may also contribute to the liver disease.

Eggs carried to the lungs as emboli gradually produce a fibrosis. Numerous cases of resulting right ventricular failure have been reported. Eggs deposited in the spinal cord produce symptoms suggestive of abscess or tumor. However, clinicians encounter different forms of schistosomiasis mansoni in various endemic areas, ranging from asymptomatic (with eggs present in the feces) to severe hepatic and pulmonary involvement. Occasionally cases in which the central nervous system was involved have been reported from Puerto Rico[21] and Africa.[22]

It is believed that numerous exposures to small numbers of cercariae cause much milder manifestations and less ultimate damage than a single exposure to many cercariae, because immunity prevents later invading worms from developing into adults.

Patients with chronic *Salmonella paratyphi* A infections and schistosomiasis mansoni have been found to present a difficult thera-

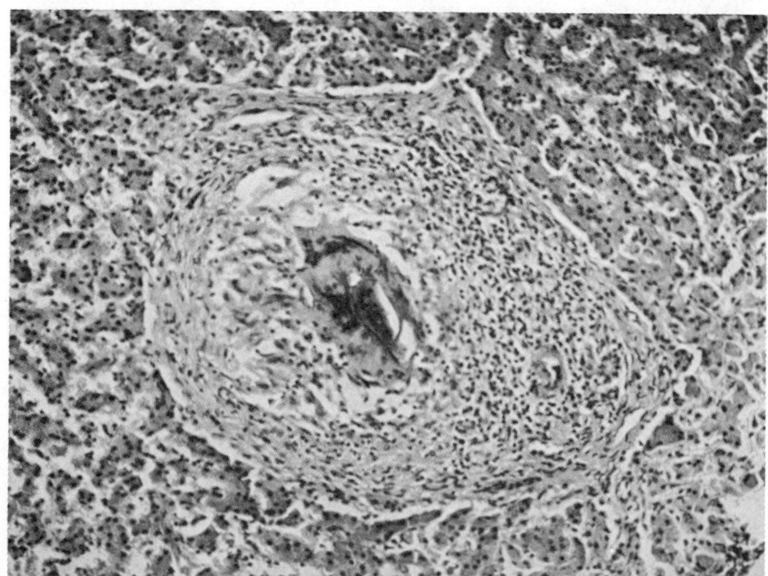

Figure 52–10. Schistosomiasis pseudotubercle in liver: foreign body reaction, cellular infiltration and early connective tissue proliferation about egg of *S. mansoni.*

peutic problem. This relationship has been shown to be due to the ability of the *Salmonella* to establish colonies on the tegument or within the tissues of *S. mansoni*.[23] (See Chapter 20, p. 179.)

Diagnosis. Demonstration of the characteristic lateral-spined egg is necessary to establish the diagnosis (Fig. 53–2, p. 571). Eggs begin to appear in the feces 6 to 8 weeks after infection. In a formed stool they are at first more likely to be found on the outside, especially in flecks of mucus or blood. If there is dysentery they should be numerous. In mild or late cases concentration techniques may be needed to locate the eggs. Sedimentation or centrifugation and washing in normal saline will keep the eggs alive and prevent hatching. The acid-sodium sulfate-Triton-ether concentration method is one of the most efficient but kills the miracidium within the egg. The modified Kato thick-smear technique is also useful.[24, 25] (See pp. 820 and 821.)

Proctoscopy may reveal small nodules, bleeding points or ulcers from which a biopsy specimen or a scraping can be obtained. It should be pressed between two slides or a slide and coverslip for observation in order to demonstrate the viability of the eggs (Fig. 52–11). In late cases this is especially valuable. If eggs cannot be found in clinically suspected cases, the complement-fixation, intradermal or the circumoval test may help to confirm the diagnosis.[6, 7]

Treatment. Stibophen (Fuadin) is widely used to treat schistosomiasis mansoni. It is given intramuscularly; the regimen consists of 4 ml every other day for a total of 80 to 100 ml. The side effects of all antimony preparations are similar; however, antimony sodium dimercaptosuccinate (Stibocaptate, Astiban) tends to be less toxic than tartar

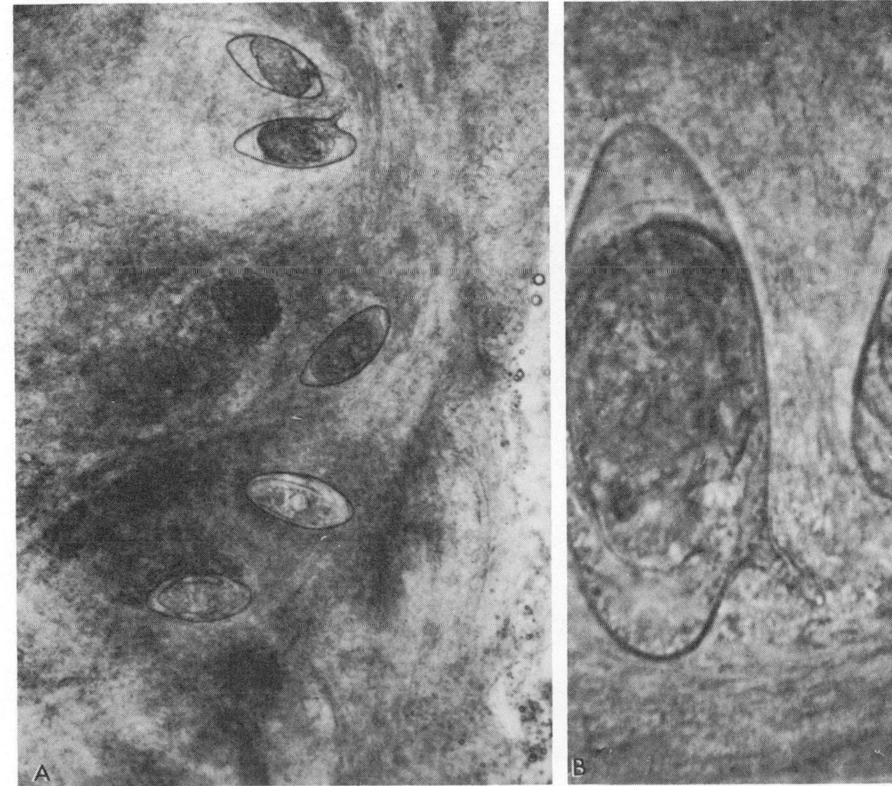

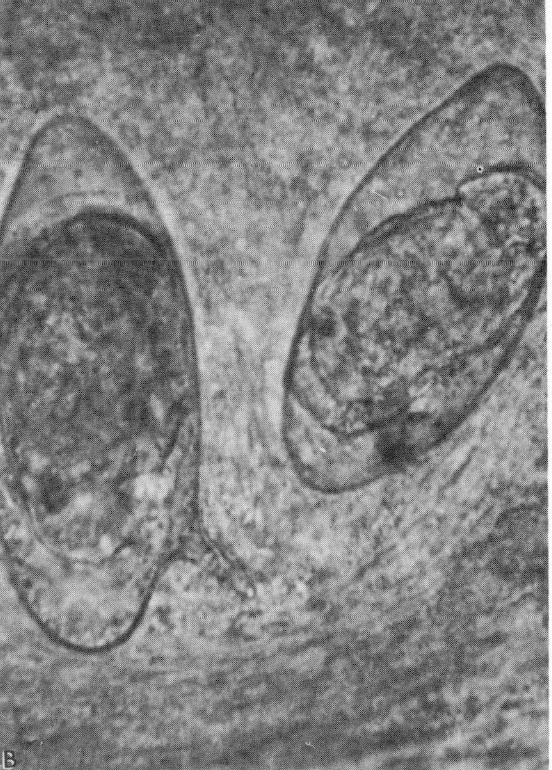

Figure 52–11. Biopsy of the colon from a case of schistosomiasis mansoni showing the typical eggs. *A*, Low power. *B*, Higher magnification. (Courtesy of Dr. Joseph H. Miller, Louisiana State University School of Medicine, New Orleans; photomicrography by Eugene Wolfe and Eugene Miscenich.)

emetic. Niridazole and hycanthone have also been used. For dosage and additional information concerning toxicity see pages 548 and 552.

Prophylaxis. *Marisa cornuarietis*, a large ampullarid snail, competes in some areas with *Biomphalaria glabrata* and offers some hope of being useful in biologic control.[26] Other species of snails and fish are also under study (p. 672). Otherwise, the prophylaxis of infection by *S. mansoni* does not differ from that for schistosomiasis haematobia (p. 552).

Schistosomiasis Japonica

Synonyms. Oriental schistosomiasis, Katayama disease, Yangtze River fever, urticarial fever.

Definition. Schistosomiasis japonica is a grave, chronic disease endemic in the Far East, with abdominal and dysenteric symptoms caused by *Schistosoma japonicum*. Man and animals are affected.

Distribution. Schistosomiasis japonica is found only in the Far East in parts of China, Japan, Taiwan, the Philippines, Lake Lindu in Sulawesi (Celebes), Thailand, Laos, Cambodia and Malaysia. The total number of human infections has been estimated at 46 million. In China large portions of the Yangtze Valley, coastal areas from the Yangtze delta to Canton, river valleys inland from Canton, the Mekong Valley in Yünnan Province and the island of Hainan compose the endemic areas (Fig. 52–3, p. 549).

In Japan the disease was limited to six small areas: the Tone River Basin, Kofu, Numazu, Fujikawa-chô on the Fuji River, Katayama and the Chikugo River on Kyushu. In 1950 the United States Army set up a control project that was highly successful.[29] In the same year a national program was initiated which has drastically reduced the prevalence of the disease; surveys in 1970 and 1971 revealed newly infected cases only in the Kofu and Tone River areas.[30]

In Taiwan the enzootic area is limited to the Changhua district on the west coast. The infection is caused by a zoophilic strain that is limited to domestic and wild animals, man being an unsuitable host.[13]

In the Philippines there are endemic foci on the islands of Luzon, Mindoro, Bohol, Samar and on much of Leyte and Mindanao (Fig. 52–3).

The Lake Lindu region of Sulawesi (Celebes),[31] Thailand,[32] Cambodia,[33,34] Laos[35,36] and Malaysia[37] are isolated endemic foci of human infection. Further studies show that some of these areas are infested by a different strain of *S. japonicum*.[35,38]

Etiology. MORPHOLOGY. Adult *S. japonicum* (Katsurada, 1904) can be distinguished from the other two human species by the absence of the tuberculated integument. Instead, the cuticula of both sexes is covered with minute spines. The male possesses seven testes; the female is characterized by a long uterus which may contain as many as 300 eggs. The eggs are broad, oval, measure 70 to 90 by 50 to 70 μm and may be distinguished by the enclosed miracidium and the barely detectable small knob on the lateral aspect of the shell (Fig. 53–2, p. 571).

DEVELOPMENT. *Schistosoma japonicum* follows the pattern of development described for *S. haematobium* and *S. mansoni*.

Epidemiology. Amphibious snails of the genus *Oncomelania* that normally inhabit the banks of irrigation ditches and canals or marshes and quiet fresh water serve as the intermediate hosts of *S. japonicum*. (See Table 66–1.) These small, slender snails, measuring not over ½ inch in length, are usually not known by the local inhabitants. Canals, irrigation ditches, marshes, overflow areas, slow-flowing streams and shallow ponds or pools where the snails live are often seeded with eggs in human feces from defecation sites, nightsoil boats or buckets (Fig. 52–12).

Human infection results from wading in the shallow water along irrigation ditches, canals, rice fields or rice seedling beds containing cercariae which have emerged from infected snails. The infection may also be

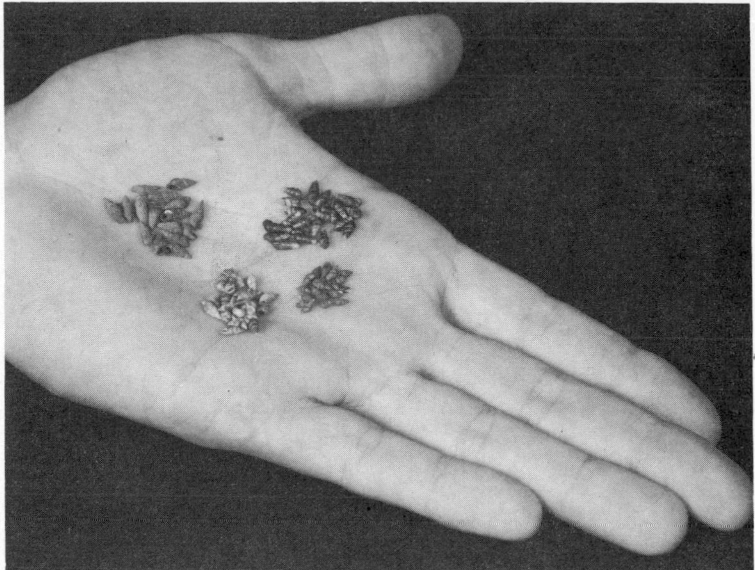

Figure 52-12. Known intermediate hosts of *S. japonicum*. Reading left to right, they are: (Top row) *Oncomelania hupensis*—China; *O. nosophora*—Japan; (Bottom row) *O. formosana*—Taiwan; *O. quadrasi*—Philippines. (Courtesy of the University of Florida College of Medicine, Gainesville.)

acquired by bathing, washing clothes or vehicles, or, less frequently, drinking the contaminated water. In many areas it is primarily a rice farmer's disease.

Schistosoma japonicum has a variety of reservoir hosts in addition to man. Dogs, cats, horses, pigs, cattle, water buffalo, deer, field and other mice and rats may become infected in endemic areas and serve as an additional source of contamination of the water. In the Mekong Basin 14.4 per cent of the persons examined were positive by skin test and then by stool for a *S. japonicum*-like infection. Miracidia successfully penetrated the snail *Lithoglyphopsis aperta* Temcharoen, 1941, and subsequently yielded cercariae that produced *S. japonicum*-like worms in experimental animals.[35, 38]

Pathology. The female *S. japonicum* extrudes about ten times as many eggs a day as *S. mansoni*. The eggs are often extruded in masses and produce abscesses in which there is a large area of necrosis surrounded by polymorphonuclear leukocytes including many eosinophils. Egg deposition begins about 4 weeks after infection and occurs in the venules of both the small and large intestine. Single eggs and those from superficial abscesses break into the lumen, and blood, pus and mucus accompany them into the fecal discharge. Proliferation of epithelium between and into abscess cavities leads to polyp formation, and in patients with advanced disease there may be hundreds of these polyps protruding into the lumen. Deeper abscesses (Fig. 52-13) ultimately heal, producing thickening of the wall, and lesions on the serosal surface (Fig. 52-14) produce fibrinous adhesions which become fibrous, causing permanent matting together of loops of intestine. Eggs carried by the portal blood stream to the liver likewise cause abscesses and scars (Fig. 52-15) which may lead to large areas of fibrosis and obstruction to the portal circulation (Fig. 52-16). The liver at first becomes enlarged but ultimately may shrink with scarring until it is no longer palpable. The spleen becomes progressively enlarged from the portal obstruction until it may occupy the entire left half of the abdomen. Ascites develops and may become massive. Varicose veins may develop in the abdominal wall or in the lower esophagus, and fatal hemorrhage may occur.

In some heavy infections eggs may be carried through anastomoses in the liver or portacaval vessels to the lungs and produce minute abscesses or pneumonic areas. In a small proportion of cases worms may migrate through anastomoses from the mesenteric to the spinal veins and ultimately reach the brain, where their eggs produce abscesses. Others have been known to migrate to the cutaneous veins of the trunk where

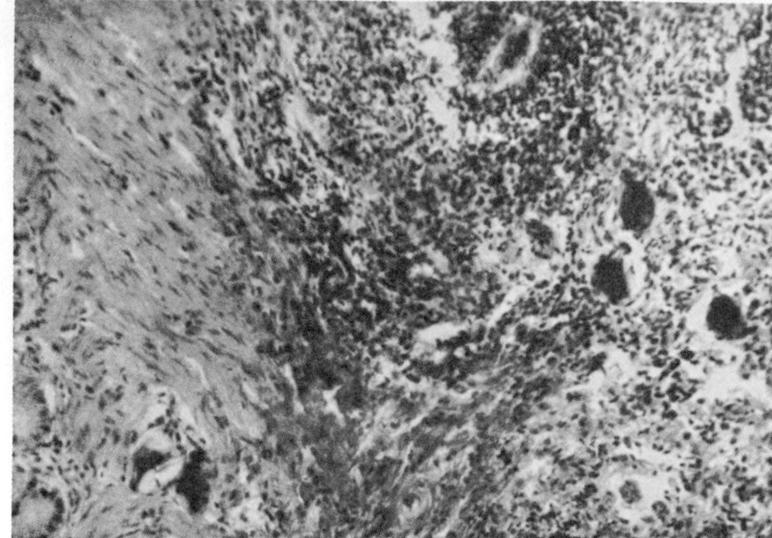

Figure 52–13. Schistosomiasis: eggs of *S. japonicum* and inflammatory reaction in wall of intestine.

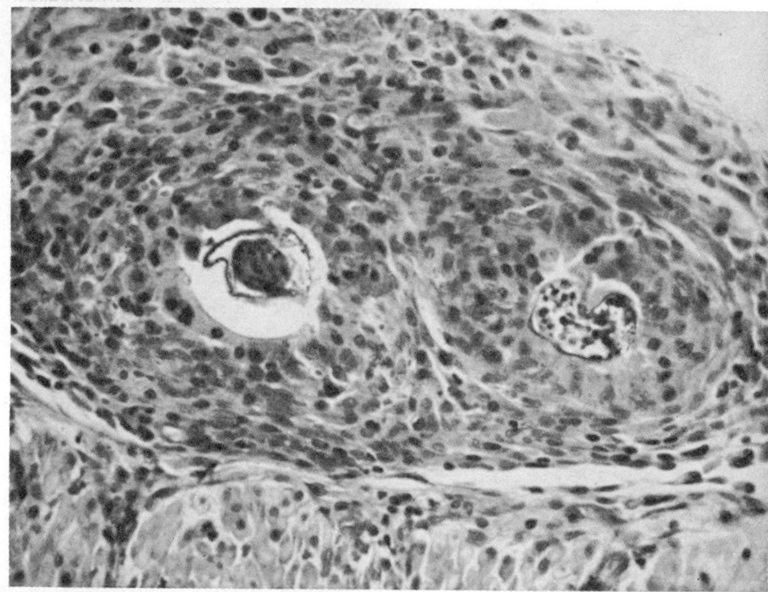

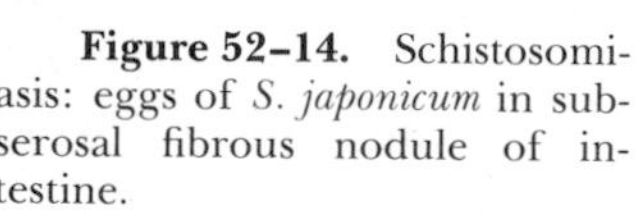

Figure 52–14. Schistosomiasis: eggs of *S. japonicum* in subserosal fibrous nodule of intestine.

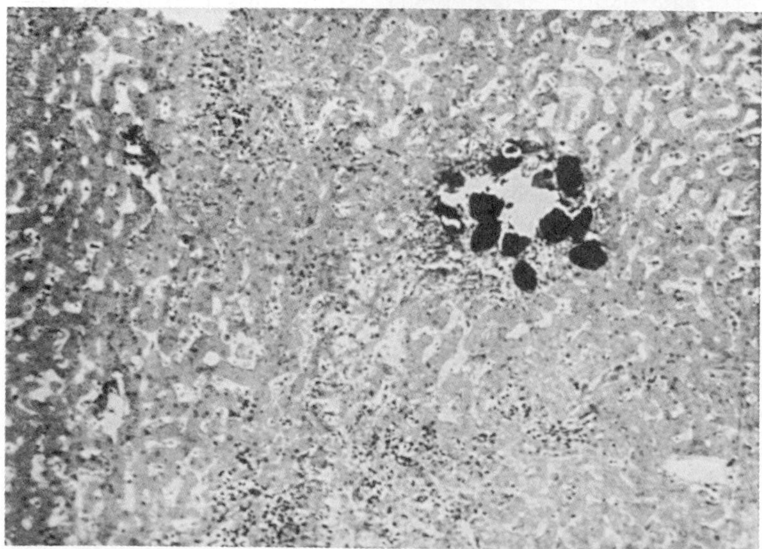

Figure 52–15. Schistosomiasis: small abscess in liver containing calcified eggs of *S. japonicum*.

their eggs were discovered in pustular lesions.

Carcinoma of the colon or liver may occur on rare occasion and has been thought to be initiated by the irritation produced by the eggs.

Clinical Characteristics. The worms mature and begin to deposit eggs about 4 weeks after infection. During the week prior to this a foreign protein reaction to the worms produces the clinical syndrome originally called Yangtze River fever. It consists of afternoon fever, malaise, dry cough and giant urticaria. The lungs show evanescent moist rales. Among infected American troops in the Philippines several showed

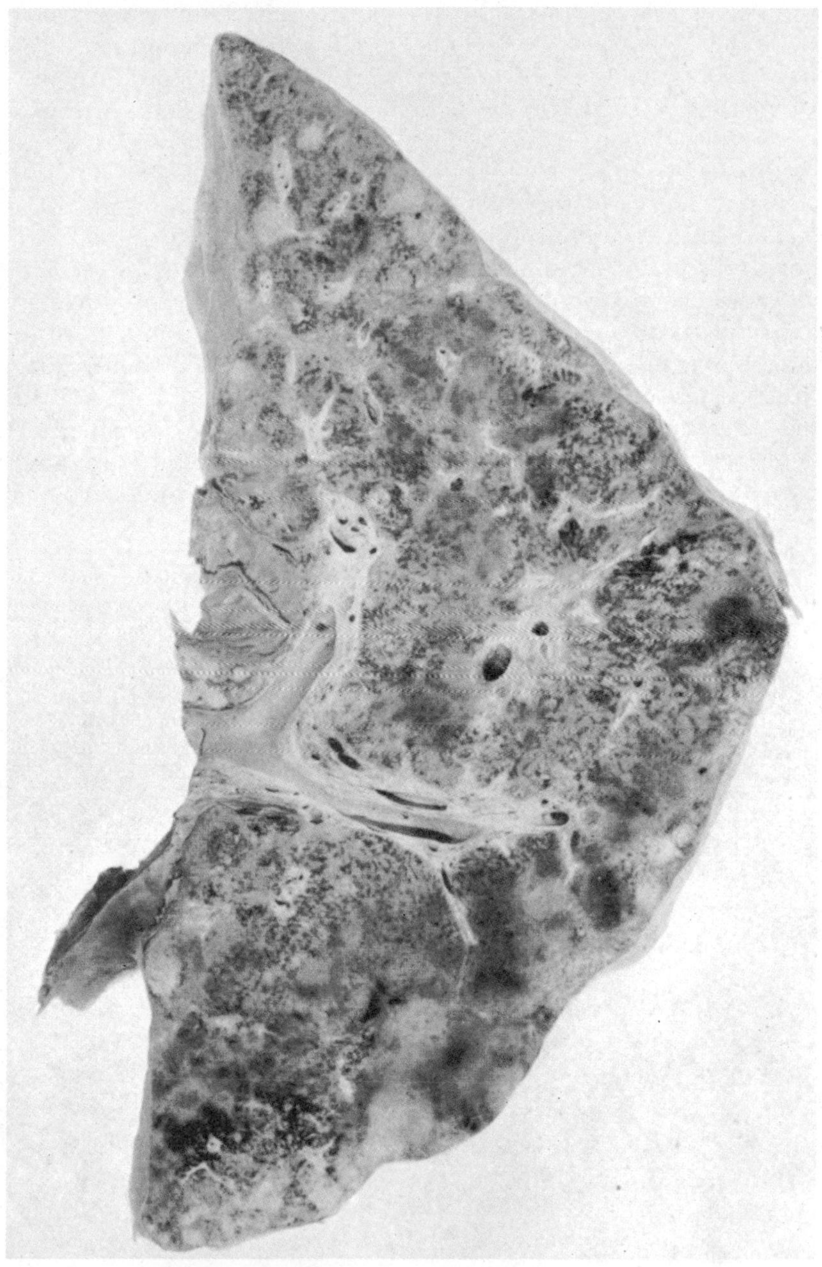

Figure 52-16. Cut surface of the liver in the case of a heavy infection by *Schistosoma japonicum*. (Courtesy of E. C. Faust and H. E. Meleney in the American Journal of Hygiene, Monograph Series No. 3, 1924.)

early neurologic symptoms—lethargy or coma, mental confusion, spastic paralysis involving one or more extremities, and abnormal superficial and deep reflexes. Only upper neurons appeared to be involved, and the spinal fluid was normal. Improvement rapidly followed the initiation of treatment, but in some cases residual signs lasted for several months. Because of the early occurrence, widespread involvement of the brain, and rapid improvement with treatment, it seems probable that these early cerebral manifestations were due to toxic edema of the brain comparable to urticaria, rather than to the deposition of eggs in the brain, as described below.

The deposition of eggs in the walls of the intestine and liver causes continued fever, abdominal discomfort, right upper quadrant tenderness and severe malaise. Eggs appear first in the formed feces, but soon there may be diarrhea with blood, pus and mucus. Increasing leukocytosis occurs with eosinophils sometimes rising to 90 per cent. This acute stage may last for 8 to 10 weeks, the fever falling gradually. The liver and spleen become palpable early and the former is tender. Heavy infections may progress to fatal hepatic failure in less than a year. Exacerbations of symptoms are frequent in lighter cases. The stage of scarring, portal cirrhosis, splenomegaly and ascites may develop gradually over many years. Poor nutrition and intercurrent infections may contribute to a fatal termination.

In a few cases, sometimes previously unrecognized, migration of worms to the brain and the deposition of eggs, usually in cortical venules, produce physical signs of lesions, often epileptiform in nature. Exploration reveals an abscess containing eggs of *S. japonicum* (Fig. 52–17). If the disease is suspected from a history of possible exposure, or if it is diagnosed either by finding eggs in the feces or by rectal biopsy, specific treatment usually produces rapid improvement and often complete recovery.

Diagnosis. Definitive diagnosis requires the identification of eggs in the feces or in a rectal biopsy specimen. The egg (Fig. 53–2) is about the size and shape of an *Ascaris* egg but differs from it in having a

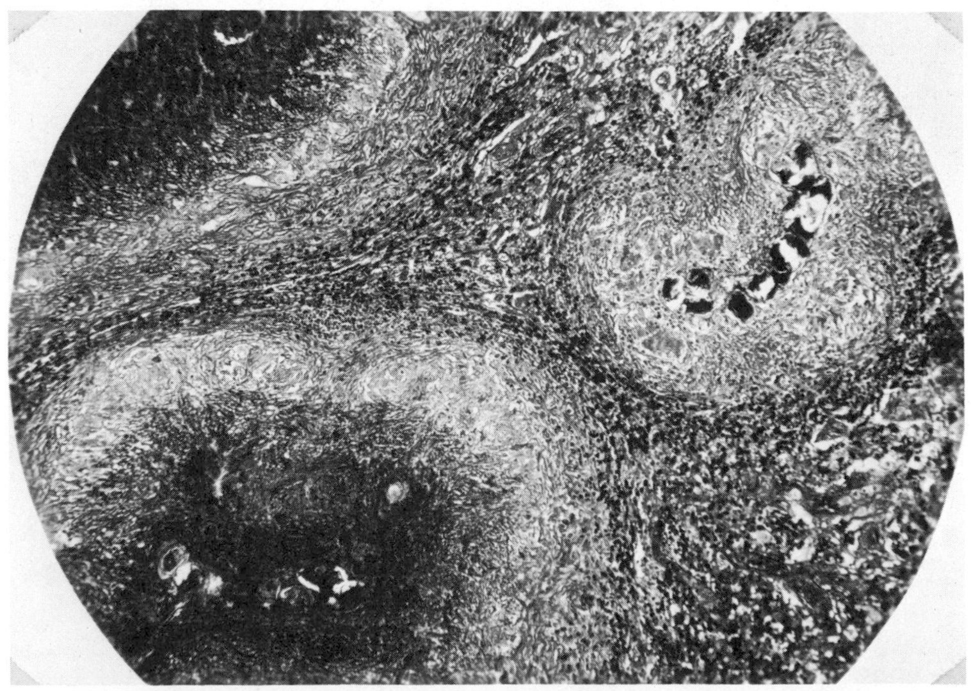

Figure 52–17. Brain abscesses caused by eggs of *S. japonicum* deposited by worms which had migrated into a cerebral vein. (Courtesy of the University of Florida College of Medicine, Gainesville.)

thin wall and usually a fully developed miracidium. The rudimentary spine is usually hidden by fecal debris sticking to the egg shell. The technique of examination of feces and rectal biopsy is the same as for the eggs of *S. mansoni* (p. 557). In the follow-up of treated cases numerous dead or calcified eggs may be found in rectal biopsy specimens; these are not an indication for further treatment. The complement-fixation and intradermal tests are of practical value when eggs cannot be found, if antigen is available. The intradermal test has been used to estimate prevalence in an endemic community where it is impractical to obtain fecal specimens. Spleen surveys have been used under similar conditions provided malaria was absent.

Treatment. *Schistosoma japonicum* is more resistant than the other species of schistosomes to therapy. Antimony potassium tartrate (tartar emetic) is the drug of choice. It must be administered intravenously *with great care.* Use a 0.5 per cent solution in 5 per cent glucose, physiologic saline, or distilled water. Sterilize by *gentle boiling (not by autoclaving)* for 5 minutes. Inject slowly, not faster than 4 ml per minute *on alternate days.* The dosage schedule follows: 8, 12, 16, 20, 24 ml; continue at 28 ml for 10 additional doses. It is best to give injections 2 to 3 hours following a light meal.

Antimony sodium dimercaptosuccinate (Stibocaptate, Astiban) gives a lower cure rate. (See p. 552 for dosage.) Stibophen (Fuadin), 8.5 mg antimony per ml, may be given daily using 8 to 10 ml per day (a very toxic amount) intramuscularly for 10 days or longer if required or well tolerated.[9]

The serious and not infrequently fatal cerebral complications constitute an imperative indication for the use of tartar emetic intravenously unless the administration of antimony is absolutely contraindicated. This will usually alleviate the central nervous system disease and should always be used in preference to surgical intervention. Permanent sequelae are twice as common in operated cases as in those receiving one or more courses of tartar emetic. (For details of treatment see preceding.)

Prophylaxis. Prophylaxis does not differ materially from that described for other schistosomiases except that there are more known reservoir hosts. The disease usually occurs in an area where human nightsoil is commonly used as a fertilizer, and the snail host is amphibious, being capable of surviving several weeks of desiccation. In addition, the vast extent of some endemic areas further complicates the picture and makes control difficult except in foci of limited size, as in Japan where molluscicides and other measures are highly effective.[29,30] On Leyte, in the Philippines, a pilot experimental control area making use of water management practices, drainage and reclamation of swamplands, channeling of streams and ponding for pisciculture demonstrated that partial control at least might be achieved.[39] It is hoped that the improved crop yields and economic gains of the proposed program will offset the expenses involved.[40]

Schistosomiasis Intercalatum

Synonyms. None.

Definition. Schistosomiasis intercalatum is an endemic intestinal disease with abdominal pain, diarrhea and other symptoms, caused by the blood fluke *Schistosoma intercalatum.*

Distribution. This distinctly African disease is found only in limited foci in West Central Africa where it occurs in man from Zaire (Kisangani = Stanleyville), Congo (Brazzaville), Central African Republic, Gabon, the Cameroons and probably Nigeria, Upper Volta and Chad.[41] It is probable that the disease will be spread to new foci by migrant African laborers as well as by the regular seasonal migration of nomads between southern and northern Cameroons, especially since potential snail vector species are widely disseminated throughout Central Africa.

Etiology. The dimensions of the adult parasites may vary with the host and be confused with other species of schistosomes. The males range in length between 11.5 and 14.5 mm and in breadth (with the gynecophoral canal folded) from 0.31 to 0.5 mm. The testes vary in number from two to seven but in most hosts the average is four. The ventral, lateral and dorsal surfaces of the male are spinose and from the testes posteriorly the cuticula is tuberculate.

Adult female worms range from 13 to 24 mm in length by 0.2 to 0.25 mm in breadth. The ovary lies between the intestinal ceca and in many specimens is spirally twisted. The intrauterine eggs measure 140 $\pm$ 10.7 μm by 36.7 $\pm$ 2.4 μm in breadth. After 80 days the gravid eggs that are passed from an experimental host average between 25 and 60 per worm with a maximum of 122 being recorded. The eggs that occur in the feces are characterized by a terminal spine that is usually slightly bent. The egg shells are Ziehl-Neelsen–positive, i.e. acid fast, when fixed in Bouin's; frequently the contained miracidium appears to be hourglass-shaped.[42]

The best criteria for identifying *S. intercalatum* as a separate species and distinguishing it from other schistosomes lie in a number of biologic characters. The most distinctive features are:

1. the Ziehl-Neelsen positive staining reaction of the egg shell in histologic sections;
2. the behavioral pattern of the cercariae, which tend to congregate near or at the surface (as do those of *S. japonicum);*
3. the tendency of the cercariae to adhere to objects;
4. the glandular secretions of the cercariae take the form of granular strings; and
5. in most of the known transmission foci *S. intercalatum* is found alone; in only a few places does it coexist with *S. mansoni* and only in the Cameroons with *S. haematobium.*[43]

Epidemiology. The epidemiology of *S. intercalatum* is essentially similar to that of *S. mansoni,* since the ranges of the two parasites overlap in a few areas. Surveys made in endemic regions reveal a prevalence rate for *S. intercalatum* of between 5.7 and 24.3 per cent.[44]

Two natural infections have been found in *Hybomys univittatus,* the one-striped mouse. However, more potential hosts need to be examined for these schistosomes from endemic foci. More recently laboratory infections of *S. intercalatum* have been produced in hamsters, gerbils, rats, mice, guinea pigs, rabbits, goats, sheep and rhesus monkeys. Other species of monkeys and the American opossum have also been infected.[43]

The proven intermediate hosts consist primarily of strains of *Bulinus (B.) forskalii.* Strains of *B. (Physopsis) africanus* were not susceptible to laboratory infections and so are not believed capable of serving as a vector.[43]

Pathology. The often-bent, terminal-spined eggs of *S. intercalatum* are deposited in the mesenteric venules and usually break through to the lumen of the intestine where they are passed in the feces. The parasite causes less reaction in the definitive host than do the other human schistosomes. There usually is no marked hepatomegaly; however, liver biopsies reveal perioval abscesses. There may be an alteration in the retention of sulfobromophthalein.

Clinical Characteristics. The symptomatology may include episodes of pain in the left iliac fossa with tenesmus. Marked digestive disturbances are frequent and blood and mucus may be present in the stool. Proctoscopy may reveal hyperplasia of the mucosa near the rectal valves, inflammation of the wall, and sometimes polyposis. These conditions are usually relieved following adequate treatment.[45]

Diagnosis. Demonstration of the characteristic, often-bent, terminal-spined eggs is necessary to establish the diagnosis. These may be demonstrated in the feces or by mucosal snips from the rectum. The eggs are Ziehl-Neelsen-positive, i.e. acid fast, while those of *S. haematobium* are not and the contained miracidium is often narrowed in the middle giving it something of an "hourglass" shape.

Treatment. Niridazole is the drug of choice. For dosage and additional information on toxicity see pages 548 and 552.

Prophylaxis. This is the same as for the other African schistosomes of man.

Schistosome Cercarial Dermatitis

Etiology and Epidemiology. The cercariae of approximately 20 species of nonhuman schistosomes, mostly adult in birds or small mammals, are known to penetrate the skin of man and produce a dermatitis. Depending upon the circumstances under which the disease is acquired, it has been variously designated as "swimmer's itch," "schistosome dermatitis," "clam digger's itch," "sawah itch" or "koganbyo." In all cases it involves the association of man and potential intermediate snail hosts infected from the droppings of bird or mammal hosts harboring the parasites (Fig. 52–18).

Schistosome dermatitis is widely distributed throughout the freshwater areas of the Americas and has been reported from Alaska, Canada, many parts of the United States, Mexico, El Salvador, Colombia and Argentina. It is highly endemic in Canada, Michigan, Wisconsin and Minnesota and occurs from sea level to over 9000 feet elevation (Colorado). Elsewhere, outbreaks have occurred in Wales, Germany, France, The Netherlands, Switzerland, Malaya, New Zealand, Africa and Japan.

It has now been reported in the brackish and coastal waters along the Atlantic seaboard, the Gulf Coast, southern and lower California and Hawaii.

The freshwater mollusks that serve as intermediate hosts include species of *Lymnaea, Physa, Polypylis, Gyraulus, Segmentina, Stagnicola* and *Chilina.* Some of the marine molluscan hosts include representatives of *Nassarius, Littorina, Haminoea, Cerithidea* and *Batillaria.*

Clinical Characteristics. There are marked differences in the responses of unsensitized and sensitized individuals to the penetration of the skin by the cercariae of nonhuman schistosomes. Initial exposures to these cercariae produce only mild, transient reactions that often pass unnoticed. Even so, many persons experience a prickling sensation as the water evaporates and the parasites penetrate the skin. Macules usually appear within 12 hours and in nonsensitized individuals soon disappear. However, in persons sensitized by previous exposures to these cercariae, the macules will be followed by papules, possibly accompanied by erythema, vesicle formation, edema and pruritus which may persist for a week or 10 days (Fig. 52–19). Reactions vary markedly, not only because of differences in susceptibility of the

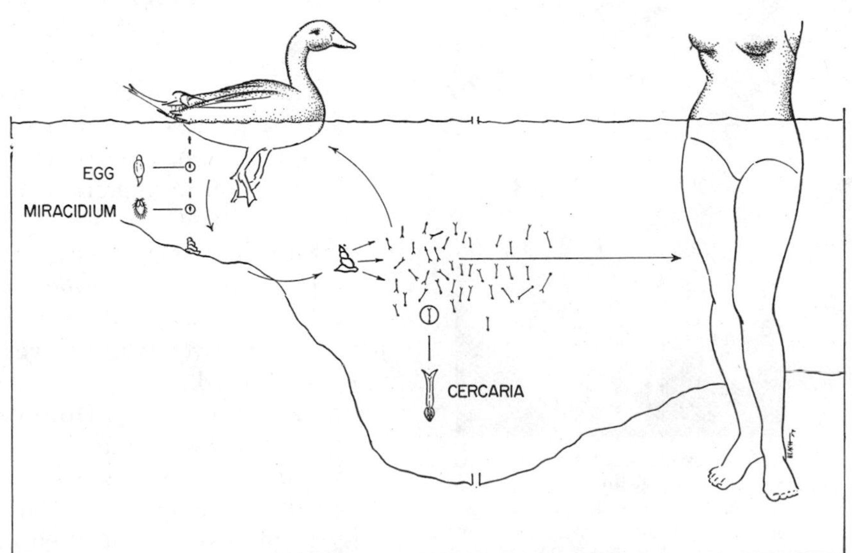

Figure 52–18. Life cycle of a bird schistosome showing how man may acquire swimmer's itch. (Partly after Dr. Max J. Miller, courtesy of the University of Florida College of Medicine, Gainesville.)

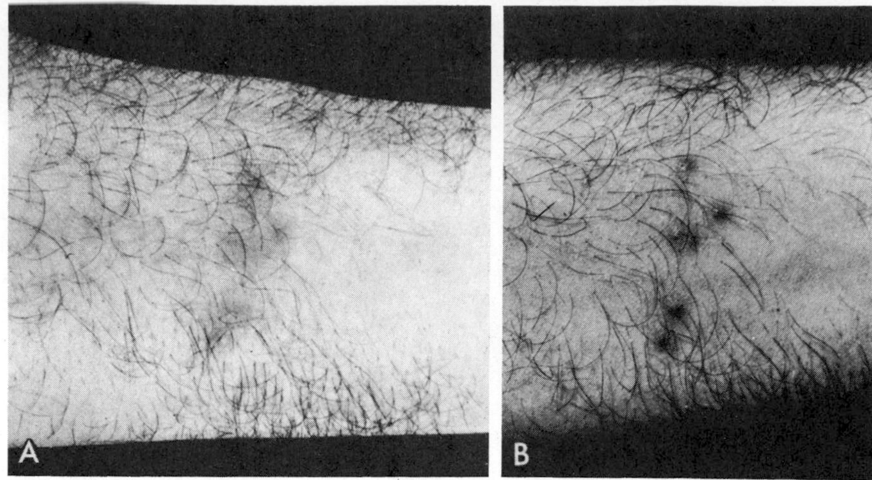

Figure 52-19. Dermatitis caused by experimental exposure to cercariae of the mammalian zoonotic schistosome, *Heterobilharzia americana*. *A*, 56 hours after exposure. *B*, 6 days after exposure. (Courtesy of Dr. E. A. Malek, Tulane University School of Medicine, New Orleans, Louisiana.)

host, but also because the nonhuman schistosome cercariae differ markedly in their ability to produce a response in the human host (Fig. 52-20).

Treatment consists of palliative topical applications accompanied in severe cases by oral or parenteral antihistamines.

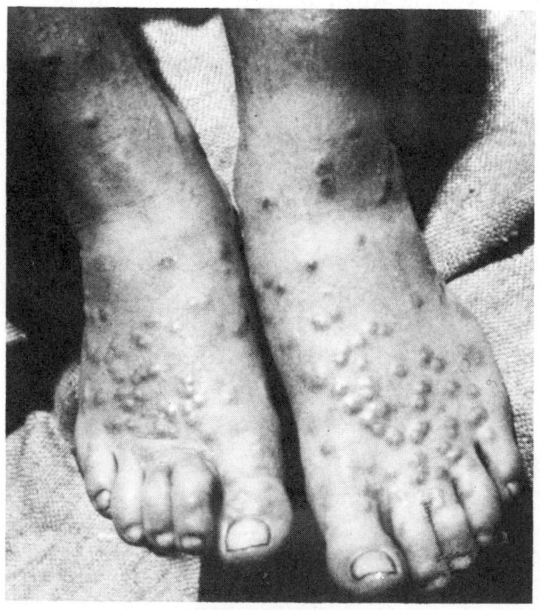

Figure 52-20. Marked reaction in sensitized amateur fisherman about 4 days after fishing in a brackish-water lagoon near Sydney, Australia. The infection was caused by cercariae of *Austrobilharzia terrigalensis*. (Courtesy of Dr. A. J. Bearup, School of Public Health and Tropical Medicine, University of Sydney, N.S.W., Australia.)

Control. Control of the freshwater snail host is possible in some areas by treating infested bathing areas with 1 lb. of 10 per cent fresh lime and 2 lb. of copper sulfate snow per 1000 square feet of bottom. Sodium pentachlorophenate should also prove effective. (See pp. 672 and 673 for other molluscicides.)

SOME POTENTIAL HUMAN SCHISTOSOMES

Several other species of schistosomes, normally parasites of mammals, may occasionally infect man. Experiments with monkeys suggest that nonpatent visceral schistosomiasis is probably produced in man as a result of infection with the cercariae of *Schistosomatium douthitti*, *Heterobilharzia americana* and *Schistosoma spindale*. Young preadult worms were recovered from livers of rhesus monkeys exposed to these schistosomes but later the worms were lost. However, in South American monkeys, cebus and squirrel, *Heterobilharzia americana* produces a patent infection with the deposition of large numbers of eggs in the tissues, and their excretion in the feces. Other zoonotic species of *Schistosoma* include *S. bovis*, *S. mattheei*, *S. margrebowiei*

Table 52–2. Geographic Distribution and Hosts of the Zoonotic Mammalian Schistosomes

Schistosome	*Geographic Distribution*	*Snail Intermediate Hosts*	*Natural Definitive Hosts*
Schistosomatium douthitti	Northern U.S.A., Alaska and Canada	*Stagnicola palustris* *Lymnaea stagnalis*	Muskrats, meadow mice
Heterobilharzia americana	U.S.A.: Florida, Georgia, Texas, Louisiana, North Carolina, South Carolina	*Lymnaea cubensis* *Pseudosuccinea columella*	Bobcats, raccoons, dogs, nutria, white-tailed deer, rabbits, opossums
Schistosoma spindale	Malaya, Sumatra, India	*Indoplanorbis exustus*	Cattle, buffalos, goats
	South Africa, Zambia and Rhodesia	*Bulinus tropicus*	Cattle, reedbucks, other antelopes
Schistosoma bovis	Southern Europe, Northern Africa, Southwestern Asia	*Bulinus (Bulinus) truncatus*	Sheep, goats, cattle, equines
	Central and South Africa	*B. (Ph.) globosus* *B. (Ph.) africanus*	Sheep, goats, cattle, equines, camels, man
Schistosoma mattheei	South Africa, Zaire	*B. (Ph.) africanus* *B. (Ph.) globosus*	Cattle, sheep, goats, zebras, impalas, man
Schistosoma margrebowiei	Zambia, South Africa		Equines, cattle, sheep, antelopes, man
Schistosoma rodhaini	Zaire, Uganda	*Biomphalaria sudanica* *B. bridouxiana*	Rodents, dogs, man

and *S. rodhaini*. These produce a patent infection in man with passage of viable eggs in the stools or urine. In the Transvaal, South Africa, for example, prevalences of 23, 35 and 40 per cent infections with *S. mattheei* were reported to occur mixed with *S. haematobium* among the inhabitants of certain villages. (See Table 52–2.) The geographic distribution and hosts of these mammalian schistosomes are also indicated in Table 52–2.

REFERENCES

1. Faust, E. C., and Meleney, H. E. 1924. Studies on schistosomiasis japonica. Am. J. Hyg. Monogr. Ser. No. 3. 339 pp.
2. Warren, K. S. 1972. The immunopathogenesis of schistosomiasis: a multidisciplinary approach. Tr. Roy. Soc. Trop. Med. Hyg. *66*:417–432.
3. Warren, K. S. 1973. The pathology of schistosome infections. Helm. Abst., Ser. A, *42*:591–633.
4. Smithers, S. R. 1972. Recent advances in the immunology of schistosomiasis. Br. Med. Bull. *28*:49–54.
5. Shennan, D. W., and Gelfand, M. 1971. Bilharzia ova in cervical smears. A possible additional route for the passage of ova into water. Tr. Roy. Soc. Trop. Med. Hyg. *65*:95–99.
6. Moriearty, P. L., and Lewert, R. M. 1974. Delayed hypersensitivity in Ugandan schistosomiasis. I. Sensitivity, specificity, and immunological features of intradermal responses. Am. J. Trop. Med. Hyg. *23*:169–178.
7. Moriearty, P. L., and Lewert, R. M. 1974. Delayed hypersensitivity in Ugandan schistosomiasis. III. Examination of serological responses and clinical states. Am. J. Trop. Med. Hyg. *23*:190–196.

7a. Phillips, J. F., Cockrill, H., Jorge, E., and Steiner, R. 1975. Radiographic evaluation of patients with schistosomiasis. Radiology *114*:31–37.

7b. Legator, M. S., Connor, T. H., and Stoeckel, M. 1975. Detection of mutagenic activity of metronidazole and niridazole in body fluids of humans and mice. Science *188*:1118–1119.

8. Davis, A. 1973. Chemotherapy in control. *In* Ansari, N. (ed.): Epidemiology and Control of Schistosomiasis (Bilharziasis). University Park Press, Baltimore. pp. 592–608.
9. Anonymous. 1974. Drugs for parasitic diseases. The Medical Letter on Drugs and Therapeutics *16*:5–11.
10. Ritchie, L. S. 1973. Chemical control of snails. *In* Ansari, N. (ed.): Epidemiology and Control of Schistosomiasis (Bilharziasis). University Park Press, Baltimore. pp. 458–532.
11. Lemma, A. 1971. Present status of Endod as a molluscicide for the control of schistosomiasis. Ethiop. Med. J. *9*:113–118.
12. Jordan, P. 1972. Epidemiology and control of schistosomiasis. Br. Med. Bull. *28*:55–59.
13. Wright, W. H. 1973. Geographical distribution of schistosomes and their intermediate hosts. *In* Ansari, N. (ed.): Epidemiology and Control of Schistosomiasis (Bilharziasis). University Park Press, Baltimore. pp. 32–249.
14. Abdel Sayed, W., Bassily, S., Mohran, Y., Wassef, S. A., and Abdel Ghaffar, Y. 1969. LDH activity in urinary schistosomiasis and its complications. Br. J. Cancer *23*:73–77.
15. Kisner, C. D. 1973. Vesical bilharziasis. Pathological changes and relationship to squamous carcinoma. S. Afr. J. Surg. *11*:79–87.
16. Norden, D. A., and Gelfand, M. 1972. Bilharzia and

bladder cancer. An investigation of urinary glucuronidase associated with *S. haematobium* infection. Tr. Roy. Soc. Trop. Med. Hyg. *66*:864–866.

17. Barlow, C. H., and Meleney, H. E. 1949. A voluntary infection with *Schistosoma haematobium.* Am. J. Trop. Med. *29*:79–87.
18. Gove, R. B. 1970. Further observations on the distribution of the eggs of *Schistosoma haematobium* in the urinary stream. Tr. Roy. Soc. Trop. Med. Hyg. *64*:431–432.
19. Cook, J. A., and Jordan, P. 1970. Excretion of *Schistosoma mansoni* ova in the urine. Tr. Roy. Soc. Trop. Med. Hyg. *64*:793–794.
20. Most, H. 1971. Schistosomiasis mansoni of Puerto Rican origin with involvement of the urinary tract (bladder). Tr. Roy. Soc. Trop. Med. Hyg. *65*:411–412.
21. Rosenbaum, R. M., Ishii, N., Tanowitz, H., and Wittner, M. 1972. Schistosomiasis mansoni of the spinal cord. Report of a case. Am. J. Trop. Med. Hyg. *21*:182–184.
22. Levy, L. F. 1970. Bilharzial involvement of the CNS. Med. J. Zambia *4*:191–199.
23. Young, S. W., Higashi, G., Kamel, R., El-Abdin, A. Z., and Mikhail, I. A. 1973. Interaction of Salmonellae and schistosomes in host-parasite relations. Tr. Roy. Soc. Trop. Med. Hyg. *67*:797–802.
24. Borda, C. E., and Pellegrino, J. 1971. An improved stool thick-smear technique for quantitative diagnosis of *Schistosoma mansoni* infection. Rev. Inst. Med. Trop. São Paulo *13*:71–75.
25. Martin, L. K., and Beaver, P. C. 1968. Evaluation of Kato thick-smear technique for quantitative diagnosis of helminth infections. Am. J. Trop. Med. Hyg. *17*:382–391.
26. Ruiz-Tibén, E., Palmer, J. R., and Ferguson, F. F. 1969. Biological control of *Biomphalaria glabrata* by *Marisa cornuarietis* in irrigation ponds in Puerto Rico. Bull. W.H.O. *41*:329–333.
27. Knight, W. B., Ritchie, L. S., Laird, F., and Chiriboga, J. 1970. Cercariophagic activity of guppy fish *(Lebistes reticulatus)* detected by cercariae labeled with radioselenium (^{75}SE). Am. J. Trop. Med. Hyg. *19*:620–625.
28. Voilker, J. 1966. Wasserwanzen als obligatorische Schneckenfresser im Nildelta *(Limnogeton fieberi* Mayr: Belostomatidae, Hemiptera). Ztschr. Tropenmed. Parasit. *17*:155–165.
29. Hunter, G. W., III, Okabe, K., Burke, J. C., and Williams, J. E. 1962. Aspects of schistosomiasis control and eradication, with special reference to Japan. Ann. Trop. Med. Parasit. *56*:302–313.
30. Yokogawa, M. 1970. Schistosomiasis in Japan. *In* Sasa, M. (ed.): Recent Advances in Researches on Filariasis and Schistosomiasis in Japan. University of Tokyo Press. pp. 231–255.
31. Hadidjaja, P., Carney, W. P., Clarke, M. D., Cross, J. H., Jusuf, A., Saroso, S., and Oemijati, S. 1972. *Schistosoma japonicum* and intestinal parasites of the inhabitants of Lake Lindu, Sulawesi (Celebes). A preliminary report. S. E. Asian J. Trop. Med. Pub. Hlth. *3*:594–599.
32. Harinasuta, C., and Kruatrachue, M. 1962. The first recognized endemic area of bilharziasis in Thailand. Ann. Trop. Med. Parasit. *56*:314–322.
33. Audebaud, G., Tournier-Lasserve, C., Brumpt, V., Jolly, M., Mazaud, R., Imbert, X., and Bazillio, R. 1968. Premier cas de bilharziose humaine observé an Cambodge (region de Kratié). Bull. Soc. Path. Exot. *61*:778–784.
34. Brandt, R. A. M., and Temcharoen, P. 1971. The molluscan fauna of the Mekong at the foci of schistosomiasis in South Laos and Cambodia. Arch. Molluskenk. *101*:111–140.
35. Sornmani, S., Kitikoon, V., Schneider, C. R., Harinasuta, C., and Pathammavong, O. 1973. Mekong schistosomiasis: 1. Life cycle of *Schistosoma japonicum,* Mekong strain, in the laboratory. S. E. Asian J. Trop. Med. Pub. Hlth. *4*:218–225.
36. Kitikoon, V., Schneider, C. R., Sornmani, S., Harinasuta, C., and Lanza, G. R. 1973. Mekong schistosomiasis: 2. Evidence of the natural transmission of *Schistosoma japonicum,* Mekong strain, at Khong Island, Laos. S. E. Asian J. Trop. Med. Pub. Hlth. *4*:350–358.
37. Murugasu, R., and Dissanaike, A. S. 1973. First case of schistosomiasis in Malaysia. Tr. Roy. Soc. Trop. Med. Hyg. *67*:880.
38. Harinasuta, C., Sornmani, S., Kitikoon, V., Schneider, C. R., and Pathammavong, O. 1972. Infection of aquatic hydrobiid snails and animals with *Schistosoma japonicum*-like parasites from Khong Island, southern Laos. Tr. Roy. Soc. Trop. Med. Hyg. *66*:184–185.
39. Hairston, N. G., and Santos, B. C. 1961. Ecological control of the snail host of *Schistosoma japonicum* in the Philippines. Bull. W.H.O. *25*:603–610.
40. Farooq, M. 1973. Review of national control programmes. *In* Ansari, N. (ed.): Epidemiology and Control of Schistosomiasis (Bilharziasis). University Park Press, Baltimore. pp. 388–421.
41. Wolfe, M. S. 1974. *Schistosoma intercalatum* infection in an American family. Am. J. Trop. Med. Hyg. *23*:45–50.
42. Becquet, R., and Saout, J. 1969. La bilharziose intestinale à *Schistosoma intercalatum* en Haute-Volta. Bull. Soc. Path. Exot. *62*:146–151.
43. Wright, C. A., Southgate, V. R., and Knowles, R. J. 1972. What is *Schistosoma intercalatum* Fisher, 1934? Tr. Roy. Soc. Trop. Med. Hyg. *66*:28–56.
44. Deschiens, R., Delas, A., Ngalle-Edimo, S., and Poirier, A. 1969. La schistosomiase à *Schistosoma intercalatum* en République fédérale du Cameroun. Bull. W.H.O. *40*:893–898.
45. Barbier, M. 1969. La bilharziose à *Schistosoma intercalatum* dépistée chez des Africains, en France métropolitaine, Étude parasitologique, clinique, thérapeutique de cinquante cas. Bull. Soc. Path. Exot. *62*:874–893.

CHAPTER 53
Trematodes Exclusive of Schistosomes

MORPHOLOGY

Introduction. The similarity in pattern, structure, and physiology of most trematodes exclusive of the schistosomes warrants their consideration as a group. Despite individual differences in their life cycles, these trematodes all gain entrance to man through the digestive tract. Each first parasitizes a snail, then encysts on vegetation or in some aquatic animal which is subsequently ingested by man.

Morphology of Adults. All trematodes of man are nonsegmented, bilaterally symmetrical and, with the exception of the schistosomes, hermaphroditic. As a rule, these parasites are leaflike, flattened dorsoventrally, range in length from a few millimeters to several centimeters and possess two suckers with which they attach themselves to the mucosa or other tissues of their host. The anterior or *oral sucker* surrounds the mouth; the ventral one or *acetabulum* is merely a holdfast device. The body surface is covered by a thin noncellular cuticle secreted by the underlying cells. In some species this cuticula may be spined.

The digestive tract opens through the oral sucker into a muscular pharynx, followed by an esophagus which bifurcates to form the two lateral intestinal ceca or crura (Fig. 53–1). In some species, such as *Fasciola hepatica,* the crura may be highly branched. The partially digested food or liquid in which the worm is bathed is taken into the digestive system, some absorbed, and the unused balance rejected by mouth (except in the rare cases where an anus exists). Respiration in those inhabiting the alimentary canal is essentially anaerobic. The so-called excretory system begins with numbers of microscopic "flame cells," or *solenocytes,* leading into minute ducts which ultimately coalesce to form two main lateral ducts emptying into

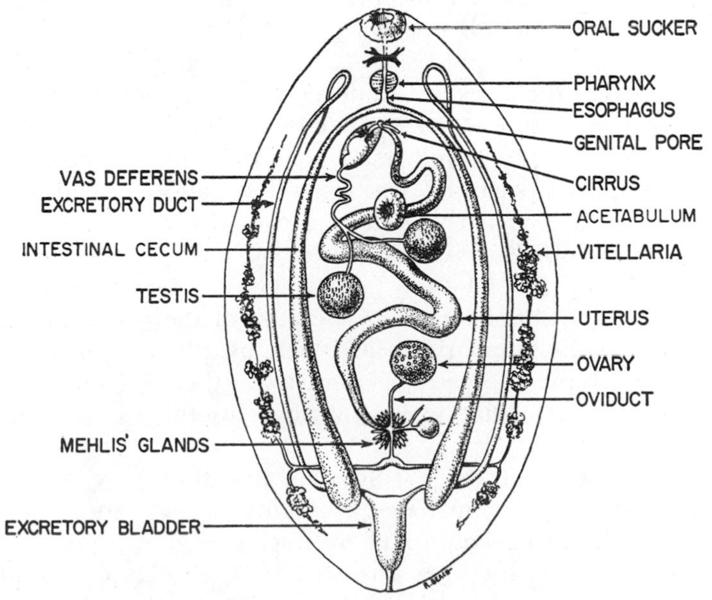

Figure 53–1. Morphology of a typical digenetic trematode. (Modified from various authors; courtesy of University of Florida College of Medicine, Gainesville.)

a posterior, terminal excretory bladder; this, in turn, opens externally through an excretory pore. The nervous system is also bilaterally symmetrical.

The reproductive systems are extremely complex. The male system usually consists of two testes drained by *vasa efferentia* into a single *vas deferens.* This empties through a ventrally situated genital pore near, and usually anterior to, the acetabulum. The terminal portion of the male system is modified to form a muscular copulatory device, or *cirrus.*

The female reproductive system includes a single *ovary* which gives rise to the *oviduct.* The oviduct complex includes a blind seminal receptacle which sometimes drains to the exterior through a dorsal *Laurer's canal,* ducts from the laterally situated yolk glands or *vitellaria,* and a *shell gland* which empties into the coiled *uterus.* This latter structure stores the eggs until they are discharged through a *genital pore* beside that of the male system into the common genital sinus. The lower portion of the uterus serves as a *vagina.* Fertilization takes place in the oviduct. In rare instances (as in the HETEROPHYIDAE), the genital pore is surrounded by a muscular genital sucker *(gonocotyl).*

Trematode Eggs. Eggs of all the trematodes, except those of the schistosomes which are spined or tuberculate, possess a lid or *operculum* which opens to allow the ciliated, free-swimming *miracidium* to emerge. As a rule, the eggs are undeveloped when passed in a stool, containing only the fertilized zygote and a yolk mass. However, in some species, such as *Clonorchis sinensis* and *Heterophyes heterophyes,* each egg contains a fully developed miracidium when evacuated by the host (Fig. 53–2).

Group Characteristics. Because of the morphologic similarity displayed by the various trematodes, a brief summary of their group characteristics may prove more useful than a key.

Members of the FASCIOLIDAE infecting man are large trematodes averaging more than 25 mm in length and producing eggs 150 by 90 μm; their cercariae encyst on vegetation. In members of the genus *Fasciola (F. hepatica* and *F. gigantica)* the dendritic testes are arranged in tandem; these, together with the intestinal ceca and vitellaria, are profusely branched, almost entirely filling the posterior two-thirds of the worm with their ramifications.

Fasciolopsis buski, which bears a superficial resemblance to *F. hepatica* in size and shape, belongs in a different taxonomic subdivision of the FASCIOLIDAE. *Fasciolopsis buski* possesses dendritic testes but has straight, unbranched intestinal crura. The eggs of the FASCIOLIDAE are undeveloped when laid and are approximately the same size. However, the operculum on the egg of *F. buski* is smaller than that on the egg of *F. hepatica.*

The HETEROPHYIDAE infecting man are all small, ovoidal, pyriform or elongate trematodes (1 to 3 mm long). They are intestinal parasites which produce minute, embryonated eggs that average nearly 30 μm in length. The chief human representatives of this family are *Heterophyes heterophyes* and *Metagonimus yokogawai.*

Clonorchis sinensis, the Oriental liver fluke, is classified in the OPISTHORCHIIDAE, which also includes other liver flukes of man and carnivores *(Opisthorchis viverrini* and *Opisthorchis felineus).* This slender trematode of man ranges between 18 and 40 mm in length. It is further characterized by dendritic testes arranged posteriorly in tandem and by the unbranched intestinal crura which extend to the posterior tip of the worm.

The lung flukes all belong to the genus *Paragonimus* and the family TROGLOTREMATIDAE. They are thicker, more opaque, broader and more generally ovoid than those described above. *Paragonimus westermani* appears to be the principal human parasite and is characterized by having straight, unbranched intestinal ceca, and lobate testes opposite one another in the posterior third of the body; the branched ovary lies to one side of the acetabulum, which is in the middle third of the body.

Other parasites of man that might be encountered in some areas include the spiny-collared worms of the echinostome group and *Gastrodiscoides hominis.*

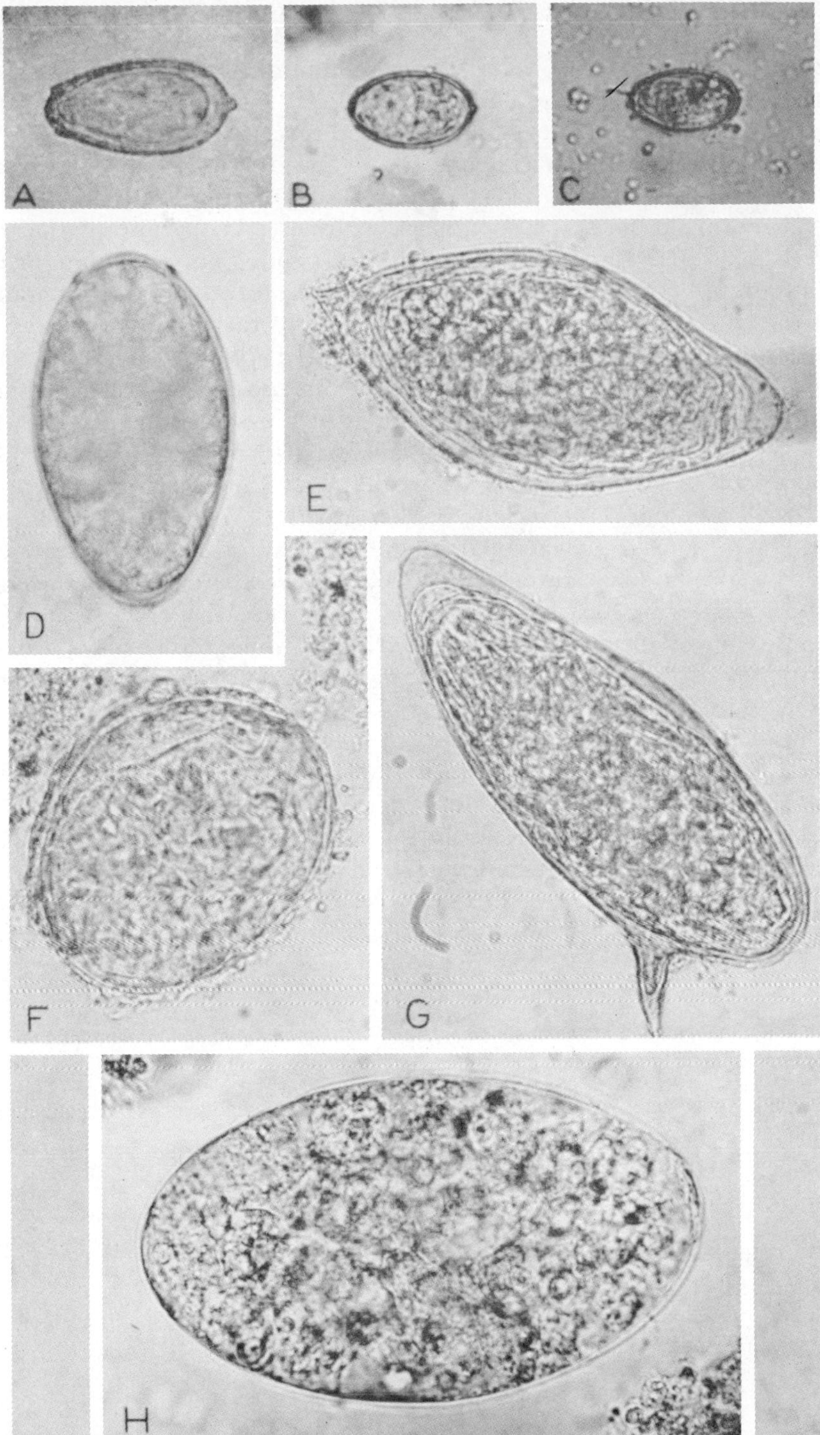

Figure 53–2. Some trematode eggs: *A,* Chinese liver fluke, *Clonorchis sinensis. B, Heterophyes heterophyes. C, Metagonimus yokogawai. D,* Lung fluke, *Paragonimus westermani. E,* Vesical blood fluke, *Schistosoma haematobium. F,* Oriental blood fluke, *Schistosoma japonicum. G,* Manson's blood fluke, *Schistosoma mansoni. H,* Large intestinal fluke, *Fasciolopsis buski.* All figures 500 × except *A,* which is 830 ×. (Fig. *A,* courtesy of Dr. E. C. Faust, in Brenemann: Practice of Pediatrics, W. F. Prior Co. Figs. *B* and *C* courtesy of Lt. L. W. Shatterly, MSC, School of Aviation Medicine, Gunter AFB, Alabama. All others courtesy of Dr. R. L. Roudabush, Ward's Natural Science Establishment, Rochester, New York; photos by T. Romaniak.)

GENERALIZED CYCLE

Oviposition. The trematodes mentioned above have similar life cycles. The eggs are liberated by the parasite at its definitive location in the host, and in most species the eggs are passed in the feces (except for those of *Paragonimus* spp. which are often coughed up into the sputum). All must reach water and, in the case of undeveloped eggs, must undergo a period of maturation before the miracidium hatches. Those that are embryonated when laid must be actually ingested by the appropriate snail before they hatch (i.e. species of *Clonorchis, Opisthorchis, Dicrocoelium, Heterophyes* and *Metagonimus*).

The Snail Host. Eggs or hatched miracidia must reach a specific snail host within a few hours if the parasites are to survive. This is accomplished either by the penetration of a susceptible species or by ingestion. In the tissues of this host the miracidium becomes transformed into a *mother sporocyst* which then produces a generation of *rediae* and, in some cases, *daughter rediae*. Finally, free-living *cercariae* develop and emerge; these, in turn, must reach a suitable plant or animal host if they are to survive. In the case of the schistosomes, the *mother sporocyst* produces long, slender *daughter sporocysts* which in turn liberate the fork-tailed, brevifurcate cercariae. In the case of *Dicrocoelium* spp., two generations of sporocysts are formed in the terrestrial snail host, from which single-tailed cercariae emerge.

The Resting or Metacercarial Stage. In the groups considered here all types of cercariae (except those of the schistosomes, p. 545) encyst on vegetation, or on or within the tissues of some aquatic animal (Fig. 53–3). The cercariae of *Dicrocoelium* spp. encyst in ants. Typically, encysting cercariae produce an inner cyst wall from secretions of their own cystogenous glands, which is soon surrounded by an outer cyst wall of host tissue. After varying intervals a reorganization or growth of these larvae leads to the formation of resting stages, or *metacercariae,* which soon are ready to infect man (Fig. 53–3).

The cercariae of *F. hepatica* seek various grasses, while those of *F. buski* encyst on water chestnuts, caltrops, hyacinths and the like. In the case of the liver flukes *Clonorchis* and *Opisthorchis* spp., and the intestinal flukes *H. heterophyes* and *M. yokogawai,* the cercariae seek certain species of fish, and most of them penetrate beneath their scales and reach the musculature before encysting. The cercariae of the lung fluke, *P. westermani,* enter freshwater crabs and crayfishes and encyst.

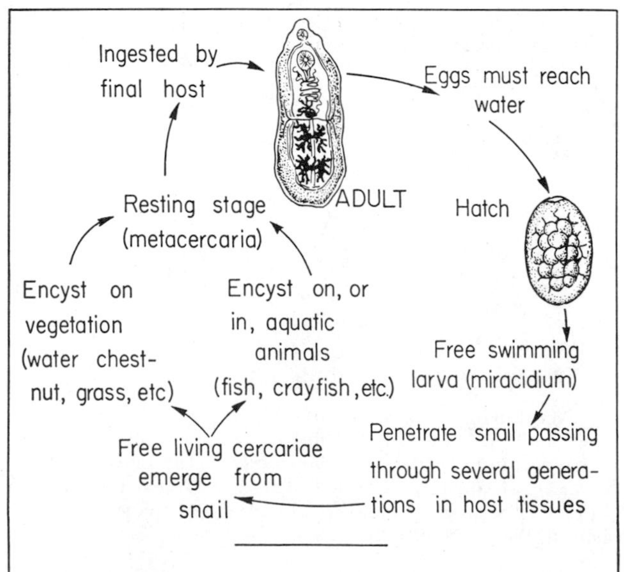

Figure 53–3. Life cycle of hermaphroditic trematodes.

Table 53–1. Reservoirs of the Intestinal, Liver and Lung Trematodes

Species of Trematode	*Hosts*	*Typical Location in Host*
Intestinal Flukes		
Fasciolopsis buski	Pigs, occasionally dogs, rabbits and man	Duodenum, jejunum
Echinostoma ilocanum	Dogs, rats, mice, and man	Small intestine
Echinochasmus perfoliatus	Dogs, cats, pigs, foxes and man	Small intestine
Heterophyes heterophyes	Cats, dogs, foxes, other piscivorous mammals and man	Small intestine
Metagonimus yokogawai	Piscivorous mammals, mice (experimental infection), pelicans and man	Small intestine
Gastrodiscoides hominis	Pigs, "mouse deer" (*Tragulus napu*), rats (*R. brevicaudatus*) and man	Cecum and colon
Liver Flukes		
Clonorchis sinensis	Dogs, cats and man	Biliary passages
Opisthorchis felineus	Dogs, cats, foxes, pigs, rats, martens, wolverines, beavers, rabbits, seals, probably others and man	Biliary and pancreatic passages
O. viverrini	Dogs, cats, civet cat, piscivorous mammals and man	Biliary passages
Fasciola hepatica	Sheep, cattle, wild rabbits, hares, other herbivorous and omnivorous mammals, and man	Liver and biliary passages
F. gigantica	Cattle, water buffalo, other herbivorous mammals and man	Biliary passages
Dicrocoelium dendriticum	Sheep, goats, deer, other herbivorous and omnivorous mammals and man	Biliary passages
Lung and Tissue Flukes		
Paragonimus westermani	Tigers, cattle, many crab- or crayfish-eating mammals and man	Lungs
P. kellicotti	Mink, many other crayfish-eating mammals and man	Lungs
P. ohirai	Brown rats, field voles, dogs, raccoons, badgers, weasels, pigs, wild boars and numerous experimental hosts	Lungs
P. iloktsuenensis	Brown rats, dogs, weasels and experimentally in white rats and mice	Lungs
P. miyazakii	Weasels, yellow martens, dogs, wild boars and experimentally in white and brown rats, cats, dogs and rabbits	Lungs
P. compactus	Mongooses, rusty spotted cats and fishing cats	Lungs
P. africanus	Mongooses (2 species), civet cats, dogs and man	Lungs
P. heterotremus (=*P. tuanshanensis*)	Cats, dogs, leopards and man; experimentally in monkeys and rabbits	Lungs and migratory swellings
P. harinasutai	Experimentally in cats and dogs	Lungs
P. mexicanus	Opossum and man	Lungs
P. siamensis	Rats (*R. rattus* and *R. berdmorei*), cats and bandicoots	Lungs
P. bangkokensis	Mongoose (*Herpestes javanicus*); experimentally in cats and bandicoot	Lungs
P. macrorchis	Rat and bandicoot (*Bandicota indica* and *B. bengalensis*)	Lungs
P. skrjabini (=*P. szechuanensis*)	*Paguma larvata*, cats, dogs and man	Lungs and subcutaneous nodules
Achillurbainia nouveli	Leopard, giant rat (*Rattus muelleri*) and man	Lungs and subcutaneous cysts

For data on other species of *Paragonimus* see Yokogawa, M. 1969. Adv. Parasit. 7:375–387.

The Final Host. In all cases, infection of man results from the ingestion of raw or inadequately cooked vegetation, fish or crustaceans which serve as the "transfer agents" or intermediate hosts for these parasites.

Location in Man. *Fasciolopsis buski, H. heterophyes, M. yokogawai* and *Echinostoma ilocanum* are intestinal parasites of man. *Clonorchis sinensis, F. hepatica, Opisthorchis* spp. and *Dicrocoelium dendriticum* localize in the biliary and pancreatic ducts; *P. westermani,* after migrating through the body, usually reaches the lung where it becomes encapsulated.

Many mammals other than man serve as reservoir hosts for the intestinal lung and liver flukes. The more important of these are summarized in Table 53–1.

Diseases Caused by Intestinal Trematodes

FASCIOLOPSIASIS

Synonym. *Fasciolopsis buski* infection.

Definition. Fasciolopsiasis is due to the presence of the giant intestinal fluke, *F. buski,* in the duodenum or jejunum, and more rarely in the pylorus or the colon of man. The parasites may produce local areas of inflammation and sometimes ulceration and hemorrhage.

Distribution. *Fasciolopsis buski* occurs commonly in pigs and man in many areas of eastern Asia, particularly in Central and South China.[1,2] The disease has also been found in Taiwan, Vietnam, Cambodia, Laos, Thailand, Burma, Assam, Bangladesh and much of the eastern half of India.[3-9]

Etiology. MORPHOLOGY. *Fasciolopsis buski* (Lankester, 1857) Odhner, 1902, the large intestinal fluke, is 50 to 75 mm long when extended. It is fleshy, often broadly ovate and possesses a spined integument. A cephalic cone such as occurs in the genus *Fasciola* is lacking, although the oral sucker and ventral sucker (acetabulum) are close together. The latter is about four times as large as the oral sucker and measures 2 to 3 mm in diameter. The intestinal ceca are unbranched; the dendritic testes lie in the posterior half of the body and are arranged in tandem. The small vitelline follicles extend from the acetabular region to the posterior tip (Fig. 53–4).

DEVELOPMENT. Although the adult parasite produces eggs ranging from 67 by 43 to 181 by 95 μm the majority are large eggs between 130 and 140 μm in length and 80 and 85 μm in breadth. These are undeveloped when passed and are capped by a small operculum. Upon reaching quiet fresh water the egg develops a miracidium in 3 to 7 weeks. After hatching, the miracidium must reach a snail of the genus *Hippeutis, Segmentina* or *Planorbis.*[3] It then transforms into a mother sporocyst; this, in turn, produces two generations of rediae. The daughter rediae produce free-living cercariae 30 to 50 days after the miracidium has penetrated the snail.

The cercariae encyst on almost any aquatic plant, although water caltrops, hyacinths, chestnuts and bamboos usually serve as "transfer hosts." As many as 1000 metacercariae have been found on a single nut or root. The metacercariae are very resistant and will survive for a year or more *if kept moist;* desiccation, however, soon destroys them. When an infected root or bulb is peeled and eaten, the metacercariae are ingested by the definitive hosts; the parasites excyst in the intestine and develop into mature flukes within 3 months.[1]

Epidemiology. Infection by *F. buski* results from the ingestion of viable metacercariae on the uncooked stems, bulbs or fruits of edible water plants. The more important plants and the areas where they are particularly prevalent appear in Table 53–2.

The red water caltrop, *Trapa natans,* is probably the most heavily infested, since it is cultivated for market in artificial ponds fertilized by nightsoil or by defecation directly into the water. The plants growing wild in the canals and rivers are less heavily infested. Both the water caltrops and water chestnuts are sold fresh in the markets during the summer months, and it is then that man becomes infected. It is a common practice to peel off the external covering with the teeth and eat the succulent inner parts raw. Many metacercarial cysts may be ingested in this way. In Thailand the following were found to be infested: the water caltrop, lotus, watercress *(Neptunia oleracea),* water "morning glory" *(Ipomoea aquatica)* and water hyacinth.[5] In Taiwan it is the caltrop, water

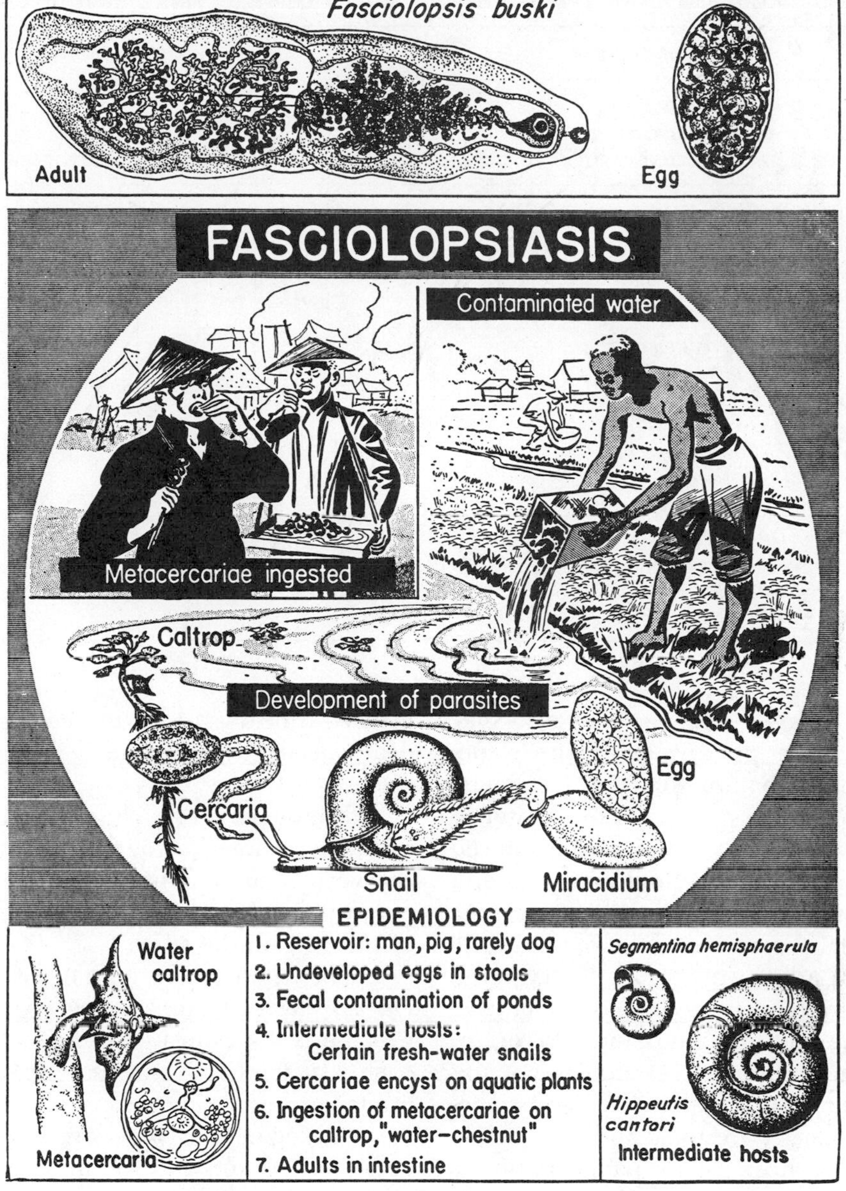

Figure 53–4. Epidemiology of fasciolopsiasis.

chestnut and a water plant, "Kung-shin-tsai" *(I. reptans).* The latter harbors the metacercariae of *F. buski* not only on its surface but also in its hollow stem.[4] (See Table 53–2.) Since desiccation destroys the parasites, only fresh plants are dangerous and infection is less frequent when these have been allowed to dry. However, in the markets, vendors of caltrops and nuts often maintain the freshness of their wares by sprinkling them with water, a custom which prevents the drying of the cysts (Fig. 53–4).

There are several different species of snails that serve as first intermediate hosts for *F. buski.* The principal snail hosts are *Segmentina hemisphaerula, S. trochoideus, Hippeutis cantori, Gyraulus convexiusculus* and *Planorbis* species.

Pathology. The parasites are usually attached to the mucosa of the duodenum or

Table 53–2. Some Species of Plants Carrying Fasciolopsis Buski: Listed by Countries

Species of Plant	*Country*			
Key x–proven carrier s–suspected carrier	China	India	Taiwan	Thailand
Red water caltrop—*Trapa natans*	x	x		
Water caltrop—*T. bicornis*				x
Water caltrop—*T. bispinosa*			x	
Lotus—*Nymphaea lotus*		s		x
Indian lotus—*Nelumbo nucifera*		x		
Water chestnut—*Eliocharis tuberosa*	x		x	
Watercress—*Neptunia oleracea*				x
Water morning glory—*Ipomoea aquatica*				x
"Kung-shin-tsai"—*I. reptans*			x	
Water hyacinth—*Eichhornia speciosa*				x
—*Euryale feroy*		s		
—*Ottelia alismoides*		s		
Water bamboo—*Zizania aquatica*	x			
—*Salvinia natans*	x			
—*Lemna polyrhiza*	x			
Water hyacinth—*Eichhornia crassipes*	x			

jejunum; in heavy infections they also may be found in the pylorus or in the colon. Localized inflammation followed frequently by ulceration occurs at the site of attachment, and when deep erosions are produced hemorrhage may occur. Intestinal stasis and obstruction may occur, especially when large numbers of worms are involved. Several thousands of adult worms may be harbored by a patient. In severe cases among children, edema of the face and trunk may also occur. The mechanism of this reaction is not understood, but it is probable that the metabolites of the worms are toxic and may be absorbed by the host. Many patients show a leukocytosis with an eosinophilia up to 34 per cent; in others there may be a lymphocytosis.

Clinical Characteristics. Light infections may be asymptomatic, or there may be diarrhea and abdominal pain which may simulate duodenal ulcer. The diarrhea often alternates with periods of constipation. Later the stools become greenish yellow and contain much undigested food. Ascites, anorexia, nausea and vomiting may occur in severe infections. In the final stage of the disease, edema of the face, abdominal wall or lower extremities, described above, usually appears. The skin becomes dry, and death occurs from cachexia or intercurrent disease.

Diagnosis. The clinical picture is not distinctive; hence, diagnosis depends upon recovery and identification of the adult worm passed in the feces or demonstration of the eggs in the stool.

The adult worm may be confused with *Fasciola hepatica* and *Fasciola gigantica* from which it is distinguished by lack of a cephalic cone, suckers of unequal size and unbranched intestinal crura.

The eggs of *F. buski* are large, ranging between 130 and 140 μm in length by 80 to 85 μm in breadth. They are unembryonated when laid and may be differentiated with difficulty from the eggs of *Fasciola hepatica* by means of the smaller operculum on the former. Eggs of *F. buski* can usually be distinguished from those of *Fasciola gigantica* as the eggs of the latter are longer, ranging from 160 to 190 μm in length. Most other operculate eggs found in the stool are smaller than those of *F. buski.*

Treatment. The drug of choice in the treatment of fasciolopsiasis is hexylresorcinol (Crystoids anthelmintic). A dose of 0.4 gm is given if the patient is under 7 years of age, 1 gm if older. (For precautions, see p. 470.) Tetrachloroethylene is also effective; a saline purge should be given 2 hours after treatment. (See p. 480.)

Prophylaxis. Prophylaxis is based upon two measures: (1) the proper cooking of all roots and "nuts" which might serve as possible "transfer agents" for *F. buski;* (2) education of foreigners to avoid sampling uncooked native dishes.

Other measures include sufficiently prolonged storage of nightsoil to insure the destruction of eggs, and the education of natives in the proper location and use of privies.

HETEROPHYIASIS

Definition. Heterophyiasis is an infection by the minute intestinal fluke, *Heterophyes heterophyes* (v. Siebold, 1852) Stiles and Hassall, 1900, in the small intestine of man.

Distribution. It is common in the Nile Delta and in Japan, southern Korea, Taiwan, central and south China, the Philippines and western India.

Etiology and Epidemiology. The parasites are small, spinose and less than 2 mm in length. The adult has a large genital sucker almost equal to and contiguous with the acetabulum. The eggs are embryonated when laid; they hatch after being ingested by the snail host. In Egypt the snail host is *Pirenella conica;* in Japan it is *Cerithidea cingula alata.* Cercariae emerging from the snail encyst in fresh- or brackish water mullets. Infection occurs when fish containing viable metacercariae are eaten raw, salted or pickled in brine.

A second species, *Heterophyes katsuradai* (Ozaki and Asada, 1925), has been recovered from patients suffering from diarrhea in Japan. The parasite is distinguished from *H. heterophyes* by its relatively enormous acetabulum. The eggs are slightly smaller, measuring 25 or 26 by 14 or 15 μm. Transmission occurs by the eating of infected raw mullet flesh.

A third species, *Heterophyes brevicaeca* (Africa and Garcia, 1935), was reported from man in the Philippines.

Pathology. They live attached to the mucosa of the small intestine where they may produce a mild irritation or a superficial necrosis of the mucosa. Eggs may be deposited in the tissues, and because of their minute size may be carried by the blood stream to other areas, especially the brain, the spinal cord and the heart muscle. Severe and fatal heart lesions may be caused by the eggs of these flukes. In the Philippines it has been estimated that over 14 per cent of cardiac deaths resulted from heterophyid myocarditis.[10]

Clinical Characteristics. Symptoms include abdominal pain frequently associated with mucous diarrhea. When eggs are distributed by the blood stream, serious clinical disease may result, with evidence of organic changes in the central nervous system and often cardiac insufficiency.

Diagnosis. Diagnosis is based upon the recovery from the stool of characteristic eggs, which are difficult to differentiate from those of other heterophyid trematodes (Fig. 53–2). They are small, operculate, ovoid, light brown in color, are not markedly "shouldered," and average 29 by 16 μm.

Treatment. Tetrachloroethylene, as employed for hookworm, is effective (p. 480); or treat as for fasciolopsiasis with hexylresorcinol (Crystoids anthelmintic). A single dose of bephenium hydroxynaphthoate also is quite effective (p. 480).

METAGONIMIASIS

Metagonimiasis is caused by the presence of a small trematode, *Metagonimus yokogawai* Katsurada, 1912, attached to the intestinal mucosa of man. Other piscivorous animals and even pelicans may serve as reservoir hosts. It is believed to be the most common heterophyid fluke of man in the Far East, being endemic in parts of China, Japan, the Maritime Provinces of the U.S.S.R. and the northern provinces in Siberia. It also occurs in man in Spain and various Balkan states. The parasite is small, usually less than 3 mm in length, and resembles *H. heterophyes* in size and shape, but differs in morphologic details. These embryonated eggs are virtually indistinguishable from those of *Heterophyes heterophyes* and measure 26 to 28 μm by 15.5 to 17 μm (Fig. 53–2). They may be ingested by several species of snails, such as *Thiara granifera* and *Semisulcospira libertina.* Infection is acquired when the flesh of improperly cooked Oriental freshwater trout or other infected freshwater fish is ingested.

Pathology. These flukes may actually invade the intestinal mucosa at the duodenal and jejunal levels causing granulomatous infiltration, inflammation and occasionally ulceration; they ultimately become encapsulated. Rarely, eggs deposited in the tissues may be carried by the blood stream and deposited in other regions.

Clinical Characteristics. Infection by this parasite usually causes few symptoms. In heavy infections, however, especially when eggs have lodged in other tissues, serious disease may result. The clinical picture in such instances will vary in accordance with the distribution and severity of the pathologic changes.

Diagnosis. The diagnosis is based upon the recovery from feces of characteristic eggs, which resemble those of *C. sinensis* in shape but are almost indistinguishable from the eggs of *H. heterophyes.*

Treatment. Treat with tetrachloroethylene, as for hookworm (p. 480), or hexylresorcinol (Crystoids anthelmintic) (p. 576). Kamala has been used in mass therapy.

ECHINOSTOMIASIS

Echinostomiasis is a general term applied to infection by several related genera and species of spiny-collared flukes which parasitize man. Their distribution is limited to the Philippines, Indonesia, Assam, Japan, Malaysia, Sumatra, India, Thailand, Taiwan, China, Rumania and U.S.S.R.

Among the species reported from man, *Echinostoma ilocanum* from the Philippines, Java and Canton, China, and *Echinochasmus perfoliatus* from Japan are the more important. Although varying in size and morphologic details, all members of the group are slender and flattened, the majority being less than 25 mm long. Identification is based on morphologic characteristics, especially the size of the eggs and the arrangement and number of spines composing the collar. Infection is acquired by eating raw or improperly cooked freshwater snails and clams containing encysted metacercariae; these snails belong to such genera as *Pila* and *Viviparus,* and the clams belong to the genus *Corbicula.* (See Table 66–1, p. 670.) Recent surveys in the Lake Lindu area of Sulawesi (Celebes) indicate the disappearance of infections of *Echinostoma lindoensis* in man. This is partly due to changes in the food habits of the population who are now eating a recently introduced fish, *Tilapia mossambica,* and partly due to the present scarcity of the clams.[11]

Pathology. The echinostomes are found attached to the mucosa of the small intestine and their presence ordinarily does not appear to be associated with marked pathologic changes. Heavy infections, however, may be accompanied by abdominal pain and diarrhea.

Diagnosis. Diagnosis depends upon demonstration of the eggs in stools from the infected individual. Echinostome infections may be differentiated from fascioliasis and fasciolopsiasis by the smaller size of the egg.

Treatment. The following drugs have been recommended for the treatment of echinostomiasis: oleoresin of aspidium, tetrachloroethylene, and hexylresorcinol (Crystoids anthelmintic) (pp. 470, 576).

GASTRODISCIASIS

Gastrodisciasis is an infection by the trematode *Gastrodiscoides hominis* (Lewis and McConnel, 1876) Leiper, 1913 in the cecum and ascending colon of man. It has been reported from man in Assam, Indochina, India and Malaysia. Pigs are reservoir hosts in Assam and India, while deer *(Tragulus napu)* serve in this capacity in Malaysia.

Clinical Characteristics. Infection of man by this parasite is associated with diarrhea, but other details of the clinical picture are unknown.

Diagnosis. The parasite may be identified readily by its pyriform shape, reddish orange color and the huge acetabulum which occupies the ventral posterior portion of the worm. The acetabulum bears a characteristic notch at its posterior extremity. Parasites range from 5 to 14 mm in length and have a conical anterior portion about 2 mm in length. The eggs are ovoidal, immature when passed and measure about 150 by 65 μm in length and breadth, respectively.

Treatment. Treat with tetrachloroethylene (p. 480) or hexylresorcinol (Crystoids anthelmintic) (pp. 470, 576).

Diseases Caused by Liver Flukes

CLONORCHIASIS

Synonym. Chinese liver fluke disease.

Definition. Clonorchiasis is caused by the presence of the Oriental liver fluke, *Clonorchis sinensis,* in the biliary passages. It may be associated with proliferation of the biliary epithelium, connective tissue hyperplasia and, in severe cases, fatty degeneration and cirrhosis of the liver.

Distribution. This fluke occurs in the Far East as a common parasite of fish-eating mammals. The highly endemic regions of human infection are Japan, Korea, China and Vietnam. Clonorchiasis is especially important in Okayama, Niigata and Miyagi Prefectures in Japan,[12] South Korea,[13] Kwantung Province of South China, Hong Kong,[14] North Vietnam and Taiwan.[15] Infection by this parasite has also been recorded in Chinese inhabitants of the United States, Cuba and India and in native Hawaiians.

Etiology. MORPHOLOGY. *Clonorchis sinensis* (Cobbold, 1875) Looss, 1907 is a slender, attenuated trematode ranging from 10 to 25 mm in length and 3 to 5 mm in breadth. The oral sucker is clearly larger than the acetabulum. Unstained specimens of *Clonorchis sinensis* placed between two slides and held to a strong light reveal the characteristic deeply lobulated testes lying in tandem in the posterior third of the worm. Anterior to the testes is the ovarian complex; the uterine mass, typically appearing brown owing to the presence of numerous eggs, fills the middle third of the worm. Laterally in the same region lie the vitellaria.

DEVELOPMENT. The operculate eggs of *C. sinensis* contain fully developed miracidia and are among the smallest passed by man. The eggs are 27 to 35 μm in length by 12 to 19.5 μm in breadth (averaging 29 by 16 μm); they are light brown in color and ovoid in shape. The edge of the convex operculum or lid fits down into a swollen lip which surrounds the lid, this portion of the shell being markedly "shouldered." There is also a definite knob or boss at the anopercular end.

The eggs, laid in the smaller bile passages, are carried down the common bile duct to the duodenum and pass in the stools. The eggs must reach water and are believed to hatch when ingested by appropriate species of snails: *Parafossarulus manchouricus* (= *P. striatulus*), *P. manchouricus* var. *sinensis*, *Bulimus fuchsianus*, *Alocinma longicornis* (= *Bithynia longicornis*) and *Hua ningpoensis*. Development within the snail requires 4 to 5 weeks and includes the production of mother sporocysts, followed by a generation of rediae. At the end of this interval typical lophocercous (tail with finfolds) cercariae break out of the rediae and emerge from the snail. These cercariae penetrate beneath the scales and into the musculature of freshwater fish, where, after a developmental period of several weeks, they produce cysts that are infective for the definitive host.

After ingestion by man or other suitable mammalian hosts the cysts in the fish muscle are digested, and the contained parasites are released in the duodenum where they become attached to the mucosa. They soon migrate to the smaller biliary radicles, especially those of the left lobe of the liver where they mature.[16] The entire cycle requires approximately 3 months.

Epidemiology. *Clonorchis sinensis* is found principally in the bile passages of dogs, cats, minks, rats and man, although other fish-eating mammals may be infected. The infective or metacercarial stage occurs in the musculature of over 40 species of freshwater fish belonging to the CYPRINIDAE, GOBIIDAE, ANABANTIDAE, OSMERIDAE[12] and SALMONIDAE. Fish ponds or canals in China are often the chief source of human infection. These pondlike areas are filled with water much of the time and, consequently, afford ideal habitats for snails and fish serving as intermediate hosts for this parasite. Man acquires the infection from the ingestion of raw, inadequately cooked, or even dried, salted or pickled flesh of infected freshwater fish (Fig. 53–5).

It appears likely that Hawaiians become infected through shipments of infected frozen, dried or pickled fish from China or Japan.

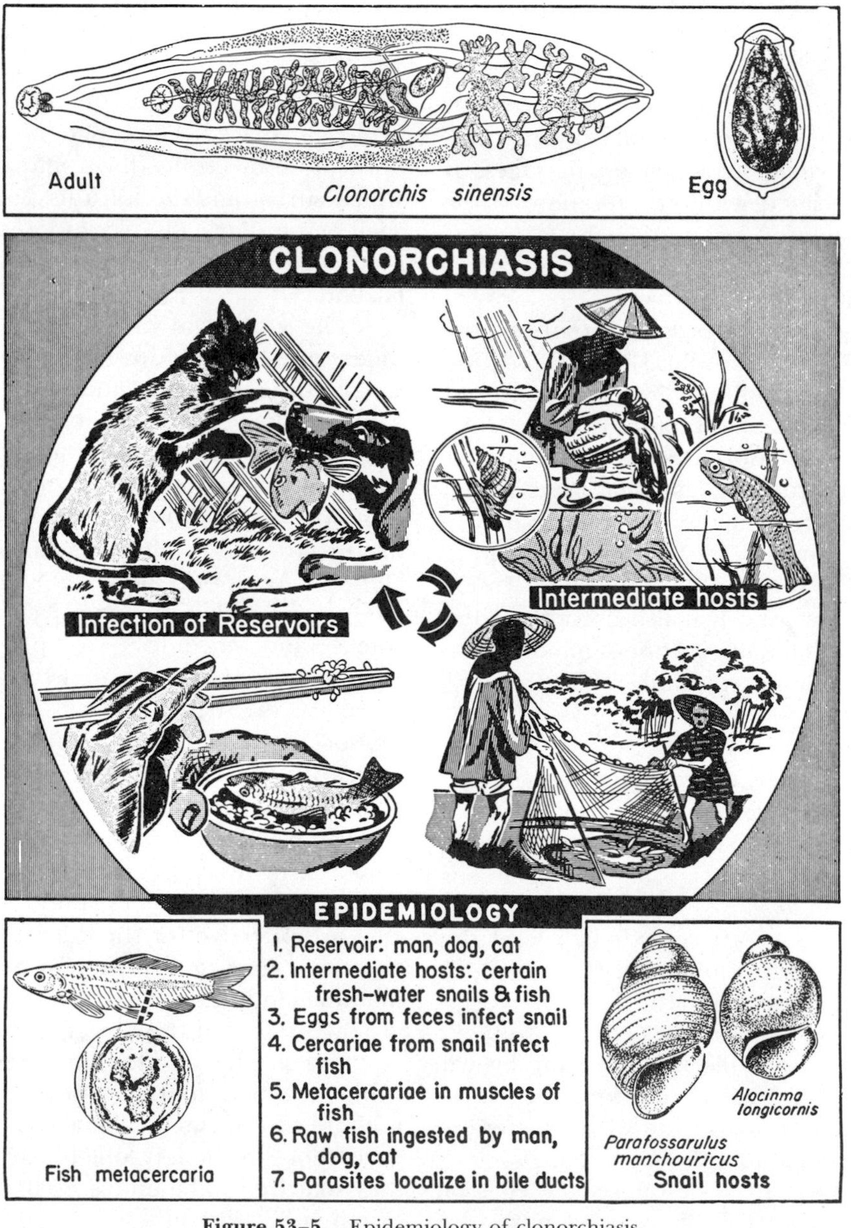

Figure 53–5. Epidemiology of clonorchiasis.

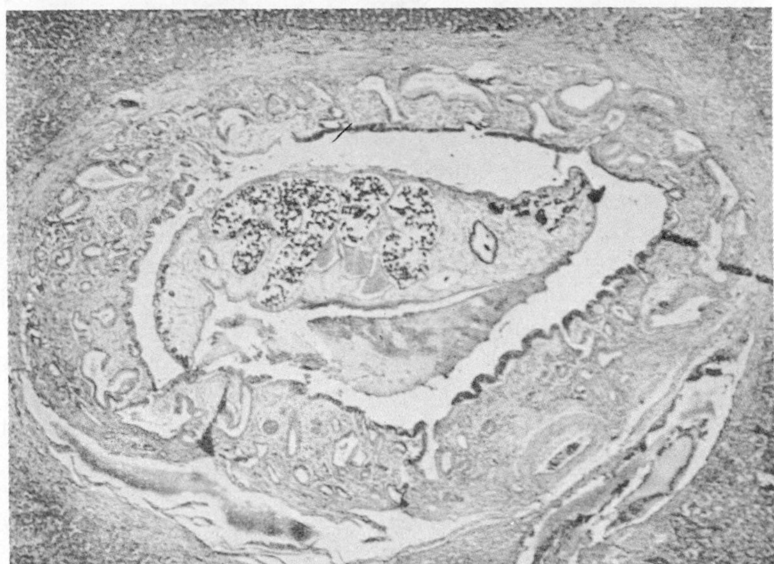

Figure 53–6. *Clonorchis sinensis* in dilated biliary duct: adult with eggs in uterus.

Pathology. Adult *C. sinensis* tend to localize in the distal bile passages, especially those of the left lobe of the liver. One result of infection is proliferation, sometimes desquamation, of the biliary epithelium, while in the larger ducts progressive dilatation, thickening of the wall and crypt formation occur. It is believed by some workers that toxic secretions of the parasite may be responsible for some of the pathologic changes that are found in ducts too small for the worm to penetrate. Liver damage, however, depends upon the number of parasites present, the age of the infection and the number of reinfections that have occurred. In endemic areas surprisingly large numbers of parasites have been found at autopsy, as many as 21,000 having been recovered from a single individual.

Frank cirrhosis is rare, although increase of periportal tissue in varying degree and infiltration with eosinophils often occur. In the parenchyma fatty changes in the liver cells and atrophy of cells in the center of the lobule are not unusual. Even in light infections significant histologic changes are usually present in the liver (Fig. 53–6).

Clinical Characteristics. Three typical stages in the development of clonorchiasis are recognized. (1) Early manifestations of the disease are fever, eosinophilia, leukocytosis and epigastric pain. (2) The second stage is characterized by diarrhea and progressive hepatomegaly; anorexia, prolonged low-grade fever, episodes of jaundice and tenderness over the liver also may be present. (3) The most advanced cases are associated with cirrhosis of the liver, ascites, anasarca, cachexia and, occasionally, extreme jaundice.

It should be borne in mind, however, that in endemic areas the majority of infected individuals harbor few worms and do not show significant symptoms.

Prognosis is good in cases of light infections. Patients rarely die from this disease alone; death, however, may occur in heavy infections of long standing when the parasites have caused serious impairment of liver function.

Diagnosis. Diagnosis depends upon the detection of the characteristic eggs in the feces, or in bile or fluid obtained by a duodenal intubation. Differentiation from eggs of closely related heterophyid flukes, especially those of *M. yokogawai* and *H. heterophyes,* is necessary. Eggs of *M. yokogawai* are yellowish in color and lighter than those of *H. heterophyes,* the lighter color being due to the thinner shell. The eggs of *C. sinensis* become narrower toward the operculate end and the shell is more distinctly "shouldered" where the operculum occurs (Fig. 53–2). Eggs of *Opisthorchis felineus* are elongate, ovoidal and about three times as long as broad. Adults must be distinguished from the broader, heavier, more ovate members of the *Fasciola* group. At autopsy the bile ducts should be examined carefully for the presence of this and other parasites of the biliary passages and liver proper.

It is necessary to differentiate infections caused by liver flukes from other types of hepatic disease, such as amebic abscess of the liver, cancer, hydatid disease and nutritional disorders like beriberi.

Treatment. Hetol at a dosage of 50 mg per kg daily for 5 to 12 days depending upon the severity of infection appears to be safe and effective for treatment of clonorchiasis.[17, 18] Dehydroemetine, in late-release tablets, was effective at the high dosage of 2.5 mg per kg every other day for 25 to 30 medication days. Side reactions including diarrhea, dizziness and weakness were observed; however, dehydroemetine was considered well tolerated and safe even in clinically serious cases.[18] Niclofolan (Bayer 9015) administered orally at a dose of 1.0 to 2.0 mg per kg for 2 or 3 days was highly effective; side effects noted were weakness and neuralgia in the sacral region and extremities.[18]

Prophylaxis. The prevention of clonorchiasis in persons residing in an endemic area can be accomplished effectively by insistence upon the thorough cooking of all freshwater fish. Foreigners should be discouraged from sampling native dishes. Other measures include the storage and treatment of nightsoil with ammonium sulfate and the education of the population to the use of privies.

OPISTHORCHIASIS

This disease is due to the presence of the trematode *Opisthorchis felineus* (Rudolphi, 1819) Blanchard, 1895, *O. viverrini* (Poirier, 1886) Stiles and Hassall, 1896, or other species in the bile ducts of man.

Distribution. *Opisthorchis felineus* occurs in many species of piscivorous mammals and man in central, eastern and southeastern Europe and the Ukraine[20] as well as regions east of the Urals and in the West Siberian Lowlands of the U.S.S.R.; there, up to 64 per cent of the people and 87 per cent of the carp were reported to be infected.[21] Infections have been reported from Japan and India but are not apparently autochthonous. *Opisthorchis viverrini* is the dominant liver fluke of man in Thailand and occurs in the north and northeastern portions of the country, where the average prevalence was 61.5 per cent and the highest 92 per cent.[6, 23, 24] *Opisthorchis viverrini* also occurs in Laos, West Malaysia and probably in other Far Eastern countries.

Etiology. MORPHOLOGY. *Opisthorchis felineus* resembles *O. viverrini* and *C. sinensis* in general shape and arrangement of the organ systems. It is a slender worm, tapering anteriorly and rounded posteriorly. The oral sucker and acetabulum are about of equal size, whereas in *C. sinensis* the oral sucker is larger. In *O. felineus* the testes are lobate and arranged obliquely; in *C. sinensis* they are more deeply lobed and are arranged in tandem. The small, elongate, ovoidal eggs are roughly three times as long as broad (about 30 by 11 μm) and contain a miracidium when the egg is laid. The operculum fits into a thickened rim of the shell; eggs may be distinguished from those of *C. sinensis* by their smaller diameter and less pronounced shouldering at the margin of the operculum. Adult specimens of *O. viverrini* resemble those of *O. felineus* in morphology, except for the testes which are more notched than those of *O. felineus*. However, the eggs of *O. viverrini* average 28 by 15 μm and resemble those of *C. sinensis* more than those of *O. felineus*.

Epidemiology. The eggs of *O. felineus* are believed to be ingested by the snail *Bulimus* (= *Bithynia*) *leachii*, where they hatch and develop, producing lophocercous cercariae in about 2 months. These penetrate several freshwater cyprinoid fish, which after a suitable developmental period for the metacercariae are infective for man and other hosts when their raw infected flesh is ingested.

In Thailand it has been demonstrated that *Bithynia goniomphalus* and two closely related species are the first intermediate hosts. Three species of freshwater fish serve as the most important second host: *Cyclocheilicthus siaja, Hampala dispar* and *Puntius orphoides.* These are all eaten in "Koi-Pla," which is made of raw fish, rice, vegetables and spices.[22,23] In West Malaysia the snail host is *Melanoides tuberculata,* while the grass carp, *Ctenopharyngodon dellus,* serves as a piscine host that is also served raw in several native dishes.[24]

Another species of *Opisthorchis* has been reported in natives of New Guinea. A related species occurs in man in Ecuador and also in reservoir hosts in the United States, Ecuador, Panama and parts of Brazil.[25]

Pathology and Clinical Aspects. The pathology and clinical aspects of opisthorchiasis are not thoroughly understood, although in general they resemble those of clonorchiasis. The degree of damage to the liver and bile ducts depends upon the mass and duration of the infection. Local injury may be expected in the distal bile capillaries and surrounding liver tissue when large numbers (several hundred) are present. In severe infections and in heavy and long continued reinfection, cirrhosis of the liver with areas of necrosis and fatty degeneration, jaundice and congestion of the spleen are not uncommon. In such cases invasion of the pancreas may occur. In addition, some cases present with cachexia, edema, malnutrition and ascites. However, these may be attributable to mixed infections with other parasites.[23]

In mild infections many patients are asymptomatic while those with moderate infections report flatulent dyspepsia, pain over the liver, diarrhea with three to four bowel movements a day, hepatomegaly and sometimes jaundice and fever. It is probable that some of these symptoms also are due to mixed infections and malnutrition.[26]

Diagnosis. See methods employed for clonorchiasis (p. 581).

Treatment. Oral dehydroemetine, 1.5 mg per kg daily, in 3 divided doses, for 10 days is moderately effective. Higher doses showed a greater effect on egg reduction but side effects were high.[19]

FASCIOLIASIS

Synonyms. Fascioliasis hepatica, "liver rot," or sheep liver fluke disease.

Definition. Fascioliasis is a disease caused by the presence of the sheep liver fluke, *Fasciola hepatica,* in the bile ducts or liver parenchyma. The disease is characterized by hyperplasia of the biliary epithelium, dilatation of biliary passages, leukocytic infiltration and periductal fibrosis. It is essentially a disease of sheep in which it produces "liver rot." Man is occasionally infected.

Distribution. *Fasciola hepatica* is widely distributed in sheep throughout the world wherever the proper snail host is present.

Etiology. MORPHOLOGY. *Fasciola hepatica* Linnaeus, 1758 is a large, brownish, flat fluke up to 30 mm in length and 13 mm in breadth. The integument of the anterior portion of the worm is covered with scalelike spines. A cephalic cone extends 4 to 5 mm anteriorly beyond the ovoid body proper. Oral and ventral suckers 1 and 1.6 mm in diameter lie at the distal and basal portions of the cone, respectively. Nearly all organs, especially the testes, vitellaria, ovary and the two main intestinal crura, are highly branched and permeate the entire body parenchyma. In adult specimens the uterus, which is confined to the anterior third of the worm, is filled with large operculate eggs usually a light brown color, ranging between 130 and 150 μm in length and 63 to 90 μm in breadth; they are undeveloped when deposited.

DEVELOPMENT. The eggs, which must reach water after leaving the host, require a developmental period of 9 to 15 days. Undeveloped eggs remain viable in moist feces up to 9 months. Upon hatching, the ciliated miracidia may attack various species of lymnaeid snails. Penetration of the snail is a combination of adhesion by the suctorial action of the anterior papilla, other mechanical activities, and the digestion (cytolysis) of the epithelial and subepithelial cells of the snail by the liberation of enzymes at the anterior tip of the miracidium. The ciliated epithelium of the miracidium is shed at the moment of penetration; thus, it is the mother sporocyst that finally gains entry into the snail. The next generations are known as rediae and daughter rediae, respectively. The latter produce free-living cercariae which emerge from the snail about 30 days after penetration by the miracidium and encyst upon aquatic vegetation or debris, or even free in shallow water, until they become metacercariae. In the absence of freezing or desiccation, the cysts remain viable for months.

Upon ingestion by the final host the parasites excyst in the intestine and migrate through the intestinal wall. Some reach the liver by the hepatic portal circulation; others pass into the peritoneal cavity and penetrate the liver capsule, ultimately reaching the bile ducts where they mature. Adult parasites have survived 3 years in rabbits and at least 5 years in sheep.

Epidemiology. Numerous ruminants, especially sheep, goats, cattle, horses and camels, as well as some carnivores, such as dogs, may harbor the adult *F. hepatica.* Numerous snails, mainly amphibious but also aquatic, including species of *Lymnaea* of the subgenera *Lymnaea, Stagnicola, Pseudosuccinea* and *Fossaria,* serve as intermediate molluscan hosts. The infective, or metacercarial, stage is so readily acquired in endemic areas through the ingestion of vegetation, such as watercress, and possibly water containing the cysts, that infections of many host species including man occur. Human fascioliasis infections often manifest themselves in the form of epidemics in many parts of the world where infections among sheep and cattle are prevalent.

Fascioliasis is geographically widespread. The parasite does not require large bodies of water for its development. Consequently, pasture lands with small or temporary ponds and sluggish brooks are a frequent source of infection.

Pathology. Infection of sheep by *F. hepatica* is characterized by extensive liver damage. Fascioliasis of man is usually a mild disease, although in the rare case of heavy infection the biliary passages are the site of hyperplasia, necrosis and cystic dilatation accompanied by leukocytic infiltration. Also, on rare occasions, the adult worms may occlude the common bile duct. The young larvae usually enter the liver from the peritoneal cavity by penetration of the capsule. In subsequent migrations they destroy liver parenchyma and produce more or less extensive necrosis and fibrosis. In very heavy infections the parasites may wander back

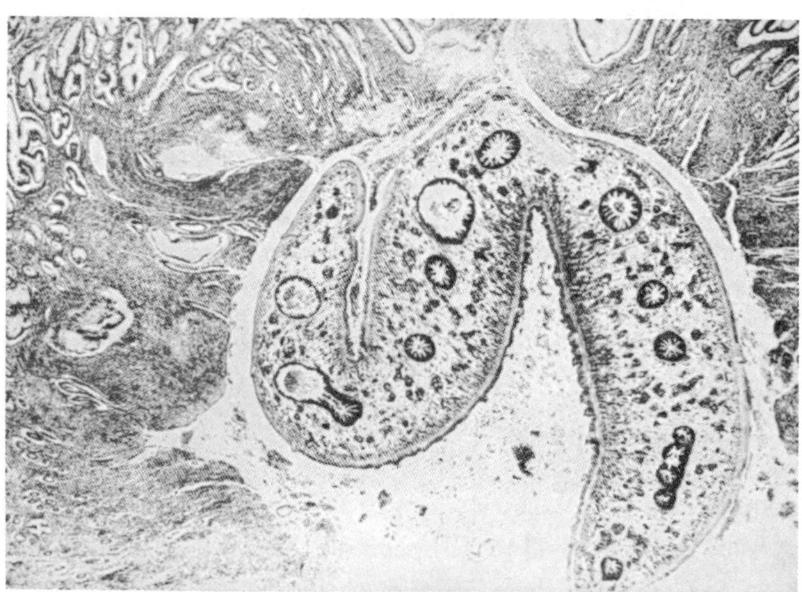

Figure 53–7. *Fasciola hepatica* in biliary duct – note marked proliferation of bile epithelium.

into the liver parenchyma to deposit their eggs, causing additional liver damage and fibrosis. Eosinophilia as high as 68 per cent has been recorded (Fig. 53–7). Ectopic human fascioliasis is of common occurrence and is of significance both pathologically and clinically.

Clinical Characteristics. The symptoms include vomiting, coughing and generalized abdominal pain. Occasionally, jaundice, urticaria, myalgia, myocardial episodes, lymphadenitis, diarrhea and fever are present. Frequently there is hepatosplenomegaly, eosinophilia and dysproteinemia.[27] A pharyngeal type of fascioliasis (halzoun) is known among the peoples of Lebanon, owing to the ingestion of infected raw livers of goats and sheep. In such cases the worms often are lodged on the mucosa of the pharynx. These exotic infections result in dyspnea, dysphagia or deafness.

Diagnosis. Diagnosis depends upon finding the large operculate eggs, 130 to 150 μm in length, in the feces or in material obtained by duodenal or biliary drainage; the eggs must be differentiated from those of *Fasciolopsis buski,* which they closely resemble. False diagnoses may be made in areas where infected livers are eaten raw. In such instances, eggs from these livers appear in the stools after passing through the intestinal tract. A differential diagnosis can be made by placing the patient on a liver-free diet for a few days. If eggs continue to be passed, the infection is genuine. *Fasciola hepatica* antigen is reported to give a specific intradermal reaction for this infection and a negative reaction with *Onchocerca volvulus* and *Taenia saginata* infections. Precipitin reactions appear to be more specific.

Infections by *F. hepatica* must be differentiated from those caused by other worms (both liver and intestinal) as well as other liver ailments accompanied by jaundice and hepatomegaly. Eosinophilia is suggestive.

The liver and its ducts should be examined carefully post mortem for the presence of this and other liver-inhabiting parasites.

Treatment. Injections of dehydroemetine have been recommended using 1 mg per kg daily intramuscularly for 10 days.[28] Emetine may also be administered giving 20 to 65 mg daily intramuscularly for 8 to 10 days. Bithionol has also been used with a regimen of 30 to 50 mg per kg on alternate days for 10 to 15 doses.[28] Because of the toxicity of emetine compounds patients should have electrocardiographic monitoring.

Prophylaxis. Drainage of pastures and perhaps the elimination of the snail host through the use of derris, copper sulfate or other molluscicides may control this disease in limited areas. The molluscicide Frescon has proved to be effective against the amphibious lymnaeid snails in several European countries (p. 672). In endemic rural areas the use of watercress should be avoided. In regions where sheep livers are eaten they should be thoroughly cooked before being consumed.

FASCIOLIASIS GIGANTICA AND MAGNA

Fascioliasis gigantica is caused by the presence of the giant liver fluke *Fasciola gigantica* Cobbold, 1856 in the liver tissues and ducts of man. Human infections have been reported occasionally from Africa and Asia. The fluke is more lanceolate and has a shorter cephalic cone, a larger acetabulum and a more anterior location of the testes than *F. hepatica.* The eggs range from 160 to 190 μm in length and from 70 to 90 μm in breadth. The snail intermediate host in Africa is *Lymnaea natalensis* and in Asia it is *L. auricularia rufescens* and *L. acuminata.* The biologic and pathologic picture is similar to that described for *F. hepatica;* patients develop fever, eosinophilia, hepatomegaly and have a raised erythrocyte sedimentation rate.[29] Treat as for *F. hepatica* infections.

Fascioloides magna, the giant liver fluke of deer, cattle and other herbivores in northern Europe and North America, has not been reported from man.

DICROCOELIASIS

Dicrocoeliasis is due to the presence of *Dicrocoelium dendriticum* (Rudolphi, 1818)

Looss, 1899 in the biliary passages of man, a condition which may be confused with fascioliasis. The small, fully embryonated, thick-shelled eggs are 38 to 45 μm in length by 22 to 30 μm in breadth. They are ingested by various species of land snails in which the eggs hatch and develop. Cercariae are released from the snail in slime balls; these are eaten by ants in which the cercariae develop into metacercariae. The parasites mature following ingestion of the ant by herbivorous definitive hosts. Spurious infections due to the consumption of infected livers have been reported; however, genuine human cases have been diagnosed from Africa, Asia and Europe. No treatment appears to be satisfactory. It is suggested that this infection be treated as for *C. sinensis.* (See p. 582.) Studies in animals infected with *D. lanceolatum* suggest that Stibophen, thiabendazole and Hetolin merit attention for human dicrocoeliasis.

Diseases Caused by Lung Flukes

PARAGONIMIASIS WESTERMANI

Synonyms. Pulmonary distomiasis; endemic hemoptysis; Oriental lung fluke disease.

Definition. Paragonimiasis is a disease of man caused by the presence of the Oriental lung fluke, *Paragonimus westermani,* and other species, encapsulated in the parenchyma of the lung.

Distribution. The human species of *Paragonimus* are widely distributed, being present in Africa, Asia, the Far East, Mexico, Central and South America. (See Table 53-3, which also lists the important foci of human infection.)

Etiology. MORPHOLOGY OF PARAGONIMUS WESTERMANI. *Paragonimus westermani* (Kerbert, 1878) Braun, 1899 is a plump, ovoid fluke lacking definitely attenuated extremities. In life it is reddish brown in color and 7 to 12 mm in length by 4 to 7 mm in breadth. Microscopic, scalelike integumental spines are present. The two, approximately equal, well defined suckers are about 0.8 mm in diameter, the ventral or acetabular sucker lying just anterior to the equatorial plane on the ventral surface. Stained specimens reveal the irregularly lobed testes situated side by side in the posterior half of the body. The long, slender excretory bladder extends from the posterior tip to the region of the

Table 53-3. DISTRIBUTION OF PARAGONIMIASIS BY COUNTRIES

Africa	Far East	Asia
Zaire Republic	*Central China	Assam
Cameroon	*Vietnam	Bengal
Republic of Dahomey	*Japan	Sri Lanka (Ceylon)
Nigeria	*Korea	Malabar
	Manchuria	Madras Presidency
	*Taiwan	Mexico
	Malay Peninsula	Central America
	*Philippines	*Costa Rica
	Indonesia	Honduras
	New Guinea	South America
	*Thailand	Colombia
	*Laos	Peru
		Ecuador
		Venezuela
		Brazil

*Indicates important endemic foci in man.

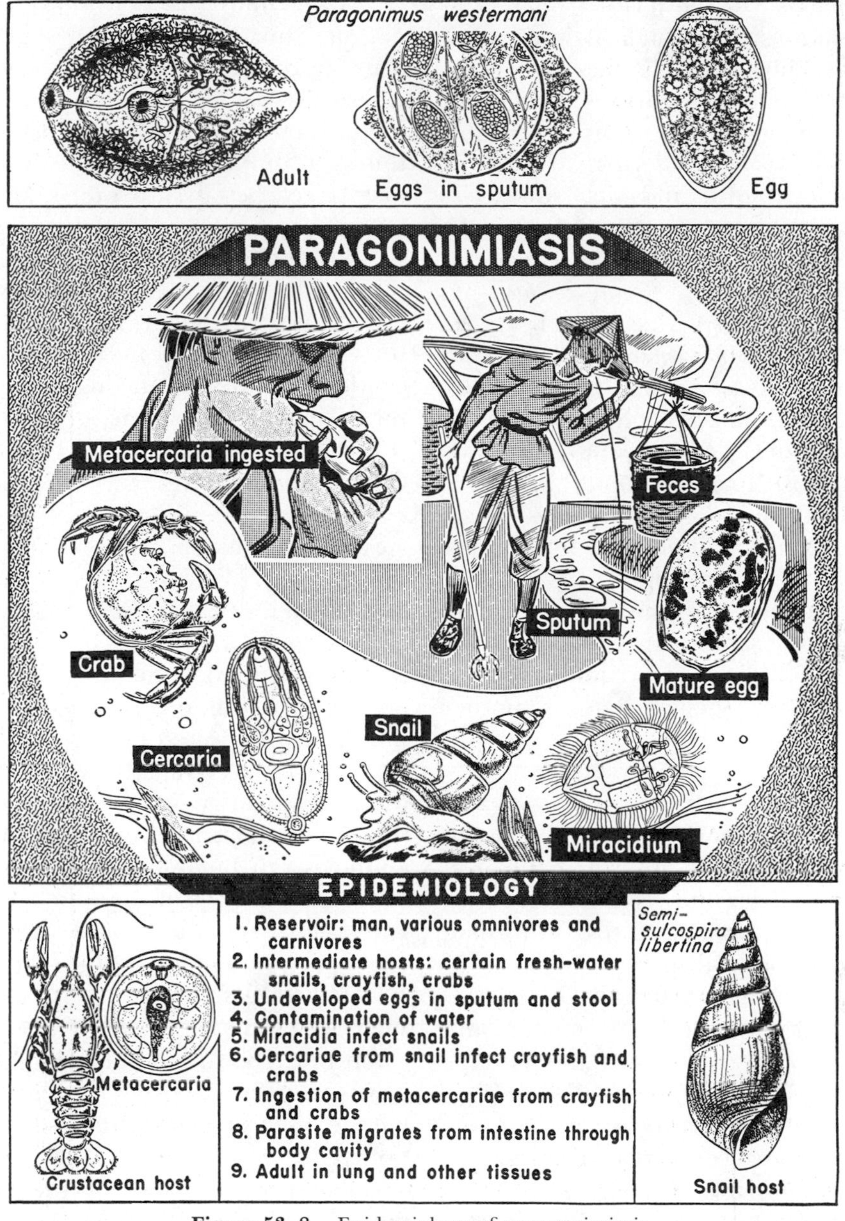

Figure 53–8. Epidemiology of paragonimiasis.

pharynx. In carefully flattened, preserved and stained specimens, the eccentric, centrally located lobate ovary can be seen to one side of the acetabulum. At the lateral margins, extending from the oral sucker to the posterior tip, are the yolk glands; the uterus occupies the central portion of the worm opposite the ovary. Anteriorly are the globose pharynx and a short esophagus which divides to form the two unbranched intestinal crura (Fig. 53–8).

DEVELOPMENT OF PARAGONIMUS WESTERMANI. The mature adults produce eggs which range between 80 and 118 μm in length by 48 and 60 μm in width, averaging 85 by 53 μm. The golden brown eggs are slightly broader at the operculate end and show some shouldering where the operculum originates. Posteriorly the shell is thicker than in the anterior half. The undeveloped eggs are passed up the respiratory tree and either expectorated in the sputum or swallowed and passed in the feces. Under satisfactory conditions they hatch in water after 17 to 28 days, liberating characteristic miracidia. These penetrate various species of snails. But the most important susceptible snails are *Semisulcospira libertina* (Gould), *S. amurensis* (Gerstfeldt) and its subspecies *gottschei* (von Martens) and *nodiperda* (von Martens), *Thiara (Tarebia) granifera* (Lamarck), *Hua toucheana* (Heude), *Brotia costula* and *B. asperata. Paragonimus* has also been recorded in *Oncomelania nosophora* (Robson) and *Syncera lutea* (A. Adams) (= *Assiminea). Pomacea luteostoma* needs confirmation as the host in Venezuela. *Pomatiopsis lapidaria* is the known host for *P. kellicotti* in North America. Hydrobiid snails of the genus *Aroapyrgus* are the snail hosts of lung flukes of animals, *Paragonimus* spp. in Central and South America, and probably also of human lung flukes in the same geographic area.

Three to 5 months are required to produce the successive generations of mother sporocyst, rediae, daughter rediae and finally the stumpy tailed, or microcercous, cercariae.

The cercariae attack crayfish and freshwater crabs, the second intermediate host, invading the muscles and viscera where they become metacercariae infective for man after a developmental period of 6 to 8 weeks. The following crustaceans (both crayfish and crabs) serve as hosts for the metacercariae of *P. westermani* in the Orient: *Cambaroides japonicus; C. similis; Eriocheir japonicus; E. sinensis; Potamon (Goethelphusa) dehaani; Potamon (Potamon) rathbuni; P. miyazakii; P. (P.) denticulatus; Procambarus clarkii; Parathelphusa sinensis; Sesarma (Holometopus) dehaani; Sesarma (Sesarma) intermedia (= S. (S.) sinensis).* In the Cameroons the metacercariae of *Paragonimus africanus* occur in the freshwater crabs *Sudanautes africanus* and *S. pelii.* In Venezuela the cercariae encyst in *Pseudothelphusa iturbei*, and *P. kellicotti* in North America encysts in members of the genus *Cambarus.*

Infection of man and other reservoir hosts results when the crustacea containing metacercariae of *P. westermani* are eaten raw. The metacercariae excyst in the duodenum and migrate through the wall of the alimentary canal into the peritoneal cavity. Most migrate through the diaphragm and penetrate into the parenchyma of the lungs where the parasites are finally encapsulated by the host. About 3 weeks are needed for this migration, even though the diaphragm may be reached in 3 to 4 days. Maturity is attained 5 to 6 weeks after ingestion.

Epidemiology. The following includes some of the carnivores and omnivores in addition to man which serve as reservoir hosts for species of *Paragonimus:* tiger, cat, wild cat, leopard, fox, wolf, dog, panther, rat (?), pig, beaver, wolverine, cattle, civet cat *(Viverra zibetha ashtoni,* and *V. indica mayori),* Chinese lesser civet cat *(Viverricula malaccensis pollida),* pencilled cat *(Nyctereutes procyonides),* fishing cat *(Felis viverrina),* mongoose *(Herpestes urva),* and Indian mongoose *(Mungos mungo)* (Table 53–1). All acquire the metacercariae through the ingestion of infected, raw freshwater crabs or crayfish. In addition, man secures the infection by eating salted or wine-soaked parasitized crustacea. While the wine kills the crabs, the metacercariae survive for several hours (Fig. 53–6). Recent outbreaks of human paragonimiasis in Japan are due to the ingestion of the raw muscles of the wild boar, *Sus scrofa leucomystax* Temminck and Schegel, which serves as a paratenic host for P. westermani.[41]

The disease is limited to areas where such dishes are common, or where crabs are eaten raw; roasting or heating the crustacea in water at 55° C (131° F) for 5 minutes will kill the metacercariae, thus preventing infection.

Pollution of water by the eggs of the parasites, especially those from reservoir hosts other than man, serves as the principal source of infection for the snails which, in turn, produce the cercariae that invade the crustacean hosts.

Pathology. The young flukes migrate through the peritoneal cavity and penetrate the diaphragm to reach the lungs. Many never reach their destination but become encapsulated and sometimes destroyed in other locations. Parasites encysted in the intestinal mucosa elicit an inflammatory reaction which sometimes terminates in ulceration, resulting in passage of eggs in the feces. Par-

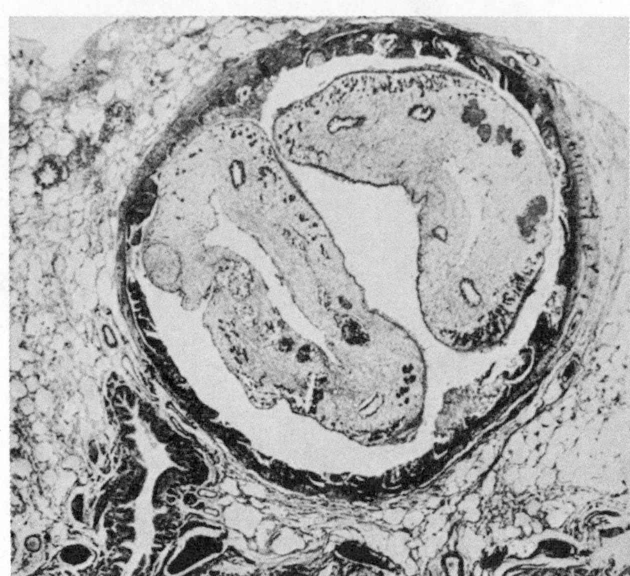

Figure 53–9. *Paragonimus westermani* in the lung of a bengal tiger. (Courtesy of Dr. T. W. M. Cameron, Macdonald College of McGill University.)

asites localizing in the body cavity usually produce an abscess. Such ectopic locations are associated with the migration route usually followed by the worms. However, some aberrant flukes have been recovered from the brain and, more rarely, the spinal cord. In such locations the patient exhibits various manifestations of damage to the central nervous system. This is fairly common in highly endemic areas such as Korea and Japan. In Korea it was found that cerebral paragonimiasis is often accompanied by intracranial calcifications which are revealed in radiographs of the skull.

The most characteristic and significant pathologic changes are found in the lungs (Fig. 53–9).

On arrival in the pulmonary tissue the parasites produce a surrounding inflammatory reaction with leukocytic infiltration, necrosis of parenchyma, and the formation of an enclosing fibrous tissue capsule. The resulting cysts, which may reach 2 cm in diameter, are more frequent in the deeper portions than at the periphery of the lung. Upon reaching maturity the encapsulated parasite starts producing eggs; eventually, the capsule swells and ruptures, usually into a bronchiole. It is the mixture of eggs, inflammatory cells and blood that is expectorated in the sputum. In other instances, tunnels or burrows lined with fibrous tissue are formed from damaged and dilated bronchioles and bronchi, and larger cysts may be formed by breakdown of adjacent tunnel walls. The lesions are often directly connected with radicles of the bronchial tree. Usually there are not more than 20 to 25 parasites in the lungs.

The cysts characteristically have a reddish or chocolate brown color while the cyst-like burrows often have a bluish tint. Each cyst contains one or more living or dead worms, together with quantities of brownish, necrotic, frequently purulent exudate composed of eggs, debris and Charcot-Leyden crystals (Fig. 53–10). Leukocytosis with eosinophilia may occur but is frequently absent.

Clinical Characteristics. The clinical picture of paragonimiasis is predominantly that of a chronic bronchitis or bronchiectasis with morning cough productive of variable amounts of gelatinous tenacious sputum which characteristically is brownish or reddish in color. Exertional dyspnea is common. The term "endemic hemoptysis" is due to the frequency with which hemoptysis occurs. When cysts are localized in close proximity to the pleura, pleural pain may be troublesome, or pleural effusion may occur. In other instances, the clinical phenomena indicate a nonresolving bronchopneumonia.

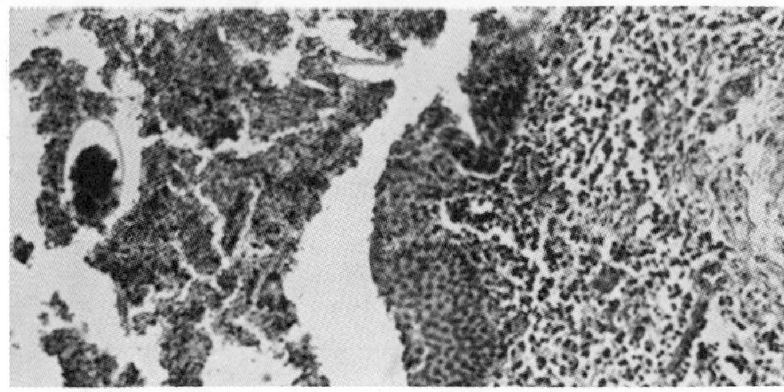

Figure 53-10. Egg of *P. kellicotti* in exudate in bronchus.

In heavy infections lung abscess may occur.

X-rays of many patients will show a patchy, cloudy infiltration of the lungs; others will reveal nodular shadows, calcified spots, or some pathology of the pleura (thickening, pleuritis or pleural effusion).

Abdominal symptoms occur when considerable numbers of parasites have localized in this region. They include pain, tenderness, rarely muscle spasm, and diarrhea that is sometimes bloody, with mucus and eggs in the stools.

The cerebral type of the disease occurs only when wandering parasites lodge in the brain. The local lesions in these cases resemble those of cysticercosis, and a Jacksonian type of epilepsy is a frequent clinical manifestation. Studies reveal that cerebral involvement occurs in 0.8 per cent of patients with active pulmonary paragonimiasis in South Korea and that there is evidence of significant mental retardation in 90 per cent of these.[30, 31]

Rarely, localization in the skin or subcutaneous tissues leads to abscess formation.

The prognosis is good in light infections; in heavy infections, however, it is grave.

Diagnosis. The clinical picture of pulmonary paragonimiasis and especially the brownish or reddish purulent sputum may be suggestive.

A positive diagnosis is made by detecting the characteristic eggs in aspirated pleural effusion, in the sputum, feces and, more rarely, the cutaneous lesions. By using the AMS III technique (acid-sodium sulfate-Triton-ether) on stool specimens, nearly 80 per cent of a known positive series were positive by stool. (See page 820 for details of technique.) While this egg is sometimes confused with that of the fish tapeworm, a careful comparison of the two makes differentiation possible. The sputum may contain egg masses that appear as rusty brown flecks, or it may be tinged with blood. Leukocytes, especially eosinophils, and Charcot-Leyden crystals also appear in the sputum. (See page 828 for details of technique for examining sputum.) Examination of at least three stool and sputum specimens on successive days increases the number of positives obtained.[32]

It is necessary to differentiate paragonimiasis from such other pulmonary diseases as lobular pneumonia, tuberculosis, bronchial spirochetosis and bronchiectasis.

The abdominal form of the disease may be confused with a variety of intestinal infections, new growth, and certain surgical lesions. The cerebral type likewise may produce a varied clinical picture.

Treatment. Bithionol (Actamer, Bitin) is the drug of choice.[32, 33] Thirty to 50 mg per kg of body weight is given every other day in divided doses for 20 to 30 days. Sputum and stools became negative in a few days and remained so for a year when follow-up studies were carried out. Side effects were minor and consisted of transient diarrhea, abdominal pain, nausea, vomiting and occasional urticarial rash. Niclofolan (Bayer 9015) reportedly is also highly effective against paragonimiasis with a single dose of 2.0 mg per kg.

Prophylaxis. Human infection may be avoided easily by thorough cooking of all freshwater crustaceans used for food. The relatively large number of reservoir and intermediate hosts in many endemic areas renders effective control by other measures impracticable or impossible at present.

OTHER PARAGONIMUS AND RELATED SPECIES

A number of other new species of *Paragonimus* and their definitive hosts have been described and are listed. (See Table 53–1). Few have been reported from man with certainty.[36] However, all should be suspect as it is probable that most would develop in man if the uncooked intermediate host, crab or crayfish, is ingested or the metacercariae are accidentally transferred to an uncooked dish. Some reported from man are described below.

Paragonimus heterotremus. Paragonimus heterotremus Chen and Hsia, 1964 (= *P. tuanshanensis* Chung, et al., 1964) has been recorded from man in Thailand, Laos and China. Immature adults may cause migratory swellings.[34, 35] The metacercariae occur in *Potamon smithianus, Parathelphusa germani,* and rarely *P. dugasti.* In addition to being found in man, this *Paragonimus* has been found in cats and dogs; experimentally it has developed in monkeys and rabbits.

Paragonimus skrjabini. This parasite, *P. skrjabini* Chen, 1959 (= *P. szechuanensis* Chung and Ts'ao, 1962), is one of many species found in China. It occurs in the masked palm civet, *Paguma larvata,* cats, dogs and man. *Tricula* sp. is the snail intermediate host.

Paragonimus africanus. A new species, *P. africanus,* Voelker and Vogel, 1965, is suggested as the causative agent of paragonimiasis of man in West Africa.

Paragonimus kellicotti. This species, P. *kellicotti* Ward, 1908, is a rare parasite of man in the Western Hemisphere. It occurs as a natural parasite in cats, dogs and pigs, with crayfish serving as the second intermediate host.

Paragonimus mexicanus. Autochthonous human cases of paragonimiasis have been reported from Mexico, Honduras, El Salvador, Ecuador, Peru and Costa Rica. However, accurate species identification was not possible due to a dearth of material. Recently *Paragonimus mexicanus* Miyazaki and Ishii, 1968 was described from an opossum from Mexico. The life cycle of *P. mexicanus* has since been worked out in Costa Rica and evidence presented that *P. peruvianus* Miyazaki et al., 1969 is a synonym of *P. mexicanus.*[37, 38] The snail host is *Aroapyrgus costaricensis,* while the freshwater crabs *Ptychophallus tristani, Ptychophallus* n.sp. and *Potamocarcinus magna* harbor the metacercariae. Adult *P. mexicanus* have been found in the lungs of cats, four-eyed opossums, raccoons and gray foxes; eggs of *Paragonimus* have been recovered from the feces of ocelots. The cycle has been confirmed in experimental animals.[37, 38]

Two other tissue-inhabiting trematodes which may be confused with *Paragonimus* are: (1) *Achillurbainia nouveli* Dollfus, which has been taken from a 10-year-old girl from South Kwantung Province of China. It was found in a cyst behind the left ear.[39] Freshwater crabs were suspect. (2) From Sarawak comes the report of a similar cyst in a boy. Only eggs were encountered; these resembled the eggs of *Poikilorchis congolensis* Fain and Vandepitte.[40]

REFERENCES

1. Barlow, C. H. 1925. The life cycle of the human intestinal fluke, *Fasciolopsis buski* (Lankester). Am. J. Hyg. Monogr. Ser. No. 4. 98 pp.
2. Hsü, H. F., and Li, S. Y. 1953. Notes on *Fasciolopsis buski* in China. Tharpar Commemoration Volume, 1953. Dept. of Zoology, National Taiwan University, Taipei, Taiwan. pp. 133–138.
3. Cross, J. H. 1969. Fasciolopsiasis in Southeast Asia and the Far East: a review. *In* Harinasuta, C. (ed.): Proc. 4th S. E. Asian Seminar on Parasit. and Trop. Med., Schistosomiasis and Other Snail-Transmitted Helminthiasis. Bangkok, Thailand. pp. 177–196.
4. Fan. P. C. 1965. Prevalence of parasitic diseases in Taiwan. J. Chinese Nursing *12*:50–61.
5. Manning, G. S., and Ratanarat, C. 1970. *Fasciolopsis buski* (Lankester, 1857) in Thailand. Am. J. Trop. Med. Hyg. *19*:613–619.
6. Manning, G. S., Sukhawat, K., Viyanant, V., Subhakul, M., and Lertprasert, P. 1969. *Fasciolopsis buski* in Thailand, with comments on other intestinal parasites. J. Med. Assoc. Thai. *52*:905–914.
7. Plaut, A. G., Kampanort-Sanyakorn, C., and Manning, G. S. 1969. A clinical study of *Fasciolopsis buski* in Thailand. Tr. Roy. Soc. Trop. Med. Hyg. *63*:470–478.

8. Bauge, R. 1954. Incidence of intestinal parasites in Hongay region, North Vietnam in February–May 1953. Bull. Soc. Path. Exot. *47*:720–729.
9. Shah, A., Gadgil, R. K., and Manohar, K. D. 1966. Fasciolopsiasis in Bombay: a preliminary communication. Indian J. Med. Sci. *20*:805–811.
10. Kean, B. H., and Breslau, R. C. 1964. Parasites of the Human Heart. Chapter X. Cardiac Heterophyidiasis. Grune & Stratton, New York. pp. 95–103.
11. Hadidjaja, P., Carney, W. P., Clarke, M. D., Cross, J. H., Jusuf, A., Saroso, J. S., and Oemijati, S. 1972. *Schistosoma japonicum* and intestinal parasites of the inhabitants of Lake Lindu, Sulawesi (Celebes); a preliminary report. S. E. Asian J. Trop. Med. Pub. Hlth. *3*:594–599.
12. Yokogawa, M. 1969. Clonorchiasis in Japan. *In* Harinasuta, C. (ed.): Proc. 4th S. E. Asian Seminar on Parasit. and Trop. Med., Schistosomiasis and Other Snail-Transmitted Helminthiasis. Bangkok, Thailand. pp. 209–218.
13. Soh, Chin-Thack. 1969. Clonorchiasis in Korea. *In* Harinasuta, C. (ed.): Proc. 4th S. E. Asian Seminar on Parasit. and Trop. Med., Schistosomiasis and Other Snail-Transmitted Helminthiasis. Bangkok, Thailand. pp. 219–229.
14. Sun, T. 1969. Clonorchiasis in Hong Kong. *In* Harinasuta, C. (ed.): Proc. 4th S. E. Asian Seminar on Parasit. and Trop. Med., Schistosomiasis and Other Snail-Transmitted Helminthiasis. Bangkok, Thailand. pp. 243–247.
15. Cross, J. H. 1969. Clonorchiasis in Taiwan: a review. *In* Harinasuta, C. (ed.): Proc. 4th S. E. Asian Seminar on Parasit. and Trop. Med., Schistosomiasis and Other Snail-Transmitted Helminthiasis. Bangkok, Thailand. pp. 231–242.
16. Sun, T., Chou, S. T., and Gibson, J. R. 1968. Route of entry of *Clonorchis sinensis* to the mammalian liver. Exp. Parasit. *22*:346–351.
17. Yokogawa, M., Tsuji, M., Koyama, H., Wakejuma, T., Ozu, S., and Ogino, Y. 1967. Chemotherapy of *Clonorchis sinensis* with 1,4-bis-trichloromethyl benzole. Ztschr. Tropenmed. Parasit. *18*:82–88.
18. Rim, H.-J. 1974. Chemotherapy for human clonorchiasis in Korea. Proc. Third Internat. Congr. Parasit. Vol. 3, 1325–1326.
19. Bunnag, G., and Harinasuta, T. 1974. Chemotherapy on human opisthorchiasis in Thailand. Proc. Third Internat. Congr. Parasit. Vol. 3, 1326–1327.
20. Gritsay, M. K., and Yakubov, T. C. 1970. On peculiarities of epidemiology and epizootiology of opisthorchiasis in the Ukraine. Medskaya Parazit. *39*:534–537. (In Russian)
21. Beer, S. A., Fedorova, S. P., Pobruz, Yu N., Nadezhdina, T. I., Novosiltsev, G. I., and Tseitlin, D. G. 1971. Peculiarities of epidemiology of opisthorchiasis in the Surgut District of the Tyumen Region. Medskaya Parazit. *40*:447–453. (In Russian.)
22. Harinasuta, C. 1969. Opisthorchiasis in Thailand: a review. *In* Harinasuta, C. (ed.): Proc. 4th S. E. Asian Seminar on Parasit. and Trop. Med., Schistosomiasis and Other Snail-Transmitted Helminthiasis. pp. 253–264.
23. Wykoff, D. E., Harinasuta, C., Juttijudata, P., and Winn, M. M. 1965. *Opisthorchis viverrini* in Thailand—The life cycle and comparison with *O. felineus*. J. Parasit. *51*:207–214.
24. Bisseru, B. 1969. Opisthorchiasis in West Malaysia. *In* Harinasuta, C. (ed.): Proc. 4th S. E. Asian Seminar on Parasit. and Trop. Med., Schistosomiasis and Other Snail-Transmitted Helminthiasis. pp. 265–270.
25. Artigas, P. de T., and Perez, M. D. 1960–62. Consideracões sôbre *Opisthorchis pricei,* Foster, 1939, *O. guayaquilensis,* Rodriguez, Gomez et Mantalvan, 1949, e *O. pseudofelineus,* Ward, 1901. Descrição de *Amphimerus pseudofelineus minutus,* n. subsp. Mem. Inst. Butantan *30*:157–166.
26. Sadun, E. H. 1955. Studies on *Opisthorchis viverrini* in Thailand. Am. J. Hyg. *62*:31–115.
27. Alekseeva, M. I., Karzin, V. V., Karnaukhov, V. K., Ozeretskovskaya, N. N., Plotnikov, N. N., and Tumolskaya, N. I. 1969. Clinical pattern and treatment of fascioliasis in man. I. Clinical features of early and chronic stages of fascioliasis. Medskaya Parazit. *38*:515–521. (In Russian)
28. Anonymous. 1974. Drugs for parasitic diseases. The Medical Letter on Drugs and Therapeutics *16*:5–12
29. Janssens, P. G., Fain, A., Limbos, P., De Muynck, A., Biemans, R., Van Meirvenne, N., and De Mulder, P. 1968. Trois cas de distomatose hépatique à *Fasciola gigantica* contractés en Afrique centrale. Ann. Soc. Belg. Méd. Trop. *48*:631–650.
30. Oh, S. J., and Jordan, E. J. 1967. Findings of intelligence quotient in cerebral paragonimiasis. Jap. J. Parasit. *16*:436–440.
31. Oh, S. J. 1968. Cerebral paragonimiasis. J. Neurol. Sci. *8*:27–48.
32. Kim, J. S. 1970. Treatment of *Paragonimus westermani* infections with bithionol. Am. J. Trop. Med. Hyg. *19*:940–942.
33. Yokogawa, M., Okura, T., Tsuji, M., Iwasaki, M., and Shigeyasu, M. 1962. Chemotherapy of paragonimiasis with Bithionol. III. The follow-up studies for one year after treatment with Bithionol. Jap. J. Parasit. *11*:103–116.
34. Miyazaki, I., and Harinasuta, C. 1966. The first case of human paragonimiasis caused by *Paragonimus heterotremus* Chen and Hsia, 1964. Ann. Trop. Med. Parasit. *60*:509–514.
35. Miyazaki, I., and Fontan, S. 1970. Mature *Paragonimus heterotremus* found from a man in Laos. Jap. J. Parasit. *19*:109–113.
36. Yokogawa, M. 1969. *Paragonimus* and paragonimiasis. Adv. Parasit. 7:375–387.
37. Brenes, R. R., Zeledón, R., and Rojas, G. 1968. The finding of *Paragonimus* sp. in mammals, crabs and snails in Costa Rica. Bol. Chileno Parasit. *23*:70.
38. Brenes, R., Zeledon, R., and Rojas, G. 1974. Personal communication.
39. Chen, Hsin-T'ao. 1965. *Paragonimus, Pagumogonimus* and a *Paragonimus*-like trematode in man. Chinese Med. J. *84*:781–791.
40. Wong, S. K., and Lie, K. J. 1965. Another periauricular abscess from Sarawak, probably caused by a trematode of the genus *Poikilorchis,* Fain and Vandepitte. Med. J. Malaya *19*:229–230.
41. Miyazaki, I., and Habe, S. 1976. A newly recognized mode of human infection with the lung fluke, *Paragonimus westermani* (Kerbert, 1878). J. Parasit. *62*:646–648.

CHAPTER 54
Cestodes

Introduction

BIOLOGY OF THE CESTODES

The cestodes, or tapeworms, include several divergent groups which may be separated not only morphologically but also on clear-cut biologic criteria. They are all flattened dorsoventrally and are creamy to white in color. The biologic criteria become evident as the life cycles of the parasites are studied; they also modify the various epidemiologic patterns. On such criteria the cestodes may be divided into two large groups. In the first the eggs must reach water; in the second this is not necessary. The broad tapeworm of man, *Diphyllobothrium latum,* and *Sparganum* spp. are the only important human parasites in the first group.* All the remaining common tapeworms of man fall in the second category. One cestode of man, *Hymenolepis nana,* requires no intermediate host, but may pass directly from person to person. Other species must have at least one intermediate host to complete the cycle. Although the members of these two groups will not be segregated as their morphology is discussed, their biology is sufficiently distinct to warrant separate consideration of their development.

MORPHOLOGY OF THE CESTODES

The Adults. The tapeworms, Cestoda or cestodes, as they are commonly called, range in size from the small *Hymenolepis nana* of 40 mm or less to the huge *Taenia saginata* and *Diphyllobothrium latum* which may measure up to 10 or 12 meters in length. Members of this entire class have morphologic and biologic characteristics that differentiate them from the other helminths.

All tapeworms have a mechanism for attaching the *scolex* or "head" to the host's intestinal wall. In the case of *Diphyllobothrium latum* and related species the scolex bears two sucking grooves or *bothria* which serve in this capacity. Other common human tapeworms possess four round and highly muscular sucking cups located on the scolex. These, in turn, may be supplemented further by a terminal, sometimes retractile protuberance known as a *rostellum.* The rostellum in a given species of tapeworm is characteristic and is often armed with small hooks, the number, the length and the arrangement of which serve as further differential aids (Figs. 54–1, 54–2).

Behind the scolex is a short, unsegmented narrow *neck* which is the region from which the partially segmented young *proglottids* develop. This region of immature proglottid formation is succeeded by a region of fully developed proglottids, each of which contains a full complement of mature reproductive organs. This gives way to a distal group of *gravid segments* which are frequently little more than sacs of eggs and which, exclusive of the scolex, represent the oldest portion of the worm. As new segments are continuously being formed at the neck, the old proglottids are pushed farther and farther from the scolex, thereby increasing the length of the parasite. The entire worm from the scolex to, and including, the gravid proglottids is termed the *strobila.*

Tapeworms differ from most other helminths in that they have no alimentary canal. Each mature proglottid possesses nerve trunks, excretory canals, a well developed musculature and a complete set of male and female reproductive organs. The gravid proglottids should be studied when making a

**Diplogonoporus grandis* is not considered here as only a few cases of human infection are known.

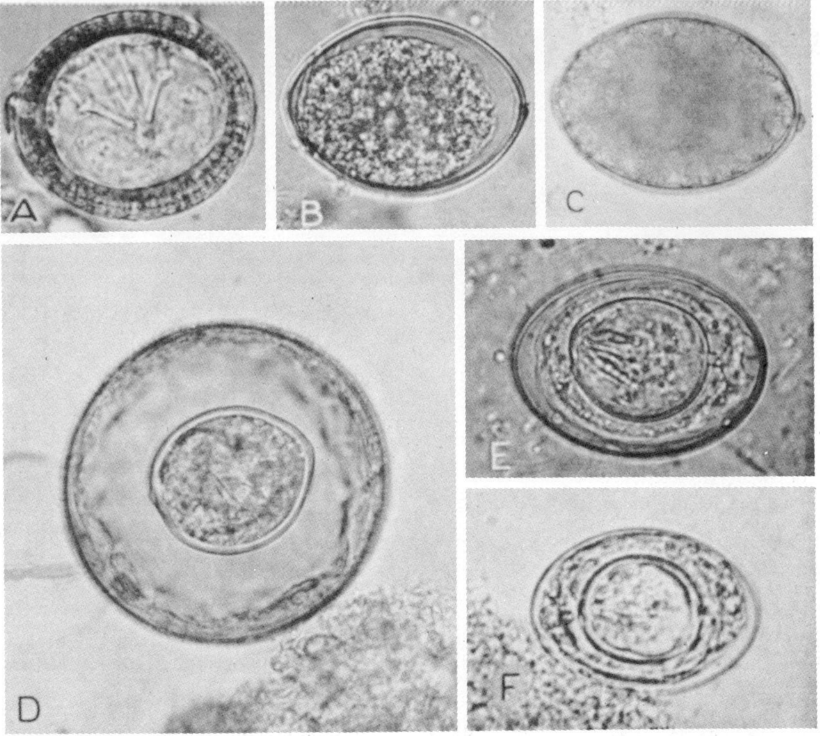

Figure 54–1. Some cestode eggs. *A,* Human tapeworm, *Taenia* sp. 750 ×. *B,* Broad tapeworm of man, *Diphyllobothrium latum.* 500 ×. *C,* Broad tapeworm of man, *Diphyllobothrium latum.* 500 ×. *D,* Rat tapeworm, *Hymenolepis diminuta.* 650 ×. *E,* Dwarf tapeworm, *Hymenolepis nana.* 750 ×. *F,* Dwarf tapeworm, *Hymenolepis nana* (note polar filaments). 750 ×. (Figs. *B* and *F* courtesy of Lt. L. W. Shatterly, MSC, School of Aviation Medicine, Gunter AFB, Alabama; all others courtesy of Dr. R. L. Roudabush, Ward's Natural Science Establishment, Rochester, New York; photos by T. Romaniak.)

diagnosis, since many of the human species are differentiated by recognition of the position of the genital pore and the branchings of the uterus (Fig. 54–2).

Eggs. Tapeworm eggs are either operculate or nonoperculate. The former are adapted for development in water *(D. latum);* the latter must reach the soil (as in the *Taenia* group). Representatives of the first or *D. latum* type are undeveloped when passed. Their lid or operculum permits the subsequent hatching of a free-swimming larva or *coracidium.* Eggs of all tapeworms in the *Taenia* group contain an inner, developed, six-hooked embryo or *oncosphere.* This is surrounded by an outer protective layer or layers, the nature and arrangement of which are frequently diagnostic of the species (Fig. 54–1).

Developmental Stages. The tapeworm eggs or larvae that are ingested by a proper host soon develop into typical stages. Upon ingestion by a copepod, coracidia of the *D. latum* group produce a *procercoid* larva that may retain the embryonic six hooks and show developing holdfast devices or bothria. This is followed by the infective stage, called a *plerocercoid* larva, found in the flesh of fish (Fig. 54–3).

Embryos of the *Taenia* group may develop several types of cysts. If the oncosphere gives rise to a single cyst containing but one scolex it is called a *cysticercus* (Fig. 54–4), or in the case of members of the genus *Hymenolepis,* a *cysticercoid.* On the other hand, if a single oncosphere produces a single cyst containing many scolices it is called a *coenurus* as in the larval stage of *Multiceps multiceps* in sheep. In instances when daughter cysts, each containing many scolices, are elaborated, a *hydatid,* or echinococcus cyst, is said to result (Fig. 54–5).

The outer surface of the worm consists of a glistening *cuticle* which is secreted by the underlying cells of the hypodermis. Beneath this lie the layers of longitudinal and circular muscles that enclose a mass of loose *parenchymal cells* in which the various organ systems (i.e. nervous, excretory and reproductive) are embedded (Fig. 54–2). Since an

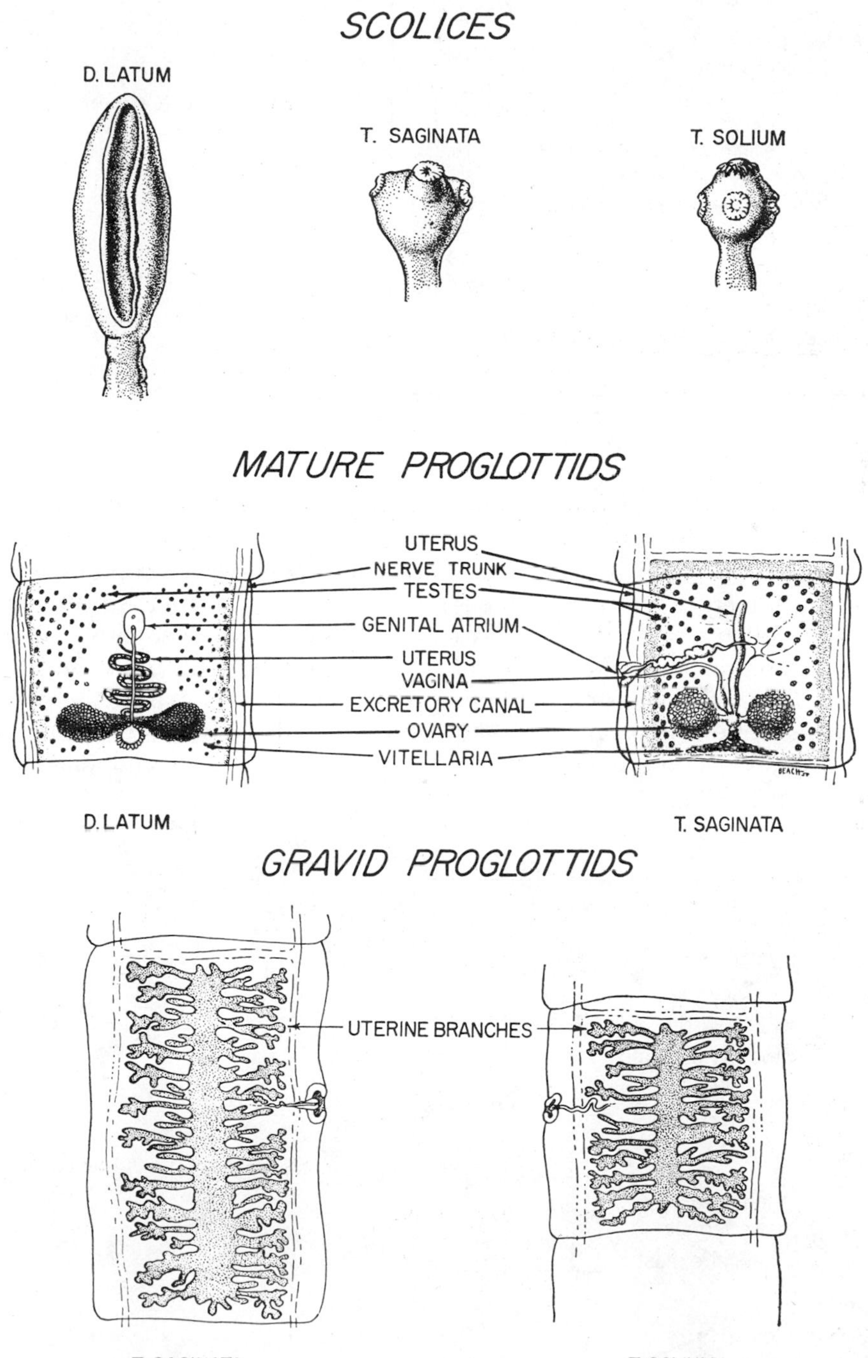

Figure 54–2. Scolices and proglottids of some tapeworms of man. The full complement of testes and vitellaria is not shown. (Modified from various authors; courtesy of the University of Florida College of Medicine, Gainesville.)

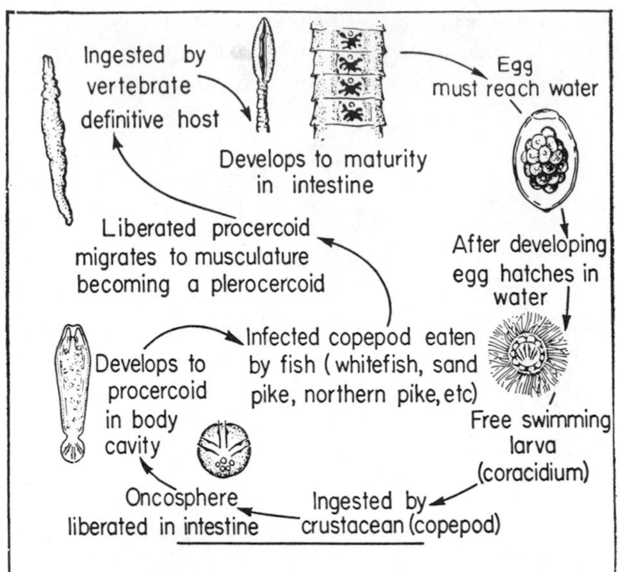

Figure 54-3. Cestode cycle—*D. latum* type.

alimentary canal is absent, nutriment must be absorbed selectively through the integument of the worm.[1] Carbohydrates are obtained from the lumen of the host alimentary canal while other required substances are absorbed from or near the intestinal mucosa. The cells of the parenchyma contain a high ratio of lipids, phospholipids and glycogen to protein;[2, 3] oxygen may be obtained from the stored glycogen.[4] Calcium is present and stored as *calcareous granules* (calcareous corpuscles) throughout the parenchyma, being particularly prominent in some larval stages (procercoids, plerocercoids). These granules probably serve to buffer acids entering the parasite's body from the outside and, possibly, to buffer acids produced during aerobic and anaerobic fermen-

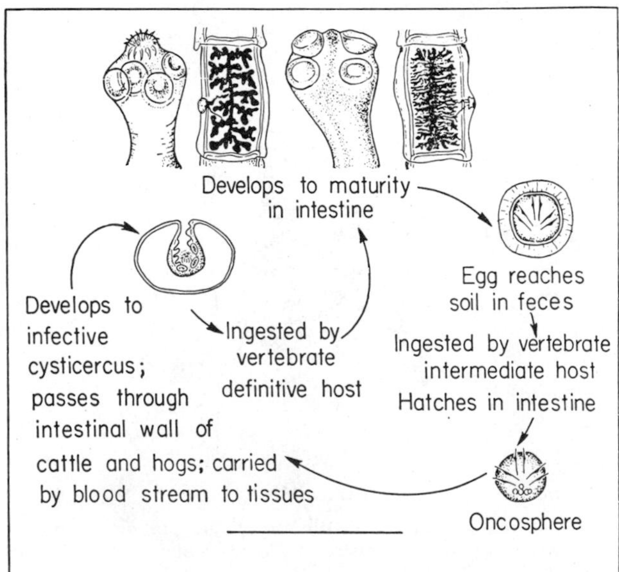

Figure 54-4. Cestode cycle—*Taenia* type.

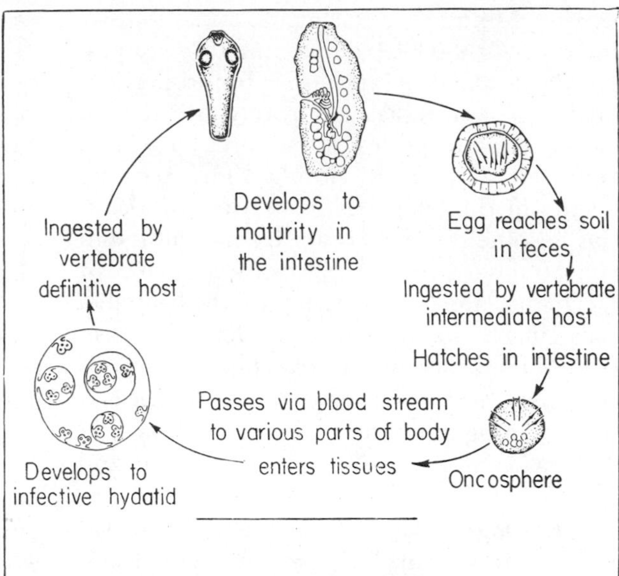

Figure 54-5. Cestode cycle—hydatid type.

tations.[5] Vitamins (especially G) and sex hormones also appear to be necessary for the normal development of cestodes.[6, 7]

THE GENERALIZED CYCLE

The developmental characteristics of the two groups mentioned earlier will be considered separately.

Nonembryonated Eggs. *Diphyllobothrium latum* is the human representative of greatest importance in this group. The undifferentiated, operculate eggs of parasites in this category develop in water, hatch, and liberate a free-swimming ciliated larva or *coracidium.* This organism is ingested by a copepod (a minute crustacean), the first intermediate host, and metamorphoses into a *procercoid* larva. The next intermediate host is a fish, in which the *plerocercoid* stage, infective for man, develops. Infection occurs when insufficiently cooked fish containing this parasite are eaten.

Embryonated Eggs. All the human tapeworms considered in this category retain the eggs in utero until they are embryonated, at which time the six hooklets, diagnostic of such tapeworm eggs, become apparent. These worms may require an intermediate host for the completion of development. In the case of *Hymenolepis nana* none is necessary, as infection is direct—the only requirement being the introduction of viable eggs into a susceptible definitive host. Eggs of the others, after reaching the ground, are ingested by the intermediate host, where development to the infective stage, usually a *cysticercoid, cysticercus* or *hydatid cyst,* takes place. When these larvae in the infective stage are ingested by man or other final hosts, the parasites reach maturity in the digestive tract.

Diphyllobothriasis

Synonyms. Broad tapeworm infection, fish tapeworm infection.

Definition. Diphyllobothriasis is the infection of man by adult *Diphyllobothrium latum.* Its presence is sometimes associated with anemia, loss of weight and debility.

Distribution. *Diphyllobothrium latum* is common in persons living in the Baltic countries, the western U.S.S.R., Finland, parts of Scandinavia and in certain endemic foci in the United States and Canada. In the latter regions the parasite occurs in northern Wisconsin, Minnesota, Michigan, and in provinces of Canada bordering on those states. In Alaska *D. latum* infection is found particularly in Eskimos, as, very rarely, are several closely related species. A few cases have been reported also from Florida. The parasite occurs in the lake regions of Italy, where it has become extremely rare in man although still abundant in fish, Switzerland, parts of Germany, and in the valley of the Danube, particularly in Rumania. It has been reported in Manchuria, Korea, Japan, portions of Siberia and in scattered areas of Africa. It is also indigenous to Chile, Argentina and Australia and possibly New Guinea and Papua.

Etiology. MORPHOLOGY. The broad tapeworm of man, *D. latum* (Linnaeus, 1758) Lühe, 1910, lives with its scolex attached to the mucosa of the small intestine. It may reach a length of 10 meters or more. The spatulate head is small and bears a deep sucking groove on either surface. Posterior to the scolex is the narrow unsegmented neck 5 to 10 mm in length; the remainder of the worm consists of 3000 or more segments or proglottids.

The chief diagnostic feature of *D. latum* is the rosette-shaped, egg-filled uterus of both the mature and gravid proglottids. The finding of the genital pore on the flattened surface in the anterior third of the proglottid is also helpful. Gravid segments are normally retained as part of the strobila, being sloughed off only as they degenerate. It has been estimated that a fully developed strobila will produce about 1,000,000 eggs in a day, but both eggs and proglottids are produced irregularly at intervals of 3 to 30 days. The eggs average from 59 to 71 μm in length by 42 to 49 μm in breadth; they are operculate and undeveloped when laid and possess a minute but distinct *boss* or thickening at the anopercular end.[8]

DEVELOPMENT. The eggs must reach water, where, after approximately 2 weeks at the optimum temperature, the egg hatches, liberating a free-swimming coracidium consisting of a typical six-hooked oncosphere invested by ciliated epithelium. The larva must be ingested by species of *Cyclops* or *Diaptomus* (copepods). About ten species are believed to act as hosts for this tapeworm. Within the alimentary tract the larva loses its ciliated epithelial layer and immediately penetrates to the body cavity of the copepod, where it develops into a procercoid larva in 10 to 21 days. During this period the oncospheral hooks appear in a tail-like *cercomer.* The cycle is continued when the infected copepod is ingested by any of 24 or more species of freshwater fish capable of serving as the second intermediate host. The larva migrates from the alimentary canal to the flesh, where it coils between the muscle fibers as a plerocercoid, or *sparganum,* often reaching a length of 6 mm or more. It becomes infective in 1 to 4 weeks, the time varying with the temperature. Frequently, these young fish, which at this stage feed upon copepods and other plankton, are captured by larger fish; the plerocercoid larvae then migrate to the flesh of these larger freshwater fish. When a viable parasite is ingested by man the larva develops to maturity in the intestine within 3 to 6 weeks. The complete cycle requires 8 to 15 weeks.

Epidemiology. In the United States the wall-eyed pike, sandpike, blue pike, great northern pike and yellow perch have been implicated as second intermediate hosts. In Africa it is the barbel; in Europe the pike, perch, salmon, Miller's thumb, trout, lake trout, grayling, white fish, ruff and eel are known hosts. Comparable species of trout or salmon serve in Japan. Although most marine fishes have not been implicated in the transmission of *D. latum,* they may carry the related species *D. pacificum,* a definitive host of which is the seal. This species has recently been involved in a small number of human cases in coastal Peru. Transmission of *D. latum* to man is accomplished by the eating of insufficiently cooked fish containing viable plerocercoid larvae, infection occurring, for example, through the sampling of "gefüllte" fish being prepared by Jewish housewives and the eating of raw pike hard roe in Russia (Fig. 54–6).

It is believed by many that bears, mink, foxes, cats, mongooses, walruses, seals, sealions, pigs and dogs serve as reservoirs in endemic areas.

Pathology. In most infections with *D.*

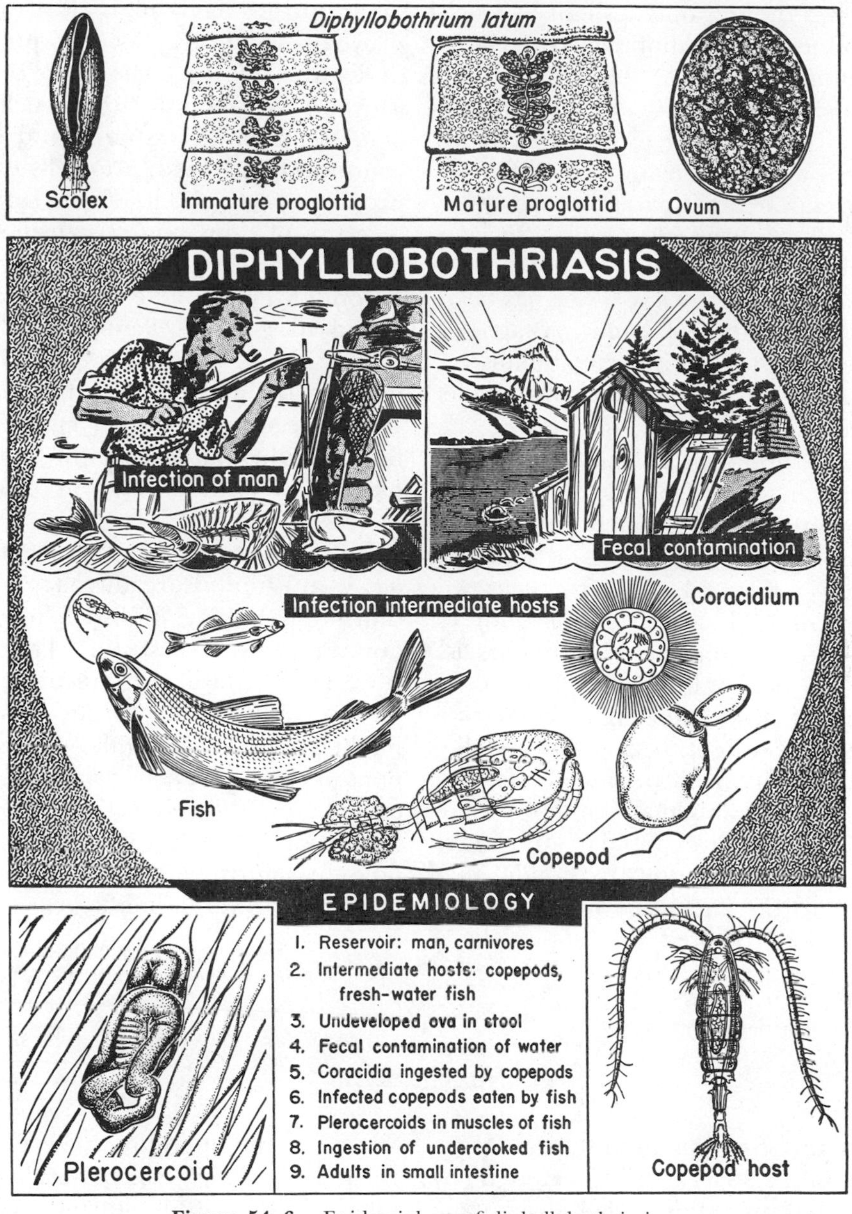

Figure 54–6. Epidemiology of diphyllobothriasis.

latum there is scant evidence of significant pathologic change, since adult worms in the intestine do not cause lesions. However, some infections with *D. latum* produce a marked anemia.

Clinical Characteristics. An infection with *D. latum* is asymptomatic in many people. Others, however, experience abdominal pain, loss of appetite, or hunger pains, anorexia, nausea, diarrhea, or loss of weight.

The anemia that occurs in some persons with *D. latum* infection is usually called "bothriocephalus anemia"; it is megaloblastic and clinically resembles genuine pernicious anemia. The fish tapeworm has been found to contain considerable amounts of vitamin B_{12} and competes with the host for this metabolite. If the parasite is located in the proximal portion of the jejunum, manifest B_{12} deficiency (pernicious anemia) may develop.[9] The absorption of this vitamin also is disturbed in nonanemic carriers of the worm.

In many cases there is only a slight leukocytosis and moderate eosinophilia. Infections may be multiple.

Diagnosis. Diagnosis depends upon the recovery of the characteristic operculate eggs in the stool. These must be differentiated from eggs of other parasites such as the lung fluke, *Paragonimus westermani,* occurring in the Orient, and a closely related tapeworm, *Diplogonoporus grandis,* which has been reported only from the Japanese. Diagnosis may be confirmed following the administration of a saline purge, which usually results in the recovery of some proglottids of the worm. These should be examined to determine the arrangement of the reproductive system, since the rosette-shaped uterus lying medially in each proglottid is diagnostic, while there is a bilateral set in *D. grandis.*

Treatment. The drug of choice for *D. latum* infection is niclosamide (phenasale, Yomesan), the patient ingesting a single dose of 2 gm (adult dose), thoroughly chewed, a short time after a light meal. No other dietary restrictions are needed. Side effects even in pregnancy are minimal. Other chemotherapeutic agents are popular in various countries. Bithionol, a diphenylsulfide, in a dose of 50 to 66 mg per kg given on an empty stomach followed in 2 hours by a saline purge, has a high cure rate but may provoke vomiting. Several phloroglucinol derivatives of the male fern *Dryopteris filix mas* and the Finnish broad-buckler fern *D. austriaca,* such as aspidin and desaspidin, continue to be used, are well tolerated and provide cures in 50 to 80 per cent of cases.[10] The use of quinacrine (Atabrine) has, however, largely been superseded. The antibiotic paromomycin sulfate has recently been found to give excellent results: 4 gm (divided into 1 gm every 15 minutes) is ingested by infected adult patients (children should receive 75 mg per kg), before breakfast.[11] Anthelmintic therapy should be supplemented by administration of folic acid for the anemia.

Prophylaxis. The prevention of *D. latum* infection is readily accomplished by thorough cooking of fish before consumption. Freezing the fish for 24 to 48 hours at 14° F (−10° C) will also effectively destroy the plerocercoid larvae. Other measures that might be practiced under favorable conditions include sewage treatment in endemic areas and the education of housewives against sampling fish while preparing it. Pet dogs in highly endemic regions should be dewormed several times a year.

Sparganosis

Synonym. Sparganum infection.

Definition. Sparganosis is caused by the presence of migrating larvae or spargana of several species of tapeworms related to *D. latum* but requiring final hosts other than man. Localization occurs primarily in the subcutaneous tissue and muscle fascia.

Distribution. The greatest number of cases of sparganosis has been reported from Japan, Korea, China, Taiwan, Vietnam and Indonesia; scattered instances are known from other areas of the world, including Holland, East Africa, Uruguay, Ecuador, Colombia, Guyana, Belize, Puerto Rico and the United States.

Etiology. Sparganosis is a disease caused by the migration of several species of related parasites which accidentally infect man; these are designated collectively as "*Sparganum mansoni*" and may be either the nonproliferating or proliferating type (Fig. 54–8). These parasites normally mature in other mammals such as dogs and cats. Morphologically indistinguishable spargana occur in subcutaneous tissue and between the muscles of frogs, snakes, birds and mammals in endemic areas, in the United States the raccoon often being heavily infected.[12] Spargana from these hosts or man cannot be identified as to species until the life cycle has been completed experimentally by feeding them to dogs or cats.

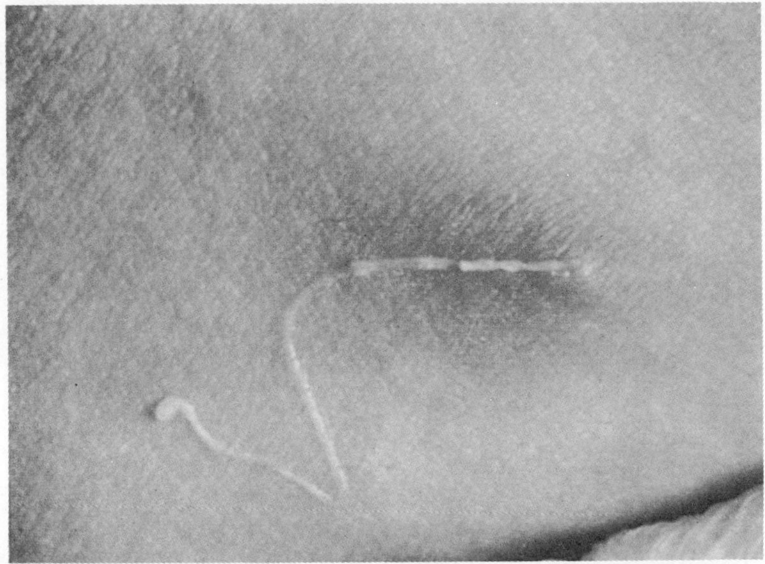

Figure 54–7. *Sparganum* extending from an incised lesion on the right posterolateral aspect of the chest. (Courtesy of Drs. J. H. Miller and S. H. Abadie, Louisiana State University School of Medicine, New Orleans.)

It has been shown in the case of *Spirometra mansonoides* (= *Diphyllobothrium mansonoides*) that the eggs hatch in water and the coracidium is ingested by a copepod. Following ingestion of the infected copepod, spargana develop in mice and rhesus monkeys, whereas adult worms mature in the definitive or final hosts, the dog, cat or bobcat. Most cases of sparganosis in the United States are nonproliferating and probably are caused by this species.[13, 14]

Sparganum proliferum (Ijima, 1905) Stiles, 1908 is a proliferating larva which is unknown in the adult stage. In the tissues of man it appears as an elongate mass with branched and sometimes proliferating processes (Fig. 54–8). Some of these may become separated from the parent worm and develop individually. These parasites invade not only the subcutaneous tissues and intermuscular fasciae but also the viscera and brain.

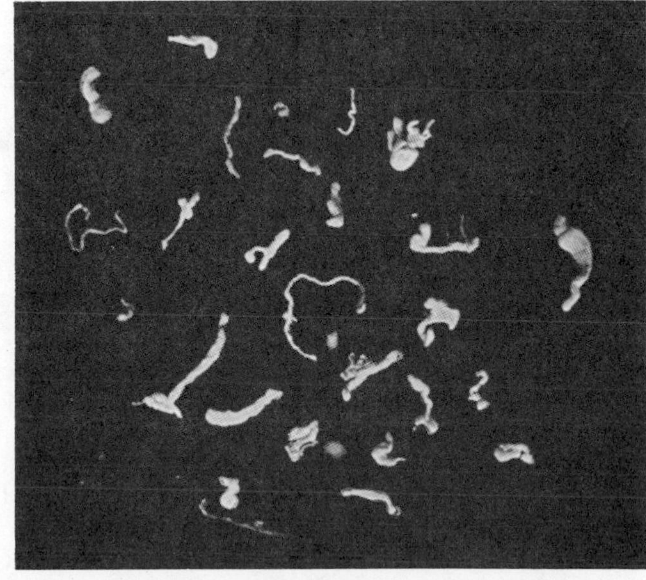

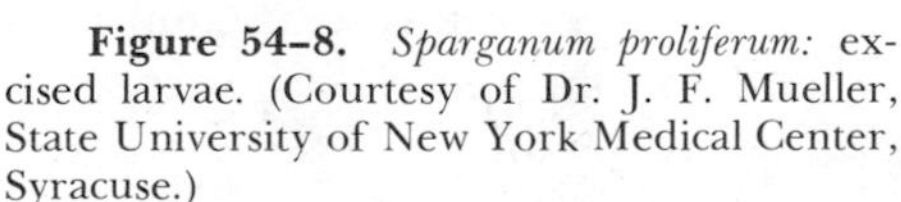

Figure 54–8. *Sparganum proliferum:* excised larvae. (Courtesy of Dr. J. F. Mueller, State University of New York Medical Center, Syracuse.)

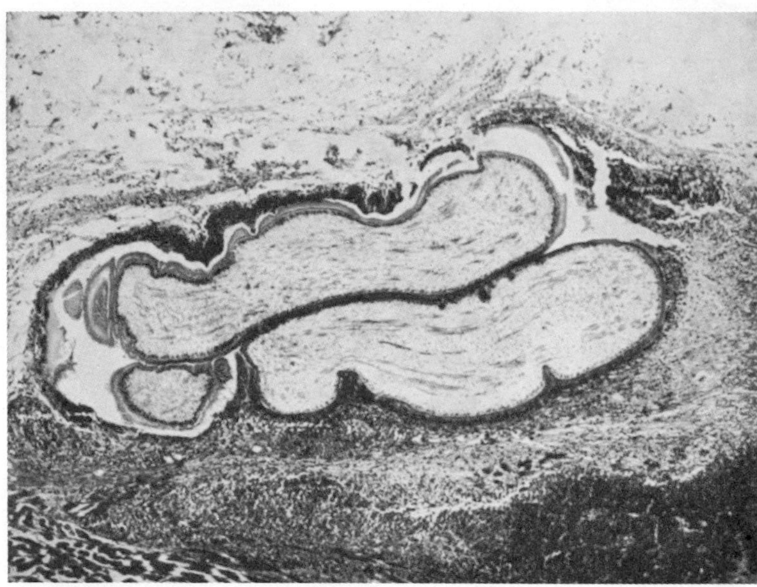

Figure 54-9. Sparganosis: larva of *Spirometra mansonoides* in tissues showing surrounding inflammation and foreign body reaction. (Courtesy of Dr. J. F. Mueller, State University of New York Medical Center, Syracuse.)

Epidemiology. Human sparganosis is acquired by the following means: (1) the ingestion of infected copepods containing the infective larvae; (2) the local application of infected vertebrates to the skin as poultices from which the larvae migrate into human tissue; or (3) ingesting infected, uncooked tadpoles, flesh of snakes, or other vertebrates as a remedy for a real or imagined ailment.

Pathology. The larvae invade primarily the subcutaneous tissues where they develop and produce considerable inflammation, swelling and fibrosis (Fig. 54-9). When opened, the lesions may be characterized by a shiny matrix within which the living larvae contract and elongate. Sometimes the parasite has degenerated and only a caseous mass remains.

In China, where infections occur in the eye as a result of the application of infected frogs as poultices, edematous conjunctivitis and corneal ulceration are seen.

Clinical Characteristics. The symptoms depend upon the number of larvae present and their location. Many cases of light infection remain asymptomatic. Infected cutaneous tissues become edematous and extremely painful to the touch. When sparganosis involves the breast and a nodule is detected by palpation, carcinoma usually is suspected until a specific diagnosis is made by examination of the surgical specimen. Lesions of the skin also may reveal acnelike nodular pustules frequently surrounded by tissue honeycombed with parasites. Actively moving spargana stimulate a moderate eosinophilic and lymphocytic infiltration. Ocular sparganosis results in redness, nodule formation, edema in the conjunctiva, excessive lachrymation, toxemia and, in cases of penetration of the retrobulbar region, corneal ulceration.

Diagnosis. Infections due to sparganosis are extremely difficult to diagnose except in areas where they are common. Consequently, they often remain undiagnosed until after surgical removal of the worm. However, the indirect fluorescent antibody test has recently been applied with success as a diagnostic aid in Japan.

Treatment. Orbital sparganosis may be treated with 2 to 4 ml of 40 per cent ethyl alcohol with Novocain (epinephrine-free) to kill the worms in situ, thus permitting ultimate resorption. Other workers recommend 0.3 to 0.45 gm per dose of novarsenobenzol intravenously for adults. This drug is given every 4 or 5 days for 2 to 6 administrations. In some instances, excision may prove more satisfactory.

Prophylaxis. Infection by this parasite can be avoided in endemic areas by the use of boiled or adequately filtered water. Education of the public against the application of freshly killed vertebrates as poultices, or the ingestion of their raw flesh, is essential if ultimate control is to be achieved.

Taeniasis Solium

Synonyms. Pork tapeworm infection, *Taenia solium* infection, cysticercosis.

Definition. Taeniasis solium is caused by the presence of the adult pork tapeworm, *T. solium,* in the intestine of man; cysticercosis is caused by the cysticerci in the tissues of man.

Distribution. The pork tapeworm has a cosmopolitan distribution, being found throughout the world wherever raw or inadequately cooked pork is eaten. Infection is rare in England, Canada and the United States. However, it is quite common in Mexico and the rest of the Latin American mainland, in Manchuria, U.S.S.R., North China, Pakistan, India and the Slavic countries of Europe.

Etiology. Morphology. The adult "measly pork" tapeworm, *Taenia solium* Linnaeus, 1758, attains a length of 2 to 7 meters. It lives attached to the intestinal wall of man. The scolex is about 1 mm in diameter and has been described as being "roughly quadrate." Anterior and central to the four suckers is a prominent terminal rostellum which bears two circular rows of hooklets. These hooklets number between 22 and 32 in an upper and lower row. The neck is short. Posterior to this structure are the immature, mature and gravid proglottids. The mature proglottids are nearly square, and, although the gravid ones are longer than broad, they do not attain the length of the corresponding proglottids of *T. saginata.* Morphologically, the mature proglottids of *T. solium* are in general similar to those of *T. saginata,* except that the testes in the former number between 150 and 200 compared with 300 and 400 in *T. saginata.* In addition, the ovary is trilobed instead of bilobed as in *T. saginata.* The uterine sac runs up the middle of the proglottid, with the ovarian complex in the posterior third of the segment. In the more elongate gravid proglottids the reproductive organs degenerate, with the exception of the uterus, which has 7 to 13 (an average of 9) main lateral branches on a side.

Eggs are spherical to subspherical in shape, 31 to 43 μm in greatest diameter, and cannot be differentiated from those of *T. saginata.* The terminal proglottids often become separated and are passed intact. Occasionally, they migrate actively from the anus when the host is not at stool.

Development. The eggs burst from the gravid proglottids either before or after the proglottids have become detached from the strobila. Eggs reaching the soil remain viable for weeks and, when ingested by hogs or man, hatch immediately. The liberated oncosphere penetrates the intestinal wall and reaches the lymphatic or circulatory system. These embryos are distributed throughout the body, most localizing in the musculature or subcutaneous tissues. Within 60 to 70 days they become metamorphosed into infective bladder worms, or *Cysticercus cellulosae,* about 5 mm in length by 8 to 10 mm in breadth.

In the usual course of events, cysticerci reach man when he ingests raw or inadequately prepared "measly pork." The larvae are digested out of the cysts, become attached to the intestinal wall and grow to maturity in 5 to 12 weeks. *Taenia solium* adults are believed to have survived as long as 25 years in the intestine of man.

Epidemiology. Man is the usual definitive host of *T. solium,* although the lar gibbon has recently been implicated,[15] and the hog is the usual intermediate host. Two forms of human infection occur. When man serves as the definitive host, the adult tape-

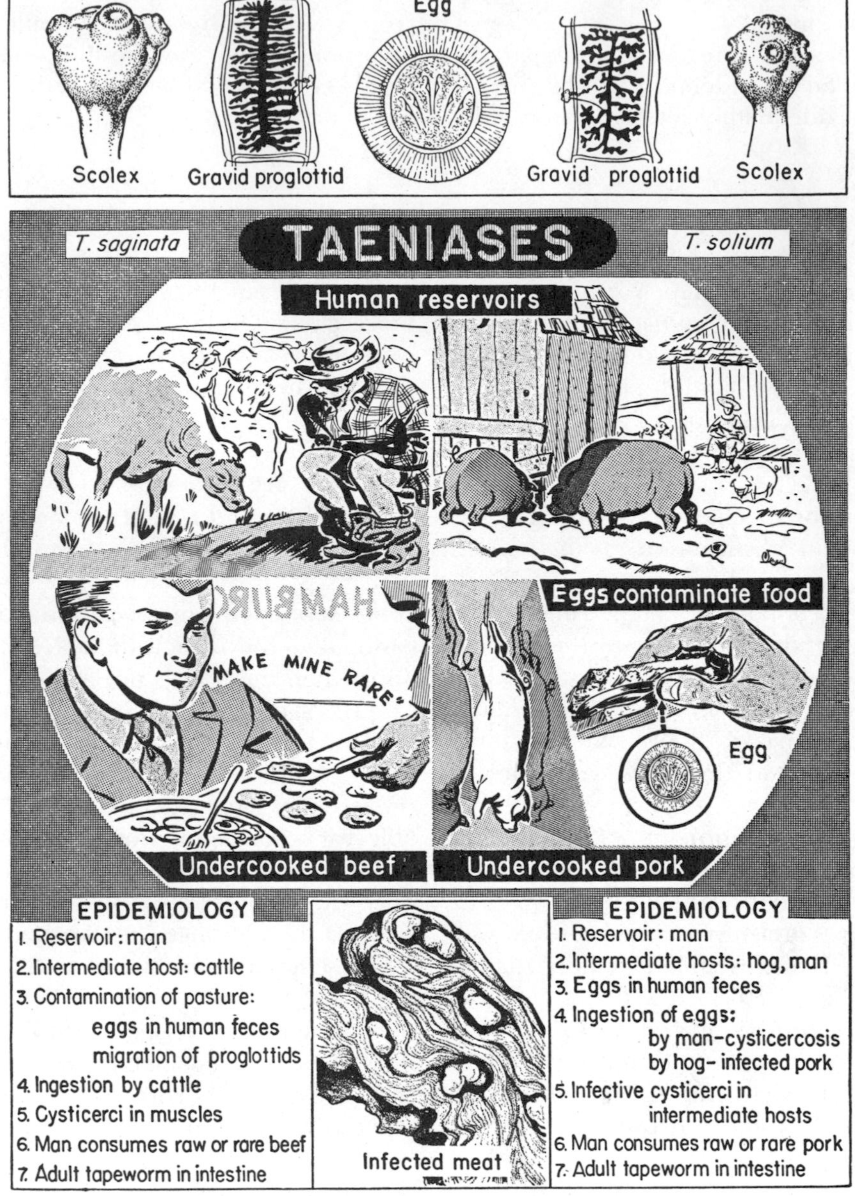

Figure 54–10. Epidemiology of the taeniases.

worm is present in the intestine. Such infection is acquired only by the ingestion of raw or insufficiently cooked "measly pork" containing viable cysticerci (Fig. 54–10).

In cysticercosis man serves as the intermediate host, and the larval stages, cysticerci, are present in his tissues. Human infection results usually from the ingestion and subsequent hatching of viable eggs. They reach the alimentary canal in food or drink contaminated by feces from a person harboring the adult worm. Autoinfection may occur when eggs are carried from feces to the mouth on the hands of infected persons. It is believed to occur also when reverse peristalsis brings egg-laden proglottids back to the stomach or duodenum where they hatch. Occasionally, other primates, dogs and sheep are infected with cysticerci.

Taeniasis solium, infection with the

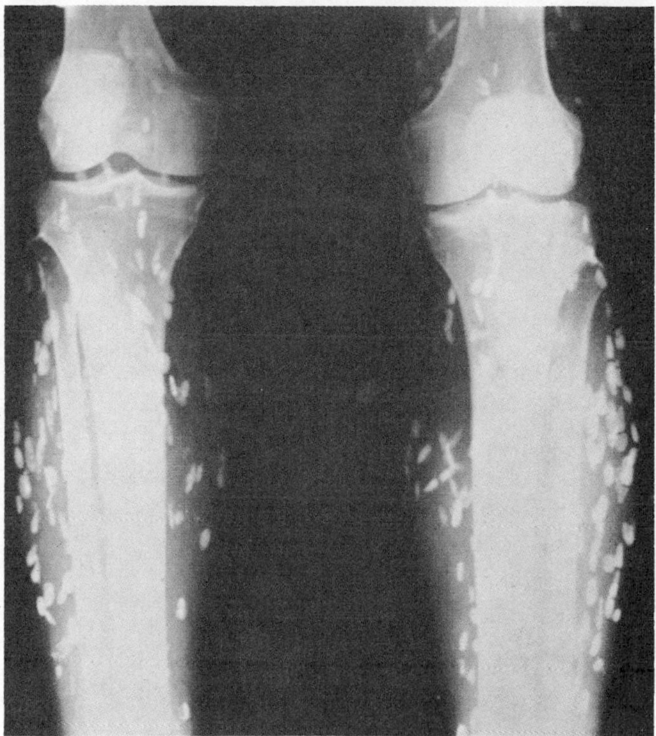

Figure 54-11. X-ray of legs showing calcified cysticerci of *Taenia solium.* (Courtesy of Dr. M. Campagna.)

adult worm, is not found among such groups as the Jews and Mohammedans, since they rarely eat pork; cysticercosis, on the other hand, may occur.

The infection is maintained in nature by improper disposal of human feces, which permits ingestion of the eggs by the normal intermediate host, the hog.

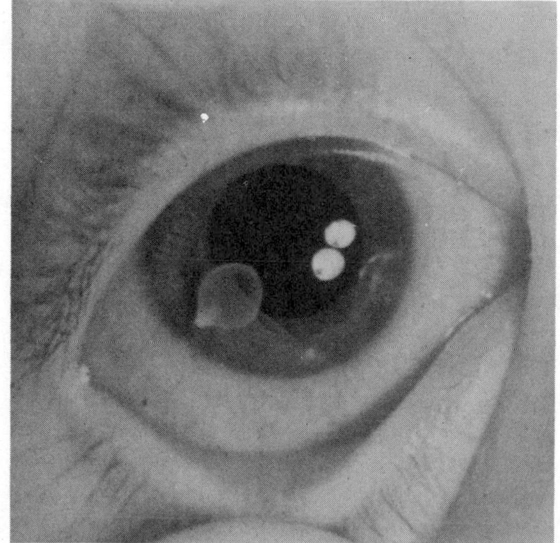

Figure 54-12. Cysticercus of *Taenia solium* in the eye. (Courtesy of Dr. A. Trejos, Costa Rica.)

Pathology. THE ADULT WORM. The mature tapeworm in the intestine seldom causes significant pathologic changes. A moderate eosinophilia may be present (up to 13 per cent).

Cysticercus cellulosae. The cysticerci may be lodged in any tissue of the body. They are most frequently found in the subcutaneous tissues, skeletal musculature, eye, brain, heart, liver, lungs and abdominal cavity (Figs. 54-11 to 54-13). The larvae cause, at first, a local surrounding inflammatory reaction, with infiltration by neutrophils, eosinophils and lymphocytes and a stimulation of fibroblast production. Subsequently, the larvae become enclosed within a fibrous capsule, or necrosis may occur followed by caseation or calcification (Fig. 54-11). Giant cells may be found about the lesions. The resulting cysts may vary from 0.5 to 2 or even 3 cm in diameter.

Clinical Characteristics. THE ADULT WORM. Common complaints include passing of "segments," abdominal or epigastric

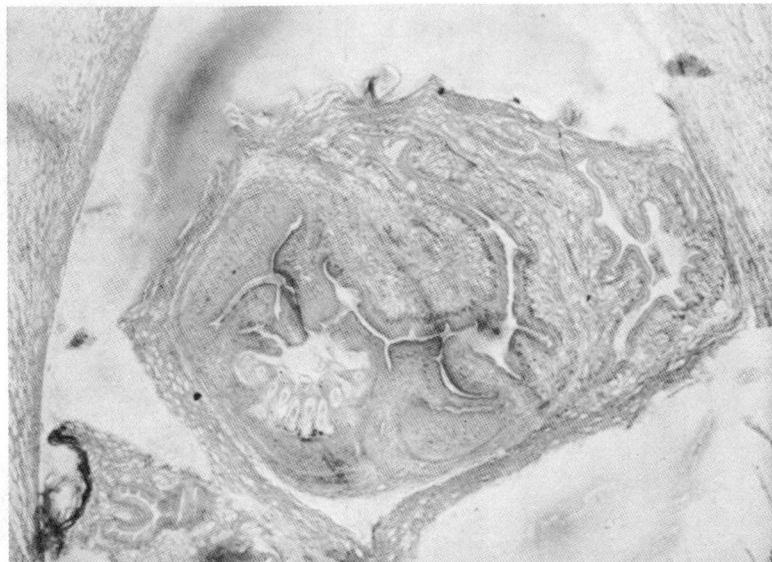

Figure 54–13. Cysticercus of *T. solium* in brain. Note slight tissue reaction of host, rostellar hooks and laterally placed suckers of parasite.

pain, increased appetite, hunger pains, weakness and weight loss.

Cysticercus cellulosae. The clinical picture of cysticercosis is extremely variable and depends upon the location and the number of cysticerci in the host. When these are few and restricted principally to the subcutaneous tissues, symptoms may be negligible or absent. When they localize in the brain, the spinal cord, the eye or the heart muscle, serious effects are common. The phenomena associated with tumor formation in the particular anatomic region are then noted. Localization in the fourth ventricle or in the cerebral cortex is frequent, and in these instances there may be epileptiform convulsions, mental changes and other phenomena that accompany brain tumors irrespective of type (Fig. 54–13). Eosinophilia is not remarkable in this infection.

Cysts may be palpable as firm nodules in the superficial tissues.

Diagnosis. THE ADULT. Differentiation between *T. saginata* and *T. solium* infections on the basis of their eggs is impossible. Therefore, it is important to differentiate between the mature proglottids, which may be pressed between two slides and held to the light. The uterus may be injected with India ink to facilitate the determination of the number of main lateral uterine branches, which range between 7 and 13 (average 9) in *T. solium* and 15 to 20 in *T. saginata.*

Cysticercus cellulosae. The occurrence of epilepsy or the clinical picture of brain tumor developing in a previously healthy individual who is known to have been in a hyperendemic area should arouse suspicion and lead to careful search of the entire body surface for the characteristic nodules in the subcutaneous tissues. Soft tissue roentgen examination of the extremities will often reveal characteristic "rice grain" or "puffed rice" calcific shadows (Fig. 54–11).

The differential white blood count is not of assistance in view of the frequent lack of eosinophilia. Precipitin tests are only group-specific, but an indirect hemagglutination test, using antigen prepared from lyophilized pig cysticerci, has helped confirm diagnosis in 85 per cent of a series of cases.[16] Progress is being made in the diagnostic application of immunoelectrophoretic and indirect fluorescence tests. Definitive diagnosis depends upon recovery of the larva by excision of a cyst and identification of species by the presence of four suckers and two rows of hooks of unequal size on the inverted rostellum.

Since cysticercosis may be due to autoinfection, stool examinations should be made for the presence of eggs in the event intestinal infection is still present. A history of tapeworm infection should be sought.

Treatment. There continues to be controversy concerning the choice of specific therapy for *T. solium* infections. Most of the drugs listed for *D. latum* (p. 600), effective also for *T. saginata,* kill *T. solium,* producing lysis of the adult worms in the intestine with release of eggs in situ. It is feared that regurgitation of *T. solium* eggs, but not the others, may result in the development of cysticercosis. Should one of these drugs be used for *T. solium,* therefore, it must be followed in 3 or 4 hours by a purgative. Niclosamide (Yomesan), administered after a light meal in a dosage of 60 mg per kg in two portions 2 hours apart and thoroughly chewed, is the drug of choice in these circumstances.[17]

Quinacrine, despite its known side effects, is preferred by some authorities because it usually produces the expulsion of *T. solium* intact without release of eggs. On an empty stomach, 200 mg (adult dose) are given at intervals of 10 minutes for 4 doses (total 800 mg), each dose being accompanied by 600 mg of sodium bicarbonate to quell nausea and vomiting. The tendency to vomit may further be reduced by administration of chlorpromazine prior to the quinacrine, and the latter may be introduced by means of a duodenal tube. This specific treatment should be followed in 2 hours by a saline purge. Stools should be examined for 12 hours to confirm passage of the scolex, dyed yellow.

Recently mebendazole has been shown to be effective in removing *Taenia* spp. Dosage schedules of 200 mg twice daily for 4 days, or 300 mg twice daily for 3 days, appear to be the most promising. No side effects were observed at these dosages.[18]

Although the treatment of cysticercosis is essentially surgical, metrifonate has recently been given for several months without intolerance to a patient with cysticercosis, and resulted in symptomatic improvement with regression or disappearance of cysts.[19]

Prophylaxis. Intestinal infection by *T. solium* is prevented by proper cooking of all pork products. Cysticerci present in pickled or salted pork may be viable; they are destroyed, however, by freezing. United States Government meat inspection provides a safeguard but not complete protection.

Sanitary disposal of human feces prevents infection of the hog and is the essential procedure in the control of taeniasis solium.

Cysticercosis may often be prevented by prompt and effective therapy of the individual harboring the adult worm, efficient methods of personal cleanliness to prevent autoinfection, and protection of food and drink against possible contamination by human feces containing eggs of *T. solium.*

Taeniasis Saginata

Synonyms. Beef tapeworm infection, *Taenia saginata* infection.

Definition. Taeniasis saginata is caused by the presence of the adult beef tapeworm, *T. saginata,* in the intestine of man.

Distribution. The beef tapeworm is cosmopolitan in distribution, being especially prevalent in Mexico, South America and some areas of Africa, Asia and the U.S.S.R.

Etiology. MORPHOLOGY. *Taenia saginata* Goeze, 1782 is a large tapeworm usually 5 to 10 meters in length. The scolex appears quadrate in cross section and carries four round suckers. The rostellum and hooks typical of *T. solium* are lacking in *T. saginata.* The neck is short, being about half as broad as the head and several times its length. Then follow the immature, mature and gravid proglottids, respectively. The mature proglottids are broader than long and contain about twice as many testes (300 to 400) as comparable proglottids of *T. solium.* The gravid proglottids are longer than broad, 5 to 7 mm in width by about 20 mm in length. There are 15 to 20 main uterine branches on either side of this median saclike structure which virtually fill the entire proglottid.

The spherical to ovoid eggs are 31 to 43

μm in diameter and cannot be differentiated from the eggs of *T. solium.* The oncosphere, containing six characteristic hooklets, is surrounded by a narrow space filled with a transparent material. This clear area, in turn, is surrounded by a thick outer shell heavily marked by radial striations. The delicate, hyaline, thin outer envelopes surrounding these eggs in utero are rarely present when the eggs are detected in the stool.

DEVELOPMENT. Eggs may remain alive on pasture for 4 months, and develop in cattle, giraffes, llamas and buffaloes. Sheep and other herbivorous animals are recorded as experimental intermediate hosts. After ingestion the outer shell membrane is digested, thus setting the embryos free in the upper part of the small intestine. These larvae migrate through the intestinal wall of the intermediate host, reach the blood or lymph streams and are carried about the body until filtered out in the striated muscles. Here they metamorphose into cysticerci. Man, the only definitive host, acquires the infection upon ingesting infected meat containing viable *Cysticercus bovis.* An incubation period of 10 to 12 weeks is required for maturation of the parasite and the appearance of eggs in the stool.

Epidemiology. Infection results from the ingestion of infected raw or poorly cooked beef (Fig. 54–10). Among certain religious groups, such as the Mohammedans, who merely sear the outside of large chunks of beef before eating it, the infection rate is particularly high. In the United States only about 0.37 per cent of federally inspected cattle have been found infected. Soil may be contaminated directly by eggs in feces or indirectly by viable proglottids. Even when the infected individual is not at stool, the latter sometimes migrate through the anus and subsequently reach the ground.

Pathology. No significant pathologic phenomena usually occur, although detached proglottids occasionally migrate to the appendix and, through occlusive or traumatic actions, initiate appendicitis. Eosinophils may be moderately or, occasionally, markedly increased (6 to 34 per cent); this may be followed by a slight neutropenia. Human infection with *Cysticercus bovis* is very rare.

Clinical Characteristics. Many cases of taeniasis saginata are asymptomatic. Patients with beef tapeworm infection usually give a history of passing proglottids. Although many infected persons exhibit no symptoms, a significant percentage of cases may have abdominal or epigastric pain, increased appetite, weakness or malaise and weight loss. Vertigo, nausea, vomiting, dyspnea, headache and diarrhea are among the infrequent manifestations in cases of taeniasis saginata.

Diagnosis. Diagnosis depends upon (1) the detection of characteristic *Taenia*-like eggs in the stool or in perianal scrapings,[20] and (2) the finding of gravid proglottids, since species identification cannot be made from eggs alone. The proglottids may be pressed between two glass slides and the number of main lateral uterine branches counted under a dissecting microscope or with a hand lens. These range in number from 15 to 20 and average 18 or 19 on each side. In *Taenia solium* there are only 7 to 13, with an average of 9 on each side.

Treatment. The specific treatment of *T. saginata* infections is similar to that of *D. latum* (p. 600), niclosamide being the drug of choice. Mebendazole also is effective in removal of *Taenia saginata* (p. 607).[18]

Prophylaxis. Beef tapeworm infections may be prevented in the United States by avoiding all beef that does not bear a proper inspection label. Adequate freezing, at −10° C (14° F) for 14 days, or salting of uninspected meat is efficacious. The eating of raw beef should be discouraged. Thorough cooking of beef prevents infection of man, and the sanitary disposal of human feces prevents infection of the intermediate host.

Unilocular Hydatid Disease

Synonyms. Echinococciasis, echinococcosis, echinococcus disease.

Definition. This is an infection by the larval form of *Echinococcus granulosus* in man or another intermediate host. It is characterized by the formation of single or multiple expanding cysts which are unilocular in character. The alveolar form of hydatid disease is caused by *Echinococcus multilocularis* (p. 615).

Distribution. Unilocular hydatid disease is prevalent in sheep raising countries where man is closely associated with heavily infected sheep dogs. Such regions are mainly temperate or subtropical. Autochthonous cases, though rare in the United States, have been reported from about 15 states (Fig. 54–14).

Etiology. THE ADULT. Adult *Echinococcus granulosus* (Batsch, 1786) Rudolphi, 1805 (= *Taenia echinococcus*) occur mainly in carnivores, such as dogs, wolves, jackals and cats. These are small tapeworms ranging from 3 to 6 mm in length and consisting of four parts: (1) The pyriform scolex is only about 0.3 mm in diameter and carries four suckers and a rostellum which bears two circular rows of hooklets varying in total number but ranging from 28 to 50 (usually 30 to 36). The scolex is continued without evidence of segmentation into a narrow neck. (2) Behind this occurs an immature proglottid. (3) More posteriorly is the single mature proglottid which is nearly twice as long as the preceding one and which contains a complete set of reproductive organs. (4) The terminal or gravid proglottid may reach 2 mm in length. It consists principally of a uterus with lateral evaginations; these become so distended with eggs that the uterus finally bursts, liberating the eggs either before or after detachment from the strobila. The eggs are indistinguishable from other *Taenia* eggs found in dogs or man. They possess thick brown shells which surround the six-hooked oncospheres. Maximum diameter of the eggs is 30 to 38 μm.

THE LARVA. Human infection results from the ingestion of the eggs of *E. granulosus.* These hatch in the duodenum, and most of the liberated oncospheres then penetrate its wall. The larvae are carried throughout the body, most being filtered out in the liver and lungs and the remainder in other tissues, where many of them are destroyed by phagocytic cells. Probably 60 to 70 per cent of the surviving larvae reach maturity in the liver. Growth at first takes place quite rapidly; on the fourth day the parasite is only 40 μm in length, but in 3 weeks it is 0.25 mm long. At the end of 5 months it has grown to about a centimeter in size. Cysts subsequently grow more slowly and frequently come to the notice of a physician as late as 20 years after the initial infection.

If a young developing unilocular cyst is comparatively uninfluenced by pressure, the following structural characteristics of the growth may be noted:

1. An external laminated cuticula (Fig. 54–15).
2. An interior germinative membrane which buds off the daughter cysts or the brood capsules (Fig. 54–15).
3. The hydatid fluid which fills the hydatid cysts and gradually produces considerable distention.
4. The germinative membrane which also lines the new budding daughter cysts.
5. The daughter cysts free in the hydatid fluid which, in turn, may produce granddaughter cysts within them (Fig. 54–16).
6. Some of the brood capsules become separated from the wall and settle to the bottom together with liberated scolices as a fine "hydatid sand."

Not all of the germinal epithelium that lines the hydatid cyst is fertile, nor are all the daughter cysts fertile.

The cycle in nature is completed when the hydatid cysts are ingested, usually by a carnivore, as, for example, when a sheep dog feeds on the discarded viscera of a slaughtered infected sheep, or a wolf preys upon a flock. The hydatid cyst contains many scolices, each of which may develop to a mature, adult tapeworm in the intestine of the carnivorous host.

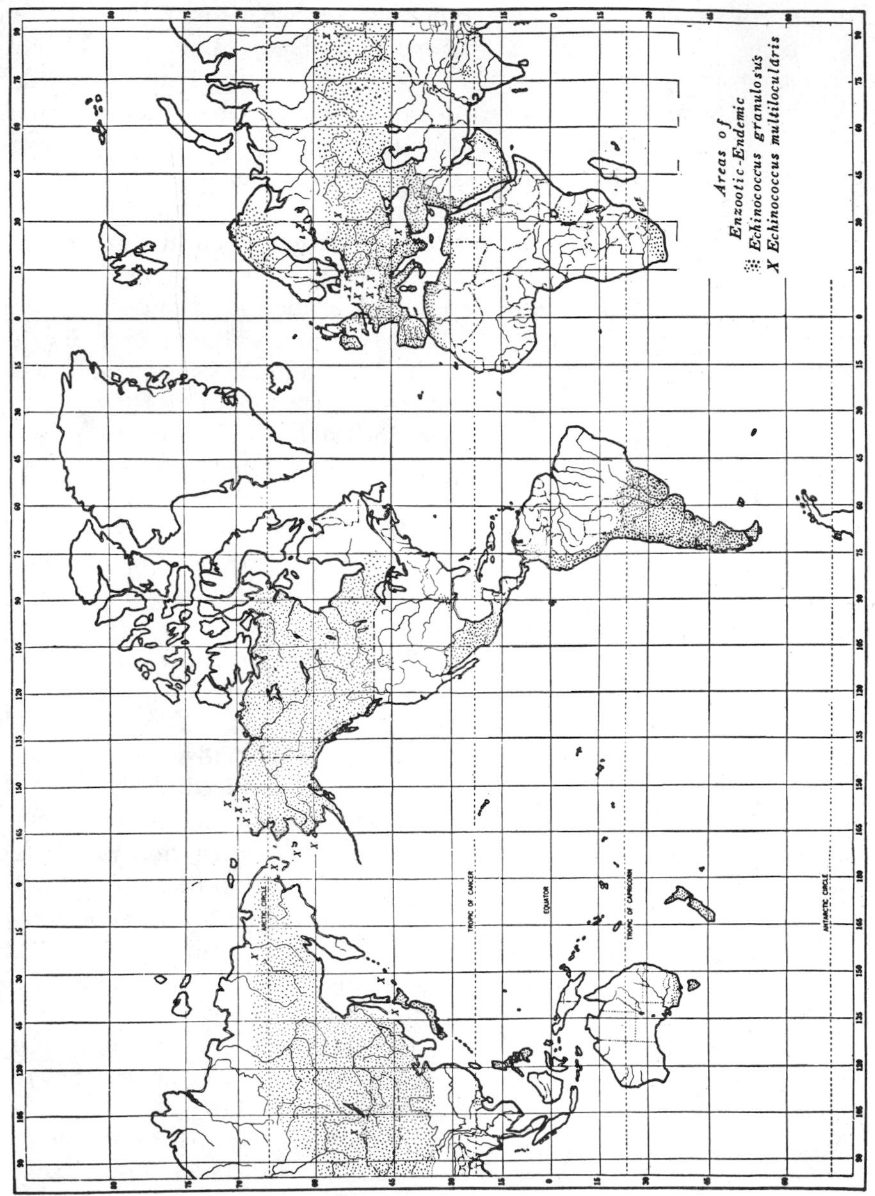

Figure 54–14. Map showing the distribution of *Echinococcus granulosus* and *E. multilocularis* in man and reservoir hosts. (From Faust, E. C., Russell, P. F., and Jung, R. C. 1970. Craig and Faust's Clinical Parasitology. 8th ed. Lea & Febiger, Philadelphia. Information from Mexico kindly provided by Dr. L. Mazzotti.)

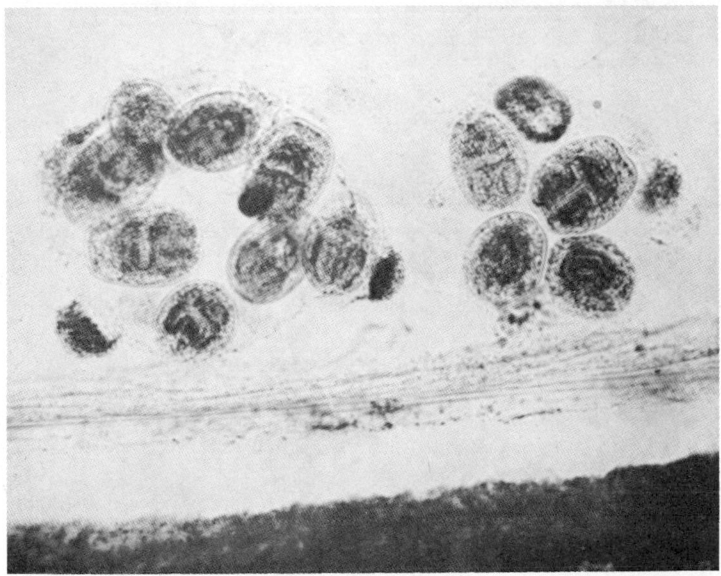

Figure 54-15. Wall of hydatid cyst: two daughter cysts budding from germinal epithelium of wall. Note contained scolices. (Courtesy of Dr. A. C. Chandler, Rice Institute.)

Epidemiology. Hydatid disease is important in many parts of the world. The dog is the common definitive host and the chief reservoir of infection, although other wild CANIDAE have been reported as carrying the adult. The common intermediate hosts are sheep, cattle, hogs and occasionally man. Eggs are deposited in the feces of the hosts carrying the adult parasites and thus contaminate the range or pasture. Herbivores grazing over this seeded area ingest the eggs. After a variable period these intermediate hosts develop characteristic hydatid cysts, the scolices of which will produce adults when they are ingested by a suitable definitive host. Human infection results from ingestion of eggs of *Echinococcus granulosus.* Such eggs reach the mouth of man by hands, food, drink or containers contaminated with feces of infected dogs (Fig. 54-17).

In sheep raising countries, sheep dogs should be regarded with suspicion, since many carry the adult tapeworms. The sheep raising districts of Australia report a high in-

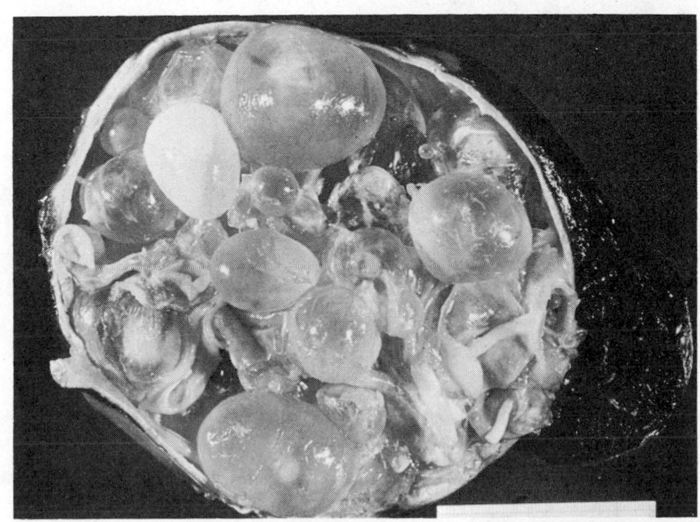

Figure 54-16. Unilocular hydatid cyst of the liver containing daughter cysts. (Courtesy of Dr. G. Carrera, Ochsner Foundation Hospital, New Orleans, Louisiana.)

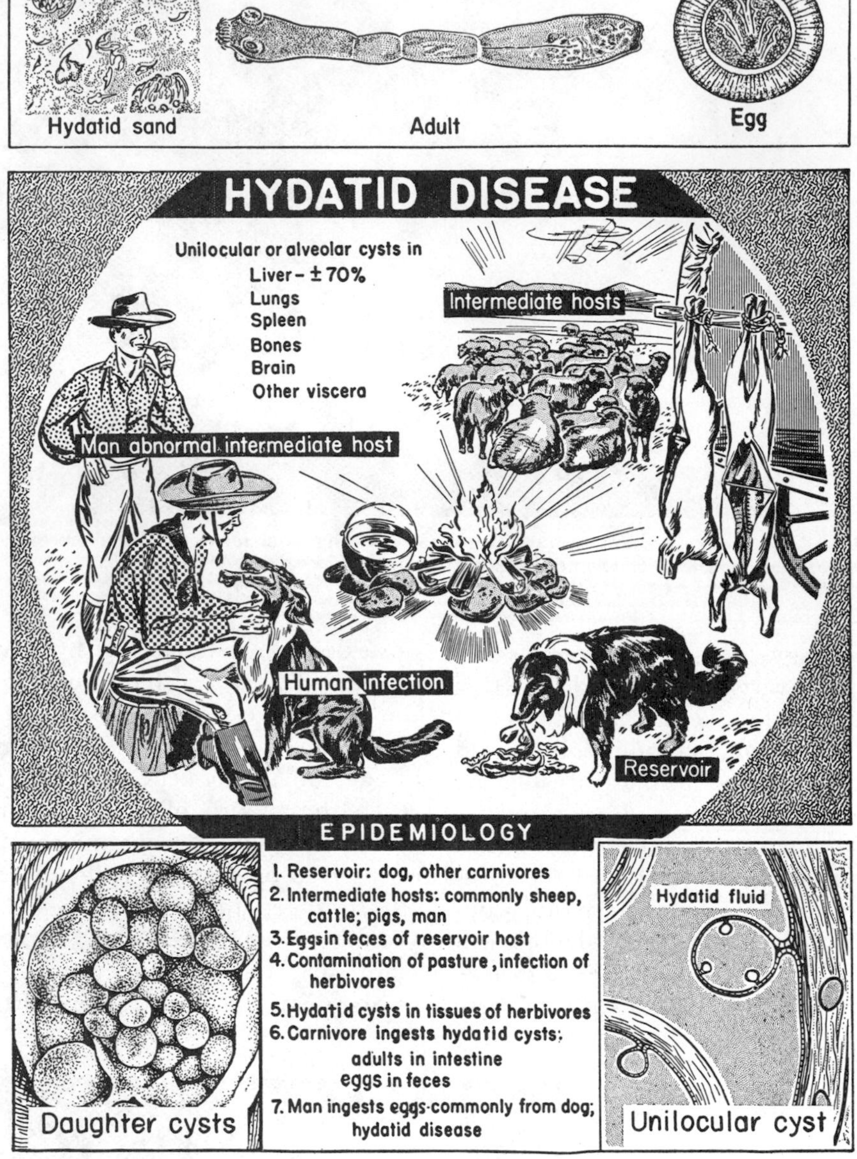

Figure 54-17. Epidemiology of unilocular hydatid disease.

fection rate in dogs (up to 50 per cent), but only 3 per cent of the human population is infected. In New Zealand about 120 human cases with about 14 per cent fatality are seen each year.

In northern Canada "sylvatic echinococciasis" exists. Wolves are highly infected and seed areas with eggs. These are ingested by such wild herbivores as the caribou and moose, and the cycle is completed when these herbivores are killed by wolves. This sylvatic cycle enters the domestic picture because the wild herbivores are slaughtered in large numbers for food. The viscera are fed to the dogs, which become infected with the adult parasite. By infecting his dogs man initiates a cycle in which he may assume the role of intermediate host, and so eventually develops echinococciasis.

The epidemiology and characteristics of the tapeworm *Multiceps multiceps*, rare in man, resemble those of *E. granulosus*. The adult worm occurs as an intestinal parasite of dogs, while larval stages encyst in sheep, usually in the central nervous system. Such cysts have been found in man very rarely, the condition, known as coenuriasis, presenting with central nervous system pressure symptoms or, should the cysts rupture, acute toxemia. A closely related species has been incriminated recently in a number of human cases in the eastern Congo and Uganda.

Pathology. The unilocular hydatid cyst produces a characteristic reaction on the part of the host. This consists at first of a localized surrounding inflammatory reaction with infiltration by eosinophils, round cells and giant cells. This is followed by fibroblast proliferation and the gradual formation of an enclosing fibrous capsule (Fig. 54–16). As progressive growth of the cyst takes place, pressure necrosis of adjacent tissue occurs.

Hydatid cysts may develop in bone, causing extensive destruction, and spontaneous fractures and nonunion are not unusual. The subsequent invasion of the soft tissues is typically associated with the deposition of calcium.

Since the oncospheres are distributed through the body by the blood, hydatid cysts may develop in any region. They are most commonly found, however, in the liver, lungs, omentum and mesentery.

Clinical Characteristics. Hydatid cysts frequently cause no symptoms during early stages, especially if localized in the liver, but later as the tumor increases in size it may give rise to both subjective and objective signs due to pressure. Most patients with unilocular hydatid disease have complaints referable to the biliary tract or complaints such as bloating, indigestion, nausea and vomiting. Histories of mild pain in the right upper abdominal quadrant, severe biliary colic and of jaundice during the attacks of pain are relatively common. Cysts frequently rupture and discharge their contents into a large bile duct. The resulting embolic obstruction of the biliary tract accounts for the colicky pain and jaundice. Unilocular cysts may suppurate and produce a clinical picture of hepatic abscess. Hydatid cysts may rupture into the peritoneal cavity, lung, pleura, bronchus and kidney. Release of hydatid fluid may produce a severe and even fatal reaction.

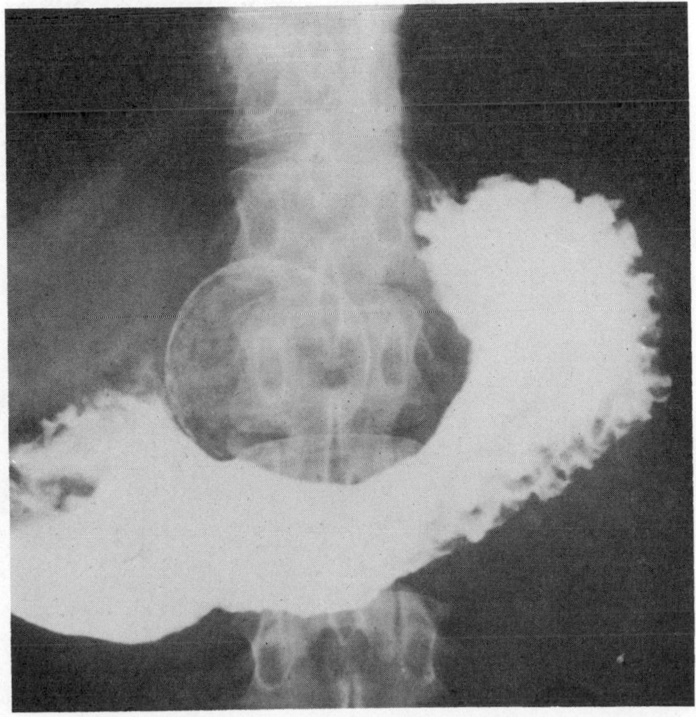

Figure 54–18. X-ray showing cannon ball shape of a calcified unilocular hydatid cyst of the liver. The patient had been given a barium meal for diagnosis of a gastrointestinal disorder and the hydatid cyst was detected coincidentally. (Courtesy of Dr. D. Harllee and the Charity Hospital of Louisiana, New Orleans.)

In about 12 per cent of the cases the lungs may be involved. Such cases are characterized by cough, hemoptysis and, sometimes, fever. When the cyst is located in bone, spontaneous fracture and deformity may result. If the brain is the site of the infection, epilepsy and blindness may become apparent.

Diagnosis. A history of signs indicative of an expanding tumor in an individual who has been in an endemic area may be suggestive. Eosinophilia, however, occurs in only 10 to 20 per cent of the cases. Hydatid thrill or fremitus may be demonstrable over large intra-abdominal cysts. This is a tremulous impulse sometimes felt on palpation of the body surface over a unilocular hydatid cyst. When present, it is a specific diagnostic sign of unilocular hydatid. Roentgen examination may likewise be of assistance; cysts in the liver or lung frequently have a cannon ball shape (Figs. 54–18 to 54–20). If cysts of the lung have ruptured into a bronchus, examination of the sputum may reveal hydatid sand. Exploratory puncture is not advised because of the hazard of anaphylactoid reaction and of contaminating uninjured tissues.

The precipitin, complement-fixation and Casoni intradermal tests are reasonably specific and are valuable diagnostic aids. However, the most useful test is the hemagglutination reaction using formalinized red cells.[21] Obviously, stool examination is of no value in human hydatid disease.

Treatment. The only effective treatment is complete excision of the cyst. Whether this is practical depends upon the location and type of cyst. Surgical intervention should be considered only in cases of unilocular cysts. In many cases the cyst may be removed intact, but such a procedure is difficult, as the fibrous capsule surrounding the cyst proper gradually gives way to normal tissue. Two procedures have been commonly used: (1) Aspiration of 10 to 15 ml of the fluid and replacement with 10 per cent formalin. This kills the scolices and brood capsules and renders the contents of the cyst harmless in the event they are accidentally scattered during removal. (2) Marsupialization, in which case the cyst, after sterilization with 10 per cent formalin, may be stitched to the abdominal wall and allowed to heal by granulation. A recently developed proce-

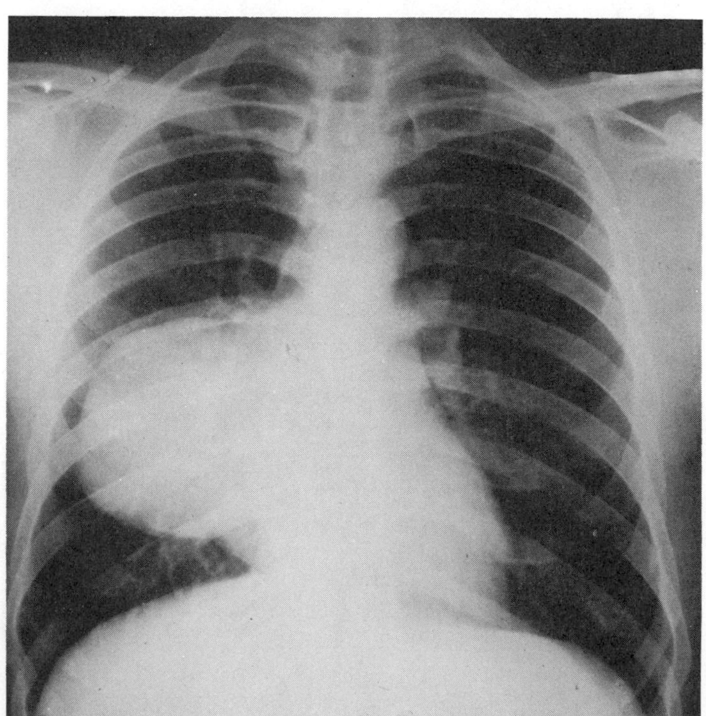

Figure 54–19. X-ray showing unilocular hydatid cyst of the lung. (Courtesy of the Veterans Administration Hospital, New Orleans.)

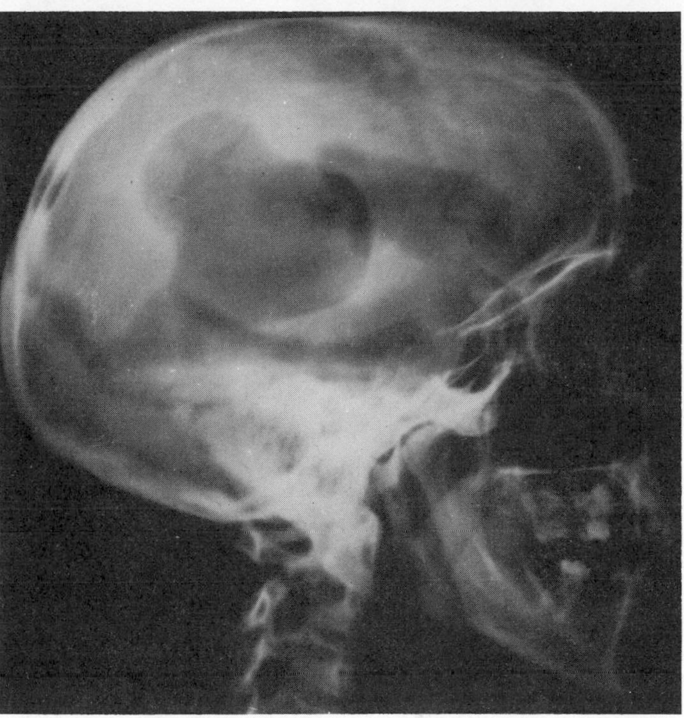

Figure 54–20. Ventriculogram showing outline of cerebral hydatid in markedly dilated left ventricle. (Courtesy of the Charity Hospital of Louisiana, New Orleans.)

dure involves sealing the operating area in the cyst wall by freezing, and destruction of scolices in the aspirated cyst by introduction of 0.5 per cent silver nitrate solution.[22] Since hydatid fluid may be released or spilled during the operation, patients may be protected from allergic or anaphylactic reaction by administration of adrenocortical steroids during and after operation.

Prophylaxis. Prophylaxis of the disease on a wide scale entails elimination of the infection in the common definitive host. Deworming of dogs with arecoline hydrobromide or other suitable veterinary taeniacides is practiced in some heavily endemic areas. Proper disposal of carcasses on sheep ranges or of entrails from slaughter houses will prevent dogs from gaining access to them. Prophylaxis, so far as sporadic human cases are concerned, involves caution against the contamination of hands, food or drink with dog feces.

Alveolar Hydatid Disease

Definition. This infection is caused by larval stages of *Echinococcus multilocularis* (Leuckart, 1863) Vogel, 1955. These invade the affected organs and destroy the host's tissues. The parasites behave very much as an infiltrating neoplasm.

Distribution. *Echinococcus multilocularis* is restricted to the Northern Hemisphere,[23] occurring in south central Europe, mainly in the neighborhood of the Alps, throughout much of the U.S.S.R., in northern Canada around Hudson Bay, in the states of Minnesota and North Dakota, and in northern and western Alaska and adjacent islands. A related species, *Echinococcus oligarthrus* (Diesing, 1863), has been identified recently as the cause of echinococcosis in man in Colombia and Panama.[24]

Etiology. The Adult. Foxes are the important hosts of the adult worms in nature, but dogs and cats also become infected. The strobila consists of a scolex, neck and single immature, mature, and gravid proglottids. It ranges in size from 1.2 to 3.7 mm. In addition to their shorter length, the adults of *E. multilocularis* can be differentiated from *E. granulosus* by other morphologic details. In the former, the uterus usually has no lateral branches, the genital pore of the gravid segment is located near the middle, and the testes are distributed from the level of the genital pore to the posterior end of the segment. The number of testes ranges from 17 to 26 and averages 22. In contrast, lateral branches of the uterus are present in *E. granulosus*, the genital pore is near the posterior end of the segment, and the testes are located both anterior and posterior to the genital pore; the testes range from 45 to 65, with an average of 56.

THE LARVA. Unlike *E. granulosus* which produces large single cysts with endogenous growth and a well defined fibrous tissue encapsulation, *E. multilocularis* forms an aggregate of innumerable small cysts. These proliferate by exogenous budding. The alveolar hydatid in human tissue appears as small, irregular cavities with thin and crumpled hyaline membranes. In some human infections the parasites are sterile and no scolices are present in the alveolar cavities. As the cysts develop, particularly in animal hosts, numerous calcareous granules (corpuscles) appear throughout the germinal membrane. The number of brood capsules and scolices then increases, filling the many alveolar cavities.

Epidemiology. The natural intermediate hosts of *E. multilocularis* are field mice and other small mammals. These herbivorous animals, and occasionally man, become infected by swallowing *Taenia*-like eggs from the feces of the carnivorous definitive hosts. The latter, in turn, are infected through preying upon microtine rodents, such as field mice, and ingesting the scolices contained in their larval cysts. In boreal regions sled dogs are the usual source of human infection, although foxes may be important under some conditions. In agricultural regions man may acquire the infection by consuming fruits and vegetables contaminated by the excreta of

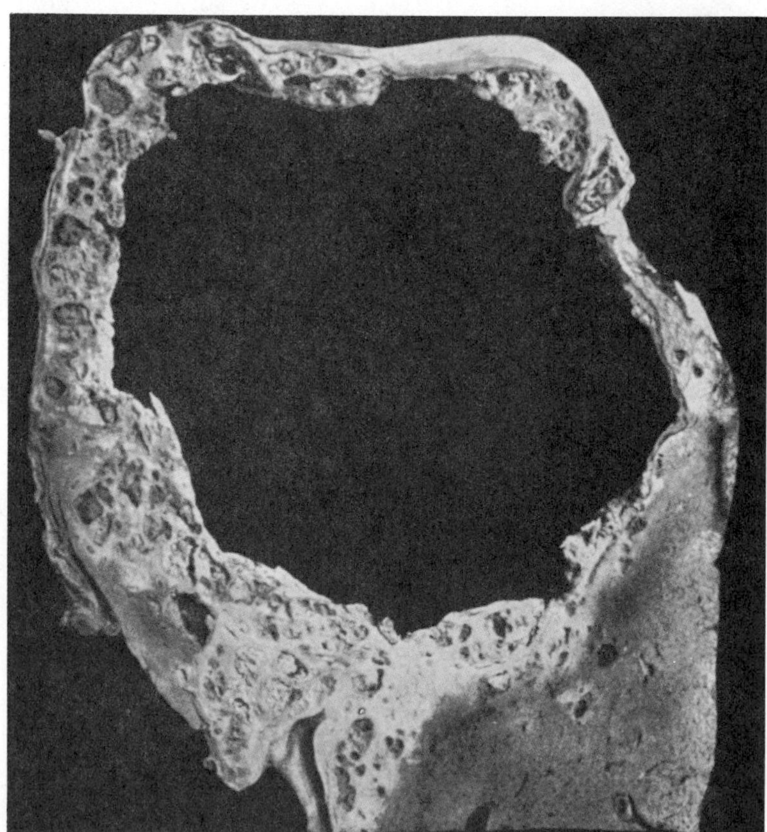

Figure 54–21. Alveolar hydatid cyst invading liver. (From Faust, E. C., Russell, P. F., and Jung, R. C. 1970. Craig and Faust's Clinical Parasitology. 8th ed. Lea & Febiger, Philadelphia.)

foxes or other canids, by handling contaminated soil, picking and eating berries grown close to the soil, and through association with infected dogs and cats. Children may acquire the infection by eating or soiling their hands with dirt in areas frequented by dogs, cats, wolves and foxes.

Pathology. The liver is involved in over 90 per cent of human infections. Larval growth is exogenous and a progressive invasion of the infected organ results, owing to the lack of a circumscribing capsule. The tissue is honeycombed by the alveolar hydatid. When the tumor has grown sufficiently, it begins to break down in the center, forming an abscess-like cavity, while the peripheral cysts continue to multiply (Fig. 54–21). The parasite resembles a malignant tumor in its behavior, even to the point of forming metastases.

Clinical Characteristics. The disease runs a chronic, afebrile course characterized by hepatomegaly and later by splenomegaly, icterus and ascites. The clinical signs are typical of intrahepatic portal tension.

Diagnosis. The differential diagnosis between alveolar echinococciasis and carcinoma of the liver is very difficult clinically. As a rule, the diagnosis is established by histologic examination of biopsy specimens. Noncalcified hepatic cysts may be detected by radioisotopic liver scanning, which also serves to define the extent of the cysts as a guide for surgical procedures. For serologic diagnostic tests see page 838.

Treatment. This consists of surgical extirpation of the involved portion of the organ. However, early diagnosis is difficult, and advanced cases usually are inoperable. Radiation therapy has not been of significant value.

Prophylaxis. Prevention includes control of dogs and cats, and measures to avoid fecal contamination of food and water supplies by dogs and other hosts of the adult worms. Since wild canids, such as foxes and wolves, may harbor the adult forms, precaution should be taken to prevent contamination by their excreta.

Other Tapeworms Infecting Man

There are records in the literature of infection of man by many other tapeworms. A few of these infections are discussed briefly in the following paragraphs.

HYMENOLEPIASIS NANA

Synonym. Dwarf tapeworm infection.

Definition. Hymenolepiasis nana is caused by the presence of *Hymenolepis nana* in the alimentary canal of man.

Distribution. This small tapeworm has a cosmopolitan distribution.

Etiology. MORPHOLOGY. *Hymenolepis nana* (v. Siebold, 1852) Blanchard, 1891 is 25 to 40 mm in length by 1 mm in breadth (Fig. 54–22). The scolex bears four small suckers and a short rostellum armed with 20 to 30 hooks arranged in a single ring. The rostellum and the hooks may be invaginated into the tip of the scolex.

DEVELOPMENT. This tapeworm requires no intermediate host. Eggs are infective for man and mice. Hatching occurs in the small intestine, where each oncosphere penetrates a villus and develops into a cysticercoid. Eventually the parasites break out into the lumen of the gut, pass farther down the tract and attach themselves between the villi, where they reach maturity. Internal autoinfection may occur and probably accounts for persistent heavy infections. There is experimental evidence which indicates that fleas and beetles *(Tenebrio* spp.) and other insects may serve as nonobligatory intermediate hosts.

Epidemiology. The worm is especially prevalent in children. Infection is acquired initially by ingestion of the infective eggs passed in the stools. The murine strain may be acquired by children; however, the important reservoir is the human one.

Pathology. There are no characteristic

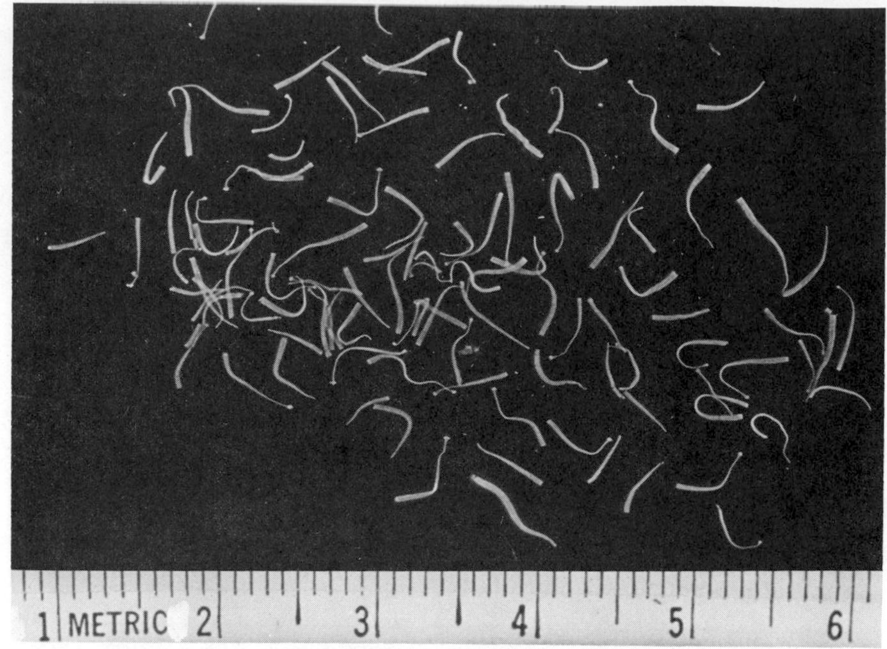

Figure 54–22. *Hymenolepis nana,* dwarf tapeworm, adults. (Courtesy of Dr. Francisco J. Aguilar, Guatemala.)

pathologic changes. A moderate eosinophilia sometimes accompanies a heavy infection.

Clinical Characteristics. Patients infected by these parasites are usually asymptomatic except when worms are present in large numbers. In such cases abdominal pain, diarrhea, anorexia, dizziness, headache, inanition and pruritus may occur.

Diagnosis. Diagnosis is based upon the following characteristics of the eggs (Fig. 54–1): (1) shape—usually ovoid; (2) size—30 to 47 μm in diameter; (3) shell—hyaline with clear area between shell and inner envelope; (4) six-hooked embryo—enclosed in an inner envelope; (5) filaments—four to eight threadlike filaments arising from each of the two polar thickenings of the inner envelope.

Treatment. No uniformly successful therapeutic is available. Anthelmintics usually must be given repetitively and continued preferably over a 2-week period in order to prevent maturation of the cysticercoid stages emerging uninterruptedly from the intestinal villi. Recrudescences may occur despite treatment. Thus, it is desirable to follow patients by stool examination for 2 months or more after treatment. Niclosamide (Yomesan) 40 to 80 mg per kg daily for 5 days has been effective in 90 per cent of children followed up for 2 months;[25] paromomycin 30 mg per kg in 2 doses 7 days apart has proved almost as good;[11] as has an acridine derivative, Acranil, in 4 doses of 0.5 gm (adult dose) given at 3-day intervals. A saline purge should be administered after these treatments. However, the infection usually does not justify use of rigorous therapeutic measures, and excessive purgation should be avoided in children.

Prophylaxis. Prophylaxis depends upon sanitary disposal of human feces. Domestic rodent control and proper protection of food will prevent infection originating from mice.

HYMENOLEPIASIS DIMINUTA

Synonym. Rat tapeworm infection.

Definition. Hymenolepiasis diminuta is caused by the presence of *Hymenolepis diminuta* in the alimentary canal of man.

Distribution. This cestode is a common and cosmopolitan intestinal parasite of rats and mice. It has been found infrequently in persons residing in Europe,

Russia, Iran along the Persian Gulf, Africa, India, China, Japan, the Philippines, New Guinea, South and Central America and the Caribbean, and the southern United States (especially Georgia, Tennessee and Texas).

Etiology. MORPHOLOGY. The rat tapeworm, *Hymenolepis diminuta* (Rudolphi, 1819) Blanchard, 1891, ranges from 20 to 60 cm in length. The scolex carries four suckers and an unarmed retractile rostellum. Mature proglottids are wider than long; each contains a central ovary flanked on one side by two testes, and on the other side by one. Eggs are nearly spherical, measuring 60 to 86 μm in greatest diameter. The yellowish outer membrane is distinct and is clearly set off from the inner membrane which invests the six-hooked oncosphere. The space between the outer and inner membranes is filled with a gelatinous substance (Fig. 54–1).

DEVELOPMENT. Since the gravid proglottids disintegrate after detachment from the strobila, eggs appear in the feces of the definitive host. Numerous insects, such as fleas, cockroaches and mealworms, may ingest the eggs and serve as intermediate hosts for this tapeworm. These animals become infective for the final hosts as soon as the cysticercoid larvae have completed their intermediate development.

Epidemiology. Infection in man occurs through the ingestion of parasitized insect hosts which are often encountered in grains and cereals. In many instances, the parasites remain viable during metamorphosis of the insect from the larval to the adult stage, as in the case of fleas which cannot feed on solids after the larval state (Fig. 54–23).

Pathology. No pathologic changes are recognized.

Clinical Characteristics. The alleged symptoms include indefinite gastrointestinal complaints, diarrhea and abdominal pain.

Diagnosis. Diagnosis depends upon detecting eggs with the following characteristics (Fig. 54–1): (1) shape—roughly spherical; (2) size—moderately large, 60 to 86 μm; (3) shell—transparent yellowish outer membrane lines shell, clear area between this zone and the thick inner envelope; (4) six-hooked oncosphere—within inner envelope, the latter sometimes bearing polar thickenings but never polar filaments.

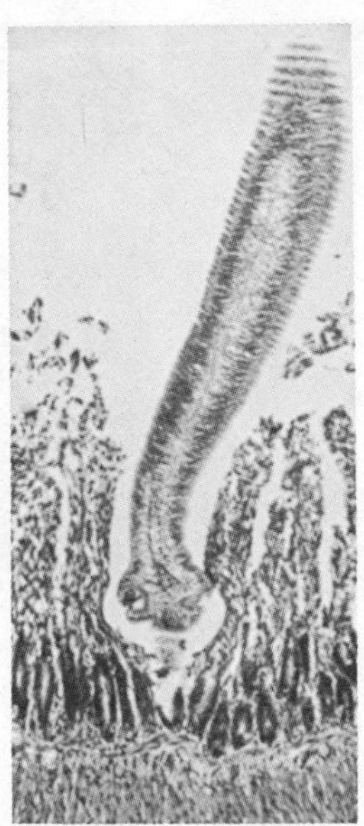

Figure 54–23. *Hymenolepis diminuta* attached to intestinal mucosa of rat.

Treatment. Same as for hymenolepiasis nana (p. 618), although it is reported that paromomycin is less effective against *H. diminuta.*

Prophylaxis. The ingestion of infected insects, especially those occurring in processed grains and cereals to which rodents have access, should be guarded against. Education and provision for adequate sanitation with reference to rodent control and food storage are important preventive measures.

DIPYLIDIASIS

Dipylidium caninum (Linnaeus, 1758) Railliet, 1892 is a common tapeworm of dogs and cats throughout the world. It has been found infrequently in humans in the United States, most European countries, the Philippine Islands, China, Rhodesia, Guatemala, Argentina, Chile and probably other Latin American countries. Eggs from feces or from disintegrated proglottids in soil may be ingested by larval fleas and develop ultimately into infective cysticercoid larvae. These larvae

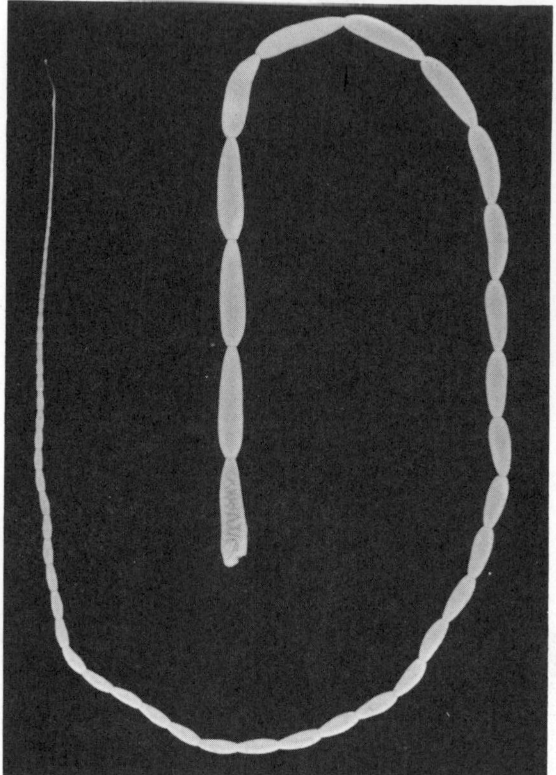

Figure 54–24. Strobila of *Dipylidium caninum*, a common tapeworm of dogs and cats. (Courtesy of the Louisiana State University School of Medicine, New Orleans.)

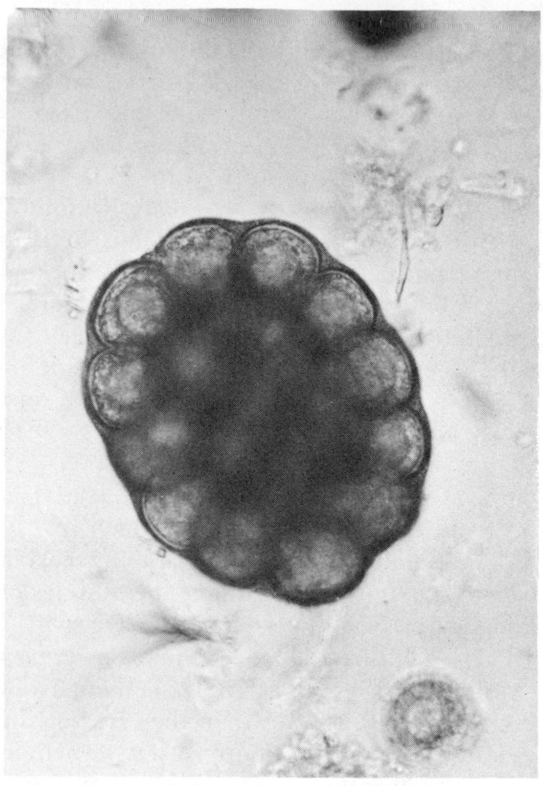

Figure 54–25. Eggs of *D. caninum* typically in a packet. (Courtesy of Dr. Stanley H. Abadie and Dr. Mark R. Feldman, the Louisiana State University School of Medicine, New Orleans.)

remain viable while the fleas metamorphose to the adult stage. Infection in dogs and cats is caused by the ingestion of infected fleas, and probably the dog louse, *Trichodectes canis*, which serve as intermediate hosts. Human infections occur primarily in children. The insects may gain access to their mouths when they fondle pets.

Diagnosis. The gravid proglottids are shaped like melon seeds and are characterized by having a genital pore on each side (Fig. 54–24). Single or multiple segments of the parasite may be passed in the stool or may migrate from the bowel. The eggs are in packets; several eggs are encased in a capsule (Fig. 54–25). The spherical capsule is red, which accounts for the pink tinge of the gravid proglottids.

Clinical Characteristics, Treatment and Prophylaxis. Essentially, the symptoms and therapy of *D. caninum* infection are similar to those of *H. nana* and *H. diminuta* infections. (See page 618 for treatment.) Use of suitable insecticidal veterinary products on dogs and cats to eliminate their ectoparasites will help to prevent human infection and reinfection of the pets.

REFERENCES

1. Daugherty, J. W., and Foster, W. B. 1958. Comparative studies on amino acid absorption by cestodes. Exp. Parasit. 7:99–107.
2. Hedrick, R. M. 1958. Comparative histochemical studies on cestodes. II. The distribution of fat substances in *Hymenolepis diminuta* and *Raillietina cesticellus*. J. Parasit. *44*:75–84.
3. Read, C. P., Rothman, A. H., and Simmons, J. E., Jr. 1963. Studies on membrane transport, with special reference to parasite-host integration. Ann. N.Y. Acad. Sci. *113*:154–205.
4. Smyth, J. D. 1947. The physiology of tapeworms. Biol. Rev. *22*:214–238.
5. von Brand, T., Mercado, T. I., Nylen, M. U., and

Scott, D. B. 1960. Observations on function, composition, and structure of cestode calcareous corpuscles. Exp. Parasit. *9*:205–214.

6. Addis, C. J., Jr., and Chandler, A. C. 1946. Further studies on the vitamin requirements of tapeworms. J. Parasit. *32*:581–584.
7. Read, C. P. 1951. Studies on the enzymes and intermediate products of carbohydrate degradation in the cestode, *Hymenolepis diminuta.* Exp. Parasit. *1*:1–18.
8. Faust, E. C. 1952. Some morphologic characters of *Diphyllobothrium latum.* Ann. Inst. Med. Trop. (Lisb.) *9*:1277–1300.
9. Gräsbeck, R., Nyberg, W., Saarni, M., and von Bonsdorff, B. 1962. Lognormal distribution of serum vitamin B_{12} levels and dependence of blood values on the B_{12} level in a large population heavily infected with *Diphyllobothrium latum.* J. Lab. Clin. Med. *59*:419–429.
10. Östling, G. 1961. Treatment of tapeworm infection with Desaspidin, a new phloroglucinol derivative isolated from Finnish fern. Am. J. Trop. Med. Hyg. *10*:855–858.
11. Wittner, M., and Tanowitz, H. 1971. Paromomycin therapy of human cestodiasis with special reference to hymenolepiasis. Am. J. Trop. Med. Hyg. *20*:433–435.
12. Corkum, K. C. 1966. Sparganosis in some vertebrates of Louisiana and observations on a human infection. J. Parasit. *52*:444–448.
13. Mueller, J. F., Hart, E. P., and Walsh, W. P. 1963. Human sparganosis in the United States. J. Parasit. *48*:294–296.
14. Swartzwelder, J. C., Beaver, P. C., and Hood, M. W. 1964. Sparganosis in southern United States. Am. J. Trop. Med. Hyg. *13*:43–47.
15. Cadigan, F. C., Jr., Stanton, J. S., Tanticharoenyos, P., and Chaicumpa, V. 1967. The lar gibbon as definitive and intermediate host of *Taenia solium.* J. Parasit. *53*:844.
16. Proctor, E. M., Powell, S. J., and Elsdon-Dew, R. 1966. The serological diagnosis of cysticercosis. Ann. Trop. Med. Parasit. *60*:146–151.
17. Perera, D. R., Western, K. A., and Schultz, M. G. 1970. Niclosamide treatment of cestodiasis. Clinical trials in the United States. Am. J. Trop. Med. Hyg. *19*:610–612.
18. Peña Chavarría, A. Personal communication.
19. Salazar Mallén, M., González Barranco, D., and Vega Vital, M. V. A. 1972. Ensayo de tratamiento de la cistocercosis, con metrifonato. Revta Invest. Salud Públ. *32*:1–7.
20. Rijpstra, A. C., Smit, A. M., and Swellengrebel, N. H. 1961. How and where to search for the ova of *Taenia saginata.* Trop. Geogr. Med. *13*:160–166.
21. Allain, D. S., and Kagan, I. G. 1961. The use of formalinized red cells in the serology of hydatid disease. J. Parasit. *47*:61–64.
22. Saidi, F., and Nazarian, I. 1971. Surgical treatment of hydatid cysts by freezing of cyst wall and instillation of 0.5 per cent silver nitrate solution. N. Engl. J. Med. *284*:1346–1350.
23. Williams, J. F., López Adaros, H., and Trejos, A. 1971. Current prevalence and distribution of hydatidosis with special reference to the Americas. Am. J. Trop. Med. Hyg. *20*:224–236.
24. Thatcher, V. E. 1972. Neotropical echinococcosis in Colombia. Ann. Trop. Med. Parasit. *66*:99–105.
25. Most, H., Yoeli, M., Hammond, J., and Scheinesson, G. P. 1971. Yomesan (niclosamide) therapy of *Hymenolepis nana* infections. Am. J. Trop. Med. Hyg. *20*:206–208.

SECTION VIII
Nutritional Diseases

JEAN MAYER
FREDRICK J. STARE

CHAPTER 55
Introduction

The science of nutrition is concerned with food and the ingredients of food necessary for health, with the physiologic action of these nutrients and with the consequences of lack of effective concentrations of the 50 or 60 known specific nutrients. The same essentials are provided by many different staples. It is possible, therefore, to provide protective diets by utilizing a variety of foods. In fact, variety of diet constitutes one of the cardinal principles of nutrition practice. Except in the case of milk for infants there is no single food which, of itself, is essential for good nutrition, and even in this instance a "soybean milk" provides a satisfactory substitute.

An adequate diet must contain sufficient amounts of protein, fat, carbohydrate, fiber, water and the essential minerals and vitamins. The absolute requirements for these substances cannot be stated, since many have interrelated physiologic functions. The amount of protein required in the diet depends upon the calories furnished by carbohydrate and fat. The requirement for the B vitamin niacin is based upon the available amount of the amino acid tryptophan; and, similarly, the need for iron is related to the ascorbic acid content of the diet.

However, we do know the relative amounts and ranges of many of the specific factors required for good health. The caloric content must meet the basal metabolic need in order to maintain weight equilibrium, and it must provide for the activity of the individual. The range for an adult may vary from 2000 to 5000 calories per day. Generally, carbohydrate provides 60 to 75 per cent of the required total, fat 10 to 40 per cent, and protein 8 to 15 per cent. Except for pregnant and lactating women, the protein requirements of adults approximate 30 gm per day, but in practical nutrition twice or more this amount is desirable. Therefore, the recommended daily allowances of the more important food constituents are based on the theoretical minimal requirements, with a substantial increment to provide for special needs and to afford a factor of safety (Table 55–1).

EFFECT OF TROPICAL CLIMATE ON NUTRITIONAL REQUIREMENTS

The opinion is frequently expressed that tropical climates cause unusual changes in nutritional requirements. Except in the matter of calories and water, there is little evidence to support this view. The widely prevalent malnutrition in such areas is largely an expression of insufficient supplies of protective foods, selectivity of diet determined by the cultural and religious backgrounds of the people and the direct and indirect effects of infection. Many people in tropical climates are unable to obtain the basic foods essential for a good diet. The problems are fundamentally agricultural and economic rather than climatic. Other

Table 55–1. Desirable Ranges for Daily Intake of Certain Nutrients

	Sedentary	*Moderately Active*	*Very Active*
Calories	1800–2000	2200–3200	3200–5000
Protein, gm	50– 100	50– 100	50– 100
Calcium, gm	0.4– 0.8	0.4– 0.8	0.4– 0.8
Iron, mg	12– 18	12– 18	12– 18
Sodium, gm	1– 5	1– 5	1– 5
Vitamin A, I.U.	3000–5000	3000–5000	3000–5000
Thiamine (vitamin B_1) mg	1– 2	1– 2	1– 2
Riboflavin (vitamin B_2) mg	2– 3	2– 3	2– 3
Niacin, mg	10– 20	10– 20	10– 20
Ascorbic acid, mg	40– 75	40– 75	40– 75

groups, because of religious beliefs or social practices, avoid available animal protein. Still others prefer polished to unpolished rice. Parasitic or other gastrointestinal infections may interfere with the absorption of specific food factors or utilize those available for their own economy at the expense of the host. Systemic infections, by their effect on the metabolism or the tissues of the host, may increase significantly the daily requirements for particular nutrients. Thus, the essential problem will vary from region to region, depending upon the practices of man and only secondarily upon the effects of climate.

Calories. Energy requirement is decreased in the tropics, since the higher environmental temperatures diminish the need for heat production. The relative importance of temperature has, however, often been overemphasized. Observers have been impressed unduly by the temporary anorexia that frequently follows sudden passage from the temperate or tropical climates. An investigation of calorie requirements was conducted during World War II using United States and Canadian troops stationed in various parts of the world. All the groups retained their usual food habits and all were engaged in the same types of duty. Under these conditions a linear correlation was observed between voluntary calorie intake and climatic environment, with the daily intake decreasing by 16 calories for each degree of increase in mean Fahrenheit temperature, or 29 calories for each degree centigrade. Since that study, additional evidence relating the voluntary intake of troops to mean annual temperature has been obtained, particularly in studies made by the Royal Air Force. On the basis of these observations and of national averages of caloric intake in various climates, the Second Calorie Requirement Committee of the United Nations Food and Agriculture Organization estimated that there is a 3 per cent decrease in caloric requirements for every 10° C of mean annual external temperature above the reference temperature of 10° C.

Protein and Fat. Available evidence indicates that high environmental temperatures introduce no change of practical importance in human protein requirements. Attention has been called to the low fat consumption in many tropical areas. This appears to be due essentially to local economic conditions. A low fat diet has been claimed repeatedly to be of value where conditions causing impaired liver function are widespread.

Vitamins. While it has been claimed that requirements for thiamine and for ascorbic acid are increased by heat, the evidence in support of this assertion is unconvincing. Similarly, claims that tropical climates per se "predispose" to rickets are obscured by lack of control of other factors, such as the availability of calcium and phosphorus. Whenever regular exposure to sunshine is prevalent, the appearance of rickets is prevented. This probably explains the infrequent occurrence of rickets in the tropics, in spite of low calcium and the possible "predisposing" effect of heat. The great preponderance of evidence indicates that vitamin requirements of healthy persons are essentially the same in temperate and in tropical climates.

Water and Minerals. Water requirements are increased roughly in proportion to the amount of sweat secreted. They may increase from 2 or 3 liters per day in a temperate climate to 13 liters or more during work in a hot environment. Under extreme conditions, the need for water may actually outstrip thirst. Wartime studies demonstrated that the best level of performance is obtained when the water lost in sweat is replaced hour by hour. While loss of minerals, sodium chloride in particular, is increased in individuals first exposed to hot climates, acclimatization is accompanied by decreased salt concentration in sweat so that salt requirements are increased only slightly. The trend in recent practice has been against providing salt to men working in the heat—either as tablets or as salinized drinking water—except possibly to unacclimatized individuals or in cases of unusual extremes of activity and temperature.

FOODS AS SOURCES OF NUTRIENTS

Rice is the single most important food of many tropical regions because it is usually more plentiful, but other predominantly carbohydrate foods, such as corn and millet, and root vegetables such as taro are used widely. Unfortunately, these are low in vitamins, minerals and protein. When refined, as they usually are by preference and for stability, they contain even less of these nutrients. Vegetable proteins are incomplete, since they lack sufficient amounts of one or more of the essential amino acids, particularly lysine. On the other hand, the proteins of legumes, the germ of grains, and of nuts are more complete. These foods are also better sources of vitamins and minerals. Hence, rice diets can be improved by including supplements of some of these "superior" vegetable and grain foods, or by enrichment with lysine. The recent research on the high-lysine corn, *opaque*-2, constitutes a major advance in protein nutrition.[1]

Animal foods, such as meat, fowl, fish, eggs, milk and milk products, provide complete protein and are generally excellent sources of minerals and vitamins. They are often unavailable in adequate quantity to many peoples in the tropics. However, inclusion of even small amounts significantly improves the diet, since they supplement the "weak links" of the incomplete vegetable diet.

Poor quality protein, along with inadequate calories, is probably the single greatest cause of nutritional ill health in the tropics. Although it may be difficult to provide certain peoples with adequate protein, qualitatively and quantitatively it is usually possible to improve conditions by more effective use of indigenous foodstuffs. Even in the absence of refrigeration, excess meat can be preserved for reasonable periods if it has been smoked, dried or pickled and is protected against flies. Invertebrates and other lower animals are often valuable protein sources, and the proteins of cereals can be supplemented with legumes, nuts and preparations of whole grains, or improved nutritionally by mixture with other cereals or by fortification with certain essential amino acids such as lysine.

Milk is of special importance in nutrition. In many areas it is unobtainable or available only in limited supply, in part because of the lack of a dairy industry and in part because of the problems associated with conservation and distribution. In the hot climates, in the absence of refrigeration, canning or drying provides the only safe means for storage and transport.

The problem of providing a satisfactory milk substitute is crucial in many regions, particularly where animal milk is not available. In some areas soybean milk, mixtures of vegetable proteins with mutually supplementary amino acid content and availability, and powdered small fish rich in protein and calcium have been used with considerable success.

Fortification of foods with one or more key nutrients may offer a partial solution. The enrichment of salt with iodine, milk with vitamin D, margarines with vitamin A, and white flour and corn meal with thiamine, riboflavin, niacin and iron, and water with the mineral nutrient fluoride have been outstanding advances in public health nutrition. Similar addition of thiamine to rice in the Philippines has resulted in a dramatic decrease in the prevalence of beriberi. Comparable improvement in the nutritional qualities of rice may be achieved by modern methods of milling, by parboiling brown rice and by making "converted" rice. However, manufacturing facilities for the latter are expensive, and parboiled rice may not be acceptable to indigenous populations because of altered flavor, color and consistency. Acceptability of food and local dietary customs are necessarily determining factors in the development of any practical nutrition program. At present, it appears that enrichment with synthetic vitamins is the most realistic approach to the problem of the predominantly rice diet. Similarly, addition of synthetic amino acids may prove to be practical in the future for supplementing the deficient proteins in regions where the complete proteins of animal origin are unobtainable in sufficient amounts.

The fluoridation of the water supply, a cheap and safe way to decrease dental caries by as much as two-thirds, has been one of the striking recent advances in public health nutrition. The amount of fluoride added (usually one part per million in temperate climates) may have to be adjusted downward in tropical areas where water consumption is substantially greater than in colder climates.

Diets typical of the tropics commonly provide only a limited choice of foods. Selection is still further restricted by the hazard of contamination by parasitic or other infectious agents. However, the daily diet should be as varied as local conditions permit. It should include animal products, fruits, greens and vegetables, particularly beans, in addition to the carbohydrate staple rice, corn or millet. Scalding of fruits that are eaten raw and light boiling of greens will afford protection against infection without impairing nutritional values. The chemical treatment of foods, such as washing in permanganate solution, is not a dependable safeguard.

GENERAL PHYSIOLOGIC EFFECTS OF INADEQUATE DIET

Investigation of the various deficiency diseases of man indicates that they are the result of the action of a variety of factors having a complex interrelationship and not the expression of single specific deficiencies. This is to be anticipated, since it is very doubtful that a defective diet is ever lacking in only one factor.

The water soluble vitamins—the whole B complex and vitamin C—are not stored in large amounts within the body and are rapidly depleted in the absence of dietary sources. The fat soluble vitamins A, D, E and K, however, appear to be stored in considerable amounts, and prolonged periods of dietary deficiency are required to deplete them.

Present indications of the roles of the vitamins in intracellular metabolism and of their probable interactions strongly suggest that lack of various of the substances may produce similar disturbances of normal physiology. It seems probable that any deficit below the physiologic requirements is associated with impairment of function and, if sufficiently great, with the appearance of symptoms. Later, if the deprivation is severe and long continued, this disturbance of function is accompanied by alteration of structure. Consequently, the deficiency is then expressed clinically by the presence of both symptoms and physical signs. It follows, therefore, that the responses to a defective diet may be protean and are the result of (1) multiple deficiencies in the diet, (2) the degree to which each essential substance is deficient, and (3) the duration of the particular deficits.

The ultimate clinical expression of inadequate diet will, therefore, vary in accordance with the type of deficiency of the diet with respect to its content of calories, biologically complete protein, mineral constituents and the various vitamins. The clinical picture will vary further in accordance with the magnitude of the deprivation, its duration and the level of energy output of the individual. Thus, under certain conditions, the indications of sodium chloride deficit may be acute and appear within a very brief period. The expression of vitamin B complex deficiency will appear much earlier than those clinical syndromes depending upon lack of the fat soluble factors; and a diet providing inadequate protein may require a prolonged period before its effects become clinically evident.

Finally, in the presence of a definite clinical syndrome, functional changes occur in the small intestine which interfere with normal utilization of the diet and, consequently, operate still further to augment existing deficiencies. Thus, there is created a vicious progressive spiral in which both a primary dietary deficit and a secondary disturbance of normal physiology causing impaired absorption contribute to progression of the deficiency state.

The operation of these varied factors upon population groups is well illustrated by studies of the nutritional status of the inhabitants of Madrid during the Spanish Civil War. These observations can be used likewise to predict with a reasonable probability of accuracy the status of groups subjected to famine or near-famine if the approximate duration of the period of deprivation is known. During the siege of Madrid the available diet consisted mainly of starches. Animal protein and good sources of the vitamin B complex were both seriously restricted. The first noticeable effects of this deficient diet were indicative of a lack of adequate amounts of the B complex vitamins. Thus, functional neurologic disturbances appeared early. Later a marked increase in the incidence of pellagra occurred, particularly during the spring seasons of the second and third years. Famine edema, however, did not appear until the third year of the war.

During World War II internees in areas of the Far East developed beriberi because the limited food available to them was polished rice devoid of thiamine and other B vitamins. Internees in Western Europe were fed on whole grain breads and potatoes, reasonably good sources of the water soluble vitamins, and few cases of the classic vitamin deficiencies developed. In western Holland, for example, during the last 6 months of the war severe starvation was frequent, but vitamin deficiencies did not develop because, with little food to metabolize, the need for the B complex vitamins which function in various metabolic reactions is minimal.

Although the most striking clinical phenomena occurring in the specific nutritional diseases may indicate a marked deficit of one particular substance or group of substances, other important deficiencies exist as well. Immediate institution of a completely adequate diet becomes, therefore, the essential procedure in the treatment of this whole group of conditions. It is frequently necessary, however, to supplement dietary therapy by administration of pharmacologic preparations of certain of the vitamins, and of ample amounts of particularly rich crude sources. Additional amounts of certain minerals and an excess of biologically complete protein are likewise often required to obtain the most complete and most rapid response to treatment.[2]

TROPICAL MALNUTRITION

No striking deviation from temperate zone requirements, except for water, is thus characteristic of tropical conditions. The tropical climate itself may play a secondary role in the evolution of certain nutritional diseases, in that climatic factors, such as wind, exposure to sun and extreme heat, may influence nutritional dermatoses. The effect of sunlight on skin appearance in pellagra is well known. Local climatic conditions may contribute to the differences in skin abnormalities associated with kwashiorkor in various regions of the world. But the essential significance of tropical nutritional diseases lies in fields other than human physiology. An obvious and well known factor is the prevalence of parasitic and infectious diseases. These will often contribute to decreased intestinal absorption, sometimes to increased requirements, and usually to some degree of anorexia. Another and more important factor is the agricultural, economic and social status of many tropical populations. Many such peoples subsist on a diet

Table 55–2. SUGGESTED GUIDE FOR INTERPRETATION OF CLINICAL SIGNS*

Dietary Obesity
- Excessive weight
- Excessive skin folds
- Excessive abdominal girth

Undernutrition
- Lethargy, mental and physical
- Low weight in relation to height
- Diminished skin folds
- Exaggerated skeletal prominences
- Loss of elasticity of skin

Protein-Calorie Deficiency Disease
- Edema
- Muscle wasting
- Low body weight
- Pyschomotor change
- Dyspigmentation of the hair
- Thin, sparse hair
- Moon face
- Flaky paint dermatosis
- Areas of hyperpigmentation

Vitamin A Deficiency
- Xerosis of skin
- Follicular hyperkeratosis
- Xerosis conjunctivae
- Keratomalacia
- Bitot's spots

Riboflavin Deficiency
- Angular stomatitis
- Cheilosis
- Magenta tongue
- Central atrophy of lingual papillae
- Nasolabial dyssebacea
- Angular palpebritis
- Scrotal and vulval dermatosis
- Corneal vascularization

Thiamin Deficiency
- Loss of ankle jerks
- Sensory loss and motor weakness
- Calf-muscle tenderness
- Cardiovascular dysfunction
- Edema

Niacin Deficiency
- Pellagrous dermatosis
- Scarlet and raw tongue
- Tongue fissuring
- Atrophic lingual papillae
- Malar and supraorbital pigmentation

Vitamin C Deficiency
- Spongy and bleeding gums
- Folliculosis
- Petechiae
- Ecchymoses
- Intramuscular or subperiosteal hematoma
- Epiphyseal enlargement (painful)

Vitamin D Deficiency
1. *Active rickets* (in children)
   - Epiphyseal enlargement (over 6 months of age), painless
   - Beading of ribs
   - Craniotabes (under 1 year of age)
   - Muscular hypotonia
2. *Healed rickets* (in children or adults)
   - Frontal and parietal bossing
   - Knock-knees or bow legs
   - Deformities of thorax
3. *Osteomalacia* (in adults)
   - Local or generalized skeletal deformities

Iron Deficiency
- Pallor of mucous membranes
- Koilonychia
- Atrophic lingual papillae

Iodine Deficiency
- Enlargement of the thyroid

Excess of Fluorine (Fluorosis)
- Mottled dental enamel

*From N. S. Scrimshaw. 1971. Assessment of nutritional status. *In* Beeson, P. B., and McDermott, W. (eds.): Cecil-Loeb Textbook of Medicine. 13th ed. W. B. Saunders Co., Philadelphia. p. 1429. Adapted from World Health Organization Technical Report Series No. 258, Expert Committee on Medical Assessment of Nutritional Status. Geneva, W.H.O., 1963. pp. 59–61.

based almost exclusively on one principal starchy staple food—rice, millet or corn, for example. Ignorance of sound nutritional practices reinforces poverty as a cause of "tropical" malnutrition.[3] The classic deficiency diseases characteristic of such diets could perhaps best be termed "diseases of society" rather than "tropical diseases," despite their geographic localization.[4, 5]

Pathologic conditions associated with malnutrition and found in the tropics may be classed in four categories:

1. Syndromes that are essentially of dietary origin, even though they may be complicated by parasitic and infectious conditions, for example, beriberi, pellagra and kwashiorkor.

2. Conditions that are probably of nutritional origin, such as tropical ulcer, sprue, pernicious anemia and certain urolithiases.

3. Conditions of unknown etiology in which nutritional factors appear to be important, such as primary carcinoma of the liver and certain pancreatic fibroses.

4. Diseases, the primary causes of which are non-nutritional, but in which nutritional factors affect directly the response to the pathogenic agent or which contribute indirectly to the development of complicating malnutrition.

Important examples of the first two categories only will be considered in this section. The recognized clinical syndromes present one part of the picture of malnutrition (Table 55–2). Nutritional diseases characteristically develop as multiple deficiencies. The signs and symptoms characteristic of several nutritional syndromes commonly appear simultaneously or in succession.[6-8]

CHAPTER 56

Pellagra

Synonyms. Mal de la rosa, mal del sole, psilosis pigmentosa, Alpine scurvy, chichism (northern South America).

Definition. Pellagra is the principal manifestation of a severe deficiency of niacin, generally complicated by deficiencies of other B vitamins. It is characterized clinically by a red, sore tongue, disturbances of the alimentary tract, symmetrical dermatitis and changes in the central and peripheral nervous systems.

Distribution. The disease has a worldwide distribution. It is generally associated with the consumption of diets containing an excessive proportion of corn (maize). The disease is more prevalent during the spring than at any other season.

Etiology. Endemic pellagra is caused by prolonged ingestion of a low protein diet containing small amounts of nicotinic acid. The amino acid tryptophan can be converted to niacin by the human organism, so that low levels of both of these nutrients must generally be present for pellagra to appear. Diets high in corn and containing little or no meat, milk, fish or other good sources of protein are pellagragenic. The importance of the amino acid composition of the diet is illustrated by the fact that wheat diets are not pellagragenic in spite of a niacin content often lower than that of corn diets.[2,4]

Lack of niacin interferes with the formation and the function of two essential respiratory enzymes, the diphosphopyridine and triphosphopyridine nucleotides. The effects of this deficiency can therefore be expected to be widespread. Less severe deficiencies of niacin produce milder symptoms.

While the lack of nicotinic acid and tryptophan in the diet are essential etiologic factors of endemic pellagra, certain organic diseases which interfere with the ingestion, assimilation or utilization of pellagra-preventing food factors contribute to the prevalence of pellagra. Among these, amebic dysentery, hookworm infection, malaria and cirrhosis of the liver are of particular importance in tropical regions. Secondary pellagra is one of the secondary deficiency diseases sometimes associated with chronic alcoholism.

As in other deficiency diseases, the phenomena characteristic of pellagra are usually accompanied by a relative lack of other essential nutrients. Cheilosis responding to riboflavin administration and peripheral neuritis responding to thiamine treatment are frequently seen as complications.

Pathology. No characteristic or constant pathologic changes are observed. In acute cases there is active inflammation of certain skin areas and of the mucosa, particularly of the mouth and pharynx. Repeated attacks lead to atrophy and pigmentation of the affected skin regions.

Clinical Characteristics. The clinical picture is variable and the disease may be acute, subacute or chronic. The onset is usually gradual, with asthenia, loss of weight, mental depression and a sore red tongue.

Dermatitis may also occur. Characteristically, it is symmetrically distributed, affecting areas that are exposed to irritation, such as the dorsum of the hands and wrists, the elbows, face, neck, the skin beneath the breasts, the perineal region, the patellar areas and the dorsum of the feet. In most instances it is restricted to parts exposed to the sun. In the early stage there is erythema resembling sunburn. This may be followed by vesiculation and bulla formation. The skin becomes thickened and roughened and, as the acute inflammation subsides, brownish pigmentation remains. Repeated attacks lead to marked atrophy of the skin (Figs. 56–1, 56–2).

Lesions of the tongue and mouth are usual. Acute glossitis and stomatitis may progress to extensive ulceration; simultaneously, there is fissuring at the angles of the mouth. The tongue is swollen, denuded of

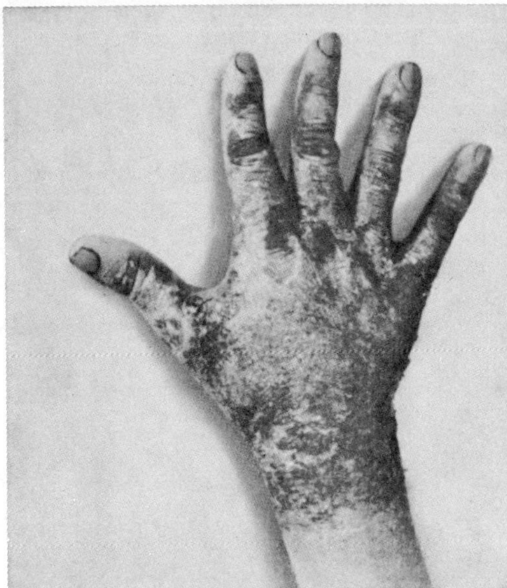

Figure 56-1

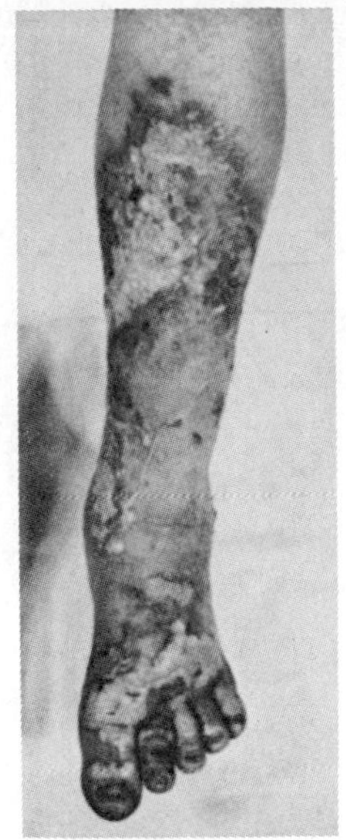

Figure 56-2

Figure 56-1. Acute pellagra—dermatitis of hand and wrist. (Courtesy of Dr. Julian Ruffin, Duke Hospital.)
Figure 56-2. Acute pellagra—dermatitis of exposed areas of leg and foot. (Courtesy of Dr. Julian Ruffin, Duke Hospital.)

its papillae and often painful and extremely sensitive (Fig. 56-3).

Hypochlorhydria or achlorhydria is common, and there may be diarrhea or alternating periods of diarrhea and constipation. The stools are not abnormal in color and contain no excess fat.

Pellagra is accompanied by a variety of symptoms referable to the nervous system. In the early stages the picture is that of neurasthenia, which increases in severity with progression of the disease. In advanced and long-standing cases true psychoses occur. In these cases, peripheral neuritis, spastic gait and other indications of organic involvement are not uncommon.

Diagnosis. The four cardinal symptoms—dermatitis, glossitis, gastrointestinal symptoms and psychic disturbances—are characteristic of the well developed acute case.

Diagnostic difficulties may be encountered in the early stages of the disease or in advanced chronic cases in which the characteristic acute phenomena are lacking. The combination of pigmentation and atrophy of exposed skin areas, smooth atrophy of the tongue, and the picture of neurasthenia should arouse suspicion. Analysis of urine

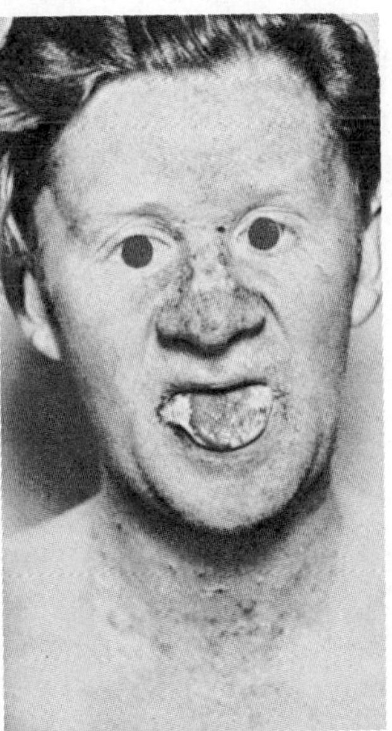

Figure 56-3. Acute pellagra—characteristic dermatitis of exposed skin of face and neck, acute glossitis. (Courtesy of Dr. Julian Ruffin, Duke Hospital.)

for *N*-1-methyl nicotinamide content may be of help. Normal excretion is usually over 3 mg per day. Levels of excretion below 1 mg reinforce the presumption of pellagra or prepellagrous state.

Treatment. 1. High protein, high vitamin diet.[3, 6]

2. Nicotinic acid or nicotinic amide, 300 to 500 mg daily in divided doses.

3. Therapeutic doses of the B complex vitamins, in particular thiamine chloride, 5 to 10 mg daily as indicated.

Prophylaxis. The prophylaxis of pellagra is based upon an adequate diet.

CHAPTER 57
Beriberi

Synonyms. Polyneuritis endemica; barbiers; kakke (China and Japan); maladie des sucreries (French Antilles); hinchazon (Cuba); inchacao or perneiras (Brazil); maladie des jambes (Louisiana); alcoholic neuritis.

Definition. Beriberi is a nutritional disease resulting from a deficiency of vitamin B_1 (thiamine) and other vitamins. It exhibits acute and chronic forms characterized by peripheral neuritis and, in severe cases, by congestive heart failure. It may occur in all age groups.

Distribution. Beriberi has been widespread in the past in the Orient and in areas of the tropics where polished rice is an important dietary staple. It has been prevalent also in Labrador, Newfoundland and Iceland where the winter diet is restricted largely to white flour and other non-vitamin-bearing foods.

Etiology. Primary beriberi is the result of prolonged subsistence on a deficient diet. Secondary beriberi may occur as a complication of other disease states attended by deficient absorption, incomplete utilization or unusual requirements for thiamine such as occur with elevated levels of metabolism.

Epidemiology. The incidence of beriberi varies with dietary habits and with the availability of foods that provide adequate amounts of essential food factors. It is seen most commonly in men and there is evidence to indicate that hard physical labor is a precipitating factor. Among women the disease occurs particularly during pregnancy and lactation. Infantile beriberi is a frequent cause of death among breast-fed infants in endemic areas. Although it is not an infectious disease, "epidemics" have been noted when outbreaks of diarrheal disease have occurred in populations subsisting on borderline diets, since diarrhea increases the physiologic requirements of the individual and diminishes the utilization of specific food factors.

Pathology. The heart and the nervous system are involved primarily. The cardiac changes are predominantly hypertrophy and subsequent dilatation. The weight of the heart is frequently considerably increased. No specific lesions have been identified, and the observed pathologic changes are often insufficient to account for the deaths from cardiac failure. The effects on tissues other than those of the nervous system are those of congestive heart failure.

Degenerative lesions without evidence of inflammation may be found throughout the nervous system. They occur in the peripheral nerves, the spinal cord, the spinal ganglia, the nuclei of the medulla and pons, and the structures of the autonomic nervous system. In the spinal cord the changes predominate in the posterior columns and in both the anterior and posterior nerve roots. There is destruction of myelin sheaths, which may be accompanied by fragmentation of the nerve fibers and atrophy of the nerve cells. Usually these changes affect only part of the fibers constituting a nerve trunk. The extent of these changes depends upon the duration and the severity of the disease. Of the peripheral nerves the sciatic is most frequently involved, and evidence of this appears early. Of the cranial nerves the vagi and the phrenics are most frequently affected. With the disturbance of innervation there is secondary atrophy of the muscles.

Clinical Characteristics. Four clinical types of the disease are recognized: dry beriberi, wet beriberi, infantile beriberi and atypical beriberi.

There are no specific phenomena that are necessarily common to all types. The clinical manifestations of the disease fall into three general categories: those referable to degenerative lesions of the nervous system; those resulting from cardiac hypertrophy and dilatation; and the secondary effects of edema and anasarca. The onset may be rapid or gradual, the condition may become chronic, and recurrences of the acute form are frequent. The disease is commonly ushered in by the development of muscle weakness, anorexia and neurasthenia. Tachycardia and cardiac enlargement usually become evident early. There is often slight anemia. As the disease becomes established, progressive peripheral nerve palsies appear.

DRY BERIBERI. The onset is usually gradual, and the outstanding symptom is progressive weakness of the muscle groups that are most used. This most commonly appears in the extensor muscles of the thighs, and a significant early symptom in many instances is inability to rise from a squatting position. With the weakness there is atrophy of the muscles. Sensory disturbances appear at the same time but are usually less prominent. These may take the form of paresthesias, hyperesthesias or hypoesthesias. In severe cases many muscle groups may be affected, and the clinical picture is that of flaccid paralysis, muscular atrophy with or without evidence of cardiac enlargement, and tachycardia.

WET BERIBERI. In wet beriberi the clinical picture is predominantly that of acute congestive failure with relatively little evidence of nervous system involvement. Signs of neuropathy, however, can be elicited in most instances. The onset is frequently rapid and acute, and the marked edema may mask the presence of significant muscle atrophy.

Electrocardiographic changes are common and characteristically consist of alterations in the T waves and prolongation of the electrical systole (Q-T). Sudden collapse is not infrequent. The exact mechanism of this form of the disease is uncertain, but it seems probable that both the heart and the peripheral vascular system are concerned.

INFANTILE BERIBERI. Breast-fed infants of mothers subsisting on a diet deficient in thiamine develop an acute condition differing markedly from the disease of adults. In the usual type the onset is preceded by a period of diminished urine secretion accompanied by progressively increasing edema. If treatment is withheld, acute cardiac failure suddenly supervenes, and death may follow rapidly. With the appearance of the acute phenomena the child cries constantly, and meningism and convulsions may occur.

In the more uncommon dry type of infantile beriberi, edema and circulatory disturbances are not prominent. There may be vomiting, constipation, anorexia, loss of weight, pallor, fretfulness and a characteristic plaintive cry of aphonia. The muscles are hypersensitive but there is usually little definite evidence of nervous system disease.

ATYPICAL BERIBERI. The clinical picture of the disease may be modified by other nutritional disorders, such as scurvy, pellagra or nutritional edema. So-called ship beriberi and land scurvy fall into this category, as does the polyneuritis of alcoholic beriberi.

Diagnosis. The essential diagnostic features are signs and symptoms of peripheral neuritis, with weakness of the most used muscle groups. Hyperesthesia of muscles, particularly the plantar muscles and the gastrocnemius, is common and significant. An important and early physical sign is reduction or loss of vibratory sensation over the affected distal portions of the extremities, with diminution or loss of distal proprioceptive sense. Tendon reflexes are later diminished and then lost. In severe cases marked muscle atrophy occurs. Measurement of thiamine excretion in the urine may provide confirmatory evidence. The range, considered to be normally 100 to 200 μg daily, is markedly reduced in clinical cases of beriberi.

The occurrence of diminished urinary secretion and edema in a breast-fed infant should immediately arouse suspicion and lead to prompt institution of specific therapy.

Beriberi must be differentiated from other types of peripheral neuritis, tabes dorsalis, postdiphtheritic paralysis and acute heart failure resulting from other causes.

The following eight criteria have been

suggested to differentiate cardiac disease due to other causes from that of beriberi:

1. Enlarged heart with normal sinoatrial rhythm.
2. Dependent edema.
3. Elevated venous pressure.
4. Peripheral neuritis.
5. Nonspecific changes in the electrocardiogram.
6. Lack of other recognized cause of heart failure.
7. Grossly deficient diet for at least 3 months.
8. Clinical improvement with reduction of heart size after specific treatment.

Treatment. 1. Thiamine chloride, 5 to 10 mg parenterally twice daily.

2. High vitamin diet supplemented by rich sources of the B complex, such as vitamin preparations, or if these are not available, brewer's yeast 180 gm daily, or tikitiki (extract of rice polishings) 90 gm daily.

The wet form of beriberi must be treated by absolute rest and high dosage of thiamine, which should be administered both intravenously and subcutaneously. The appropriate measures for the management of acute congestive failure should be used as they may be indicated.[5]

Infantile beriberi should be treated by appropriate alteration of the mother's diet and the infant should receive large doses of thiamine parenterally.

Prognosis. Deaths from the acute form of wet beriberi are not infrequent. The chronic form may leave permanent disability, such as muscle weakness or flaccid paralysis due to nerve cell degeneration. Recovery from the disease in adults is slow. The muscle weakness and neuritis frequently persist for months. Infantile beriberi, on the other hand, responds very rapidly and completely when treatment is adequate.

Prevention. Like other deficiency diseases, beriberi should be prevented rather than treated. Increasing the variety of foods consumed, parboiling of rice and enrichment of rice with thiamine (rice is usually also enriched with riboflavin, niacin and iron) have all been used successfully in the prevention of beriberi.[5] The Japanese army has also used thiamine pills as preventive agents for soldiers fed white rice.

CHAPTER 58
Sprue

Synonyms. Psilosis, Ceylon sore mouth, Cochin-China diarrhea.

Definition. Sprue is a chronic afebrile relapsing disease characterized by sore tongue, flatulence, steatorrhea, progressive emaciation, cachexia and anemia. The latter is at first hypochromic, becoming hyperchromic and, in the terminal stages of untreated cases, occasionally aplastic.

Distribution. It occurs predominantly in the Far East in India and Sri Lanka (Ceylon), and in the Western Hemisphere in Puerto Rico. It occurs sporadically in the United States and other parts of the world with the exception of Africa, where it is extremely rare.

Etiology. The exact etiology is unknown. The fully developed syndrome is the expression of mixed multiple nutritional deficiencies, among which folic acid deficiency appears to play the dominant role. The fact that daily administration of pteroylglutamic (folic) acid relieves the symptoms of sprue might be interpreted to indicate that sprue is a specific deficiency disease. The etiology is confused, however, and some of the epidemiologic data have suggested that the primary mechanism may be of infectious origin. Despite this, nutritional considerations dominate both the etiologic and the therapeutic aspects of the disease.

Digestion of protein, carbohydrate and fat is normal, but there is incomplete absorption of fatty acids and glucose. This dysfunction is associated with flatulence and bulky, gaseous, acid stools which contain large amounts of unabsorbed fatty acid crystals. There is likewise excessive loss of calcium in the form of insoluble calcium soaps in the feces. Hypochlorhydria is the rule and achlorhydria occurs occasionally.

It has been suggested that the basic defect—loss of ability to absorb fatty acids, glycerol and glucose—is due to failure of phosphorylation and to loss of phosphorus as the result of failure of phospholipid formation.

Epidemiology. It has not been possible to explain adequately the geographic distribution of the disease. Its incidence is not associated with any particular type of diet or dietary deficiency. It is a disease characteristically of the white race, affecting especially individuals in the upper economic levels and persons long resident in endemic areas.

Pathology. There is no specific or characteristic pathologic process. The findings at post mortem are limited essentially to wasting and atrophy of the various organs and of the body as a whole.

In the advanced stage showing macrocytic anemia, the bone marrow is characteristically hyperplastic as in pernicious anemia. In still later cases the marrow may be aplastic and contain little active hemopoietic tissue.

Clinical Characteristics. The clinical picture varies greatly and the onset is gradual and insidious. In the majority of cases, however, the three cardinal symptoms—sore tongue and mouth, flatulent indigestion and diarrhea—are present when the disease is fully established. These features appear simultaneously or in succession in any order.

Mouth lesions are prominent in most instances and usually precede the appearance of diarrhea. At first, they consist of small, painful, aphthous ulcers on the tongue and buccal mucosa. Later, the tongue becomes acutely inflamed and denuded. Extension of the lesions into the pharynx and the esophagus may cause severe dysphagia. Salivation may be troublesome.

Flatulence, at first mild and intermittent and frequently relieved by evacuation of a stool, gradually becomes continuous and increasingly severe. Eventually, extreme and persistent abdominal distention may be a source of much distress to the patient.

In the early stages the diarrhea is usually intermittent and frequently mild, coming in the early morning accompanied by a sense of urgency. Gradually, the stools become increasingly voluminous, gassy, foul and light yellow or gray.. At first, there may be only one evacuation each day; later, the number increases and the stools become more fluid and irritating.

Spontaneous remissions of symptoms are characteristically followed by increasingly severe relapses. The latter result in progressive papillary atrophy of the tongue, weight loss and increasing asthenia. In the early stages of the disease there is commonly a moderate microcytic anemia.

In advanced cases emaciation is often extreme. The tongue is characteristically smooth, fiery red, painful and extremely sensitive to heat and condiments. There is marked mental depression and severe anorexia. Paresthesias of the extremities may be present. The patient often complains of epigastric distress and flatulence. The skin, especially of the face and the flanks, frequently exhibits muddy pigmentation. The abdomen is markedly distended and individual coils of intestines are visible. In some instances, there may be evidence of subacute combined degeneration of the cord. Stools are frequent, liquid, white or yellowish white in color, abnormally bulky and gassy. Evacuation may be painful owing to excoriation of the anus. At times, severe tetany may occur and, in some instances, there may be bleeding resulting from lack of vitamin K.

In the advanced case the anemia is macrocytic and may be severe. Gastric analysis will reveal hypoacidity or anacidity but not achylia. There is a large excess of fat and fatty acids in the stools but no evidence of failure of fat splitting or of incomplete digestion of starch and protein. The fecal nitrogen is not elevated. The blood calcium is frequently low; the phosphorus content is normal or somewhat low. Hypoproteinemia is common in severe cases. The glucose tolerance test after the ingestion of 1.5 gm of glucose per kg of body weight reveals a flat blood sugar curve with the maximum rise seldom exceeding 40 mg per 100 ml. Intravenous administration of 0.2 gm of glucose per kg of body weight, however, gives a normal blood sugar curve. Vitamin A tolerance tests reveal a flat curve indicative of poor fat absorption.

Roentgen examination of the small intestine reveals characteristic functional disturbances. The barium tends to accumulate in dilated coils. The mucosal pattern is much coarser than normal, and the progress of the opaque meal is slow and intermittent. Barium enema may reveal a markedly dilated and atonic colon.

Diagnosis. The characteristic case, with glossitis, hyperchromic anemia and steatorrhea, presents little diagnostic difficulty. The typical clinical phenomena, however, may not all be present, a feature which has led to the clinical classification of "complete" and "incomplete" sprue. The differential diagnosis entails differentiation from chronic pancreatitis, carcinoma of the pancreas, pernicious anemia, gastrojejunocolic fistula and regional enteritis. The following features are characteristic of sprue:

1. Steatorrhea with normal splitting of fat and normal digestion of starch and protein.

2. Flat glucose tolerance curve on oral administration.

3. Normal glucose tolerance curve on intravenous administration.

4. In severe cases, macrocytic anemia with megaloblastic arrest of the bone marrow.

Treatment. 1. High protein, high vitamin, low fat diet. In cases with marked flatulence it may be necessary to restrict starches and sugars.

2. Daily intramuscular injection of 15 mg of folic acid, followed by maintenance dose of 5 mg by mouth when the patient's condition permits.

3. Parenteral administration of vitamin K, or oral administration of a water soluble vitamin K preparation.

4. If folic acid is not available, brewer's yeast 60 gm, or tikitiki extract of rice polishings 30 gm, should be given daily by mouth, and concentrated aqueous liver extract 5 ml intramuscularly each day.

When treatment is effective, it is followed by rapid healing of the mouth lesions and progressive improvement in the intestinal features. Stools become less frequent, the volume is diminished, the consistency is improved, the color returns toward normal, and the amount of unabsorbed fatty acids decreases. Lack of gastrointestinal and of hematologic response to folic acid should lead to doubt of the diagnosis. The response to vitamin B_{12} should then be tested.[6, 7]

Prognosis. The prognosis depends to a large extent upon the duration and severity of the disease prior to the institution of adequate therapy. Mild cases ultimately may be able to resume a normal diet without medication. More commonly, fats in the diet must be restricted permanently and parenteral injections of aqueous liver extract continued at intervals of 1 to 2 weeks. The character of the stools, the amount of unabsorbed fatty acids in the feces and the presence or absence of flatulence provide satisfactory guides to therapy.

CHAPTER 59

Protein-Calorie Malnutrition: Kwashiorkor and Nutritional Marasmus

Kwashiorkor and nutritional marasmus constitute the most important and widespread nutritional deficiency disease syndromes in the world today. In the former, the main deficiency is one of protein; in the latter, of calories. There are, however, many intermediate cases which are difficult to fit into either category. There are also many children who are deficient in protein or calories or both, who have failed to grow normally, and who are on the brink of one or other of these diseases yet could not properly be diagnosed as having either syndrome.

Over the past two decades kwashiorkor has been recognized and studied in many parts of the world, and now has been accepted as one disease with only slight local variations. During this period the emphasis has been on protein deficiency, and worldwide effort has been made to increase the quantity of protein available in many countries and especially to improve the quality of protein in the diets of children.

More recently, the equal importance in young children of a shortage of calories as part of an overall deficiency of food, including protein-rich products, has been realized. Together, all these conditions fall under the title protein-calorie deficiency disease.

Kwashiorkor and nutritional marasmus should be regarded as the two poles of this syndrome. It should be clear, however, that the majority of clinical cases, though lying between the two extremes, nevertheless are nearer to one pole or the other. There is some overlapping which leads to descriptive terms such as "marasmic kwashiorkor"; however, most cases can be labeled as one or the other disease. A good example is "sugar baby" kwashiorkor in which there is little evidence of calorie deficiency.

Kwashiorkor

Synonyms. Malignant malnutrition (South Africa), fatty liver disease of children (West Indies), fatty liver of Brahmin children (India), bouffissure d'Annam (Vietnam), sindrome pluricarencial infantil (Central America). The syndrome merges into other nutritional syndromes, such as Mehlnährschaden.

Definition. Kwashiorkor is a nutritional syndrome in which a deficiency of good quality protein appears to be a dominant factor. It is found among many poor populations, especially among children 1 to 4 years of age. Characteristically, the following occur: retarded growth and maturation; muscle wasting; edema; mental changes including apathy, misery and sometimes irritability; anorexia; diarrhea, sometimes vomiting; alteration in color and texture of the hair, skin changes including depigmentation and sometimes a dermatosis; marked fatty infiltration of the liver; anemia; reduction of serum protein and alteration of the albumin-globulin ratio.

Distribution. The various synonyms for the disease testify to its widespread character. It is found wherever tropical peoples subsist on starchy staple foods without adequate protein supplements. It has been studied particularly thoroughly in Central and South America, in Jamaica, India, Mexico, and in Central and South Africa. However, it is found as well in North Africa, the Near East and in many areas of Asia besides India. Its prevalence within populations can be extremely high. It has been claimed that practically every child in certain African and Central American regions, for example, has or has had some degree of protein malnutrition bordering on kwashiorkor.

Etiology. Lack of proteins, particularly complete proteins, seems to be responsible principally for the characteristic pathologic changes. These appear to be the result of a deficiency of good quality protein in general rather than a deficiency of a single amino acid. The disease is not observed during the period of breast feeding so long as the supply of maternal milk is adequate. It closely follows weaning and transfer of the child to starch gruels, when maternal milk is replaced by low grade and dilute foodstuffs.

The reason for the lack of protein varies widely. It may be due to an overall lack of protein-rich foods in the country or for the particular family, or it may be due to poverty and, therefore, the inability to purchase protein-rich foods which are generally more expensive than predominantly carbohydrate foods. More often the cause is ignorance of the fact that foods contain different nutrients and that children require a variety of these for growth and development. The majority of persons in many countries regard food as something to fill the stomach and cannot conceive that illness can be caused by dietary deficiencies in a child who is never hungry. A further factor in the etiology of kwashiorkor is an unfair distribution of available protein foods within the family.

A common train of events is the sudden weaning of a child, between 1 and 2 years of age, onto a starchy diet. This weaning often takes place as soon as the mother finds that she is pregnant again. The child who has had an extraordinarily close physical and psychological relationship with his mother may be sent to live with a relative in order to make the weaning process "easier." The child, as well as being suddenly placed on an unaccustomed and often unsuitable diet deficient in protein, has also suffered a psychological trauma. Both these events may cause a reduction in appetite and lead directly to kwashiorkor.

In recent years, the importance of infections, particularly infectious diarrhea, in the causation of both kwashiorkor and marasmus has been established. A child entering his second year of life has lost his maternally inherited immunity, and because he is now able to propel himself, comes into contact, often for the first time, with many possible sources of infection. It is during this period that gastroenteritis, measles, hookworm, schistosomiasis and a host of other diseases may attack him. Any of these may

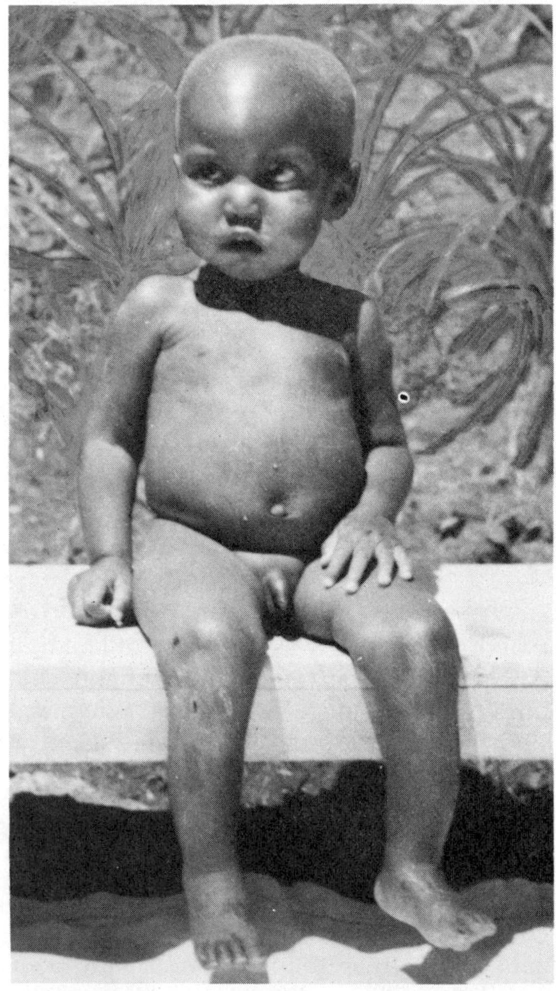

Figure 59-1. Kwashiorkor in young native of the former Belgian Congo. Note the white hair, skin discoloration and general edema. (Courtesy of Dr. Louis Van den Berghe; photo courtesy of IRSAC by Macot.)

serve to tip the balance in a child on a poor diet who is poised on the brink of protein-calorie malnutrition. The role of diarrhea is particularly important because this interferes with the absorption of nutrients, and it may cause increased loss of valuable nitrogen in the stools. The diarrhea is all too often treated at home with a bland carbohydrate diet or even by starvation rather than by the proper use of modern antibiotics and by proper electrolyte and fluid therapy.

Pathology and Clinical Characteristics. The following signs, symptoms and pathologic findings are observed (Fig. 59–1):

RETARDATION OF GROWTH AND MUSCLE WASTING. This begins at the late breast feeding, weaning and postweaning ages. It is fundamental to kwashiorkor but is also common to other conditions such as undernutrition due to lack of available calories or to anorexia, marasmus and atrophy. The muscles are always wasted.

In spite of the serious growth retardation and reduction of muscle bulk, the child with kwashiorkor does not always look emaciated or starved. If he has been provided with a nearly adequate supply of calories in the form of starch or sugar while he was deprived of protein, his subcutaneous fat may be appreciable and is never so lacking as in marasmus. Edema frequently masks the wasting and growth failure, sometimes giving a superficial appearance of good nutrition.

EDEMA. This is always present in kwashiorkor. It usually starts in the feet and lower legs but may affect any part of the body including the face.

PSYCHIC CHANGES. Children with kwashiorkor are usually apathetic and anorexic. They appear extremely miserable and may be irritable.

DIARRHEA AND GASTROINTESTINAL DISORDERS. Frequent loose stools are a common finding. Mucosal lesions and atrophy, diarrhea and deficient intake may all be part of a vicious circle. Pancreatic fibrosis is commonly observed and examination of duodenal fluid reveals a reduction in pancreatic enzymes. Serum amylase is reduced.

HAIR CHANGES. The texture of the hair is frequently altered. That of an African child, for example, loses its luster and sheen and may alter in color with a reduction of pigmentation. If there are periods of better nutrition, the hair may grow normally, but a further period of malnutrition may cause another band of discolored hair.[9, 10] This leads to the so-called "flag sign" in the hair which is commonly seen in Central America but not in Africa (Fig. 59–2). The hair is often sparse and sometimes it can be plucked out painlessly and easily.

DEPIGMENTATION AND DERMATOSES. The skin, particularly of the face, may be depigmented. This must be distinguished from hypopigmentation caused by admixture with people of lighter color or inborn mutations (half albinos). Skin depigmentation resulting from kwashiorkor can be patchy or diffuse and, in some cases, may cover the entire body.

Dermatoses do not appear to be the same in various regions of the world and, therefore, probably have several different

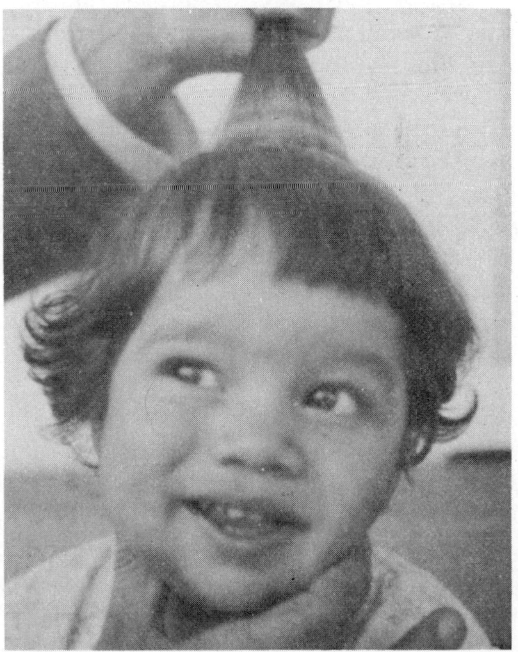

Figure 59–2. Flag sign. Three year old child with hypoproteinemia, who in the last 8 months experienced periods of malnutrition, leaving stripes of hypopigmentation. (Courtesy of Dr. A. Peña Chavarria, San Juan de Dios Hospital, San José, Costa Rica.)

origins. The most common form is an eruption of sharply defined black varnished patches on areas exposed to irritation (diaper area, buttocks, back, limb flexures) and not confined to areas exposed to sunlight (hands and face), thus permitting differentiation from pellagra. The hyperpigmented areas may become dry, cracked and scaled, and may peel. In extreme cases they may blister and resemble second degree burns.

Fatty Infiltration of the Liver. The liver may or may not be palpable but is universally found to be extremely infiltrated with fat, frequently to such an extent that the normal lobulation is hardly recognizable.

Anemia. Examination of the blood nearly always shows moderate anemia. Severe anemia when present may be the result of malaria, hookworm or some other disease which is also present. The erythrocytes are usually normocytic or slightly macrocytic and the hemoglobin around 9 gm per 100 ml. The anemia is thought to be the result, at least in part, of a lack of the protein necessary to synthesize red blood corpuscles.

Serum Proteins. There is always a marked reduction in the level of serum protein. This is due mainly to the low serum albumin, which may average 1.5 gm per 100 ml (normal level 3.5 gm per 100 ml), but may be below 1 gm per 100 ml. The level of serum globulin is not usually affected; the gamma globulin is often raised, possibly as the result of infection. The reduction in serum albumin may be a factor in the production of edema. The level of serum albumin rises as successful treatment proceeds.

Mortality in Untreated Cases. Mortality in the untreated syndrome is high. Recent studies suggest that the heavy mortality is associated with irreversible biochemical changes. In the absence of proper treatment the mortality is seldom less than 30 per cent, and in some areas goes up to 100 per cent.

Treatment. Well planned treatment is based on an understanding of the primary factor in the etiology—primary deficiency of good quality proteins, often associated with calorie and vitamin deficiency. The degree of severity of the case, the nature and extent of dehydration and electrolyte imbalance, and the presence and extent of intestinal parasitosis and other infections are also important considerations.

The main treatment for kwashiorkor is dietary. In children whose general condition is fair, a complete and balanced diet is given from the outset. It is adjusted to the age of the child but consists largely of skim milk and other animal proteins. Some fat, preferably in the form of a vegetable oil, can be included as a source of calories.

Hospital admission is advised for severe cases, as judged by the general condition of the patient, amount of edema, extent of the dermatosis, hemoglobin level, severity of diarrhea, vomiting and dehydration and, perhaps most important, the ability and willingness of the child to feed. Once again, dried skimmed milk should form the basis of treatment. A mixture of this with added vegetable oil and casein is ideal. If the child is extremely ill or if he cannot or will not take this mixture from a feeding cup or spoon, the same mixture is best given through an intragastric tube. This should be about 1 mm in diameter, 2 feet in length and made of polythene. The tube can be left safely in situ for 5 days. The milk mixture can be either given by continuous drip or administered intermittently. It should aim to provide about 120 calories and 7 gm of protein per kg of body weight per day. Marked dehydration following severe diarrhea and vomiting may require the preliminary administration of intravenous (or failing this, intraperitoneal) electrolyte solutions. In any event, if diarrhea is a prominent symptom, it will be desirable to administer by the oral route 0.5 gm of potassium chloride in water 3 times a day. Penicillin or some other antibiotic should be given from the outset to combat infection. In areas where malaria is endemic, an antimalarial such as chloroquine is also highly desirable.

If anemia is severe or shock is present, a blood transfusion might prove lifesaving. Moderate anemia can be treated with ferrous sulfate, 300 to 600 mg orally per day.

There is no place in the treatment of

kwashiorkor for the routine administration of vitamins; these should be given only if there is clinical evidence of a deficiency. Thus, for example, if xerophthalmia is found to be present, vitamin A should be prescribed, or if the anemia is believed to be the result of a lack of folic acid or vitamin B_{12}, these would form part of the treatment. Subclinical vitamin and mineral deficiencies will be combated adequately by the balanced diet that forms a part of the treatment.

Treatment of intestinal parasitosis is best left until the condition of the child has begun to improve.

A severe case of kwashiorkor can be expected to respond to the above regimen quite rapidly. The diarrhea and gastrointestinal symptoms subside, diuresis brings about rapid reduction in edema and, as anorexia disappears, the mood of the child begins to change. At this stage, treatment can be pursued as described for mild cases and later a more varied diet can be given. This should, if possible, include foods that are locally available and to which the child has access. The mother's cooperation in the diet regimen as the child improves should form an integral part of therapy and should be combined with nutrition education. In order to prevent both the recurrence of the disease in the recovering child and its occurrence in siblings, it is important to convince the mother that the disease was caused by a dietary deficiency and has been cured, not by medicines, but by the administration of proper foods.

Prognosis in Treated Cases. The short term prognosis of mild cases given full treatment is good. The frequency of multiple episodes is high when home conditions are unfavorable. Recurrences take place not only in children taken home by parents before the cure is complete but also, less commonly, in children who leave the hospital "clinically cured." Relapse usually occurs 3 to 6 months after the child has left the hospital. The clinical state during relapse is usually similar to and often more serious than that at first admission. The mortality rate in such cases continues high.

The prognosis of successfully treated cases over a longer or life-span period is not known. It is unlikely, from their world distribution, that cirrhosis and primary carcinoma of the liver on the one hand and kwashiorkor on the other are related in any direct cause and effect manner. Adult cirrhosis may well result from the effects of continued protein deficiency and parasitosis, infection and toxic factors on a liver already damaged in childhood by kwashiorkor. A similar situation may exist with respect to primary carcinoma of the liver.

Prophylaxis. Proper prevention is based on:

1. Increasing the supply of proteins, both animal and vegetable. This entails development of milk-producing livestock—cattle, sheep and goats—and the expansion of fisheries and fish farming. Proper mixtures of vegetable protein must also be developed, in particular by increasing availability of pulses, nuts and green vegetables.

2. Eliminating the "hungry months," during which incidence of kwashiorkor increases, by developing cash crops and other additional sources of income.

3. "Supplementary feeding" programs directed at infants and young children, with emphasis on foods providing adequate amounts of good quality protein.

For the prevention and treatment of the syndrome of infantile protein malnutrition (infantile protein syndrome, IPS) in countries where the production of milk and protein food of animal origin is scarce and expensive, the use of an easily assimilable vegetable mixture for children is effective and recommended. For example, INCAP (Institute of Nutrition for Central America and Panama) has developed a vegetable mixture called "Incaparina." This mixture has a nutritional value similar in quantity and quality to cow's milk. The principal source of this mixture is flour made from cottonseed to which has been added other nutrients to increase its caloric value to that of cow's milk. Incaparina is inexpensive and is well accepted.[6, 7]

4. Education. With the best intentions, young mothers in poor tropical countries commit many grave faults in providing nutri-

tion for their children. However, when proper nutrition education programs are put into effect, it is found that changes in traditional patterns of infant and small child feeding can be introduced fairly rapidly. Maternity and child health centers have had considerable influence on nutrition habits. Family dietary habits can be influenced also through schools, although in underdeveloped areas many girls do not attend school.

5. Social welfare. In poor areas there are unusually substantial numbers of small children who suffer from simple neglect. This situation can be remedied through the work of strong social agencies, which must be well versed in the nutritional requirements of this age group.

Nutritional Marasmus

Definition. This is a severe form of protein-calorie malnutrition. In kwashiorkor the main deficiency is one of protein; in marasmus the child is receiving inadequate food, including calories, a form of starvation. It occurs usually during the first 3½ years of life but, in contrast to kwashiorkor, is especially common during the first 12 months. Typically, there is hunger, failure of growth and lack of nearly all subcutaneous fat.

Distribution. Nutritional marasmus is seen mainly in the same geographic areas as kwashiorkor, but its actual distribution is worldwide. Outside the developing countries, it occurs either secondary to some other disease or under grossly abnormal social or family circumstances.

Etiology. The disease is caused by a lack of sufficient calories and other nutrients in the diet of a young child. For one of a variety of reasons, the child is getting neither adequate supplies of breast milk nor any alternative suitable food.

A common cause is failure of lactation in a woman who is part of a society in which there is no suitable alternative to breast feeding. Abandonment of a young infant or death of the mother may be causes. In some tropical areas, the increasing tendency to bottle feed rather than to breast feed infants for prestige or other reasons is becoming a potent cause of nutritional marasmus. Because of the high cost of milk products, the mixture given by bottle is frequently overdiluted, thus causing caloric deficiency. Finally, because adequate facilities and knowledge regarding preparation and sterilization of bottles and the feeding mixture do not exist, infective diarrhea frequently supervenes and leads to marasmus.

An overall lack of food in a family, prolonged starvation as a form of treatment for diarrhea and diseases that hinder proper absorption of food may all be causes of marasmus.

Clinical Characteristics. In all cases, the child fails to grow and is much lighter and shorter than is normal for his age. In severe cases, the main feature is emaciation. There is always obvious wasting of the muscles, the limbs being extremely thin. The skin, especially around the buttocks, is loose and wrinkled, but, when taken up between the forefinger and thumb (or when measured with skinfold calipers), will reveal almost complete absence of subcutaneous fat. The abdomen, in contrast to the emaciated chest and limbs, is protuberant. The face is drawn and monkeylike.

In contrast to kwashiorkor, the marasmic child is not disinterested or irritable and usually has a good appetite. In fact, constant mouth action or sucking of hands or clothing indicates that he is ravenously hungry.

Diarrhea and anemia are frequently but not always present. Edema and dermatosis are absent although, in severe cases, pressure zones over bony prominences may be found.

The hair may show changes, but these are more frequently alterations in texture than in color.

Treatment. The treatment is as described for kwashiorkor. It is, however, especially important to make certain that adequate calories and protein are provided to allow for weight gain and growth. It is also necessary to see that the child is not discharged from the hospital back to the same environment that led to the disease. Thus, if the mother of the infant is dead, some arrangement should be made to supply dried skim milk or some other preparation to feed the child during the critical months before he can eat the normal family diet.

Prophylaxis. This is similar to prevention of kwashiorkor and rests on the provision of an adequate diet for each member of every family. This is dependent on the food supplies and economic status of each country. Nutrition and health education of all sections of the community are vital. Encouragement should be given to breast feeding as the normal mode of infant feeding.

Because of the importance of diarrhea and other infectious diseases in the etiology of protein-calorie malnutrition, all measures designed to improve public health will serve to reduce the incidence of malnutrition. Conversely, the improvement of nutrition will lower the incidence of disease, including diarrhea.[8, 11, 12]

CHAPTER 60

Nutritional Edema

Synonyms. War edema, famine edema, prison edema.

Definition. This condition is a nutritional disorder that follows long-continued subsistence on a diet deficient in biologically complete protein. It is characterized by changes in the concentration of the plasma proteins, altered osmotic tension of the blood and anasarca.

Distribution. This disease occurs particularly in famine areas. It was widely prevalent in Central Europe during and immediately after World War I and has occurred in India, Mauritius, Fiji and Java, and in Spain during the Spanish Civil War. It occurs endemically as a complication of other nutritional diseases.

Etiology. Nutritional edema develops when the diet is limited in total calories and the average protein content is less than 40 gm per day. The appearance of the clinical syndrome is preceded by a prolonged period of negative nitrogen balance. In the early stages, the total plasma protein is unchanged, the albumin somewhat reduced and the globulin correspondingly increased. Later, the total protein is reduced, and there is inversion of the normal albumin-globulin ratio accompanied by disturbances of osmotic relationships and by water retention within the tissues.

The normal values for the plasma proteins are:

Total protein	6.5 to 8.5 gm per 100 ml
Albumin	4.2 to 5.7 gm per 100 ml
Globulin	1.3 to 3.0 gm per 100 ml

Clinical Characteristics. The development of the characteristic clinical picture is usually preceded by progressive weight loss due to the limited caloric intake. As the chemical imbalance is established, further weight loss is checked by water retention and may be followed by an actual weight gain.

In the early stages there is marked pitting edema of the lower extremities; later, this becomes generalized and, if progressive, lead to anasarca.

Diagnosis. The occurrence of edema in individuals subjected to famine conditions is suggestive. The diagnosis is based upon fluid retention in the absence of congestive heart failure or significant renal disease and is confirmed by determination of the plasma proteins and demonstration of inversion of the albumin-globulin ratio.

Treatment. The treatment of nutritional edema is essentially the institution of a high protein, high vitamin diet which should be arranged to provide 120 to 150 gm of animal protein per day and to restrict salt and fluids.

Epidemic Dropsy

Epidemic dropsy is believed to be nutritional edema complicating other nutritional disorders such as pellagra and beriberi. It has appeared in mass outbreaks, especially in India. The condition is often accompanied by the neurologic symptoms and signs of beriberi and by erythematous skin lesions, followed by pigmentation of exposed areas that is suggestive of endemic pellagra.

CHAPTER 61
Simple Goiter

Synonym. Endemic goiter, simple colloid goiter.

Definition. The term goiter denotes an enlargement of the thyroid gland. "Simple" goiter denotes such an enlargement, without either hypothyroidism or hyperthyroidism. It is also called "endemic" because of its widespread character in many parts of the world.

Distribution. The endemic form of goiter occurs in the following types of terrain: in mountainous areas of Europe, Asia, North and South America, and Africa; on glacial plains such as the Great Lake area and certain areas of New Zealand; and in certain areas where the water consumed is unusually hard. Also, it occurs in areas where consumption of goitrogens is unusually high.

Formerly it was believed that goiter was found only far from the sea. It is now recognized that proximity of the sea by itself is of no consequence unless seafood is consumed. In the W.H.O. 1960 survey, 200,000,000 people were estimated to have goiter.

Etiology. The principal cause of endemic goiter is a dietary deficiency of iodine. As long as the soil content of iodine is adequate, enough iodine (about 100 to 200 μg per person per day) is usually ingested to prevent goiter. Mountainous areas, glacial areas where glaciers crushed virgin rocks never exposed to atmospheric iodine and leached soluble iodine salts out of the virginal soil, and alluvial plains where the iodine is periodically leached out of soils usually hold a flora (and a fauna) deficient in iodine. A contributing factor in the etiology is the presence of goitrogenic substances in foods; cabbage, turnips, cabbage seeds, mustard seeds, and rape seeds are high in such substances as thio-oxazolidine, a highly goitrogenic compound. Thiourea, thiouracil, and other thio-compounds are similarly goitrogenic. Hardness of drinking water is also a factor. Addition of limestone to the water, or pumping water out of deep limestone wells, has been shown also to be a contributing factor in various parts of England. Stress and pregnancy are precipitating factors.

Clinical Characteristics. In the majority of cases, there are no clinical effects due to either mild hypofunction or mild hyperfunction. In some cases, simple goiter may be treated surgically because of unsightliness or because of pressure on adjacent structures.

Complications are rare and include hypothyroidism, cretinism, deaf mutism and hyperthyroidism. Such complications are more prevalent in areas where simple goiter is endemic.

Treatment. At its inception, simple goiter usually responds well to the daily administration of small therapeutic doses of iodine. By the time goiter is clearly developed, regression is at best limited. Prevention is therefore particularly important.

Prevention. The most important factor in prevention is the administration of small doses of iodine either in "iodized" salt or through injection of iodated oil. When salt is iodized, if both table and cooking salt are treated, the recommended amount is 10 parts of potassium iodide per million parts of sodium chloride. If only table salt is iodized, the recommended amount is 3 to 5 times higher. In some areas, potassium iodate is used in preference to potassium iodide because of its greater stability.

The iodization of salt has recently lost some favor because, in industrialized countries, "convenience" foods are usually so high in sodium (as a result of salting with "noniodized" salt) that one hesitates to advise the use of supplementary table salt. The answer here is the use of iodized salt in such foods, in fact in the preparation of all foods. In some developing areas, the salt supply comes from a multiplicity of avenues and is difficult to control. Injection of iodized oil has been used in some areas on a limited basis. Other measures that can be useful are elimination of goitrogenic feeds from the diet of milch cows (the goitrogens are transmitted into the milk), and decrease of the proportion of goitrogenic foods in human diets. However, by far the most effective and economical way to prevent simple goiter is by the universal use of iodized salt in the preparation of all food, both in the home and commercially.

CHAPTER 62

Osteomalacia

Synonym. Adult rickets.

Definition. Osteomalacia is a calcium-phosphorus deficiency disease characterized by a negative balance of calcium and phosphorus and by deficient calcification of all osteoid tissue. It is a disease primarily of women, particularly during pregnancy and lactation, and increases in severity with each successive pregnancy.

Distribution. It is widely endemic in north India, China and Japan, and occurs sporadically in Central Europe.

Etiology. Osteomalacia and rickets are the same disease. Continuous resorption and new bone formation occur, and there is failure of calcification of newly formed osteoid tissue because of insufficient absorption of calcium and phosphorus from the diet.

Failure of calcium-phosphorus absorption may be due to deficient diet, abnormal dietary calcium-phosphorus ratio, steatorrhea or vitamin D deficiency. Usually several of these factors are operative, particularly lack of calcium and phosphorus in the diet and insufficient vitamin D. The elevated mineral demands of pregnancy and lactation upon the maternal organism are important factors in the progression of the disease.

Pathology. The abnormal ossification produces gross progressive skeletal deformities, especially of the pelvis, thorax, spine and long bones. The bones become soft and flexible, and the deformities are more frequently the result of bending than of fracture. The bone cortex is thin; the trabeculae are greatly reduced in number or may be absent. Microscopic examination reveals deficient calcification. Osteoclasts are present in normal numbers while osteoblasts are very numerous.

Clinical Characteristics. The symptomatology is dominated by weakness, bone pains and, often, generalized aching. Bony tenderness is common, and severe tetany may occur. Symptoms are particularly acute during pregnancy and lactation. The process characteristically remains relatively stationary in intervals between pregnancies.

Progression of the disease leads to great deformity and disability. Distortion of the bony pelvis causes difficult labor or makes parturition impossible.

Diagnosis. The marked deformities, particularly of the lower extremities, the thorax and the spine, are suggestive in endemic areas. Roentgen examination of the skeleton reveals generalized osteoporosis, and the vertebrae often show biconcave deformity, the so-called "fish vertebrae." The diagnosis is established by blood chemistry findings. In severe cases the serum calcium and phosphorus are low and the serum alkaline phosphatase is increased. In mild cases the calcium may be normal or only slightly reduced, whereas the phosphorus is below normal levels and the phosphatase is slightly increased.

Differential diagnosis entails differentiation from other osteoporotic diseases; particular difficulty is encountered with the osteoporotic form of hyperparathyroidism. The blood chemistry findings in the latter condition are distinctive, however. The serum calcium is elevated, the phosphorus is low, and the phosphatase is above normal levels.

Treatment. Treatment of the disease can protect only against further deformities. It consists of the institution of a diet high in calcium and phosphorus and the administration of 10,000 to 50,000 units of vitamin D daily. Recent research suggests that sodium fluoride in doses of 20 mg given 3 times a day with meals favors calcification.

CHAPTER 63

Vitamin A Deficiency and Tropical Macrocytic Anemia

Vitamin A Deficiency

Distribution. Vitamin A deficiency is widely prevalent in the tropics, especially in those regions where other nutritional deficiency conditions are common.

Etiology. It usually occurs as a primary response to a diet that provides an insufficient supply of the vitamin; or, less frequently, it may be a secondary complication of diseases that are associated with defective absorption of fats.

Clinical Characteristics. Vitamin A deficiency is characterized by skin changes, reduced adaptability to darkness, eye lesions and lesions of the nervous system. In many regions of Africa and India a majority of children present skin changes that respond to vitamin A administration, and many hospitalized patients show evidence of xerophthalmia. The characteristic signs of vitamin A deficiency are as follows:

SKIN CHANGES. Synonyms: toad skin, phrynoderma, shark skin, keratosis pilaris, lichen pilaris, lichen spinulosus, Darier's disease.

The usual changes in the skin include dryness and roughness followed by eruption of hyperkeratotic papillae. When the hyperkeratotic changes do not respond to vitamin A treatment, they presumably have a different origin in spite of their similarity in appearance. The hair becomes dry and brittle and the nails develop transverse or longitudinal ridges.

EYE CHANGES. Adaptability to darkness is impaired, producing so-called "night blindness." There may be photophobia, xerosis and Bitot's spots. In extreme cases, keratomalacia may lead to corneal ulceration, panophthalmitis and loss of the eyes.

NERVOUS SYSTEM CHANGES. The susceptibility of the nervous system to vetches *(Lathyrus* sp.*)* is increased by vitamin A deficiency. The clinical syndrome lathyrism is common in parts of India and has been reported from other regions of the world. It is characterized by a spastic paraplegia.

Treatment. Effective treatment of the conditions due to lack of vitamin A requires daily administration of large doses of from 50,000 to 100,000 International Units.

Prevention. Special efforts should be made, in areas where even a few cases of vitamin A deficiency have been noted, to increase the intake of foods containing vitamin A and carotene. The replacement of white corn by yellow corn and the introduction of red palm oil are among such measures. Use can be made of the fact that vitamin A is stored for long periods in the liver; preventive administration of large doses of vitamin A (100,000 International Units or more) is a wise measure in areas where the likelihood is small that the diet of children will be improved rapidly.

Tropical Macrocytic Anemia

Tropical macrocytic anemia appears to be a response of the hemopoietic system to a nutritional deficiency. Although it may resemble certain aspects of sprue, there is no interference with intestinal absorption. Like sprue, it responds satisfactorily to treatment with folic acid.

Adequate documentation of this section would require more references than there is scope for in this book. Readers interested in delving deeper into the problems of nutrition in general, and tropical diseases in particular, should read the textbook *Human Nutrition and Dietetics* by Passmore.[2] Another good textbook on nutrition is *Modern Nutrition in Health and Disease* by Goodhart and Shils.[13]

REFERENCES

1. Mertz, E. T. 1970. High-lysine corn. Proc. 3rd. Internat. Congr. Food Sci. and Technol. pp. 305–309.
2. Passmore, R. 1973. Human Nutrition and Dietetics. 5th ed. The Williams & Wilkins Co., Baltimore. 1000 pp.
3. Scrimshaw, N. S., and Béhar, M. 1961. Protein malnutrition in young children. Science *133*:2039–2047.
4. Scrimshaw, N. S. 1964. Ecological factors in nutritional disease. Am. J. Clin. Nutr. *14*:112–122.
5. Anonymous. 1964. Recommended Dietary Allowances. 6th ed. Food and Nutrition Board. National Research Council. Publ. 1146, Washington, D.C. 59 pp.
6. Scrimshaw, N. S., Taylor, C. E., and Gordon, J. E. 1959. Interactions of nutrition and infection. Am. J. Med. Sci. *237*:367–403.
7. Scrimshaw, N. S., Béhar, M., Pérez, C., and Viteri, F. 1955. Nutritional problems of children in Central America and Panama. Pediatrics *16*:378–397.
8. Scrimshaw, N. S., Bruch, H., Ascoli, W., and Gordon, J. E. 1962. Studies of diarrheal disease in Central America. IV. Demographic distributions of acute diarrheal disease in two rural populations of Guatemalan highlands. Am. J. Trop. Med. Hyg., *11*:401–409.
9. Peña Chavarria, A., Goldman, L., Saénz Herrera, C., and Cordero Carvajal, E. 1946. Canities and alopecia in children with avitaminosis. J.A.M.A. *132*:570–572.
10. Peña Chavarria, A., Saénz Herrera, C., and Cordero Carvajal, E. 1948. Sindrome carencial de la infancia. Rev. Med. de Costa Rica *15*:125–139.
11. Gordon, J. E., Pierce, V., Ascoli, W., and Scrimshaw, N. S. 1962. Studies of diarrheal disease in Central America. II. Community prevalence of *Shigella* and *Salmonella* infection in childhood. Am. J. Trop. Med. Hyg. *11*:389–394.
12. Pierce, V., Ascoli, W., León, R. de, and Gordon, J. E. 1962. Studies of diarrheal disease in Central America. III. Specific etiology of endemic diarrhea and dysentery in Guatemalan children. Am. J. Trop. Med. Hyg., *11*:395–400.
13. Goodhart, R. S., and Shils, M. E. 1973. Modern Nutrition in Health and Disease. 5th ed. Lea & Febiger, Philadelphia. 1250 pp.

SECTION IX
Miscellaneous Conditions

CHAPTER 64
Effects of Heat

R. K. MACPHERSON
JOHN P. O'BRIEN

The most direct and elemental hazard of the tropics is the heat itself, and in prolonged periods of excessively high air temperatures heat illness may reach epidemic proportions, as in the heatwave in India in May 1972 when several hundreds died from the direct effects of heat. Heat illness is, nevertheless, a relatively rare event among well acclimatized people living in the tropics. In temperate climates, it is true, even modest increases in temperature are commonly accompanied by an increase in the death rate.[1, 2] This excessive mortality occurs chiefly among the aged and chronically ill, but such deaths are usually not accompanied by any of the characteristic symptoms of heat illness and the cause of death remains obscure.

Theoretically, heat illness can result from the breakdown of any one of the physiologic mechanisms concerned in the regulation of body temperature. Attempts have, therefore, been made to devise complicated "rational" classifications of heat illness based on the determination of the immediate cause—such as "water-deficiency heat exhaustion," "exercise-induced heat exhaustion," and the like. It is now agreed, however, that heat illness usually presents as one of a few easily recognized syndromes and the following simple classification of heat illness, or some minor variant of it, is now generally accepted.

Acute

Heat exhaustion
Salt-deficiency syndrome
Heat cramps
Heat stroke

Subacute or Chronic

Miliaria
Anhidrotic asthenia
Heat neurasthenia

Heat Exhaustion

Synonym. Heat prostration.

Definition. Acute heat exhaustion may be formally defined as a state of peripheral circulatory failure resulting from exposure to hot conditions, often associated with or provoked by dehydration, with possibly some accompanying salt deficiency.

Heat exhaustion, or more properly acute heat exhaustion, is the commonest form of acute heat illness. It is usually what is meant when a patient is reported to have "collapsed from the heat." It occurs typically in those performing arduous muscular work in the heat—long-distance runners, soldiers on route marches, and manual workers in hot industries—when to the stress of the environment there is added a heavy metabolic heat load. It can also occur in those merely sitting at rest provided the prevailing conditions of temperature, humidity and air movement impose a sufficiently heavy burden on the temperature-regulating mechanisms of the body.

The term "heat syncope" is sometimes used to describe a syncopal (fainting) attack occurring in hot surroundings. It would appear not to differ from orthostatic syncope, except insofar as its onset has been precipitated by the vasodilatation accompanying exposure to environmental warmth.

Clinical Characteristics. Dizziness and nausea, which may proceed to vomiting, and headache that may be intense and throbbing in character, are common and often early complaints. Abdominal pain, colicky in nature, a sense of pressure or "pounding" in the chest and muscular weakness are also common. Mental processes are slowed and emotional disturbance and disorientation in time and place may be present. Thirst, at first marked, is seldom a complaint in the later stages and the sufferer may even be reluctant to drink.

When collapse is imminent, the patient presents a characteristic appearance. Sweating is profuse and the face exhibits a peculiar lavender cyanosis with marked circumoral pallor. Signs of dehydration, such as sunken cheeks and a dry tongue, may be obvious. The pulse, though strong, is often so rapid as to be uncountable—rates in excess of 200 beats per minute are not unusual. The systolic pressure is usually well maintained, but the diastolic pressure may fall to very low levels resulting in a greatly increased pulse pressure. Body temperature is characteristically only moderately elevated, perhaps to 38 or 39° C (100.4 or 102.2° F), the exact level appearing to depend more on the rate of working than the severity of the environment. If at this stage the sufferer ceases work but remains standing or, if having been seated, stands up, loss of consciousness accompanied by a profound slowing of the pulse may rapidly ensue.

Advanced age, alcohol and adiposity appear to be important predisposing factors. To these must be added inadequate fluid intake, chronic salt deficiency, lack of physical fitness and ill health. Any disorder of the sweating mechanism, including damage to the skin by sunburn, the miliarias or tinea imbricata—all of which materially reduce the effective sweating area and hence the heat tolerance—will hasten the onset of heat exhaustion on exposure to hot conditions (p. 662). For the young and fit the most important predisposing factor is lack of acclimatization. Adequate acclimatization will insure tolerance of conditions which otherwise would result in failure.

Treatment. Remove the patient as rapidly as possible to a cooler environment (an air-conditioned room is ideal), take off his clothing to promote loss of heat, and allow him to rest in a recumbent position. Cooling should be assisted by cold sponging and fanning if the body temperature does not fall promptly. Give cold water to drink, commencing with quite small amounts a sip at a time, but increasing the quantity as the patient's condition improves until 200 to 300 ml have been taken. As sweat is hypotonic with respect to extracellular fluid, the water will serve to correct in part both the volume and osmolarity of the extracellular fluid. The patient should then be encouraged, while still under observation, to drink *slowly* at least a liter of either cold, dilute (0.1 to 0.2 per cent) salt solution, or, preferably, cold fruit juice to which 0.2 per cent salt has been added. Fruit juice is certainly more palatable, and appears to be more effective in restoring a feeling of well-being, possibly due to its potassium content.*

Recovery is usually rapid and uneventful, but if syncope has occurred the patient should continue to rest and be protected from heat for 24 hours. However, recovery is complete since the physiologic failure which produced the event is readily reversible.

Prophylaxis. The list of contributory causes should provide adequate guidance for prophylaxis, even if in the case of some, such as age, little can be done except to advise caution in exposure to heat stress.

---

*If available, Gatorade, a medically balanced beverage for replacement of fluid and salts, which is available in markets in some countries, may be substituted.

Salt-Deficiency Syndrome

Synonyms. Salt-deficiency heat exhaustion, heat exhaustion type I.[3]

Definition. Salt-deficiency syndrome is a condition produced by an inadequate salt intake and characterized by an intense lethargy, accompanied to a varying degree by giddiness, anorexia, nausea, vomiting and muscle cramps; in its most severe form, it can lead to complete prostration. As the body's requirement for salt, except that necessary to replace salt losses in the sweat, is negligible, salt-deficiency syndrome is essentially a disease affecting those exposed to extremely hot environments, either natural, as in the tropics and subtropical deserts, or artificial, as in hot industries.

Pathology. The pathogenesis of the condition is simple up to a point. Loss of sodium chloride in the sweat leads to a depletion of the reserves of sodium and chloride in the body with a fall in concentration of these ions in the extracellular fluid. The kidney attempts to preserve normal osmolarity by the excretion of water so that the volume of both compartments of the extracellular fluid, the plasma and interstitial fluid, is diminished. It is probable, however, that the increased plasma protein concentration results in the decrease in plasma volume being proportionately somewhat less than the decrease in interstitial fluid. It is also probable that the persisting hypotonicity of the extracellular fluid results in the transfer of water into the cells with an increase in volume and decrease in tonicity of the intracellular fluid.

The decrease in the volume of the extracellular fluid accounts for the signs of dehydration, and the circulatory insufficiency is plainly the result of the decreased blood volume, but the characteristic lethargy is less easy to explain. As in Addison's disease it is probably the result of sodium deficiency, but potassium loss may contribute, since this can be considerable at high rates of sweating. The cramps are probably due to the deficiency of sodium ions, but the transfer of water into muscle cells referred to may contribute. The cause of the nausea and vomiting remains obscure.

Clinical Characteristics. The onset is gradual, depending on the rate at which the salt stores of the body are depleted, but usually extends at least over a period of some days. The initial complaint is always of apathy, tiredness, and weakness, a state which has been described with great vividness by McCance.[4] Giddiness on standing up suddenly is perhaps the next most common complaint and, in severe cases, it may proceed to syncope. Headache is also frequent, as is nausea which, as the condition worsens, leads to vomiting and a rapid exacerbation of the condition. In the well developed form, muscle cramps are common and may cause intense suffering.

On examination the patient appears anxious and ill and exhibits a varying degree of dehydration which in severe cases may be extreme. He is rational, but listless and resents questioning. The skin is cool to the touch and there may be visible sweating. The body temperature is within the normal range for the time of day and the prevailing environmental temperature. In the recumbent position, although the pulse rate may be a little fast, the blood pressure is generally well maintained. Standing up, however, usually provokes a fall in blood pressure accompanied by a rapid increase in pulse rate. In severe cases, especially those in which the vomiting has been intense or there has been accompanying severe diarrhea from any cause, the patient may present in a state of oligemic shock. Death, however, is rare, and should not occur in a patient who has presented for treatment.

Diagnosis. The cardinal sign is diminished or absent excretion of sodium and chloride in the urine. The Fantus test for urinary chloride is particularly useful for the quick screening of suspected cases of salt depletion.[5] In the presence of suggestive symptoms a value of less than 2.0 gm of sodium chloride per liter of urine is strong presumptive evidence that the patient is suffering from salt deficiency.

Serum sodium and serum chloride are diminished but to a lesser extent than in whole blood. Blood volume is diminished and the hematocrit increased. Plasma protein concentrations are raised and the blood urea is often elevated. The urine volume, at first normal if the patient continues to drink, is diminished in the later stages as anorexia inhibits fluid intake and vomiting increases fluid loss, and the specific gravity is increased.

Treatment. Administration of both water *and* salt is required to restore normal blood volume. In the seriously ill patient, intravenous physiologic saline is indicated, but the usual precautions in its use must be observed.

In the conscious and cooperative patient simpler means will suffice. He should be put to rest in cool surroundings (preferably an air-conditioned room) and given salted fluids to drink. He may be persuaded to drink iced physiologic saline, but this can be nausea-provoking unless very cold. It is better to add salt in a corresponding amount, or less if this concentration is not tolerated, to any fluid which the patient may fancy. Iced salted fruit juice, which has the advantage that it contains considerable quantities of potassium, is usually well accepted. Tomato juice, in particular, will remain palatable even after the addition of large quantities of salt.*

As soon as the patient can take and retain solid food, he should be encouraged, or compelled if necessary, to add additional salt to his meals in copious amounts—up to 10 gm per day. As the usual diet, containing a substantial amount of meat, provides 10 gm of sodium chloride per day, this regimen will secure a total daily intake of about 20 gm. Recovery is then usually rapid and uneventful.

Prophylaxis. The salt content of sweat varies greatly between individuals, but commonly ranges from 0.4 to 6.0 gm per liter. The concentration diminishes with acclimatization so that acclimatized people tend to be at the lower end of the range. The concentration, however, always rises after prolonged heavy sweating. For those engaged in heavy work in hot conditions the rate of sweating can amount to 1 liter (or even more) per hour, although half a liter per hour would be regarded by most people as heavy sweating. In the light of these facts it is apparent that a daily intake of the 10.0 gm of salt contained in the usual diet may be insufficient for those working hard in hot conditions, and in such circumstances a supplementary salt intake may be necessary. In the past salt tablets, because of their convenience, have often been used for this purpose, but they have many disadvantages. They are often taken irregularly or in inadequate dosage, or alternatively they may be consumed needlessly or in excessive amounts; they are seldom taken with an appropriate water intake and, indeed, their consumption may deflect attention from the need to maintain an adequate water intake in the heat. Finally, their rate of disintegration and absorption in the gut is unpredictable and may be greatly delayed.

Acclimatized men and women, e.g. those who live in hot climates or are habitually engaged in hot industries, have usually adjusted their salt intake to their needs and require no supplement to their ordinary daily dietary intake. Unacclimatized men and women, e.g. new arrivals in hot climates, those working in hot industries for the first time or those who return to such conditions after an absence, may need to supplement their dietary salt intake for a period of 7 to 14 days until acclimatization is established. As additional salt is best taken with meals when fluids are also consumed in quantity, this requisite is best met by conscientiously adding extra salt to food both during cooking and during consumption. In the course of time, the need will diminish with acclimatization and a satisfactory dietary pattern will be established as a habit.

However, there are occasions when the taking of sufficient salt with meals may not be possible, as, for example, in conditions of very unusual or very severe heat stress such as prolonged physical exertion at temperatures in excess of 40° C (104° F). In such circumstances the necessary salt intake should

*If available, Gatorade, a medically balanced drink of fluids and salts, may also be used. Salt tablets should not be used.

be secured by adding salt to the drinking water in the proportion of one teaspoon (4 gm) to the gallon. This gives a concentration of approximately 0.1 per cent NaCl. The water should be as cool as possible. Concentrations above 0.1 per cent are distasteful to most people and may provoke nausea, but those with gross salt loss may tolerate or even enjoy concentrations of up to 0.2 per cent if the water is very cold. Salt must *never* be taken if, for any reason, the intake of water is restricted.

Heat Cramps

The salt deficiency syndrome just described and heat cramps have much in common. Both occur in men who have been working and sweating profusely in the heat and both are relieved by the administration of sodium chloride. They differ, however, in that heat cramps occur in those who are apparently otherwise well and their occurrence is associated with the ingestion of salt-free water in large amounts. Furthermore, cramps may occur after work has ceased, and in the case of men working in hot industries in a temperate climate, after a return to cooler surroundings. Acclimatization appears to afford no special protection to susceptible individuals. Actually, heat cramps seem to be largely a matter of individual susceptibility, with some people much more prone than others.

Little has been added to our knowledge of heat cramps since the classic observations of Moss more than 50 years ago.[6] He noted the intensity of the pain, "the lump the size of a cricket ball" in affected abdominal muscles, the association with the drinking of water in large amounts and the "chloride-free" urine. Nor has our knowledge of the pathogenesis of the condition been increased much. It is clear that the loss of "chloride" in the sweat is the cause, but whether this loss produces its effect as a result of the consequent hyponatremia or from the passage of water into the muscle cells as a consequence of the hypotonicity of the extracellular fluid (the water intoxication theory) still remains uncertain. One observation by Moss which has escaped the attention of subsequent authors is that some miners added "cream of tartar" (acid potassium tartrate) to their drinking water as a cramp preventive. This suggests that potassium loss may be involved.

Treatment and Prophylaxis. The ingestion of sodium chloride in adequate amounts gives rapid relief. Prophylaxis should follow the lines already indicated for the taking of supplementary salt. Some workers have made the empirical observation that if they do not drink while working they do not suffer from cramps. This practice is to be discouraged because it leads to inefficiency in the heat-regulating system of the body. Those at risk should be encouraged to consume salted water (0.1 per cent NaCl) freely.

Heat Stroke

Definition. Heat stroke is a grave disease, usually of sudden onset, which occurs when, as a result of exposure to severe heat, there is a failure of the temperature-regulating mechanism of the body. It is characterized by hyperpyrexia (often extreme) and a cessation of sweating. The mortality rate is high and in those who survive there may be permanent and often incapacitating sequelae.[7,8,8a]

Etiology. The basic cause of heat stroke is a failure of the heat-regulating center. It is accompanied by failure of the sweating mechanism, but it remains to be established whether the hyperpyrexia and the resulting pathologic changes ensue as a result of the cessation of sweating, or whether the anhidrosis is only one of the signs of the failure of the heat regulating center; but this is a matter of academic rather than practical interest. Some authorities have described cases of "heat stroke" in which sweating was present, but it is generally agreed that the absence of sweating is mandatory for the diagnosis.

Pathology. Serum sodium is variable depending on the previous sweating history and may be within the normal range. Serum potassium is low at first but may rise later. There is an intense metabolic acidosis, and a rise in serum bilirubin; patients who survive may become jaundiced. The blood urea is elevated. Prothrombin time is prolonged and there is hypofibrinogenemia which is gross in severe cases. The levels of serum glutamic oxaloacetic transaminase, creatinine phosphokinase and lactic dehydrogenase are elevated, indicating widespread tissue damage.

The most characteristic finding at autopsy is widespread hemorrhages of every degree in almost all organs. Diffuse neuronal damage occurs throughout the brain and involves the cortex, the basal ganglia and the brain stem. Strangely, lesions in the region of the hypothalamus have not been described. A constant feature is the extensive damage to Purkinje's cells which are sometimes completely destroyed. The liver shows extensive centrilobular degeneration.

Clinical Characteristics. The onset may be typically sudden. The patient may be said to have fallen as though felled by a blow—hence the term heat *stroke.* Careful questioning will, however, usually reveal that there was at least a brief prodromal period, when the patient exhibited some impairment of intellect or was observed to behave in an irrational way. He may exhibit marked euphoria and exert himself violently despite the prevailing heat. Rarely there may be a prodromal period extending over days during which the patient complains of a variety of symptoms—malaise, dizziness, nausea, abdominal pain and muscular cramps. The duration of the exposure to heat may be quite brief; in severe heat, exposure for less than an hour has proved fatal.

On examination the patient is obviously ill. There is always some defect of consciousness, from mere clouding of the mind with disorientation to deep coma. The skin is hot and dry though the clothing may still contain some sweat. The body temperature is grossly elevated—40 to 44° C (104 to 111° F). The pulse is rapid. The blood pressure is variable, but tends to be low. The respiration rate is raised and the hyperpnea may be extreme. Vomiting and incontinence are usual. Meningismus and convulsions, sometimes with opisthotonos, are constant features. Their severity seems to be related to the height and the duration of the hyperpyrexia. Albumin, casts and red cells are present in the urine.

As the condition of the patient deteriorates a shock-like state may supervene with a falling blood pressure, rapid, thready and irregular pulse and a cold cyanotic skin. Rales may become apparent in the lungs.

Diagnosis. It cannot be assumed that every hyperpyrexial comatose patient is suffering from heat stroke and other causes of hyperpyrexia must be excluded. In the tropics the most likely condition to be confused with heat stroke is cerebral malaria. If there is any doubt, first take adequate blood films for diagnosis, and if the result is not immediately forthcoming, administer antimalarial therapy and at the same time proceed to cool the patient. The administration of antimalarials will not prejudice the outcome if the patient is indeed suffering from heat stroke, nor will effective cooling have a pejorative effect if the hyperpyrexia arises from a cause other than heat stroke.

Treatment. The first and essential requirement is to reduce the body temperature. The patient's chance of survival depends upon the speed with which this is achieved. The individual should be removed or protected from the heat, the clothing should be taken off, and the patient cooled by the best available means. Immersion in iced water accompanied by massage of the extremities to promote venous return is most effective, but in the absence of such facilities any means at hand should be used. Spraying with cold water (or wrapping in a cold, wet sheet) with vigorous fanning to promote evaporation is effective in a dry environment; it is of little use if the air is very humid. In areas where heat stroke is common, a slatted couch fitted with iced-water sprays and a drain should be provided, as it will greatly facilitate the cooling process. The rectal temperature should be constantly monitored and cooling stopped when the temperature falls to 38.5 to 39° C (101.3 to 102.2° F) in order to avoid overcooling as a result of the "after drop." Secondary rises in temperature are to be watched for, and in such cases the cooling should be repeated. No drugs have yet been shown to be specifically effective in the treatment of heat stroke and indeed some, such as atropine, are dangerous. Convulsions must be controlled as they add greatly to the metabolic heat load, and for the same reason any shivering which may accompany cooling must also be avoided. Control is best achieved by direct but slow intravenous injection of diazepam (Valium) up to 10 mg, repeated if necessary. Anxiety and restlessness in the conscious patient may also be controlled by this drug.

Subsequent treatment follows usual intensive-care practice. The metabolic acidosis and any hypokalemia should be corrected as rapidly as possible. A good airway must be maintained. Cyanosis is best combatted by the nasotracheal administration of oxygen; a mask should not be used as this may result in the inhalation of vomitus. The bladder should be catheterized if necessary and the urinary output monitored. Blood volume should be restored, but fluids should be administered with care so as not to overload the circulation as judged by the central venous pressure.

The characteristic hemorrhages of heat stroke are thought to be the result of extensive intravascular coagulation caused by the liberation of tissue thromboplastins as a result of the widespread damage to tissue cells. It is, therefore, recommended that if evidence of bleeding is found, adequate doses of heparin (2 mg per kg intravenously every 6 hours) should be administered.[8]

Prognosis. One attack is believed to predispose to another, and as effective thermoregulation may be slow to re-establish itself, evacuation to a cool climate should be considered. Cerebral, and the usually more obvious cerebellar, damage may be permanent and disabling.

Prophylaxis. The predisposing causes of heat stroke are the same as those of heat exhaustion (p. 653). Adequate acclimatization substantially reduces the risk of heat stroke. Education of the population is desirable and those at special risk should be instructed to watch their fellows for the mental confusion, perhaps accompanied by hyperactivity, which is the commonest warning sign.

Miliaria

In the miliaria group of diseases, of which miliaria rubra (prickly heat) is the best known, the essential lesion is blockage of the sweat pores. If most or all of the sweat pores of a given area of skin become blocked by miliaria, the area becomes devoid of sweat, a condition called anhidrosis (Greek *hidros* = sweat). As extensive areas or even the whole integument may be rendered anhidrotic in this manner, the deleterious effects of the miliarias on heat control are obvious.

Three forms of miliaria exist: miliaria crystallina, miliaria rubra and miliaria profunda.

MILIARIA CRYSTALLINA

Synonym. Sudamina.

The superficial layers of the stratum corneum may inhibit the proper release of sweat on the skin surface under various circumstances, the most common being the post-sunburn state. In this state, the stratum corneum which is about to "peel" acts like a plastic membrane and retains the sweat as innumerable, small, superficial or "crystalline" sweat vesicles.

Severe sunburn may also reduce sweating during its acute, erythematous phase, but in this case the ducts are probably compressed and blocked in the dermis by severe dermal edema. Other diffuse skin diseases such as ichthyosis, diffuse eczema or tinea, exfoliative dermatitis and psoriasis, to name but a few, may also impair sweating by a variety of mechanisms which need not be considered further.

MILIARIA RUBRA AND MILIARIA PROFUNDA

Synonyms. Prickly heat, heat rash and lichen tropicus are synonyms for miliaria rubra.

Definition. Miliaria rubra is an acute inflammatory disorder of the skin associated primarily with blockage of the sweat pores. It is most common in the hot, moist tropics. Following the acute phase, there is a stage of chronic blockage known as miliaria profunda.

Etiology. Many factors are now known to lead to blockage of the sweat pores. In miliaria rubra, the most important are probably maceration of the keratin of the stratum corneum and infection of the pores, especially by staphylococci (Fig. 64–1 *A*). Lipid depletion of the stratum corneum may play an ancillary role.[9-16]

Pathology. The sequence of changes is precipitated by the blockage of the sweat pores. Pressure built up within the ducts by the retention of sweat causes dilatation and finally rupture of the ducts at the level of the stratum malpighii. Vesicles containing sweat are thus produced in the malpighian layer (miliaria rubra) (Fig. 64–1 *B*). Congestion of dermal vessels and leukocytic infiltration occur.

In the course of the next 10 or more days, a keratin (parakeratotic) mass or "plug" arises and comes to fill the vesicular space, bringing about a much deeper obstruction of the sweat duct (Fig. 64–1 *C*). The sweat duct now ruptures a second time to produce another vesicle, but because the obstruction is now deep, this second or "pro-

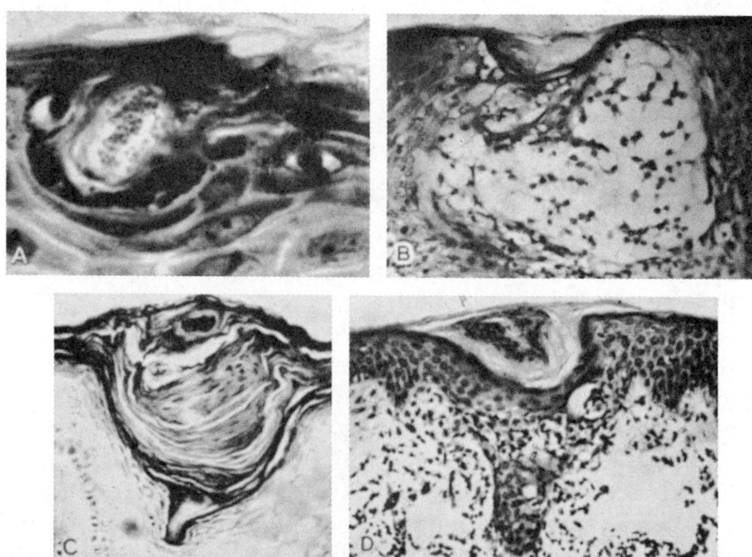

Figure 64–1. Stages in the development of miliaria. *A,* Staphylococci in a pore (the large space slightly to the left of center) from a case of miliaria. This may be the earliest lesion. *B,* Miliaria rubra showing the vesicle in the epidermis. The closed sweat pore is in the surface depression. *C,* At a later stage a large darkly stained parakeratotic plug replaces the vesicular space and causes deep blockage. *D,* Miliaria profunda, the final stage, showing the parakeratotic plug on the surface and large empty spaces in the dermis representing deep extravasation of sweat. (Courtesy of Dr. J. P. O'Brien in (*A*) J. Invest. Dermatol. *15*:105, 1950; (*B* and *D*) Br. J. Dermatol. & Syph. *59*:125, 1947; (*C*) original.)

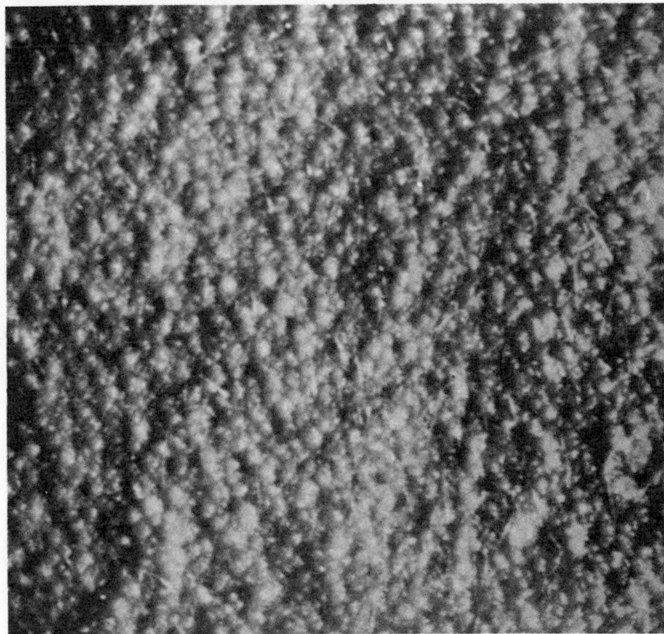

Figure 64–2. An enlarged picture of human skin showing miliaria profunda. Notice the gooseflesh-like appearance. (Courtesy of Drs. G. O. Horne and R. H. Mole. *In* Tr. Roy. Soc. Trop. Med. Hyg., *44*:465–471, 1951.)

funda" vesicle is also deep and lies within the dermis (Fig. 64–1 *D*).

The stage of superficial vesiculation (miliaria rubra) in relation to a single gland is brief but the profunda stage is prolonged, persisting for weeks. Characteristically, lesions in all stages of development coexist. When all the pores of an area of skin are obstructed, the area becomes completely dry (anhidrotic), and the lesions are, for the most part, in the chronic profunda stage.

Clinical Characteristics. The rash of miliaria rubra is largely confined to the clothed areas. It consists of innumerable tiny, superficial, glistening vesicles on a red base and is accompanied by intense itching. The early vesicles are succeeded by red papules and these, in turn, by the deep vesicles of the profunda stage. Profunda vesicles are not red or shiny, not pruritic and resemble closely the white papules of "gooseflesh" (Fig. 64–2). Recurrent episodes of miliaria rubra represent the progressive involvement of more and more gland groups. Various pyodermas (especially furuncles), chronic dermatitis and anhidrotic asthenia are frequent sequelae.

Treatment. A cool environment for all or part of the day is of great benefit. For local treatment of miliaria rubra, chlorhexidine gluconate (Hibitane) is the antibacterial agent of choice. It should be made up in a light cream or oil-containing lotion in the proportion of 0.5 gm to 100 gm of base. Salicylic acid 1.0 gm may be added to assist desquamation. The preparation is applied to the affected areas 3 times a day. If the rash is very diffuse and pustular, the systemic use of erythromycin stearate (infants and children) or tetracycline (adults) may also be considered.

Prophylaxis. The patient should be given general advice about skin care. Clothing should be loose, light and clean; it should also be as scanty as protection from the sun and as other circumstances allow. Infants indoors may wear only a diaper. Heavy continuous sweating should be avoided. If facilities exist, the spending of 8 to 12 hours a day in an air-conditioned atmosphere is helpful. The occasional use of a light lanolin cream or lotion is recommended. Hexachlorophene soap is useful. Routine use of powders is not desirable except in intertriginous areas such as the groin.

Anhidrotic Asthenia

Synonyms. Anhidrotic heat exhaustion, thermogenic anhidrosis, heat exhaustion type II.

Definition. Anhidrotic asthenia is a subacute disorder of temperature regulation caused by the blockage of many of the sweat glands of the body by miliaria rubra and miliaria profunda. It is the most common major heat disorder under military conditions in both the wet and dry tropics, but is less apparent in civilian populations.

Etiology. The sweat glands involved by miliaria remain blocked for some weeks after the acute inflammation subsides. When extensive blockage occurs, physiologic adaptation to heat is disturbed. Other causes of blockage are acute sunburn and diffuse skin diseases, such as exfoliative dermatitis. Persons who have too few sweat glands, a condition called congenital ectodermal dysplasia, suffer the same general symptoms when exposed to heat.

Clinical Characteristics. After severe or recurrent miliaria rubra persisting for some weeks, the general symptoms of anhidrotic asthenia supervene and characteristically take the form of excessive fatigue in response to physical exertion. The patient notices over a period of a week or more that exercise in the heat of the day, especially in sunshine, causes fatigue, frontal headache, giddiness, dyspnea, palpitation and, in severe cases, tremor and syncope. These are essentially the symptoms of classic heat exhaustion lacking only the characteristic heavy sweating usually present in that condition. With rest in the shade the symptoms mostly subside in ½ to 3 hours. In between periods of exercise a sense of well-being is largely restored; however, there may be polyuria. The disease lasts a few weeks, after which the ability to sweat and to undertake exertion may gradually improve.

Diagnosis. Anhidrotic asthenia may be readily diagnosed by the following signs, *provided* the patient is examined after exertion.

1. Relative or complete anhidrosis (absence of sweating) on the trunk and limbs. This is assessed partly by eye, partly by hand.

2. The presence of diffuse miliaria rubra or, more often, miliaria profunda, and the associated anhidrosis are the cardinal signs.[3, 9–14] In desert heat the whole syndrome may come on more acutely while the skin is still at the miliaria rubra stage.

3. *Excessive* sweating, probably compensatory, of the forehead and face.[14] The palms and soles sweat normally. In the desert, the anhidrosis may be more diffuse.[3]

4. Marked tachycardia and tachypnea and a slightly raised temperature—up to 38° C (100.4° F).

5. Features absent in typical cases are hyperpyrexia, dehydration, salt deficiency, cramps, vomiting, coma and immediate danger to life.

Complications. The disease may precipitate a more acute heat disorder, especially heat stroke. This risk is greater in the desert.

Treatment. The patient should avoid exercise and be placed in a cool or air-conditioned environment. Evacuation from the tropics should rarely be necessary. During recovery, exercise tolerance and sweat secretion should be checked regularly.

Inasmuch as the anhidrosis and miliaria profunda are due mainly to keratotic plugging of the pores (Fig. 64–1 *C*), restoration of sweating may be hastened if adequate desquamation can be brought about by repeated applications to the anhidrotic skin of 10 per cent salicylic acid in 70 per cent ethyl alcohol.[16] First paint a small area and discontinue the treatment if there is any untoward local reaction. Also discontinue the treatment if the patient later develops salicylism. Following desquamation inunction of a light lanolin cream or lotion should be made on the treated areas once a day. Desquamation may need to be repeated.

If adequate desquamation cannot be brought about, one must await the natural shedding of the obstructive plugs. This may take some weeks. While ample inunction of lanolin cream may increase sweating (and exercise tolerance) during this period, it is unwise to discharge the patient from supervision until sweating is normal without the use of lanolin.[16]

Prophylaxis. It is important to prevent and treat miliaria rubra and to avoid sunburn.

Hot Climate Neurasthenia

Synonyms. Tropical fatigue, chronic heat neurasthenia, hot climate fatigue, tropical neurasthenia.

In the past this term or one of its variants was frequently used to describe a condition commonly occurring in the tropics in which the sufferer complains of a wide spectrum of symptoms such as loss of appetite, loss of energy, loss of weight (though the patient is often overweight), inability to sleep at night, vague pains of wide distribution including headache and backache, dizziness on standing up, "blackouts" and loss of memory. All of these the patient attributes to the prevailing heat and none is accompanied by convincing physical signs. The condition is commonest in troops serving in the tropics in time of war and in civilians in remote areas devoid of the amenities of civilization. It is least common in those living with their families in well integrated communities leading useful and interesting lives and enjoying a high standard of living. This entity appears to be largely a disease of expatriate Europeans and to be rare among the indigenous people themselves.

There was once a widely held view that continuous exposure of Europeans, or those of European descent, for long periods to a tropical climate resulted in a progressive deterioration in both physical and mental health. It was for this reason that tours of duty in tropical areas were restricted to comparatively short periods and generous home leave granted. Therefore, it is understandable why the syndrome referred to was called hot climate neurasthenia. However, this is no longer the popular diagnosis that it once was. Indeed, many physicians practicing in the tropics would deny that any such disease exists and would hold that the condition described differs in no way from similar conditions seen in temperate climates. This is probably so, but it would appear unwise to assert that climate plays no part in the patient's illness.

Irrespective of the climate in which it is lived, life imposes stresses, mental and emotional as well as physical, many of which relate to deep and intimate personal problems. Nevertheless, most people manage to cope. However, stresses are additive and when the general burden of life is compounded with the constant discomfort of a hot climate, some succumb who in a kinder environment would survive. To this extent the diagnosis is justified.

Confusion arises in attributing the illness solely to the climate. In fact the actual precipitating cause may have been something quite different. Because the weather is respectable and can be talked about (it is an acceptable opening to any polite conversation), the sufferer attributes his illness to the heat and fails to refer to some other and probably more important factor in his illness which is socially less acceptable and which may escape detection by the physician.

Treatment consists in the exclusion of a physical basis for the complaints. Care should be taken not to prolong the investigation unnecessarily. This should be followed by reassurance and psychiatric support on conventional lines.

Living in Hot Climates

Heat illness is in a large measure preventable by the application of a few common sense rules of behavior, with which all those who live or work in a hot environment should be familiar.

Avoid unnecessary exposure to heat stress. Walk in the shade rather than in the sun. Seek the cooling breeze but shelter from hot winds. Relegate the tasks requiring the greatest expenditure of energy to the coolest part of the day. At all costs be careful to avoid potentially dangerous situations such as walking for help during the heat of the day from a broken-down vehicle in the desert.

Within doors clothing should be as scanty as is compatible with modesty or the requirements of social conventions. Out-of-doors the clothing worn should be the minimum required for adequate protection of the body, including protection from hot winds, particularly in desert conditions, and from the heat and light of the sun. Special care should be taken by those with fair complexions to protect themselves from excessive exposure to direct sunlight, since this can result not only in sunburn but in chronic degenerative and neoplastic change in the skin. The skin is particularly vulnerable in tropical climates and must be kept meticulously clean and as dry as possible, and any damage by physical or chemical agents guarded against.

Attention should be given to the diet largely in the direction of the avoidance of overeating, and the body weight should be reduced if it is excessive. Care should be taken at all times to secure an adequate intake of water and salt. In hot climates alcohol has some value as a sedative when taken in small quantities at the end of the day. Excessive consumption of alcohol in the tropics can be disastrous in many ways, not the least of which is its effect on the ability to withstand heat stress.

Housing and working accommodation specifically designed to meet the prevailing climatic conditions, hot-wet or hot-dry as the case may be, is of the utmost importance in mitigating climatic stress. Ancillary aids such as fans and evaporative coolers (in desert climates) are of great value also. Air conditioning, contrary to some opinions, is not the complete answer to heat stress; but wisely used it is a powerful adjunct to health in the tropics.

The risk of heat illness is greatest on first exposure to hot conditions when acclimatization is lacking. Acclimatization will occur with time, but it is a sensible thing to accelerate its acquisition by cautious graduated exposure to exercise in the heat and thereafter to maintain it conscientiously at a high level of effectiveness. Besides the unacclimatized, the very young and the very old are specially vulnerable and for them the precautions advised should be carefully observed.

REFERENCES

1. Macpherson, R. K., Ofner, F., and Welch, J. A. 1967. Effect of the prevailing air temperature on mortality. Br. J. Prev. Soc. Med. *21*:17–21.
2. Ellis, F. P. 1972. Mortality from heat illness and heat-aggravated illness in the United States. Environ. Res. *5*:1–58.
3. Ladell, W. S. S., Waterlow, J. C., and Hudson, M. F. 1944. Desert climate: physiological and clinical observations. Lancet *2*:491–493; 527–531.
4. McCance, R. A. 1936. Medical problems in mineral metabolism. Lancet *1*:823–830.
5. Fantus, B. 1936. Fluid postoperatively: a statistical study. J.A.M.A. *107*:14–17.
6. Moss, K. N. 1923. Some effects of high air temperatures and muscular exertion upon colliers. Proc. R. Soc. Lond. (Biol.), Series B, *95*:181–200.
7. Malamud, N., Haymaker, W., and Custer, R. P. 1946. Heat stroke. A clinico-pathologic study of 125 fatal cases. Mil. Surg. *99*:397–449.
8. Eichler, A. C., McFee, A. S., and Root, H. D. 1969. Heat stroke. Am. J. Surg. *118*:855–863.

8a. Baller, G. A., and Boyd, A. E., III. 1975. Heat stroke: a report of thirteen consecutive cases without mortality despite severe hyperpyrexia and neurologic dysfunction. Mil. Med. *140*:464–467.

9. O'Brien, J. P. 1950. The etiology of poral closure: an experimental study of miliaria rubra, bullous impetigo and related diseases of the skin. J. Invest. Dermatol. *15*:95–156.
10. Leeming, J. A. L. 1972. Miliaria. *In* Marshall, J. (ed.): Essays in Tropical Dermatology. Vol. 2. Excerpta Medica, Amsterdam. pp. 169–182.
11. Shelley, W. B. 1974. Miliaria. *In* Consultations in Dermatology. Vol. 2. W. B. Saunders Co., Philadelphia. pp. 288–294.

12. Leithead, C. S., and Lind, A. R. 1964. Heat Stress and Heat Disorders. Cassell & Co., London. 253 pp.
13. Sulzberger, M. B., and Herrmann, F. 1954. The Clinical Significance of Disturbances in the Delivery of Sweat. Charles C Thomas, Springfield, Illinois. 212 pp.
14. Allen, S. D., and O'Brien, J. P. 1944. Tropical anhidrotic asthenia. Med. J. Aust. *2*:335–337.
15. Sargent, F., II, and Johnson, R. E. 1960. Observations on experimental anhidrosis. Lancet *1*:1018–1021.
16. O'Brien, J. P. 1947. A study of miliaria rubra, tropical anhidrosis and anhidrotic asthenia. Br. J. Dermatol. *59*:125–158.

CHAPTER 65
Tropical Ulcer

JOHN P. O'BRIEN

Tropical Ulcer

Synonyms. Ulcus tropicum, Naga sore, tropical sloughing phagedena.

Definition. This is a chronic, often progressive, sloughing ulcer, usually occurring on the lower extremities. It may extend deeply, with destruction of underlying muscles, tendons, periosteum and bone. Numerous spirochetes and fusiform bacilli as well as other bacteria are generally present in the lesions.[1]

Distribution. Tropical ulcer is widespread throughout the tropical areas of the world and is particularly prevalent in the wet tropics.

Etiology. Tropical ulcer is a clinical entity of uncertain etiology. Spirochetes and fusiform bacilli are often present in the developing lesion. It is improbable that they penetrate the unbroken skin. The ulcer commonly develops at the site of an injury or abrasion.

Both the spirochetes and the fusiform bacilli are obligate anaerobes which can be cultivated on artificial media. The spirochetes, which are morphologically identical with *Borrelia vincentii* (Blanchard) Bergey et al. 1925, are slender and delicate and present a variable number of shallow irregular turns. *Fusobacterium fusiforme* (Veillon and Zuber) Hoffman 1957 is a coarse, plump, banded or beaded gram-negative rod with tapered ends. Other bacteria present may include staphylococci, streptococci and various gram-negative organisms.

Recent studies indicate that malnutrition, especially deficiency of protein and vitamins, may be important in the etiology of tropical ulcer.

Pathology. The pathologic change in tropical ulcer is essentially a necrosis of the skin and subcutaneous tissues in which many microorganisms are demonstrable. The process tends to extend by continuity to adjacent structures. The walls and base are composed of infected indolent granulation tissue, in chronic cases bounded by dense fibrous scar tissue. Squamous cell carcinoma can occur as a rare complication.

Clinical Characteristics. Tropical ulcer occasionally develops in the absence of visible abrasion of the skin. In such instances it is preceded by vesicle formation, or it may appear first as an inflamed papule which breaks down to produce a rapidly extending phagedenic ulcer (Fig. 65–1).

Pain, fever, toxemia and marked disability are characteristic. In most instances, the ulcer enlarges rapidly and may reach a diameter of 5 to 10 cm. The base of the ulcer is composed of necrotic tissue and unhealthy granulations. The edge is not greatly indurated or raised but may be undermined.

Diagnosis. Laboratory examination is desirable to exclude cutaneous diphtheria (p. 244), cutaneous leishmaniasis (p. 423) and other specific ulcerations, such as those caused by *Mycobacterium ulcerans*[2] and blood dyscrasias.

Treatment. General measures, particularly complete bed rest and a balanced diet, are important. Specific treatment falls into two phases: (1) the control of infection and (2) the subsequent promotion of healing.

For the control of infection large intramuscular doses of penicillin combined with local cleansing and mild antiseptic dressings such as a 1:1000 aqueous solution of acriflavine should be used. Topical penicillin is not recommended. As an alternative to penicillin, one may give oral tetracycline (two capsules of 250 mg every 6 hours between meals for 7 days).

After gross infection has been controlled, the ulcer should be covered with soft

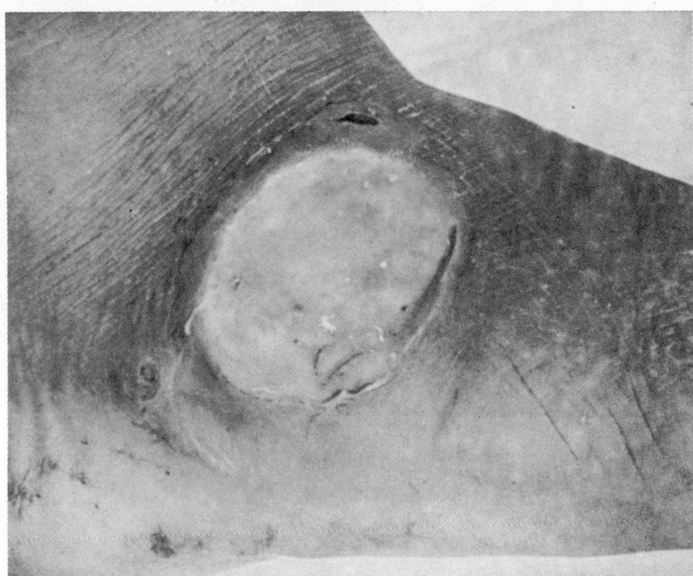

Figure 65–1. Tropical ulcer. (Courtesy of Dr. Hardy A. Kemp, Veterans Administration.)

paraffin gauze and the limb immobilized by a light plaster of Paris cast or, less effectively, by adhesive tape. Skin grafting is of great value and should be combined with immobilization.

Prophylaxis. Prevention involves cleanliness of the skin, adequate protection from minor injuries, and prompt treatment of all trauma, such as scratches, small abrasions or insect bites. An adequate diet is essential.

REFERENCES

1. Basset, A. 1969. Tropical phagedenic ulcer. *In* Simons, R. D. G. Ph., and Marshall, J. (eds.): Essays on Tropical Dermatology. Vol. I. Excerpta Medica, Amsterdam. pp. 25–33.
2. Quinn, J. V., and Crotty, J. M. 1963. *Mycobacterium ulcerans* infections in the Northern Territory. Med. J. Aust. *2*:317–319.
3. Jopling, W. H. 1968. Treatment of Tropical Diseases. 2nd ed. John Wright & Sons, Bristol. p. 136.

SECTION X

Medically Important Animals

CHAPTER 66

Medically Important Mollusks

EMILE A. MALEK

INTRODUCTION

Certain mollusks have become of increasing medical importance because of the direct or indirect injury that they are capable of inflicting, or because of their role as intermediate hosts of helminthic parasites of man or animals. In the great majority of instances the medically important members of this phylum are restricted to the freshwater snails. The exceptions include: the fatally venomous cone shells of the Indo-Pacific; certain squids and octopuses that may inflict a poisonous bite; the marine blue mussels that have been a source of *Gonyaulax* food poisoning (Table 20–2, p. 180); the freshwater clams that serve as second intermediate hosts of *Echinostoma* (p. 578); marine snail hosts of dermatitis-producing cercariae; certain species of land snails that serve as first intermediate hosts of the fluke *Dicrocoelium*, a common parasite of the biliary tract of mammals (p. 585); and other species of land snails and slugs that are intermediate hosts of the zoonotic nematodes *Angiostrongylus* spp., parasites of rats, other rodents and dogs (p. 538).

ROLE OF MOLLUSKS AS DIRECT AGENTS OF HUMAN DISEASE

Five species of the marine cone shells are known to inflict a venomous sting that, in some cases, proves fatal to man within 4 hours. Venomous specimens are known only from the coral reefs of the Indian and Pacific oceans. The venom is injected through a puncture made in the victim's skin by a half-inch long, needlelike, hollow tooth. Care should be exercised in handling live specimens over 2 inches in length. The cones are heavy shells with a long, narrow aperture, usually of attractive coloration, and covered with a thin or thick, horny periostracum (Fig. 66–4).

Octopuses must be large to be dangerous, and such specimens are very infrequently encountered in shallow water. The secretion from the salivary gland of most octopuses is a proteolytic ferment, and the bite of the creature can cause considerable pain and local swelling.

Blue mussels and certain other bivalves found along the open coast, especially the West Coast of North America, are likely to cause paralytic poisoning if eaten during the summer months. A number of human deaths have been reported from this source, which is due to bivalves that have ingested certain planktonic organisms *(Gonyaulax)*. The toxin is water soluble and is not destroyed by boiling. Mollusks can also acquire other pathogenic organisms and transmit them to man when ingested. An outbreak of cholera in Naples, Italy in the summer of 1973 was attributed to eating mussels and other bivalves from the Bay of Naples in the Mediterranean.

Table 66–1. SOME IMPORTANT HUMAN DISEASES CARRIED BY MOLLUSKS

Disease	*Etiologic Agent*	*Important First Intermediate Snail Hosts*	*Geographic Range of Mollusk*	*Molluscan Family**	*Second Intermediate Host*
Schistosomiasis haematobia	*Schistosoma haematobium*	*Bulinus (Bulinus) truncatus*	North Africa, Southwestern Asia, Portugal	Planorbidae	None
		Planorbarius metidgensis	Portugal		
		Bulinus (Physopsis) africanus	Central, East and South Africa		
		B. (Ph.) globosus			
		B. (B.) truncatus rohlfsi	West Africa		
		B. (B.) guernei			
		B. (B.) senegalensis			
		B. (Ph.) jousseaumei			
		Ferrissia sp.	India	Ancylidae	
Schistosomiasis mansoni	*Schistosoma mansoni*	*Biomphalaria alexandrina*	Egypt	Planorbidae	None
		B. ruppellii	Southwestern Asia		
		B. ruppellii	Central and South Africa[3]		
		B. sudanica			
		B. bridouxiana			
		B. pfeifferi			
		B. pfeifferi gaudi	West Africa		
		B. glabrata	West Indies, Brazil, Venezuela, Surinam		
		B. straminea (=*centimetralis*)	Brazil, Venezuela		
		B. tenagophila	Brazil		
Schistosomiasis japonica	*Schistosoma japonicum*	*Oncomelania quadrasi*	Philippine Islands	Hydrobiidae	None
		Oncomelania formosana	Taiwan		
		Oncomelania nosophora	Japan and China		
		Oncomelania hupensis	China		
		Oncomelania lindoensis	Celebes (Indonesia)		
		Pomatiopsis lapidaria	U.S.A. (experimental)		
	Schistosoma japonicum–like schistosome	*Lithoglyphopsis aperta*	Laos		
		?	Thailand, Cambodia		
Schistosomiasis intercalatum	*Schistosoma intercalatum*	*Bulinus (B.) forskalii*	Gabon, United Republic of Cameroon, Central African Republic	Planorbidae	None

Fasciolopsiasis	*Fasciolopsis buski*	*Segmentina hemisphaerula*	Eastern Asia	Planorbidae	Encysts on water plants
		Hippeutis cantori	Eastern Asia		
		Gyraulus convexiusculus			
		Segmentina trochoides	Eastern Asia		
Hetrophyiasis	*Heterophyes heterophyes*	*Pirenella conica*	Egypt	Potamididae	Mullet and Nile bolti fishes
		Cerithidea cingulata alata	Japan		Mullet
Metagonimiasis	*Metagonimus yokogawai*	*Semisulcospira libertina*	North China; Japan	Pleuroceridae	Salmonoid, cyprinoid fishes
		Thiara granifera	S. E. Asia to Hawaii	Thiaridae	
Echinostomiasis	*Echinostoma ilocanum*	*Gyraulus convexiusculus*	Philippines, Java	Planorbidae	*Pila conica, Viviparus javanicus*
		Hippeutis umbilicalis	Philippines	Planorbidae	*Pila conica*
		G. prashadi	India	Planorbidae	*Pila conica*
	Echinochasmus perfoliatus	*Parafossarulus* sp.	Japan	Hydrobiidae	Fish
	Echinostoma lindoensis	*Gyraulus convexiusculus*	Indonesia	Planorbidae	*Corbicula lindoensis, C. subplanta*
Clonorchiasis	*Clonorchis sinensis*	*Hua ningpoensis*	China	Pleuroceridae	Freshwater cyprinoid fishes
		Bulimus fuchsianus	China	Hydrobiidae	
		Alocinma longicornis	China and India	Hydrobiidae	
		Parafossarulus manchouricus	China and Japan	Hydrobiidae	
Opisthorchiasis	*Opisthorchis felineus*	*Bulimus (Bithynia) leachii*	Northern Europe	Hydrobiidae	Cyprinoid fishes
Fascioliasis	*Fasciola hepatica*	Several species of *Lymnaea*	Worldwide	Lymnaeidae	Encysts on grass and herbs
Paragonimiasis	*Paragonimus westermani*	*Semisulcospira libertina*	North China; Japan	Pleuroceridae	Freshwater crabs and crayfish
		Semisulcospira amurensis	North China; Korea		
		Thiara granifera	Taiwan to Hawaii	Thiaridae	
		Hua toucheana		Pleuroceridae	
	Paragonimus africanus	*Potadoma freethii*	United Republic of Cameroon	Thiaridae	Freshwater crabs
	Paragonimus uterobilateralis	?	Nigeria		Freshwater crabs(?)
	Paragonimus spp.	*Brotia costula*	Malaysia	Thiaridae	Freshwater crabs
		B. asperata	Philippines	Thiaridae	
		Oncomelania nosophora	Japan	Hydrobiidae	
		Assiminea (=*Syncera*) spp.	China	Assimineidae (=Synceridae)	
		Tricula sp.	China	Hydrobiidae	
		Aroapyrgus spp.	Central and South America	Hydrobiidae	

*Of first intermediate snail host.

ROLE OF MOLLUSKS AS CARRIERS OF DISEASE

All species of trematodes parasitic to man have gastropod snails as obligatory intermediate hosts. The various species of trematodes have each become adapted to a single, or at most a few, species of snails. However, penetration by the trematode miracidia takes place in both susceptible and nonsusceptible snail hosts. In a susceptible snail host the development is completed to the cercarial stage; in a nonsusceptible host the miracidium may begin development but later is walled off and dies as a result of an intense snail tissue reaction due to innate resistance. Immune reactions which may be attributed to cellular or humoral acquired resistance by infection or those acquired by injections have been observed in a few cases among invertebrate organisms. The presence of a schistosomal miracidial immobilizing substance in tissue extracts of the snail *Biomphalaria glabrata,* subsequent to infection with *Schistosoma mansoni,* has been demonstrated. Spontaneous miracidial immobilization may also occur in the presence of extracts from noninfected snails and even in water, but differences occur in the degree of immobilization between these and extracts from infected snails. Acquired humoral reaction, for example by antibody production, has yet to be demonstrated unequivocally in mollusks. In fact, the current belief is that the synthesis of antibodies or antibody-like molecules does not occur in the phylum MOLLUSCA.

The most important human diseases carried by mollusks are listed in Table 66–1, and the mollusks are illustrated in Figures 66–1 through 66–6.

Snail Control. Trematode infections may be controlled by breaking the life cycle at one or more points: at the egg-miracidial and cercarial stages by preventing human and animal excreta from reaching man's supply of water; by protection of the population against contact with cercariae; by abstaining from eating food that harbors viable encysted metacercariae; by controlling the snail intermediate host; and by chemotherapeutic measures that kill the adult worms in the definitive host.

The custom of eating certain foods and polluting bathing or drinking water may be a part of the culture and consequently very difficult to change. In the absence of effective and satisfactory therapeutic drugs, snail control appears to be the most practical measure at present.

The approaches to snail control are environmental, chemical and biological. Environmental measures disturb the habitat of the snail hosts. Examples of such control measures include the clearance of mud and vegetation, drying canals that usually harbor the aquatic snails, the installation of proper drainage by filling lowlands, lining canals with concrete and changing the agricultural methods and practices of the people. The use of predators, parasites and competitors has been advocated for the biologic control of the medically important snails. The voracious ampullarid snail *Marisa cornuarietis* has been used in small test areas in Puerto Rico as a biologic control for *Biomphalaria glabrata.* It competes with this snail for food and engulfs the *B. glabrata* eggs and young snails on vegetation. Species of the American genus *Helisoma* have also been found to compete with *B. glabrata.*[1] The use of these biologic methods may be feasible only in certain snail habitats such as small ponds.

Certain chemicals having a molluscicidal activity are available in quantities and are actually in use in control operations in some endemic areas.[2, 3] These compounds are copper sulfate, sodium pentachlorophenate or Santobrite (NaPCP), copper pentachlorophenate, niclosamide (Bayer 73 or Bayluscide), Frescon (WL 8008) and Yurimin. Copper sulfate is used primarily in Egypt, the Sudan and Rhodesia. Its efficacy is reduced considerably in the presence of organic and inorganic compounds in the water; consequently, in field operations it is applied at 30 ppm in order to secure more satisfactory results. Some organo-copper compounds have been developed and proved promising as molluscicides that do not portray the undesirable characteristics of copper sulfate.

Sodium pentachlorophenate applied at a concentration of 10 ppm for 8 hours kills both aquatic and amphibious snails and their eggs but is easily affected by sunlight or by water with a low hydrogen ion concentration. Copper pentachlorophenate is obtainable by mixing solutions of copper sulfate and NaPCP at a ratio of 1:2 and is effective also against both aquatic and amphibious snails.

Bayluscide (5-chlorosalicylic acid [2-chloro-4-nitroanilide]) is produced by Bayer Company, Germany; it is ovicidal and of low toxicity to mammals and has the advantage of not being markedly affected by physical and chemical factors in the snail habitat. Its activity exceeds that of other available molluscicides. The wettable powder, however, is not a satisfactory formulation because it has to be continually stirred when admixed with water, and nozzles of dispensing equipment become clogged by the sediment. An emulsifiable concentrate (25 per cent active ingredient) has been formulated and has overcome the difficulty in applying the wettable powder formulation.

The molluscicide dinitro-o-cyclohexylphenol also has been used in certain areas, while ICI 24223 (isobutyl-triphenylmethylamine), and the herbicides Aqualin and Sevin, have also been tested in experimental plots.

Frescon (WL 8008) is produced by the Shell Company in England. It is *N*-triphenylmethylmorpholine (*N*-tritylmorpholine). A liquid formulation in tetrachloroethylene provides good performance and is easily handled in the field. It is stable to heat, sunlight and alkalis. It has proved effective against the freshwater and amphibious snail hosts of the schistosomes in Africa, the Americas and the Orient, and against the amphibious snail hosts of fascioliasis in Europe. Yurimin (P-99) (3, 5-dibromo-4′-hydroxy-4′-nitrobenzene) is a Japanese product that proved effective against *Oncomelania nosophora,* the snail host of *Schistosoma japonicum.* The compound is more effective in alkaline than in acid water, is not affected by photochemical action, and its lethal concentration to snails is a little higher for fish.

Molluscicides may be applied as solids in jute bags or wire-mesh containers, or in liquid form by compression sprayers or by dripping from special containers.

Control by chemical molluscicides is satisfactory in certain areas but has failed elsewhere. Such failures may be attributed to differences in the methods of application, the strain of snail, the chemical composition of the water, or the hydrography of the areas treated.

Among the drawbacks of the currently available molluscicides are their cost, especially when periodic reapplications are necessary, their lack of residual effect and the piscicidal action of some of them in areas where fish constitute the chief source of animal protein. Better results may be obtained when molluscicides are applied in combination with concreting irrigation ditches (where feasible), clearance of mud and vegetation, or other environmental means of control.[2, 3]

STRUCTURE, CLASSIFICATION AND BIOLOGY OF MEDICALLY IMPORTANT MOLLUSKS

Field surveys and control operations directed against snails of medical importance require accurate identification of the various species of mollusks that may be encountered. This is frequently difficult. Although several important species of molluscan intermediate hosts are easily identified, there are many medically unimportant species possessing shells which superficially resemble those of species that carry pathogenic parasites. In addition, there are several major subfamilies, genera and species, the systematics and nomenclature of which are still unsettled. The systematics of these snails has been based mainly on shell characteristics, which of themselves exhibit individual variations due to several factors, one of which is the water in their habitat. Consequently, many invalid

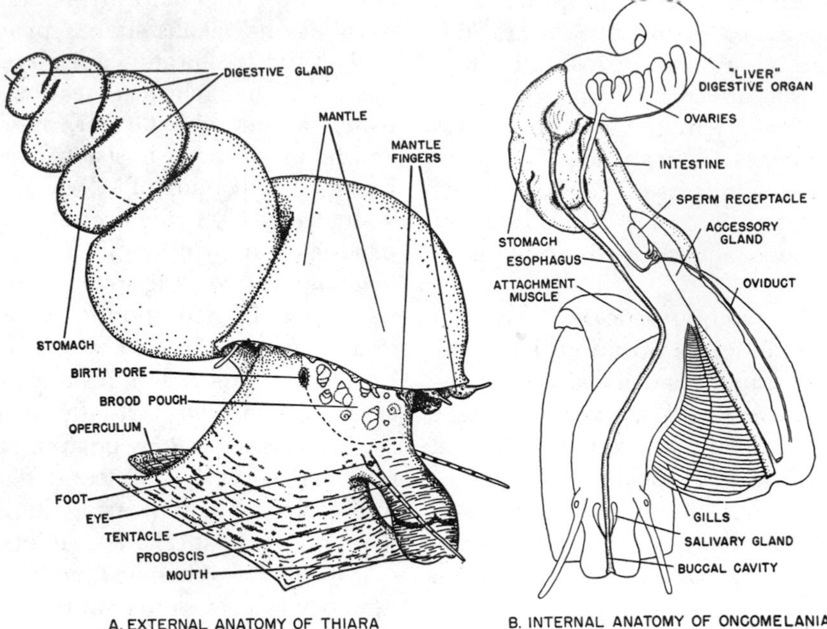

Figure 66–1. Gross anatomy of the prosobranch snail. *A, Thiara granifera* (left) is the Oriental host of *Paragonimus; B, Oncomelania quadrasi* (right) is the Philippine host of *Schistosoma japonicum.* (Redrawn from Abbott.)

species have been created; it is the nomenclature of these lower taxa that is in a state of confusion. Today the morphology of the snail is also used in determining species. Utilized in making identification among the prosobranch snails are such features as: the shape of the tentacles, copulatory organ, other reproductive organs; the verge; the number of gill branches or lamellae; and the number and shape of the radular teeth (Figs. 66–1*A* and *B*, 66–2, 66–3).[4] In the pulmonate snails the shape of the tentacles, the presence or absence of a renal ridge, the structure of the hermaphroditic reproductive organs (especially the copulatory organ, the vagina, the prostate, the spermathecal sac and duct), and the number and shape of the radular teeth all play a role of speciation.[5]

Other complications include the possibility of hybridization occurring among some snail hosts which results in the production of intermediates. Further confusion arises from the existence of different host-specific strains in the medically important species which vary not only in their susceptibility to infection with the same strain of the trematode but also in their response to molluscicides. More recently, paper chromatography and electrophoresis have been employed as additional aids in the determination of species. Serologic techniques have also been used to compare the precipitating activity of the various hemolymph antigens in the presence of specific snail "antisera." Genera and some congeneric species have been differentiated by gel diffusion methods.[6]

The phylum MOLLUSCA consists of six classes:

1. GASTROPODA: snails, slugs, whelks, conchs and others.

2. PELECYPODA [LAMELLIBRANCHIA]: clams, mussels, oysters.

3. CEPHALOPODA: squids, octopuses.

4. SCAPHOPODA: dentaliums and other tusk shells.

5. AMPHINEURA [LORICATA]: chitons, or coat-of-mail shells.

6. MONOPLACOPHORA: represented by the primitive living *Neopilina,* and several fossil forms.

All of these possess a fleshy mantle

which generally secretes a calcareous shell. The buccal mass, except in the PELECYPODA, contains a radular ribbon of hard denticulate teeth.

Mollusks are either bisexual, hermaphroditic or capable of changing sex one or more times during their life span. The eggs may be shed freely into the water, laid in capsules or brooded within the parent.

Class Gastropoda

SUBCLASS PROSOBRANCHIATA

The subclass PROSOBRANCHIATA [STREPTONEURA] are the operculate snails, which possess a horny or calcareous *operculum* that is usually attached on the upper hind surface of the foot. The visceral nerve loop is crossed, forming a figure 8, and most have lamellate gills attached to the inside of the mantle. The majority are bisexual, but a few are hermaphroditic, parthenogenetic or capable of changing sex. This subclass is generally divided into three orders, two of which are of medical importance:

1. MESOGASTROPODA [PECTINIBRANCHIATA]: This subclass contains the majority of the medically important freshwater snails. They are characterized by comblike gills which are attached to the mantle along their entire length.

2. NEOGASTROPODA: marine snails, including the venomous cone shells. They are characterized by one to three transverse rows of strong radular teeth.

ORDER MESOGASTROPODA

Family Hydrobiidae. The family HYDROBIIDAE [AMNICOLIDAE, BITHYNIIDAE] comprises two subfamilies, the HYDROBIINAE (Fig. 66–2) and the BULIMINAE. These are of considerable medical importance, since the former contains the only known intermediate hosts of *Schistosoma japonicum* and the latter the majority of the first intermediate hosts of the biliary flukes *Clonorchis* (p. 579) and *Opisthorchis* (p. 582).

The members of this family are small, aquatic or amphibious gastropods with slender or subspherical shells that rarely exceed a length of 10 mm. The sexes are separate. The males possess an external copulatory organ, known as the *verge* (=penis), attached to the right side of the body and appearing as a single or multipronged finger. The mantle edge is smooth. The operculum is either horny or calcareous. Eggs are laid singly in gelatinous packets and may be covered with mud or tiny pebbles.

SUBFAMILY HYDROBIINAE. Members of the subfamily HYDROBIINAE are characterized by: (1) thin, horny and paucispiral opercula; (2) males having a fleshy verge which may be frilled along its edge.

Genus Oncomelania Gredler. This is one of two genera known to serve as intermediate hosts of *Schistosoma japonicum* (Fig. 66–2). It comprises five species in all of which the

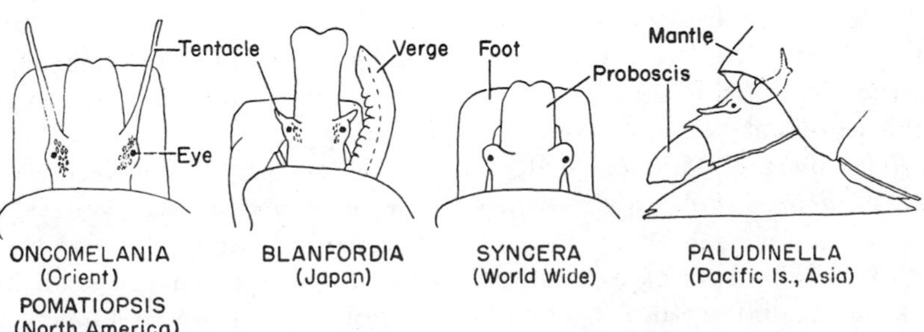

Figure 66–2. Anatomy of small, brown hydrobiid snails with a horny operculum. *Oncomelania* and *Pomatiopsis* are hosts of Oriental schistosomiasis; the other genera are not carriers. (Redrawn from Abbott.)

outer lip of the aperture is strengthened by a *varix* or thickening of the rim. The verge is a simple prong. The most characteristic feature is a streak of small, yellowish granules over each eye, forming a false "eyebrow." The five species are:

1. *Oncomelania hupensis* Gredler.

SYNONYMS. *Oncomelania schmackeri* Moellendorff, *longiscata* Heude, *elongata* Bartsch, *yaoi* Bartsch, *multicosta* Bartsch and *anhuinensis* Li.

DISTRIBUTION. This species is common in the canals in the Yangtze River basin in the provinces of Kiangsu, Chekiang, Anhwei, Kiangsi and Hupeh. It is the principal host of *Schistosoma japonicum* in China (Fig. 66–4).

The adults are gray-brown to waxy yellow in color. They are 7 to 10 mm in length and have six to nine whorls. Each whorl has 10 to 30 small axial ribs, and nuclear whorls may be tinged with rose.

All oncomelanids are regarded by some malacologists as subspecies of *O. hupensis.*

2. *Oncomelania nosophora* Robson.

DISTRIBUTION. It is common in or along small creeks, irrigation ditches, rice paddies or unflooded river bottoms in China, south of the Yangtze, and on Honshu and Kyushu islands, Japan. It is the only known host of *S. japonicum* in Japan.

The adults are dark to light chestnut brown. They measure 5 to 12 mm in length, are smooth, and have six to nine whorls.

3. *Oncomelania formosana* Pilsbry and Hirase.

DISTRIBUTION. This species is common in rice paddies and irrigation ditches in the western half of Taiwan. It is the only host of *S. japonicum* in Taiwan.

The adults are light chestnut brown in color, relatively smooth and 4 to 6 mm long. The length of the last whorl is always greater than that of the whorls above.

4. *Oncomelania quadrasi* Moellendorff.

SYNONYM. *Oncomelania hydrobiopsis* Rensch.

DISTRIBUTION. This species is common in small creeks and among the vegetation above the waterline of slow flowing streams in eastern Leyte, eastern Mindoro, Mindanao, Samar and Sorsogon Province, Luzon Island, Philippines. It is the only known intermediate host of *S. japonicum* in these islands.

The adults are translucent chocolate-brown, sometimes covered with a thin, black, encrusting slime, relatively smooth and 3 to 5 mm in length. The last whorl is always longer than those in the spine. *Oncomelania quadrasi* resembles and may be confused with *Syncera.*

5. *Oncomelania lindoensis* Davis and Carney.

DISTRIBUTION. This species is common in uncultivated areas surrounded by actively worked rice fields in the Paku area of Lake Lindu, Sulawesi (Celebes), Indonesia. The habitat is submerged periodically by irrigation and frequent rains. It is the snail host of *S. japonicum* in this area of Indonesia.

Genus Lithoglyphopsis Thiele. "The rock-loving snail." Species of this genus occur in China and Southeast Asia. *Lithoglyphopsis modesta* is in China, but another species, *L. aperta,* has only recently become recognized to be of medical importance in Southeast Asia. A strain of *S. japonicum* in Laos and Cambodia utilizes *L. aperta* as intermediate host. The snail was found naturally infected with *S. japonicum* in Khong Island, Laos (on the Mekong River), and the snail is also a good laboratory host for this strain. This strain of *S. japonicum* does not infect any known species of *Oncomelania.*

Lithoglyphopsis aperta is a small hydrobiid snail, 3 to 4 mm in height, with a light brown or white glossy shell. The aperture is pear-shaped, the body whorl is broad and large and is much higher than the spire. On Khong Island the snail is found attached to submerged rocks, twigs, leaves and other solid objects, but the snail is not found on the sandy shores of the north end of the island.

A recently discovered autochthonous case of *S. japonicum* in Malaysia has not been investigated further as to extent of the disease in the area or the snail host. The snail host of *S. japonicum* in Thailand is not known with certainty, but is probably also a hydrobiid.

Genus Blanfordia. Members of this genus are restricted to the Japanese islands. Despite their close resemblance to *Oncomelania,* they have never been implicated as carriers of schistosomiasis. There are four species, of which *B. simplex* Pilsbry from Honshu is the commonest. The shells are not so slender as those of *Oncomelania* species. The verge is a simple prong with strong serrations on the inner concave edge. There are yellow color granules close to the eyes. The eye peduncles are well developed, with a short, stubby, triangular tentacle projecting forward. The gill lamellae are only 10 to 12 in number.[7] Two other genera, *Tricula* and *Fukuia,* also resemble *Oncomelania* closely but do not serve as intermediate hosts for *S. japonicum.*[8]

Genus Pomatiopsis. This is an American genus with shells and animals that closely resemble those of *Oncomelania.*

DISTRIBUTION. This genus is found in woodland swamps and on low river banks in the United States from Minnesota east to New York, south to Alabama, Louisiana and Texas, and on the Atlantic seaboard from Pennsylvania south to Georgia.

There are ten described species. The commonest, *Pomatiopsis lapidaria* Say, has been shown to be the natural host of *Paragonimus kellicotti,* the North American lung fluke of animals, and it is an experimental intermediate host of *Schistosoma japonicum; P. cincinnatiensis* has also been shown to be a host for *Paragonimus kellicotti.*

Genus Fukuia. Two species are known in this Japanese genus, which is not of medical importance. The shells resemble those of *Oncomelania* but are more ovate, much thicker, glossy, reddish brown and without a thickened outer lip. The spiral sculpturing consists of numerous microscopic, incised lines.[8]

The verge is a single prong bearing a rather large buttonlike gland on the upper side. The tentacles are very short. Yellow granules are present behind the eyes.

Genus Aroapyrgus. Several species of this small hydrobiid mollusk are known from Central and South America, where they occur in narrow and shallow streams. The shell is smooth, translucent and averages 3 mm in height. The verge is large and simple (devoid of any papillae and unbranched). The females are ovoviviparous. Species of *Aroapyrgus,* for example *A. colombiensis* and *A. costaricensis,* are known to serve as the first intermediate hosts of lung flukes of animals, *Paragonimus* spp. in Central and South America,[9] and probably also of human lung flukes in the same geographic area.

SUBFAMILY BULIMINAE. The subfamily BULIMINAE contains the majority of the first intermediate hosts of the human biliary flukes *Clonorchis* (p. 579) and *Opisthorchis* (Fig. 66–3 and p. 582). The following genera, sometimes treated as subgenera of the genus *Bulimus* (formerly *Bithynia*), are all of medical importance.

1. *Bulimus* (north temperate regions).
2. *Alocinma* (India and China).
3. *Parafossarulus* (eastern Asia).

Members of this subfamily are characterized by: (1) a thick calcareous operculum; (2) a verge with a lateral fingerlike appendage; (3) a small, cup-shaped skin flap attached to the right side of the head just behind the right tentacle. The genera are distinguished by shell characteristics.

Genus Bulimus. 1. *Bulimus fuchsianus* (Moellendorff).

DISTRIBUTION. This species is especially common in southern China, where it serves as the principal snail host of *Clonorchis sinensis* (Fig. 66–3 and p. 579).

The adult shell is greenish brown and about 10 mm long. It is rather fragile and smooth, with a dull finish and fragile outer lip. The whorls are well rounded.

2. *Bulimus misellus* (Gredler). This is a common, medically unimportant Asiatic species (Fig. 66–3).

The adult shell is 5 to 7 mm in length with five well rounded whorls. It is distinguished from *B. fuchsianus* by its smaller, more slender shell.

3. *Bulimus (=Bithynia) leachii* (Linn.)

DISTRIBUTION. This is a common species in north European lakes and ponds and has become established in the north central and northeastern United States. It is one of the principal snail hosts of the liver fluke *Opisthorchis felineus* (p. 582).

The shell is yellowish, greenish or

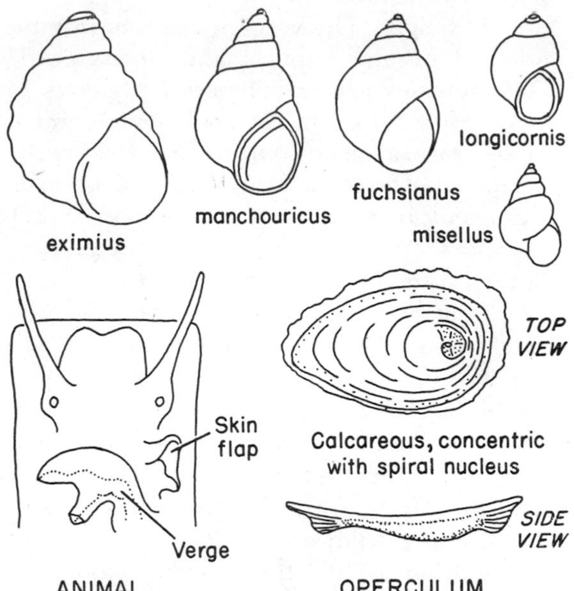

Figure 66–3. The bulimoid snails of the Orient serve as the main hosts of *Clonorchis* and *Opisthorchis.* (Redrawn from Abbott.)

brownish and 5 to 11 mm long. The operculum is calcareous.

Genus Alocinma. 1. *Alocinma longicornis* Benson.

DISTRIBUTION. This snail is common in canals and ponds in China, where it serves as one of the intermediate hosts of *Clonorchis sinensis* (Fig. 66–3 and p. 579).

The adult shell is 5 to 8 mm in length, smooth and globular, with a short blunt apex.

Genus Parafossarulus. 1. *Parafossarulus manchouricus* (Bourguignat).

SYNONYM. *Bithynia striatula* Benson.

DISTRIBUTION. This species is common in ponds in China, Taiwan, Korea and Japan (Fig. 66–3). It is the principal intermediate host of *Clonorchis sinensis* in Japan and the second most important in China. It likewise carries *Opisthorchis felineus* and *Echinochasmus perfoliatus* (p. 582).

The adult shell is yellowish to greenish brown and 7 to 10 mm long. There are spiral raised ridges of varying strength on the whorls. The calcareous operculum is not withdrawn into the shell.

2. *Parafossarulus eximius* (Frauenfeld). This largest of all Chinese bulimoid snails is common in lakes and ponds in eastern and central China. It is not of medical importance (Fig. 66–3).

The shell is reddish brown in color, reaching a length of 17 mm. There are three to four strong spiral cords on each whorl.

Family Assimineidae (Synceridae). This is a large family of small snails found mainly in tropical and subtropical areas, some members of which closely resemble schistosomiasis carriers such as *Oncomelania.* The group is of little medical importance, although *Assiminea lutea* Adams is reported to be a host of the zoonotic rodent lung fluke *Paragonimus iloktsuenensis* in southern China (p. 573). These snails are amphibious or terrestrial, with shells less than 8 mm in length and with a translucent horny, paucispiral operculum. The animals of *Assiminea* (formerely *Syncera*) have very short, stubby tentacles welded to the eyestalk, and the shell has a single, microscopic, spiral thread just below the suture of the whorls.

Family Thiaridae (Melaniidae). The THIARIDAE is a widely distributed and diversified family of operculate snails living in fresh and brackish water. A number of species are the main snail hosts for *Paragonimus, Metagonimus, Haplorchis* and *Diorchitrema.* The shells are usually 1 to 3 inches in length, black or brown and fairly slender; the young are brooded in a neck pouch, and the animal is characterized by a digitate mantle edge.

Genus Thiara. Thiara (Tarebia) granifera

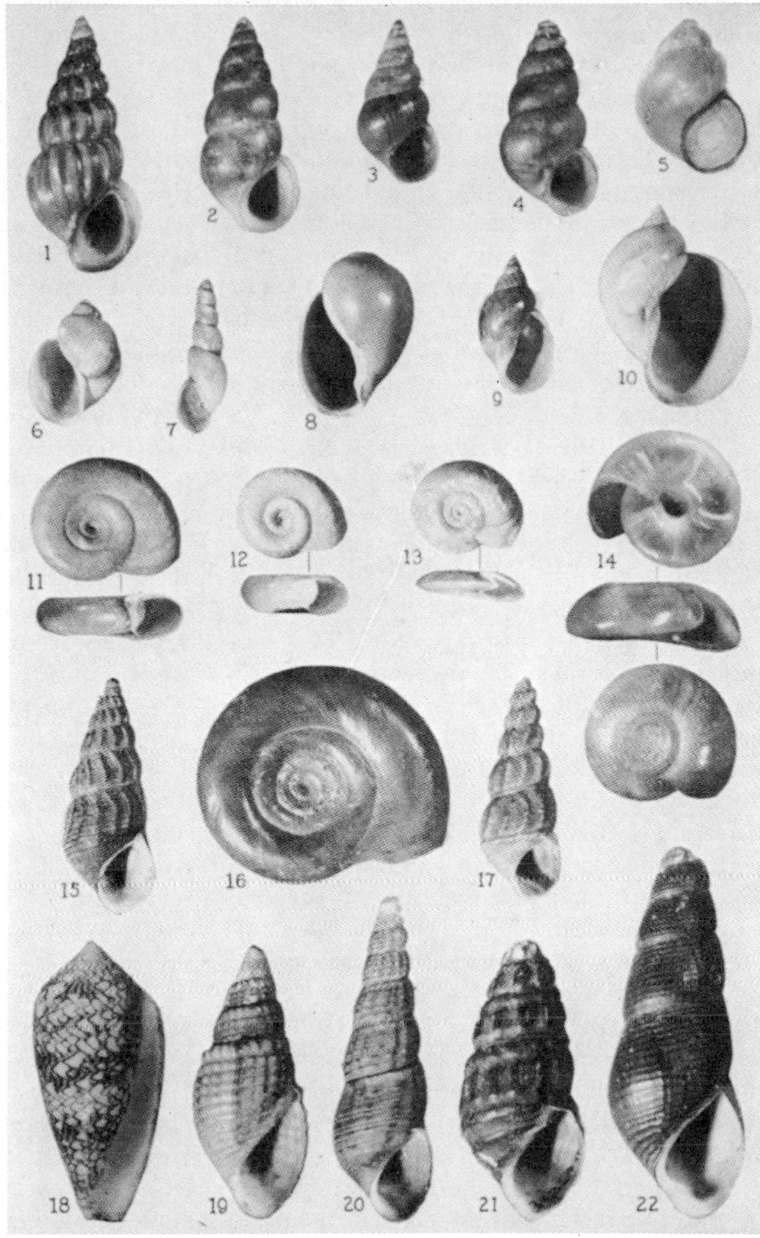

Figure 66–4. Medically important mollusks. *1, Oncomelania hupensis* Gredler (China). *2, O. nosophora* Robson (China and Japan). *3, O. quadrasi* Moellendorff (Philippines). *4, Pomatiopsis lapidaria* Say (United States and Canada) (1–4 all 4×). *5, Bulimus tentaculatus* (L.) (United States; northern Europe) (3×). *6, Bulinus truncatus* (Audouin) (Africa and Asia Minor). *7, Bulinus forskalii* (Ehrenberg) (Africa). *8, Bulinus (Physopsis) africanus* (Krauss) (Africa). *9, Lymnaea ollula* Gould Hawaii and China). *10, Lymnaea auricularia* L. (northern Eurasia). *11, Biomphalaria alexandrina* (Ehrenberg) (northern Africa). *12, Biomphalaria pfeifferi* (Krauss) (southern Africa). *13, Hippeutis cantori* (Benson) (China). *14, Segmentina hemisphaerula* (Benson) (eastern Asia) (5×). *15, Goniobasis silicula* Gould (northwest United States). *16, Biomphalaria glabrata* (Say) (West Indies and South America). *17, Hua ningpoensis* (Lea) (China). *18, Conus textile* L. (Indo-Pacific reefs). *19, Thiara (Tarebia) granifera* (Lamarck) (Southeast Asia; Pacific Islands). *20, Thiara (Melanoides) tuberculata* (Müller) (Africa to Southeast Asia; Pacific Islands). *21, Semisulcospira amurensis* (Gerstfeldt) (northern China; Korea). *22, Semisulcospira libertina* (Gould) (Japan to Formosa). (Numbers 6 to 22 are $1\frac{1}{2}\times$, except 14.)

(Lamarck). This common species lives in fast flowing streams in Southeast Asia, Indonesia, Taiwan and the western Pacific Islands, where it serves as the first intermediate host for *Paragonimus westermani, Metagonimus yokogawai, Diorchitrema formosanum* and *Haplorchis taichui* (Fig. 66–4). The snail formerly was established in Lithia Spring, Florida. It has been introduced into Puerto Rico where it is now very abundant. Adults are 6 to 40 mm long, elongate-turrate, yellowish to reddish brown, have whorls with four to six spiral rows of round to quadrate small beads and a fragile outer lip. The mantle edge has several prominent, fleshy digitations, four of which may be seen projecting beyond the shell lip on the left side. Mature specimens have shelled young in a brood pouch under the skin behind the head. The operculum is two-thirds the size of the aperture, horny and blackish brown. *Melania obliquegranosa* is a synonym.

Thiara (Melanoides) tuberculata (Müller) is common in warm, sluggish water from Africa to subtropical Asia and the western Pacific Islands. The animal is similar to that of the above species (Fig. 66–4). The shell is 1 to 2 inches long and slender, with well rounded whorls and sculpturing of numerous axial and spiral threads. It is brownish and sometimes mottled with reddish brown. This species is a host for *Diorchitrema formosanum* and is suspected to be a minor host for *Clonorchis sinensis.*

Family Pleuroceridae. Members of this family lay eggs or brood the young in a uterine pouch; they are characterized by having a smooth mantle edge that is never digitate. Among its genera are *Semisulcospira, Hua* and *Goniobasis.*

Semisulcospira libertina (Gould). This species is considered to be the main intermediate snail host of *Paragonimus westermani* in the Orient (Fig. 66–4). It has an insular distribution that extends from Japan and Korea to Taiwan. The shell is 3/4 to 2 inches in length, is somewhat spindle-shaped and has slightly flattened, fairly smooth whorls. Length of the aperture is about half the total length of the shell. The whorls have numerous fine, spiral threads. It is brownish to yellowish brown, but sometimes heavily flushed with greenish blue. The edge of the mantle is smooth and the uterus on the inside of the mantle may be filled with many equal-sized, small young. The males lack a verge.

Semisulcospira amurensis (Gerstfeldt) is common in fast flowing streams in northern China and Korea (Fig. 66–4). It is an intermediate host of *Paragonimus westermani.* This species has many minor races in Korea. The shell is 1/2 to 1 inch in length, dark brown to greenish brown, and usually heavily sculptured, with two or three very strong cords on the base of the shell. Blunt axial ribs and low nodules are sometimes present. The animal is similar to the above species; the operculum is opaque brown, horny and paucispiral.

Hua (Namrutua) ningpoensis (Lea) is very common in canals and small rivers of central and southern China, where it serves as one of the main intermediate hosts of *Clonorchis sinensis* (Fig. 66–4). It was formerly known as *Melania cancellata* Benson. The operculum is translucent, thin, horny and paucispiral. The shell is about 1 inch in length and slender; the upper two-thirds of each whorl have even, strong, slightly curved, axial ribs, and there are three or four smooth, spiral cords on the base of the shell. The animal lays eggs. The mantle edge is wavy but without digitations.

Goniobasis silicula (Gould). This is the only known snail host of *Troglotrema salmincola* Chapin, the trematode associated with "salmon poisoning" in northwestern United States (Fig. 66–4). It is common in lakes and creeks of Washington and Oregon. The shell is 1/2 to 1 inch long, brownish to greenish, slender, and has rounded whorls. Strong axial ribs are usually present on the first few whorls, and the numerous spiral threads are strongest on the last whorl. It is erroneously listed in the literature as *Galbaplicifera silicula.*

Family Potamididae (=CERITHIIDAE). These are slender, operculated snails found on mud flats in brackish water areas. The genera *Pirenella* and *Cerithidea* are known to serve as the first intermediate hosts of *Heterophyes heterophyes* in Egypt and Japan, respectively. *Cerithidea cingulata* is characterized by its small aperture, which terminates in a siphonal canal at the base. *Cerithidea scalariformis,* commonly known as the "ribbon horn shell," is the intermediate host of the bird schistosome *Austrobilharzia penneri* in Florida.

Batillaria minima, the "black horn shell," another member of this family, is common on the muddy coasts of Florida. It is the intermediate host of the bird schistosome *Ornithobilharzia canaliculata.*

Families Viviparidae and Pilidae. These are the large apple snails of ponds and lakes. A number of cercariae have been found in them, and a few trematodes of medical importance have been associated with these families. In *Viviparus* the operculum is horny, with a concentric nucleus near the margin. Females brood pea-sized young in the uterus. In the males the right tentacle is truncate or recurved and serves as the penis. The eyes are on large, bulbous swellings at the base of the tentacles. The central tooth of the radula is quadrate and denticulate only on the top edge. In the PILIDAE, which have similarly large, 3-inch shells, the operculum is calcareous, the tentacles are very long and slender and the penis arises from the right side of the mantle edge. The females lay clusters of pea-sized calcareous eggs on reeds just above the surface of the water. The genera *Pila* and *Pomacea* belong in this last family but are of little medical importance. *Pila conica,* on the Philippine Islands, and *Viviparus javanicus,* on Java, are second intermediate hosts of the human echinostome *Echinostoma ilocanum* (p. 578). *Pila* eggs in Thailand are hosts for the nematode *Angiostrongylus cantonensis.*

Marisa cornuarietis is a discoidal species belonging to the family PILIDAE; it has been tested successfully in certain ponds in some Caribbean Islands for the biologic control of such medically important planorbid snails as *Biomphalaria glabrata.*

SUBCLASS PULMONATA

These mollusks have a pulmon or lung, are hermaphroditic and are mainly freshwater or terrestrial.

ORDER BASOMMATOPHORA

These are mostly freshwater snails and comprise many medically important species of snails.

Family Planorbidae. The planorbid snails are worldwide in distribution and play an important part in the life cycle of many trematodes. The foot of a planorbid is elongate, truncate in front, and usually tapers to a point behind. Above and in front of the foot is a short, broad, fleshy velum which bears the head and two tentacles. The small, black eyes, as in other basommatophorans, are situated at the inner bases of the tentacles. The respiratory opening and pseudobranch or false gill are on the left side of the body. The genital openings are also on the left side. There is no operculum. The animals are monoecious and lay gelatinous globs in which the eggs are embedded (Fig. 66–5).

SUBFAMILY PLANORBINAE. *Biomphalaria glabrata* (Say). This species is the main intermediate host of the human intestinal schistosome *Schistosoma mansoni* in the West Indies and South America (Figs. 66–4, 66–5). It is the largest species in those areas and in some sites reaches a diameter of a little over an inch. The shell is smooth and made up of slowly widening whorls that are either rounded or slightly angular in cross section. The color of the animal is gray or black, and the mantle is mottled with brown or cinnamon. Among the synonyms of this species are *Planorbis guadaloupensis, P. olivaceus* and *P. antiguensis.*

Several species belonging to the genus *Tropicorbis* Pilsbry and Brown, now placed under *Biomphalaria,* occur in the neotropics; some are actual transmitters of *Schistosoma mansoni,* while others are potential or nonpotential hosts. It is often difficult to distinguish all these species on the basis of shell characteristics only and even on the basis of anatomy,[10] and specialists have to be consulted.

Among other planorbids in the endemic areas of the Western Hemisphere besides the medically important ones are species of *Drepanotrema* Crosse and Fischer and *Helisoma* (Swainson). In addition to anatomical characteristics, *Drepanotrema* can be differentiated by having a small shell generally of several flat whorls. A young *Helisoma* has an angled shoulder and a large aperture; shells of adult *Helisoma* are usually higher than those of *Biomphalaria* (= *Australorbis* Pilsbry and *Tropicorbis*) and have distinct axial sculpture.

In Africa and southwestern Asia several species of *Biomphalaria* are all transmitters of *Schistosoma mansoni.* Among these are *B. alexandrina* occurring in the Nile Delta; *B. pfeifferi* and related species *(bridouxiana, rhodesiensis, nairobiensis, rüppellii* and *gaudi*) occurring in Africa south of the Sahara; and *choanomphala, smithi* and *stanleyi* restricted to certain great lakes in central Africa.[11] In

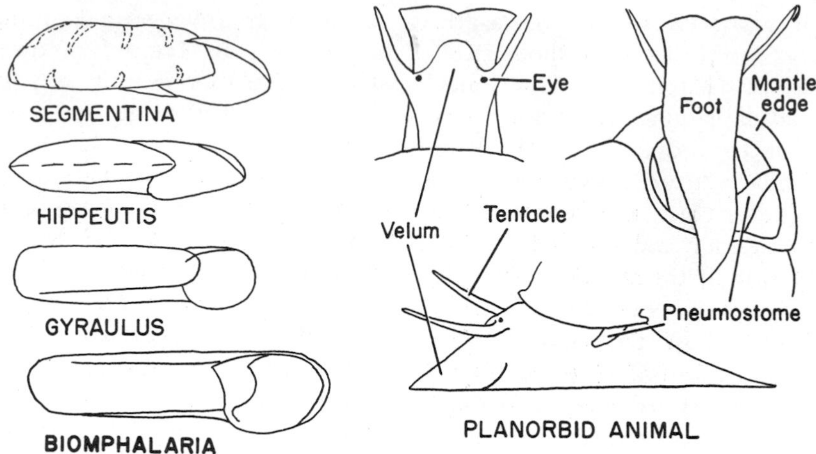

Figure 66–5. *Segmentina hemisphaerula* and *Hippeutis cantori* (above) are Oriental hosts of *Fasciolopsis buski; Gyraulus* is the second intermediate host of *Echinostoma; Biomphalaria glabrata* (above) is the tropical American host of *Schistosoma mansoni.* (Redrawn from Abbott.)

southwestern Asia the transmitter is *B. rüppellii.*

Biomphalaria alexandrina (Ehrenberg) has been called *Planorbis boissyi* Potiez and Michaud. The shells are typically planorboid. An adult specimen from Egypt has five whorls, a diameter of 14 mm and a height of 3.5 mm. The upper side of the shell is slightly concave but almost flat, and the apex is not very deep. The upper part of the aperture is usually arched and may be a little higher than the next to the last whorl. The aperture is more or less evenly oval in cross section. A dissected specimen of this species is shown in Figure 66–6.

Biomphalaria pfeifferi (Krauss). This is similar to *B. alexandrina* but is generally not so flat (diameter 12 mm, height 4.2 mm) and is much more concave at the top, with a deep apex. The upper part of the aperture is generally less arched, and the aperture has a tendency to be more pinched or triangular in cross section. In both species, the young shells may have small, whitish teeth or folds within the aperture. The intermediate hosts of *S. mansoni* in the Western Hemisphere (i.e. *Australorbis* and *Tropicorbis*) and those in Africa (i.e. *Biomphalaria)* are congeneric, and The International Commission on Zoological Nomenclature has decided (Opinion 735, 1965) in favor of the name *Biomphalaria.*

Subfamily Segmentininae. *Segmentina hemisphaerula* (Benson). In eastern Asia, this small, common species serves as one of the intermediate hosts of *Fasciolopsis buski* (Figs. 66–4, 66–5) and the bird schistosome *Gigantobilharzia sturniae* in Japan. The adult shell is "fat," with a height of about 3 mm and a diameter of 7 to 9 mm. It is glossy reddish brown to light brown, and the umbilicus is very deep. The internal calcareous lamellae are visible through the shell. *Planorbis nitidellus* von Martens is a synonym.

Hippeutis cantori (Benson). In eastern China, this species is one of the main intermediate hosts of *Fasciolopsis buski* (Figs. 66–4, 66–5, and p. 574). The adults are fairly large (8 to 10 mm in diameter) but rather flat (1 to 2 mm in height). The spire is slightly concave, the umbilicus very wide but not very deep. The periphery of the last embracing whorl may be sharp; there are no internal shell folds. It is a glossy translucent brown and is common in ponds and lakes. A similar species, *H. umbilicalis* Benson, is fatter (6 by 2 mm), with a neatly indented spire and a much narrower umbilicus. It is of no known medical importance.

Subfamily Bulininae. *Genus Bulinus* Müller. Members of this genus are the main intermediate hosts of *Schistosoma haematobium* in Africa and the Near East. *Bulinus* is readily recognized by its glossy, up to 13 mm long, left-handed or sinistral physoid shells. The mantle is without digitations (Fig. 66–4). The genus comprises the subgenus *Physopsis,*

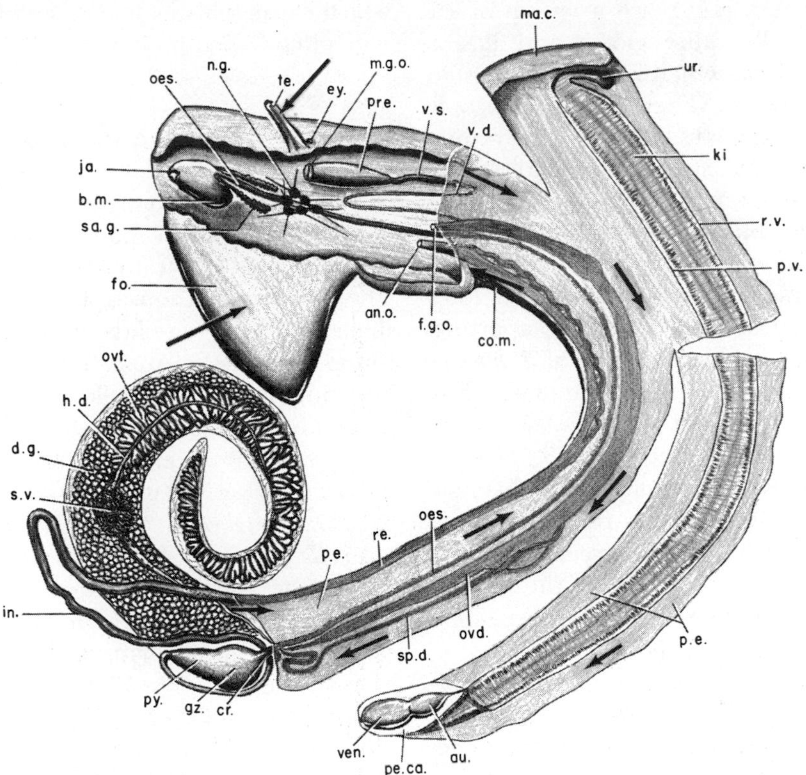

Figure 66–6. A dissected *Biomphalaria alexandrina* (Ehrenberg). (Courtesy of Dr. E. A. Malek, Laboratory Guide and Notes for Medical Malacology, Burgess Publishing Co., Minneapolis.[5]) Key to abbreviations used with figures: an.o., anal opening; au., auricle; b.m., buccal mass; co.m., columellar muscle; cr., crop; d.g., digestive gland; ey., eye; f.g.o., female genital opening; fo., foot; gz., gizzard; h.d., hermaphroditic duct; in., intestine; ja., jaw; ki., kidney; ma.c., mantle collar; p.e., pulmonary epithelium; pe.ca., pericardial cavity; m.g.o., male genital opening; n.g., nerve ganglia; oes., oesophagus; ovd., oviduct; ovt., ovotestis; pre., preputium; py., pylorus; p.v., pulmonary vein; re., rectum; r.v., renal vein; sa.g., salivary gland; sp.d., sperm duct; s.v., seminal vesicle; te., tentacle; ur., ureter; v.d., vas deferens; ven., ventricle; v.s., vergic sac. Arrows show sites of penetration of the miracidia of *Schistosoma mansoni*, the route of migration of the daughter sporocysts to distal organs, and the route of migration of the cercariae proximad on their way to emerge from the snail, at the pseudobranch and neighboring tissues.

in which the columella is truncate, the sculpture of the shell consists of spirally arranged rows of small transverse impressions or nodules, and there is a distinct ridge on the ventral surface of the kidney; in the subgenus *Bulinus* the columella is usually straight, the shell is costulate and there is no renal ridge.

Species of the subgenus *Physopsis* (*globosus, africanus, jousseaumei* and *nasutus*) are transmitters of the human urinary schistosome *S. haematobium* and some animal schistosomes. Among the subgenus *Bulinus* the species *truncatus, truncatus rohlfsi, coulboisi, guernei, senegalensis* and *cernicus* are transmitters of *S. haematobium* and other animal schistosomes.

1. *Bulinus (Bulinus) truncatus* (Audouin). This is a widespread species found in the northern part of Africa and in Asia Minor (Fig. 66–4). Probable synonyms of this species are *Bulinus contortus* Michaud and *B. brocchi* Ehrenberg. The adults are about 8 to 13 mm in length, sinistral, brownish and not very glossy. Microscopic axial growth lines are irregular. The columella is thin and is not rolled back to form a ridge, callus or tube, and not abruptly truncate at the base. Three to four whorls are present.

2. *Bulinus (Physopsis) africanus* (Krauss). This and related species are the main carriers of *S. haematobium* in South, East, West and Central Africa (Fig. 66–4). It is similar

to *B. truncatus* but may reach a length of 16 mm. It is usually quite glossy and has a reflected columella which is strongly twisted and truncate below. There are microscopic sculpturing of growth lines and very fine, punctate dots or short, crowded, wavy threads. The spire may be high or low.

3. *Bulinus (Bulinus) forskalii* (Ehrenberg), formerly referred to in the literature as *Pyrgophysa forskalii,* has a shell with a long and slender spire and a narrow aperture (Fig. 66–4). It is a potential host of *S. haematobium* and a primary host of animal schistosomes. The host of *S. haematobium* in Mauritius is a related species, *B. (B.) cernicus* and not *B. (B.) forskalii,* while in Gambia and Senegal *B. (B.) senegalensis,* a related species, is the transmitter of *S. haematobium. B. (B.) forskalii* is also the transmitter of the human intestinal schistosome *Schistosoma intercalatum* in Gabon and the Cameroons.

Family Lymnaeidae. The genus *Lymnaea,* a group of dextrally coiled pond snails, is of moderate importance, and some of its species, such as *L. auricularia* Linné (and its varieties), *L. ollula* Gould and *L. bulimoides* Lea, serve as the first intermediate hosts of *Fasciola hepatica.* "Swimmer's itch" or schistosome dermatitis is caused by nonhuman schistosomes; in many areas of the United States the snail hosts are species of *Lymnaea* (p. 565). Identification of the lymneid mollusks generally requires the services of an expert. The head and eyes resemble those of the planorbid snails, but the genital openings are on the right side of the body. There is no operculum (Fig. 66–4).

Family Ancylidae. These limpets, with a caplike (patelliform) shell, have a worldwide distribution. *Ferrissia tenuis,* in a small locus near Bombay, India, is claimed on epidemiologic grounds to be an intermediate host of *Schistosoma haematobium.*

Family Physidae. This family contains several species of anoperculate, sinistrally coiled, freshwater snails with spiral shells. They are hermaphroditic and possess a radula consisting of many teeth in V-shaped rows. One important genus is *Physa.* Several species of this genus serve in many areas as hosts of nonhuman schistosomes, some of which cause schistosome dermatitis or "swimmer's itch." (See p. 565.)

ORDER STYLOMMATOPHORA

The slugs and garden snails are characterized by their two pairs of head tentacles, with the eyes at the tips of the second pair. There are many thousands of species of land snails, but only relatively few have been found to serve as snail hosts to trematodes infecting man. The following families and genera have been shown to carry *Dicrocoelium dendriticum:* PUPILLIDAE (Chondrina) (=*Torquilla*); FRUTICICOLIDAE *(Bradybaena);* HELICELLIDAE (*Helicella, Cochicella*); CIONELLIDAE (*Cionella*).

In the Pacific, mainly in Tahiti and Hawaii, the nematode *Angiostrongylus cantonensis,* the rat lungworm, is of great zoonotic importance (p. 538). The infection is also of importance in other Pacific Islands, Malaysia, Taiwan, Thailand and probably in other parts of the world. The terrestrial snails *Achatina fulica, Bradybaena similaris, Subulina octona, Pupina complanata;* the slugs *Deroceras laeve, Girasia peguensis, Vaginulus plebius, Veronicella alte;* and the aquatic snails *Indoplanorbis exustus, Pila ampullacea* and *Pila gracilis* are among the natural intermediate hosts of *A. cantonensis.* In addition, several species of terrestrial and aquatic snails can be infected experimentally.

Angiostrongylus costaricensis is a nematode of rats and other rodents in Central America. Slugs of the species *Vaginulus plebius* harboring the infective third-stage larvae are infective to humans when they are ingested, and the parasite localizes in the mesenteric arteries (p. 539). Another species, *Angiostrongylus vasorum,* is a parasite of dogs and foxes in Europe and Asia and of dogs in Uganda, Australia and South America. It utilizes the slug *Arion rufus* as the molluscan intermediate host. A number of other species of mollusks can be infected experimentally, among which are the slugs *Deroceras agreste* and *D. laeve,* the terrestrial snail *Vitrea diaphana,* and the aquatic snails *Anisus leucostomus* and *Lymnaea tomentosa.*

REFERENCES

1. Cheng, T. C. 1969. An electrophoretic analysis of hemolymph proteins of *Helisoma duryi normale* experimentally challenged with bacteria. J. Invertebr. Pathol. *14*:60–81.
2. Hunter, G. W., III, Okabe, K., Burke, J. C., and Williams, J. E. 1962. Aspects of schistosomiasis control and eradication, with special reference to Japan. Ann. Trop. Med. Parasit. *56*:302–313.
3. Malek, E. A. 1961. The ecology of schistosomiasis. *In* May, J. M. (ed.): Studies in Disease Ecology. Hafner Publishing Co., New York. pp. 261–327.
4. Abbott, R. T. 1948. Handbook of medically important mollusks of the Orient and Western Pacific. Bull. Mus. Comp. Zool. Harvard College *100* (3):245–328.
5. Malek, E. A. 1962. Laboratory Guide and Notes for Medical Malacology. Burgess Publishing Co., Minneapolis, Minnesota. 154 pp.
6. Burch, J. B., and Lindsay, G. K. 1970. An immunocytological study of *Bulinus* s.s. (Basommatophora, Planorbidae). Malacol. Rev. *3*:1–18.
7. Abbott, R. T., and Hunter, G. W., III. 1949. Studies on potential snail hosts of *Schistosoma japonicum.* I. Notes on the amnicolid snails *Blanfordia, Tricula* and a new genus, *Fukuia* from Japan. Proc. Helm. Soc. Wash. *16*:73–86.
8. Hunter, G. W., III, and Abbott, R. T. 1949. Studies on potential snail hosts of *Schistosoma japonicum.* II. Infection experiments on amnicolid snails of the genera *Blanfordia, Tricula* and *Fukuia.* Proc. Helm. Soc. Wash. *16*:86–89.
9. Malek, E. A., and Little, M. D. 1971. *Aroapyrgus colombiensis* n.sp. (Gastropoda:Hydrobiidae), snail intermediate host of *Paragonimus caliensis* in Colombia. Nautilus *85*:20–26.
10. Malek, E. A. 1969. Studies on "tropicorbid" snails *(Biomphalaria:* Planorbidae) from the Caribbean and Gulf of Mexico areas, including the Southern United Sates. Malacologia 7:183–209.
11. Mandahl-Barth, G. 1958. Intermediate hosts of *Schistosoma.* African *Biomphalaria* and *Bulinus.* W.H.O. Monogr. Ser. No. 37. 132 pp.

CHAPTER 67

Selected Animals Hazardous to Man

H. L. KEEGAN

The following discussion covers a miscellaneous group of animals that commonly injure man, either mechanically or otherwise. Except for leeches it does not include direct parasites or vectors of disease, since these are discussed elsewhere. Arthropods in all categories are omitted for the same reason. Similarly, although the spines of sea urchins and other echinoderms may cause painful injuries, such accidents are relatively uncommon, and the group is given excellent coverage in other publications.

No attempt is made here to furnish keys for the identification of fish and snakes; rather, information is given concerning the recognition and treatment of injuries caused by the dangerous species and the methods of protection against them.

Coelenterates

Swimmers, fishermen, shell collectors, surfers and scuba divers share the hazard of skin contact with dangerous jellyfish, corals and sea anemones. Some of these coelenterates, all salt water species, may produce symptoms in man which range from mild discomfort to severe pain, allergic reactions and even death. Although some of the medically important species occur in temperate zones, most accounts of severe reactions come from subtropical or tropical waters.

Even though, at first glance, the jellyfish, corals and sea anemones may seem unrelated, these animals are alike in having radial symmetry and possessing tentacles armed with stinging structures called *nematocysts.* In this phylum (COELENTERATA or CNIDARIA) there are two basic structural types and individuals. These are: *polyps,* which are usually stationary and have the form of an elongated cylinder fastened to the substrate at one end, and with mouth and tentacles at the free end; and *medusae,* free-swimming, bowl-, bell- or saucer-shaped jellyfish with marginal tentacles. Both polyps and medusae may be represented in the life cycle of a single species. Some colonial coelenterates may include several types of individuals.

One of the most widely distributed of the medically important coelenterates is *Physalia,* the Portuguese man-of-war. This colonial species floats by means of a brilliantly colored air bladder and possesses tentacles that may be many yards in length (Fig. 67–1).

True jellyfish of several species are known to cause severe reactions in man in Pacific waters from Japan southward to Australia. Among these, locally known as "sea wasps" or "sea nettles," but with no widely accepted common names, are species of *Carybdea, Chiropsalmus, Dactylometra* and *Chironex.*

Accidents caused by contact with sea anemones and corals include both stings from nematocysts and cuts from coral. The general problem of coelenterate sting has been reviewed thoroughly.[1]

Nematocysts are extremely small, intracellular structures, each of which consists of a capsule containing a hollow, coiled, intraverted thread. These are discharged to the exterior by eversion. Some types may penetrate the skin of man, injecting a toxic substance. The nematocysts are contained in cells, known as *cnidoblasts,* which are most abundant on the tentacles, where they are grouped in warts, knobs or spiral ridges.

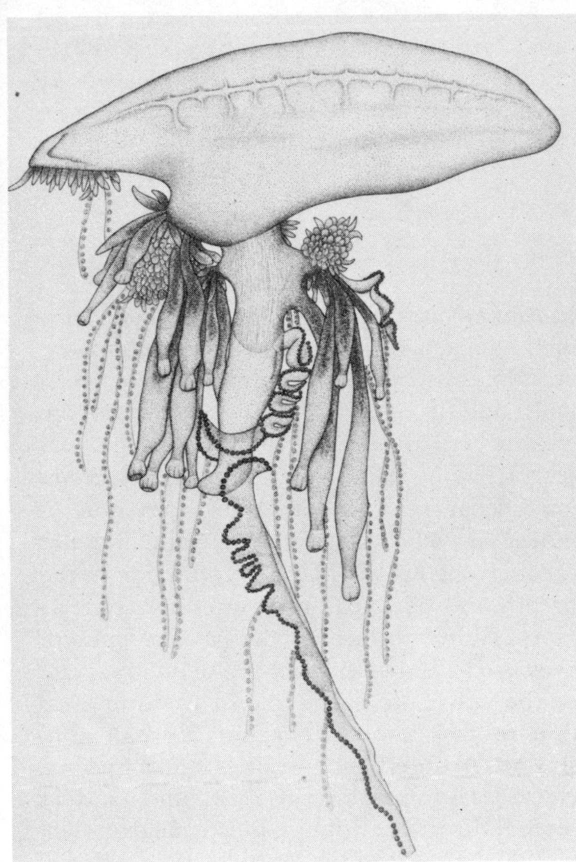

Figure 67-1. *Physalia,* the Portuguese man-of-war. (Courtesy of Commanding Officer, 406th Medical General Laboratory, U.S. Army Medical Command, Japan.)

The cause of discharge is not entirely clear, but appears to be a selective response to mechanical stimulation.

Clinical Characteristics. Symptoms following contact with venomous coelenterates show considerable variation. Contact with one of the more potent species often is followed immediately by intense, burning pain. Lines of contact with the tentacles often appear as purplish, swollen wheals. These either disappear in a few hours or vesiculate. In some instances, a massive blister develops along the entire line of contact. Systemic effects may be absent or may be delayed for as much as an hour after the sting has occurred. Such effects include muscle spasms, particularly in the abdomen, back and diaphragm. The patient may have great difficulty in breathing and be nauseated. Profuse lacrimation and nasal and bronchial secretion can occur. Some workers have reported cardiac arrhythmias, tachycardia and dyspnea and generalized muscular weakness following jellyfish stings. Miscellaneous symptoms, which are observed at times, include anxiety, swelling of the extremities, profuse perspiration, erythema, elevated temperature, vertigo, mental confusion, rapid pulse and moderate dilation of the pupils. There is often residual stiffness, and sometimes residual skin discoloration and disturbance of sensation.

One of the chief dangers from sting by highly venomous jellyfish is that, even in shallow water, the victim may drown when afflicted by cramps and respiratory muscle spasm. Although deaths from jellyfish stings have been reported from several areas, the most complete series of case histories has come from Australian workers concerning fatal cases along the coast of North Queensland. In several instances, the victim did not survive more than 10 minutes following the sting. The symptoms in these cases were those of anaphylactic shock. Although *Physalia* is a common cause of jellyfish sting in many areas, there are few records of human fatalities caused by this species.

Treatment. Measures for treatment of jellyfish sting have been directed toward relief of pain, muscle spasms and dyspnea. As a first step, any adhering jellyfish tentacles should be removed as quickly as possible. This may be done with a towel, clothing, or even sand. Injection of adrenaline (epinephrine) subcutaneously (7 minims) has been found effective by Australian workers. Noradrenalin should be administered to combat cardiac weakness. Intravenous injection of 10 ml of 10 per cent calcium gluconate, repeated as needed, provides relief of muscle spasms. Some workers have found cortisone therapy helpful. In severe cases, artificial respiration and administration of oxygen may be necessary. Codeine, morphine, sodium phenobarbital, Benadryl and atropine have been used with varying success in treatment of jellyfish sting.

Prophylaxis. Persons swimming or wading in jellyfish-infested waters should keep a close lookout for these organisms. As some of the dangerous species are nearly transparent, they are often difficult to detect, particularly if they are submerged. Enclosure of beach areas with nets or fences has been tried in some areas. Where water is smooth and clear, jellyfish may be removed with dip nets. Particular care should be taken following storms at sea, as many jellyfish, especially specimens of the Portuguese man-of-war, may be stranded on beaches.

Leeches

These annelids possess single anterior and posterior suckers, which are used for locomotion and attachment. At the center of the anterior sucker is the mouth, which, in most bloodsucking species, possesses three semicircular cutting plates, each armed with up to a hundred or more tiny teeth. In sucking blood, leeches secrete an anticoagulant, *hirudin,* the action of which often continues even after the animals have engorged and dropped off the host.

Although some leeches are found in salt water, all of the bloodsucking species of medical importance live in fresh water or are terrestrial. Aquatic bloodsucking leeches are widely distributed in temperate as well as tropical regions; land leeches, with a few exceptions, are confined to the subtropics and tropics and are particularly numerous in portions of Central, East, and Southeast Asia.

Most widely distributed of the aquatic bloodsucking leeches are species of the genus *Hirudo.* Other aquatic leeches of medical importance are the buffalo leeches of genus *Poecilobdella,* and the nasal leeches of genera *Dinobdella* and *Limnatis.* Species of the latter two genera enter the nares when humans or animals are drinking from ponds or streams. In some areas of the Middle East and North Africa these have been reported to be important causes of anemia in children.

When a person or animal enters leech-infested water, the leeches quickly swim toward the source of water disturbance. Upon reaching the host, the leech will immediately adhere with the anterior sucker, then begin "exploring" the skin surface in measuring-worm style. When a suitable attachment site has been reached, the skin of the host is quickly perforated, suction begins and is continued until the leech is engorged. During engorgement a leech may take up to several times its own weight in blood.

Land leeches are found on damp ground or vegetation and are often numerous along game or cattle trails. They are quickly aroused when the vegetation is moved or when a person or animal walks through the area. The carbon dioxide in the breath and perhaps other stimuli are attractants. Although leeches possess five pairs of eyes on the dorsal surface at the anterior end of the body, the exact role of these in location of blood meals has not been demonstrated. Aroused land leeches "stand up" in a characteristic reaching attitude and sway in several directions when a host is nearby (Fig. 67–2). If sufficiently stimulated, they will inch their way toward the host, often stopping to "reach and sway" en route. Upon the slightest contact with a host they attach with the anterior sucker, then commence exploring for a suitable attachment site. In doing this they may enter any opening in the clothing and have been known to go through the eyelets of boots, or through the fabric in loosely woven cloth. They often crawl between the boot and sock and feed by penetrating the sock mesh. In such instances, the bite may go unnoticed until the wearer takes off his boots to find that a "wet feeling" inside the boot is from his own blood.

Clinical Characteristics. Effects of bloodsucking leeches on man are both physical and psychological. Leeches may cause extensive blood loss by their bites. Infection of these lesions occurs frequently. The psychological factor may be of even greater importance. The unexpected discovery of saclike engorged leeches on the skin, the prolonged bleeding from attachment sites following removal of leeches, and the exaggerated

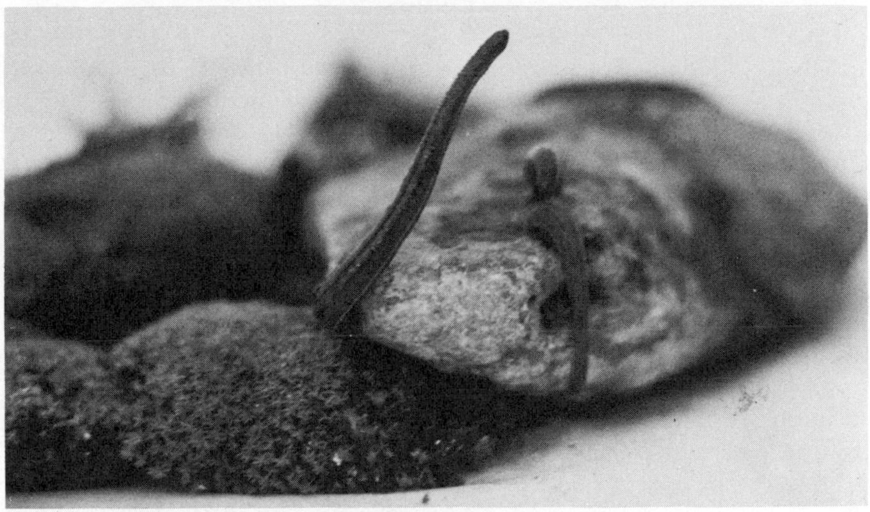

Figure 67-2. A land leech, *Haemadipsa japonica,* in "searching" attitude. (Courtesy of Commanding Officer, 406th Medical General Laboratory, U.S. Army Medical Command, Japan.)

stories of entry of leeches into the nose or urethra combine to produce an effect that may greatly affect the efficiency of persons working in leech-infested territory. There is no evidence that leeches transmit disease agents to man.

Treatment. A leech attached to the skin may be dislodged by the simple expedient of pulling it off by hand. Otherwise, it can be induced to detach by touching it with a lighted cigarette, a few drops of insect repellent, or even a pinch of table salt. Oozing of blood from points of leech attachment may be controlled with a styptic pencil. Calamine lotion or other soothing medication may be helpful in relieving the itching caused by leech bites. This may last 2 or 3 days following bites by some of the land leeches. Removal of leeches from the nasopharynx or from the urethra is seldom an easy matter for the patient. In such cases, manual removal of the leech with forceps either with or without application of pain-killing medication is the usual technique. In one instance, a nasal spray of a 1:1000 solution of adrenaline hydrochloride induced a leech to detach. Treatment of infections caused by scratching of leech bites may be necessary.

Prophylaxis. Protection against aquatic and terrestrial bloodsucking leeches is best afforded by wearing protective clothing and by the use of insect repellents on the skin and clothing. Even without repellents, the possibility of leech attachment is greatly reduced if trouser bottoms are tucked inside sock tops in properly laced boots. The repellent formulation M-1960, which at present has restricted availability, has proved effective in protecting wearers of treated clothing against attacks by aquatic and land leeches. However, commercially available insect repellents, particularly those containing diethyltoluamide, also give adequate protection if applied to skin and, especially, to clothing, in either aerosol or lotion formulations. Unfortunately, diethyltoluamide is soluble in water; thus frequent reapplications may be necessary if the wearer is wading or swimming, is caught in heavy rain, or must walk through wet vegetation.

Area control of leeches with insecticides has not been attempted except on an experimental basis. It has been found that leeches captured in farming areas of Japan, Korea and Taiwan are highly tolerant to several insecticides, including DDT. Whether this tolerance is natural or acquired is not known.[2]

Fishes

This discussion is limited to consideration of puncture wounds and lacerations caused by venom-bearing spines of some fishes and to illness following ingestion of the flesh of others. Bites by sharks, morays and such freshwater fishes as the piranhas may result in severe wounds, or even death, or may be complicated by secondary infection and should be treated appropriately.

Poisoning by Contact. Ichthyoacanthotoxism is the specific term used to designate intoxication resulting from injuries produced by the piercing spines of venomous fishes. Most of these occur in salt water. The venom-bearing spines, which are grooved, and which may be serrate, usually are located in the dorsal, pectoral or pelvic fins, but may be present in other areas such as the top of the head and the cheeks. Venom-secreting tissues line the grooves of the spines, or saclike venom glands may be present at the base of each spine. An integumentary sheath may enclose each of the spines, particularly those of the dorsal fin. Pressure on the spine forces back the sheath and venom flows along the spinal groove into the wound. These sharp, sturdy spines can easily penetrate a glove or soft-soled shoe. Even slight penetration may cause agonizing pain.

The various categories of venomous fishes include stingrays, catfishes, stonefishes, wasp fishes, rock cods, butterfly cods and miscellaneous species such as spinefeet and bastard stonefishes.[3]

Stingrays are flat, disk- or kite-shaped animals that possess a long tail armed with one or more barbed spines. These fish habitually lie partially buried on the bottom in shallow water and are a serious menace to waders. Several species of bottom-dwelling catfishes possess serrate venom-bearing spines on dorsal and pectoral fins. The stonefishes are grotesque in appearance and often bear a close resemblance to weed-covered rocks or pieces of bottom debris. They are extremely difficult to detect as they lie half buried in bottom mud or sand or among rocks. Unlike most fishes, they do not swim away when approached but may lie motionless unless touched. Some species possess as many as 13 venom-bearing spines in the dorsal fin (Fig. 67–3).

Other important relatives of the stonefish are the scorpion fish, and species of genus *Pterois*, known as lion fish, zebra fish and butterfly fish. Many of these fish greatly resemble their surroundings and, like the stonefish, are bottom dwellers. When disturbed, many of these fish will turn to confront the intruder with the tips of their dorsal spines. Others actually may "butt" an offending object, bringing spines on their head and opercula into play.

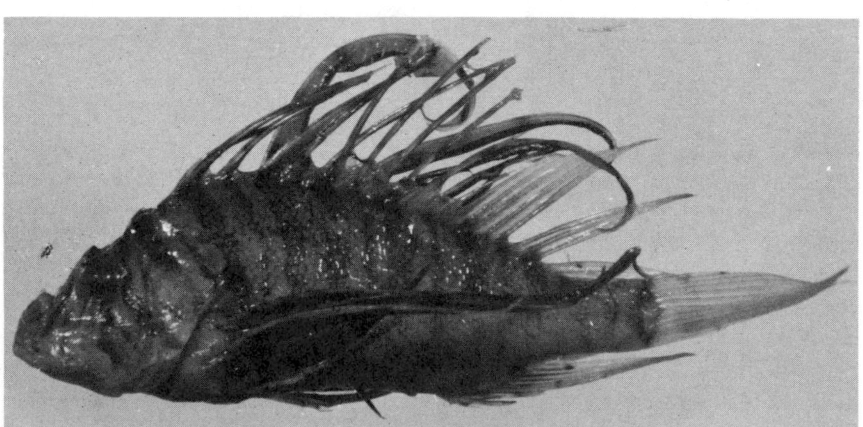

Figure 67–3. A stonefish, *Synanceja verrucosa*, from the Solomon Islands. (Courtesy of Commanding Officer, 406th Medical General Laboratory, U.S. Army Medical Command, Japan.)

Clinical Characteristics. Wounds produced by the large, barbed caudal spines of stingrays are either punctures or lacerations. If the sting breaks off in the tissue, its removal is extremely difficult because of the posteriorly directed barbed spines. This laceration, plus effects of the venom, produces immediate, excruciating pain, which may be localized or radiating in nature. The area about the wound at first has an ashen appearance, later becoming cyanotic, followed by redness and swelling. Primary shock may occur. Deaths from severe stings have been reported. Often similar symptoms immediately follow catfish stings. In extreme cases tissue necrosis, due to the effect of the venom or secondary infection, may be so severe as to result in the loss of a limb. Stonefish stings ordinarily are severe, and as with stings by other venomous fish, immediate pain is the usual response. This may be followed by edema, paralysis, and loss of sensation in the injured limb. General effects may include syncope, impairment of all sensations, involvement of respiration, and coma. Abscess formation, necrosis and gangrene may delay convalescence. Dyspnea and general weakness may last for several months following a sting.

Treatment. The treatment of venomous fish stings should be directed toward achievement of three objectives: alleviation of pain, combating effects of venom, and prevention of secondary infection. The wound should be cleansed by irrigation with cold salt water and, if possible, by suction; the injured limb should be soaked in hot water for 30 minutes to an hour; the wound should be infiltrated with 0.5 to 2.0 per cent procaine; lacerated wounds should be closed with a dermal suture and protected with an antiseptic and a sterile dressing. In severe cases, opiates and barbiturates will be required for pain. A prophylactic course of antibiotic may be employed, since secondary bacterial infections usually occur. Administration of tetanus toxoid, or antitoxin if indicated, is an advisable precautionary procedure. Care must be exercised to treat primary and secondary shock, maintain cardiovascular tone, and prevent further complications. Respiratory stimulants may be required.

It is recommended that in stonefish stings a tourniquet be applied immediately, the wound scrubbed with water, and as much of the venom removed as possible by incision and suction. It also has been recommended that 0.5 to 1.0 ml of a solution of 1 grain per ml of emetine hydrochloride be injected along the track of each puncture. Care should be taken to remove any foreign bodies imbedded in the wound. The wound should be left open to permit drainage. A stonefish antivenin, which is said to be highly effective in treatment, is now produced at the Commonwealth Serum Laboratories, Melbourne, Australia.

Poisoning by Ingestion. Ichthyosarcotoxism is the specific term used to designate intoxication resulting from the ingestion of the flesh of poisonous fishes. Illness and death of humans after eating marine fishes of many species is a relatively common occurrence, particularly in tropical regions. Prevention of such accidents is complicated by the fact that it is often impossible to determine the harmless or poisonous nature of a fish by its appearance. While fish of some species are always poisonous, other fish, of ordinarily edible species, may be poisonous only at certain times or in certain places. Both edible and poisonous examples of the same species may sometimes be collected together.

One of the foremost authorities on this problem listed several categories of poisonous fishes.[4] These included: some species of sharks and rays; several of the scombroid fishes such as tuna, bonito, mackerel and skipjack; the puffers and pufferlike fish; and the large number of fishes such as sea bass, herring, jack, surgeonfish, trunkfish, porgie, anchovy, wrasse, snapper, barracuda and moray eels.

The chief danger from consuming shark meat appears to lie in the liver. Flesh of the scombroid fishes is usually dangerous only if the recently captured fish are allowed to remain at room temperature or out in the sun for several hours. Properly refrigerated or canned specimens are safe to eat. The symptoms of poisoning are histaminelike in nature, consisting of severe headache, flushing of the face, congestion of the soft tissues of the eyes, nausea, vomiting, giant urticaria and erythema. Patients usually recover in a period of 8 to 12 hours. Puffers offer a constant hazard. The powerful toxin present in these fish is concentrated in the viscera and gonads. The common puffer in Japanese waters, *Fugu rubripes,* and the Atlantic coast puffer, *Sphaeroides maculatus,* are considered delicacies by gourmets in their respective areas. Both require special preparation in order that they may be eaten without danger. In Japan "fugu" cooks must be licensed by the government.

CLINICAL CHARACTERISTICS. Numbness of the lips, tongue, and tips of the fingers and toes usually develops within 30 minutes after ingestion of the toxic flesh. These symptoms may be followed by nausea, vomiting, headache, dizziness and generalized weakness, to the extent that the patient is incapable of standing. The power of speech becomes impaired and dyspnea is marked. In severe cases within 2 hours the patient may be completely paralyzed because of relaxed muscles and be unable to speak although conscious. Just prior to death the patient becomes unconscious. Death occurs in severe cases as a result of respiratory paralysis within 1 to 24 hours after ingestion of the fish. The mortality rate is estimated at 60 per cent in this type of ichthyosarcotoxism, even with the best medical care. If the patient survives 24 hours, the prognosis is considered to be good.

The condition known as ciguatera poisoning is caused by consumption of the flesh of a great variety of ordinarily edible reef and shore fishes. This type of poisoning has been reported from many areas and is particularly common in the central and south Pacific Ocean and the West Indies. The toxin that produces this type of ichthyosarcotoxism is believed to be related to the feeding habits of the fish. It is thought that herbivorous species acquire or elaborate the toxin after feeding on certain plants and that carnivorous fish acquire the toxin by feeding on the herbivorous species.

Tingling followed by numbness usually develops almost immediately or within a period of 30 hours after ingestion of the toxic flesh. Nausea, vomiting, diarrhea and abdominal pain are present in about 75 per cent of the patients. Joint aches, malaise, chills, fever, prostration, headache, profuse sweating, pruritus, metallic taste, generalized motor incoordination, muscular weakness and myalgia are common. Sensory disturbances are present in most cases, the patient complaining of hot objects being cold and cold objects as hot or like "electric shock." Convulsions and severe paralysis are less common. Although the mortality rate has been estimated to be only about 2 to 3 per cent, complete recovery from the weakness and myalgia sometimes takes weeks or months.

Seven species of moray eel, *Gymnothorax,* are known definitely to be toxic; they are *G. buroensis, G. flavimarginatus, G. javanicus, G. meleagris, G. petelli, G. pictus* and *G. undulatus.* Symptoms of tingling and numbness about the lips, tongue, hands and feet usually develop within 20 minutes to 8 hours after ingestion of the flesh of the eel. These symptoms may be followed by nausea, vomiting, laryngeal spasm, aphonia, excessive mucus production, foaming at the mouth, conjunctivitis, paralysis of the respiratory muscles, motor incoordination, violent clonic and tonic convulsions, abnormal deep and superficial reflexes, and coma. The mortality rate is estimated to be about 10 per cent. The excessive mucus production, laryngeal spasm, violent convulsions, and respiratory distress present difficult problems in management of these patients. The acute symptoms generally subside within 10 days.

TREATMENT. An attack of fish poisoning does not impart immunity and there is no known specific antidote. The treatment is purely symptomatic. Gastric lavage and catharsis should be instituted at once. Ten per cent calcium gluconate administered intravenously has proved effective at times. Patients with violent convulsions caused by moray eel poisoning present difficult nursing problems. Sedation, rest and quiet are essential, since the convulsions are precipitated by noise. Paraldehyde and ether inhalation have been effective in controlling the convulsions. Respiratory stimulants are advisable in cases of respiratory depression. In patients in whom excessive production of mucus is a factor, aspiration and constant turning are essential. Atropine has been found to make the mucus more viscid and difficult to aspirate and is not recommended. If laryngeal spasm is present, intubation or tracheotomy may be necessary. Oxygen by inhalation and intravenous fluids supplemented with vitamins given parenterally usually are beneficial. If the pain is severe, opiates will be required. Morphine in small divided doses is recommended. Cool showers will relieve the severe itching. Fluids given to patients suffering from the paradoxical sensory disturbance (temperature upset) should be slightly warm or at room temperature. Vitamin B complex supplements are advisable.

PROPHYLAXIS. The only reliable method for identification of poisonous fishes is the injection of tissue extracts intraperitoneally into mice or the feeding of viscera and flesh to cats or dogs. Viscera (liver, intestines and roe) should never under any circumstances be eaten. If one must eat fish in a tropical area, the majority of poisonous fishes may be avoided by following these rules: never eat brightly colored fish; never eat fish that have a leathery skin or whose skin is warty or tuberculated; never eat fish that have a bony exoskeleton; and never eat fish that the natives in the area will not eat.

Lizards

Of all the lizards only two species are venomous: the Gila monster of southern Arizona and New Mexico, and the beaded lizard of southern Mexico and Central America. Some of the larger carnivorous lizards, such as the monitors and tejus, may cause severe lacerations by their bites, but such accidents usually occur when these reptiles are unwisely handled. Although bites by the two venomous species, both of genus *Heloderma,* are rare, results of such accidents may be quite severe. When these animals bite they maintain a firm grasp, and it is sometimes most difficult to dislodge them. There is no commercially produced antivenin against *Heloderma* venom, and treatment is symptomatic. There has never been a thorough evaluation of first aid measures for *Heloderma* bite.

Snakes

Medically important snakes are distributed widely in tropical regions. Large pythons, anacondas and boas are found within the tropics. Although some of these snakes can produce severe lacerations with their long teeth and are capable of injuring a person seriously by constriction, such accidents seldom occur. The chief danger from snakes lies in the effects of bites by the venomous species.

Venomous snakes, of course, are found in both tropical and temperate regions. Temperature and isolation have apparently prevented spread of either venomous or nonvenomous species to such areas as Hawaii, New Zealand, New Caledonia, Ireland and Madagascar, as well as the Arctic regions. However, many snake-free tropical islands of the Pacific and Indian oceans have sea snakes in their fringing surf. Distribution of venomous snakes of the world is indicated in Table 67–1.

In the most recent survey of the worldwide scope of the snakebite problem, it was estimated that deaths from snakebite yearly number between 30,000 and 40,000 and that the majority of these occur in Africa and in semitropical and tropical portions of Asia.[5] A number of species of dangerously venomous snakes occur in India and the countries of

Table 67–1. Geographic Distribution of Venomous Snakes of Medical Importance

Area	*Species*
Western Europe	Several true vipers of genus *Vipera.*
Eastern Europe	Several species of *Vipera.* The western fringe of the range of a pit viper, *Agkistrodon halys.*
Middle East	Several species of true vipers of genera *Vipera, Cerastes,* and *Pseudocerastes* (asps or sand vipers); *Echis* (saw-scaled vipers), *Atractaspis, Bitis.* The North African cobra, *Naja haje,* and the desert cobra, *Walterinnesia.*
North Africa	As in Middle East. Fewer true vipers.
Central Africa	Many elapids and true vipers. Elapids include the cobras, *Naja* and *Boulengerina;* the mambas, *Dendroaspis,* and *Hemachatus,* the ringhals. Vipers include species of *Bitis, Causus, Vipera,* and *Echis.*
South Africa	Important elapid snakes include cobras, mambas, and true vipers of genera *Causus* and *Bitis.* One dangerous rear-fanged snake, *Dispholidus,* the boomslang.
North Asia (Asiatic Russia, Mongolia)	Three true vipers, two species of *Vipera* and one of *Echis;* one pit viper, *Agkistrodon halys.*
Central Asia (Afghanistan, India, Pakistan, Sri Lanka, Kashmir, Nepal)	A wide variety of elapids, true vipers, and pit vipers. Important elapids are cobras, *Naja* and *Ophiophagus* (the king cobra); and kraits, *Bungarus.* True vipers of importance are species of *Vipera* and *Echis.* Two pit vipers of genus *Agkistrodon* occur in the area, and several pit vipers of genus *Trimeresurus* are present. These vary considerably in habit.
East Asia (Tibet, China, Korea, Japan, Ryukyu Islands, Taiwan)	Important species in warmer parts of the area include cobras, kraits, and the habus and related species of *Trimeresurus.* Four species of *Agkistrodon* are present, but none is found in the Ryukyu Islands; only one, *A. acutus,* occurs on Taiwan; and only *A. halys* is found in Japan and Korea.
Southeast Asia	Many species of venomous snakes in this region. Only one true viper, *V. russelli;* many species of *Trimeresurus;* and at least three species of *Agkistrodon.* Cobras and kraits of considerable importance.

Southeast Asia. In contrast, only one species of venomous land snake occurs in Korea and the main Japanese islands. Even in areas where venomous snakes are relatively common, snakebite may be a rarity. Newcomers to the tropics are often surprised at the scarcity of snakes of any kind in jungle areas. It is significant that a large proportion of snakebite cases and deaths occur in rural areas, where people are bitten while working barefooted in the fields, or while walking at night or early morning through fields or along roads without benefit of the protection given by boots or shoes.

The venomous snakes of the world are classified in five families. The Elapidae are characterized by possession of two comparatively short, permanently erect, deeply grooved fangs, one on either side of the mouth at the front of the upper jaw. Prominent members of this family are cobras and mambas in Africa, the cobras and kraits in Asia, the tiger snake and its allies in Australia, and the coral snakes of the New World.

Members of family Viperidae each possess two relatively long, hollow fangs at the front of the upper jaw. These fangs, which are attached to movable bones, are erected during a bite, but at rest are folded against the palate when the mouth of the snake is shut. Among the well-known species are the common vipers of Europe and the Middle East; the Gaboon viper, Rhinoceros viper and puff adder of Africa; the saw-

Table 67–1. Geographic Distribution of Venomous Snakes of Medical Importance (*Continued*)

Area	*Species*
Australia, New Guinea, and the Melanesian Archipelago	All of the many species of venomous land snakes in this area are elapids. Among the important species are the death adder, *Acanthophis;* the brown snake, *Demansia;* the tiger snake, *Notechis; Denisonia,* the copperhead; and *Pseudechis,* the black snake. All of the above dangerously venomous.
Canada and the United States	The most important venomous snakes in this region are the rattlesnakes, of genera *Crotalus* and *Sistrurus;* and the copperheads and moccasin of genus *Agkistrodon,* all pit vipers. Few accidents are caused by the three subspecies of the coral snake, *Micrurus fulvius,* which occur in the southeastern States and as far west as Texas.
Mexico and Central America	Most snake bites throughout this region are caused by pit vipers of genera *Crotalus* and *Bothrops. B. atrox,* the fer-de-lance, and *C. durissus,* the tropical rattlesnake, are of particular importance. Many coral snakes of genus *Micrurus* occur in both Mexico and Central America. Although most of these possess potent venom, coral snakebite is less common than bites by the pit vipers. This is due to the secretive habits of these reptiles.
Tropical South America	Many species of *Bothrops* and the tropical rattlesnake rank high in medical importance among snakes of the area. Of particular interest are *B. alternata, B. jararaca, B. atrox,* and *B. jararacussu.* Largest of the pit vipers, the bushmaster, *Lachesis muta,* is actually not an important cause of snakebite in man. Dangerously venomous species of coral snakes also are found in this area. Availability of specific antivenin is essential for successful management of bites by these snakes.
Southern South America	*B. alternatus, B. neuwiedi, B. jararaca,* and *B. jararacussu* are of greatest importance in this area.

scaled viper of Africa and West and Central Asia; and Russell's viper of Central and Southeast Asia. None of the Viperidae occur in the New World.

The family Crotalidae includes both Old and New World species. Members of this family differ from the true vipers only in the presence of a pit on either side of the head between the eye and the nostril (Fig. 67–4). Among the better known snakes of this family are the rattlesnakes, copperheads, moccasins, fer-de-lance, bushmaster and their relatives in North, Central and South America; the mamushi of Japan and Korea; and the habus and related species of East and Southeast Asia.

The Hydrophiidae, or sea snakes, differ from all other snakes in that the tail is vertically compressed and paddle- or oar-like in appearance. While sea snakes are common in shallow waters along coastal margins in many areas of the Pacific, they have been of medical importance in only two regions—one along the western coast of Malaya, the other along coastal areas of Vietnam. Although 52 species of sea snakes are recognized, and all of them are venomous, very few of these have been known to bite man. The fangs, like those of the cobras, are comparatively small and are grooved and permanently erect.

Although most species of family Colubridae are nonvenomous, some possess relatively small, grooved fangs in the rear of the upper jaw. These rear-fanged snakes occur in North and South America as well as in Asia and Africa. Although little is known concerning the venom of most of these

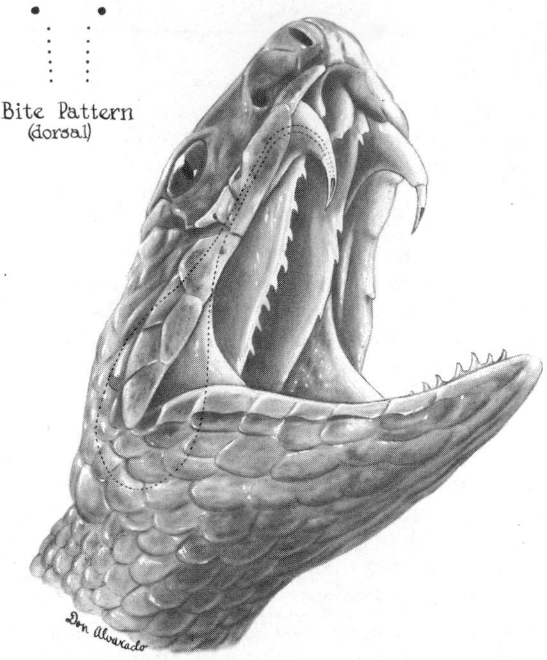

Figure 67–4. Head of a rattlesnake, showing hollow fangs with slitlike opening near the tip, outline of the venom gland, teeth in both upper and lower jaws, pit lying between but below the level of the eye and nostril, and the vertical, elliptical, catlike pupil. The two fang marks and the teeth marks from the upper jaw are shown in the inset of the dorsal bite pattern. (Courtesy of the Louisiana State University School of Medicine, New Orleans.)

snakes, some, such as *Dispholidus typus,* the boomslang of South Africa, are dangerously venomous.

Table 67–1 presents information concerning distribution of some of the more important species in major areas of the world. More detailed information concerning venomous snakes is contained in two cited publications.[6, 7]

Clinical Characteristics. Symptoms following snakebite vary according to the size and species of the snake involved. Location of the bite, as well as the size and physical condition of the person bitten, is also an important factor. It is generally believed that snake venoms are either hemorrhagic or neurotoxic in their effect; however, many venoms have both neurotoxic and hemorrhagic elements. The symptomatology varies considerably following bites by most venomous snakes.

The following criteria are diagnostic of envenomation following a bite by North American pit vipers—fang puncture wounds, plus any of the following: prompt and progressive swelling, pain and ecchymosis (bruiselike discoloration). These same criteria, with some modifications, could be considered as diagnostic of bites by pit vipers and vipers in other areas. Symptoms resulting from bites by these snakes include the criteria listed above plus: nausea, vomiting, hemoptysis, bleeding from fang punctures; development of serous or sanguineous blisters, limb discoloration, respiratory and visual difficulty, bleeding from the gums, and shock. Criteria diagnostic of envenomation by elapid snakes are the presence of fang puncture wounds plus any of the following: blurring of vision; ptosis, a feeling of thickened tongue, slurring of speech and tingling sensation; soft tissue swelling at the puncture point; drowsiness and lassitude; nausea and vomiting; burning pain at the site of injury. Pain and swelling occasionally may be absent after bites by certain elapids.[8]

It should be understood that envenomation and severe symptoms do not always occur after a person has been bitten by a venomous snake. Even a large venomous snake may bite but inject little or no venom. Venoms of some species rarely produce severe illness in man. In a series of 250 cases of snakebite by the Malayan pit viper *Agkistrodon rhodostoma,* it was found that one-half of the patients had slight or no envenomation; one-third had moderate envenomation; and only one-sixth were seriously ill.[8] An additional and interesting finding was that only four of 33 cases of Malayan cobra bite showed neurotoxic symptoms. These patients developed flaccid paralysis of only a few days' duration. Contrary to experience in other areas, the most prominent features of envenomation in this series of cases were local effects, including severe necrosis. More recently, it was reported that of 2433 patients hospitalized for snakebite in the United States, 27 per cent had no venom poisoning, and an additional 37 per cent had minimal envenomation with only local symptoms. Only 14 per cent of the patients had suffered severe envenomation.[9]

The following criteria may be considered as diagnostic of severe envenomation by the sea snake *Enhydrina schistosa,* a common species in Malayan waters: generalized muscle aches, pains, and stiffness on movement commencing 1/2 to 1 hour after the bite; moderate or severe pain on passive movement of arm, thigh, neck, or trunk muscles 1 to 2 hours after the bite; myoglobinuria within 3 to 6 hours after the bite. Dusky yellowness precedes by an hour the red-brown color of myoglobinuria. Onset of pain and other symptoms may be delayed for several hours following bites by some elapids, including the North American coral snakes. It is therefore essential that treatment be started as soon as it has been determined that a person has been bitten by a dangerously venomous elapid snake.

Treatment. It is advisable that first aid measures by persons without some medical training be confined to immobilization of the affected part in a position below the heart; application of a *lightly* constricting tourniquet 2 to 4 inches closer to the heart than the site of the bite (and reapplication of the tourniquet if swelling progresses up the arm or leg); and, lastly, transportation of the bitten person to the nearest source of professional medical assistance, or obtaining assistance from the nearest medical source.[8] Persons with some medical training should carry out procedures mentioned above and, in addition, if the patient is seen within 1 hour following the bite, should institute incision and suction. Incisions should be not more than 1/2 inch in length and should be made through the skin parallel to the line of the extremity and over the site of the fang marks. Care must be taken to avoid excessively deep incisions; incisions over the bony parts may sever nerves or tendons. Controversy remains over the value, or lack of it, of incision and suction as first aid measures. It is the consensus that both incision and suction are useless if instituted more than an hour or so following a bite by a venomous snake. Every effort should be made to supply the proper antivenin for the patient. In the absence of a physician, when it has been determined that serious envenomation has occurred, the patient should be tested for sensitivity to horse serum. If no sensitivity is evident, antivenin should be given intravenously as soon as possible after onset of symptoms. Several ampules may be necessary to control the envenomation. Infiltration of tissues of fingers or toes with antivenin may prove damaging. Except in extreme emergency, untrained persons should not attempt such measures as incision and suction and administration of antivenin.

During most of the early hospitalization period, immobilization of the bitten limb in a position of function should be continued. Ice bags may be applied locally to relieve pain. Active and passive exercise to prevent contracture should be started as soon as the patient's condition permits. In serious cases, specific antivenin should be given intravenously. Electrolyte balance should be maintained. Use of corticosteroids should be restricted to prevention of late manifestations of allergy following administration of antivenin. In severe cases of viper bite, blood transfusions may be necessary. A tetanus toxoid booster should be given on admission, if this was not previously given as a first aid measure. Antibiotics should be used if the case is severe. Paralysis may follow bites by such elapid snakes as cobras and kraits. In such cases, tracheotomy and intermittent positive pressure artificial respiration may be necessary. Since renal shutdown sometimes occurs as a result of massive envenomation, daily tests such as blood urea nitrogen (BUN), carbon dioxide combining power, and serum potassium levels are indicated in severe cases.

Many problems remain in the field of snakebite treatment. One of the most important of these is the improvement of antivenins. Even when specific antivenins are administered, several ampules of 10 ml or more each may be required in treatment of severe cases. Even though antivenins may save lives, they often do not prevent local necrosis, which may be crippling. Many antivenins produced today are of rather narrow specificity and neutralize only the venoms that were used in their preparation. Relationship of snake species involved is not a safe criterion for judging potential value of an antivenin in snakebite treatment.

Antivenin (Crotalidae) Polyvalent (Wyeth) contains protective substances against the venoms of the crotalids (pit vipers) of North and South America. This antivenin has therapeutic value for envenomation by the rattlesnakes (*Crotalus* spp. and *Sistrurus* spp.), cottonmouths and copperheads (*Agkistrodon* spp.) of the United States, and Old World species of *Agkistrodon (e.g. Agkistrodon halys* Pall. and *Agkistrodon halys blomhoffi* Boie of Korea and Japan); the fer-de-lance (*Bothrops atrox* Linn.) and other species of *Bothrops,* the tropical rattler [*Crotalus durissus terrificus* (Laurenti) and allied species], the cantil [*Agkistrodon bilineatus* (Wied.)], and the bushmaster *(Lachesis mutus* Linn.) of Central and South America; and the habu (*Timeresurus* spp.) of the Pacific Islands and Southeast Asia. It must be noted that the Wyeth product is not as effective in neutralization of venoms of the Asian pit vipers as are specific antivenins now produced in Japan and on Okinawa.

The desirability of the use of cryotherapy has been debated for some time. Its improper use can be severely damaging to tissues, especially when a tourniquet is employed. Some authorities recommend the use of cold for relief of pain. It has been demonstrated in the laboratory that cold slowed down spread of viper venom in experimental animals. Advisability of use of corticosteroids, antihistamines and other substances in treatment of snakebite has been a matter of some controversy for years. It has been found that the administration of adrenocorticotropic hormone (ACTH), cortisone, hydrocortisone and antihistamines against snake venoms, given at higher but sublethal doses, actually increased toxicity of pit viper venom for mice.

Recently, workers in Japan and in the United States have reported that dihydrolipoic acid and EDTA each have shown promise in prevention of local necrosis due to snakebite. Although coral snake antivenins have been produced for some time in Brazil and in Costa Rica, it was not until 1968 that an antivenin became available against venom of the North American coral snake *Micrurus fulvius.* This product, developed as a public service by Wyeth Laboratories, has been distributed to selected hospitals and health care centers in states where the coral snake occurs. In addition, a supply is available at the Center for Disease Control, Atlanta, Georgia.

Prophylaxis. Persons who must go into the field where venomous snakes occur should wear protective clothing, including stout boots with trouser legs tucked into them. Particular care should be taken at night, when many snakes emerge from daytime hiding places and are found in fields, along roads, and even in housing areas. Many accidents occur when persons try to catch venomous snakes, or when they handle supposedly dead specimens carelessly. Even the recently severed head of a snake should be handled with caution.

Bats

The vampire bats of the American tropics and other species of both tropical and temperate regions are of public heath importance because they sometimes transmit rabies to man (p. 48) and also because soil enriched with bat guano is a source of histoplasmosis infection of man (p. 292). Additionally, more than a score of viruses have been recovered from bats, although the role of bats in the transmission of these agents to man is not well understood.[10]

Vampire Bats. Vampire bats occur in tropical parts of Mexico, and Central and South America including Trinidad. They are small creatures, only 3 inches long, and have incisors modified for cutting skin. Their undisturbed bite is painless and they feed on blood.

In parts of Mexico, vampire bats transmit a modified form of rabies virus to cattle, causing a disease in these hosts long familiar to the ranchers as derriengue. It has been estimated that several hundred thousand cattle a year die of vampire-borne rabies in Latin America. Human rabies deaths caused by bites of vampire bats, although not frequent, are reported from Mexico, Trinidad, Guyana, Brazil, Bolivia and Argentina. There is limited evidence that vampire bats may be involved in the transmission of Venezuelan equine encephalitis in some circumstances.

Screened quarters or bed nets afford protection against the nocturnal visits of vampire bats. Their numbers can be reduced by destroying them when their daytime roosts can be found in caves and hollow trees near human habitations.

Other Bats. Within recent years rabies-infected insectivorous and frugivorous bats of a number of species have been found in temperate as well as tropical regions. Human cases of rabies have been reported in the United States when curious persons have picked up apparently disabled bats or, occasionally, after a bat has made an unprovoked attack. There is evidence that these bats infect each other, as young flightless bats associated only with older bats in roosts have been found infected. Geographic spread of the virus may be effected by migratory bat species, since the course of the disease and the period of liberation of the virus in saliva are often prolonged. It has been demonstrated experimentally that foxes and coyotes developed rabies after exposure to the air in a cave with a large colony of bats, and two human rabies fatalities have been reported following such exposure in a cave in Texas densely populated with Mexican free-tailed bats *(Tadarida brasiliensis)*.

Bites by bats, even though of nonhematophagous species, should be carefully avoided. Bats found alive in the open in daytime should be treated with great caution. If possible, they should be pushed into a container with a stick and sent to a qualified laboratory for examination for rabies. Persons already bitten should proceed as in the case of dog bite. (See p. 49.) Random attacks by rabid insectivorous bats may be unavoidable. However, roosting colonies of those species in buildings or in caves may be controlled by screening or plugging the openings by which they enter in the first instance, or by the use of insecticides in both cases. Bats that have been exposed to DDT or other insecticides may display tremors and lack of coordination. In the past this has led to submission of large numbers of specimens to laboratories for examination for rabies.

Histoplasma capsulatum has been frequently isolated from soils with a high organic content such as that found under bird or bat roosts. Numbers of human cases of histoplasmosis have been reported in persons exposed to bat guano both in caves and in association with bat colonies in houses. These episodes have occurred in the United States as well as the New and Old World tropics. Care should be exercised in these situations to avoid inhalation of dust from guano or soil-guano mixtures.

The role of nonhematophagous bats in the natural history of a number of viruses other than rabies is as yet obscure. There have been more than a dozen arboviruses isolated from bats as well as several uncharacterized viruses. Agents such as Rio Bravo and Montana myotis leukoencephalitis viruses in the United States and Dakar bat, Mt. Elgon and Entebbe viruses in Africa have been isolated from bat salivary glands, implying a possible transmission route by bite.

One suggested mechanism for the overwintering of certain of the arboviruses of temperate regions is that bats infected in the fall maintain the infection at low levels during the period of reduced metabolism while hibernating. They again experience viremias capable of infecting vector mosquitoes in the spring.

REFERENCES

1. Southcott, R. V. 1963. Coelenterates of medical importance. *In* Venomous and Poisonous Animals and Noxious Plants of the Pacific Region. A Symposium Volume from Proceedings of the 10th Pacific Congress, Pergamon Press, Oxford, England. pp. 41–45.
2. Keegan, H. L., Toshioka, S., and Suzuki, H. 1968. Blood sucking Asian leeches of families Hirudidae and Haemadipsidae. Special report, 496th Medical Laboratory, U.S. Army Medical Command, Japan. 130 pp.

3. Halstead, B. W., and Mitchell, L. R. 1963. A review of the venomous fishes of the Pacific area. *In* Venomous and Poisonous Animals and Noxious Plants of the Pacific Region. A Symposium Volume from Proceedings of the 10th Pacific Congress. Pergamon Press, Oxford, England. pp. 173–202.
4. Halstead, B. W. 1959. Dangerous Marine Animals. Cornell Maritime Press, Cambridge, Maryland. 146 pp.
5. Swaroop, S., and Grab, B. 1954. Snake bite mortality in the world. Bull. W.H.O. *10*:35–76.
6. Werler, J. E., and Keegan, H. L. 1963. Venomous snakes of the Pacific area. *In* Venomous and Poisonous Animals and Noxious Plants of the Pacific Region. A Symposium Volume from Proceedings of the 10th Pacific Congress. Pergamon Press, Oxford, England. pp. 219–325.
7. Minton, S. A. (ed.). 1971. Snake Venoms and Envenomation. Marcel Dekker, Inc., New York. 188 pp.
8. Seeley, S. F. 1963. Special Communication—Ad Hoc Committee on Snake-bite Therapy Report. Toxicon *1*:81–87.
9. Parrish, H. M. 1966. Incidence of treated snakebites in the United States. Pub. Hlth. Rept. *81*:269–276.
10. Constantine, D. G. 1970. Bats in relation to the health, welfare, and economy of man. *In* Wimsatt, W. A. (ed.): Biology of Bats. Vol. 2. Academic Press, New York. pp. 319–449.

SECTION XI
Medically Important Arthropods

CHAPTER 68
Introduction

HAROLD D. NEWSON

The phylum ARTHROPODA contains more species than all the other phyla of the animal kingdom and its members are highly diversified and widely distributed. They are characterized as possessing bilateral symmetry, metameric segmentation, jointed appendages and a hard chitinous exoskeleton. However, not all of these characteristics are readily apparent in every group included in this phylum. Digestive, vascular, excretory and nervous systems are developed in most groups and reproduction usually is sexual although parthenogenesis may occur. Five classes of arthropods are of significant medical importance: CHILOPODA—centipedes; CRUSTACEA—crabs, crayfish, lobsters, shrimp and related groups; PENTASTOMIDA—tongue worms; INSECTA—insects; and ARACHNIDA—spiders, scorpions, ticks and mites. Representatives of these classes are illustrated in Figure 68-1.

CLASS CHILOPODA

Centipedes are wormlike in appearance, have a distinct head with a pair of antennae, and their individual body segments are somewhat flattened. They vary in length from 5 to 25 cm and have a single pair of well developed legs on most of their body segments. Most species feed upon insects and small animals. A pair of poisonous claws, located on the first segment posterior to the head, is used in obtaining food and for self defense. Few of the smaller species can penetrate human skin with these claws; those that can inflict a bite seldom produce more than localized pain, erythema and, occasionally, induration. Larger species, however, may inflict very painful bites that produce local necrotic lesions and mild systemic reactions such as headache, fever and nausea. Extreme fear concerning the toxicity of these bites to humans is not warranted. One death, of a 7-year-old child, has been reported due to a centipede bite; however, the overwhelming majority of published records indicates that they rarely cause more than an immediate localized pain that rapidly diminishes, much like a bee sting. Injection of a local anesthetic in the vicinity of the bite wound usually will provide immediate relief from even severe pain. Necrotic lesions, should they develop, may require surgical dressings. Systemic reactions normally are alleviated by bed rest and treatment with analgesics.

CLASS DIPLOPODA

Millipedes may be confused with centipedes, since their superficial appearance is similar. They differ in that their bodies are more cylindrical than centipedes and most apparent body segments possess two pairs of appendages. The members of this group are

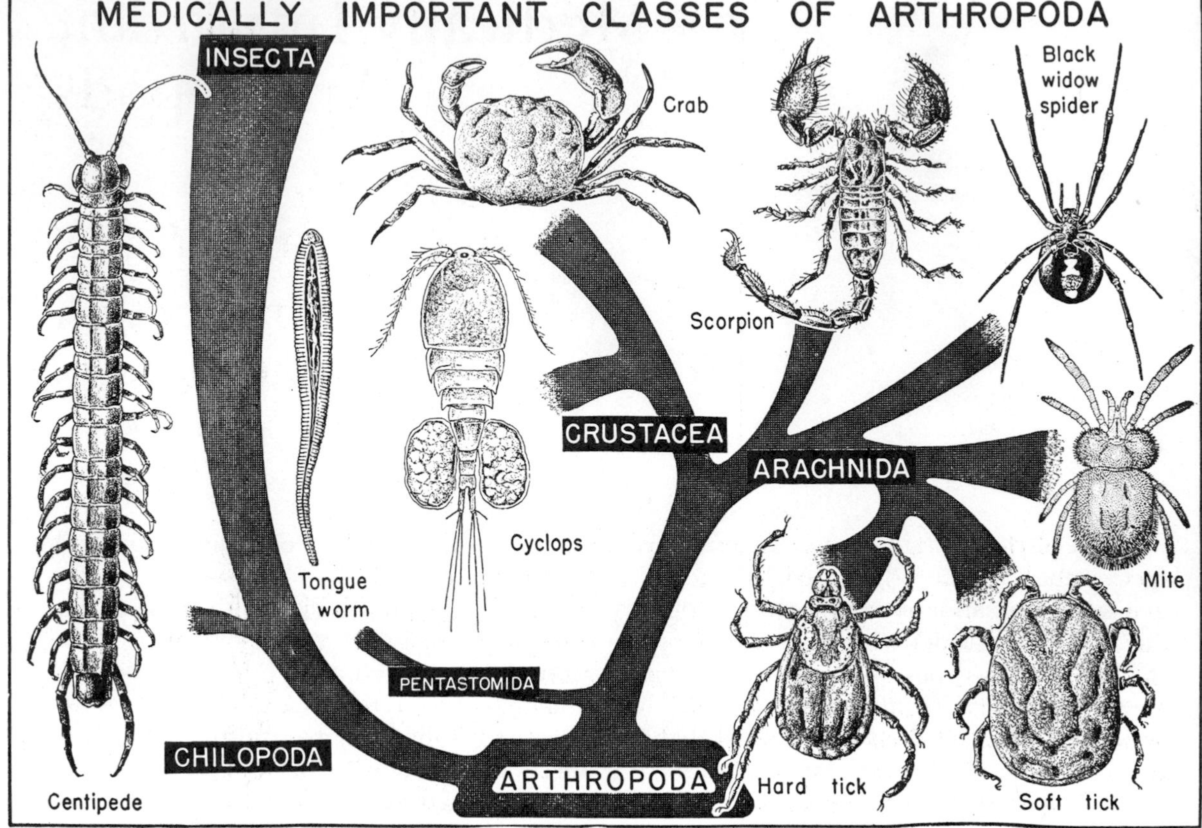

Figure 68–1. Medically important classes of ARTHROPODA—selected examples.

vegetarians and lack the poisonous claws of the centipedes. Some millipedes produce secretions that can cause contact vesicular dermatitis, but human cases are rare.

CLASS CRUSTACEA

Several aquatic species of crustaceans are involved in the life cycles of certain human and animal parasites. Freshwater copepods of the genera *Cyclops* and *Diaptomus* are intermediate hosts for the broad tapeworm, *Diphyllobothrium latum* (p. 598). *Cyclops* spp. also serve similar roles in the development of the Guinea worm, *Dracunculus medinensis* (p. 521), and the animal nematode, *Gnathostoma spinigerum* (p. 533). The ingestion of *Cyclops* infected with the procercoid form of several animal cestodes may produce sparganosis in humans (p. 602). Species of freshwater crabs and crayfish are second intermediate hosts of the lung fluke, *Paragonimus westermani,* and serve as the source of human infections in areas where infected crustacean hosts are eaten raw (p. 588). Details concerning these parasitic relationships are given in earlier sections of the book and in Table 68–1.

CLASS PENTASTOMIDA

The adults of these degenerate wormlike arthropods parasitize the nasal passages of reptiles, birds and mammals but rarely occur in humans. Human infections of both

(*Text continued on p. 711*)

Table 68–1. Human Diseases Transmitted by Arthropods

Disease	*Etiologic Agent*	*Geographic Distribution*	*Vector*	*Reservoir*	*Location of Etiologic Agent in Man*	*Diagnostic Procedures*
HELMINTHIC DISEASES						
Loiasis	*Loa loa*	Tropical Africa, especially Congo River basin	Mango flies (*Chrysops dimidiata* and *C. silacea*)	Man	Subcutaneous tissues; microfilariae in blood	Clinical picture; worm beneath skin; blood exam., day
Filariasis	*Wuchereria bancrofti, Brugia malayi*	Tropical Africa, Asia, Australia, South America, Pacific and Caribbean Islands	Mosquitoes (*Culex, Aedes, Anopheles* and *Mansonia* spp.)	Man	Lymph nodes and vessels; microfilariae in blood	Clinical picture; worms in lymph nodes; microfilariae in blood or chyle
Onchocerciasis	*Onchocerca volvulus*	Africa, Mexico, Central America, Venezuela, Colombia, Brazil	Blackflies (*Simulium* spp.)	Man	Nodules and tumors; microfilariae in skin, eyes	Biopsy of skin and nodule; puncture of tumors and nodules
(1) Ozzard's filariasis (2) Dipetalonemiasis	(1) *Mansonella ozzardi* (2) *Dipetalonema perstans*	(1) Latin America (2) Latin America and Africa	Midges (*Culicoides* spp.)	Man	Microfilariae in peripheral blood; occasionally pathogenic	Blood smear
Dracunculiasis	*Dracunculus medinensis*	Africa, India, U.S.S.R., Middle East	*Cyclops* spp.	Man	Loose connective tissue	Roentgenograms
Diphyllobothriasis	*Diphyllobothrium latum*	Northern Europe, northern U.S.A., U.S.S.R.	Copepods (*Diaptomus* and *Cyclops*)	Man, dog, cat, fox, bear, others	Intestine	Fecal examination
Sparganosis	Spargana of several species of tapeworms, e.g. *Spirometra mansonoides*	Asia, scattered areas including Holland, Guyana, U.S.A., Colombia, Uruguay, Angola	*Cyclops* spp.	Man,* frogs, snakes, birds, mammals	Subcutaneous tissues	Excision (?)
Dipylidiasis	*Dipylidium caninum*	Europe, Asia, U.S.A., Africa, Pacific Islands, Chile	Fleas and possibly lice of dogs	Man, dog	Intestine	Fecal examination
Hymenolepiasis diminuta	*Hymenolepis diminuta*	India, U.S.S.R., Japan, Italy, U.S.A., Chile	Fleas, cockroaches, mealworms	Man, rat, mouse	Intestine	Fecal examination
Hymenolepiasis nana	*Hymenolepis nana*	Cosmopolitan	Fleas (?), mealworms (?)	Man, mouse	Intestine	Fecal examination
Paragonimiasis	*Paragonimus westermani, P. ohirai, Paragonimus* spp.	Far East, Asia, Africa, C. and S. America	Freshwater crabs and crayfish	Man, carnivores	Primarily lungs	Examination of sputum and feces
PROTOZOAL DISEASES						
Malaria	*Plasmodium vivax, P. malariae, P. falciparum, P. ovale*	Worldwide (see exceptions in certain Pacific Islands, Arctic, Antarctic)	Mosquitoes (*Anopheles* spp.)	Man	Erythrocytes; hepatic parenchyma	Blood smear
African sleeping sickness	*Trypanosoma gambiense, T. rhodesiense*	Africa	Tsetse flies (*Glossina* spp.)	Man, game	Peripheral blood, lymph nodes, spinal fluid	Stained blood smear or fresh preparation; lumbar puncture; lymph node puncture

*Maturity not reached in man.

Table continued on the following page

Table 68–1. Human Diseases Transmitted by Arthropods (*Continued*)

Disease	*Etiologic Agent*	*Geographic Distribution*	*Vector*	*Reservoir*	*Location of Etiologic Agent in Man*	*Diagnostic Procedures*
Chagas' disease (South American trypanosomiasis)	*Trypanosoma cruzi*	South America, Central America, Mexico, U.S.A.	Kissing bugs (*Triatoma, Panstrongylus, Rhodnius, Eutriatoma* spp.)	Armadillo, opossum, dogs, cats, rodents, others	Peripheral blood, heart muscle	Blood smear and culture (NNN); complement-fixation; animal inoculation; xenodiagnosis
Kala-azar (visceral leishmaniasis)	*Leishmania donovani*	China, India, Mediterranean, South America, Central America	Sandflies (*Phlebotomus* and *Lutzomyia* spp.)	Man, dogs, jackals	Spleen, liver, bone marrow, reticuloendothelial system	Sternal marrow biopsy, splenic puncture, blood culture (NNN)
Old World cutaneous leishmaniasis (Oriental sore)						
Rural—moist	*Leishmania tropica var. major*	Mediterranean, Asia Minor, India, China	Sandflies (*Phlebotomus* spp.)	Gerbil	Skin lesions	Smear and culture of lesions (NNN)
Urban—dry	*Leishmania tropica var. minor*			Dog, man		
New World cutaneous leishmaniasis						
Chiclero ulcer	*Leishmania mexicana*	Latin America	Sandflies (*Lutzomyia* spp.)	Forest rodent	Skin and mucous membrane lesions	Smear and culture of lesions (NNN)
Espundia	*Leishmania braziliensis*					
Uta	*Leishmania braziliensis*			Forest rodent		Montenegro intradermal test
Leishmaniasis tegumentaria diffusa	(Anergy of host)			Dog		
			SPIROCHETAL DISEASES			
Relapsing fever, louse-borne	*Borrelia recurrentis*	Europe, Asia, Africa	Human body louse (*Pediculus humanus humanus*)	Man	Peripheral blood	Direct and dark field exam., and animal inoculation of blood
Relapsing fever, tickborne (see Table 15–1, p. 140)	*Borrelia duttonii, Borrelia* spp.	Africa, America, Europe, Asia	Soft ticks (*Ornithodoros* spp.)	Ticks, rodents and other mammals	Peripheral blood	Direct and dark field exam., and animal inoculation of blood
Yaws	*Treponema pertenue*	Tropics	Eye gnat (*Hippelates* sp.), flies (*Musca* spp.)	Man	Skin lesions	Clinical picture, Kahn test
			BACTERIAL DISEASES			
Bubonic plague	*Yersinia pestis*	Cosmopolitan	Rodent fleas, especially *Xenopsylla* spp.	Rats and wild rodents	Blood stream, lymph nodes	Lymph node puncture, blood culture
Tularemia	*Francisella tularensis*	United States, Canada, Japan, Russia, Europe, Turkey	Hard ticks (*Dermacentor andersoni* and *D. variabilis*); deer fly (*Chrysops discalis*)	Rabbit and other wild animals	Blood stream, lymph nodes, skin lesions	Clinical picture, agglutination, animal inoculation
Verruga peruana (Oroya fever, bartonellosis)	*Bartonella bacilliformis*	Peru, Colombia, Ecuador: altitude 520–3200 m.	Sandflies (*Lutzomyia* spp.)	Man	Erythrocytes, reticuloendothelial system	Clinical picture, blood smear and culture, perhaps biopsy of skin lesion
Catarrhal conjunctivitis	Koch-Weeks bacillus (?)	Tropical and temperate regions, especially Egypt	Eye gnats (*Hippelates* spp., *Siphunculina* spp.); mechanical transmission	Man	Conjunctiva	Clinical picture, smear of exudate

RICKETTSIAL DISEASES

Epidemic typhus, Brill-Zinsser disease	*Rickettsia prowazekii*	All continents except Australia	Human body louse (*Pediculus humanus humanus*)	Man	Intracellular (intracytoplasmic)	Clinical picture, Weil-Felix test, specific complement-fixation and agglutination
Murine typhus	*Rickettsia typhi*	All continents	Rat fleas, especially *Xenopsylla cheopis*, also *X. astia* and *Nosopsyllus fasciatus*	Rats	Intracellular (intracytoplasmic)	
American spotted fever	*Rickettsia rickettsii*	Canada, United States, Mexico, Panama, Colombia, Brazil	Ticks: *Dermacentor andersoni, D. variabilis, Amblyomma americanum.* In Mexico, *Rhipicephalus sanguineus* and *A. cajennense.* In South America, *A. cajennense* principally	Rodents (?), ticks	Intracellular (intranuclear)	Clinical picture, Weil-Felix test, complement-fixation
Fièvre boutonneuse (including Kenya typhus, South African tickbite fever and Indian tick typhus)	*Rickettsia conorii*	Mediterranean, Crimea, Africa, India	Ticks: *Rhipicephalus sanguineus, R. evertsi, Amblyomma hebraeum, Haemaphysalis leachi* and probably others, in appropriate geographic areas	Ticks, dogs (?), wild animals (?)	Initial lesion and lymphatics, endothelial cells	Clinical picture, Weil-Felix test
Queensland tick typhus	*Rickettsia australis*	Queensland	*Ixodes holocyclus (?)*	Small marsupials (?)	Intracellular (intranuclear)	Clinical picture; Weil-Felix test; complement-fixation
Asian tick typhus (Siberian tick typhus)	*Rickettsia sibirica*	Siberia, Armenia, Central Asia, Mongolia	Ticks: *Dermacentor silvarum, D. nuttalli, Haemaphysalis concinna, H. asiaticum* and others	Ticks, rodents (?)	Blood (and probably tissues)	Clinical picture, Weil-Felix test
Scrub typhus (tsutsugamushi disease)	*Rickettsia tsutsugamushi*	Various Asiatic-Pacific areas	Trombiculid mites (chiggers): *Leptotrombidium deliense* group	Mites, field rats and other small mammals	Intracellular	Clinical picture, Weil-Felix test
Q fever	*Coxiella burnetii*	Australia, North America, Panama, Europe, Middle East, Africa, China (?)	Rickettsiae present in certain ticks, but tick transmission to man is rare	Ticks, cattle, sheep, goats, and probably certain wild animals	Intracellular	Isolate rickettsiae; complement-fixation and agglutination with Q rickettsial antigen; no Weil-Felix
Rickettsialpox	*Rickettsia akari*	Northeastern United States, Korea, U.S.S.R	Mite: *Liponyssoides sanguineus*	House mice (*Mus musculus*), wild rodents	Intracellular (intranuclear)	Clinical picture; isolate rickettsiae; complement-fixation
Trench fever	*Rochalimaea quintana*	Europe	Human body louse (*Pediculus humanus humanus*)	Man	Blood, urine	Clinical picture, no Weil-Felix

Table continued on the following page

Table 68–1. HUMAN DISEASES TRANSMITTED BY ARTHROPODS (*Continued*)

VIRUS DISEASES* Revised by Dr. H. Trapido

Disease	*Etiologic Agent*	*Geographic Distribution*	*Vector*	*Reservoir*	*Location of Etiologic Agent in Man*	*Diagnostic Procedures*
Eastern equine encephalitis	Arbovirus, Group A	United States, Canada, Mexico, Panama, Jamaica, Dominican Republic, Trinidad, S. America to Argentina	Mosquitoes [In U.S. principally *Aedes sollicitans* (epidemic) and *Culiseta melanura* (enzootic); others in tropics]	Wild birds	Central nervous system	
Western equine encephalitis	Arbovirus, Group A	United States, southern Canada, Mexico, Guyana, Brazil, Argentina	Mosquitoes (In western U.S. *Culex tarsalis;* others in South America)	Wild birds	Central nervous system	
Venezuelan equine encephalitis	Arbovirus, Group A	South America, Trinidad, Panama, Central America, Mexico to S. Texas and S. Florida	Mosquitoes [Enzootic, *Culex* (*Melanoconion*) spp.; epidemic, many species of several genera]	Rodents, perhaps also wild birds and bats. Equines are amplifying hosts	Blood and central nervous system	Attempt virus isolation as early as possible in clinical course; serologic tests with paired acute and convalescent sera
Mayaro	Arbovirus, Group A	Trinidad, Brazil, northern South America, Panama and Central America	Mosquitoes (*Haemagogus* .spp. and others)	Rodents (?)	Blood	
Sindbis	Arbovirus, Group A	Africa, East and S.E. Asia, Philippines and Australia	Mosquitoes (*Culex univittatus, C. antennatus* and others)	Wild and domestic birds and mammals (?)	?	
Chikungunya	Arbovirus, Group A	Africa, India, S.E. Asia and Philippines	Mosquitoes (*Aedes aegypti, Ae. africanus, Culex* spp., and *Mansonia* spp.)	Non-human primates (?)	Blood	
O'nyong-nyong	Arbovirus, Group A	East Africa	Mosquitoes (*Anopheles funestus* and *An. gambiae*)	?	Blood	
Ross River	Arbovirus, Group A	Australia	Mosquitoes (*Aedes vigilax*)	?	?	
Yellow fever – urban	Arbovirus, Group B	South and Central America, Africa	Mosquitoes (*Aedes aegypti*)	Man	Blood early in clinical course, liver and kidney	Clinical picture in severe cases; autopsy findings; virus isolation; serologic tests with paired acute and convalescent sera
Yellow fever – jungle	Same virus as above	South and Central America, Africa	Mosquitoes (*Haemagogus* spp. and *Sabethes chloropterus* in S.A.: *Aedes simpsoni* and *Aedes* spp. in Africa)	Monkeys and perhaps other jungle mammals	Same as above	

Dengue: Types 1–4	Arbovirus, Group B	Tropics and subtropics. With hemorrhagic syndrome in S.E. Asia and Philippine Islands	Mosquitoes [*Aedes aegypti* and other *Aedes (Stegomyia)* spp.]	Man (?)	Blood early in clinical course	Attempt virus isolation as early as possible in clinical course; serologic tests with paired acute and convalescent sera
Japanese B encephalitis	Arbovirus, Group B	Far East and S.E. Asia, including Indonesia and India	Mosquitoes (*Culex tritaeniorhynchus, C. gelidus* and others)	Wild birds, pigs, others (?)	Central nervous system	
Murray Valley encephalitis	Arbovirus, Group B	Australia, island of New Guinea	Mosquitoes (*Culex annulirostris, C. bitaeniorhynchus, Aedes normanensis*)	Wild birds (?)	Central nervous system	
West Nile fever	Arbovirus, Group B	Africa, Middle East, South Asia and southern Europe	Mosquitoes (*Culex univittatus, Culex pipiens, C.* spp., *Mansonia metallica*); ticks (*Argas reflexus hermanni*)	Wild birds	Blood	Attempt virus isolation as early as possible in clinical course; serologic tests with paired acute and convalescent sera
St. Louis encephalitis	Arbovirus, Group B	United States, Jamaica, Trinidad, Panama, Brazil	Mosquitoes (In U.S. *Culex p. quinquefasciatus, C. tarsalis, C. nigripalpus;* in tropics *Culex nigripalpus* and others)	Wild birds	Central nervous system; blood (rarely)	
Ilheus	Arbovirus, Group B	Brazil, Trinidad, northern South America, Panama, and Central America	Mosquitoes (*Psorophora ferox, P.* spp., *Aedes* spp., *Culex* spp. and others)	Wild birds (?)	Blood	
Russian spring-summer encephalitis	Arbovirus, Group B	U.S.S.R.	Ticks (*Ixodes persulcatus* and others)	Wild and domestic mammals	Central nervous system	
Central European tick-borne encephalitis	Arbovirus, Group B	Central Europe	Ticks (*Ixodes ricinus* and others)	Wild mammals and birds, goats	Central nervous system	
Kyasanur forest disease	Arbovirus, Group B	India	Ticks (*Haemaphysalis spinigera* and others)	Wild mammals and birds	Blood	
Omsk hemorrhagic fever	Arbovirus, Group B	Western Siberia	Ticks (*Ixodes persulcatus* and others)	Wild mammals and birds	Blood	
Louping ill	Arbovirus, Group B	Scotland, England, Ireland	Tick (*Ixodes ricinus*)	Wild mammals and birds; sheep	Central nervous system	
Powassan	Arbovirus, Group B	Canada, northern United States	Ticks (*Ixodes* spp.)	Wild mammals	Central nervous system	
Negishi	Arbovirus, Group B	Japan	Ticks (?)	?	Central nervous system	
Oropouche	Arbovirus, Group Simbu	Brazil, Trinidad	Mosquitoes (*Culex p. quinquefasciatus* and others?)	?	Blood	
Bwamba	Arbovirus, Group Bwamba	Africa, south of the Sahara	Mosquitoes (?)	Monkeys (?)	Blood	
California encephalitis (California, La Crosse and Tahyna types)	Arbovirus, Group California	United States (California and La Crosse types), Europe and Africa (Tahyna type)	Mosquitoes (*Aedes triseriatus* for La Crosse type; *Aedes melanimon* and *Culex* spp. for California type; *Aedes* spp. for Tahyna type)	Wild mammals	Central nervous system	

Table continued on the following page

Table 68–1. Human Diseases Transmitted by Arthropods (*Continued*)

Disease	*Etiologic Agent*	*Geographic Distribution*	*Vector*	*Reservoir*	*Location of Etiologic Agent in Man*	*Diagnostic Procedures*
Naples and Sicilian sandfly fevers	Arboviruses, Group sandfly fever	Old World tropics and subtropics	Sandflies (*Phlebotomus papatasi* and others)	Sandflies, man (?)	Blood	
Candiru, Chagres, and Punta Toro fevers	Arboviruses, Group sandfly fever	Brazil and Panama	Sandflies (*Lutzomyia* spp.)	?	Blood	
Vesicular stomatitis, Indiana type and others	Arboviruses, Group vesicular stomatitis	Tropics, subtropics and temperate regions	Sandflies (*Lutzomyia* spp. for Indiana type in American tropics; arthropod transmission inconclusive elsewhere)	Tropical forest mammals for Indiana type; cattle, horses, pigs for others	Blood (rare)	Attempt virus isolation as early as possible in clinical course; serologic tests with paired acute and convalescent sera
Rift Valley fever	Arbovirus, Ungrouped	Africa	Mosquitoes (*Eretmapodites* spp., *Aedes* spp. and others)	Cattle (?), sheep (?)	Blood	
Colorado tick fever	Arbovirus, Ungrouped	Northwestern United States	Ticks (*Dermacentor andersoni* and others)	Wild rodents and porcupine	Blood	
Congo (Crimean hemorrhagic fever)	Arbovirus, Ungrouped	Africa and southern U.S.S.R.	Ticks (*Hyalomma* spp. and *Amblyomma* spp.)	?	Blood	
MISCELLANEOUS						
Enteric diseases: typhoid, bacillary and amebic dysentery, diarrheas, Asiatic cholera, certain helminthic infections		Differs in various regions	Houseflies (*Musca domestica*) et al. frequenting human excrement and food; mechanical transmission	Man	Intestines	Clinical picture, stool exam. and culture
Human bots (myiasis)	*Dermatobia hominis*	American tropics	Flies, mosquitoes, blood-sucking arthropods	Various mammals, birds	Superficial layers of skin	Appearance of lesion; excision

*Additional arboviruses known to have produced naturally acquired human disease thought to be transmitted by mosquitoes are: Bussuquara (Brazil, Colombia, Panama), Spondweni (Africa), Wesselsbron (Africa), Zika (Africa, Malaya) of Group B; Bunyamwera (Africa), Ilesha (Africa), Germiston (Africa), Guaroa (South America, Panama and Central America) of the Bunyamwera Group; Apeu, Caraparu, Itaqui, Madrid, Marituba, Murutucu, Oriboca, Ossa, and Restan, all of Group C from Brazil, Trinidad, Surinam and Panama; Guama and Catu of the Guama group from Brazil, Trinidad and Panama. Other ungrouped arboviruses associated with human disease are: Quaranfil from Africa, isolated from argasid ticks; Nairobi sheep disease from Africa for which the vector is unknown; Kemerovo from western Siberia and Egypt, isolated from the tick *Ixodes persulcatus*. For further information on these and other arthropod-borne viruses which may infect man see Theiler and Downs.[7]

Table 68–2. ENVENOMIZATION (INCLUDING ALLERGIES)

Common Name	*Scientific Name (or Group)*	*Distribution*	*Important Effects on Man*	*Remarks*
Mites:				
Chiggers	*Eutrombicula alfreddugesi* and other trombiculine larvae	Tropics and warmer temperate regions	Intense itching; dermatitis; purplish ecchymoses	Avoid by use of protective clothing (impregnated with miticides, e.g. diethyltoluamide or dimethyl phthalate); application of miticidal insect repellents
Cheese and flour mites	Several genera of ACARIDAE (TYROGLYPHIDAE)	Worldwide	Dermatitis; allergic phenomena from contact with bodies of dead mites	Infestation usually limited to handlers of dry food products
Rat and bird mites	*Ornithonyssus* spp. and others	Worldwide	Dermatitis; intense itching; hemorrhagic areas	Infest persons who work or loiter in rat and bird infested premises
Grain itch mites	*Pyemotes ventricosus*	Widespread	Dermatitis and fever	Infest threshers and persons who sleep on or work with straw
Ticks:				
Soft ticks	*Ornithodoros* spp.	All continents	Local and systemic reactions: some species (*O. coriaceus*) extremely venomous	Avoid rest houses, rodent burrows, mountain homes
Hard ticks	*Dermacentor andersoni*	Western Canada Western U.S.A.	Tick paralysis	Removal of ticks very important; otherwise usually fatal (applies to all three)
	D. variabilis	Central and Eastern U.S.A.	Tick paralysis	
	Ixodes spp.	Widespread	Tick paralysis	
	Amblyomma spp.	Tropical and subtropical		
Widow spiders	*Latrodectus mactans*	The Americas	Abdominal rigidity; intense pain	See p. 714
	Latrodectus spp.	Widespread		
Other venomous spiders	*Loxosceles reclusus*, *L. unicolor*, *L. laeta* and other *Loxosceles* spp. (?)	N. America S. America	Necrotic lesion, fever, rash, hemoglobinuria Gangrenous spot	Corticosteroids and antihistamines may be useful
	Lycosa raptoria	S. America, esp. Brazil	Necrosis, pain, swelling	Necrotic arachnidism
	Phoneutria fera	Brazil	Central and peripheral nervous symptoms	Specific antiserum, symptomatic treatment with analgesics and antihistamines in early stages
	Atrax formidabilis *A. robustus*	Australia	Severe symptoms which may result in death.	
	Chiracanthium spp.	United States	Painful localized symptoms	
Scorpions	Order: SCORPIONIDA	Tropics and subtropics	Painful sting; neurotoxin and hemolysin injected; sometimes fatal	Specific antiserum is helpful; other treatment empirical
Centipedes	Class: CHILOPODA	Warmer regions	Painful bite; local necrosis; generalized symptoms	Give sedatives; apply dilute ammonia, locally; local anesthetic
Insects:				
Mayflies	Order: EPHEMEROPTERA	Worldwide	Asthmatic paroxysms from inhalation of insect fragments	Desensitization perhaps feasible
Caddis flies	Order: TRICHOPTERA	Worldwide	Asthmatic symptoms from inhalation of hairs and scales	Desensitization perhaps feasible
Kissing bugs (cone noses)	Fam: REDUVIIDAE	Worldwide	Painful bites, with more or less local edema and inflammation	Symptoms vary with species; may be due to Chagas' disease
Blister beetles (and others)	Fam: MELOIDAE	Worldwide	Severe blisters (from cantharidin)	Symptoms result from crushing insects on skin; apply soothing lotions (applies to all four families)
	Fam: STAPHYLINIDAE	Worldwide	Delayed blistering effect	
	Fam: PAUSSIDAE	Worldwide		
	Fam: OEDEMERIDAE	Mid-Pacific and Caribbean Islands	Severe blistering	
Caterpillars (with urticating hairs and spines)	Order: LEPIDOPTERA (several families)	Worldwide	Pain, urticaria, rash and generalized symptoms on contact with hairs or spines	Codeine; alkaline compresses useful; supportive treatment sometimes necessary
Bees, wasps, certain ants	Order: HYMENOPTERA (several families)	Worldwide	Painful stings; local swelling, sometimes anaphylaxis (certain ants *bite* rather than sting)	Apply soothing lotions; administer epinephrine subcutaneously for anaphylaxis

Table 68–3. Dermatoses of Arthropod Origin

Common Name of Arthropod	*Scientific Name (or Group)*	*Distribution*	*Effects on Man*	*Remarks*
Itch Mites (scabies) (Also, see Mites, Table 68–2.)	*Sarcoptes scabiei*	Worldwide	Burrows in skin, causing chronic dermatosis (acariasis)	Transmitted by direct contact. Benzyl benzoate, Eurax, Kwell are effective.
Hard ticks	*Ixodes* spp.	Worldwide	Cause extreme annoyance	Protective clothing helpful. DDT effective against larval forms. Vectors of certain rickettsial and viral diseases.
	Dermacentor spp.	Worldwide		
	Amblyomma spp.	Widespread		
	Hyalomma spp.	Old World		
	Haemaphysalis spp.	Old World		
Springtails	Order: Collembola (Several species)	Worldwide	Sharp bites, followed by pruritus	Ordinarily phytophagous. Introduced into houses (and hospitals) on garden vegetables and flowers.
Lice:				
Head lice	*Pediculus humanus capitis*	Worldwide	Hair becomes matted, with fetid odor	Kwell or Eurax; delousing spray or powders (DDT, lindane, etc.). Body louse vector of epidemic typhus, relapsing fever and trench fever.
Body lice	*P. humanus humanus*	Worldwide	Reddish papules; pruritus, followed by induration and pigmentation	
Pubic lice	*Phthirus pubis*	Worldwide	Intense irritation; attacks not necessarily limited to pubic region	
Bedbugs	*Cimex lectularius*	Worldwide		No proved role in disease transmission; (mechanical vectors under experimental conditions).
	Cimex hemipterus	Tropical and subtropical	Periodic blood suckers; some persons suffer from bites, others immune to attack	
	Cimex (Leptocimex) boueti	South America, Africa, New Guinea		
Fleas:				
Human flea	*Pulex irritans*	Worldwide	Marked dermatitis frequent	
Dog flea	*Ctenocephalides canis*	Worldwide	Marked dermatitis frequent	Apply soothing lotions. Vectors of important disease agents. Avoid contact.
Cat flea	*Ctenocephalides felis*	Worldwide	Marked dermatitis frequent	
Tropical rat flea	*Xenopsylla cheopis et al.*	Spreading from tropics	Marked dermatitis frequent	
Other rodent fleas	*Xenopsylla* spp.	Widespread	Marked dermatitis frequent	
Chigoe flea (jigger)	*Tunga penetrans*	Tropical Africa and America	Burrows in skin; introduces tetanus, gas gangrene, other organisms	Remove flea aseptically. Dilute lysol bath before and after removal recommended.
Flies (all types):				
Punkies	*Culicoides* spp.	Worldwide	Nodular, inflamed swelling, becoming vesicular	Attack in daytime; fierce biters. Transmit certain helminth infections.
Black flies	*Simulium* spp.	Worldwide	Hemorrhagic punctures; pain, swelling, general discomfort	Vectors of onchocerciasis.
Sandflies	*Phlebotomus* and *Lutzomyia* spp.	Widespread in warmer regions of the world	Stinging bite, followed by itching; whitish wheals	Night biters. Prefer ankles, wrists. Vectors of several diseases.
Mosquitoes	Family: Culicidae	Worldwide	Swelling, itching, annoyance, according to susceptibility of individual	Over 1500 species, of various biting habits. Vectors of several diseases.
Horse and deer flies	Family: Tabanidae (*Tabanus, Chrysops*)	Worldwide	Painful bite; no poisonous aftereffects	Daytime biters. Vectors of loiasis, tularemia.
Snipe flies	Family: Rhagionidae	Europe, Australia, the Americas	Painful bite; no poisonous aftereffects	Daytime biters: few species attack man. Not vectors of disease.
Stable flies (dog flies)	*Stomoxys calcitrans*	Worldwide	Painful bite; no poisonous aftereffects	Fills to capacity in 3–4 minutes. May be mechanical vector of disease.
Tsetse flies	*Glossina* spp.	Africa	Painful bite; no poisonous aftereffects	Cyclical vectors of various trypanosomes of man and animals.

the larval and nymphal stages are much more common and have been reported from Europe, Africa, Central and South America. Sources of human infections are, presumably, egg-infested food and water. The four-legged larvae that hatch from ingested eggs penetrate the intestinal wall and encyst in the lungs, liver, spleen, mesenteric glands, eye and other organs.

CLASSES INSECTA (HEXAPODA) AND ARACHNIDA

Most of the species of arthropods related to human health and well-being are included in these two classes. The role which the major groups of insects and arachnids play in human health problems is discussed in some detail in subsequent chapters.

Medical Importance of Arthropods

The relationships of arthropods to human health are almost as numerous and diverse as the many species involved. Adult and immature arthropods may play important roles in the transmission, development and survival of bacterial, rickettsial and viral pathogens as well as protozoan and metazoan parasites (Table 68–1; and Sections I to IV, VI and VII). In some of these instances the arthropod is involved only in the mechanical transfer of a pathogen, while in others it serves as an essential biologic host during the propagation or progressive maturation, or both, of an etiologic agent. The accommodation of some agents to their arthropod host is such that the pathogens remain viable through the host's progression from one developmental stage to the next (transstadial transmission). Also, pathogens may pass into the eggs of an infected host and thus be transmitted to the succeeding generation (transovarian transmission). In these types of associations the arthropod acts not only as a vector but also as a reservoir of the disease agent and greatly enhances its potential for survival and dissemination.

Arthropods also may injure humans directly in a variety of ways, such as by envenomization, vesication, bloodsucking, irritation or invasion of tissues and the stimulation of allergic responses (Tables 68–2 and 68–3). The abnormal fear of insects (entomophobia), mites (acarophobia), spiders and other arthropods may cause acute anxiety and annoyance in certain individuals that, in some cases, can lead to nervous disorders with sensory hallucinations. Arthropodophobia or, if no actual arthropod is involved, "delusory parasitosis" can become a very serious problem requiring psychiatric as well as medical treatment.[1]

The clinical management of arthropod-borne diseases normally may be accomplished satisfactorily with very little knowledge of the vector species. The development of effective disease control programs or comprehensive epidemiologic investigations, however, will inevitably require an accurate identification of the arthropod vector and some knowledge concerning its behavior and natural biologic relationships.[1-7]

Information on control of various arthropods, and for treatment of parasitosis of man by some of them, is presented in Chapter 72, especially in Table 72–1, page 794.

REFERENCES

1. James, M. T., and Harwood, R. F. 1969. Herms's Medical Entomology. The Macmillan Co., New York. 484 pp.
2. Smith, K. G. V. (ed.). 1973. Insects and Other Arthropods of Medical Importance. British Museum (Natural History), London. 561 pp.
3. Baker, E. W., and Wharton, G. W. 1952. An Introduction to Acarology. The Macmillan Co., New York. 465 pp.
4. Imms, A. D. 1957. A General Textbook of Entomology. 9th ed. Revised by O. W. Richards and R. G. Davies. Methuen & Co., Ltd., London. 885 pp.
5. Maramorosch, K. 1962. Biological Transmission of Disease Agents. Academic Press, New York. 192 pp.
6. Philip, C. B., and Burgdorfer, W. 1961. Arthropod vectors as reservoirs of microbial disease agents. Ann. Rev. Entomol. *6*:391–412.
7. Theiler, M., and Downs, W. G. 1973. The Arthropod-Borne Viruses of Vertebrates. Yale University Press, New Haven. 578 pp.

CHAPTER 69

Class Arachnida

HARRY HOOGSTRAAL

The primarily terrestrial ARACHNIDA[1,2] are chelicerate arthropods lacking antennae, mandibles and wings. The head and thorax are fused and most adults have four pairs of legs. Five of the 11 subclasses—SCORPIONES, UROPYGI, ARANEAE, SOLIFUGAE and ACARI—are considered here.

Subclass Scorpiones
Scorpions

The scorpion's large anterior pedipalps carry stout pinching claws (Fig. 68–1, p. 702). The conspicuously segmented abdomen is broad anteriorly but narrowed posteriorly as a "tail" tipped by a bulbous enlargement and a poisonous sting. Only the sting endangers man. Some species carry the tail over the back, others drag it behind. Few of the approximately 650 scorpion species inject sufficient poison to cause human concern. Scorpions are chiefly tropical and subtropical in distribution.

About 1600 persons, mostly children, stung by *Centruroides suffusus* Pocock died in the Mexican State of Durango over a 36-year period. In Belo Horizonte, Brazil, 1328 stings to children, mostly by *Tityus serrulatus* Lutz and Mello, resulted in 145 deaths. The mortality rate among young Egyptian children is nearly 60 per cent when stung by *Leiurus (Buthus) quinquestriatus* Hemprich and Ehrenberg. In the southwestern United States, the important species is *Centruroides sculpturatus* Ewing (=*C. gertschi* Stankhe). Dangerous scorpions also occur in Trinidad, North Africa, Turkey, southwestern Asia, Manchuria and Malaya. Large tropical species reach 8 inches in length but are not always the most poisonous.

Behavior. Scorpions feed at night on spiders or insects. During daytime, they hide beneath stones, logs or bark and under buildings or lumber. In houses, scorpions may rest in shoes or clothing.

Venom. Scorpion venoms, as most venoms, are complex mixtures capable of producing several or many biologic changes, sometimes concomitantly and sometimes in sequence over a period of time. They may affect almost all body tissues. None should be considered entirely hemolytic, neurotoxic or cardiotoxic.

Clinical Characteristics. Most scorpions produce only minor local reactions in man. In some cases there is intense, burning pain with minimal localized swelling and redness. However, the venom of a few species causes local vesicles, but this is relatively uncommon. Other scorpion venoms produce deleterious changes in the nervous system, particularly the peripheral nervous system. Weakness of the affected extremity, numbness, increased cerebrospinal and blood pressure, sweating and restlessness sometimes follow the stings of certain species. There may also be anxiety, nausea, vomiting and abdominal pain. The venoms of some scorpions appear to have a specific effect on presynaptic transmission, giving rise to muscle weakness and paralysis, including respiratory paralysis.

Treatment and Control. The immediate aim of therapy is to maintain vital functions and delay venom absorption and dissemination. In severe respiratory embarrassment, artificial respiration and oxygen therapy may be lifesaving measures. The affected area may be covered with crushed ice to reduce pain and cause some localized vasoconstriction, but long-term immersion in ice is to be avoided. Patients should be observed for 24 hours, and children should be hospitalized. Antivenins available in high risk areas are listed in Dreisbach's *Handbook of Poisoning*,[3] which should be consulted for medical aspects of scorpion stings (and also spider bites). Muscular spasm and fibrillation are best controlled intravenously with muscle relaxants or 10 per cent calcium gluconate. Convulsions are usually controlled with phenobarbital intravenously, or paraldehyde orally or intramuscularly. Respiratory depressants should be used with caution to avoid respiratory failure. The parasympatholytic effects of atropine may be beneficial. Hypotension may require treatment with vasopressor agents or corticosteroids, but hypertension is often a more common finding.

Scorpions are controlled by residual insecticides, screening and "scorpion-proofing" houses.[4] (See Table 72–1, p. 794.)

Subclass Uropygi
Whip Scorpions

The stingless whip scorpions occur from southern United States to Panama, in northeastern South America, and in parts of Asia. Their anterior legs are slender and whiplike. Some also have a whiplike abdominal appendage. Whip scorpions defend themselves by emitting an acetic and formic acid repellent with a vinegary odor responsible for the common Latin American names "vinegorone" or "vinegarroon." This repellent may irritate sensitive skin but is quite harmless.

Subclass Araneae
Spiders

More than 30,000 spider species have been described. A slender pedicel joins the cephalothorax and unsegmented abdomen. Each jaw (chelicera) contains a poison gland opening near the apex. Segmented pedipalps preceding the four pairs of legs suggest a fifth pair. "Silk" issues from six or eight ventral spinnerets near the abdominal tip.

In the subclass, the order ARANEIDA contains the suborder ORTHOGNATHA (MYGALOMORPHA) with *paraxial* chelicerae (moving vertically or forward and backward) and the suborder LABIDOGNATHA (ARANEOMORPHA) with *diaxial* chelicerae (moving laterally in and out). A third obscure suborder occurs in Malaya.

Spiders in all except two small families have poison glands for killing prey but few produce a venom harmful to people or attempt to bite people, even when handled roughly. Medical interest centers in the families THERAPHOSIDAE and DIPLURIDAE (ORTHOGNATHA), and HETEROPODIDAE, THERIDIIDAE and LOXOSCELIDAE (LABIDOGNATHA). Families of lesser medical concern, and the order SOLPUGIDA, are mentioned later. The general problems of spider bites and treatment have been discussed by Russell and colleagues.[5]

FAMILY THERAPHOSIDAE
TARANTULAS

The immense hairy spiders commonly known as tarantulas are mostly sluggish and attack humans only when extremely provoked. However, the common, large, black *Sericopelma communis* Cambridge of Panama is poisonous and much feared. The venom of other tarantulas is seldom harmful, but the powerful chelicerae of large species may produce a painful wound. Species of the Western Hemisphere use their hind legs when annoyed to brush urticating hairs off the dorsum of the body. These hairs can cause temporary discrete, punctate, pruritic lesions about 1/2 hour after touching human skin, and irritation after scratching may recur for several weeks.

FAMILY DIPLURIDAE FUNNEL-WEB SPIDERS

Two tarantula-like Australian funnel-web spiders, *Atrax robustus* Cambridge and *Atrax formidabilis* Rainbow, injure humans and *A. robustus* has caused several deaths.

FAMILY HETEROPODIDAE BANANA SPIDERS

The genus *Heteropoda* occurs in Old World and New World tropics. *Heteropoda venatoria* (Linnaeus), the banana spider abundant in tropical American seaports, occasionally is found with fruits shipped to the United States. It is sometimes confused with the tarantula but differs by its smoother body, longer legs and diaxial jaws. The bite is painful and occasionally serious enough to require hospitalization.

FAMILY THERIDIIDAE WIDOW SPIDERS

The mostly sedentary, comb-footed, widow spiders spin irregular webs near the ground. The tarsus of the fourth pair of legs bears a comb of strong, toothed setae. Most if not all widow spiders, genus *Latrodectus,* have a poisonous bite that is sometimes fatal to man. Widow spiders are recognized (Fig. 68–1) by the black, brown or gray globose abdomen and a ventral red, orange, yellow or white hourglass marking. The ventral ornamentation is reduced in some mature specimens. Immatures and males have other ornamentation dorsally on the abdomen and sometimes on the legs. Female bodies are about 1/2 inch long; males are somewhat smaller.

Latrodectus geometricus Koch is cosmotropical but most widespread in Africa. *Latrodectus mactans* (Fabricius), commonly referred to as the Black Widow spider, occurs in warm areas of all continents. *Latrodectus pallidus* Cambridge lives among shrubs in North Africa and the Middle East. *Latrodectus curacaviensis* (Muller) is common in temperate regions of North and South America. *Latrodectus hystrix* Simon occurs in Aden and Yemen, and *Latrodectus dahli* Levi in Iran and Socotra.

Widow spiders ordinarily bite only for food but may bite people in self-defense, when frightened in the web or on the ground. Females guarding egg sacs are particularly aggressive.

Clinical Characteristics. The bites of widow spiders usually cause instant pain. A cramping pain beginning within 10 minutes often extends successively to the abdomen, legs, chest and back when the bite is on the legs. The larger muscle groups, especially those of the abdomen, often become rigid.

Acute symptoms persisting for 12 to 48 hours include elevated temperature, blood pressure and spinal fluid pressure. Conversely, the temperature, pulse and blood pressure may be subnormal and shock may follow. Hypertension is important in patients with heart diseases. There may be leukocytosis. Nausea, vomiting, excessive perspiration, and respiratory embarrassment are common. Chills, hyperactive reflexes, priapism, and tingling in the fingertips and toetips may occur. Very few cases end in death.

Clinical manifestations of widow spider bites may be similar to those of perforated peptic ulcer, acute abdomen or acute appendicitis.

Treatment and Control. Patients should be hospitalized to insure adequate nursing. Ice is applied immediately to the bite area to reduce pain. Russell and colleagues[5] consider the muscle relaxant methocarbamol (Robaxin) to provide the most effective relief. They administer 10 ml intravenously over a 5-minute period and follow with another 5 to 10 ml in a drip of 250 ml of 5 per cent dextrose in water. If the muscle pains and cramps, headache and nausea are relieved, oral methocarbamol, 500 mg every 6 hours for 24 hours, can then be given. Other muscle relaxants, including orphenadrine citrate (Norflex), have been used. Ten ml of 10 per cent calcium gluconate, administered intravenously, relieves the muscle pains and spasms caused by *Latrodectus* venom. Several doses at 3- to 4-hour intervals may be needed to control the muscle pain, but this drug is not useful against nausea and vomiting. Some physicians use meperidine hydrochloride (Demerol) or morphine sulfate, repeated as required.

Pain of mild cases is usually controlled with acetylsalicylic acid, phenacetin, and caffeine (APC) and codeine. Hot baths may give some relief. The patient should be mildly sedated and should rest for 12 hours. Symptoms rarely persist for more than 2 days.

Patients with a history of hypertensive heart disease should be hospitalized immediately, given the appropriate antivenin, mildly sedated, and watched closely for any significant increase in blood pressure. In a hypertensive crisis, appropriate measures for reducing blood pressure should be instituted.

Black Widow Spider Antivenin relieves symptoms and signs and speeds recovery, if given promptly. An antivenin against any *Latrodectus* species affords some protection against the venom of other species of the genus; all contain horse serum requiring the usual precautions.

Insecticides and crushing the spiders and egg sacs are control measures. (See Table 72–1, p. 794.)

FAMILY LOXOSCELIDAE FALSE HACKLED BAND SPIDERS

The nocturnal, band-spinning spiders of the genus *Loxosceles* have six eyes arranged in a semicircle. They live beneath stones, boards or debris, in holes, under tree bark, in wall crevices, and in caves in temperate and tropical zones of the world. The dense body hairs of living *Loxosceles* are usually grayish, tawny or brown but in preservative become yellow, orange or reddish. Other six-eyed diaxial spiders differ from *Loxosceles* by the following combination of characters:

1. median pair of eyes anterior to the two lateral pairs;
2. chelicerae basally fused and each bears a pincerlike fang;
3. thoracic furrow conspicuous and longitudinal;
4. carapace flat;
5. sternum somewhat pointed posteriorly; and
6. two tarsal claws on each leg.

Loxosceles laeta (Nicolet) inhabits crude buildings in parts of South America northward to Guatemala. A severe systemic reaction, including hemolytic anemia, sometimes follows the bite. An antivenin against the toxin of this species is produced by the Instituto Butantan in São Paulo, Brazil. Some authorities dispute the usefulness of antivenins against *Loxosceles* bites. *Loxosceles reclusa* Gertsch and Mulaik, *L. unicolor* Keyserling, and *L. arizonica* Gertsch and

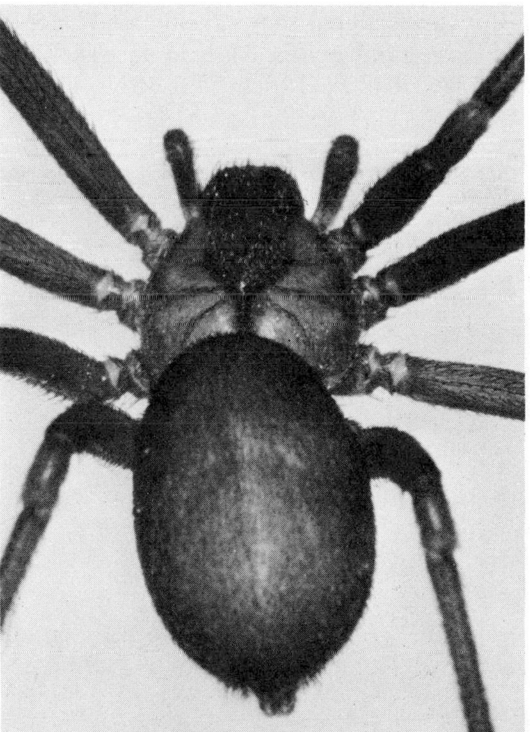

Figure 69–1. The distinguishing mark of *Loxosceles reclusa,* the brown recluse spider, is the darker violin-shaped band over the dorsal cephalothorax. (Courtesy of Drs. C. J. Dillaha, G. T. Jansen, W. M. Honeycutt, and C. R. Hayden in J.A.M.A., *188*:33–36, 1964.)

Mulaik, the brown spiders of the United States, have a venomous bite similar to that of *L. laeta.*[6] These spiders bear a distinctive violin-shaped pattern on the cephalothorax (Fig. 69–1). Over 60 cases of presumed *Loxosceles* bites were reported in Texas between 1959 and 1962. In Mississippi, where *L. reclusa,* the brown recluse spider, is widely distributed, physicians may excise the affected area if they see the patient within 8 hours and are certain that the bite is caused by *L. reclusa.*

Indoors, brown spiders hide in clothes, in boxes, beneath furniture, behind baseboards, or in corners and crevices. Outdoors they live in weedy shelters and among rocks. These hunting spiders, which do not use their nondescript whitish or grayish web to catch food, usually run for cover when disturbed.

Reactions are local or both local and systemic.[7] Initial pain is followed by a whitish lesion with an erythematous halo. Painful blisters and edema may develop into purple and black gangrenous skin and necrosis (Fig. 69–2). A depressed ulcer, left after about 2 weeks when the eschar sloughs off, gradually fills with scar tissue. Systemic symptoms are coma, chills, fever, malaise, weakness, nausea, joint pains and various eruptions. Biochemical alterations cause acute thrombocytopenia, leukocytosis, hemolytic anemia, hemoglobinemia, hemoglobinuria, hematuria, proteinuria and bilirubinemia. These changes may lead to shock and death.

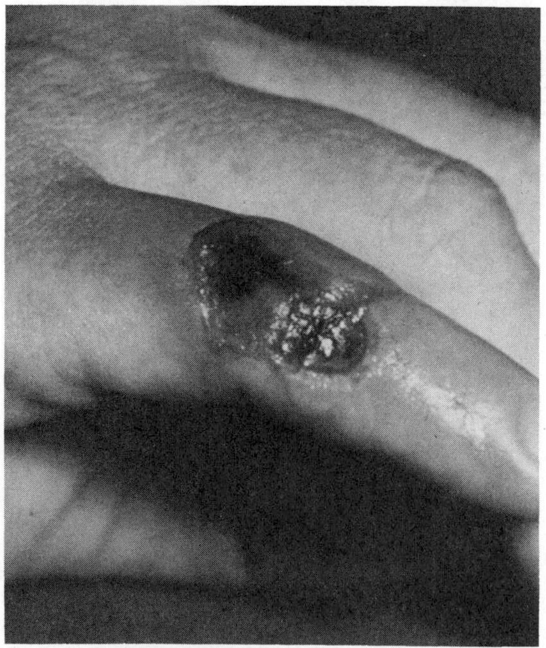

Figure 69–2. Local necrosis of finger following the bite of the brown recluse spider, *Loxosceles reclusa;* it was considered originally to be a vascular occlusion. (Courtesy of Drs. C. J. Dillaha, G. T. Jansen, W. M. Honeycutt, and C. R. Hayden in J.A.M.A., *188*:33–36, 1964.)

Systemic reactions are particularly severe in small children. Prompt administration of corticosteroids prevents local necrotic development and appears to protect against some systemic effects. Fresh whole blood transfusions are given in cases of severe hemolysis and thrombocytopenia.

OTHER LABIDOGNATH SPIDERS

The South American orb-weaving cat-headed spider, *Mastophora gasteracanthoides* (Nicolet), family Araneidae, causes necrotic spot among vineyard workers.

A wolf spider, *Scaptocosa raptoria* (Walck.), family Lycosidae, with a potent venom causes necrosis in Brazil.

In the family Clubionidae, *Chiracanthium inclusum* (Hentz) of California and *Chiracanthium diversum* Koch of Hawaii produce local envenomization.

The large, solitary, aggressive South American wandering spider, *Ctenus* (= *Pheneutra*) *ferus* (Perty), family Ctenidae, does not construct a web or have a permanent home. Several hundred bites are reported annually in the state of São Paulo, Brazil, and death of children under 6 years old has been reported. The bite causes swelling, usually pain (which may become severe), and weakness in the involved extremity sometimes leading to mild paralysis. Systemic manifestations may be cardiac irregularity, respiratory difficulty, and paralysis of the eyelids and extraocular muscles. An antivenin is produced by the Instituto Butantan, São Paulo.

A lynx spider, *Peucetia viridans* (Hentz), family Oxyopidae, shoots a corrosive fine spray that can cause a painful burn on the eyes.

Order Solpugida
Sun Spiders or Wind Scorpions

These spiderlike arachnids, which differ from true spiders in having the segmented abdomen broadly jointed to the cephalothorax, inhabit mostly drier areas of the tropics and subtropics. The extremely large chelicerae can inflict a painful bite but have no poison glands. The effect is transitory except when the bite is deep and secondary infection occurs.

Order Acarina
Ticks and Mites

Acarina are distinguished from other Arachnida and from insects by the general absence of body segmentation. Acarina lack antennae and wings; the thorax and abdomen are fused in all except some adult mites. Like spiders and scorpions, adult ticks and mites have four pairs of legs, but larvae only three pairs (or fewer in some mites).

SUPERFAMILY IXODOIDEA TICKS

In ticks[8,9] the *capitulum* ("head") consists of a proximal *basis capituli* bearing a pair of dorsal cutting *chelicerae;* a ventral, characteristically toothed *hypostome* that anchors the tick to its host; and lateral, paired sensory *palpi.* The "mouth" opens between the bases of the chelicerae and hypostome. Eyes are simple or absent. Slightly over 800 tick species exist almost from pole to pole. All are obligate ectoparasites.

The superfamily Ixodoidea contains three families.[9] A primitive, poorly known family, Nuttalliellidae, is confined to southern Africa. "Soft or argasid ticks," Argasidae, lack a hard dorsal shield (scutum). The nymphal and adult capitulum is situated ventrally and adults of most species are only slightly dimorphic (Fig. 69–3). "Hard or ixodid ticks," Ixodidae, have a scutum covering the entire dorsum in males but only the anterior part of the dorsum in females, nymphs and larvae. Thus, ixodid males and females are quite dimorphic. The capitulum of each stage arises anteriorly on the body (Fig. 69–4).

Biologic patterns differ distinctly in the two chief families of ticks, as do their interrelationships with humans and pathogens. In the family Argasidae, most immatures and adults are confined to specific, sheltered habitats such as caves, burrows, bird rookeries or marine bird colonies. In many situations, argasids feed only during the host nesting season, but in stables or structures housing chickens or pigeons they may feed throughout the year. In the family Ixodidae, most adults, and also immatures of many species, are more widely scattered by hosts wandering through forests and grasslands. Thus hosts are often continuously available to tropical ixodids. However, a few members of each family have biologic patterns more or less like those of the other family.

FAMILY ARGASIDAE SOFT TICKS

About 160 species are contained in the genera *Argas* (55 species), *Ornithodoros* (100), *Antricola* (4), and *Otobius* (2). Another genus from Central America is about to be described. *Antricola* of tropical and subtropical American bat caves has no known medical importance.

Sheltered burrows, caves, stables and other buildings, usually in steppes, savannas or semideserts, harbor *Borrelia*-infected *Ornithodoros* species, which are notorious sources of human relapsing fever (Chapter 15, p. 137). *Ornithodoros marocanus* Velu of the Iberian and Moroccan areas parasitizes swine and other domestic animals in buildings and

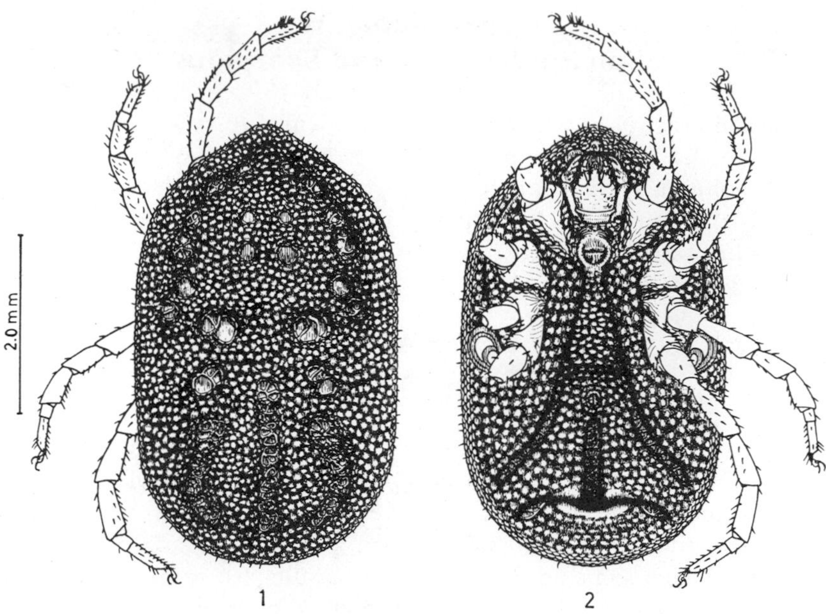

Figure 69–3. A "soft or argasid" tick (family ARGASIDAE), *Ornithodoros muesebecki* Hoogstraal. This parasite of marine bird nesting colonies in the Arabian Sea, Arabian Gulf and Seychelles is infected by Zirqa virus. Humans bitten by these ticks suffer from fever, headache, itch and erythema. Adult (female), (1) dorsal and (2) ventral views. (Courtesy of Dr. Harry Hoogstraal, U.S. Naval Medical Research Unit No. 3.)

stone enclosures, where it also bites people. *Ornithodoros erraticus* (Lucas) of northern Africa and the Near East has similar habitats but is also associated with a wider range of burrow-inhabiting wild vertebrates. In eastern Africa, members of the *Ornithodoros moubata* complex attack people and domestic animals dwelling together in houses and hunters venturing into burrows of large mammals. *Ornithodoros tholozani* Laboulbène and Mégnin [= *O. papillipes* (Birula) and *O. crossi* Brumpt] inhabits caves, stables and caravansaries from northern Africa to Central Asia and is much feared by shepherds and travelers. *Ornithodoros talaje* (Guerin-Meneville) attacks humans and domestic animals in houses and stables, and wild animals in burrows, from central and western United States well into South America.

The pajaroello, *Ornithodoros coriaceus* Koch, inflicts painful bites to hunters and hikers resting under trees where deer bed in California and Mexico. Pajaroello toxin may produce a vesicular lesion followed by necrosis and ulceration. *Ornithodoros savignyi* (Audouin) inflicts similarly irritating bites to people resting in the shade of trees where camels and cattle shelter in African semideserts. Indeed, numerous argasid species bite humans when the opportunity arises even though their normal host range in nature is limited.

About 20 different viruses are known to circulate in about 25 argasid species. (See Section I and Table 68–1, p. 707.) Some of these viruses cause mild or severe human disease; others are under study in this respect. The African *Argas arboreus* Kaiser, Hoogstraal and Kohls of heron rookeries is infected by Quaranfil virus (Quaranfil group), which was first isolated from blood of a febrile child near Cairo. The same virus infects *Argas hermanni* Audouin inhabiting pigeon houses in Afghanistan and Nepal. *Argas hermanni* is also an overwintering reservoir of West Nile virus, which has caused outbreaks of illness among newcomers to the Near East. In India, *Ornithodoros chiropterphila* Dhanda and Rajagopalan and its cave-dwelling bat hosts function in the epidemiology of Kyasanur Forest disease. Candidates for study of human febrile episodes are Zirqa virus infecting *Ornithodoros muesebecki* Hoogstraal in the Arabian Gulf, and Punta Salinas virus infecting *Ornithodoros amblus* in Peru. Petroleum industry employees, orni-

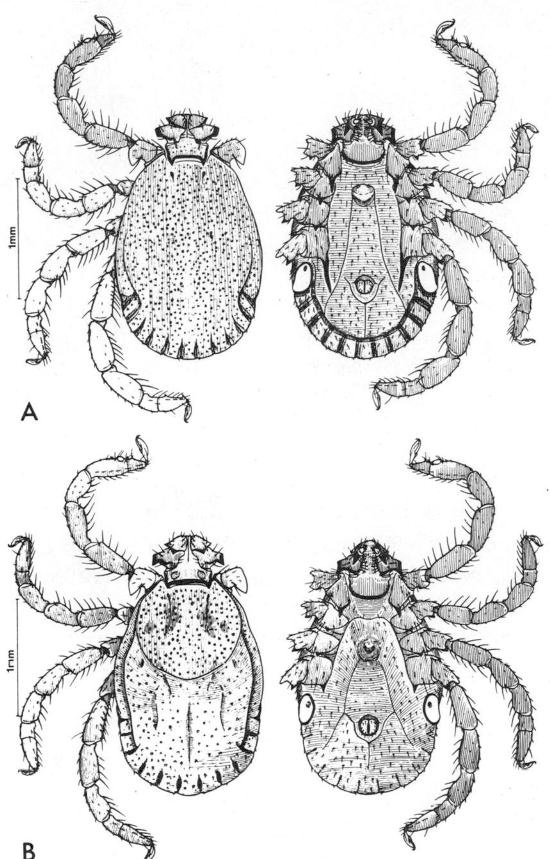

Figure 69–4. A "hard or ixodid" tick family (IXODIDAE), *Haemaphysalis spinigera* Neumann, the principal vector of Kyasanur Forest disease virus in India. Dorsal (*left*) and ventral (*right*) views of (*A*) male and (*B*) female. (Courtesy of Dr. Harry Hoogstraal, U.S. Naval Medical Research Unit No. 3.).

thologists, egg gatherers, guano diggers, and other visitors to marine bird colonies are bitten by these two tick species and afterward suffer from similar syndromes. Colorado tick fever virus has been isolated from *Otobius megnini* Cooley and Kohls, an ear-infesting parasite of domestic animals that also invades human ears and has been transported from western North America to several warmer areas of the world.

Experimentally, certain argasid species are able to maintain and transmit *Francisella tularensis* (tularemia), *Coxiella burnetii* (Q fever), *Rickettsia rickettsii* (Rocky Mountain spotted fever), Kyasanur Forest disease virus, and other pathogenic organisms. Some Old World argasids cause tick paralysis in domestic birds and mammals.

Life History. Argasids also differ from ixodids by feeding rapidly. Each postembryonic stage (larva, nymph, adult) completes the blood meal in 30 minutes to 2 hours (except some larvae that feed for several days and the nonfeeding larvae of *O. savignyi* and *O. moubata*).[8,9] Larvae feed once, nymphs and adults two or more times. Argasid nymphs may have two to eight instars but usually three or four (ixodid nymphs molt to adults, not to other nymphal instars). Nymphs typically feed fully once in each instar, or two or three times if taking incomplete meals, and then molt. Complex factors influence argasid nymphal instar numbers.[9] The life cycles of *Otobius* and a few species in specialized *Ornithodoros* subgenera are atypical. The type and range of argasid hosts have been indicated previously.

After each of the five to 12 or more blood meals during its lifetime, the argasid retreats to a shelter in a rock or wood crevice, or just below the soil surface, for digestion and development. Fed females mate and oviposit in the shelter site. Parthenogenesis is uncommon. Argasids oviposit several batches of 20 to 700 eggs that are individually and totally smaller than the single egg batch of ixodids.[9] Tropical argasids complete the life cycle in several months to a year, but elsewhere the cycle may continue through as many as 10 years.

FAMILY IXODIDAE
HARD TICKS

About 640 ixodid species are known. Members of most of the 13 ixodid genera have been reported to maintain infectious agents in nature, but only the six genera most directly involved in the epidemiology of human infections and injury will be discussed here. (See Sections I, II and Table 68–1, p. 703.) Typical capitula of several ixodid genera are shown in Figure 69–5.

Genus Ixodes. The 250 *Ixodes* species occur in arctic, temperate and tropical climates; 10 have yielded about a dozen different viruses.[9] *Ixodes persulcatus* Schulze is the chief vector of Russian spring-summer

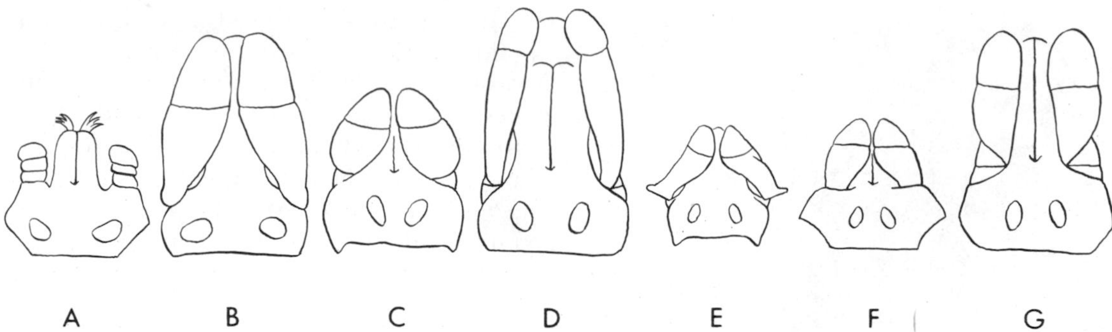

Figure 69–5. Typical capitula (Ixodidae), females, dorsal view: *A, Boophilus; B, Ixodes; C, Dermacentor; D, Amblyomma; E, Haemaphysalis; F, Rhipicephalus; G, Hyalomma.* (Courtesy of Dr. R. A. Cooley, Rocky Mountain Laboratory, U.S.P.H.S.)

encephalitis, *I. ricinus* L. of tick-borne encephalitis (Central Europe) and louping ill (British Isles), and *I. granulatus* Supino of Langat virus (Malaysia). Kyasanur Forest disease virus has been isolated from *I. petaurista* Warburton and from *I. ceylonensis* Kohls in India. Other viruses are from *Ixodes* in temperate zones. *Ixodes holocyclus* Neumann causes tick paralysis in Australia, and *I. acutitarsus* Karsch and other *Ixodes* species are irritating pests of humans in the Himalayas and elsewhere in the tropics.

Genus Haemaphysalis. Among the 150 haemaphysaline species, mostly of Old World temperate and tropical zones, at least eight Indian species participate in the epidemiology of Kyasanur Forest disease. Others transmit Russian spring-summer and tick-borne encephalitis virus and several viruses that cause fevers in humans in Asian and African tropics. Haemaphysalines also transmit the *Rickettsia* spp. of spotted fever group typhus diseases in Africa, Asia and the Americas.

Genus Amblyomma. About 100 *Amblyomma* species occur in the tropics and subtropics of the world. Four are known to carry seven different viruses. The African *A. variegatum* (Fabricius) is commonly infected by Crimean-Congo hemorrhagic fever virus, and several other viruses have been recovered from this species in West Africa. *Amblyomma* ticks transmit rickettsiae of the spotted fever group in the Americas and in Africa. Immatures and sometimes adults of several species are severe pests of humans in Asian and American rural areas and forests.

Genus Dermacentor. Of the 31 *Dermacentor* species, several in temperate America (Fig. 8–2, p. 113) and Eurasia transmit spotted fever group rickettsiae, Colorado tick fever virus and various members of the Russian spring-summer encephalitis virus complex. In the Indian subregion, *D. auratus* Supino causes severe distress when it bites humans and is also infected by Kyasanur Forest disease virus.

Genus Hyalomma. Twenty-one *Hyalomma* species (with nine subspecies) occur in warmer unforested areas of Africa and Eurasia where five participate in the epidemiology of Crimean-Congo hemorrhagic fever and at least one is also infected by Thogoto virus, which may be fatal in humans. Seven *Hyalomma* species are known to be infected by nine different viruses. Q fever (*Coxiella burnetii*) is frequently isolated from some species. Numerous immatures of the four subspecies composing the *H. marginatum* complex are carried intercontinentally by northward and southward migrating birds, and adults and immatures of other species are carried far and wide by camel caravans and by nomadic and migrating wild and domestic mammals. These movements appear to be largely responsible for the extensive dissemination of certain arboviruses.

Genus Rhipicephalus. About 50 of the 65 *Rhipicephalus* species are native to Africa, the others to southern Europe, Asia and Indonesia. *Rhipicephalus sanguineus* (Latreille) has been carried to all continents with domestic dogs and survives in heated buildings far north of the tropics. Several species have been found infected by six different viruses, including Crimean-Congo hemorrhagic fever, Thogoto and Kyasanur Forest disease. *Rhipicephalus* ticks are also vectors of spotted fever group rickettsiae and some are unpleasant pests of humans.

Life History. Ixodids pass through the same developmental stages as argasids but in a different manner and nymphs molt only to adults. Some males do not feed. The life histories of a number of *Ixodes* species are atypical of the family. About six species in three genera are parthenogenetic. Mating while feeding on the host is necessary to stimulate females to complete the blood meal, which usually requires 3 to 7 days. Males remain on the host and may mate several times before dying. Females drop to the ground after finishing feeding. A few days later (or after overwintering) they begin the several-day oviposition process, after which they die. The single batch usually contains 3000 to 6000 eggs, but 18,497 eggs have been counted from a female *Amblyomma maculatum* Koch. In the tropics, eggs of most species develop within 3 weeks. Several days later, larvae begin to feed for 2 to 7 days. Afterward they molt, either on the same host or after having dropped to the ground. Nymphs repeat the feeding and dropping schedule but most, except in the genera *Boophilus* and *Margaropus* (parasites of ungulates), drop to the ground to molt to the adult stage. Thus most ixodid tick species feed on three hosts, some on two hosts, and a few on one host. Tropical ixodids have one, two or three generations a year, but in northern climates a 3-year or even a 4-year cycle is common. Most species have a marked host preference, but those that accept a wider range of hosts are the most important ixodid reservoirs and vectors of agents infecting humans and domestic and wild animals. The larvae, nymphs, and adults of a single ixodid species may all feed on the same type of host. However, in many species the hosts of immatures and of adults differ dramatically, e.g. rat for immatures and elephant for adults, or lizard and cow, or bird and tiger.

Tick Paralysis

Ticks known to cause tick paralysis in humans and other animals number about 20 species in the genera *Argas, Ornithodoros, Ixodes, Haemaphysalis, Dermacentor, Amblyomma* and *Rhipicephalus*.[10] Female ticks are most frequently cited but males and immatures may also cause this syndrome. The ascending flaccid paralysis may start soon after the tick attaches, but usually 1 or 2 days later. The condition gradually worsens. With initial symptoms primarily of ataxia and areflexia, tick paralysis should be considered under the acute causes of ataxia in children and adults. In its second phase with progressive motor weakness, it mimics Landry-Guillain-Barré syndrome. Removal of the tick(s) often, but not always, results in rapid improvement. Children with ticks feeding in the hair and on the back are common victims. It is believed that the paralysis is caused by a toxin introduced when the tick bites, although the nature of the toxin is not fully understood. There is no evidence that an infectious agent causes this illness.

Weakness, stumbling and falling are followed by hyperesthesia and paresthesia in the extremities. Flaccid paralysis gradually ascends to the trunk, arms, tongue and pharynx; the voice changes and swallowing becomes difficult or impossible. Convulsions and respiratory changes may lead to stupor and death. The temperature is only slightly elevated. Leukocyte and erythrocyte counts and the spinal fluid, hemoglobin and urine are usually normal.

Prompt removal of the tick is often the most effective curative measure. No food should be given if swallowing is difficult and the head should be turned to assist drainage. Sedatives and narcotics are not indicated. Oxygen, a respirator, or other artificial respiration may be required.

Differential diagnosis includes poliomyelitis, polyneuritis, myelitis, infectious neuronitis, syringomyelia, spinal cord tumor and botulism.

Avoiding Tick Bites

In the tropics, immature or adult ticks are active at most seasons and in a wide variety of biotopes. Exceptions are marine bird colonies, where ticks are inactive, unless disturbed, when nesting birds are absent. Caves, huts and corrals are likely sources of tick infestation, as are vegetation along game trails, in riparian forests and bordering pastures, and soil under shade trees and shrubs in semideserts. Keeping trousers tucked into boots, shirts within tight belts, and sleeves buttoned helps prevent tick entry to the body, but the exposed neck and head may be attacked. Some ticks attach rapidly, others after a good deal of wandering. Frequent inspection of the body, especially skin folds and hairy and moist areas, is advised. Tiny larvae, or "seed ticks," may not be felt until they fill with blood a day or more after having attached. In Kyasanur Forest disease foci, many people are unaware of ticks on their bodies. Early removal of feeding ticks is recommended in the hope of avoiding pathogen transmission. Chemicals and repellents to prevent attachment are listed in Table 72–1, pages 794 and 800.

Removal of Attached Ticks

Remove ticks with forceps, a bent twig, or fingers covered by paper or a leaf. Pull gently at first, then with more force, directly outward from the body. Pull from as close to the skin as possible to avoid leaving the capitulum imbedded. Avoid crushing the tick and prevent tick secretions from contacting skin cuts and abrasions and the eyes and mouth. Chemicals such as camphorated phenol, 0.6 per cent pyrethrins in methyl benzoate, chloroform or mineral oil may be applied to the tick to facilitate its removal by gentle pulling after an interval of about 20 minutes.

Confusion Between Arthropod Bites and Other Skin Lesions

The usual reaction to attachments or bites of ticks, chiggers, mosquitoes and unidentified arthropods is a dense dermal infiltrate characterized by numerous eosinophilic leukocytes, plasma cells and histiocytes. This reaction may be mistaken for Hodgkin's disease, mycosis fungoides, atypical lymphoblastoma, histiocytosis, and the heterogeneous group of eosinophilic granulomas. The lesions are often associated with pseudoepitheliomatous hyperplasia, which may be confused with squamous cell carcinoma; however, the association with an eosinophilic dermal infiltrate and with epidermal inclusion cysts provides helpful differential clues.

The reaction to arthropod bites may persist, generally with no appreciable histologic difference, for 3 weeks to 2 years. A single cutaneous lesion with a histologic picture suggestive of Hodgkin's disease or another lymphoblastoma is suspect as the site of an arthropod bite until conclusively proved otherwise.

Control of Ticks

Information on control of ticks is presented in Table 72–1, page 794.

Acarina Other Than Ticks
Mites

More than 200 families, 1700 genera and 30,000 species of mites have been described and possibly half a million more species are estimated to exist.[11, 12] Most species are free-living but thousands of species parasitize plants or animals. The degrees and patterns of parasitism vary. Some are parasitic in all active stages (scabies mites), others only during the larval stage (chiggers). Cheese mites are fortuitous parasites.

The mites of medical importance are:

1. those causing a dermatitis (Dermanyssidae, Pyemotidae, Acardidae and Demodicidae);
2. chiggers, larvae of the family Trombiculidae, some of which cause a dermatitis or transmit the rickettsiae of scrub typhus;
3. the itch mite, *Sarcoptes scabiei* (De Geer) (Sarcoptidae);
4. the house mouse mite, *Liponyssoides sanguineus* (Dermanyssidae), vector of rickettsialpox;
5. those associated with fungi and pollens and causing house dust allergy, *Dermatophagoides* spp. (Tyroglyphidae), and producing an irritating poisonous fluid,

Holothyrus coccinella Gervais (HOLOTYRIDAE); and

6. others, such as the tropical rat mite, which may transmit the agents of murine typhus, Q fever, tularemia and plague, but which are considered unimportant as vectors. Although several arboviruses have been isolated from mites as noted below, mites are not presently thought to participate significantly in the epidemiology of these disease agents.

FAMILY DERMANYSSIDAE DERMANYSSID MITES

Ornithonyssus bacoti (Hirst) (formerly treated as genera *Bdellonyssus* and *Liponyssus*), the tropical rat mite, is associated with wild and domestic rodents and other mammals and birds throughout the world. Humans living on rodent-infested premises suffer from the irritating bite, which may cause a painful dermatitis. The tropical rat mite is the intermediate host of *Litomosoides carinii*, a filarial nematode parasite of rodents, and is a serious pest of laboratory animals. Experimentally it can transmit the agents of plague and rickettsialpox.

Ornithonyssus sylviarum (C. and F.), the northern fowl mite, is worldwide in temperate zones. This mite of wild and domestic birds occasionally bites humans and rodents and has been found to be infected with the viruses of western and eastern equine encephalitis, Newcastle disease and ornithosis. The *Bartonella*-like agent of hemolytic-uremic syndrome, a fatal human illness, was isolated from *O. sylviarum* collected in a patient's bedroom. The bite of this mite may cause immediate irritation and subsequent erythema, induration and pruritus.[13]

Dermanyssus gallinae (De Geer), the chicken mite, a cosmopolitan parasite of chickens, other domestic birds, and many wild birds, is an annoying pest to humans. The painful bite sometimes causes a papular urticaria. It has been found naturally infected with the viruses of St. Louis, western and eastern encephalitides.

Liponyssoides (= Allodermanyssus) sanguineus (Hirst), the house mouse mite (Fig. 69–6), is infected by *Rickettsia akari*, the agent of rickettsialpox, and transmits this pathogen to humans. (See p. 123.) The bite also causes a rash in humans. Originally described from Egyptian rodents, *L. sanguineus* distribution is localized in Africa, Asia, Europe and North America.

FAMILY PYEMOTIDAE (= PEDICULOIDIDAE)

The widely distributed *Pyemotes (= Pediculoides) ventricosus* (Newport) is predaceous on the larvae of numerous insects and also parasitizes humans. When the tiny, elongate female is pregnant, the abdomen becomes enormously distended and globoid. In this ovoviviparous species, the eggs hatch, the

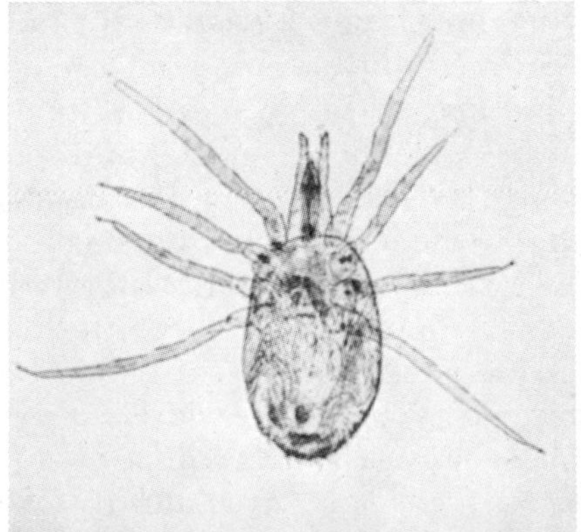

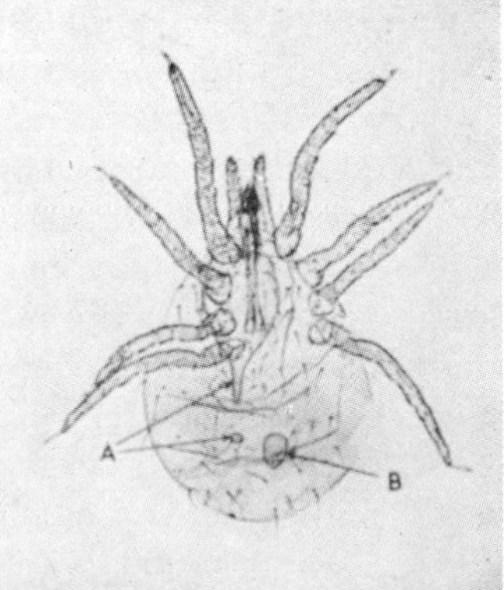

Figure 69–6. Photomicrographs of *Liponyssoides sanguineus* (Hirst), the mite vector of rickettsialpox; adult ♀ (left, 108 ×), and nymph (150 ×, with 2 dorsal shields (*A*) and anal plate (*B*), retouched for emphasis). (Courtesy of the Rocky Mountain Laboratory; photo by N. J. Kramis.)

young mites develop to maturity, and the newly adult females are often fertilized within the body of the mother before escaping to the outside. *Pyemotes ventricosus* causes numerous epidemics of straw itch, a vesiculopapular dermatitis of farmers, potters, packers, and broom and strawboard factory workers who handle wheat, barley or straw. Persons sleeping on straw mattresses also are often affected. Mite-laden dust from harvesting machines may be carried considerable distances. The dense dermatitis, sometimes covering the entire body, has been confused with chickenpox, smallpox and scabies. A relatively high fever is common and numerous other signs accompany severe cases.

The burning of grain stubble is recommended to destroy the mites and insect larvae on which they feed. Pyrethrins and piperonyl butoxide can be used on straw, and clothing impregnated with acaricides gives effective protection against these mites (pp. 130 and 794).

FAMILY ACARIDAE (= TYROGLYPHIDAE) FLOUR AND MEAL MITES

Members of this cosmopolitan family infest cereals, grains and other stored products. The hypopial (second nymph) stage attaches to insects, mollusks or millipedes, which serve as disseminators. Several species cause a dermatitis similar to that produced by *Pyemotes ventricosus.* The spore-eating *Tyrophagus castellanii* (Hirst) causes copra itch in copra handlers. The grain-eating *Acarus siro* Linn. causes vanillism in vanilla pod handlers. Some species infest the human urinary and intestinal tracts and may be introduced on contaminated catheters. When *Tyrophagus longior* (Gervais) is ingested, especially in cheese, it may be found in the feces, but apparently does not produce a true intestinal infection. The characteristic pungent flavor of Attenburger Milbenkäse is due to mites. Contact with the excrement or powdered bodies of these mites may result in allergic phenomena. *Glycyphagus domesticus* (De Geer) in the closely related family Glycyphagidae causes the well known grocers' itch.

FAMILY DEMODICIDAE HAIR FOLLICLE MITES

Adults of the microscopic, vermiform *Demodex folliculorum* Owen, the follicular or face mite, have a transversely striated abdomen and four pairs of stubby legs (Fig. 69–7). Many may be found "head down" in hair follicles and sebaceous glands (Figs. 69–8, 69–9) of the face, nose, lips, forehead, and main collecting ducts of the nipples. *Demodex folliculorum* has been reported in about 13 per cent of skin biopsies and to infest numerous if not most humans. Despite lack of visible infestation, these mites may cause formation of comedones (blackheads), ingrown hairs, dilated hair follicles, and a slightly raised, firm, erythematous, scaly skin nodule that slowly enlarges for many months. An ointment containing the gamma isomer of benzene hexachloride (Kwell) is therapeutically useful. Closely related species of *Demodex* cause mange in dogs and other animals.

FAMILY TROMBICULIDAE CHIGGERS

Chiggers (red bugs, harvest mites, bête rouge) are the larvae of mites of the family Trombiculidae; nearly all parasitize vertebrates. In some areas the term chigger, probably a corruption of chigoe, is also applied to the burrowing flea. Chiggers are almost microscopic (Fig. 69–10). Adults may exceed 1 mm in length but are usually smaller and sometimes are brilliantly colored (Fig. 69–10). Nymphs and adults are predators on small arthropods and on their eggs. Many hundreds of species have been described. Mostly tropical and subtropical, they occur from Alaska to New Zealand and from sea level to over 16,000 feet altitude. Eggs are deposited in light soil. The hexapod larvae attach to vertebrates, including humans,

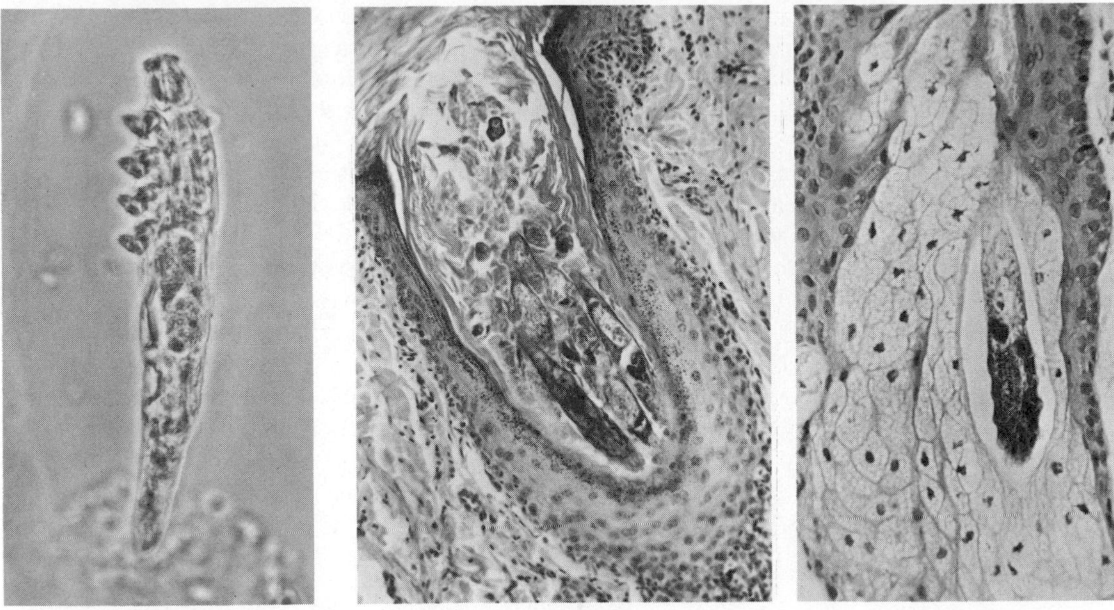

Figure 69-7. Photomicrograph of *Demodex folliculorum* (Simon) adult showing vermiform shape and four of the eight molelike legs (phase contrast microscopy).

Figure 69-8. Longitudinal section of several mites surrounded by keratin in a hair follicle. The anterior portion of the mites is directed toward the base of the follicle.

Figure 69-9. Longitudinal section of *D. folliculorum* in a sebaceous gland. (All three courtesy of the Louisiana State University School of Medicine, New Orleans.)

but do not burrow into the skin. After prolonged feeding, the engorged larvae fall to the ground and molt. Nymphs and adults are predaceous. In temperate zones there is one, or possibly two, generations a year, but in the subtropics and tropics the generations are continuous.

The bites of chiggers are not felt at the

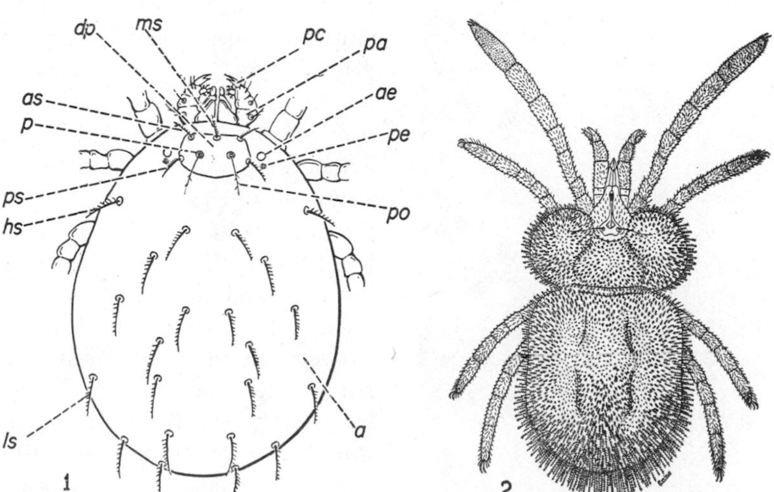

Figure 69-10. *Eutrombicula alfreddugesi. 1,* Larva (North American chigger), greatly enlarged. *a,* abdomen; *ae,* anterior eye; *as,* anterolateral seta; *dp,* dorsal plate; *hs,* humeral seta; *ls,* lateral seta I; *ms,* median seta; *p,* pseudostigma; *pa,* palpus; *pc,* palpal claw; *pe,* posterior eye; *po,* pseudostigmatic organ; *ps,* posterolateral seta. *2,* Adult. (Modified from Ewing.)

time of attachment. In sensitive individuals, intense itching and severe dermatitis result from the host's reaction to chigger secretions and usually occur several hours after the bites. The mites attack the ankles and legs and/or migrate upward. The lesions are numerous at sites where the clothes fit tightly and the movement of the chiggers is impeded, e.g. by elastic at top of socks, at waistline and thighs by the belt and underwear, at the edge of the brassiere, in the groin and other locations. Extravasation of blood from subcuticular capillaries causes bluish or purple ecchymoses (Fig. 69–11). Loss of sleep and secondary infection result in work loss, reduced efficiency, and avoidance of recreational areas. The affliction occurs in areas of every continent, but in Africa humans reportedly seldom experience intense reaction to chigger bites. *Eutrombicula alfreddugesi* (Oudemans) and *Eutrombicula splendens* (Ewing) are common in the eastern half of the United States (Fig. 69–10). Seasonal activity varies from late summer in Minnesota and Massachusetts to the entire year in southern Florida.

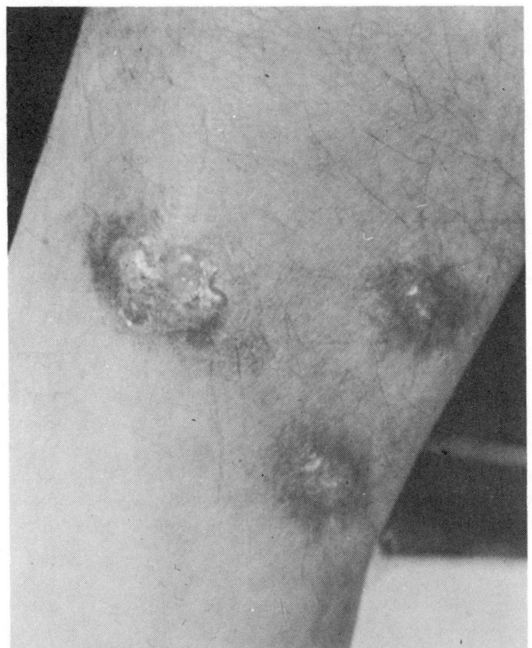

Figure 69–11. Dermatitis of leg resulting from reaction of chigger bites. (Courtesy of the Louisiana State University School of Medicine, New Orleans.)

Rickettsia tsutsugamushi transmitted from rodents to humans by chiggers causes scrub typhus (tsutsugamushi disease, flood fever) in Japan, Taiwan, Philippines and other Pacific islands, New Guinea, Indonesia, Australia, much of continental Asia from Malaya, Korea, and the Soviet Far East to India and the Himalayas.[14, 15] The rickettsiae survive through the nonparasitic nymphal and adult stages and are passed transovarially to the next generation of the mite. (See Chapter 12, p. 125.)

Scrub typhus foci, characterized by abundant food for rodents, occur in such varied tropical and temperate environments as primary and secondary jungle, grasslands (lalang), plantations, abandoned gardens, agricultural fields, temperate coniferous forests, mountain meadows and alpine deserts.

Numerous species of *Leptotrombidium* (= *Trombicula*) are involved as vectors of *Rickettsia tsutsugamushi* in different foci (Fig. 12–1, p. 125 and p. 126).

Mites are suspected on epidemiologic grounds of being involved in transmitting the agent of epidemic hemorrhagic fever. (See p. 91.)

Prevention of attachments by chiggers is more important than treatment. After the larval mites have attached, only palliative measures for local reaction and for the pruritus are of value. Therefore, use of clothing impregnated with a miticidal compound, such as benzyl benzoate, dibutyl phthalate or dimethyl phthalate, which are not removed completely by laundering or leached by water, is effective in preventing chigger bites. Diethyltoluamide preparations, such as OFF and DEET, are also effective if sprayed on clothing and exposed skin, but are removed rapidly by water. Table 72–1 (p. 794) contains additional information on prevention of attachments by chiggers and for area control of mites.

After exposure in areas infested by mites, promptly soap well and shower. Rub the skin briskly with a coarse towel. Topical application of an antipruritic and antihistaminic preparation may ameliorate the discomfort. Some persons recommend use of

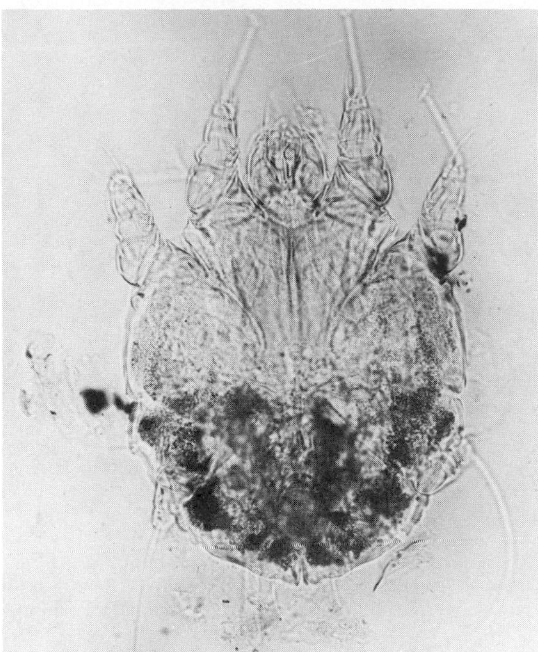

Figure 69–12

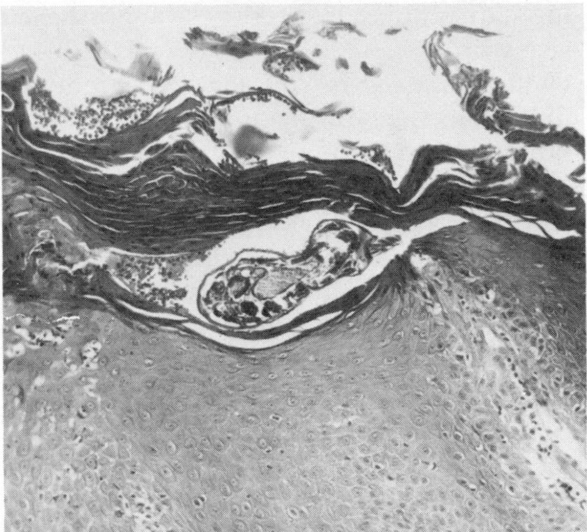

Figure 69–13

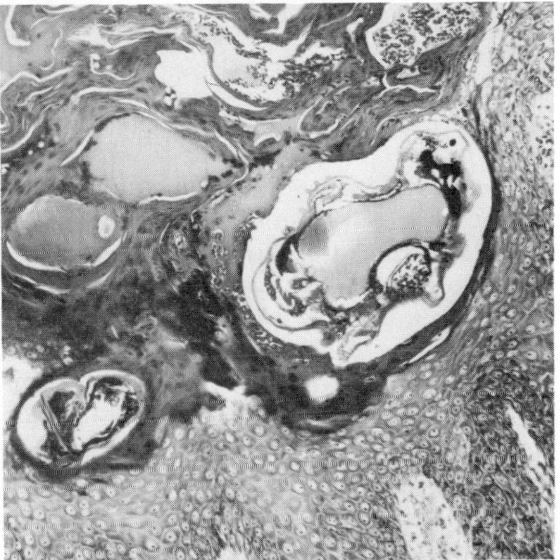

Figure 69–14

Figure 69–12. Adult mite, *Sarcoptes scabiei hominis.*

Figure 69–13. Adult *Sarcoptes scabiei hominis* in a burrow. Note spinose wall.

Figure 69–14. Section of scabies lesion showing mite and its spinose wall. (All three courtesy of the Louisiana State University School of Medicine, New Orleans; photographs by Eugene Wolfe.)

antihistamines orally. Field personnel and rural dwellers have stated that application of clear nail polish to individual lesions, in the absence of other preparations, afforded considerable relief.

FAMILY SARCOPTIDAE ITCH MITES

The burrowing sarcoptid itch mites produce diseases in many species of birds and mammals. *Sarcoptes scabiei hominis* Mégnin (= var. *scabiei* De Geer of authors) causes scabies in humans (Figs. 69–12, 69–13, 69–14). Different varieties cause sarcoptic mange in sheep, goats, pigs and other domestic and wild animals.

Scabies. Human scabies is also called 7-year itch, Norwegian itch, sarcoptic acariasis and gale (French). Physiologic variations in the host-parasite relationship reduce or prevent the survival of ectopic varieties of *S. scabiei* in atypical hosts. For example, the subspecies parasitizing cats does not establish itself successfully in humans but that of dogs may cause severe pruritus and prolonged papular eruption in humans.

Human scabies is produced almost exclusively by *Sarcoptes scabiei hominis* (Fig. 69–12). Clinical scabies is sporadic or common in numerous environments among crowded populations with poor sanitation.

Scabies mites are most readily spread through close bodily contact, especially when sleeping with an infected person. Interdigital infections are frequent, thus shaking hands is also a common method of transfer, especially when children play games requiring prolonged handclasping. Clothing and bedding are less important in spreading sarcoptid mites. Some workers consider the young, newly impregnated female mite to be most successfully passed to a new host; others assign the larva or the nymph to this role.

The pathologic responses to scabies mites are characteristic of previous sensitization. Wastes or other substances liberated by the parasites into the epidermis promote erythema and edema. The tissues become waterlogged and eosinophils tend to infiltrate the lesion. A vesicle gradually develops and ruptures, often giving rise to secondary infections. Most mite burrows are very superficial in the stratum corneum and lesions heal without scar formation (Figs. 69–13, 69–15). Some patients exhibit a mild eosinophilia during acute stages of the infection.

Severe itching, the cardinal symptom of scabies, is most intense shortly after a warm bath or going to bed, when the gradual warming of the body induces greater mite activity. Loss of sleep resulting from scabies has caused many lost man-days during military operations. A follicular eruption may occur in sensitive persons. Scratching serves to kill some scabies mites and to inoculate others into new sites, and allows development of secondary infection.

Untreated scabies cases often terminate spontaneously after several months. As sensitization develops, each new mite is immediately surrounded by transudates that reduce its normal activity. Some cases become chronic but parasite numbers are fewer than in the acute stage. Norwegian itch or crusted itch is a severe form of the disease accompanied by hyperkeratosis (Fig. 69–14).

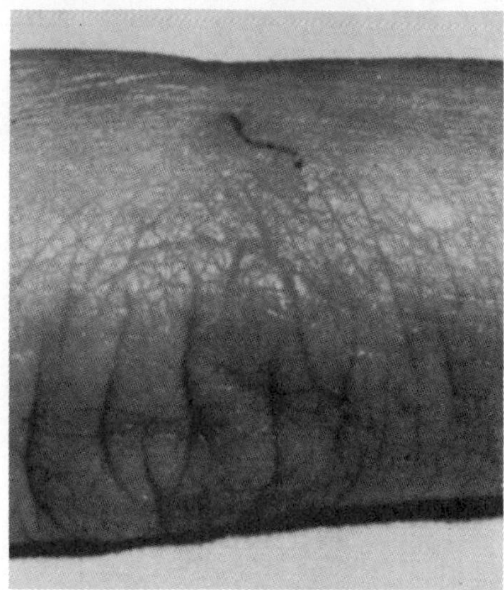

Figure 69–15. Superficial cutaneous track in a case of scabies. (Courtesy of A. Rook, D. S. Wilkinson, and F. J. G. Ebling (eds.): Textbook of Dermatology, 1968. F. A. Davis Co., Philadelphia.

Definitive diagnosis of scabies, based on demonstration of the mite, is often difficult. Under a hand lens the typical scabies mite burrow, a tortuous channel a few millimeters long, appears as a fine line on the skin (Fig. 69–15). The burrow orifice may be marked by a black plug of crusted serum and mite feces. Toward the blind end of the tunnel, where the female is situated, the skin is erythematous and a small vesicle is frequently found. This region should be incised with a fine-pointed scalpel or sharp needle and the contents placed on a glass slide with a 10 per cent potassium hydroxide solution to clear cutaneous scales and other debris. Then add a coverslip and examine microscopically. Finding a mite in any stage of the life cycle is diagnostic. Mite eggs are sometimes observed.

When the mite cannot be demonstrated in adult patients, a dermatologic diagnosis may be made if the lesions are distributed in characteristic places – interdigital spaces (Fig. 69–16), wrists, extensor aspects of elbows, axillae (particularly folds), abdomen and belt line (especially umbilical region), scrotum,

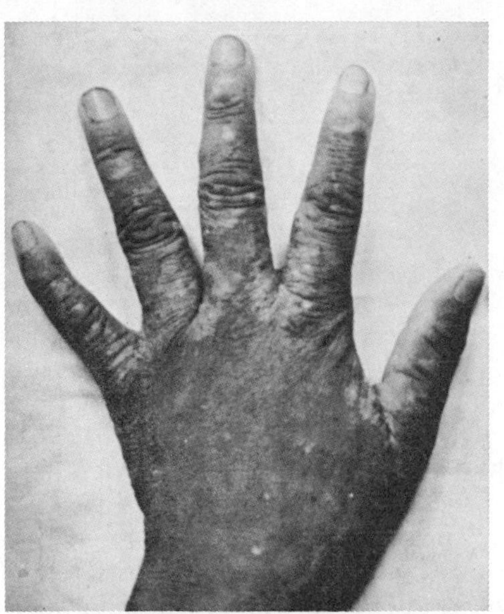

Figure 69–16. Scabies—showing advanced lesions and characteristic distribution.

penis, and areolae of the nipples. In severe cases, lesions may extend around the trunk to the middle back. The upper back, face, scalp, palms, and soles are rarely involved in adults, but all the body surface of infants is susceptible to mite invasion.

A history of primary lesions between the fingers and close contact with members of the family group and other persons having characteristic symptoms is suggestive of scabies.

Several other dermatologic conditions may superficially resemble scabies. However, it is generally safe to rely on the characteristic scabies lesion distribution, which is rarely mimicked by other diseases. (See Table 72–1, p. 795 for treatment.)

Acarophobia

Delusion of dermal parasitosis by mites, or acarophobia, can be a serious psychiatric condition. Unsuccessful attempts to remove imaginary parasites may lead to much mutilation and excoriation. The condition may be manifested by folie à deux, a psychosis shared by two persons.

Irritation and Allergy

Holothyrus coccinella Gervais (HOLOTHYRIDAE) produces an irritant poisonous fluid. This family of large predators occurs in Australia, New Guinea, Sri Lanka, Seychelles and Mauritius. House dust allergy, caused by *Dermatophagoides* spp. (TYROGLYPHIDAE) associated with fungi and pollens, is reported from temperate Europe, America and elsewhere.

REFERENCES

1. Savory, T. 1964. Arachnids. Academic Press, New York, 291 pp.
2. Snow, K. R. 1970. The Arachnids. An Introduction. Routledge & Keegan Paul, London. 84 pp.
3. Dreisbach, R. H. 1974. Handbook of Poisoning. 8th ed. Lange Medical Publications, Los Altos, California. 517 pp.
4. Ennik, F. 1972. A short review of scorpion biology, management of stings, and control. Calif. Vector Views *19*:69–79.
5. Russell, F. E., Wainschel, J., and Gertsch, W. J. 1973. Bites of spiders and other arthropods. *In* Conn, H. F. (ed.): Current Therapy. 25th ed. W.B. Saunders Co., Philadelphia. pp. 868–870.
6. Russell, F. E., Waldron, W. G., and Madon, M. B. 1969. Bites by the brown spiders *Loxosceles unicolor* and *Loxosceles arizonica* in California and Arizona. Toxicon *7*:109–117.
7. Williams, R. E. 1972. Necrotic arachnidism. *In* Hoeprich, P. D. (ed.): Infectious Diseases. Harper & Row, Publishers, Hagerstown, Maryland. pp. 917–920.
8. Balashov, Yu. S. 1972. Bloodsucking ticks (Ixodoidea)—vectors of diseases of man and animals. [English translation.] Misc. Publ. Entomol. Soc. Am. *8*:161–376.
9. Hoogstraal, H. 1973. Acarina (ticks); and Viruses and Ticks. *In* Gibbs, A. J. (ed.): Viruses and Invertebrates. North Holland Publishing Co., Amsterdam. pp. 90–103; 349–390.
10. Gregson, J. D. 1973. Tick Paralysis—An appraisal of natural and experimental data. Can. Dep. Agr. Monogr. No. 9., Ottawa. 109 pp.
11. Krantz, G. W. 1970. A Manual of Acarology. Oregon State University Bookstores, Corvallis. 336 pp.
12. Baker, E. W., and Wharton, G. W. 1952. An Introduction to Acarology. The Macmillan Co., New York, 465 pp.
13. Yunker, C. E. 1973. Mites. *In* Flynn, R. J. (ed.): Parasites of Laboratory Animals. Iowa State University Press, Ames. pp. 425–492.
14. Audy, J. R. 1968. Red Mites and Typhus. Athlone Press, London. 191 pp.
15. Traub, R., Wisseman, C. L., and Ahmad, N. 1967. The occurrence of scrub typhus infection in unusual habitats in West Pakistan. Trans. Roy. Soc. Trop. Med. Hyg. *61*:23–57.

CHAPTER 70

Class Insecta (Hexapoda)

R. H. Grothaus
D. E. Weidhaas

INTRODUCTION

Insects constitute the most abundant form of life on earth, accounting for about 800,000 of the known animal species.[1] They thrive in a variety of ecosystems nearly everywhere in the world. Insects have dwelt on earth for 250 to 300 million years, which provides an indication of their ability to adapt to adversity and divergent environments.

The class Insecta is of great general importance to man. However, only those insects that directly affect man's health and well-being or transmit disease will be considered in this text.

Insects share the characters common to all members of the phylum Arthropoda (Chapter 68). In addition, insects are characterized by a segmented body, with the segments grouped into three specific regions: the head, thorax and abdomen. The head bears the mouthparts, one pair of antennae, and the eyes. Three pairs of legs are located ventrally on the thorax (lacking in some immature insects); wings, when present, are located on the dorsum of the thorax. The abdomen is usually elongate with five to ten visible segments; appendages, when present, are found on the posterior tip.[2]

Some 26 to 33 orders of insects are recognized today. Only four of these orders are of major medical importance to human health. However, several other orders are of some medical importance and will be discussed in proportion to their importance. The order of presentation will, in general, be from the simplest to the most highly evolved groups.

List of Medically Important Orders

1. Collembola (Springtails)
2. Orthoptera (Cockroaches, Walking Sticks)
3. Ephemeroptera (Mayflies)
4. Trichoptera (Caddis flies)
5. Mallophaga (Biting lice)
*6. Anoplura (Sucking lice)
*7. Hemiptera (Bugs)
8. Coleoptera (Beetles)
9. Lepidoptera (Butterflies, Moths)
*10. Diptera (Flies, Mosquitoes)
*11. Siphonaptera (Fleas)
12. Hymenoptera (Ants, Bees, Wasps)

*These orders are of outstanding medical importance.

Order Collembola
Springtails

The Collembola are small (3 mm or less) wingless insects with chewing mouthparts. They are called springtails because of the springlike structure at the tip of the abdomen (Fig. 70–1). Springtails are usually found in litter and other decaying organic material. However, *Entomobrya nivalis* (Linn.) (cosmopolitan) and *E. tenuicauda* Schött (Australasian) are reported to cause a pruritic dermatitis in man. Affected patients complain of sharp, biting sensations followed by irritation and papules similar to mosquito bites, with pruritus. One American species, *Orchesella albosa* Guthrie, has been reported as infesting man without causing dermatitis.

Order Orthoptera
Blattidae – Cockroaches

Of the ORTHOPTERA, only the cockroaches (family BLATTIDAE) are believed to be concerned in the transmission of disease. They are cosmopolitan in distribution. These insects frequent filthy places and are known to feed on both excrement and sputum. Soon after, they may be found on human food, where, both by their feces and by regurgitation, they discharge some of their flora. Cockroaches have been associated experimentally with a variety of bacteria, including species of *Streptococcus, Salmonella* and *Vibrio;* several viruses, including poliomyelitis virus; and protozoa. There is also evidence to indicate that cockroaches serve as intermediate hosts of certain helminths.

Cockroaches are fast running, flattened, nocturnal insects with long, slender antennae and semitransparent brownish wings (in the wing-bearing species) (Fig. 70–1). The head is turned so far under that the mouthparts are actually directed backward. Mouthparts are of the chewing type. Not all species enter buildings.

Life History. Cockroach eggs are deposited in a leathery capsule that may often be seen protruding from the body of the female. Eventually she either glues the capsule to some object or merely drops it. The 20 or 30 eggs (*Blattella*) hatch into tiny nymphs, which resemble the adults except that they have no wings. A gradual metamorphosis ensues. Cockroaches have scent glands that secrete an oily liquid responsible for their characteristic odor. See Table 72–1 for control.

ORTHOPTERA of the family PHASMIDAE (walking sticks) have been known to discharge an irritating fluid, which in the case of *Anisomorpha buprestoides* (Stoll) is capable of being squirted a distance of 2 feet. If introduced into the eye, it causes excruciating pain.

Order Ephemeroptera
Mayflies

This order contains species known as mayflies. The species *Hexagenia bilineata* (Say) used to occur in such numbers along the shores of Lake Erie that many people developed an allergic condition from breathing fragments of the cast insect skins. Hypersensitivity and severe asthmatic paroxysms have been recorded (Table 68–2). Changing ecologic conditions have resulted in reduced numbers of these insects (Fig. 70–1).

Order Trichoptera
Caddis Flies

TRICHOPTERA, or caddis flies, are likewise causative agents of allergic symptoms at times. The hairs and scales from their mothlike bodies cause the allergic reactions.

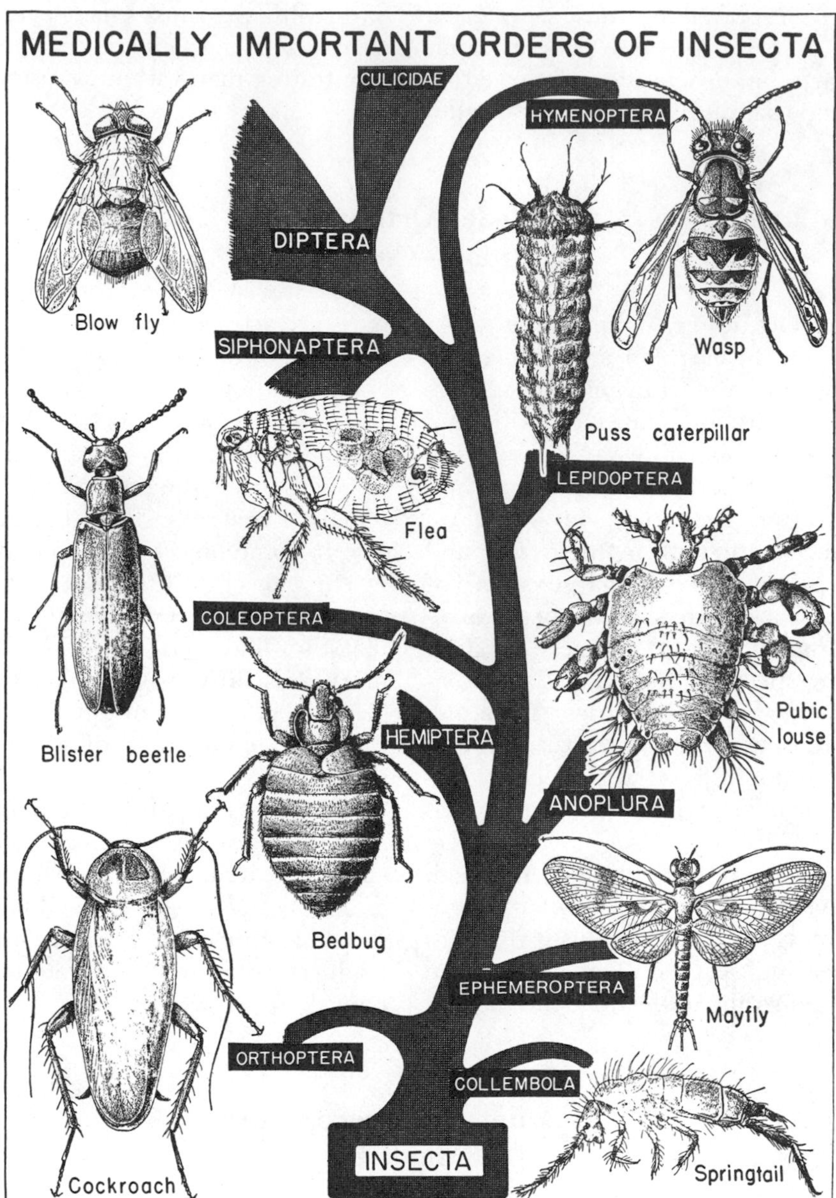

Figure 70–1. Some important orders of insects.

Order Mallophaga
Biting Lice

MALLOPHAGA, or biting lice, are mentioned here merely to distinguish them from the sucking lice discussed below. MALLOPHAGA abound on birds and many species of mammals. They have chewing mouthparts and feed chiefly on dandruff, scurf or dried blood. They are exceedingly irritating when abundant and constitute a considerable problem for the veterinarian. Poultry handlers are frequently annoyed by them, but the irritation is of short duration since these species will not remain on human hosts. The biting dog louse, *Trichodectes canis* De Geer, is an intermediate host of the dog tapeworm, *Dipylidium caninum* (Linn.), a species occasionally found in man.

Order Anoplura
Sucking Lice

The ANOPLURA (sucking lice) are of major medical importance. They are primary vectors of three important infections of man: epidemic (louse-borne) relapsing fever, epidemic typhus and trench fever. In addition, they frequently cause adverse skin responses, particularly in sensitized individuals.

The order ANOPLURA includes six families and over 400 species. One family, PEDICULIDAE, contains the parasites of man. Sucking lice are characterized by the lack of wings, a dorsoventrally flattened body and retractile piercing-sucking mouthparts. The head is narrow and pointed with eyes reduced or lacking (well developed in human species). The legs are highly modified for grasping hair (Figs. 70–1, 70–2).

The species infesting man include: *Phthirus pubis* (Linn.), the crab louse (Fig. 70–1); *Pediculus humanus humanus* (Linn.), the body louse (Figs. 70–2; 6–2, p. 104); and the subspecies *Pediculus humanus capitis* De Geer, the head louse. These insects are cosmopolitan in distribution. However, body louse infestations frequently occur in greater numbers in cooler climates where people utilize wool clothing.

Biology of Human Lice. Pubic or crab lice are small (1.5 to 2 mm) crablike insects with strong grasping legs. Their normal habitat includes the pubic regions but may include facial hair, axillae, and body surface when the infestation is heavy. Both the body and crab lice have similar life histories. Adult female crab lice and head lice attach eggs individually to hairs, while body lice deposit eggs on the fibers or in the seams of clothing. Eggs (nits) hatch in 7 to 10 days. Three molts occur as the immature lice increase in size through gradual metamorphosis. The egg to egg cycle takes from 3 to 4 weeks, depending on the species and environmental conditions. Female crab lice deposit about 30 eggs in a lifetime, whereas head lice deposit 50 to 150. The body louse may deposit as many as 300 eggs. Adult lice live 2 to 4 weeks after reaching maturity.

The head and body lice (Fig. 70–2) are longer and less crablike than the pubic louse (Fig. 70–1). They range in size from 2 to 3 mm. Head lice are typically found on the head around the occiput and ears. Body lice are most commonly found where the clothing comes in tight contact with the body (armpits, waist, neck, shoulders and crotch).

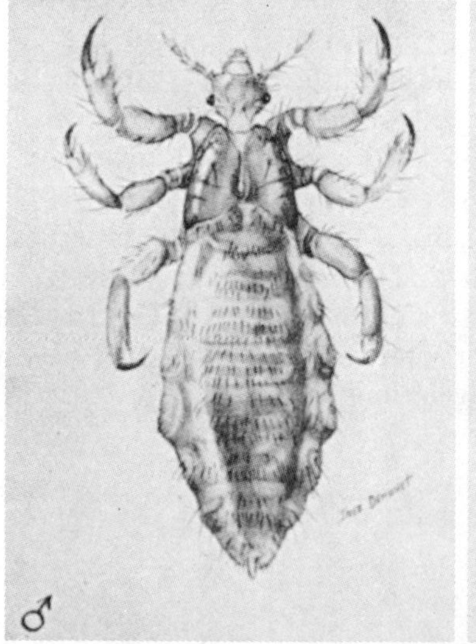

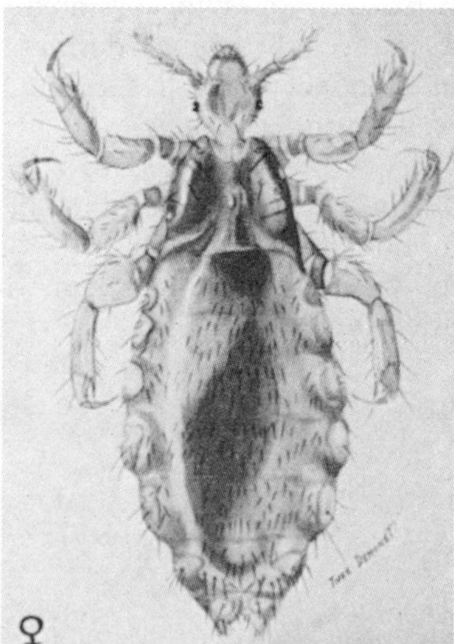

Figure 70–2. *Pediculus humanus humanus* male and female. (Courtesy of the National Institutes of Health, U.S. Public Health Service.)

The seams of clothing appear to be the preferred habitat when feeding is not taking place. Both body and head lice are disseminated through contact with infested clothing or lousy people. Pubic lice are most frequently disseminated through sexual contact, but other means are possible. Nursing care personnel handling infested patients may acquire infestations with lice. In recent years a resurgence of louse infestations has occurred in the more affluent countries because of changing life styles. Communal living, poor hygiene and crowded conditions all provide for increased dissemination of lice.

Disease Vectors. Of the three species of lice, only the body louse is of major importance as the vector of epidemic typhus (Chapter 6, p. 102), trench fever (Chapter 14, p. 135), and louse-borne relapsing fever (Chapter 15, p. 137). The infections are normally acquired by scratching to relieve the itching caused by the bite, thereby rubbing infected feces or crushed louse fragments into scratches or skin abrasions. The bite is of doubtful importance in disease transmission.

Pediculosis. The bites of lice often cause intense discomfort, not only when the insect is feeding but also during the hours that follow. In the case of sensitized persons, symptoms may persist for many days. Typically, a small reddish papule appears at the site of each feeding puncture. Intense pruritus follows and scratching frequently results in a "weeping" dermatitis, predisposing to secondary infection. Both diffuse swelling and erythema may occur, especially if many lice have fed in a restricted area. Healing is usually accompanied by induration and mild fissuring of the skin, with the deposition of a bronze pigment that persists indefinitely.

It has been shown that repeated exposures are necessary for the development of dermal hypersensitivity and that the feces of the louse are involved in this reaction. The pruritus is part of the syndrome of hypersensitivity. As for the bite itself, the reaction appears to involve two components—a purpuric reaction, which depends on the act of feeding, and an inflammatory reaction, dependent on sensitization. If one remains infested over an extended period, the bronze pigmented condition of the skin known as "vagabond's disease" results. Systemic symptoms have been recorded, including general malaise, mental depression and a rash somewhat like that of rubella.

Untreated pediculosis of the scalp results in a condition in which the hair becomes matted together by exudate from the pustular lesions and the entire mass develops a fetid odor. The severity of the condition is often aggravated by the presence of mycotic infections.

At times, peculiar bluish or slate-colored macules, which do not itch or disappear on pressure, occur in association with *P. pubis.* These macules are about 0.5 cm in diameter and are located chiefly on the sides of the trunk and on the inner aspects of the thighs.

Hair casts and globules (pseudo-nits) attached to the hair shafts have been confused with nits, with resultant erroneous diagnoses. This has led to incorrect reports of "outbreaks of pediculosis capitis" involving as many as several thousand students. Microscopic examination of the objects readily serves to differentiate the pseudo-nits from eggs of lice. When microscopic diagnosis is not possible, one should be suspicious of diagnoses of head louse outbreaks among well groomed persons when no adults or nymphs are found or when accepted treatment remedies for their control fail, as they may prove to be pseudopediculosis.

Treatment. Refer to Table 72–1, page 795, for treatment for infestations by lice and for methods of louse control.

Order Hemiptera
True Bugs

The insects in this order are both winged and wingless. Two pairs of wings are present in the winged species; the first pair is thick and leathery basally and membranous apically. The HEMIPTERA are characterized by piercing, sucking mouthparts arising anteriorly from the head. The proboscis is typically flexed back under the head and thorax when at rest. Insects of this order undergo gradual metamorphosis.

There are over 50,000 described species in the order HEMIPTERA; most are phytophagous in habit. Two families contain blood-feeding species of considerable medical importance: the CIMICIDAE (bedbugs) and the REDUVIIDAE (assassin bugs, conenose bugs or kissing bugs). Members of several other families also inflict painful bites even though their feeding habits are predaceous or phytophagous in nature.

FAMILY CIMICIDAE
Bedbugs

Life History and Feeding Habits, Including Effects of Bites. Bedbugs inhabit houses, barracks and other abodes, secreting themselves in crevices of walls, floors and furniture. They are flattened insects with an oval contour and a reddish color. Adult bedbugs are about 6 mm in length. They are wingless in all stages.

Bedbugs normally prefer to feed at night. Engorgement seldom requires more than 10 to 15 minutes. After feeding they return to their hiding places. Lesions produced by bedbug bites are usually firm, conical papules. If sensitivity is marked, large hemorrhagic bullae may form. The grouping of lesions in pairs or triplicates fairly close together and often linear in distribution is a characteristic feature. The bites may become erythematous and swollen and are sometimes characterized by severe and prolonged itching. Scratching may result in secondary infection. These insects have been experimentally incriminated as carriers of human disease, but there is no direct evidence that they transmit infection from man to man under natural conditions.

Female bedbugs deposit their eggs singly, gluing them to solid supports in the crannies that harbor the insects by day. A single female may deposit over 500 eggs in batches of 10 to 60 over a period of several months. The average is probably near 200. The eggs require about a week for development at optimum temperature. Newly hatched bedbugs resemble adults in miniature and are known as nymphs. When human hosts are not available, bedbugs will feed readily on other mammals. The normal life span is from 6 to 8 months.

Two common species of bedbug attack man: *Cimex lectularius* (Linn.) in most temperate regions and *C. hemipterus* (Fabr.) in the tropics, especially Asia. These species are almost identical in appearance. Closely related forms attend other warm-blooded vertebrates, such as bats, but these very rarely feed upon man. Bat bedbugs, *C. pillosellus* (Horvath), are easy to recognize by reason of the abundant hair on the body. In Africa man is attacked by still another species, *Leptocimex boueti* (Brumpt), whose long antennae and long legs (especially the last pair) distinguish it from related forms (Figs. 70–1, 70–3).[3] For control of bedbugs see Table 72–1, page 796.

FAMILY REDUVIIDAE
Kissing Bugs

Life History and Feeding Habits—Relation to Chagas' Disease. This family contains over 3000 species. Most species (assassin bugs) feed on the body fluids of other insects. However, more than 75 feed on mammals, including man. Some species are vectors for *Trypanosoma cruzi*, the causative agent of Chagas' disease in the Americas (p. 441). Some authors treat the kissing bugs as

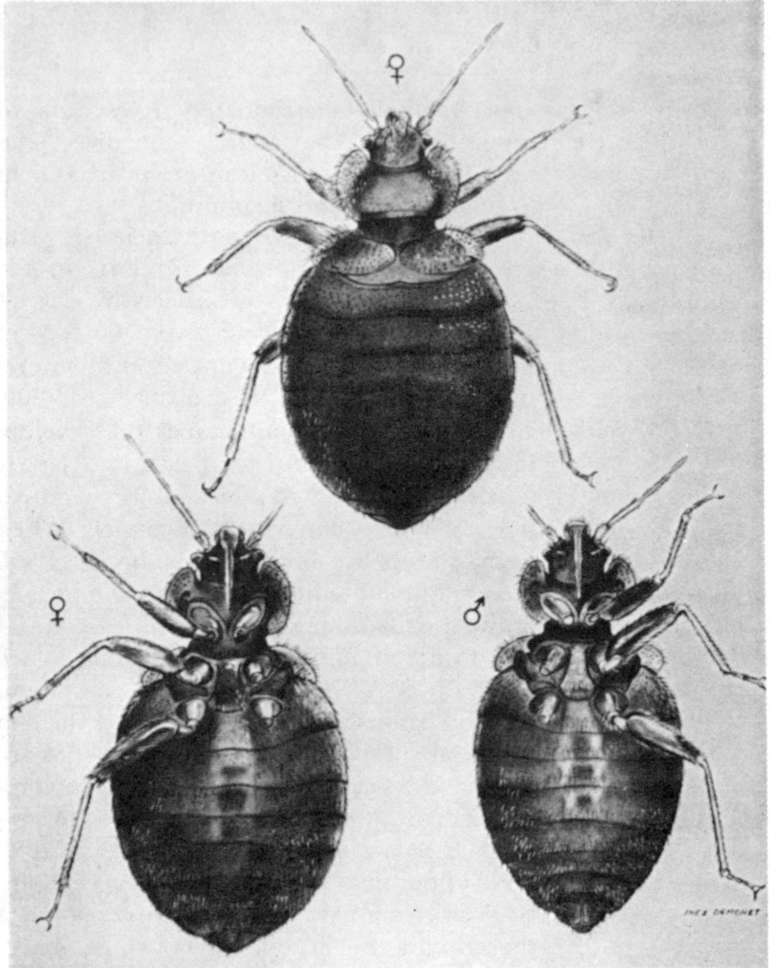

Figure 70–3. Bedbug, *Cimex lectularius.* (Courtesy of the National Institutes of Health. U.S. Public Health Service.)

a distinct family, the TRIATOMIDAE (Fig. 70–4).

Both adults and nymphs are nocturnal, remaining in cracks in the walls of houses or other suitable sites during the day. Feeding usually takes place while humans are sleeping. The bite is commonly on the cheeks near the eye, hence the name "barbeiros." Less commonly the mouth area is the site of the bite (kissing bugs). In many of the blood-feeding species the bite is benign, but there are notable exceptions. Considerable edema around the eye (Romaña's sign) is usually associated with the early stages of Chagas' disease and this is frequently caused by the reaction to the bite, rather than the parasite. Most assassin bugs, such as *Reduvius personatus* (Linn.), the masked hunter, and *Arilus cristatus* (Linn.), the wheel bug, cause painful bites when humans are accidentally attacked. The bites may cause nausea, palpitation and generalized urticaria.

Most kissing bugs have a 1- or 2-year life cycle. Females deposit their eggs (2 mm long) singly or in small clusters in cracks and other sites in and around the normal resting places. Eggs per female vary from a few to over 2000. The incubation period varies from 8 to 30 days, depending on environmental conditions, and the nymphs pass through five instars.

Other Vectors and Potential Vectors. The accompanying tables (Tables 70–1, 70–2) list various species believed to be capable of transmitting Chagas' disease in the areas where that disease exists (Mexico, Central

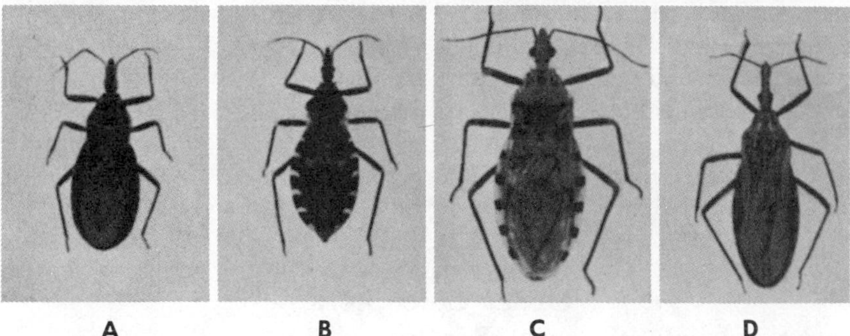

Figure 70–4. Four species of REDUVIIDAE. *A, Triatoma protracta; B, Triatoma sanguisuga; C, Panstrongylus geniculatus; D, Rhodnius lescens.* (Herms' Medical Entomology. 6th ed. By permission of The Macmillan Company.)

Table 70–1. REDUVIID BUGS REPORTED AS VECTORS OF *Trypanosoma cruzi* IN MEXICO, CENTRAL AND SOUTH AMERICA

Location	*Species of Bug*
Mexico	*Triatoma sanguisuga* (LeConte), *Rhodnius prolixus* Stal, *T. hegneri* Mazzotti, *T. barberi* Usinger
Guatemala	*Triatoma dimidiata* Latr.
Panama	*Eratyrus cuspidatus* Stal, *Rhodnius pallescens* Barber, R. *prolixus* Stal, *Panstrongylus geniculatus* Latr., *T. dimidiata.*
Argentina	*Eutriatoma sordida* Pinto, *Psammolestes coreodes* Berg., *T. infestans* Klug
Bolivia	*Eutriatoma sordida, T. infestans*
Brazil	*Panstrongylus megistus* (Burmeister), *T, brasiliensis* Neiva, *E. sordida* Pinto, *T. chagasi* Brumpt and Gomez, *T. vitticeps* Stal
Chile	*Mepraia spinalai* Porter, *T. infestans*
Colombia	*Rhodnius prolixus, R. pictipes* Stal
Costa Rica	*Triatoma dimidiata, R. prolixus*
Paraguay	*Eutriatoma sordida, T. infestans*
Uruguay	*Eutriatoma sordida, T. infestans*
Venezuela	*Eratyrus cuspidatus, E. nigromaculatus* Stal, *Panstrongylus rufotuberculatus* Champ., *Psammolestes arthuri* Pinto, *Psammolestes geniculatus* Latr., *R. prolixus, T. maculata* (Erichson)
Ecuador	*Triatoma dimidiata*

Table 70–2. REDUVIID BUGS NATURALLY INFECTED WITH *Trypanosoma cruzi* (U.S.A.)

Species	*Geographic Location*	*Host Animals or Hiding Place*
Triatoma protracta (Uhler)	New Mexico California Arizona	*Neotoma* sp. (wood rats)
Triatoma rubida uhleri Neiva	Arizona California	*Neotoma* sp.
Triatoma gerstaekeri (Stal)	Texas	*Neotoma* sp.
Triatoma heidmanni Neiva	Texas	Dwellings–bedding
Triatoma protracta woodi Usinger	New Mexico Texas	*Neotoma* sp.
Triatoma sanguisuga (Le Conte)	Texas	*Neotoma* sp.
Triatoma sanguisuga ambigua Neiva	Texas	*Neotoma* sp.
Triatoma recurva (Stal)	Arizona	*Neotoma* sp.

and South America). It should be mentioned that *Triatoma infestans* has recently gained considerable prominence as a vector in those countries where it occurs. Table 70–2 shows those species that have been found naturally infected with *Trypanosoma cruzi* within the boundaries of the United States. The construction of housing in the United States generally does not permit easy access or favorable conditions for potential vectors of *T. cruzi.* This and other factors that limit human contact with reduviid bugs probably are important reasons that Chagas' disease is rare in the United States.[4, 5]

Order Coleoptera
Beetles

This is the largest order in the class INSECTA, containing over 250,000 species. The species distribution is worldwide. These insects are characterized by the presence of two pairs of wings; the anterior pair is rigid and horny. This pair of wings, called *elytra,* usually meets in a straight line down the back. The shell-like elytra serve as a cover for the second pair of wings, which are membranous. The mouthparts are of the chewing type. Metamorphosis is complete, with the insect passing through egg, larval, pupal and adult stages.

Although not of major medical importance, COLEOPTERA affect the health of man in several ways:

1. by vesicating and poisonous effects;
2. as parasitic larvae (canthariasis) and adults (scarabiasis);
3. as intermediate hosts of helminthic parasites; and
4. by mechanical transmission of infective organisms.

VESICATING AND POISONOUS EFFECTS

Certain beetles in the families MELOIDAE, STAPHYLINIDAE and OEDEMERIDAE contain powerful dermal toxicants in their body fluids. The blister beetles (MELOIDAE) contain cantharidin (Spanish fly), which produces a dramatic blistering effect when rubbed on the skin. The irritating substance of STAPHYLINIDAE (rove beetles) of the genus *Paederus* is chemically different from cantharidin and is called pederin. Several species in these families have become well known for their vesicating properties. *Lytta vesicatoria* (Linn.), the Spanish fly, is common in southern Europe. *Epicauta vittata* (Fabr.), *Epicauta pennsylvanica* (De Geer) and *Epicauta cinerea* (Foster) are common in the United States. *Zonabris nubica* (de Marseul), *Epicauta tomentosa* Maeklin, *Epicauta sapphirina* Maeklin and *Paederus crebrepunctatus* Eppelsheim are important in Africa; the fluid from crushed beetles of the latter species produces a conjunctivitis known as "Nairobi eye." *Sessinia collaris* (Sharp) and *Sessinia decolor* Fairmaire (coconut beetles) are important on the Pacific Islands. *Oxicopis vittata* (Fabr.) is found in Puerto Rico. Species of STAPHYLINIDAE cause severe problems in Japan; *Paederus fuscipes* Curt causes difficulty in Thailand.[6]

When blister beetles are irritated or brushed from the skin, they release fluid that causes a tingling, burning sensation in about 10 minutes, followed by mild erythema. In 2 or 3 hours the bullae or vesicles appear as flat-topped collections of fluid. In 8 to 10 hours, the bullae develop into slightly flaccid blisters. They are typically asymptomatic. Diagnosis is not difficult. The bullae are frequently linear in arrangement; multiple bullae may coalesce to form a single linear lesion. The bullae are usually found on exposed portions of the body, lack erythema and are all in the same developmental stage. A lack of a central puncture permits differentiation from bites. The latent development of lesions aids in differentiation from chemical and thermal lesions. The condition is most often seen during the summer in temperate climates.

Large bullae may be drained and protected with an occlusive dressing using an antibiotic ointment. Lesions in areas unlikely to be traumatized resolve in 3 to 5 days and the overlying epidermis flakes off in about 1 week. Protection of the affected area is adequate treatment in these cases.

CANTHARIASIS AND SCARABIASIS

Infection of man by larval beetles is known as canthariasis. Scarabiasis refers to infection of man by adult beetles. Intestinal, urinary, ocular, nasal, aural and cutaneous varieties have been recorded. These conditions are rare, as they follow the accidental entrance of eggs, larvae or adults into the human body. An intense diarrhea occurred among children in Sri Lanka that apparently was due to intestinal infection with coleopterans.

BEETLES AS HOSTS TO HELMINTHIC PARASITES

Various species belonging to different families are known to serve as intermediate hosts of helminth parasites of man and animals. This relationship is no doubt largely caused by the ingestion of fecal matter containing eggs by many cereal and omnivorous feeders as well as the purely coprophagous beetles. Included are the infective stages (cysticercoids) of the rat and mouse tapeworms *Hymenolepis diminuta* and *H. nana,* as well as the larvae of the nematode *Gongylonema pulchrum* Molin and the spiny-headed worm *Macracanthorhynchus hirudinaceus.*

MECHANICAL TRANSMISSION OF MICROORGANISMS BY BEETLES

Adults of Staphylinidae (rove beetles), Silphidae (carrion beetles) and Histeridae feed upon dead animal matter of one form or another. They may thus convey pathogens (1) upon their bodies, legs or mouthparts or (2) by way of the alimentary tract. Species of Dermestidae, or carpet beetles, feed on such material chiefly in the larval stage. Anthrax bacilli have been found in the feces of *Dermestes vulpinus* F. that had developed to maturity on skins of animals known to have had the disease.

Dung beetles ("tumble bugs," dung-burying beetles and other coprophagous species) of the family Scarabaeidae are attracted to human feces. Certain species form balls of feces and roll them away for burial (food storage); other dung beetles bury feces directly and produce mounds of disturbed soil at the site of deposition. The larger coprophagous species excrete considerable amounts of fecal material during their feeding and burrowing activities. This, as well as transport of mammalian feces to a distance, may be a factor in the dissemination of microorganisms present in human and animal stools. Stools may be buried by numbers of dung beetles within a few hours after deposition. The rapid removal of stools by these beetles may have indirect influence on the degree of pollution and worm infestation of soil by maintaining defecation sites in acceptable condition for repeated use and thus enhancing the infection potential of particular spots. Hookworm and *Ascaris* eggs ingested by dung beetles usually are destroyed by mastication owing to the grinding action of the beetle's mandibles. However, when soil conditions are favorable for their development, hookworm larvae develop wherever beetles bury infected feces. The activities of the beetles thus result in lateral dispersion of hookworms in the soil. Conversely, beetles work against effective dissemination of *Ascaris* eggs both by destroying them through ingestion and by burying them.

Order Lepidoptera
Butterflies and Moths

Species in this order are characterized by the presence of numerous scales on the body and wings and by the nature of their mouthparts, which consist of a sucking tube that is coiled beneath the head when not in use. Two pairs of wings are usually present. The metamorphosis is complete. Their larvae (caterpillars) may be wormlike or covered with hairs, according to the species concerned. Most moths pupate inside a silken cocoon spun by the larva just prior to transformation.

The order is of minor medical significance but, as with the beetles, certain important medical problems exist.

URTICATING HAIRS

There are several groups of caterpillars (Figs. 70–5 to 70–7) and a few adults that bear hairs capable of causing envenomization in humans. The hairs may be simple or hollowed, but all are associated with poison-secreting cells or glands (Figs. 70–8, 70–10). Individuals contacting these hairs are usually pierced by the hair fragments, resulting in urticating or allergic responses.

Lepidopterism. This term is applied to poisonous accidents caused by adult lepidopterans. This syndrome has only recently been recognized as being relatively widespread in South America. The genus *Hylesia* (SATURNIIDAE) is responsible for epidemic outbreaks of dermatitis in South America. Each adult carries thousands of urticating spines or hairs (flechettes) that are shed as the moth flies and rubs against leaves and other obstacles. When large numbers of moths are present, airborne clouds of hairs settle on skin, bed sheets and other sites, resulting in dermatitis and other toxic responses. Dermatitis usually occurs on the exposed parts of the body and occasionally on the abdomen. It appears a few minutes after contact with urticating hairs. The first signs include immediate intense itching, followed by the appearance of papules, then erythematous patches, swelling, induration and burning pain; less frequently monomorphic eruptions, single or with stiff micropapules, follow. When moths are contacted directly, extensive urticariform eruptions with bullae may occur.

TREATMENT. The rapid use of 50 per cent sodium hyposulfite lotion usually eliminates itching and enhances the disappearance of cutaneous lesions. The use of oral antihistamines is also recommended. Adrenocorticotropic hormone (ACTH) has been used with some success. Treatment should bring about regression and relief in 1 to 3 days; normal regression occurs in 6 to 14 days.

Erucism. This term applies to poisoning by caterpillars. Unlike lepidopterism, erucism usually occurs through direct contact of individuals with caterpillars possessing venomous hairs (Figs. 70–8, 70–10). The most common response is a simple inflammatory dermatitis; erythema is constant (Figs. 70–9, 70–11). Local swelling often ensues. The pathologic change caused by the dermatitis, e.g. due to *Automeris io,* is a rapidly developing edema of the corium and subcutaneous tissues without necrosis. A sharp stinging sensation or intense burning pain for up to 6 or more hours, followed by numbness, usually occurs. Lymphadenopathy, leukocytosis and eosinophilia are present in some cases. The manifestations, sudden in onset, normally disappear within 24 hours, except for the occasional linear series of lesions depicting the pattern of the offending hairs, which may persist longer (Figs. 70–9, 70–11). In more severe cases nausea and fever occur. Muscle spasm, with difficulty in respiration, rarely may ensue, particularly if the sting is on the neck.

Caterpillars of at least 10 families and more than 50 species of LEPIDOPTERA possess urticating hairs. A number of species are of medical importance in various parts of the world. In the United States, larvae of *Megalopyge opercularis* (J. E. Smith), the puss

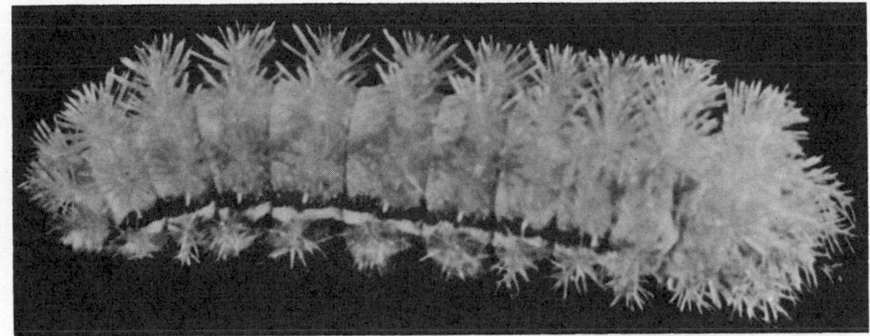

Figure 70–5

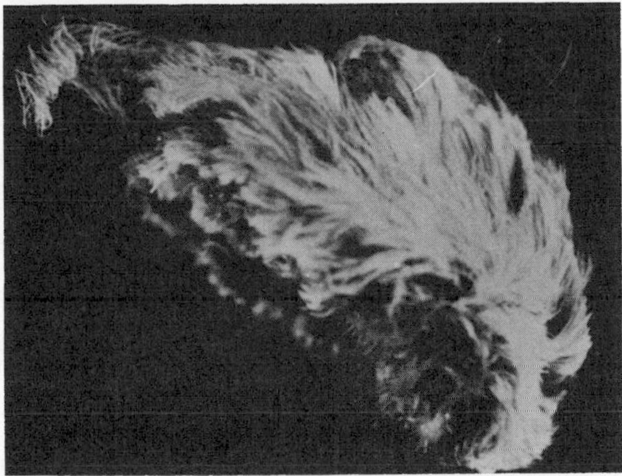

Figure 70–6

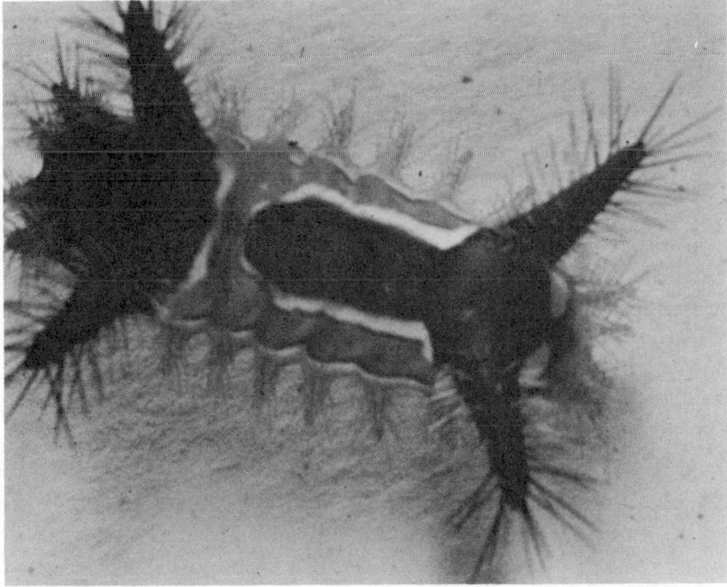

Figure 70–7

Figure 70–5. Larva of *Automeris io*, the io moth.

Figure 70–6. Larva of *Megalopyge opercularis*, the puss caterpillar.

Figure 70–7. *Sibine stimulea* larva, the saddle-back caterpillar. (All three courtesy of the Louisiana State University School of Medicine, New Orleans.)

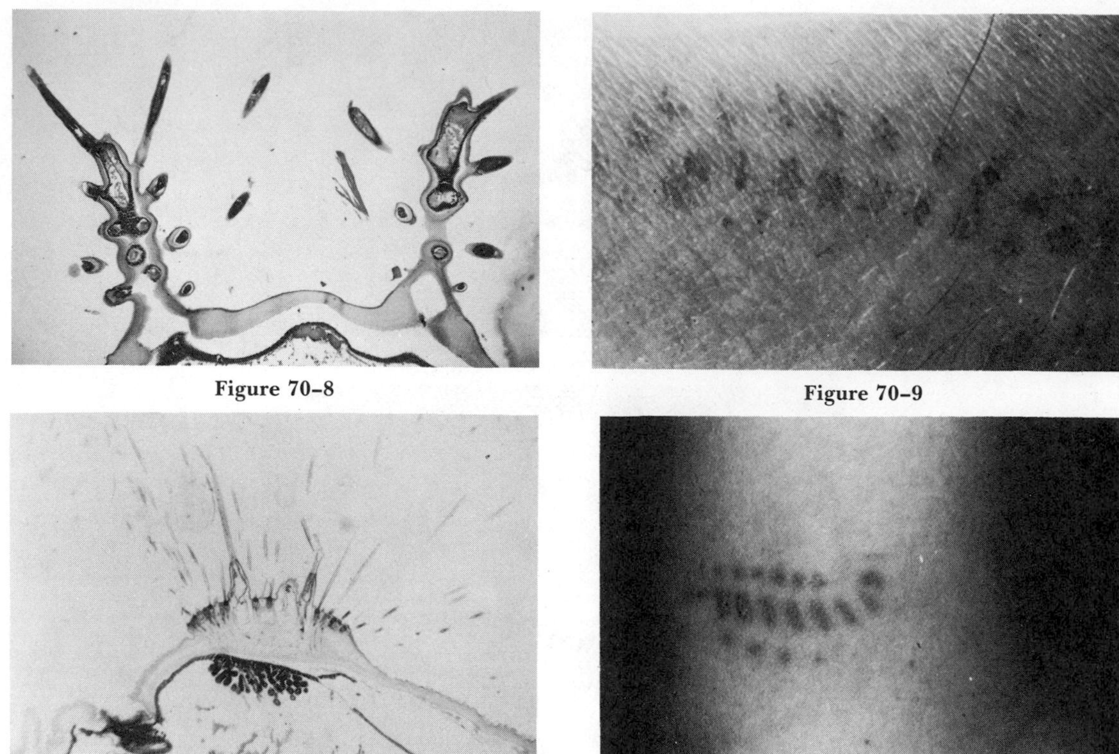

Figure 70–8 Figure 70–9 Figure 70–10 Figure 70–11

Figure 70–8. Cross section of *Automeris io* caterpillar showing hairs and poison-secreting cells in the hairs.

Figure 70–9. Lesions on arm following contact with *Automeris io* larva; pattern of the offending hairs is depicted in the linear series of lesions.

Figure 70–10. Cross section of *Megalopyge opercularis* caterpillar; note poison-secreting cells at the base of the hairs.

Figure 70–11. Lesions on arm from contact with *M. opercularis* (puss caterpillar). (All four courtesy of the Louisiana State University School of Medicine. New Orleans; photography for Figs. 70–8 and 70–10 by Dr. Mark Feldman.)

caterpillar (Fig. 70–6); *Automeris io,* (Fabricius), the io moth (Fig. 70–5); *Nygmia phaeorrhoea* (Donovan), the brown-tail moth; *Sibine stimulea,* the saddle-back caterpillar (Fig. 70–7); and *Hemileuca oliviae,* the range caterpillar, are among the important offending species. Larvae of another flannel-moth, *Megalopyge lanata,* are a common cause of a painful dermatitis in Panama. Numerous species of urticating and venenating caterpillars, including *N. phaeorrhoea,* are found in Europe. A species of *Hylesia* is important in parts of Brazil. Additional clinically important species occur on the other continents.

TREATMENT. Codeine usually is required for relief of pain. Calcium gluconate or Benadryl administered intravenously have afforded relief. Oral antihistamines may be beneficial. Acetylsalicyclic acid usually does not allay severe pain from envenomization. Alkaline compresses may be applied to the lesion: bicarbonate of soda, ammonia water, and lime water with 7 per cent zinc oxide and 1.5 per cent phenic acid. Creams with antihistamines and Novocain are also helpful. When symptoms persist for more than 2 days, corticosteroids should be considered.

SCOLECIASIS

This term is applied to the rare condition in which lepidopterous larvae manage to survive in the alimentary canal. The most authentic record relates to a case of poisoning from ingesting the larva of *Pieris* sp. (cabbage worm) with raw cabbage.

LEPIDOPTERA AS HOSTS OF HELMINTH PARASITES

The rat tapeworm, *Hymenolepis diminuta*, may pass its cysticercoid stage in several species of MICROLEPIDOPTERA (p. 619).

Order Diptera

This is the most important order of insects from a medical point of view. Malaria, yellow fever, dengue, kala-azar, Oriental sore, espundia, African sleeping sickness, several types of filariasis, Carrión's disease, pappataci fever and several of the viral encephalitides are transmitted by dipterous vectors. In addition, cholera, typhoid, amebiasis, shigellosis and various diarrheas, conjunctivitis and occasionally trachoma are distributed by the activities of flies.

For an account of the medically important DIPTERA by families, see Chapter 71, page 754.

Order Siphonaptera
Fleas

Fleas are laterally compressed, highly chitinized, small, wingless ectoparasites of mammals and birds.[2] The common species vary from 1.5 to 4.0 mm in length.

The mouthparts are adapted for piercing and sucking. The hind legs are modified for jumping. The impregnated chigoe flea is exceptional in that it burrows into the skin.

The head bears inconspicuous annulated antennae that normally lie in grooves. The eyes are simple, when present. The thorax is divided into three segments, and the abdomen is variously stated to consist of 10 to 12.

The *ctenidia*, or combs, bold backward-pointing rows of spines, are characteristic structures. The genal comb is located just above the mouthparts and the pronotal comb dorsally on the first thoracic segment. Their presence or absence in either location or both locations is important in identification. Other taxonomic characters are the shape of the head, the cranial grooves, the male terminalia, the receptaculum seminis in the female, and the location and arrangement of certain bristles, spinelets and spurs (Figs. 70–1, 70–12).

Life History. Flea eggs are glistening white and are deposited dry among the hairs of the host or in the nest. The larvae are wormlike, have 13 segments and biting mouthparts. There are three larval instars. They feed chiefly on organic debris. At the end of the feeding period the larva spins a cocoon and pupates. The time required for completion of the entire life cycle varies from about 3 weeks to several months. Some species may live for several months without feeding, thus enabling them to act as "reservoirs" of *Yersinia pestis* in the prolonged intervals between blood meals.

More than 1900 species and subspecies of fleas have been described. These are grouped into six or more families, of which the PULICIDAE, DOLICHOPSYLLIDAE (CTENOPSYLLIDAE) and TÚNGIDAE are of special medical importance.

The family PULICIDAE includes: *Ctenocephalides felis* (Bouché) and *Ctenocephalides canis* (Curtis), the cat and dog fleas; *Pulex*

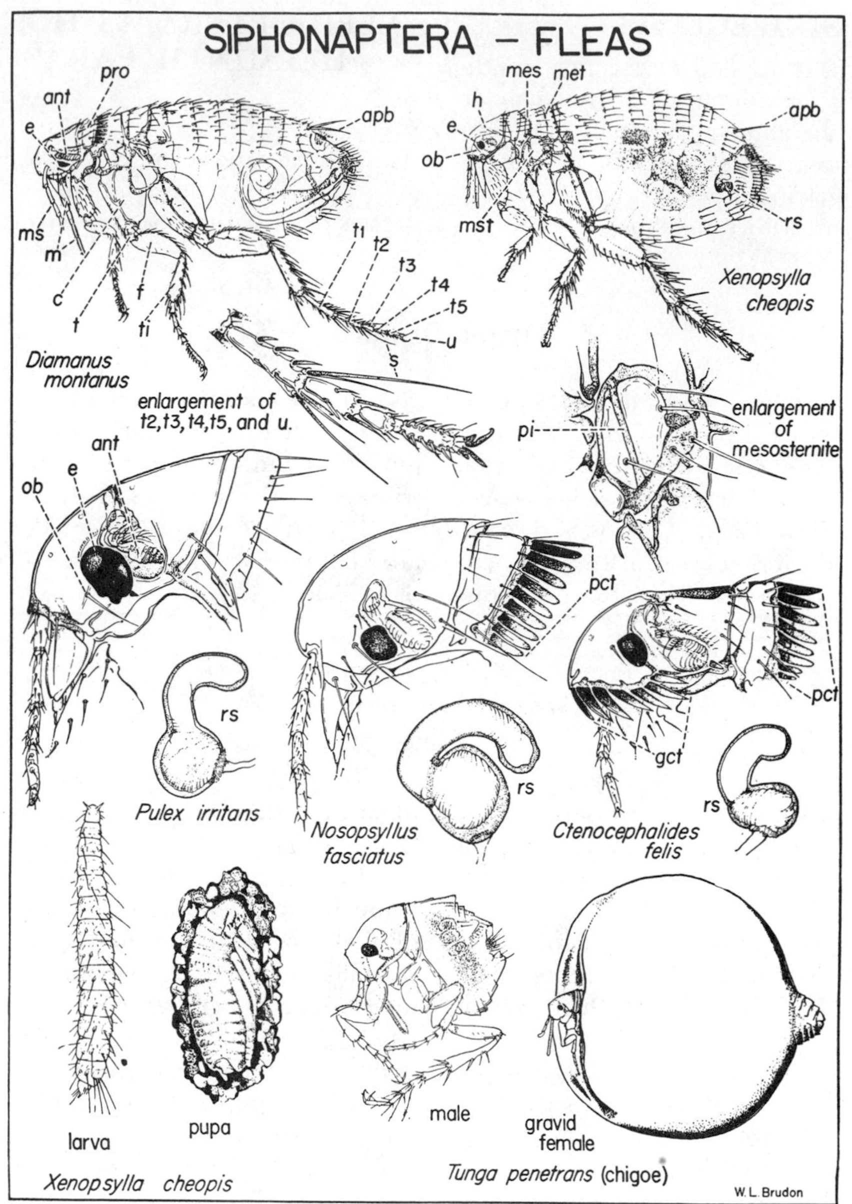

Figure 70–12. SIPHONAPTERA. Certain characters used in identification: *ant,* antenna; *apb,* antepygidial bristle; *c,* coxa; *e,* eye; *f,* femur; *gct,* genal ctenidium; *h,* head; *m,* mouthparts; *ms,* maxillary palpus; *mes,* mesothorax; *met,* metathorax; *mst,* mesosternite; *ob,* ocular bristle; *pct,* pronotal ctenidium; *pi,* perpendicular incrassation of mesosternite; *pro,* pronotum; *rs,* receptaculum seminis; *s,* spine at tip of second tarsus; *t,* trochanter; *ti,* tibia; *t1* to *t5,* tarsus 1, 2, 3, 4, 5; *u,* ungues.

irritans Linn., the human flea; and several species of *Xenopsylla* and *Hoplopsyllus.*

Ctenocephalides felis and *C. canis* are cosmopolitan. In both species, genal and pronotal combs are present. The genal comb consists of eight spines and the pronotal of 16. *Pulex irritans* has been reported from all of the major zoographic regions but is absent from some large cities. *Xenopsylla cheopis* (Roth.) is widely disseminated in many countries. It has been recorded from many of the United States and has become established as far north as Michigan and Minnesota. *Pulex irritans* and *X. cheopis* are similar in that they both lack genal and pronotal combs. However, in *X. cheopis* there is one rodlike thickening of the mesosternite extending anterodorsally and another extending nearly perpendicularly. In *P. irritans* the perpendicular rod is absent. In addition, the ocular bristle of *X. cheopis* arises in front of and just above the middle of the eye, whereas in *P. irritans* it arises near the lower anterior margin (Fig. 73–12). Other important species of *Xenopsylla* are *X. braziliensis* (Baker), *X. eridos* (Roth.), *X. nubicus* (Roth.), *X. piriei* Ingram, and *X. astia* Roth., all of which are implicated in plague transmission.

The family Dolichopsyllidae contains medically important species of several genera. Among these are a ground squirrel flea, *Diamanus montanus* (Baker); the temperate zone rat flea, *Nosopsyllus fasciatus* (Bosc); the South American cavy flea, *Rhopalopsyllus cavicola* (Weyenb.); and two rodent fleas from the Russian steppes and Manchuria, *Ceratophyllus tesquorum* (Wagner) and *Oropsylla silantiewi* (Wagner), respectively. All are vectors of *Y. pestis* among rodents, and *N. fasciatus* is also a vector of murine typhus among rats.

The family Túngidae is represented by two important genera, *Echidnophaga* Olliff and *Tunga* Jarocki. *Echidnophaga gallinacea* (Westwood), the stick-tight flea, is widely distributed in tropical and subtropical regions, including Australia. In the United States it has been listed from 22 states and is reported as permanently established as far north as Virginia and Kansas. It is a serious pest of poultry in the south and attacks many species of vertebrates including dogs, cats, rats and man. When feeding, the female attaches firmly to its host. Thus, rats and wild birds may function in its dispersal. Although it is reported as relatively rare on rats in the United States, it is said to occur in large numbers on rats in the Malagasy Republic. *Yersinia pestis* has been recovered from these fleas taken from the burrowing owl, *Speotyto cunicularia* (Molina), in the western United States.

Tunga penetrans (Linn.), the burrowing flea, is widely distributed in the tropical regions of America and Africa. It is commonly known as the jigger, sand flea or chigoe. In Latin America it is also known as *nigua* and *bicho do pê*. The fertilized female burrows into the skin of the feet, often beneath the nail, or in other parts of the body, where its abdomen becomes greatly distended by blood and developing eggs. There is intense itching and inflammation and, not uncommonly, secondary infection. In Central America tetanus and gas gangrene occur frequently. Autoamputation of the toes has

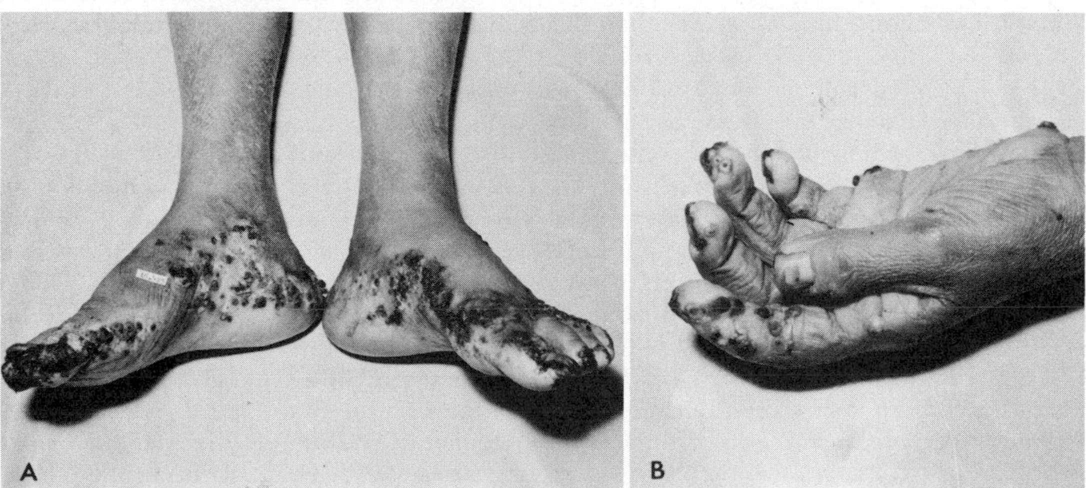

Figure 70–13. Lesions due to *Tunga penetrans*, the chigoe or burrowing flea. (Courtesy of Dr. Rodolfo Cespedes, Hospital San Juan de Dios, San José, Costa Rica.)

been attributed to infection with this flea in Angola (Fig. 70–13).

Surgical removal of the intact flea is recommended. This involves enlarging the entrance hole of the flea using a sterile needle, followed by gentle pressure on the sides of the aperture. The flea is thus forced out. The wound is then cleansed and an antiseptic dressing applied. On the other hand, excellent results are reported from the use of an initial Lysol bath, followed by puncturing each flea with a needle. A second Lysol bath kills the liberated eggs and sterilizes the wound. Five other species of *Tunga* are known, one of which appears in Brazil and one in China.

Relation to Disease. Fleas serve as vectors of *Rickettsia typhi,* the causative agent of murine typhus, from rat to rat and from rat to man. They are "reservoirs" of *Yersinia pestis,* the causal agent for bubonic plague, and transmit this organism from rat to rat, rat to man and man to man; and in campestral plague from wild rodent to wild rodent, from wild rodent to rat and from both to man. They are also intermediate hosts of several tapeworms.

The bites of some fleas are extremely annoying and result in a dermatitis. Individual fleas may produce multiple bites in the course of feeding. Thus, flea bites occur in irregular groups of several to a dozen or more. They occur predominantly on covered parts of the body, especially about the belt line, shoulders and hips, where clothing fits snugly, and also on the legs. Severe reactions are more frequent in children. Most persons initially allergic to flea bites cease to have any significant reaction to subsequent bites within a year or more. Flea bites are not seasonal in most areas. Like other insect bites, those of fleas are discrete and when seen early may show a small central hemorrhagic punctum. The location and grouping of flea bites are important diagnostic features. Desensitization by the use of flea antigen, which is commercially available in the United States, has been reported to be helpful.

Although the flea fauna is, to some extent, characteristic for certain hosts, host specificity is not marked. The fleas that most frequently bite man are said to be *Ctenocephalides canis* and *C. felis,* the dog and cat fleas, and *Pulex irritans,* which is a common parasite also of swine and prairie dogs *(Cynomys). Xenopsylla cheopis* and *Nosopsyllus fasciatus* are typically parasites of rats. Both are widespread and the former bites man readily. On the other hand, *Diamanus montanus* and *Hoplopsyllus anomalus* are parasites of certain ground squirrels. Neither is reported as a frequent parasite of man, but an interchange of parasites between rats and ground squirrels is not uncommon.

Bubonic plague is transmitted to man primarily by the bite of the tropical rat flea, *X. cheopis.* It has been suggested that the human flea, *P. irritans,* may serve to convey the infection from person to person. Although many fleas feeding on an infected rat take up plague organisms, only a few become effective vectors for transmitting the disease to other rodents or to man. In the stomach of effective vectors, the plague organisms, *Yersinia pestis,* multiply somewhat as in a culture tube until they obstruct the part of the alimentary canal of the fleas known as the proventriculus. This may require as long as 2 or 3 weeks. When this obstruction occurs, the flea encounters difficulty in obtaining another blood meal. In endeavoring to do so, it is likely to regurgitate plague organisms into the wound made by the piercing organs. This so-called "blocked flea" remains infective during its life, but this often is shortened by the very existence of the blocking. Blocked fleas may live several weeks. (See Chapter 25, p. 224.)

Intensive studies in widely separated endemic areas have served to amplify rather than simplify the already complex ecology of *campestral (sylvatic) plague.* In the western United States about 30 species of rodents and two species of lagomorphs have been found plague-infected, and more than 30 species of fleas are capable of harboring *Y. pestis.* Of the two species of fleas most frequently found on the ground squirrel, *Spermophilus beecheyi* (Richardson) [=*Citellus beecheyi* (Richardson)], *Hoplopsyllus anomalus* and *D. montanus,* the latter is by far the more efficient vector. This flea has been recovered from pack rats *(Neotoma)*, prairie dogs *(Cynomys)*, tree squirrels *(Tamiasciurus)*, ground squirrels *(Spermophilus)*, ground hogs *(Marmota)*, and from *Rattus norvegicus* (Berkenhout) and *Rattus rattus* (Linn.). *Xenopsylla cheopis*, the common vector in classic plague, has also been recovered from Beechey ground squirrels. The stick-tight flea, *Echidnophaga gallinacea*, with a wide variety of hosts including the burrowing owl, *Speotyto cunicularia*, has been found naturally infected. (See Chapter 25 and Fig. 25–2).

On epidemiologic grounds, *P. irritans* was under suspicion as the vector in the Paris epidemic (1921). On similar grounds it has been indicated as a vector in the mountainous regions of Ecuador where *X. cheopis* does not occur. In some areas in the western United States, the prairie dog *(Cynomys* spp.), a natural host of this flea, constitutes an important rodent reservoir.

Xenopsylla cheopis is considered the most common flea vector of murine typhus. (See Chapter 7, page 110.)

Information on control of fleas and on flea repellents is presented in Chapter 72. (See Table 72–1, p. 797 and p. 800.)

Order Hymenoptera
Bees, Wasps and Ants

This order includes the bees, wasps and ants. Except for wingless forms, and a few primitive families, these insects are characterized by the presence of four membranous wings and a "pinched" abdomen. The mouthparts are formed for chewing or for both chewing and sucking, but never for sucking blood. The abdomen in the female is usually provided with a sting, piercer or saw. The metamorphosis is complete (egg, larva, pupa, adult) (Fig. 70–1).

HYMENOPTERA are of medical interest for two reasons: (1) the poisonous effects of their stings;[6,7] (2) as mechanical vectors of parasites (of very slight importance).

THE POISONOUS EFFECTS OF STINGS

The sting of the female hymenopteran is really a modified ovipositor, composed (in the honeybee) of a central shaft, two lateral lancets or *darts* and two finger-like *stingpalpi*. The darts are provided with sharp, recurved teeth.

In most species the poison glands are of two types. The acid-secreting gland, a paired structure, produces a toxin that is capable of paralyzing other insects. Those species that provision their nests with living prey have only this gland.

The second gland, usually single, produces an altogether different substance, alkaline in nature. Like the acid secretion, this substance is only mildly irritating in itself, but when the two are combined, as occurs at the time of the sting, typical and painful symptoms ensue. In cases in which the stinger remains in the wound the muscles continue to contract for some minutes, thereby forcing the shaft deeper into the subcutaneous tissue and causing a greater amount of poison to be discharged.

The composition of bee venom (apitoxin) is not understood thoroughly. Formic acid, once thought to be an active principle, is reportedly not a constituent. A non-nitrogenous substance related in its action to saponins, an active principle of snake poisons, has been isolated. Histamine has been shown to be a constituent. Through electrophoresis and paper chromatography, it is known now that bee venom contains a number of basic and acid components of which two principal ones are basic. One of these, a protein termed "melittin," contains the hemolytic factor and also causes general and local effects. The other basic component contains the most powerful dehydrogenase inhibitor known—more powerful than that of cobra venom—and a hyaluronidase, which may assist spread of the venom. Bee venom is hemolytic; the factor responsible has been separated into two components: a lecithinase, which transforms lecithin into hemolytic lysolethicin, and another which has a direct hemolytic action.[7]

Bee venom has been shown to have four characteristic toxic effects. The hemolytic effect (similar to rattlesnake poisoning) resembles that of sapotoxins and explains the occasional occurrence of hemoglobinuria and melena in bee sting victims. The venom also elevates the coagulation time either by preventing the formation of thrombokinase or by interfering with its action. A neurotoxic effect is evident from the paralysis produced by the venom in some species. Finally, the histamine effect, produced by this component of the venom, accounts for the local reaction of redness, flare and wheal of the skin. The venom of bees also has been shown to cause localized muscular necrosis, edema and cellular infiltration at the site of the sting in unsensitized tissues.

Local swelling is always characteristic and especially so if the sting should be in the vicinity of the eye or mouth. A sting on the tongue has been known to endanger life by reason of the great amount of collateral edema produced. It is estimated that some 500 stings at or about the same time are necessary for a lethal dose of poison. In certain instances, however, individuals become sensitized, after which a single sting may produce alarming and occasionally fatal results. The severity of allergic manifestations depends upon the degree of hypersensitivity. Some of the manifestations, in order of frequency, are generalized urticaria, angioedema, shock with respiratory and cardiac impairment, cyanosis, asthma with wheezing or choking, nausea, vomiting, chest pain and, occasionally, fever and convulsions. The venom poisoning may produce a leukemoid blood picture with immature white cells in peripheral blood and leukocytosis.

In fatal cases, symptoms of cyanosis, shock and respiratory difficulty last about 30 minutes and death results from anaphylactic shock. Autopsy usually reveals laryngeal edema with obstruction by both bullous folds and mucus, pulmonary emphysema, acute pulmonary and cerebral edema, cardiac dilatation and visceral congestion.

The whole question of allergy in relation to bee venom is somewhat confused, since bees frequently carry various pollens and other substances that they have picked up while visiting flowers and other sources of food. These, rather than bee venom, may be responsible for the hay fever and asthmatic symptoms reported by persons handling hives, bee frames or honey, or in other ways having contact with bees. Such facts argue for the utilization of whole bee extract rather than venom alone in desensitizing procedures.

Gel diffusion studies indicate that the yellowjacket, yellow hornet, black hornet, wasp and honey bee contain common antigens. In addition, each insect contains several antigens specific for the individual genus. Homologous antigen produces fatal anaphylactic shock in experimental animals, whereas heterologous antigens produce lesser degrees of shock or none. The antigens vary in their ability to produce sensitization; yellowjacket is the most potent sensitizer, whereas black hornet antigen is the least potent. Some individuals with little sensitivity to the above venenating insects may be extremely reactive to the venom of fire ants. When a severe allergic reaction to an insect sting occurs and the offending insect can be identified accurately, desensitization with antigen from the appropriate species may be safe. Testing for sensitivity to antigens of other insects also may be desirable. If the insect causing the severe reaction cannot be identified, or if there is a possibility of sensitivity to other stinging insects, desensitization with a combined antigen, including at least bee, wasp, yellowjacket and hornet extracts, appears to be advisable. Antigen of the fire ant should be employed or added if reactions to stings or sensitivity tests indicate the need.

The honeybee *Apis mellifera* Linn. falls in the family APIDAE; bumblebees (various species of *Bombus*) belong in the BOMBIDAE. Both, however, are included in the superfamily APOIDEA. Unlike the honeybee and some wasps, representatives of *Bombus* do not leave the stinging apparatus in the wound but may withdraw and insert the stinger repeatedly. Certain South American bees are stingless but nevertheless cause great discomfort by biting and twisting with their mandibles. When aroused they tend to attack the scalp in large numbers. Some inject an irritating saliva at the point of the bite.

Besides the APOIDEA, the following five superfamilies of HYMENOPTERA contain stinging forms:

Certain of the FORMICOIDEA, true ants, may possess dangerous stings; fire ants, harvester ants and numerous tropical species, e.g., the bulldog ant, *Myrmecia gulosa,* are to be avoided for this reason. The VESPOIDEA include wasps, hornets, yellowjackets, velvet ants, mud daubers and mason wasps; all are capable of stinging. Less often encountered are thread-waisted wasps of the insect-destroying SPHECOIDEA. The BETHYLOIDEA and ICHNEUMONOIDEA include various wasplike insects, most of them of little medical concern.

Treatment of Hymenopterous Stings. The necessity and extent of treatment depend largely on the severity of the stinging and of the patient's reaction. Although bee stings usually are just an inconsequential nuisance, they occasionally may be disastrous.

1. If the sting remains in the tissue, as is usually the case with the worker honeybee, it should be removed by scraping with a knife blade or scalpel. If the protruding end of the sting is grasped with forceps or fingers, the squeezing effect will inject more venom under the skin.

2. For local treatment of stings, ice and elevation are usually sufficient to minimize pain and swelling. Early use of oral antihistamines (e.g., Benadryl) and fluorinated steroid creams (e.g., Kenalog and Synalar) may be helpful in more severe local reactions. In delayed local allergic responses, appearing approximately 24 hours after the initial sting, a 4- to 5-day course of tapering systemic corticosteroids may be extremely effective.

3. Individuals known to be sensitive to stinging insects should be provided with an emergency kit containing a tourniquet and a sterile pre-loaded syringe of epinephrine hydrochloride 1:1000. Epinephrine (0.1 to 0.5 ml) should be administered subcutaneously and that dose repeated every 5 to 15 minutes if necessary. The epinephrine solution must be periodically examined to determine whether the solution has turned brown, which is an indication that it has become oxidized and useless.[8] First aid treatment with such a kit is important but should not be considered a substitute for prompt physician care.

4. Anaphylaxis is a true medical emergency requiring prompt and decisive therapy. Hypotension, upper and lower respiratory obstruction, and aspiration of stomach contents into the lungs are the primary considerations when formulating a therapeutic approach.

IMMEDIATE THERAPY. *Tourniquet.* If anatomically feasible, application of a tourniquet proximal to the site of the sting with sufficient tension to obstruct venous return will decrease absorption of the antigen.

Epinephrine. 0.1 to 0.3 ml of 1:1000 epinephrine should be injected subcutaneously (proximal to the tourniquet) and an equal amount should be injected at the site of the sting unless anatomically contraindicated. If the patient is in shock, 1 to 2 ml of 1:10,000 aqueous epinephrine should be administered intravenously and repeated every 5 to 15 minutes if necessary.

Oxygen. Myocardial irritability is markedly increased by a combination of hypoxemia, hypotension and vasoactive amines. Early use of oxygen may decrease myocardial irritability and prevent ventricular fibrillation, which is a major cause of death in anaphylaxis.

Antihistamines. Diphenhydramine (Benadryl) may be administered intravenously (2 mg per kg in children, 100 mg in adults). Early use may be of value in the prevention of additional histamine release, but should be considered of secondary importance and should not delay more important therapeutic steps.

SUPPORTIVE THERAPY. *Intravenous Fluids.* A secure large caliber intravenous line should be promptly established. Saline or other plasma volume expanders should be infused rapidly in an effort to maintain blood pressure.

Aminophylline. Severe bronchospasm may be relieved by aminophylline given intravenously, 7 mg per kg diluted in 2 equal volumes of saline and injected over a 5- to 10-minute period being efficacious. For maintenance thereafter, a dose of 9 mg per kg may be infused during 24 hours. The use of aminophylline is hazardous in elderly patients and in those with cardiovascular disease, particularly hypertension.

Corticosteroids. Steroids have little effect in the early crucial minutes of anaphylaxis and should be considered more for recovery phase treatment. Intravenous infusion of hydrocortisone 7 mg per kg (or equivalent) followed by 7 mg per kg per 24 hours should be given when other major therapeutic steps have been accomplished.

Metaraminol Bitartrate (Aramine). If blood pressure does not respond to volume expanding fluids, Aramine, 0.5 to 5 mg (0.4 mg per kg) may be added to the intravenous fluids, but cardiac side effects should be monitored closely.[9]

Airway. If an adequate airway cannot be maintained by the use of an oral airway and drug therapy as outlined above, endotracheal intubation or tracheostomy may be necessary.

Position. Head down with legs elevated is a desirable position from the standpoint of treating shock, but may not be well tolerated because of respiratory distress. Aspiration of vomitus into the lungs is a potential hazard and may be avoided by having the patient on his side.

LONG-TERM THERAPY. *Hyposensitization.* A hyposensitizing series of injections appears to impart significant protection from severe reactions when patients are stung again.[10] Sensitive persons should be encouraged to undergo this procedure.

The Fire Ant

VINCENT J. DERBES
RODNEY C. JUNG

Many hymenopterans attack humans, but few with the aggressive viciousness of the imported fire ant, until recently named *Solenopsis saevissima richteri* Forel. It is now recognized that two species are involved: the black imported fire ant, *Solenopsis richteri* Forel, apparently introduced to the United States from Argentina or Uruguay in the 1920s; and the red imported fire ant, *Solenopsis invicta* Buren, introduced from Brazil in the 1940s. The latter is now the dominant species in the fire ant infested region of the southeastern United States.[11] Their similarity to the indigenous fire ant, *S. geminata* (F.), may have allowed them to be overlooked for some years. Entomologists attribute their rapid spread to flying and crawling, drifting downstream on logs, traveling aboard cars, trucks, trains and airplanes, and to being transported in nursery stock. Today they are scattered over ten southern states.

Pathogenesis. The ant first attaches itself with the mandibles, pulling on the skin and pinching and raising it slightly, thus causing a definite sensation of pain before the sting is inserted. It then arches its back at the peduncle and inserts the stinger, maintaining this position usually for 20 to 25 seconds. It may then remove the stinger and, using the head as a pivot, rotate and reinsert the stinger in two or three additional sites (Fig. 70–14). This clustering of stings is useful in diagnosis. A flare of 25 to 50 mm follows almost immediately. Within a minute a wheal appears and grows to 2, 3 or even 10 mm in diameter. This persists for about 1 hour, regardless of local therapy. Small prominences may be seen at the site of stings 1½ to 2 hours later. Within 4 hours it is evi-

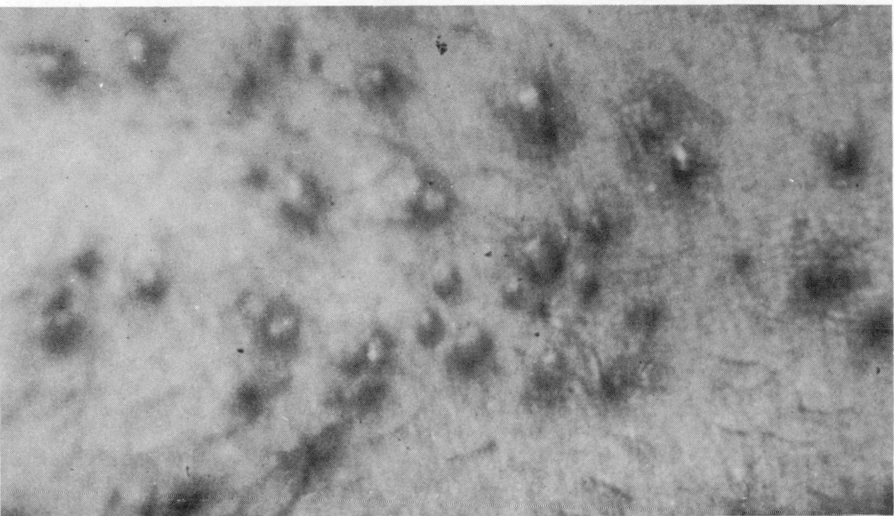

Figure 70–14. Clusters of pustules on arm at sites of fire ant stings.

dent that these elevations consist of quite superficial vesicles containing thin, clear fluid. Loss of this fluid by rupture or drying produces depressed centers. Eight to 10 hours later the vesicular fluid is noted to be cloudy, and soon becomes purulent. After 24 hours the sting sites are slightly umbilicated pustules, sometimes surrounded by a narrow red halo. In other instances there is a large, red, edematous, painful area. Such areas are often seen clinically, for multiple stings are the rule. The pustule remains 3 to 10 days; it then ruptures and a crust is formed. Cultures of pustules consistently produce negative results except for occasional contaminants, and organisms are not seen in sections of biopsied tissue (Fig. 70–15).

On the lower extremities particularly, pigmented macules persist for days or weeks. One may see residual fibrotic nodules

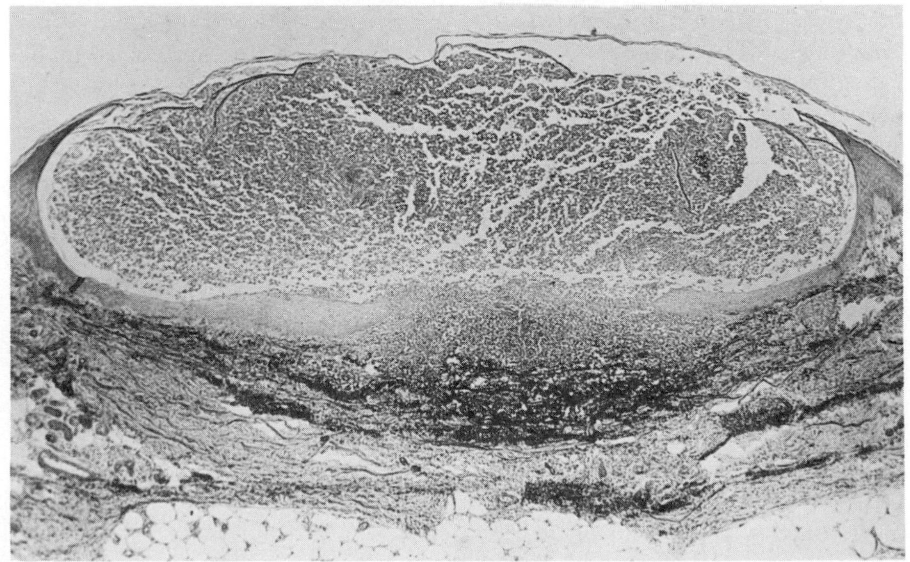

Figure 70–15. Section of biopsied pustule caused by fire ant sting. (Courtesy of Dr. Vincent J. Derbes and Dr. Rodney C. Jung, Tulane University School of Medicine, New Orleans.)

of 2 or 3 mm diameter, especially in older persons. These are of the type that has been described under the designations dermatofibroma or histiocytoma cutis. Frequently at the sites of ant stings, particularly on the lower extremities, patients tend to develop patches of infectious eczematoid dermatitis, which may be persistent.

Reactions to the stings of the fire ant are of two types: local and systemic. The local changes (immediate punctum, wheal and flare, sterile pustule) suggest strongly that a powerful necrotizing toxin is responsible. Such a substance, *solenamine,* has been isolated, purified, and identified as the probable active constituent of fire-ant venom.[12] Recent work by Adrouny[13] makes it appear likely that solenamine consists of a binary mixture of constant composition with the following structures postulated: (a) 2-methyl-3-hexadecyl-pyrrolidine, (b) 2-methyl-3-hexadecyl-3-pyrroline. Thus, the two structures differ by a mere bond. The pure substance, when injected into the skin, produces lesions comparable to those produced by the whole venom.[14] The structural formula proposed by Adrouny was disputed by MacConnell, Blum and Fales, who presented evidence that the component of lowest molecular weight (for which they offered the name solenopsin A) is *trans*-2-methyl-6-*n*-undecylpiperidine-3, or its mirror image.[15]

Systemic reactions after ant stings are febrile and allergic. The fever is seldom severe; 24- to 48-hour elevations to 38°C (100.4°F) are customary. The allergic reactions are first manifested by increasing local response to ant stings—larger and larger areas of local edema, erythema and discomfort. The pustular elements do not similarly increase in size, again suggesting that allergy plays no role in the production of the pustule. Patients may develop generalized urticaria and bronchial asthma shortly after being stung. This reaction to the ant sting must be relatively uncommon, at least at present, although it is extremely frequent after bee stings.

Histopathologic examination of a 72-hour pustule discloses a thin roofed lesion containing many eosinophils, leukocytes, plasma cells, lymphocytes and cells with small pyknotic nuclei. The floor of the pustule is an edematous epidermis, except at its center, where the epidermal floor is completely absent and the cellular infiltrate breaks through to extend profusely into the underlying necrotic tissue. Mantles of cellular infiltrate also extend laterally and more deeply about the dilated blood vessels and the nearby sweat glands (Fig. 70–15).

These histopathologic changes are not like those generally seen following other insect stings or bites. The inflammatory reaction is much more severe. The consistent formation of a pustule is a differentiating feature, and the necrosis is of a degree that often leads to scar formation.[16]

Treatment. The allergic manifestations that result from stings of the fire ant may be treated in the usual way with antihistaminic drugs, epinephrine and its congeners, the various corticosteroid agents and ACTH. The pustules are entirely refractory to these agents and to antibiotic drugs, as would be expected from the sterile nature of these lesions. Whole bee extract has been used with beneficial results to desensitize patients allergic to the stings of bees, wasps and ants. Extracts of the fire ant have also been employed in patients with systemic reactions following the sting of this insect. The changes produced in the skin by the sting of the fire ant are necrotic, and it is not likely that these could be prevented by desensitization.

REFERENCES

1. Askew, R. R. 1971. Parasitic Insects. American Elsevier Publishing Co., Inc., New York. 316 pp.
2. Borror, D. J., and De Long, D. M. 1970. An Introduction to the Study of Insects. 3rd. ed. Holt Rinehart and Winston, Inc., New York. 812 pp.
3. James, M. T., and Harwood, R. F. 1969. Herm's Medical Entomology 6th ed. The Macmillan Co., New York. 484 pp.
4. Usinger, R. L. 1944. The Triatominae of North and Central America and the West Indies and Their Public Health Significance. Pub. Hlth. Bull. No. 288. 83 pp.
5. Rickman, R. E., Folkes, D. L., Olsen, L. E., Robb, P. L., and Ryckman, A. E. 1965. Epizootology of *Trypanosoma cruzi* in Southwestern North America. Parts I–VII. J. Med. Entomol. *2*:87–108.
6. Frazier, A. C. 1969. Insect Allergy, Allergic and

Toxic Reactions to Insects and Other Arthropods. Warren H. Green, Inc., St. Louis, Missouri. 493 pp.
7. Biicherl, W., and Buckley, E. E. 1971. Venomous Animals and Their Venoms. Academic Press, New York. 537 pp.
8. Mark, M. B. 1969. Stinging insects: allergy implications. Pediat. Clin. North Am. *16*:177.
9. Committee on Drugs, Anaphylaxis. 1973. Pediatrics *51*:136–140.
10. Houser, D. D., and Caplin, I. 1967. Insect sting allergy. A clinical review. Am. J. Dis. Child. *113*:498–503.
11. Smith, D. R. 1972. Two species of imported fire ant in the United States (Hymenoptera: Formicidae). Co-op. Econ. Insect. Rept., U.S.D.A., *22*:103–104.
12. Adrouny, G. A., Derbes, V. J., and Jung, R. C. 1959. Isolation of a hemolytic component of fire ant venom. Science *130*:449.
13. Adrouny, G. A. 1966. The fire ant's fire. Bull. Tulane Univ. Med. Fac. *25*:67–72.
14. Jung, R. C., Derbes, V. J., and Burch, A. D. 1963. Skin response to a solenamine, a hemolytic component of fire ant venom. Dermatol. Trop. *2*:241–244.
15. MacConnell, G., Blum, S., and Fales, M. 1970. Alkaloid from ant venom: Identification and synthesis. Science *168*:840–841.
16. Caro, M. R., Derbes, V. J., and Jung, R. C. 1957. Skin responses to the sting of imported fire ant, *Solenopsis saevissima* var. *richteri* Forel. Arch. Dermatol. *75*:476–488.

CHAPTER 71
Order Diptera

HAROLD D. NEWSON

Members of this order, the true flies, are involved in the transmission of more human and animal pathogens than any other group of arthropods. Some are external bloodsucking parasites; others develop as larvae within the human host; and still others are mechanical or biologic vectors of protozoal, viral, bacterial and helminthic diseases. The distribution of the group is worldwide.

Characterization. The winged members of the order have only one pair of wings. The second pair is represented merely by a pair of knobbed structures, the *halteres* (see Fig. 71–5), which are believed to function in the maintenance of equilibrium. The mouthparts, when developed, are always suctorial, but only in comparatively few groups is there adaptation for piercing skin. The metamorphosis is complete, consisting of four stages—egg, larva, pupa and adult. Only a small percentage of the known species are of medical interest.

Classification. Most taxonomists divide the DIPTERA into three suborders: NEMATOCERA, BRACHYCERA and CYCLORRHAPHA. Adults of the first two groups escape from the pupal case through a T- or Y-shaped suture, whereas the Cyclorrhapha adults push off the terminal portion of the puparium to produce a circular opening through which they exit. Other characteristics used in the classification and identification of DIPTERA are the shape and arrangement of bristles and terminal body structures. For most clinical purposes recognition of the major family-level groups will be adequate. Identification to the level of genus and species, should it be desired, usually will require the services of a specialist.

Suborder Nematocera

This, the most primitive of the three suborders, includes mosquitoes, midges and many similar forms. Four families of NEMATOCERA contain medically important species by reason of the blood-feeding habits of the females and their roles as vectors of some of the most important arthropod-borne diseases.

FAMILY CERATOPOGONIDAE (HELEIDAE) PUNKIES, NO-SEE-UMS

This family contains many genera, but only three, *Culicoides*, *Leptoconops* and *Lasiohelea*, include species that feed on the blood of man.[1] Of these, *Culicoides* is the most widespread and abundant. The adult flies may be recognized by their small size (0.6 to 5.0 mm in length), and their somewhat pubescent (finely hairy) wings, which in most species display a characteristic spotting (Fig. 71–1). The larva is elongate, eel-like and legless. The pupa resembles that of a mosquito, except that the abdomen is kept extended instead of curled under. Adults are variously known as "punkies," "no-see-ums" or "sandflies," the first two names being preferred.

Life History. Larvae are found in a wide range of aquatic, semiaquatic and moist habitats.[2] They include coastal salt marshes; inland pools; moist sandy, adobe and alkaline soils, as well as those rich in organic matter; humus and leaf refuse in tree holes and the axils of large leaves, and the rotting stems of fibrous and woody plants. They are

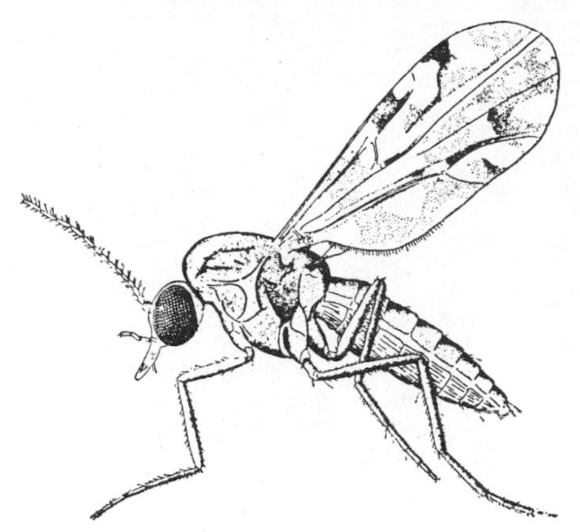

Figure 71–1. *Culicoides* sp. Female specimen. (After Dampf. From Herms: Medical Entomology. By permission of The Macmillan Co.)

probably unselective in their feeding, utilizing principally organic fragments.

Adult activity for most species is either crepuscular or nocturnal, although a few species are active diurnally. Both sexes will feed on nectar, but only females take blood. Each species has a range of vertebrate hosts on which it will feed, with a definite preference being shown for one or more of these. Except for a few autogenous species, maturation of eggs requires a blood meal. The flight of *Culicoides* is slow and occurs only under calm conditions. Most species are thought to have a very limited range of flight, but some are known to be capable of traveling extensive distances from their breeding sites.

Medical Importance. The bites of these minute flies cause intense itching, usually accompanied by transient local swelling and erythema. Secondary infections may occur as a result of scratching to relieve the itch. In certain individuals the bites may become vesicular, rupture and produce an open exudative lesion that persists for several days or weeks.

Members of the genus *Culicoides* serve as intermediate hosts for at least three species of human filarial parasites. In parts of Africa and South America, *Dipetalonema perstans* passes 7 to 9 days as a developing larva in the body of the fly (p. 517). *Culicoides austeni* Carter, Ingram and Macfie and *Culicoides grahami* Austen are important vectors of this parasite and also serve in Africa as an intermediate host for *Dipetalonema streptocerca* (p. 518). In the Caribbean and in South America, *Culicoides furens* (Poey) is the vector for *Mansonella ozzardi* (p. 516). This parasite is also transmitted by *Culicoides paraensis* (Goeldi), and possibly by *Culicoides debilipalpis* Lutz, in Argentina. The viruses of eastern equine encephalitis in Georgia and of Venezuelan equine encephalitis in Ecuador have been isolated from undetermined species of *Culicoides*, but the findings are not thought to be of epidemiologic significance. *Culicoides* species are, however, known to be the vectors of two important viral diseases of livestock—African horse sickness and blue tongue disease of sheep.

FAMILY SIMULIIDAE BLACK FLIES

This family contains approximately 1200 species, known variously as "black flies," "buffalo gnats" or "turkey gnats," and is found throughout many parts of the world. The adults are small (1 to 5 mm long), usually dark, compactly built flies with a rounded, humped back and short broad wings that have the heavy veins concentrated near the anterior margin (Fig. 71–2). The mouthparts are adapted for bloodsucking in the female but are more or less rudimentary in the male. The larva has a cylindrical body, usually somewhat swollen posteriorly. The last segment is provided with a sucking disk surrounded by a series of parallel rows of small hooks. The head usually is equipped with a pair of large, fan-shaped structures (mouth brushes) used for straining food from the water. The pupa is rather short and compact, and the abdomen is provided with various hooklets for holding the pupa in the cocoon. Usually, the cocoon is a well defined wall-pocket or boot-shaped structure and often possesses characters of value in specific identification.

Life History. Eggs are laid on a variety of solid surfaces in water or at its edge. They may be deposited in masses or scattered loosely over the water surface. Larvae almost invariably prefer running water, but occur in

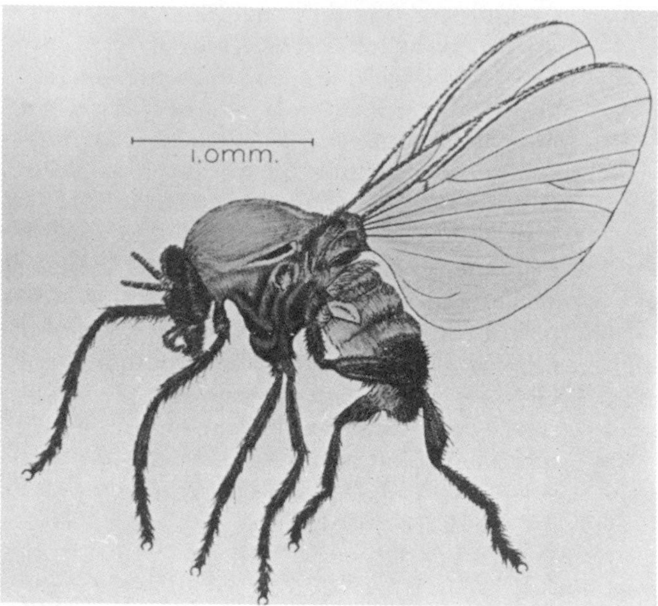

Figure 71–2. *Simulium ochraceum*, the most important vector of onchocerciasis in Guatemala. (Courtesy of Dr. Herbert T. Dalmat, Smithsonian Misc. Pub., vol. 125, no. 1. 425 pp.)

such diverse habitats as small swiftly flowing streams, large rivers and temporary or semipermanent waterways. Attachment sites utilized by the larvae include rocks, submerged logs, aquatic and emergent vegetation and a variety of aquatic animals such as mollusks, insects and river crabs. When mature the larva spins a cocoon, attaches it to the surface on which it is resting and pupates within it. The emerging adult surfaces in an air bubble and is able to fly immediately upon reaching the water surface. Adult flight ranges of 7 to 10 miles are common and some Nearctic species are known to travel very long distances from their emergence sites. Females of most species require a blood meal for ovarian development. Certain species attack man readily, while others prefer other mammalian or avian hosts. Males are not blood feeders. Adults are active primarily during daylight but may be attracted to lights at night.

Medical Importance. There is perhaps no other insect of equal size that can inflict a bite as painful as that of the black fly. When feeding, they will attack the ears, nostrils, eyes and the skin on any exposed portion of the body. They make a conspicuous puncture that remains swollen, indurated and hemorrhagic long after the fly has fed (Fig. 71–3).

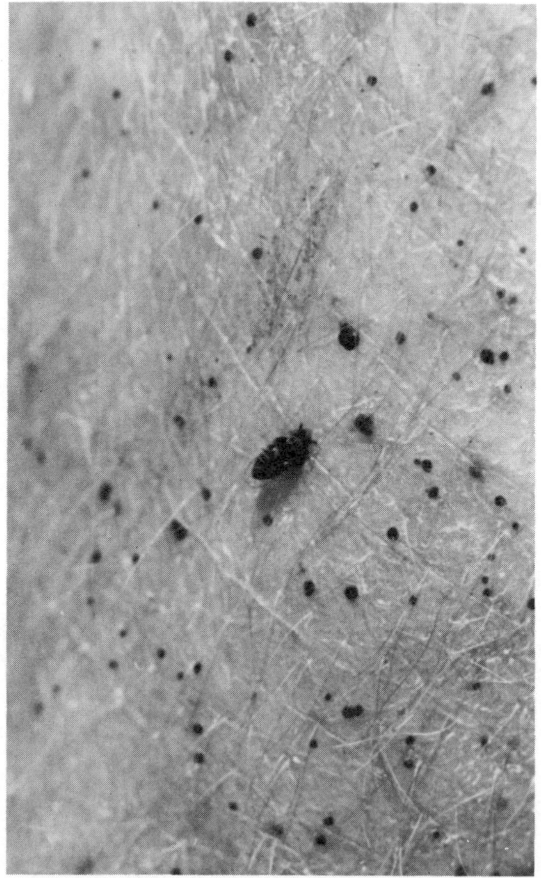

Figure 71–3. Blood encrusted lesions following *Simulium* bites. A *Simulium* is seen feeding. (Photograph courtesy of Dr. Harold Trapido, Louisiana State University School of Medicine, New Orleans.)

Individual reactions to these bites are quite variable. In some persons they produce extreme swelling and toxemia, whereas in others the effects are minimal. In sensitized individuals the bite itself may be painless, but soon much pain, intense itching, swelling and general discomfort may occur. Lesions may develop that become confluent, vesicular, excoriated, weeping and crusted. These may persist for days or a few weeks. Satellite adenopathy is a common feature. An apparent desensitization to the bites may develop in some individuals, whereas others become more sensitized as a result of repeated exposure to the bites of black flies. Black flies are most annoying in the North Temperate and Subarctic Zones, appearing in enormous numbers when conditions favor their development. At times domestic animals have been killed by them. Death seems in most cases to be the consequence of a toxemia caused by the bites or the result of anaphylactic shock, although debility resulting from blood loss and suffocation brought about by inhalation of the flies may be a contributing cause.

As Vectors of Disease. The most important pathogen transmitted by simuliid flies is *Onchocerca volvulus,* a filarial parasite edemic in certain parts of Africa, Mexico and South and Central America (p. 508). The principal vector species in Africa are *Simulium damnosum* Theobald and *S. neavei* Roubaud. The most important vector in Central America, in the light of host preference, feeding habits and epidemiologic information, seems to be *S. ochraceum* Walker (Fig. 71–3), with *S. metallicum* Bellardi and *S. callidum* (Dyar and Shannon) also involved. In Venezuela the main vector is thought to be *S. metallicum,* and in a small recently discovered focus in Colombia, *S. exiguum* Roubaud. Black flies are also the vectors of *Leukocytozoon* infections of poultry and wild waterfowl in North America.

FAMILY PSYCHODIDAE SANDFLIES, MOTH FLIES

This important family, the species of which are known variously as "moth flies," "owl flies" or "sandflies," is characterized by small size, long legs and the presence of abundant hair on both wings and body. The wing venation is also characteristic, having a series of more or less parallel veins and lacking cross veins except near the base (Fig. 71–4).

There are two subfamilies of medical importance: the Psychodinae, the "moth flies" or "owl midges," whose wings are held rooflike over the body and whose larvae are commonly aquatic; and the Phlebotominae, "sandflies," whose wings are held at a 45 degree angle from the body and whose larvae are never aquatic.

None of the Psychodinae feed on blood, but some species of this subfamily are recognized human pests and at least one has been associated with human myiasis. Sev-

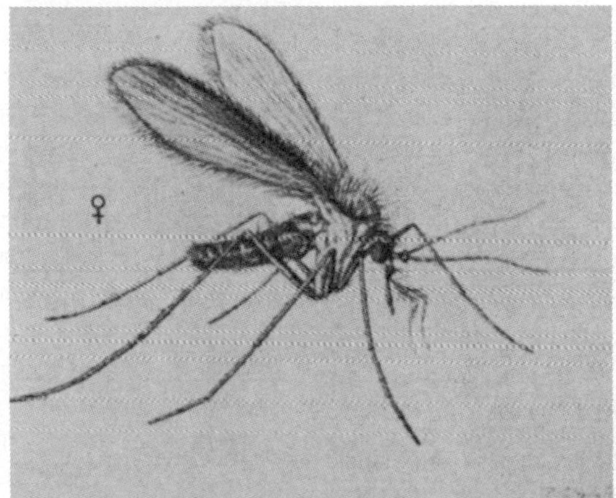

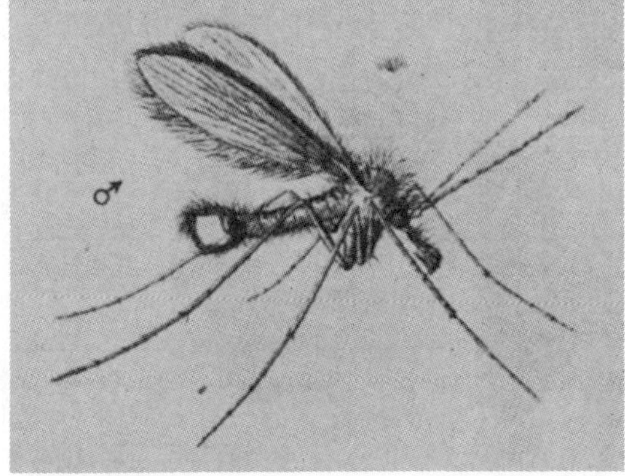

Figure 71–4. Female and male of *Phlebotomus papatasi,* the vector of sandfly fever. (Courtesy of A. B. Sabin, C. B. Philip, and J. R. Paul in J.A.M.A. *125*:603–606, 1944.)

eral species breed in sewage disposal plants, cesspools, and the drains of household sinks and washbasins. The great numbers that may originate from these sources become particularly annoying when present in or around human habitations. The one recorded case of urinary myiasis caused by *Psychoda* is believed to have resulted from larvae migrating from the rectum, after being ingested with garden soil, rather than originating in the urinary tract. Species in the subfamily PHLEBOTOMINAE have much greater medical significance, since the females all are blood feeders (males are not) and several are vectors of human pathogens. The ensuing portions of this section are concerned only with this subfamily.[3,4]

Life History. The eggs are laid in small batches in the breeding places, which are characteristic for each species. The breeding places typically are dark and humid, and contain a supply of organic matter that serves as food for the larvae. Such places may be found in rock piles, cracks in walls, beneath debris of various kinds, in hollow trees and in animal burrows. Adult phlebotomines are weak fliers and remain active only in the near absence of air currents. They are nocturnal and rest during the day in protected locations such as animal burrows, termite mounds, leaf litter on forest floors, deep cracks in the soil and the dark moist areas of human and animal habitations. When disturbed the adults fly in a short hopping motion, but they are capable of longer sustained flights and, with consistent prevailing winds, can travel rather extensive distances from their sites of origin. The females of some species feed on cold-blooded animals, whereas others obtain blood meals from a variety of warm-blooded animals, including man.

Medical Importance. The bites of phlebotomine sandflies often cause considerable annoyance and discomfort. When biting, the females seek out the ankles, wrists, knees and elbows, showing a preference for areas where the skin is particularly delicate or tightly drawn. Bites produce a painful, stinging sensation followed by itching that persists for some time. Firm whitish wheals, which may become pustular and edematous if scratched, are characteristic. If no secondary infection ensues, the irritation usually subsides in a few days, though systemic manifestations, nausea and rise in temperature may be experienced after numerous bites.

AS VECTORS OF DISEASE. Species of the genera *Phlebotomus* in the Old World and *Lutzomyia* in the New World (subfamily PHLEBOTOMINAE) serve as vectors of sandfly fever (in the Old World), several other arbovirus infections (in the American tropics), kala-azar, cutaneous leishmaniasis, mucocutaneous leishmaniasis, Carrión's disease and possibly tropical ulcer. *Lutzomyia verrucarum* (Townsend) is the chief vector of Carrión's disease in South America, while *Phlebotomus papatasi* Scopoli is the proved vector of sandfly fever in the Mediterranean region. Numerous species are involved in the transmission of the different forms of leishmaniasis. (See Table 42–2, p. 413.)

FAMILY CULICIDAE MOSQUITOES

The CULICIDAE, or mosquitoes, constitute the single most important family of insects from the standpoint of human health. From time immemorial they have been known as intolerable pests, but they also serve as vectors for a number of serious human diseases. Distributed throughout the world, mosquitoes are absent only from Antarctica, Arctic and Antarctic islands, and some isolated oceanic islands. They occur everywhere on the continents except in areas with permanent snow or ice, but the numbers of species, of which there are about 2600, are greatest in the tropics.[5]

Two characteristics distinguish adult mosquitoes from all other DIPTERA. Their mouthparts are elongate and adapted for piercing, and they have scales on the wing veins, head, thorax, legs and, in most groups, the abdomen. The diagnostic characteristics for the adult stage are illustrated in Figure 71–5. All larvae are aquatic and differ from other aquatic insects in being legless and having a bulbous thorax that is

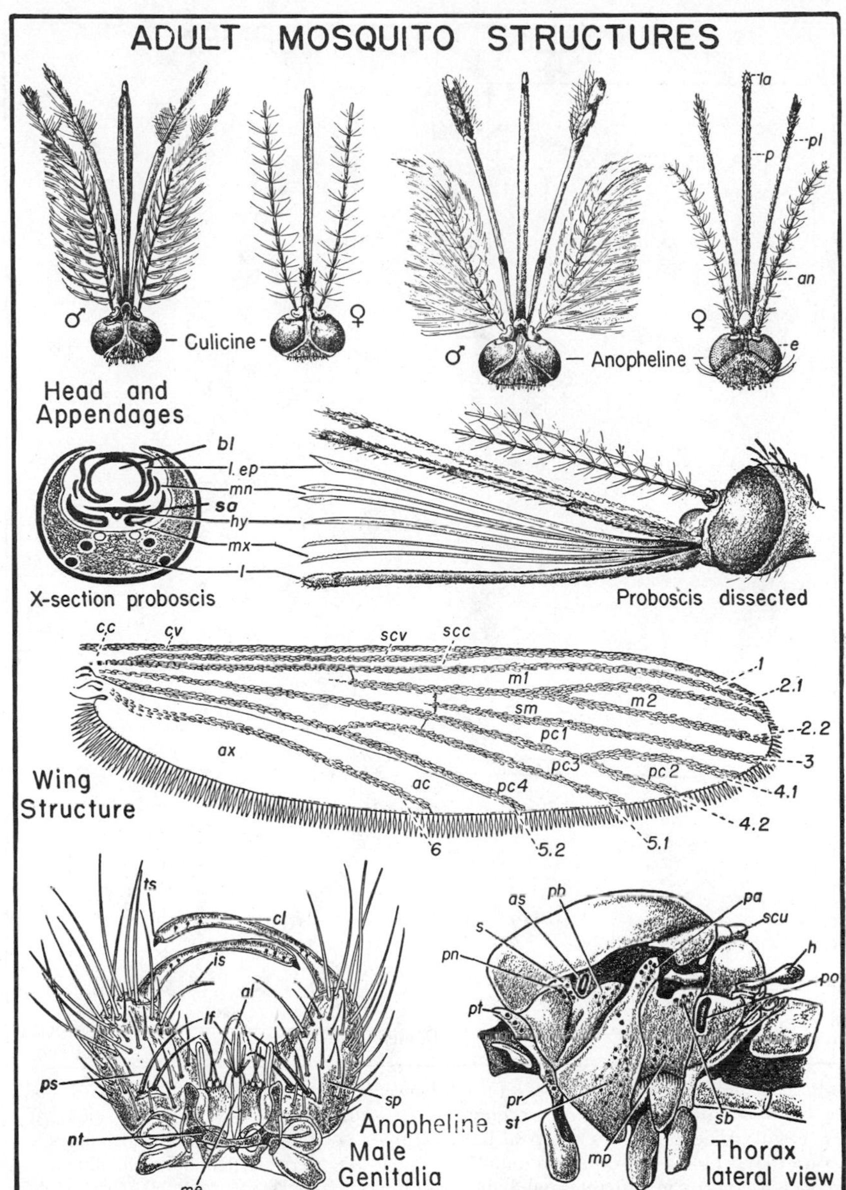

Figure 71–5. Adult mosquito structures: *ac,* anal cell; *al,* anal lobe; *an,* antenna; *as,* anterior thoracic spiracle; *ax,* axillary cell; *bl,* blood canal; *cc,* costal cell; *cl,* clasper; *cv,* costal vein; *e,* eye; *h,* halter; *hy,* hypopharynx; *is,* internal spine; *l,* labium; *la,* labellum; *lep,* labrum-epipharynx; *lf,* leaflets of mesosome; *m1, 2,* marginal cells by number; *me,* mesosome; *mn,* mandible; *mp,* mesepimeral bristles (lower); *mx,* maxilla; *nt,* ninth tergite; *p,* proboscis; *pa,* prealar bristles; *pb,* postspiracular bristles; *pc1, 2,* posterior cells by number; *pl,* palpus; *pn,* pronotal bristles; *po,* posterior thoracic spiracle; *pr,* prosternal bristles; *ps,* parabasal spines; *pt,* prothoracic bristles; *s,* spiracular bristles; *sa,* salivary canal; *sb,* subalar bristles (upper mesepimerals); *scc,* subcostal cell; *scu,* scutellum; *scv,* subcostal vein; *sm,* submarginal cell; *sp,* side piece; *st,* sternopleural bristles; *ts,* terminal spine of clasper; *1, 2.1, 2.2, 3, 4.1, 4.2, 5.1, 5.2, 6,* longitudinal veins by number.

broader than either the head or abdomen. Unlike larvae of other DIPTERA, they have a complete head capsule and only two functional spiracles, located near the posterior end of the abdomen. The form and location of various body structures and the length, shape and number of branches of body hairs are used in the specific identification of the larval and pupal stages. These are illustrated in Figures 71–6 and 71–7.

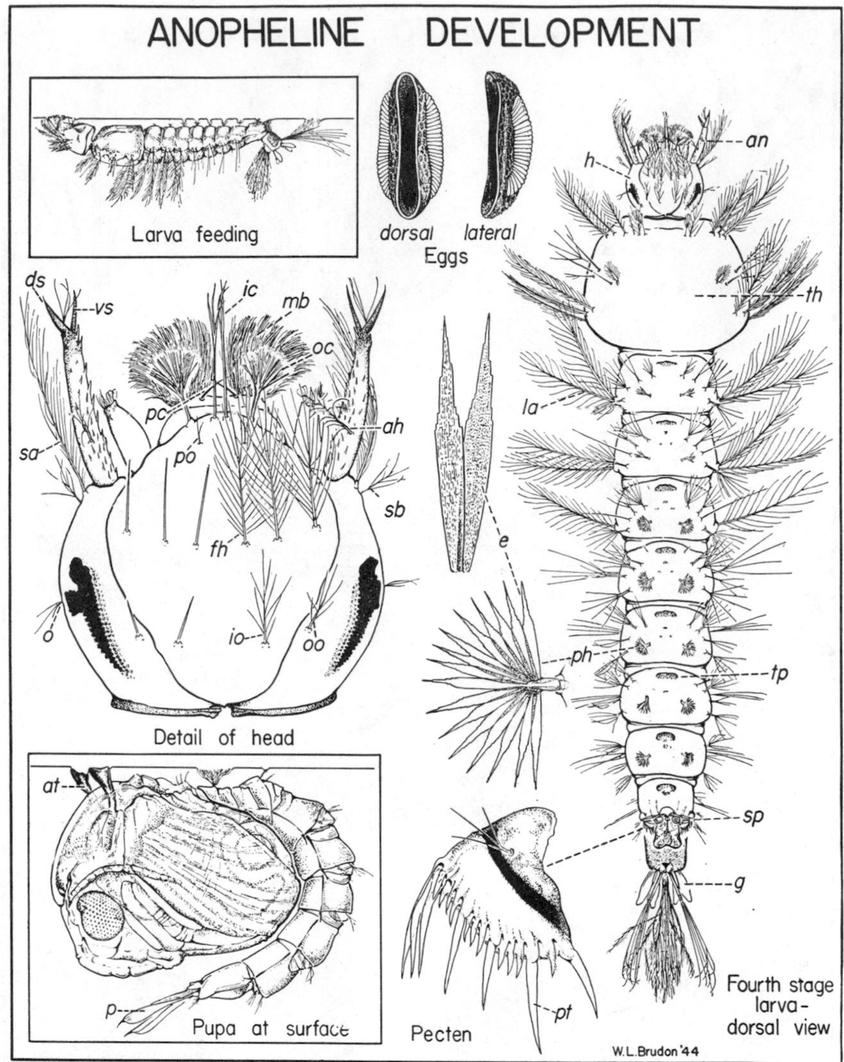

Figure 71–6. All figures except eggs pertain to *Anopheles maculipennis* Meigen. Eggs (dorsal and lateral) are from *A. gambiae* Giles. *ah,* antennal hair; *an,* antenna; *at,* air trumpet; *ds,* dorsal saber; *e,* element of palmate hair; *fh,* frontal hairs; *g,* gill; *h,* head; *ic,* inner clypeal hair; *io,* inner occipital hair; *la,* lateral hair; *mb,* mouth brush; *o,* orbital hair; *oc,* outer clypeal hair; *oo,* outer occipital hair; *p,* paddle; *pc,* preclypeal hair; *ph,* palmate hair; *po,* posterior clypeal hair; *pt,* pectin tooth; *sa,* subantennal hair; *sb,* sub-basal hair; *sp,* spiracle; *th,* thorax; *tp,* tergal plate; *vs,* ventral saber.

The family Culicidae may be subdivided in several ways, but for purposes of this discussion it will be regarded as consisting of three subfamilies: Anophelinae, Toxorhynchitinae and Culicinae. These may be separated according to the characters given in Table 71–1.

The subfamily Toxorhynchitinae includes the single genus *Toxorhynchites* (formerly *Megarhinus*), in which all of the species are large iridescent forms, very striking in appearance. The genus is small, containing about 68 species and subspecies. Adult females are not blood feeders and have no medical importance. The larvae, however, are large and predaceous upon other mosquito larvae that may be present in their normal habitats, water accumulations in some artificial containers, and both dead and living plants (tree rot holes, bamboo stumps and leaf axils and pitchers). These locations are also favored by a number of very impor-

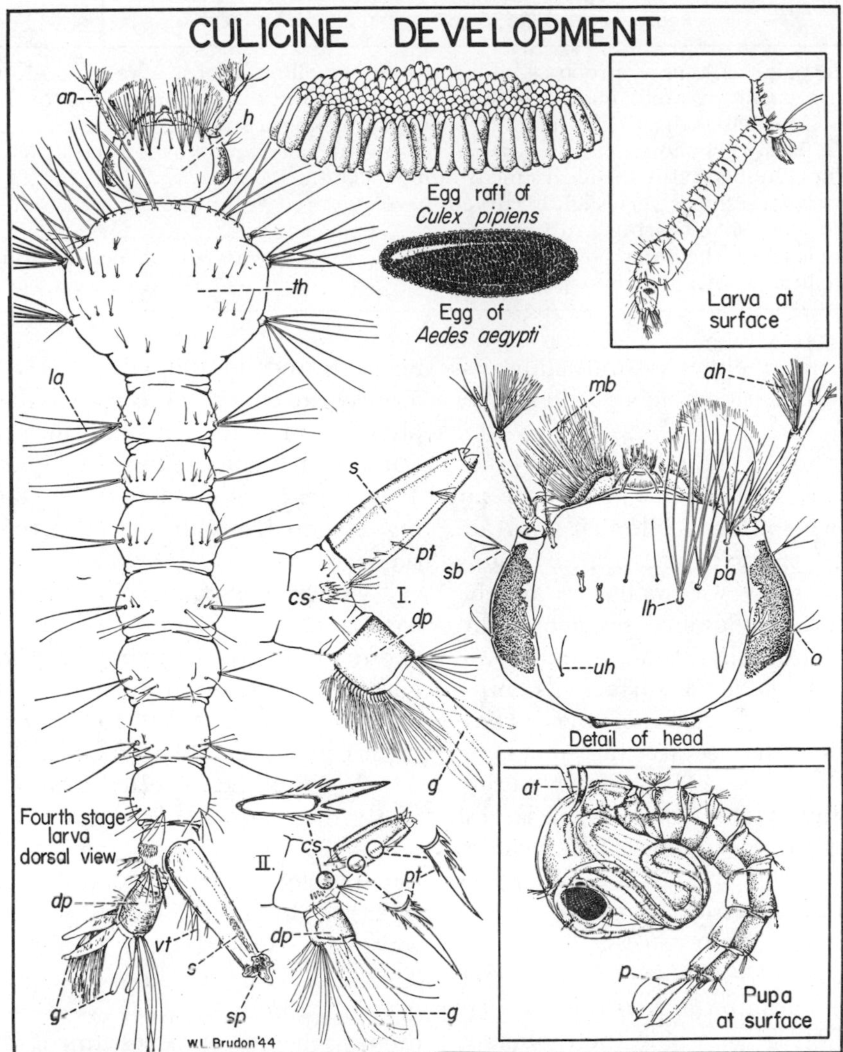

Figure 71–7. All figures except as noted pertain to *Culex pipiens* Linn. Anal segments: I, *Psorophora confinnis* (L.-Arr.); II, *Aedes aegypti* (Linn.); *ah,* antennal hair; *an,* antenna; *at,* air trumpet; *cs,* comb scales; *dp,* dorsal plate; *g,* gill; *h,* head; *la,* lateral hairs; *lh,* upper head hairs; *mb,* mouth brush; *o,* orbital hair; *p,* paddle; *pa,* preantennal hairs; *pt,* pecten tooth; *s,* siphon; *sb,* sub-basal hair; *sp,* spiracular apparatus; *th,* thorax; *uh,* sutural hairs; *vt,* ventral tufts; unlabeled tuft between *lh* and *pa,* lower head hair.

tant vector species, so when coexistence occurs the *Toxorhynchites* larvae may be instrumental in their suppression.

The subfamily ANOPHELINAE includes three genera, more than 400 species and subspecies and is widely distributed around the world, particularly in the tropics. Nearly all the species belong to the genus *Anopheles,* which is virtually worldwide, while the genus *Chagasia* occurs in Central and South America, and the remaining genus, *Bironella,* is confined to the Australasian Region. Neither of these last two genera is of medical importance.

The anopheline egg is boat-shaped and usually possesses paired lateral floats formed out of a portion of the transparent outer covering of the egg. The upper surface is flattened and is usually margined with a more or less striated or beaded structure, the frill. *Anopheles* eggs have a tendency to cluster together with the ends in contact, forming triangular, polygonal, or stellate patterns on the surface of the water. The

Table 71–1. KEY TO SUBFAMILIES OF CULICIDAE

1	(2)	Female palpi as long as proboscis or nearly so; scutellum almost always evenly rounded; wings usually spotted; male palpi long, clubbed at the tip; abdomen not covered with flat scales. Proboscis, head, thorax and abdomen forming a straight line.............. *Anophelinae*
2	(1)	Female palpi very short; scutellum variable; wings usually without spotting; male palpi long but not clubbed at tip. Profile distinctly humpbacked.............. 3
3	(4)	Proboscis straight or very slightly curved, never tapered from base to apex; scutellum trilobed, each lobe bearing a tuft of setae .... *Culicinae*
4	(3)	Proboscis rigid, the outer portion tapered and curving downward to a conspicuous degree; scutellum evenly rounded and scaled.............. *Toxorhynchitinae*

egg stage of anophelines is sufficiently distinctive to be of considerable value in species determination.

The anopheline larva differs from other mosquito larvae in lacking a siphon or air tube posteriorly on the abdomen. Instead, the two large spiracles are approximately flush with the body wall well back on the dorsal surface of abdominal segment eight, and are surrounded by five flaps. When the larva rests or feeds at the surface, its entire spiracular structure perforates the surface film, a condition that requires the larva to lie horizontally.

The subfamily CULICINAE is the largest natural group of mosquitoes and includes approximately 2200 species and subspecies distributed among about 30 to 35 genera. Best known are *Culex, Aedes, Psorophora, Culiseta, Mansonia, Haemagogus* and *Wyeomyia.* There is wide variation in structure, biology and relation to disease within the subfamily.

Culicine eggs are laid singly *(Aedes, Psorophora)* or in masses that float on the water *(Culex, Uranotaenia, Culiseta* and some *Mansonia).* None, however, is provided with specialized floats as in the case of anopheline eggs.

Culicine larvae are distinctive in possessing an elongate siphon or air tube on the dorsoposterior surface of the eighth abdominal segment. At its extremity are the two spiracles, surrounded by five outwardly directed flaps. As in the anophelines, the flaps and spiracular openings penetrate the surface film, but because of the length of the siphon the larva itself rests well below the surface, the typical posture approximating an angle of 45° to the surface. Culicine larvae are not, therefore, surface feeders. An exception to the usual structure and behavior is found in the genera *Mansonia* and *Ficalbia,* in which some species have the siphon adapted for thrusting into the underwater stems and leaves of aquatic plants. They thus remain below the surface, obtaining oxygen from air spaces in the plant tissue.

Culicine pupae are distinctive on the basis of the form and the branching of hairs and the shape of the trumpets. *Mansonia* and *Ficalbia* are again distinctive in that their trumpets are adapted for piercing plants from which they obtain their air supply.

As would be expected in such an extensive group, adult culicines display wide diversity in appearance. Many are inconspicuously colored, being a uniform dull brown, whereas others are brightly marked with white or silver scales in a variety of patterns. They differ from the anophelines in the form of the palpi (see Table 71–1) and in the humpbacked posture assumed when biting or at rest.

Life History. SUBFAMILY ANOPHELINAE. The female *Anopheles* deposits her eggs singly or in small groups on the surface of the water, utilizing a wide range of aquatic habitats for this purpose.[6] Depending upon the temperature, the eggs normally hatch in 1 to 3 days. The larvae feed just beneath the water surface where they ingest all forms of microscopic animal and plant life as well as other floating particles that come within range of their mouth brushes. They probably also utilize food materials in solution in the water. In general, it seems that microorganisms, particularly bacteria and yeasts, are the basic food materials.

The nonfeeding pupal stage requires but 2 to 3 days for the emergence of the adult. Male mosquitoes emerge before the females and live a comparatively shorter time than do the females. Copulation occurs soon after the females have completed their emergence. Following this, they begin their quest for blood. Blood source preferences vary widely among the different species but include most types of vertebrates. The majority of anopheline species are either crepuscular or nocturnal in habits. All anophelines apparently require a blood meal before they can develop eggs, and females continue to seek blood meals and to lay new batches of eggs throughout their lives. Breeding is continuous during the warm seasons of the year. In northern climates, anophelines overwinter as fertilized females, although at least one species (*A. walkeri* Theobald) may also overwinter in the egg stage.

SUBFAMILY CULICINAE. The life history of culicine mosquitoes is generally similar to that of the ANOPHELINAE.[7] The discussion that follows stresses those features in which the CULICINAE are more or less unique. Culicine eggs are laid either on water surfaces or on moist surfaces just above water lines. The first type hatch within a few days of laying, just as the ANOPHELINAE. The second type will not hatch until they are flooded at normal growing season temperatures. If flooding occurs when temperatures are too low, hatching will not occur until the eggs are once again conditioned by being exposed to the air. The hatching stimulus is a critical reduction of the oxygen level in the aqueous medium flooding the eggs. Such a decrease is generally brought about by the development of microorganisms in the flooding medium. A great range of aquatic habitats are utilized by culicine larvae, having but one feature in common, i.e. protection from excessive water motion. Larvae do not occur in the open in large bodies of water, nor in open flowing water. Some species, such as *Aedes aegypti* (Linnaeus), are known commonly as "domestic species" because they breed in cisterns, barrels, tin cans, discarded tires and related small artificial containers near dwellings or gathering places of man.

Medical Importance. The nature and appearance of mosquito bites are too well known to require extensive discussion here. The bites tend to be irregularly distributed over exposed parts, especially the face, neck, hands, legs and ankles. Mosquitoes are able to bite through thin and loosely woven clothing. Children, especially babies, may be bitten severely because of their inability to defend themselves from mosquito attacks. Numerous mosquito bites may produce dermatitis, severe itching and acute discomfort in some individuals. Bites also may become secondarily infected if scratched. The topical application of any soothing lotion or solution normally relieves the itching, while secondary infections usually respond favorably to treatment with an appropriate disinfectant or topical antibiotic.

Mosquitoes serve as vectors of filariasis, dengue, yellow fever, the malarias and several of the arboviral fevers and encephalitides. All of these diseases are discussed in detail elsewhere in the text. Only species of the genus *Anopheles* serve as vectors of the human malaria species. Most anophelines that bite humans should be regarded as potential vectors of malaria, although only about 50 species actually are known to transmit the disease in nature and less than 30 are considered really "good" vectors under ordinary circumstances. The principal vectors of the human malarias are named in Table 38–1 along with their distribution and details of their life history.

Species of *Culex, Aedes, Mansonia* and *Anopheles* (see Tables 49–1 and 68–1) serve as vectors of human filariasis. *Aedes aegypti* (Linn.), *A. albopictus* (Skuse), and members of the *A. scutellaris* (Walker) complex transmit dengue. Yellow fever, shown in 1900 to be conveyed by *A. aegypti,* is now known to be transmitted by a number of other species, of which *Haemagogus spegazzinii* Brethes and its subspecies *falco* Kumm are well known in connection with the problem of "jungle yellow fever" in tropical South America. *Culex tritaeniorhynchus* Giles is a natural vector of Japanese B encephalitis, and *C. tarsalis* Coquillett transmits western equine encephalitis in the United States. The *Culex pipiens* complex includes the vector of St. Louis encephalitis. A number of species belonging to *Culex, Aedes* and *Culiseta* have been shown to be vectors of eastern equine encephalitis.

Suborder Brachycera

Although entomologists recognize at least 17 families in this suborder, only the TABANIDAE (horsefly family), RHAGIONIDAE (snipe flies) and STRATIOMYIDAE (soldier flies) will be discussed here.

FAMILY TABANIDAE HORSEFLIES, DEERFLIES

This large family (about 2500 species), known variously as horseflies, deerflies, three-cornered flies, green-headed flies, gadflies, mangrove flies, mango flies, seroots, clegs, thunder flies and breezes, is widely distributed throughout the world. All species are blood suckers, but only the females bite. The males feed on plant juices or, in rare instances, on the juices of soft-bodied insects. The family includes more than 60 genera, but the great majority of species fall in either the genus *Tabanus* (horsefly group) or the genus *Chrysops* (deerflies). These two important genera represent separate subfamilies.

The genus *Tabanus* alone includes over 1000 species and is represented in almost every part of the world. These are large, heavy bodied flies, with a wingspread ranging up to 2½ inches. All members of the genus have the third antennal segment furnished with a conspicuous angular projection. The wings are usually uniform in color (Fig. 71–8).

The genus *Chrysops* also has a worldwide distribution. These are smaller flies, rarely exceeding ½ inch in length. The wings are marked with a dark band across the middle and frequently display a second spot at the tip (Fig. 71–9).

The genus *Silvius*, rare in North America, is abundantly represented in the Australian life zone. *Haematopota*, scantily represented throughout the world, is especially abundant in Africa and in the Orient. *Diachlorus* is represented best in South America.

Life History. Most species of TABANIDAE deposit their eggs in the vicinity of water, in many cases gluing them to foliage overhanging a swamp or stream. Marginal or emergent rocks are sometimes used, while a few species actually prefer dry situations for oviposition. From 100 to 700 eggs are deposited in a single cluster and covered by a waterproof secretion. Hatching occurs in 5 to 7 days. The soft bodied, cylindrical larvae drop to the ground (or into the water) and develop in either mud, moist earth, leaf mold or rotting logs, depending on the species concerned. Some species (especially *Chrysops*) feed on organic matter of vegetable origin, but others (most species of *Tabanus*) feed on insect larvae, earthworms, snails, crustacea and the like. A few are cannibalistic. There are four to nine larval molts, and development requires several

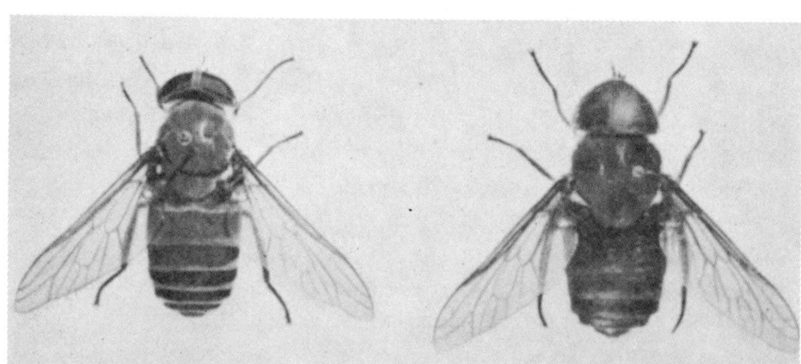

Figure 71–8. The American horsefly, *Tabanus americanus* Ford. Female *(left)* and male *(right)*. 2 ×. (Courtesy of Dr. C. B. Philip, Rocky Mountain Laboratory, U.S.P.H.S.)

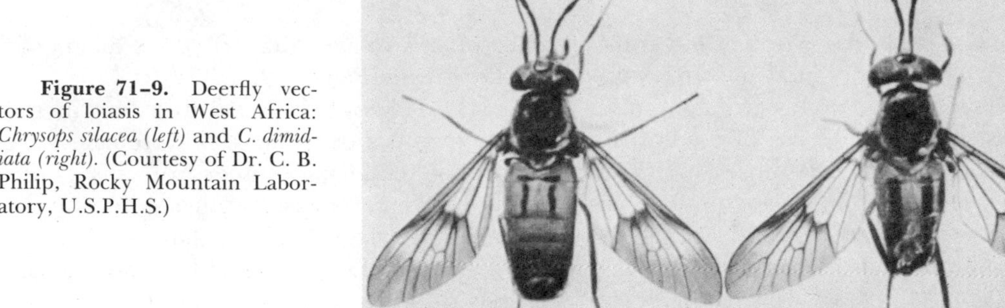

Figure 71-9. Deerfly vectors of loiasis in West Africa: *Chrysops silacea (left)* and *C. dimidiata (right)*. (Courtesy of Dr. C. B. Philip, Rocky Mountain Laboratory, U.S.P.H.S.)

months. The pupal stage lasts from 5 days to 3 weeks, larger species tending to require the longer period. The lifespan of adult tabanids is relatively long, usually extending from 4 to 8 weeks.

Medical Importance. The TABANIDAE have strong, bladelike mouthparts that can inflict a deep, painful wound. The bite is not poisonous, but owing to the size of the puncture the site may continue to bleed for some time after the fly has taken its blood meal. The saliva probably functions as an anticoagulant, but differs from that secreted by mosquitoes (and other NEMATOCERA) in being nonirritating to man.

Two species of mango flies, *Chrysops silacea* Austen and *C. dimidiata* v.d. Wulp, are biologic vectors of the African eye worm, *Loa loa*, in various tropical regions of western and central Africa. (See Chapter 49, p. 514.)

Tabanid flies function also as mechanical vectors of certain important human and animal pathogens. The chances for this type of transmission are greatly enhanced when the flies feed on a succession of animal hosts in securing a single blood meal. If disturbed while biting they usually proceed at once to a second host, carrying on the wet proboscis any microorganisms present in the blood of the first. Both anthrax and tularemia may be transferred in this manner. Following the contamination of its mouthparts with these pathogens, some *Chrysops* may remain infective for 8 to 14 days.

FAMILY RHAGIONIDAE (LEPTIDAE)

These are small to medium sized flies with small heads, large eyes, long legs and a tapering abdomen. The females of several species are vicious biters and can be serious human pests. They land silently on exposed parts of the body and inflict a sudden, painful bite before their presence is known. Their potential medical importance, as vectors, is presently undetermined, but their habits suggest they may be involved in the epidemiology of some zoonoses. Species that have a reputation of being especially annoying to man are included in the genera *Atherix, Rhagio, Spaniopsis* and *Symphoromyia.*

FAMILY STRATIOMYIDAE

In addition to the two brachycerous families discussed above, the STRATIOMYIDAE, or soldier flies, are sometimes listed as of medical interest, although for very different reasons. The adults are of no medical importance but the larvae, which develop normally in decaying fruit, vegetables or animal matter, are sometimes ingested with contaminated food and produce intestinal myiasis. The patient suffers some gastric and intestinal disturbances, which may require treatment. *Hermetia illucens* (Linn.) is the species most frequently involved.

Suborder Cyclorrhapha

These are better known flies and constitute a very large group. Even conservative taxonomists recognize no fewer than 43 families, of which at least 13 are of medical importance. Some of the more important members of the CYCLORRHAPHA are discussed under the headings of (1) biting flies and (2) nonbiting flies.

BITING FLIES OF THE CYCLORRHAPHA

The important biting flies of this suborder belong to one of two genera, *Glossina* or *Stomoxys,* both of which are members of the family MUSCIDAE.

Genus Glossina. These are the tsetse flies, best known because of their role in the transmission of trypanosomes.[8] The genus includes 21 species, some of which have several subspecies. All occur only in tropical Africa, except for *Glossina tachinoides* Westwood, which has been recorded from the southern Arabian peninsula.

Tsetse flies are for the most part slender, wasplike insects of brownish coloration. The better known forms are very slightly larger than houseflies. The proboscis is elongate and extends forward from the head like a bayonet when not in use. It is bulbous at the base and normally is enclosed by the palpi, each of which is grooved internally, so that the two palpi, taken together, form a protective sheath. When engaged in feeding, the fly lowers the proboscis until the tip makes contact with the skin. The palpi, however, continue to extend horizontally. The wings of tsetse flies are folded, scissorlike, above the abdomen when not being used for flight, and in most species extend a considerable distance beyond the caudal extremity of the fly. The fourth longitudinal vein is curiously bent rather near its base, where it is tied to vein three by a very short cross vein. This causes the *discal cell* to assume a peculiar shape, resembling somewhat the outline of a butcher's cleaver. The presence of this cleaver-shaped cell is diagnostic for the group (Fig. 45–2, p. 432).

LIFE HISTORY. Tsetse flies bite in the daytime and both males and females are voracious feeders. Members of this genus feed upon mammals, reptiles and, rarely, birds. While some species have rather restricted host preferences, others seem to be largely opportunistic. Man is not considered to be a preferred host even though he is attacked freely by some tsetse species.

A female *Glossina* does not deposit eggs but extrudes a single fully grown larva every 10 or 12 days throughout her adult life. During the intrauterine period the larvae feed upon fluids from special uterine glands and obtain atmospheric oxygen through their exposed posterior spiracles. The female requires three blood meals to complete the development of one larva and may produce a total of from eight to ten larvae. Preferred larviposition sites may include various types of soils in shaded locations, but manure and putrid materials are avoided. The larvae are unable to crawl but do manage to burrow a few centimeters beneath the surface, where pupation usually takes place within an hour. Three to 4 weeks are usually sufficient for transformation, although at cool temperatures an even longer period may be required.

The several species show marked differences in their choice of environment. *Glossina palpalis* breeds by preference on the shores of rivers and lakes, usually in dense undergrowth. It is found over an enormous range but is most abundant in West Africa and in the Congo region. Although it has been stated that *G. palpalis* is primarily a reptile feeder, it also feeds on many warm-blooded animals, such as mongoose, waterbuck, bushbuck, hippopotamus, monkey, pig and goat. Humans are not considered to be among the favorite hosts but are, none the less, readily fed upon. *Glossina morsitans* requires more open country, such as glades or plains where four-footed game animals may be found. Logs, rocks or trees

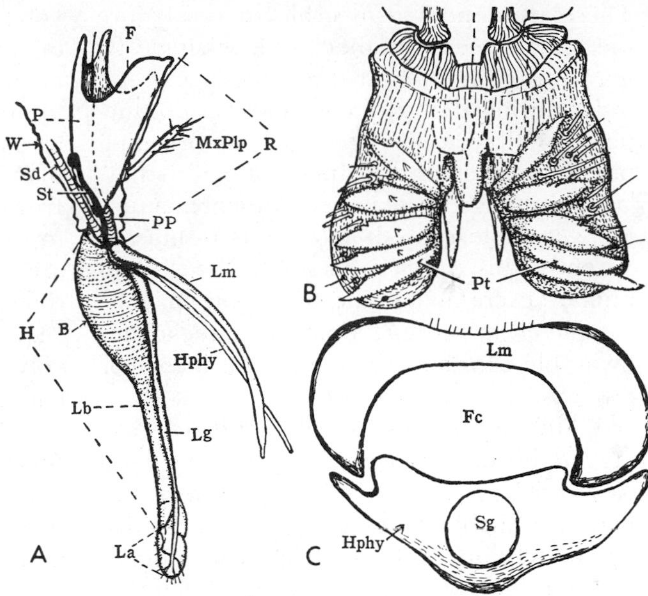

Figure 71–10. Mouthparts of the biting stable fly *(Stomoxys)*. *A*, Side view of the proboscis. *B*, The labella of the proboscis with the prestomal teeth exposed. *C*, Cross section of the labrum and hypopharynx near the middle of the proboscis. *B*, swollen base of the labium; *F*, fulcrum; *Fc*, food channel; *H*, haustellum; *Hphy*, hypopharynx; *La*, labellum; *Lb*, labium; *Lg*, labial gutter; *Lm*, labrum; *MxPlp*, maxillary palpus; *P*, pharynx; *PP*, prepharynx; *Pt*, prestomal teeth; *R*, rostrum; *Sd*, salivary duct; *Sg*, salivary duct in hypopharynx; *St*, stipes; *W*, chitinous membrane. (From Matheson, R.: Medical Entomology. 2nd ed. 1950. Comstock Publishing Co., Ithaca, N.Y.)

must be in the vicinity, however, to provide breeding and resting places for the flies. This species also has an extensive distribution but is of greatest importance in Rhodesia, Zaire, Zambia, the Democratic Republic of the Congo and the Sudan. *Glossina swynnertoni* Austen tolerates still dryer situations than *G. morsitans*. It feeds by preference on wild game.[9]

Medical Importance. Not more than three or four members of this genus are important vectors of human disease. *Glossina palpalis* is the principal vector of *Trypanosoma gambiense*, with *G. tachinoides* in all probability being a natural vector also. *Trypanosoma rhodesiense*, however, is transmitted by *G. morsitans*, *G. pallidipes* and *G. swynnertoni*. *Glossina morsitans*, the "original" tsetse fly, and *G. swynnertoni* are vectors of nagana, an important and usually fatal trypanosome disease of domestic animals. (See Chapter 45, p. 430.)

The transmission of trypanosomes by tsetse flies may be either mechanical or biological, although it is doubtful if the first is ever involved in the infection of the human host. Experimental work has shown that the flies are capable of transmitting the trypanosomes mechanically for not more than 2 days after feeding on an infected animal. They then become noninfective and there intervenes a period of some 20 days or more during which the parasites undergo cyclical development within the fly's alimentary tract. Only those that succeed in reaching the salivary glands pass through the crithidial stage and so finally become infective, metacyclic forms. It has been demonstrated that trypanosomes are usually injected in large numbers as soon as the fly's proboscis penetrates the skin. Thus, a *Glossina* that merely "probes," without remaining to feed, may nevertheless transmit infection. Adult tsetse flies live from 90 to 250 days or longer.

Genus Stomoxys. The best known species is the biting stable fly, dog fly or beach fly, *Stomoxys calcitrans* (Linn.). It enjoys practically a worldwide distribution. This species resembles the housefly, *Musca domestica* Linn., but may be distinguished by the fact that the proboscis, instead of being expanded distally into a conspicuous pair of oral lobes, is slender at the tip and adapted as an organ for piercing and sucking (Fig. 71–10). The stable fly is also more robust than the housefly and has a broader abdomen.

Life History. Both males and females are voracious blood feeders, taking two or more feedings a day during warm weather. The adult female requires a number of blood meals before she is able to develop her eggs.

These are deposited in small batches before the female seeks another meal. A single fly may engage in at least three egg-laying episodes during the season, with a total production of well over 600 eggs. Favorite breeding places are wet, rotting piles of hay, straw, lawn clippings or seaweed. Animal manure and vegetable rubbish also are used, but apparently this species does not develop in human excrement. The life cycle may be completed in as short a time as 2 weeks; unfavorable conditions may prolong it to 7 or 8 weeks.

The adult flies usually tend to congregate in sunny places in the vicinity of stables and barnyards, where blood meals are readily available. They appear to feed indiscriminately on cattle, horses, small animals and man. On dark days (and also at night) they seek shelter in houses, barns and sheds. Before and during storms they are prone to bite fiercely, thereby creating the erroneous impression that meteorologic conditions have caused the housefly to become a biter.

MEDICAL IMPORTANCE. There is little evidence that these flies are involved in the transmission of human disease. They may act occasionally as mechanical vectors, particularly if the fly is interrupted while feeding upon an infected animal and immediately thereafter attacks a human host. Although the larva of *Stomoxys* has been reported from a lesion on the foot of a stable boy in South Africa, the genus is not considered a significant myiasis-producing group.

Stomoxys flies are important as biting pests, and when present in great numbers have been known to render areas quite uninhabitable.

NONBITING FLIES OF THE CYCLORRHAPHA

Nonbiting flies of this suborder may assume medical importance either as mechanical vectors of pathogenic organisms (adults) or by inflicting direct injury to the human host through invasion of the host's tissues or organs (larval stage). The potential for involvement as a vector depends upon the type of association with humans and the degree to which the concerned species depends upon the human environment for its survival. The degree of dependence upon humans may vary significantly for any given species from one part of its geographic distribution to another, but in general, those flies that are most dependent upon humans for their biotic needs (breeding and feeding requirements) are also most likely to be involved in the transmission of human pathogens.[10,11]

The relationship of the human myiasis-producing species is somewhat different in that their involvement is a function of their parasitologic adaptation as well as their relationship to humans.[12,13] Some are obligate parasites, the majority are facultative parasites and still others have only chance involvement as agents of human myiasis. The last type of association is most common in enteric infestations and some workers question whether this is a true myiasis or merely the ability of a parasite to survive in the human alimentary tract. Whatever the biological association, each species has a preferred location and, from the clinical viewpoint, the categorization of this type of relationship may be the most useful.

Cutaneous myiasis. Cyclorrhapha larvae involved may: (1) spend their entire life off the host except when taking a blood meal *(Auchmeromyia luteola);* (2) emerge from eggs deposited on the human host, penetrate the skin and complete larval development within a stationary furuncular lesion *(Cordylobia anthropophaga, Dermatobia hominis);* or (3) hatch, penetrate the host's skin and migrate extensively without completing larval development (*Gasterophilus* and *Hypoderma* spp.).

Traumatic myiasis. Larvae invade existing wounds or lesions, rarely intact skin *(Wohlfahrtia, Chrysomyia, Cochliomyia, Phormia, Lucilia, Calliphora* and, rarely, *Stomoxys).*

Nasal, stomatic, ocular and aural myiasis. Oestrus, Rhinoestrus, Cochliomyia, Chrysomyia and various facultative genera.

Gastrointestinal myiasis. Fannia, Piophila, Eristalis, Megaselia, Musca, Muscina and *Sarcophaga.*

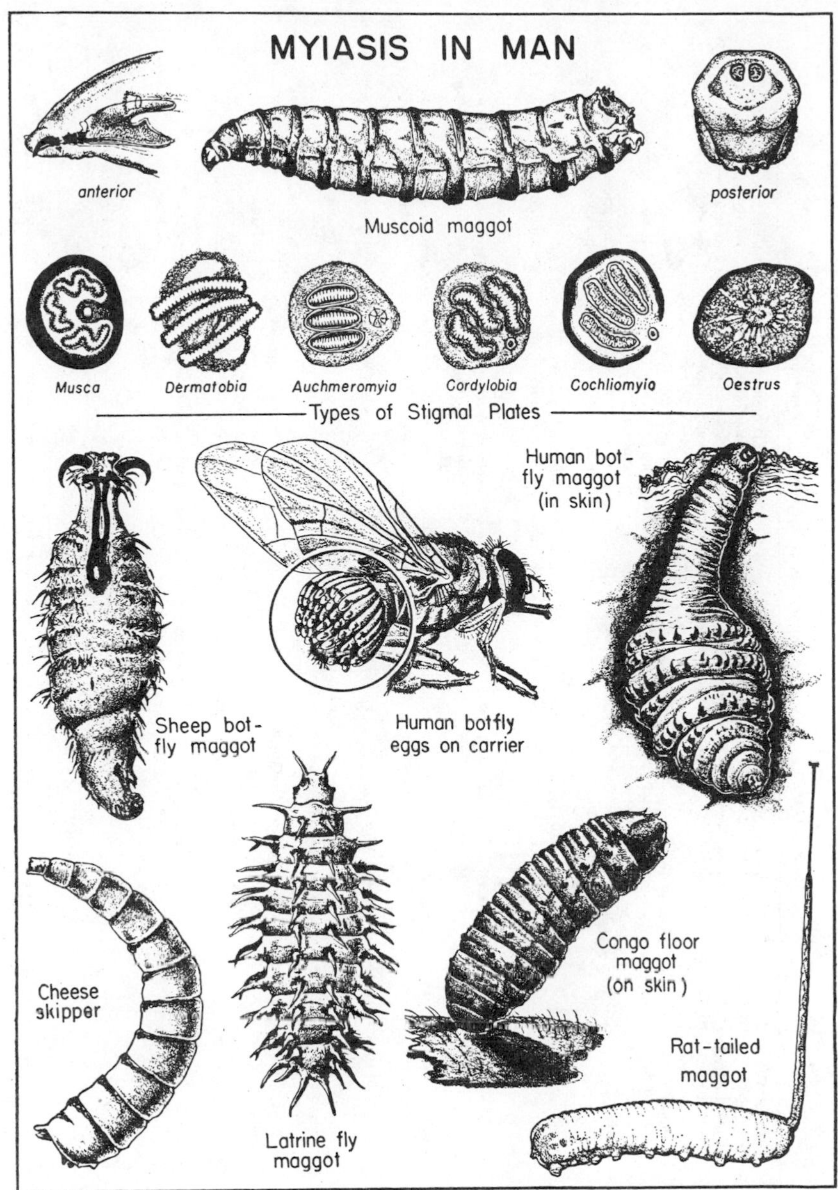

Figure 71–11. Dipterous larvae causing myiasis in man.

Genitourinary myiasis. Direct oviposition in external genitourinary apertures (*Fannia* and *Sarcophaga*) or through migration from alimentary tract (*Psychoda*).

A summary of information concerning important myiasis-producing species is given in Table 71–2, and the diagnostic features of some of the larvae are illustrated in Figure 71–11. More details are presented in the following sections.

FAMILY MUSCIDAE

INCLUDING ANTHYOMIIDAE OF SOME AUTHORS; HOUSEFLY, AND OTHERS

This family includes the housefly, *Musca domestica,* and a considerable number of related forms. Almost every conceivable medical relationship exists within the group. *Stomoxys* and *Glossina,* as obligate blood feed-

Table 71–2. Types of Myiasis in Man

Common Name of Species	Scientific Name (or Group)	Geographic Distribution	Relation to Host	Clinical Picture	Recommended Procedure	Remarks
OBLIGATORY MYIASIS						
Congo floor maggot	*Auchmeromyia luteola*	Tropical Africa	Sucks blood at night only	Perforation of skin	Avoid contaminated ground and native huts	Larvae hide in ground during daytime
Tumbu fly	*Cordylobia anthropophaga*	Tropical Africa	Young larvae invade unbroken skin (often of feet)	Furuncular swelling, with sloughing	Avoid contact with soil; mineral oil hastens emergence of larvae from tissue	Larvae leave normally after 8 to 9 days
Human botfly	*Dermatobia hominis*	Tropical South America, Central America, Mexico	Larvae invade exposed areas of skin	Throbbing pain, pruritus, oozing of blood	Adhesive tape; petroleum jelly on cotton; surgical removal	Fly glues eggs to mosquito or other "carrier"
Horse botflies	*Gasterophilus* spp.	Worldwide	Larvae wander beneath skin; galleries small, superficial	Shifting, swollen skin lesions (creeping eruption); not serious	Remove larvae, using aseptic precautions	Three species are normal parasites in gut of horse
Cattle botflies (oxwarbles)	*Hypoderma* spp.	Worldwide	Larvae beneath skin; galleries large, deep; rarely cause ophthalmomyiasis interna	Larvae less motile than above; lesions sometimes furuncular; may be serious	Remove larvae, using aseptic precautions	Are normal parasites in backs of cattle
Sheep botfly	*Oestrus ovis*	Worldwide	Pharynx, nose, conjunctival sac	Great irritation; may cause optic atrophy	Remove from eye by instruments; from nares by irrigation	Are normal parasites in head passages of sheep
Head botfly of horses	*Rhinoestrus purpureus*	Southern and eastern Europe; N. Africa; Asia Minor	Conjunctival sac	Inflammation of conjunctiva or lachrymal duct	Remove with aseptic precautions	Russian gadfly, normal in head passages of horse
Rodent botfly	*Cuterebra* sp.	Widespread (specific record from Virginia, U.S.A.).	Maxillary sinuses	Pain, congestion	Remove with aseptic precautions	Human infection very rare
Primary screw worm fly	*Cochliomyia hominivorax*	Western Hemisphere (tropical, subtropical and warm temperate)	Larvae invade nose, ears, sinuses, wounds (rarely unbroken skin)	Produce festering, deep, disfiguring wounds	Remove by aid of irrigations (chloroform in milk or oil)	A serious infection
Old World screw worm fly	*Chrysomyia bezziana*	Oriental and Ethiopian life zones	Gums, nares, ears, conjunctiva, sinuses, vagina or lesion anywhere on body	Erode bone; produce foul-smelling lesions	Remove with aseptic precautions	Usually leave wound in 7 to 14 days
Flesh flies	*Wohlfahrtia magnifica*	Mediterranean, Near East, U.S.S.R.	Invades nose, ears, wounds of all types	Produces disfiguring wounds	Remove by aid of irrigations	May cause death (All are larviparous)
	W. vigil	Nearctic	Invades unbroken skin	Furuncular lesions	Remove, with aseptic precautions	Parasitizes babies especially in neck region (All are larviparous)
	W. meigenii (New World form)	Western U.S.	Invades unbroken skin	Furuncular lesions	Remove, with aseptic precautions	Parasitizes babies especially in neck region (All are larviparous)
FACULTATIVE MYIASIS						
Common screw worm fly	*Cochliomyia macellaria*	Western Hemisphere widespread	Invades lesions, wounds (especially if malodorous)	Often complicates lesions of primary screw worm fly	Remove by irrigation, or mechanically	Normal in decaying flesh; really "saprozoic"
Green bottle flies	*Lucilia sericata* *Lucilia* spp.	Worldwide	Invade wounds, cutaneous ulcers, malodorous apertures	Complicate existing lesions; induce purulent conditions	Removal, with aseptic precautions	Usually attack only diseased tissue; formerly used in surgery, treatment of osteomyelitis
Blue bottle flies	*Calliphora* spp. *Cynomyia* spp.	Worldwide	Invade wounds, cutaneous ulcers, malodorous apertures	Complicate existing lesions; induce purulent conditions	Removal, with aseptic precautions	Usually attack only diseased tissue

Black blow flies	*Phormia regina* *Phormia* spp.	Worldwide	Invade wounds, cutaneous ulcers, malodorous apertures	Complicate existing lesions; induce purulent conditions	Removal, with aseptic precautions	Usually attack only diseased tissue; formerly used in treatment of osteomyelitis
Flesh flies	*Sarcophaga* spp.	Worldwide	Invade wounds, cutaneous ulcers, malodorous apertures; may penetrate unbroken skin	May produce serious disfigurement	Removal, with aseptic precautions	Many species are larviparous
Stable fly	*Stomoxys calcitrans*	Worldwide; (specific record from S. Africa)	Probably invades open wound	Aggravates existing lesion	Removal, with aseptic precautions	Very rare in man
Nonbiting stable fly	*Muscina* spp.	Worldwide	Probably invades open wound	Aggravates existing lesion	Removal, with aseptic precautions	Presumably a secondary invader
Houseflies	*Musca* spp.	Worldwide	Probably invades open wound	Aggravates existing lesion	Removal, with aseptic precautions	Presumably a secondary invader
ACCIDENTAL MYIASIS—INTESTINAL						
Houseflies	*Musca crassirostris*	India	Inhabit various portions of gastrointestinal tract	Symptoms variable; distress, pain, anorexia, nausea, vomiting, cramps, diarrhea, melena	Vermifuges and purges sometimes effective; (spontaneous passage of larvae rather common)	Infection acquired by eating or drinking *or* by flies depositing eggs or larvae on anus during defecation
Houseflies	*M. domestica*					
Green bottle flies	*Lucilia* spp.					
Blue bottle flies	*Calliphora* spp.					
Flesh flies	Fam. SARCOPHAGIDAE					
*Latrine flies	*Fannia scalaris*	More or less generally distributed throughout the world				
*Lesser housefly	*F. canicularis*					
Nonbiting stable fly	*Muscina stabulans*					
Cheese skippers	*Piophila casei*					
Rat-tail maggot	*Tubifera (Eristalis)* spp.					
Other syrphid flies	*Helophilus* sp.					
Soldier fly	*Hermetia illucens* (Fam. STRATIOMYIDAE)	Records few and scattered	Inhabit various portions of gastrointestinal tract	Symptoms variable; distress, pain, anorexia, nausea, vomiting, cramps, diarrhea, melena; rarely, ulcerative colitis	Vermifuges and purges sometimes effective; (spontaneous passage of larvae rather common)	Infection acquired by eating or drinking *or* by flies depositing eggs or larvae on anus during defecation
Flies of the screw worm group	*Cochliomyia putoria* *C. chloropyga*					
Wood gnats	*Rhyphus fenestralis* (Fam. ANISOPODIDAE)					
Fruit flies	*Drosophila* sp. *Calobata* sp. (Fam. MICROPEZIDAE)					
Humpback fly	*Megaselia (Aphiochaeta) scalaris* (Fam. PHORIDAE) *M. rufipes*	West Indies; N.A.; Zaire; Democratic Republic of the Congo; India, Burma; widespread (except Australian region)	Gastrointestinal tract; larvae, pupae and flies passed in feces	Intestinal distress	Vermifuges and purges helpful	Also recorded from wounds *M. scalaris* more common in man than *M. rufipes*
ACCIDENTAL MYIASIS—GENITOURINARY						
Houseflies	*Musca domestica*	Records few and scattered	Urinary tract, including bladder; genital passages of females	Obstruction, dysuria, hematuria, pyuria, strangury	Careful removal by use of cystoscope sometimes successful; (spontaneous passage of larvae is common)	Infection acquired by migration of larvae from intestinal tract *or* by flies depositing eggs or larvae on genital aperture, especially of females
Cheese skippers	*Piophila casei*					
Moth flies	*Psychoda* sp.					
Rat-tail maggots	*Eristalis* sp.					
Other syrphid flies	*Syrphus* sp. *Sepsis* sp. (Fam. SEPSIDAE)					
Latrine flies	*Fannia* spp.					
Green bottle flies	*Lucilia* sp.					
Nonbiting stable flies	*Muscina* sp.					
Flesh flies	*Sarcophaga carnaria* *Sarcophaga* sp.					
Blue bottle flies	*Calliphora* sp.					

*Most commonly reported causative agents of intestinal myiasis in man.

ers, were discussed earlier, while the two most important nonbiting genera are included here.

Genus Musca. The best known species in this large genus is the housefly, *Musca domestica* Linn. While there are many other species included in this genus, only a very few have the habits of *M. domestica* that make it of such great potential medical importance, i.e. its filth breeding habits and its intimate association with humans and their habitations.[14] The most important of these are *Musca sorbens* in Africa, the Orient, Pacific Islands and Australia; and *M. domestica vicina*, in India and North Africa.

LIFE HISTORY. The curved, whitish eggs are deposited in manure, garbage and other organic materials. Horse manure seems to be preferred, but cow, pig and chicken manure, as well as human excrement, often are used. Hatching is somewhat temperature-dependent but usually occurs within 8 to 24 hours. The larvae grow rapidly, molt three times and, under favorable conditions, reach maturity in 6 or 7 days. The pupal stage is completed in 4 to 5 days, so under optimum conditions the adults may emerge approximately 10 days after the eggs have been deposited. This relatively short development period combined with the prolific fecundity of the flies gives them a reproductive potential of awesome proportions. When adequate food and suitable environmental conditions are present, these flies normally remain near their breeding sites. They are strong fliers, however, and can migrate in considerable numbers up to 4 miles from their source. Their maximum flight range seems to be approximately 20 miles, but they may be transported even further in garbage-hauling vehicles.

MEDICAL IMPORTANCE. The external body structures and the feeding and behavioral habits of the housefly and other closely related *Musca* species give them a truly formidable potential for the transmission of pathogens. There is laboratory evidence indicating that flies may be responsible for the transmission of the etiologic agents of many diseases. Cholera, typhoid, amebic and bacillary dysentery, various diarrheas, tetanus, anthrax, trachoma, yaws and certain helminth eggs are among those involved. The larvae, living in contaminated human feces and other types of organic materials, may ingest large numbers of these organisms with their food. The more durable ones, such as *Ascaris* eggs, and the spore-forming bacteria may remain viable in the fly through its metamorphosis and thus infect the adult stage. The body surfaces, legs and tarsi of adult flies have many hairs that entrap infected materials as they walk over the surfaces and feed upon human feces and animal manure. The pathogens that are picked up or ingested may remain viable for days or weeks. When the fly subsequently lands upon and walks over human food or eating utensils, it redeposits these pathogens either through the infected material on its body or in its feces, as it defecates while feeding.

The most important mechanism for transmission, however, is in the feeding habits of the fly and the structure of its mouthparts (Fig. 71–12). When the feeding fly places its oral disk against the food surface, it regurgitates a portion of the crop contents to liquefy the food. This contaminates the food and adjacent surfaces with whatever pathogens the fly has on its mouthparts or has recently ingested. When the particle has been liquefied, the mixture of vomitus and food is sucked up through the pseudotrachea into the food channel, but many pathogenic organisms may remain on the contaminated surfaces.

A fly population will be infected with pathogenic organisms in inverse proportion to the degree of sanitation practiced in its immediate environment. In regions where human feces are readily available, the fly population becomes heavily laden, both externally and internally, with whatever infective organisms the human population may be harboring.

Although flies of other genera *(Fannia, Muscina)* and also of other families (CALLIPHORIDAE, SARCOPHAGIDAE) frequently breed and feed in filthy material, such species do not as a rule enter houses or visit human

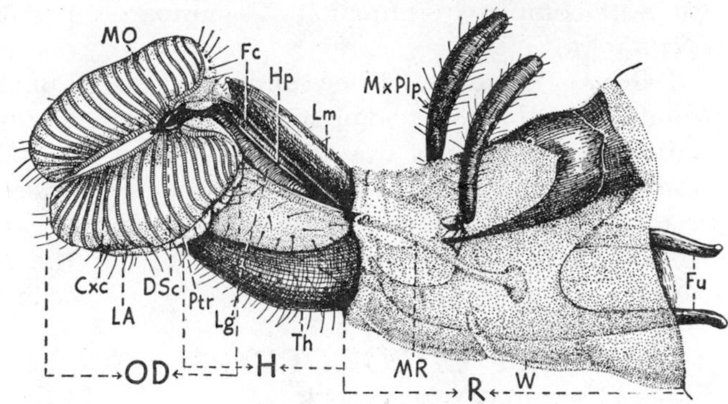

Figure 71–12. Mouthparts of a nonbiting fly, the housefly *(Musca)*. *R*, Rostrum; *H*, haustellum; *OD*, oral disc; *MO*, mouth opening; *Cxc*, a main collecting channel of the pseudotracheae; *DSc*, distal sclerite; *Fc*, food channel between the hypopharynx *(Hp)* and the labrum *(Lm)*; *Fu*, fulcrum seen in outline beneath the chitinous membrane *(W)*; *Hp*, hypopharynx; *LA*, labella; *Lg*, labial gutter; *Lm*, labrum; *MR*, maxillary rods (stipes); *MxPlp*, maxillary palpi; *Ptr*, pseudotracheae; *Th*, theca; *W*, membrane of proboscis. (From Matheson, R.: Medical Entomology. 2nd ed. 1950. Comstock Publishing Co., Ithaca, N.Y.)

food as frequently as does the housefly. They are, therefore, less likely to become important carriers of human disease agents.

Genus Fannia. This genus sometimes is considered to be in the family ANTHOMYIIDAE. However, for convenience in this discussion it will be treated as part of the family MUSCIDAE, in the larger sense, along with *Musca, Glossina* and *Stomoxys.* Two species, each with worldwide distribution, are of importance to human health; *Fannia canicularis* (Linn.), the so-called lesser housefly, and *F. scalaris* (Fabr.), the latrine fly.

Fannia canicularis is a small, grayish fly distinguishable from the housefly by wing characters, its antennal characteristics and three dorsal thoracic stripes. The legs are black and the halteres distinctly yellow. They do not, however, tend to congregate on human food as eagerly as do houseflies. The eggs of this species are laid on either decaying vegetable matter or animal manure, including human excrement. Piles of grass, especially lawn clippings, furnish an ideal breeding site. The eggs hatch in 24 hours and the larvae require at least 7 days for development. They may be very readily identified by the large spinelike processes borne both dorsally and laterally by practically every segment of the body (Fig. 71–11). The lateral processes are double or multiple. Unlike typical muscoid maggots these larvae are greatest in diameter at the middle; both anterior and posterior extremities are bluntly tapered. The entire larva is noticeably flattened dorsoventrally. The pupal stage lasts approximately 1 week.

Fannia scalaris, the latrine fly, is very similar to *F. canicularis,* but is usually a bit larger. It seems to prefer excrement to vegetable matter as a site for oviposition.

The larvae of both species repeatedly have been recorded as causing both intestinal and urinary myiasis in man. The parasites apparently gain access to the human host through the ingestion of food soiled with human or other excrement containing eggs or developing larvae, or by exposure of the anus or genitals in such a manner as to give the flies an opportunity to deposit eggs in or near these apertures. This might occur either while the person is using an open privy or while resting or sleeping in a more or less unclothed condition. Urinary myiasis, as caused by these species, probably originates by the external route rather than by migration through the tissues from the alimentary canal. Infection of the genitourinary tract is more common in females than in males.

SYMPTOMS OF INFECTION BY FANNIA LARVAE. *Gastric Myiasis.* The presence of a considerable number of larvae in the stomach usually causes nausea, sharp pain and vertigo. Sometimes violent vomiting results in the expulsion of some of the larvae, and the diagnosis of myiasis can thus be made.

Intestinal Myiasis. Pain, diarrhea and hemorrhage from the anus sometimes result from the presence of larvae in the intestinal tract. A certain number of larvae eventually may be expelled in the feces spontaneously.

Genitourinary Myiasis. Victims of infection in these organs have been known to manifest albuminuria, dysuria, hematuria and pyuria. Spontaneous passage of the larvae, with complete termination of symptoms, is common.

Genus Muscina. The genus *Muscina* (nonbiting stable fly) is sometimes of medical importance. Larvae of this genus have been found infesting open wounds (probably as secondary invaders) and have been taken from the human intestinal tract.

FAMILY CHLOROPIDAE EYE GNATS

Most of the important flies in this family are in the genus *Hippelates* (Fig. 71–13), often called eye gnats or eye flies because of their predilection for feeding on the lachrymal secretions of their hosts. These flies are small (0.5 to 2.5 mm in length) and feed avidly on blood, pus and mucus, lachrymal and sebaceous secretions. While unable to bite and penetrate human skin, they have minute rasping structures on the labellae that are thought to be able to produce microincisions suitable for the entrance of certain pathogens. Their preferred sites for oviposition and larval development are loose, cultivated soils with high organic content.

There is extensive circumstantial evidence that *Hippelates* flies are involved in the transmission of epidemic conjunctivitis and yaws, although experimental evidence supporting this contention is scarce. *Hippelates collusor* and *Hippelates pusio* are common human pest species in parts of the United States and Mexico and probably transmit the causative organism of conjunctivitis in those areas. *Siphunculina funicola,* also known as the eye fly, probably has a similar role in India, Sri Lanka, Java and other parts of the Orient. Motile *Treponema pertenue* were often present in the "vomit drops" of *Hippelates flavipes* in Jamaica, so it is thought that it may have been a mechanical vector of yaws in that country. (See Chapter 17, p. 155.)

FAMILY SYRPHIDAE HOVERFLIES

The rat-tail maggots of the genera *Eristalis (Tubifera)* and *Helophilus* are capable of adapting themselves to the human intestinal tract. Nasal myiasis due to larvae of this group also has been recorded. The drinking of water from foul ditches or puddles probably is responsible for most cases of human infection. In nature the maggots hang head downward in the water, the posterior extremity of the elongate tail-like portion piercing the surface film. They thus derive oxygen from the atmosphere, but are otherwise completely submerged. (See Fig. 71–11.) The adult flies often show a remarkable resemblance to bees.

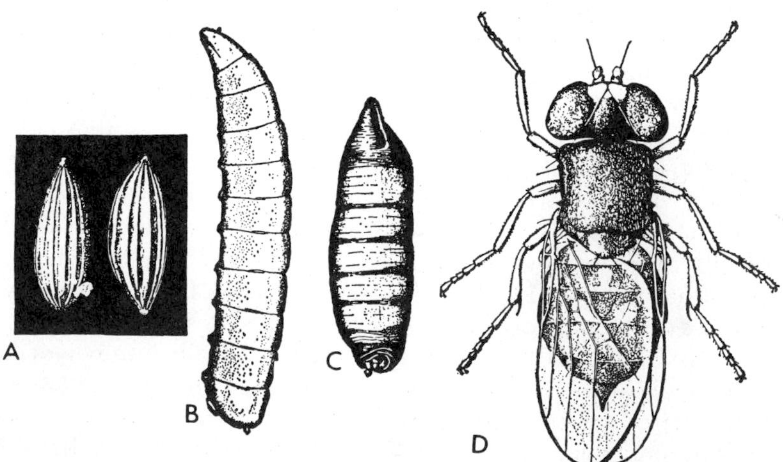

Figure 71–13. The eye gnat, *Hippelates pusio. A,* eggs; *B,* larva; *C,* pupa; *D,* adult. (Courtesy of Dr. D. G. Hall, Am. J. Hyg.)

FAMILY DROSOPHILIDAE
FRUIT FLIES

Known variously as fruit flies, pomace flies or banana flies, most members of this family breed in spoiled fruit, grape pomace and similar organic matter. The accidental ingestion of their larvae may result in infection of the alimentary tract. Both adults and larvae are very small (3 to 4 mm long).

FAMILY PIOPHILIDAE
CHEESE FLIES

The larva of *Piophila casei* (Linn.), the well known "cheese skipper," has been recorded repeatedly as causing intestinal myiasis in man. The maggot, which attains a length of more than 5 mm, is rather conical, being pointed anteriorly and truncate posteriorly (Fig. 71–11). Occasionally, the larvae will pupate and develop into adults in the intestine of man. The patient usually suffers a severe colic, with headache, vertigo and nausea. The feces may contain blood.

FAMILY GASTEROPHILIDAE
BOTFLIES (IN PART)

These are the botflies of horses, asses and related hosts. The larvae usually live within the alimentary tract of their normal equine hosts, attached by their mouth hooks to the gastric or intestinal mucosa. The exact location varies with the species concerned. The adult flies of this group range from 9 to 18 mm in length and are characterized by stout bodies rather densely clothed with fine hair. They resemble honeybees somewhat.

Life History. These flies are unable to bite; in fact, they take very little food of any kind. They are nevertheless exceedingly annoying to horses. They glue their triangular (stalked) eggs to the hairs of the host animal, hatching being stimulated (at least in certain species) by friction against the teeth or tongue, as the horse bites or licks its legs. The egg of each species has a distinctive shape. Even the newly hatched larvae possess rather conspicuous, backwardly directed spines on most of the body segments. Later instars are larger, with a greater relative diameter and heavier spines. After completing their development the larvae are passed in the animal's feces and fall to the ground. Pupation takes place in dry horse dung or loose soil. The flies copulate soon after emergence, and in a temperate climate oviposition normally takes place in early summer. The life cycle requires about a year.

Medical Importance. Symptoms of Parasitism in Man. When eggs are laid on the human host, the first-stage larvae burrow into the skin as far as the stratum germinativum, after which they wander aimlessly, producing a form of cutaneous myiasis. They may survive for months. A tortuous inflammatory line marks the path of migration. The condition is commonly termed "larva migrans." *Gasterophilus intestinalis* (De Geer) is the species most commonly involved, though *Gasterophilus haemorrhoidalis* (Linn.) and *Gasterophilus nasalis* (Linn.) also infect human hosts occasionally. Intense itching usually accompanies the infection, and secondary sepsis from scratching is not uncommon.

Diagnosis and Treatment. The larva is usually found just in advance of the inflammatory line. It may be rendered visible by the application of a small amount of mineral oil, which causes the skin of the patient to become transparent. By use of a lens the backwardly directed spines, segmentally arranged, may be demonstrated readily, thereby establishing the dipterous nature of the parasite. Hookworm larvae have no such structures. Surgical extraction is relatively easy.

FAMILY OESTRIDAE
BOTFLIES (CONCLUDED)

For practical purposes, the botflies other than the Gasterophilidae may be grouped in a single family, the Oestridae. As in the Gasterophilidae, it is only the larval stage that is of medical importance. Most species normally parasitize animals other than man, humans being attacked only rarely. The following genera will be discussed: *Dermatobia, Oestrus* and *Hypoderma*.*

Genus Dermatobia. The only recognized species is the so-called human botfly, *Dermatobia hominis* (Linn. Jr.). This species is native to Central and South America and Mexico, where its larvae are found parasitic in the skin of various birds and mammals, including man. Domestic cattle are very frequently parasitized. The young larva is sometimes called *ver macaque,* later instars being known under the designation *torcel,* or *berne.* Another common name is *ver moyocuil.* The adult fly is approximately 15 mm long and is generally a brownish gray color. The abdomen, however, is of a distinctly bluish cast, especially when viewed in reflected light. The legs and face are orange-yellow.

LIFE HISTORY. The adult fly does not seek its host directly, almost always utilizing some species of insect for the transmission of its eggs. Mosquitoes of the genus *Psorophora (Janthinosoma),* particularly *P. lutzii* (Theobald) and *P. ferox* Humboldt, seem to be favorite carrier hosts in Central America and northern South America. In Brazil biting flies, such as *Stomoxys* and *Siphona (Haematobia),* are vectors, and even *Musca* and *Anthomyia,* as well as certain species of ticks, are found with *Dermatobia* eggs glued fast to their bodies. The *Dermatobia* female usually captures the mosquito (or other species) in flight and, while hovering, manages to fasten some 15 to 25 whitish eggs to the abdomen of the carrier host without causing any injury to the latter. During oviposition the victim is held with the head forward and the dorsal surface close against the botfly's thorax. Upon release the burdened carrier then goes its own way, in the case of bloodsucking forms to seek a blood meal from an appropriate warm-blooded host, in the case of nonbloodsucking species perhaps to rest on vertebrate skin (Fig. 71–11).

The eggs, which contain fully developed embryos, are stimulated to hatch by the warmth of the host's body, the eggs being so placed that the end through which the larva emerges is directed away from the body of the carrier host. In penetrating the skin of the vertebrate host, the young larvae frequently make use of the feeding puncture of the carrier species, but are capable of perforating the unbroken surface with their own mouthparts.

The larvae, once established, do not migrate but remain in situ, where they give rise to a boil-like swelling, open at the top. The larva, whose anterior segments become robust, is markedly attenuated posteriorly, particularly for the duration of the second instar. The caudal extremity bears a pair of large, functional spiracles that remain in contact with the exterior, thus insuring an adequate supply of air (Fig. 71–11). The parasites become larger, fatter and considerably more grublike as time goes on. Conspicuous, backwardly directed spines adorn most of the forward segments. Development requires about 50 days, after which the parasites extricate themselves from the host tissue, drop to the ground and pupate.

MEDICAL IMPORTANCE. *Symptoms of Infection.* There is usually no sensation during the actual penetration of the skin by the first-stage larvae. During the first week there may be pruritus, particularly at night, and by the second week a serous exudate frequently is observed. After this the lesion begins to resemble a small furuncle, which increases in size and becomes exceedingly painful by the beginning of the fourth week, continuing so until larval development is complete. Muscular soreness and stiffness may be continuously present, and the attempts of the parasite to rotate on its own axis frequently result in excruciating pain at the point of infection. There is considerable destruction of local tissue, and the lesion may even resemble a local streptococcal infection with associated lymphangitis. Inguinal lymphadenitis likewise may be evident, particularly if the lesion is

*It is recognized that *Dermatobia, Cuterebra, Pseudogamates* and *Rogenhofera* are considered by certain authors as constituting a separate family, the CUTEREBRIDAE, with *Hypoderma* serving as the type of another natural group, the HYPODERMATIDAE. In the interest of simplification, however, the CUTEREBRIDAE and HYPODERMATIDAE are included here with the OESTRIDAE, in the broader sense.

located on or near the ankle. Prior to the emergence of the larva, the swelling may attain the size of a pigeon's egg, but emergence itself seems to involve almost no pain or sensation of any sort.

Treatment and Removal of the Larva. Several methods for removal of the parasites have been employed. Natives squeeze out the larva after opening the boil and applying tobacco juice. When there are many lesions, mineral oil, Vaseline, or even butter may be smeared over the openings. This cuts off the larval air supply by blocking the spiracles, and stimulates premature extrusion, which may be facilitated by dilatation of the opening with forceps and pressure at the base of the tumor. A good modern technique involves the following steps:

1. Injection of a 2 per cent aqueous solution of procaine with a hypodermic needle both in and around the lesion as a preliminary procedure. Larva and host are thus both anesthetized.

2. The larva is then exposed by a linear incision. The parasite may be removed by forceps. Irrigation with sterile saline, followed by packing with a one-to-one mixture of sulfanilamide and sulfathiazole, is recommended.

3. If little or no secondary infection is present, the wound may be closed with interrupted dermal sutures; otherwise it is best to apply a tight, dry dressing without suturing.

Genus Oestrus. The larval stages of *Oestrus ovis,* the common sheep bot, usually develop in the nostrils and frontal sinuses of sheep and goats. Occasionally, the adult flies deposit first-stage larvae in the human eye where they give rise to a painful and dangerous ophthalmomyiasis. (See Fig. 71–14 for an example of ophthalmomyiasis.) The species is worldwide in distribution, occurring wherever sheep and goats are raised.

LIFE HISTORY. The fly normally deposits living maggots in the nostrils of sheep and goats. The young larvae work their way into the nasal and frontal sinuses, where they may accumulate in such numbers as to cause their hosts considerable pain, and sometimes death. Larviposition may take place any time during the summer or early fall, the larvae remaining within the host until the following spring when they have completed their development (Fig. 71–11). They then wriggle out of the nostrils of the host and fall to the ground, pupate, and emerge as adults in 3 to 7 weeks.

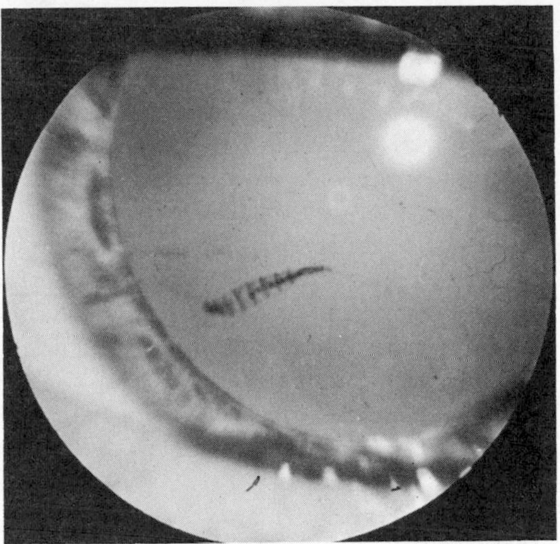

Figure 71–14. Fly larva in vitreous, species undetermined. (Courtesy of Dr. E. W. Hunt, Jr.)

MEDICAL IMPORTANCE. *Symptoms of Ophthalmic Infection in Man.* In humans this parasite usually affects the conjunctiva of the eye and produces a painful form of conjunctivitis. Since man is an atypical host the larvae do not progress beyond the first stage, so the symptoms usually persist for only a limited period of time. Typically, the patient reports being struck in the eye by an insect or small foreign object, with pain and inflammation developing a few hours later. Upon examination, this type of myiasis resembles cases of acute catarrhal conjunctivitis and may be diagnosed as such, since the small size and transparency of the first-stage larvae make them difficult to see, and they may be easily missed.

This parasite may also cause oral or nasal myiasis, but these types are less common than the ocular form. The larvae may occasionally invade the nasal cavities and frontal sinuses to produce swelling and severe pain. Symptoms may last from 3 to 10 days, or longer.

Similar types of ocular and nasal myiasis

in humans also may be caused by *Rhinoestrus purpureus,* a head maggot of horses in parts of Europe, Asia and Africa. Symptoms are the same as those produced by *Oestrus ovis* and, similarly, larval development in humans does not progress beyond the first stage.

Human myiasis caused by *O. ovis* or *R. purpureus* is most common where humans live in close association with the normal hosts. However, it can occur anywhere these parasites have been established in the domestic animal populations.

Treatment. Apply an appropriate anesthetic to the eye, then remove larvae by either irrigation or forceps.

Genus Hypoderma. These are the cattle botflies or ox-warbles. Two species are especially well known, *Hypoderma lineata* (Villers) and *Hypoderma bovis* Linn. Both occur widely in Europe, Asia and North America, the second being restricted to somewhat more northerly latitudes. The grubs are found normally in tumorous swellings on the backs of cattle, but may occur as parasites of horses and sometimes occur in man.

LIFE HISTORY. The hairy, beelike fly deposits up to 800 eggs, usually on the hairs of the host. The hatched larvae bore through the skin, migrate through the tissues and eventually localize beneath the skin of the back. Later they escape through the skin and drop to the ground to pupate. The life cycle requires a full year.

MEDICAL IMPORTANCE. *Symptoms of Infection in Man.* The act of oviposition usually goes unnoticed. Several days later progressive soreness and swelling develop. As the larvae migrate through the subcutaneous tissues, severe discomfort, itching, pain and cramps may be experienced. The larval wanderings may be extensive and are usually in an upward direction, although they may temporarily pass down an arm or leg and then retrace their course. The path of the larval movement is marked by localized swollen or painful areas or indefinite reddish lines, much less distinct than those produced by *Gasterophilus.*

When the larva is mature enough, usually several months after the initial skin penetration, it moves toward the skin surface and produces an indurated skin swelling, most often on the upper chest or back, or on the head or neck. The swelling becomes domelike, with a central opening through which the larva breathes.

The pain and discomfort associated with this parasite may be severe, and the patient can temporarily lose the use of an invaded limb. Occasionally, early stage larvae enter the eye and may cause retinal detachment or other ocular damage. (See Fig. 71–14.)

Treatment. If the open dermal lesion has formed, the larvae may be squeezed out. Otherwise, surgical removal is required. When ocular involvement has occurred, larvae located in the anterior chamber may be removed surgically, but parasitism of the posterior chamber may necessitate removal of the eyeball.

FAMILY CALLIPHORIDAE* BLOWFLIES AND OTHERS

This widely distributed family is made up of medium to large, robust, rather bristly flies, characterized for the most part by metallic green, blue or yellowish coloration, at least on the abdominal segments. None of these species is a bloodsucker in the adult stage; all, however, may function as mechanical vectors of various disease organisms by means of their feces, vomitus or body hairs. Many of their larvae produce myiasis in man, some as obligatory and others as facultative or accidental parasites. The following genera are of major medical importance: *Auchmeromyia, Cordylobia, Cochliomyia (= Callitroga), Chrysomyia, Lucilia (= Phaenicia), Phormia, Calliphora.*

Genus Auchmeromyia. The genus is well known from the Congo floor maggot, *Auchmeromyia luteola* (Fabr.), a common species in tropical Africa. The large, brownish

*This family is separated with difficulty from the family SARCOPHAGIDAE (flesh flies); in fact, the two are sometimes combined under the family name METOPIIDAE. The latter name, however, is rare in medical literature, and it is felt that separate treatment of the groups will serve the purpose of this work better.

yellow flies deposit batches of eggs on the floor of native huts, on sleeping mats or on dry sand previously contaminated with human excreta. The larvae are extremely resistant to dryness and can survive long periods (30 days) without food. They remain hidden during the day but become active at night, when they wander about in search of a blood meal. With their mouth hooks and body spines they perforate the skin of persons sleeping on the ground. With the anterior segments more or less embedded in the tissues, they engorge (Fig. 71–11). This process requires from 15 to 20 minutes. They then detach and once more go into hiding in the soil or dust. If hosts are available for nightly feeding, larval development may be accomplished in as brief a period as 2 weeks; otherwise, as long as 3 months may be required. Pupation takes place on or in the ground and requires about 12 days. Parasitism is obligatory with this species. This type of myiasis differs from all others in that the larva remains external in its parasitic relationship and spends long periods apart from its host.

PROPHYLAXIS. Avoid sleeping on the ground, especially the floors of native huts. Sleeping mats carried from village to village by native travelers undoubtedly distribute eggs and larvae. The use of repellents applied both to the skin and to the mats has been suggested.

Genus Cordylobia. *Cordylobia anthropophaga* (Grünberg) is a large, brownish yellow fly, found only in Africa south of the Sahara, where it is known as the Tumbu fly. The female deposits her eggs in polluted soil or on clothing that bears an odor of perspiration. The larvae hatch in 24 to 48 hours and proceed to seek an appropriate mammalian host. After penetrating the unbroken skin (usually the feet in man), they develop very much like *Dermatobia hominis,* the location of each parasite being marked by the presence of a furuncular swelling. Sloughing and even gangrene may occur, particularly when a number of parasites localize in a restricted area. Fortunately, only 8 to 10 days are required for development, after which the larvae leave the host and drop to the ground. Pupation takes place in the soil. The adults emerge from 22 to 24 days later.

TREATMENT AND PROPHYLAXIS. The application of mineral oil usually will cause the larvae to loosen their hold and leave the host, regardless of the stage of development. Since rats constitute the principal wild animal reservoir for these parasites, rodent control is of importance in holding the species in check. Animals that have supported an infection appear to be relatively immune to subsequent attacks.

Genus Cochliomyia (= Callitroga). These are the screw worm flies of the Western Hemisphere. The adults are metallic green in color, somewhat resembling ordinary green bottle flies *(Lucilia),* but may be recognized by the dark stripes on the dorsal surface of the thorax. Two species are of medical interest, *Cochliomyia hominivorax* (Coquerell) and *Cochliomyia macellaria* (Fabr.), of which the first, though less common, is of far greater importance.

Cochliomyia hominivorax is the primary screw worm of animals and man and is found in the southern United States and throughout the American tropics. The flies are attracted by any open wound or discharging aperture, depositing their eggs in batches on the skin close by. A single fly may deposit as many as 300 eggs in 5 minutes' time. The larvae may enter the wound or, in thin-skinned animals such as rabbits and guinea pigs, penetrate the unbroken skin. It is believed that they cannot perforate the unbroken skin of man. This species does not confine its activity to necrotic areas, preferring to burrow deep into healthy tissue, sometimes penetrating cartilage and even bone. Deep, festering, extremely malodorous wounds are characteristic of the infection. Nasal and aural infections due to this species are truly dangerous; penetration of the brain, especially by way of the middle ear, may occur occasionally.

The larvae require up to 3 weeks for development, depending on the conditions encountered. Pupation takes place in the soil. Transformation requires from 1 week (in summer) to nearly 2 months (in colder weather).

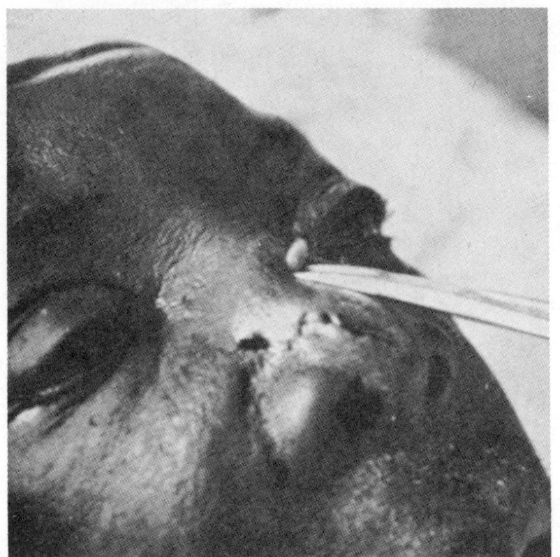

Figure 71–15. Infection with *Cochliomyia hominivorax.* Over 230 screw worm larvae were removed from this patient's nasal passages. (Courtesy of Dr. W. E. Dove and associates, Bureau of Entomology and Plant Quarantine, U.S. Department of Agriculture.)

SYMPTOMS OF INFECTION IN MAN. Nasal involvement is the most common form of infection, but it frequently goes undiagnosed for some time. There may be much local swelling, and the patient usually complains of intense pain and a sensation of "crawling." Delirium is not uncommon. Rarely, some of the larvae may be sneezed out or emerge spontaneously. With proper illumination the physician usually can see the larvae in situ with their mouthparts embedded deep in the tissues, the posterior extremity and its spiracles exposed to insure a supply of air (Fig. 71–15).

TREATMENT OF NASAL MYIASIS. 1. Anesthetize the larvae and the mucous membrane by applying benzol, ether or chloroform, either on a cotton pledget or with an atomizer. Block nostrils with dry cotton for 2 or 3 minutes.

Irrigation with 20 per cent chloroform in sweet milk or 15 per cent chloroform in light mineral or vegetable oil is also an effective method of accomplishing anesthesia.

2. Remove the larvae with forceps and have the patient blow his nose. Special care should be taken to avoid rupturing exposed blood vessels.

3. Give aftercare appropriate to any similar wound.

Two or three applications of the anesthetic may be necessary in the case of extensive infection.

PROTECTION OF THE INDIVIDUAL. Persons who sleep during the day in regions where screw worms occur should be protected by screens or bed nets. Such protection is especially important for patients with dermal lesions of any type or who have active nasal catarrh or discharges from the eyes. Blood-stained clothing or bandages also are attractive oviposition sites, so these items should be removed. Patients in hospitals, particularly surgical wards, are highly vulnerable unless protected by screens or bed nets.

Genus Chrysomyia. This genus is similar to *Cochliomyia* in that all species are medium-sized flies of bright metallic coloration. The genus is confined to Africa, Australia, parts of Asia and various islands, including the Philippines. *Chrysomyia bezziana* (Villeneuve), known generally as the Old World screw worm fly, is similar in its habits to *Cochliomyia hominivorax,* being not only an important pest of domestic animals but also the causative agent of serious and disfiguring myiasis in man, especially in Asia. The maggots may occur in any portion of the body, but ophthalmic infections are particularly serious. Erosion of bone is not uncommon. The larvae develop very rapidly and are ready for pupation on the sixth or seventh day. The adult fly is characterized by the presence of transverse abdominal bands.

Genus Lucilia (Green Bottle Flies). These are medium-sized, metallic green or bluish flies. The genus is very widespread. The females normally deposit their eggs on meat or dead animals. Not infrequently, however, they utilize open wounds or malodorous body apertures. *Lucilia sericata* (Meigen), sometimes referred to as the genus *Phaenicia,* is an important sheep maggot in the British Isles and elsewhere, damaging healthy tissue and endangering the life of animals. The same species, because of its abundance and filth-feeding habits, is frequently important in the mechanical transmission of enteric infections. Larvae of this genus have been known to cause various types of myiasis in man, including cutaneous, intestinal and genitourinary infections.

Genus Phormia (Black Bottle Flies). Flies of this group may be either shiny black, blue or green. A well known species is the black blowfly, *Phormia regina* (Meig.), normally a breeder in decaying meat but capable of causing traumatic myiasis in man.

Genus Calliphora (Blue Bottle Flies). These are rather large flies of various metallic coloration, the common pattern consisting of a grayish thorax and an abdomen of some shade of blue. As in related genera, blue bottles breed usually in the bodies of dead animals and doubtless have some sanitary value in hastening the destruction of putrefactive material. The larvae of some forms, however, develop as parasites on nestling birds. *Calliphora vicina* Robineau-Desvoidy (= *C. erythrocephala* Meig.) and *Calliphora vomitoria* (Linn.) are the best known members of the genus. *Calliphora livida* Hall is less common. All three may be of some importance in the distribution of filth-borne infections. As with *Lucilia,* larvae of this genus may cause nasal, cutaneous, gastrointestinal or genitourinary myiasis in man.

FAMILY SARCOPHAGIDAE* FLESH FLIES

This family includes a considerable number of small to large flies, most of which present a remarkable uniformity of appearance. The prevailing color is gray, although a golden pollinose sheen is not infrequently observed on the abdominal segments. Dark longitudinal lines characterize the dorsal surface of the thorax. In almost all species the dorsal surface of the abdomen presents a striking "checkerboard" appearance. Two genera, *Sarcophaga* and *Wohlfahrtia,* are of medical importance.

Genus Sarcophaga. This is a very large genus, the adults of which are either filth feeders or flower feeders. The larvae are found in a variety of situations, many feeding on the bodies of dead insects, carrion or animal excrement. *Sarcophaga haemorrhoidalis* (Fallén) is a proved agent of intestinal myiasis, the eggs or larvae presumably being ingested along with food (fruit, meat) to which flies have access. Other species are undoubtedly capable of similar adaptation. *Sarcophaga carnaria* (Linn.) seems to prefer the vaginal orifice for oviposition.

As in the following genus, larvae have been taken from wounds, cutaneous ulcers, nasal passages and sinuses, the adult flies being attracted in all cases by a malodorous discharge. *Sarcophaga dux* Thomson may cause tissue myiasis, and *Sarcophaga ruficornis* (Fabr.) has been recovered from wounds. *Sarcophaga fuscicauda (peregrina)* Böttcher has been known to cause extensive traumatic myiasis of the face.

Genus Wohlfahrtia. This genus is very similar to the genus *Sarcophaga* except that the checkerboard pattern of the abdomen gives way to something like a black spotting in most of the species. *Wohlfahrtia vigil* (Walk.) and *Wohlfahrtia opaca* (Coquillet) in North America, also *Wohlfahrtia magnifica* (Schin.) in Europe and the Near East, are frequent causative agents of myiasis of the integument and sense organs. All three are larviparous, and first-stage maggots of *W. vigil* and *W. opaca* (= *W. meigenii*), at least, are capable of penetrating the unbroken skin.

TREATMENT AND REMOVAL OF SARCOPHAGID LARVAE. Proceed as outlined for similar infections by larvae of MUSCIDAE, OESTRIDAE, GASTEROPHILIDAE and CALLIPHORIDAE.

*See note on family CALLIPHORIDAE, page 778.

REFERENCES

1. Fox, I. 1955. A catalogue of the bloodsucking midges of the Americas *(Culicoides, Leptoconops* and *Lasiohelae)* with keys to the subgenera and Nearctic species, a geographic index and bibliography. J. Agr. Univ. Puerto Rico *39*:214–285.
2. Kettle, D. S. 1962. The bionomics and control of *Culicoides* and *Leptoconops.* (Diptera, Ceratopogonidae = Heleidae.) Ann. Rev. Entomol. 7:401–418.
3. Adler, S., and Theodor, O. 1957. Transmission of

disease agents by phlebotomine sand flies. Ann. Rev. Entomol. *2*:203–226.
4. Hoogstral, H., and Heyneman, D. 1969. Leishmaniasis in the Sudan Republic. Am. J. Trop. Med. Hyg. *18*:1091–1210.
5. Stone, A., Knight, K. L., and Starke, H. 1959. A Synoptic Catalog of the Mosquitoes of the World (Diptera, Culicidae). Thomas Jay Foundation Vol. VI. Entomol. Soc. Am., Washington, D.C. 358 pp.
6. Russell, P. F., West, L. S., Manwell, R. D., and Macdonald, G. 1963. Practical Malariology. 2nd ed. Oxford University Press, London, 750 pp.
7. Foote, R. H., and Cook, D. R. 1959. Mosquitoes of Medical Importance. Agricultural Handbook No. 152. Agricultural Research Service. U.S. Department of Agriculture, Washington, D.C. 158 pp.
8. Buxton, P. A. 1955. The Natural History of the Tsetse Flies: An Account of the Biology of the Genus *Glossina* (Diptera). London Sch. Trop. Med. Mem. 10. H. K. Lewis & Co., London. 816 pp.
9. Weitz, B. 1963. The feeding habits of *Glossina*. Bull. W.H.O. *28*:711–729.
10. Lindsay, D. R., and Scudder, H. I. 1956. Nonbiting flies and disease. Ann. Rev. Entomol. *1*:323–346.
11. Greenberg, B. 1971. Flies and Disease. Vol. I. Princeton University Press, Princeton, N.J. 856 pp.
12. James, M. T. 1947. The Flies That Cause Myiasis in Man. U.S. Department of Agriculture, Misc. Publ. No. 631, Washington, D.C. 175 pp.
13. Zumpt, F. 1965. Myiasis in Man and Animals in the Old World. Butterworths, London. 267 pp.
14. Sacca, G. 1964. Comparative bionomics in the Genus *Musca*. Ann. Rev. Entomol. *9*:341–358.

CHAPTER 72

Control of Arthropods of Medical Importance

REVISED BY R. H. GROTHAUS
AND D. E. WEIDHAAS

Measures for the control of arthropods are of three types—mechanical or cultural, biologic and chemical. Chemical control measures are the most widely used, although they rarely provide a permanent solution to a problem, as mechanical measures sometimes do. Biologic control measures have been highly successful against some agricultural pests, but are only now finding a place in the control of medically important arthropods. Most recently, the combination of all control techniques into an "integrated pest management" approach has gained in professional popularity. This approach is leading to the deemphasis of chemical control as the primary technique for suppression of undesirable arthropods.

MECHANICAL AND CULTURAL CONTROL

Mechanical and cultural methods play an important part in the control of arthropods injurious to man. Some mosquito problems may be solved by elimination of the larval habitats by various types of water management—ditching, draining, impounding or filling. These are often called permanent control measures, although filling is the only method that requires no attention after installation. Proper measures for the disposal of sewage, garbage and manure are of the utmost importance in the prevention of fly breeding. Elimination of trash piles, rat harborages and birds' nests near human habitations will reduce annoyance from such pests as scorpions, centipedes and various bird and mammal parasites. Screens are an important protective measure against flying insects. The first step in any insect control campaign, be it nationwide or restricted to a single building, should be a survey to determine the source of breeding and infestation. If the breeding places can be reduced or eliminated by mechanical means, such measures should be taken first. If breeding cannot be eliminated, attention should be given to other integrated control measures.

BIOLOGIC CONTROL

Although biologic control measures have had only limited use in the past, in recent years the concern for environmental damage consequent to the use of insecticides has brought about a resurgence of interest and research support aimed at the discovery and development of effective biologic control methods. Many of these are still in laboratory research stage, but increasing numbers of field trials are currently being undertaken. Information on entomopathogenic microorganisms, including viruses, bacteria, protozoans and fungi, and the nematodes that attack insects, is growing at a rapid pace.[1,2] Mass production of the mermithid nematode *Reesimermis nielseni* has already been achieved, and field trials against culicine vectors have been undertaken in Southeast Asia.[2] Also under intensive investigation are methods of control through genetic manipulation of populations of such important disease vectors as *Aedes aegypti* and *Culex pipiens quinquefasciatus* as well as anopheline species. Techniques for the mass production and distribution of gamma irradiated (cobalt-60) sterile males of the screwworm fly, *Cochliomyia hominivorax* (Coquerell), are well established.[3] These flies are released from the air over infested areas, in numbers that exceed those of the native population. Males of this species mate repeatedly, females only once. Females that mate with sterile males lay infertile eggs, and hence are eliminated as far as maintenance of the species is concerned. The application of this technique has led to the eradication of the screwworm fly from a large area of the southeastern United States.

Aside from the use of parasites, as above, biologic control is also concerned with the propagation and distribution of predators on the target pest or vector arthropod. The classic example of this approach is the long practiced technique of introducing small fish such as *Gambusia affinis,* which are voracious feeders on mosquito larvae.

CHEMICAL CONTROL

The use of chemical control has greatly increased since World War II, as has the development of synthetic contact insecticides. Prior to that period, most chemicals had to be ingested to be effective (stomach poisons). Fumigants such as methyl bromide were available, but limited in use. New chemicals such as DDT functioned as both contact (killing on touch) and stomach poisons, while a few also released toxic vapors.

Although the synthetic insecticides have proved to be valuable tools for the suppression of vector-borne diseases, criticisms against their use have arisen.[4] Some of the compounds have been found to accumulate in the environment and cause damage through food chain organisms. As a result of this problem, some countries have drastically limited the use of certain "hard" pesticides. Other countries still rely on the "hard" pesticides as the only practical method of suppressing devastating diseases such as malaria. Table 72–1 is a comprehensive guide for the chemical control of disease vectors and does not reflect national restrictions. *All chemical listings should be checked with the control recommendations of the country in question. If the listing in this text does not conform to a particular country's permitted use laws, the listing should be disregarded.*

Types of Insecticides. Most modern insecticides are either inorganic compounds, botanicals, chlorinated hydrocarbons, or organophosphorus or carbamate compounds. Inorganic compounds, including arsenicals, fluorine compounds and other chemicals, were most widely used before World War II. The botanicals are represented by the pyrethrins, which are obtained from pyrethrum flowers. During and after World War II the chlorinated hydrocarbons, DDT, lindane, chlordane, dieldrin, methoxychlor and others, came into widespread use. Because of their low cost and greater effectiveness, it was possible to carry out extensive control programs. Later, the organophosphorus compounds, including such materials as malathion, dicapthon, parathion, Diazinon and others, came into general use.[5, 6] More recently, research has concentrated on the development of synthetic materials with juvenile hormone activity that inhibit the development of the target arthropod in its immature stages. This approach has been fostered by the effort to circumvent the resistance that has developed to the conventional insecticides among many arthropod pests and vectors, and the desire to lessen the impact on the environment consequent to the use of broad spectrum insecticides.[7]

Residual Action of Insecticides. Since the advent of DDT much emphasis has been placed on the residual action of insecticides. It is only with compounds such as DDT, which not only remain unchanged on treated surfaces for long periods but which are *effective by contact at extremely low concentrations,* that the full value of residual action can be realized.

Residual sprays differ from contact sprays or space sprays in that they are applied to surfaces on which the insects are expected to walk or rest at some later time. Contact sprays are applied with the objective of striking and killing the insects present at the time of treatment. The insecticides used in residual sprays must therefore be durable, chemically stable under all conditions of temperature and humidity, and effective in minute quantities so that the insects will pick up a toxic dose through brief body contact.

Resistance to Insecticides. Individual insects within a species vary in their susceptibility to an insecticide, just as they vary in other respects. When an insecticide application fails to kill all the insects in a population, the survivors will represent the most resistant fraction of the population, and their progeny may be more resistant than an average group. Such resistance is enhanced by cross breeding among the survivors. This has occurred with many of the insects of medical importance exposed to the chlorinated hydrocarbons, and is now occurring with the organophosphorus compounds.[8]

The resistance problem has reached such magnitude that it is now necessary to obtain information concerning specific insect resistance from workers in each locality or country. This is necessary to insure that the insecticide of choice is still effective against the insect in question in the place where its use is contemplated.

Methods of Application of Insecticides. Insecticides may be applied as sprays, aerosols (including fogs and smokes), ultra low-volume concentrates (ULV), dusts, granules or baits.[9-13] Sprays may be applied either for immediate contact or for residual action as solutions or suspensions. The latter may be prepared from emulsions or wettable powders. The solvent most commonly used for indoor sprays is deodorized kerosene, which is noninjurious to nearly all of the materials found in the home. Fuel oil is the usual solvent for solution sprays to be applied outdoors. When used as recommended, for example in airplane sprays at 1 to 4 quarts per acre, it is not injurious; however, excessive dosages may injure foliage.

The emulsifiable concentrates used to make emulsion sprays usually contain 25 to 50 per cent of an insecticide and 5 to 10 per cent of an emulsifier in a noninjurious solvent. They may be used in homes on surfaces that water will not injure, in animal shelters and on foliage. They are economical, reduce transportation problems in large scale programs, and leave satisfactory residues on most surfaces.

Wettable powders usually contain 50 to 75 per cent of the insecticide on an inert carrier with a wetting agent. They are economical and easy to transport. They are more satisfactory than solutions or emulsions for the treatment of clay, mud or concrete surfaces and are useful for treating foliage, barns or other surfaces.

Aerosols are extremely fine particles of insecticides that remain suspended in the air for considerable periods. They may be produced by liquefied gas generators (the common aerosol "bomb"), by smoke generators, or as fine mists mechanically generated. They are applied indoors or outdoors for immediate contact action only, although they do leave minimal residual deposits in closed buildings. When used outdoors they are dependent on air currents to carry them to the insects, and can be used only under satisfactory meteorologic conditions.

Ultra low-volume (ULV) concentrates are chemicals released at or near technical grade with little or no solvents added. Malathion (95 per cent) is a common mosquito adulticide. It is usually released as a fine aerosol at the rate of 3 to 6 oz per acre. The use of the ULV technique has been well accepted because of the reduced volume of nonbeneficial solvents and other additives released into the environment. It has also reduced the need for bulky tanks on spray equipment. The use of ULV equipment on aircraft has greatly reduced "down time," bringing about considerable cost savings in some control programs.

Dusts, consisting of low concentrations (usually 10 per cent or less) of insecticides in an inert carrier such as talc or pyrophyllite, are useful for the application of mosquito larvicides on open water under suitable wind conditions, for the control of adult mosquitoes by direct contact action, for the treatment of poultry manure to prevent fly breeding, as louse powders, and in other special problems. They do not cling well to most vertical surfaces, but may have residual action on horizontal surfaces, as in the treatment of cockroach harborages.

Insecticide granules are usually made with an inorganic carrier such as attapulgite, montmorillonite or vermiculite. The granules may range in size from 16-mesh to 60-

mesh, depending upon the application equipment, terrain and cover. They usually contain fairly low concentrations of insecticide, 10 per cent or less, and are usually dispersed at rates of 5 to 20 lb per acre. In medical entomology the granules are especially useful for aerial treatments of vegetated marshes for the control of mosquito, tabanid or *Culicoides* spp. larvae. Granules penetrate the foliage better and can be dispersed when wind conditions are too unfavorable for the use of dusts or sprays.

Baits have been used widely for the control of houseflies, and to a lesser extent for the control of cockroaches and ants. They consist of an insecticide in a favored food material and may be exposed at fixed stations or dispersed as granules or sprinkled droplets.

DISPERSAL EQUIPMENT. The dispersal equipment used to apply the insecticidal formulations described previously may be either hand or power operated, depending on the scale of operations and the relative availability of hand labor, funds for purchase of equipment, and access roads. All the formulations can be applied with ground equipment and some can be applied also from airplanes.[14, 15]

ANOPHELINE CONTROL

ANTIADULT MEASURES

Screenings. All buildings should be screened properly with electrogalvanized 18-to-the-inch mesh wire. In tropical areas near the sea it is necessary to use wire of a noncorrosive material such as bronze, aluminum or plastic. Screen doors should open outward, should be of sturdy construction and should be located on the windward side of buildings.

Particular attention should be paid to the closing of cracks in floors and walls. Knot holes, openings under the eaves, and spaces created by outlets for pipes and wires should also be sealed.

Insecticides. Chemical control of adult mosquitoes in buildings or shacks is conducted in various ways through the use of contact or residual sprays.[11, 12] In closed or mosquito-proofed structures, the interior should be sprayed twice daily with a contact spray, preferably in the early evening and again before sunrise if an attempt is being made to prevent all biting. In many regions it has proved possible to prevent new cases of malaria by treatments of all houses and buildings with residual insecticides, even though anophelines were not eradicated from the areas.

Aerosols or regular sprays kill mosquitoes upon contact at the time of application. The aerosol formulations of the small commercial or military dispensers or "bombs" are frequently changed to meet new developments in insecticides and insecticide resistance. The active ingredients most frequently utilized are pyrethrins extracted from pyrethrum flowers, *Chrysanthemum cinerariaefolium,* and/or a synthetic counterpart. These are often augmented by a synergist or activator, such as piperonyl butoxide or *N*-octyl sulfoxide. Some of the newer organic insecticides may also be present, although aerosols have little residual action regardless of the ingredients. Freon is commonly selected as the solvent and propellent.

Sprays used for contact action only may contain activated pyrethrins, activated allethrin or a thiocyanate.

Outdoor areas also may be freed of pest mosquitoes by spraying, but such methods are seldom included in anopheline control programs. Ground or aerial sprays containing malathion, methoxychlor, naled, dichlorvos, propoxur or fenthion provide immediate control and some degree of residual action, whereas fogs, smokes and mists furnish immediate control only.

ANTILARVAL MEASURES

The females appear to be quite selective in their egg-laying habitats, utilizing only those waters best adapted for the development of the larvae and pupae of the species concerned. Thus, *Anopheles quadrimaculatus* Say seldom oviposits in densely shaded or in wholly unshaded waters. A certain amount of aquatic vegetation also seems necessary for the proper development of *A. quadrimaculatus.* This depends not so much upon the amount of foliage present as upon the "intersection line" where air, water and plant surface meet each other. *Anopheles freeborni* Aitken, common in southern California, tends to avoid impounded waters. *Anopheles albimanus* Wied. is a hardy species of the American tropics ovipositing in the fresh, sunlit pools of streams, swamps and marshes in humid regions. *Anopheles bellator* Dyar and Knab, a forest mosquito, lays eggs in rainwater in the leaf axils of bromeliad plants high up in the branches of trees. *Anopheles aquasalis* Curry favors brackish water but will tolerate either sunlight or shade. *Anopheles superpictus* Grassi favors seepages, small trickles and occasional small pools. *Anopheles gambiae* Giles seeks sunlit pools, usually of rainwater that has settled in borrow pits, hoofprints and natural depressions, and avoids all moving water. *Anopheles funestus* Giles, however, prefers pools of permanent character. *Anopheles minimus* Theobald is found in slowly running water, in streams, springs, ditches and rice fields. Studies on this species have shown that the larvae will develop in water far more heavily polluted than the female will use for oviposition.

One of the most important aspects in the field control of malaria is the elimination of man-made anopheline larval habitats. In endemic regions much acute malaria may be traced directly to such artificial sources as wheel ruts and borrow pits, to the obstruction of streams and irrigation ditches, to improper management of irrigation water and to similar artificial collections of standing or impounded water. The measures included within this category have as their objectives either the elimination of collections of water suitable for larval development or alteration of the conditions in such a way as to render the water unsuitable. These procedures include filling, drainage, flow regulation, alteration of the salt content, oiling or dusting, edging, control of sun or shade and the use of fish predatory upon the larvae. Many of the following antilarval measures are employed less extensively since the advent of residual insecticides used for the control of adult mosquitoes. However, such measures may give "permanent" control and greater reliance may have to be placed on them in the event that the insecticide resistance problem is not overcome.

Filling. This method of eliminating larval habitats is permanent but expensive. Wheel ruts, borrow pits and small swamps should be filled whenever possible.

Drainage. If permanent fills are not feasible, drainage to eliminate larval sources may be undertaken. Open drainage ditches or subsoil drains may be utilized to remove residual surface water or surplus underground water that may cause surface seepage. Open drains are maintained more satisfactorily if they are lined with rocks or concrete. Subsoil drainage is effected by lining ditches with baked unglazed or concrete tiles. Ditching by dynamite is an efficient, rapid and cheap method. The distance between borings and the amount of dynamite necessary will vary with the type of soil and quantity of moisture present.

Salinity. Lagoons and marshes of brackish water along the sea coast are often important mosquito sources. Some anopheline larvae require water with moderate salt content; others cannot develop in brackish collections. Such areas frequently may be controlled completely by the introduction of tide gates eliminating the salt water or by the construction of channels permitting a freer flow of sea water, thus increasing the salinity.

Channeling and Fluctuation. In regions with marked rainy and dry seasons there is considerable fluctuation of water levels in streams. This is an important factor in areas where malaria vectors develop in nearly dry stream beds. Such localities can be controlled by ditching to concentrate the flow into a single channel or by constructing dams equipped with automatic siphons or hand operated sluices to flush these mosquito sources periodically.

Fluctuation of the water level in a series of reservoirs also has been used successfully to control the development of mosquitoes. Lowering of the level may strand larvae and eggs and destroy them by desiccation or force larvae to open water where they are accessible to predators. Subsequent raising of the water level drives larvae out of pockets where they were temporarily free from attack.

Edging. The removal of vegetation from the margin of a stream, lake or reservoir is an important control measure. Such a procedure tends to clear and straighten the channel of small streams or irrigation ditches and so destroys potential larval habitats. Similar clearing of the shore line about lakes or ponds removes littoral protection for larvae even though the water level may fluctuate.

Shade. Certain anopheline larvae flourish in sunlit water, whereas others must have shade. The elimination of trees and brush along the banks of streams and other small pools of water to provide free entry of sunlight will eliminate the larvae requiring shade. Conversely, planting along the banks of streams and ditches will eliminate those that need sunlight. These measures, however, should not be undertaken until a complete survey of the anophelines of the area has been made, since alteration of the sun and shade factors, while eliminating one species, may lead to the establishment of others that thrive under the altered conditions.

Larvicides. Larval sources that cannot be eliminated by filling or draining may be controlled by the judicious use of larvicides.[10, 11] A number of materials are effective for this purpose. Against nonresistant species, DDT is the most effective. (The use of DDT for this purpose is now banned in the United States.) It can be applied at the rate of 0.05 to 0.4 lb in 1 gallon of fuel oil per acre with hand applications, or in 2 to 3 quarts per acre with airplane applications. If the mosquitoes are resistant to chlorinated hydrocarbons, malathion may be applied at 0.5 lb per acre. Parathion 0.063 to 0.1 lb per acre has also been used but is more hazardous to mammals. Fenthion at 0.05 to 0.1 lb per acre is being used in some localities. If control is extremely difficult because of excessive organic content of the water or for other reasons, these rates may be increased considerably in situations where injury to fish, wildlife and domestic animals is not a problem. Any of these insecticides may be applied as dusts or granules. Older methods of control, such as the application of oil or Paris green, also may be utilized, particularly if resistance is an acute problem. Compounds with juvenile hormone activity that inhibit development of larvae have begun to be used.[7]

Biologic Measures. The introduction of top minnows such as *Gambusia* spp., which feed upon mosquito larvae and pupae, is a very efficient method of control for use in lakes, ponds and circumscribed collections of water, especially where aquatic vegetation is not abundant.

Biologic control of this nature represents merely an extension of the natural control factors that are in operation at all times. Not only fishes, but also water bugs (NOTONECTIDAE) and other aquatic predators (for example, dragonfly nymphs) play an important, though sometimes unappreciated, role in limiting the numbers of mosquito larvae. The use of entomopathogenic parasites is receiving increasing attention.[1, 2]

Species Elimination. In some areas it may be found less expensive in the long run to attempt the complete elimination of a malaria-carrying species rather than continue indefinitely the application of measures that rarely succeed in accomplishing more than a general reduction of the mosquito fauna for a given season. The extermination of *Anopheles gambiae* in Brazil is an excellent example of a species-elimination program completed on a relatively large scale. No such plan should be undertaken, however, without complete knowledge of the habits and ecologic relationships of the species concerned, lest time, money and manpower be wasted in what may later prove to have been a hopeless effort.

CULICINE CONTROL

ANTIADULT MEASURES

Most of the environmental control measures described for both adult and larval anopheline mosquitoes are applicable to the culicine group or may be modified to meet the particular situation. The following information is offered as a guide to some of the problems of control.

As with anophelines, the adults of some forms (including most species of *Aedes*) live only through the summer season. Others (*Culex* spp.) usually hibernate as adults. Domesticated species, as might be expected, feed eagerly on human blood and seem to prefer it. Semidomesticated and wild species vary in their feeding preferences. *Culiseta* spp. attack man rather rarely. *Culex apicalis* Adams is believed to feed exclusively on the blood of frogs and other poikilothermic vertebrates. There is a long list of forest and open country species that subsist normally on the blood of wild mammals and birds, but which transfer to man as soon as he becomes available.

Feeding hours tend to be rather constant for the various groups. *Aedes aegypti* (Linn.) and *Aedes albopictus* (Skuse) are daylight biters. *Culex pipiens* Linn. and *Culex pipiens quinquefasciatus* Say feed either at night or in darkened rooms. *Aedes stimulans* Walker, *Aedes excrucians* Walker and several others prefer late afternoon for feeding, but *Aedes spencerii* Theobald attacks in bright sunshine.

Culicines in general show a greater flight range than anophelines. *Aedes sollicitans* Walker has been known to migrate as much as 40 miles, *Aedes vexans* Meigen, at least 10. *Aedes cantator* (Coquillett) and *Aedes taeniorhynchus* Wied. are also known for their migrations. Some, such as *Aedes aldrichi* Dyar and Knab, restrict their migrations to wooded areas. Domesticated and semidomesticated species, however, remain fairly close to their breeding grounds.

The same contact and residual sprays used to control anophelines in buildings will also control culicine adults. In addition, since many culicine species breed in tremendous numbers and cause severe annoyance, operations are often conducted to eliminate them from outdoor areas. Entire cities or military installations are often treated from the air or with ground equipment. Such applications provide only temporary relief but are helpful where the area to be protected is surrounded by extensive breeding areas that cannot be treated with larvicides. Malathion, naled and fenthion are the insecticides used most commonly for this purpose. Sprays, dusts, smokes and fogs have all been used with good effect (Table 72–1, p. 797).

ANTILARVAL MEASURES

All members of the four genera, *Culex, Mansonia, Uranotaenia* and *Culiseta,* deposit their eggs in rafts on the surface of the water (Fig. 71–7). In the case of *C. pipiens* each female, fresh from hibernation, lays 100 to 400 eggs in a single mass.

In most other genera of culicines the eggs are laid singly in water, near water, or where water is likely to be. Species of *Psorophora* deposit eggs directly upon the ground. Protected by heavy, spiny coats, they may remain dormant for months or even years but hatch quickly when water finally becomes available. Larval development is then very rapid, requiring, as a rule, only a few days.

Most species of *Aedes* leave their eggs during the summer in the bottoms of dried out pools, swamps and marshes. Such eggs remain dormant throughout the fall and winter (even if submerged), not hatching until the following spring. A few species of *Aedes,* however, produce at least two broods a year. *Aedes varipalpus* (Coquillett) and *Aedes triseriatus* Say usually seek tree holes in which to deposit their eggs. *Aedes aegypti,* being a domestic species, oviposits on or just above the surface of water in various small containers near the habitation of man. These eggs, unlike certain species mentioned above, hatch very quickly. Where temperature permits, breeding of *A. aegypti* goes on throughout the year. This species cannot survive outside of tropical and subtropical latitudes, though it may be carried into temperate regions and reproduce successfully during the summer months.

It is convenient to classify culicines into three general groups on the basis of the type of habitat selected for oviposition:

1. Domesticated species, e.g. *A. aegypti, C. pipiens* and *C. p. quinquefasciatus,* which may select small water sources in and about human dwellings.

2. Semidomesticated species, which may select water sources close to human habitations or in other situations as opportunity affords.

3. Wild species, which avoid the habitations of man, being found in salt, brackish or fresh water marshes, in swamps, woodlands, prairies or other natural situations. The greater number of culicine species are classed as "wild." In temperate regions, wild culicines may be further divided into "spring breeding" and "summer breeding" forms. In North America, *Aedes stimulans, Aedes canadensis* Theobald and *Aedes cinereus* Meigen are examples of the first group; *A. sollicitans, A. taeniorhynchus* and *A. cantator,* of the second.

Most of the larvicides that are effective against anophelines are used for the control of culicines, and such water management procedures as ditching, impounding, draining and filling are the principal measures for the control of many species. Efficient irrigation practices can reduce or eliminate some of the worst culicine problems.

The most important culicine is *A. aegypti,* which is known to be the principal vector of dengue and the only vector of urban yellow fever. It also serves as a vector of filariasis and certain of the arboviral diseases.

Aedes aegypti. Control of *A. aegypti* centers around measures that are applicable to urban communities, as this mosquito is a domesticated species. Its larvae are found in cisterns, barrels, clogged or defective roof gutters, tin cans, buckets, discarded automobile tires, stacks of scrap metal or any artificial container in which water remains for several days. Furthermore, this species may oviposit inside houses in water pitchers, slop jars, flower bowls and the like. Ornamental garden pools, unless adequately stocked with fish, are potentially dangerous. Flower vases in cemeteries are often the source of mosquitoes.

In all such instances the larvae may be controlled by the judicious application of larvicides or by the emptying and removal of small water containers. In many tropical cities it is part of the public health program (for the control of yellow fever and dengue) to maintain crews of especially trained inspectors to enter all dwellings at frequent intervals in order to detect and destroy larvae of *A. aegypti.* Eradication programs are based on treating all possible water surfaces, containers, and adjacent surfaces, especially walls, with insecticide solution, suspension or emulsion. Depending on the life of the residual action, treatments may be spaced 3 or more months apart.

Control of Other Culicines. As previously mentioned, there are other culicine species that serve as vectors of filariasis and a number of arboviral encephalitides and fevers in tropical and temperate regions of the world. (See Table 68–1, p. 703.) In addition to these, many species of *Culex* and *Aedes* are exceedingly important as human pests. Some coastal regions are virtually uninhabitable by reason of the tremendous number of salt marsh breeding forms.

Control measures against other culicines are similar to those already described for *Aedes* and *Anopheles.*

The genus *Mansonia* presents a special problem in that the larvae and pupae of these mosquitoes secure their oxygen from the subsurface stems of aquatic plants such as water lettuce *(Pistia)* and are therefore not readily affected by surface treatment. Development is slow, requiring nearly a year. In areas where both plants and mosquitoes are abundant, control may best be achieved by destruction of the plants.

FLY CONTROL

Two principles are important to keep in mind: (1) If possible, begin early in the season before the fly population abounds. (2) Concentrate primarily on sanitation to prevent larval development rather than on destruction of the adult fly.

The elimination of fly sources involves at least three separate problems.

The Disposal of Animal Manure. The following procedures are recommended:

1. Daily spreading of the manure on agricultural land. Where possible this is the best method of all, since it allows no larval development and utilizes the fertilizer at the most favorable time for benefiting the soil.

2. Storage of the manure in fly-tight boxes or pits, preferably of concrete with wooden doors above, which of course are kept closed except when material is being put into the pit. A fly trap should be placed at the top to catch the flies of the inevitable small infestation.

3. The piling of the manure in cubes or "ricks" with vertical sides. The heat of decomposition drives the maggots to the surface where they may be treated in various ways.

4. Treatment by use of chemicals:

   a. In the absence of resistance and where permitted by law, most of the chlorinated hydrocarbons serve as effective larvicides. Chlordane, BHC (lindane) and toxaphene are effective at concentrations ranging from 0.5 to 5 per cent. They should be applied at the rate of 1 or 2 gallons per 1000 square feet. Continued use of these compounds, however, is likely to result in the rapid development of resistance.

   b. Several of the organophosphorus insecticides will control housefly larvae that are resistant to chlorinated hydrocarbons. The most effective is Diazinon.

5. "Maggot trap" method of storage. A slatted platform is arranged over a concrete pit that contains a certain amount of water. Heavy wetting of the manure will drive the maggots out, whereupon they fall into the water and are drowned. Third-stage maggots, seeking a place in which to pupate, will likewise be captured. There should be frequent cleaning or flushing of the pit. This is especially necessary in malarious areas, where a neglected pit provides an ideal situation for the development of certain species of mosquitoes.

It is needless to say that stables should be constructed properly and should receive thorough daily care.

Disposal of Human Excrement. This involves:

1. The installation of a sanitary sewage disposal system (if possible).

2. The screening of all privies and latrines, with special attention to cracks, ventilation devices and other apertures likely to be overlooked.

3. Sprinkling of borax over exposed feces at least every 3 or 4 days. Use enough to make the surface appear white.

4. Covering of feces with earth, as under field conditions where straddle trenches are in use. It is well to add oil, if possible, as flies will emerge through a considerable depth of loose soil.

Disposal of Garbage. 1. For temporary storage of garbage, watertight metal cans with accurately fitting covers should be used.

2. For ultimate disposal nothing is superior to incineration.

3. Conservation uses (require special care and supervision). These fall into four general categories:

   a. Reduction in special industrial plants, with salvage of useful chemical substances. This is practical only in very large municipalities where volume warrants the capital outlay. A market for the commercial products is also necessary.

   b. Grinding of bones for fertilizer.

   c. Feeding of edible portions to swine. Hog farms are always a menace in the matter of fly production and should be located beyond flight range of the community or camp.

   d. Composting, with a view to future agricultural use. This is very desirable in certain Asiatic countries from an economic standpoint. Skillful supervision is necessary to prevent fly development.

4. Burial of all garbage is usually very satisfactory if there is thorough compaction of both the garbage and the soil covering. The latter should be not less than 1 foot in depth, preferably 2 feet.

Measures Against the Adult Flies. In spite of conscientious efforts to prevent the development of the larvae, at least a few flies will succeed in attaining maturity. Again (especially in the military service), the medical officer may find himself confronted with a problem of fly-borne disease in a region where he has had no opportunity to face the situation early in the season and, consequently, finds a large number of flies already on hand. The following procedures are of proven value:

SCREENS. In humid climates copper, bronze, alloy or plastic must be used to avoid corrosion. In a very dry climate, however, galvanized screening is usually adequate. Painting of the screens also provides protection against weathering. A mesh of 14 wires to the inch will exclude houseflies, but it is better to use at least 18-mesh because of the desirability of controlling smaller insects at the same time. Accurate fitting of both screen doors and window screens is important. Doors should open outward. Foods likely to attract flies, such as hung meats, should, of course, be screened well.

FLY TRAPS. A tremendous reduction in the fly population may be effected by the judicious placing of fly traps of suitable construction. A conical type, made of screen and baited with molasses, milk or waste fruit, works very well. The flies enter from below and, as a result of their tendency to fly upward toward the light, pass through the narrow aperture at the apex of the cone into an upper chamber from which they are unable to escape. Frequent emptying of traps is desirable. Captured living flies should be killed before removal either with hot water or by means of a spray. Fly traps function best when set in the sun and protected from the wind.

SPRAYS. The application of sprays, by either hand or power sprayers, is a useful procedure when flies are abundant. Such sprays are of two types, which may be combined, if desired.

Aerosols. "Bombs" containing pyrethrum, Freon and a synergist may be employed to produce a floating vapor, consisting of exceedingly fine particles, very useful in killing insects in a small, enclosed space. The interiors of airplanes may be treated effectively in this way.

Space or Contact Sprays. These act as contact poisons and are especially useful indoors. (See p. 785.)

Residual Sprays. In these sprays the toxic agent is applied to walls of buildings, both inside and out, to screens and in the vicinity of garbage cans, privies, manure piles and other places where flies congregate. (See p. 784.) Some of the organophosphorus compounds, particularly malathion and Diazinon, provide effective control of houseflies when applied as residual insecticides. However, the periods of protection obtained without retreatment are short, ranging from a few days to several weeks. In a few localities flies have developed resistance to these compounds.

BAITS. The most effective formulations contain fast-acting organophosphorus compounds. Malathion, Diazinon, Dipterex and others are used in dry or liquid baits. Dry baits may consist merely of granulated sugar with the insecticide, or of the insecticide and sugar applied to corn meal, sand or other granular material. Liquid baits consist of 10 per cent of molasses or syrup in water with the insecticide. These baits are scattered or sprinkled liberally on floors or other surfaces where flies congregate to feed or rest. They cause spectacularly quick reductions but must be reapplied every day while infestations persist.

Attempts to provide longer lasting bait treatments have been made by applying heavy syrup baits that dry to a varnish-like surface on sites where flies rest. Bait stations consisting of 4-inch square paddles covered with a mixture of sugar, sand, insecticide and gelatin have also been used. These do not provide such rapid reduction as the scatter baits, but when used in adequate numbers have given reasonably good control for periods of several weeks or months.

CONTROL OF OTHER ARTHROPODS

Methods for the chemical control of and treatment for parasitosis by various arthropods of medical importance are summarized in Table 72–1.[16–18] It must be remembered that priority should be given to sanitation measures to eliminate the larval habitats of the pests wherever possible.

REPELLENTS AND ACARICIDES

Individuals who must remain exposed to arthropods in infested areas can obtain complete freedom from some species and a high degree of protection from the others by using adequate amounts of the proper repellents applied in the approved manner. Some repellents have little or no odor and give protection for 2 to 8 hours when applied to the skin and for several days or weeks when applied to the clothing.

True repellents differ from insecticides in that they do not kill the insects, but discourage them from biting or landing on treated surfaces. The materials recommended for use against chiggers function as acaricides, causing rapid knockdown and death of the mites before they have a chance to bite.

Repellents are marketed commercially as liquids, pressurized sprays (aerosols), salves, sticks and powders. Liquids are usually the most economical, but pressurized sprays have the advantage of being convenient for application to both skin and clothing.

Mosquito and Biting Fly Repellents. Experiments against various species of mosquitoes and biting flies from Panama to Alaska have shown diethyltoluamide to be outstanding as an all-purpose repellent for application to the skin.[17] Chlorodiethylbenzamide is also highly effective against a wide range of species, and ethyl hexanediol, dimethyl carbate, dimethyl phthalate, and Indalone are all good general repellents that are outstanding against certain species.

Repellents suitable for application to the clothing are required by troops or others exposed to heavy mosquito infestations, since mosquitoes easily bite through untreated clothing of normal weight. The use of clothing treatments does not eliminate the need for skin applications, however. All the repellents mentioned in Table 72–1 may be used on clothing, but some of the best clothing treatments are not recommended for skin applications. The most effective repellents recommended for treatment of clothing are diethyltoluamide and butyl ethyl propanediol. The latter should not be applied directly to the skin.

APPLICATION TO CLOTHING. A simple method of applying a repellent to clothing is to shake about a dozen drops into one hand, rub the hands together, and rub lightly on the parts of the socks, shirt, or trousers that fit tightly and where bites occur. This procedure is repeated until the areas to be treated have been covered. If preferred, a light spray may be applied to the areas of clothing where the insects are biting.

Shirts, stockings, or other garments may be impregnated with a solution or emulsion of a repellent, as described for use against chiggers. Treated garments will remain effective through 2 to 3 days of ordinary wear, but not after washing or prolonged soaking in water.

USE AGAINST CHIGGERS. For protection against chiggers (red bugs), the materials should be applied to the clothing rather than to the skin. A treatment of clothing with any of the mosquito repellents will remain effective for several weeks unless the clothing is washed or soaked in water. Benzyl benzoate will also protect against chiggers and will remain effective in clothing after two launderings. Benzyl benzoate may be injurious at high dosages; the recommended dosage should not be exceeded, and it should not be used on the skin.

The simplest way to treat clothing is to apply a spray. However, if a bottled repellent is used, liberal applications are made by hand along all openings of the clothing, such as inside the neck band, the fly and cuffs of trousers and the tops of socks. Benzyl benzoate should not be applied by this method.

IMPREGNATION METHOD. The best method of obtaining complete protection under all conditions of exposure is to impregnate all the outer clothing that will be worn in the field with a solution or emulsion of the repellent. About 1/15 ounce is used

(*Text continued on p. 801*)

Table 72–1. THE CHEMICAL CONTROL OF ARTHROPODS OF MEDICAL IMPORTANCE

Arthropod	*Place of Treatment*	*Chemical and Type of Formulation*	*Application Instructions*	*Precautions*
Scorpions	Rooms	Residual sprays applied as emulsion concentrates, solutions, wettable powders or powders in inert dusts: a. Malathion 5% in spray b. Lindane 0.5% in spray, 1% in dust c. Dieldrin 0.5% in spray, 1% in dust	If infestations are heavy, treat indoor hiding places at 200 mg of malathion, 20 mg of lindane, 20 mg of dieldrin/sq ft. Around homes, treat baseboard, moldings, underneath sinks, cracks and corners, interior surfaces of roofs made from palm fronds or straw, foundations, joists as well as the ground and rough outbuildings.	Avoid scorpions that fall from high places, as they may sting the person applying the insecticides.
Black widow spiders	Houses and outbuildings	Residual sprays as emulsion concentrates, solutions or wettable powders: a. Chlordane 2–3% b. Lindane 0.2–0.5% c. Dieldrin 0.5% d. Malathion 2%	Same as for scorpions.	Care should be taken to avoid falling spiders irritated by the spray, for they sometimes bite.
Ticks (most species)	1. Animals	1. Washes, sprays or dips as emulsions: a. DDT 1% b. Malathion 0.5% c. Lindane 0.05% d. Rotenone 0.05%	Use indicated concentrations for washes or sprays, but reduce the concentration to half for dips. Washes usually produce better control than sprays because of better penetration through the hair.	In dipping animals do not submerge the head. Do not exceed the concentrations recommended or young animals may be injured. DDT should not be used on cows, as it may appear in the milk.
		2. Powders in inert dusts: a. DDT 5–10% b. Malathion 4–5% c. Lindane 1% d. Rotenone 3–5% e. Carbaryl 5%	Dust infested parts of animal thoroughly and stroke against the hairs with the hand to get maximum penetration	It is usually necessary to treat the house or premises as well as the animals to get control. Do not treat kittens with carbaryl.
	2. Buildings	Residual sprays in oil solutions or emulsion concentrates: a. Propoxur 1% b. Chlordane 2% c. Malathion 2% d. Lindane 0.5% e. Chlorpyrifos 0.5% f. Diazinon 0.5% g. Carbaryl 2%	Treat woodwork, floor and wall cracks, behind pictures and draperies in the house with a coarse spray. In the kennel, spray should be applied until it starts to run off. Particular attention should be paid to cracks and crevices.	Do not allow children or pets in treated areas until surfaces are dry. If one application does not give sufficient control, apply another in 3 weeks. These treatments are too strong for use on animals.
	3. Outdoors on ground and vegetation	Residual sprays in emulsion concentrates, wettable powders, or powders in inert dusts: a. Chlordane 1% in spray, 5–10% in dust b. Dieldrin 1% in spray, 5–10% in dust c. Carbaryl 5% d. Lindane 0.1% in spray	Thoroughly spray or dust infested areas at the rate of 1–3 lbs of chlordane or dieldrin/acre once or twice a year as needed.	Large area treatments could prove hazardous to wildlife so treat only when necessary to protect people and animals from ticks and the diseases they carry. Do not apply insecticides to crop or grazing areas.
Mites (chiggers, red bugs, harvest mites) (*Eutrombicula, Leptotrombidium* spp.	1. Clothing	Mosquito repellents that are toxic to mites: a. Benzyl benzoate b. Diethyltoluamide (OFF, DEET) c. Dimethyl phthalate	These materials can be used on clothing as barrier treatments by applying a thin layer ½ in wide along all openings of the clothing and the socks. They are rapid acting and good until clothing is washed. They can also be used to impregnate outer clothing by dipping or spraying the items in a diluted emulsion or solution. Apply approximately 1/15 oz of repellent/sq ft. The simplest method of applying clothing treatments is to pour a small amount of undiluted repellent in the hands, rub the hands together, then make liberal applications to the clothing or socks by rubbing them with the hands.	

Table 72–1. THE CHEMICAL CONTROL OF ARTHROPODS OF MEDICAL IMPORTANCE *(Continued)*

Arthropod	*Place of Treatment*	*Chemical and Type of Formulation*	*Application Instructions*	*Precautions*
Mites (cont.)	2. Outdoors by spraying vegetation	Residual sprays prepared as wettable powders or powders in inert dusts: a. Chlordane 1% spray, 5% dust b. Toxaphene 1% spray, 5% dust c. Lindane 0.1% spray, 1% dust	Spray or dust area with sufficient material to obtain a deposit of 2 lb of chlordane or toxaphene or 0.25–1 lb of lindane/acre. Treat ground and low vegetation in area being protected.	Do not apply in areas where grazing animals are pastured.
Scabies *Sarcoptes scabiei hominis*[18]	Body	1. 1% gamma benzene hexachloride (lindane; Kwell cream, lotion and shampoo)	Warm soap and water bath at night. (Use soft brush.) Apply lotion or cream from neck downward, esp. to hairy areas, groin and perineal region; allow to dry. Reapply lotion or cream on following morning. Second bath in evening. Change underclothing, bedclothing and linens, sterilizing them by boiling or laundering. No therapy for 24 hrs. Then repeat 24-hr treatment identical to first. Kwell shampoo may be used if scalp is involved.	Keep liquid away from eyes and mucous membranes. Avoid overtreatment.
		2. Crotamiton (Eurax cream and lotion)	Massage gently; reapply 24 hrs later; cleansing bath 48 hrs after second application.	Do not use on severely inflamed areas or on head.
		3. Benzyl benzoate (25%)	Apply by spray or hand over body.	Do not apply to head. Avoid overtreatment.
Cockroaches *Periplaneta, Blattella* and *Supella* spp.	Enclosed spaces, as kitchens, pantries or store rooms	1. Residual sprays in oil solutions or emulsion concentrates: a. Propoxur 1% b. Diazinon 0.5% c. Dichlorvos 0.5% d. Chlorpyrifos 0.5% e. Malathion 5% f. Ronnel 2% g. Trichlorfon 1–2%	These liquids can be applied with a sprayer or brush to the hiding places and runways of cockroaches. A coarse spray rather than a mist should be used to wet the surface thoroughly. Pay particular attention to warm humid places, as around steam tables, heating pipes, cracks and crevices, as they are favored hiding places for cockroaches. Use in limited areas only. Instead of spraying entire walls or floors, treat only places used by cockroaches.	Avoid contamination of food, water and food-handling equipment. Cover treated tables or shelves with paper before using them again. Sprays should be applied with caution around open flames or electrically operated machinery, as the solvents used in preparing them frequently are flammable.
		2. Powders in inert dusts: a. Malathion 4–5% b. Diazinon 2–5% c. Silica Gel 100%	Dust behind baseboards, under cabinets and furniture, cracks and crevices, other out-of-sight areas, or in the vicinity of open flames or electrically operated machinery. These powders can be applied to such areas much easier than sprays with puff dusters of the bulb, plunger or bellows type.	Dusts are unsightly in well kept homes so are recommended only for out-of-sight locations and in areas where there is danger of sprays causing a fire.
		3. Baits: a. Kepone 0.125% b. Propoxur 2%	Chemical mixed with food product is placed in small containers and set in locations where it can be found easily by cockroaches, or scattered in places protected from human contact.	Kepone bait is a stomach poison and acts very slowly. A week or more may pass before control is apparent.
Lice (cootie, grey-back) *Pediculus humanus humanus* and *Pediculus humanus capitis;* pubic louse (crab) *Phthirus pubis*[18]	1. Head	1% gamma benzene hexachloride (lindane, Kwell shampoo)	Clean scalp with ordinary shampoo. Apply Kwell shampoo for at least 4 min; rinse well and dry. Use fine-toothed comb to remove remaining nits. Repeat process in 7 days. Treat combs and brushes with Kwell shampoo.	Keep medication from eyes and mucous membranes. Avoid overtreatment.

Table continued on the following page

Table 72–1. The Chemical Control of Arthropods of Medical Importance *(Continued)*

Arthropod	*Place of Treatment*	*Chemical and Type of Formulation*	*Application Instructions*	*Precautions*
Lice (cont.)	2. Body	1% gamma benzene hexachloride (lindane, Kwell shampoo)	Sterilize personal clothing and bedclothes by laundering, dry cleaning and ironing. Lather trunk and extremities with Kwell shampoo (4 min); rinse thoroughly. Repeat therapy in 7 days.	Avoid overtreatment.
	3. Pubic and other areas	1. 1% gamma benzene hexachloride (lindane, Kwell lotion or cream)	After bathing, apply Kwell cream or lotion liberally to all areas of suspected infestation. (Do not apply to eyelashes.) Leave medication on 24 hrs; repeat in 4 to 7 days in hairy infestations.	Pediculosis of eyelashes may be treated with 0.25% physostigmine ophthalmic ointment twice daily for 10 days; after application lice and/or nits may be removed carefully with a toothpick or cotton-tipped applicator. (Rule out narrow angle glaucoma before use of anticholinesterase agents.)
		2. Crotamiton (Eurax) cream or lotion	See scabies (above)	Avoid overtreatment.
		3. Benzyl benzoate emulsion, 25%	See scabies (above)	Avoid overtreatment.
	4. On body and clothing	Powders of pyrophyllite or other inert dust: a. DDT 10% b. Malathion 1% c. MYL (0.2% pyrethrins, 2% sulfoxide, 2% 2,4-dinitroanisole, 0.1% phenol S [an antioxidant]) d. Allethrin (0.3% allethrins, 3% sulfoxide) e. Abate 2%	Thoroughly dust between inside garment and the skin itself by inserting duster in all openings of clothing. Use 1 to 1.5 oz per individual. If only 1 or 2 persons are being treated, applications can be made with a sifter top can. Body lice are most frequently found in seams of clothing and particular attention should be paid to these areas inside of shirts and trousers. One application of DDT or malathion is usually sufficient unless frequent re-exposure occurs. Abate is effective against DDT- and malathion-resistant lice. The MYL and allethrin powders act rapidly but have short residual action so should be applied three times.	Avoid excessive inhalation and contamination of food during application.
	5. Clothing impregnation	DDT-water emulsion concentrate	Dilute to 2% DDT. Use ordinary laundry facilities to apply 1 pt/suit of underwear.	Rinse laundry facilities with clean water after treatment has been completed.
Bedbugs (Chinches) *Cimex* spp.	Enclosed spaces, as barracks or rooms	Residual sprays in oil solutions or emulsion concentrates: a. DDT 5% b. Lindane 0.1–0.5% c. Malathion 1% d. Ronnel 1% e. Dichlorvos 0.5% f. Diazinon 0.5%	If the infestation is a light one, spray only the bed. Wet the slats, springs and frame and lightly spray the entire mattress, paying particular attention to the seams, tufts and folds. When the infestation is heavy also treat upholstered furniture, the floors and the walls to a height of several feet. Thoroughly wet the walls and floor.	Allow the bed to dry thoroughly before using, at least 2 hrs drying time for all insecticides and 4 hrs for dichlorvos. The mattress should never be soaked with the spray. Do not treat bedding to be used by an infant. Use only 0.1% lindane on mattress or bedding.
Assassin bugs, cone nose bugs, china bedbugs, or kissing bugs. *Triatoma, Rhodnius, Panstrongylus,* and *Eratyrus* spp.	Houses	Residual sprays as emulsion concentrates, solutions or wettable powders: a. Dieldrin 2% b. Lindane 1%	Treat walls and ceilings of houses with 125 mg of dieldrin or 50 mg of lindane/sq ft.	Wettable powders are generally employed where the presence of visible residues is not objectionable. In expensive homes emulsions or solutions are preferable, as they leave no unsightly deposits.

Table 72–1. THE CHEMICAL CONTROL OF ARTHROPODS OF MEDICAL IMPORTANCE *(Continued)*

Arthropod	*Place of Treatment*	*Chemical and Type of Formulation*	*Application Instructions*	*Precautions*
Fleas (*Xenopsylla* spp., *Nosopsyllus* spp., *Pulex irritans, Ctenocephalides* spp., others)	1. Rooms	1. Solutions in kerosene, fuel oil or in emulsion concentrates: a. DDT 5% b. Chlordane 2% c. Malathion 0.5–3% d. Diazinon 1% e. Methoxychlor 5% f. Lindane 1% g. Trichlorfon 1% h. Ronnel 1%	Apply spray to floor and baseboards and to walls to a height of 1 foot using 1 gal of solution/1000 sq ft of surface. Apply a light spray to furniture, rugs and other fabrics.	Do not apply in excessive amounts to furnishings, as it may stain fabrics or rugs.
		2. Powders in inert dusts: a. DDT 10% b. Malathion 4–5% c. Dieldrin 1.5% d. Diazinon 2% e. Lindane 1%	Apply dusts in small quantities under grain bins, along runs or other places rats use. Also dust lightly over floor and furniture with hand or rotary type duster.	Avoid inhalation and contamination of foods.
	2. Animals	Powders in inert dusts: a. Malathion 4% b. Rotenone 1% c. Pyrethrins 0.2% + 2% synergist d. Lindane 1% e. Methoxychlor 10% f. DDT 5% g. Coumaphos 0.5% h. Carbaryl 2%	Apply the dust to domestic animals with any small duster, using 1 to 5 tablespoons of powder. The amount applied should vary with the size of the animal. Pay particular attention to back, neck, and top of head and rub powder thoroughly into hair.	Do not apply DDT, chlordane or lindane to cats or puppies. Avoid getting the insecticide into the eyes, nose, mouth of all animals and keep the animals from licking themselves.
Fire ants	Infested yards	1. Granules containing 2.5%, 5%, or 10% heptachlor	Broadcast granules evenly over infested area. Apply 2 treatments at 3-month intervals using 1/4 lb of insecticide/acre each time.	Avoid contamination of animal food, including fodder.
		2. Baits containing insecticide, oil and diluent: a. Mirex 0.075% in soy bean oil and corn cob grits	The bait should be scattered over the infested area at the rate of 1.7 to 6.8 gm of insecticide, 5 to 20 lbs of bait/acre. It can be scattered by hand or with the assistance of conventional seeding or dusting equipment. A colony may be killed within 1 week, or more than 16 weeks may be needed to eliminate it.	Avoid contamination of the bait with other insecticides, for quantities as low as 0.01 to 0.001% can make baits unattractive or kill the ants before the bait has been distributed throughout the colony.
Mosquito adults	1. Enclosed spaces, as barracks, rooms, barns, airplanes and the like	1. Aerosols: Pyrethrins 0.25% + piperonyl butoxide or sulfoxide 2%	Spray into air from aerosol bomb for 4 sec/1000 cu ft. Spray two or three times this amount for aircraft disinsectization.	None
		2. Space sprays in oil solutions or emulsion concentrates: a. Methoxychlor 3% b. Naled 1% c. DDT 3–5% d. Dichlorvos 0.5% e. Malathion 2–5% f. Resmethrin 1–2%	Spray into air from dispenser that gives fine atomization, making sure that all portions of the room are treated. Best results are obtained if doors and windows are kept closed during spraying and for 5–10 min afterwards.	Avoid contamination of food, drinking water or household utensils. These items should be removed or kept covered. Naled can irritate the eyes, so direct contact with spray should be avoided.
		3. Residual sprays in oil solutions, emulsion concentrates or wettable powders: a. DDT 5% b. Methoxychlor 5% c. Dichlorvos 0.5% d. Dieldrin 0.5% e. Lindane 0.5% f. Malathion 3–5% g. Propoxur 0.5–1%	Spray on interior walls and ceiling of buildings (1 qt/250 sq ft). Used primarily against house-infesting *Anopheles* and *Aedes* that are involved in disease control campaigns. Pay particular attention to dark corners and under or behind furniture, for mosquitoes prefer resting in such places.	Wettable powders are generally employed where the presence of visible residues is not objectionable.

Table continued on the following page

Table 72–1. The Chemical Control of Arthropods of Medical Importance *(Continued)*

Arthropod	*Place of Treatment*	*Chemical and Type of Formulation*	*Application Instructions*	*Precautions*
Mosquito adults (cont.)	2. Outdoors by spraying vegetation or other resting places	Residual sprays applied as wettable powders: a. DDT 5% b. Dieldrin 1–5% c. Lindane 1–5% d. Fenthion 1–5% e. Malathion 3–5% f. Propoxur 0.5–1%	DDT and fenthion should be applied at dosages of approximately 1–3 lbs/acre, but dieldrin and lindane can be used at 0.5–2 lbs/acre. Spray all low vegetation as well as under buildings, employing a power sprayer to treat large areas and garden or hand sprayers for small areas.	Do not use oil or emulsion sprays on vegetation, as they may be phytotoxic. Use with care where fish and wildlife may be endangered and do not apply to food or feed crops.
	3. Outdoors with space spray or fog	Applications from airplanes, mist blowers or thermal aerosol machines as oil solutions or emulsion concentrates: a. Methoxychlor 0.2 lb/acre b. Naled 0.02–0.1 lb/acre c. Carbaryl 0.2–1 lb/acre d. DDT 0.2 lb/acre e. Dichlorvos 0.05–0.1 lb/acre f. Pyrethrins 0.002–0.0025 lb/acre g. Lindane 0.1–0.2 lb/acre h. Fenthion 0.1 lb/acre i. Malathion 0.075–0.2 lb/acre	Insecticides are usually applied from airplanes on a lb/acre basis and dispensed at the rate of 2–4 qts of diluted spray/acre. When the applications are made with ground equipment, the spray and fog formulations are usually prepared at designated concentrations of the insecticide and dispersed from equipment mounted on a vehicle moving at specified speeds. The principal insecticides and the concentrations employed per gal for space spray and fog applications dispersed from vehicles moving at 5 mi/hr are malathion 6–8 oz, naled 2 oz and fenthion 2 oz. These sprays usually furnish only temporary relief. Treatments should be applied as close to dawn or dusk as possible, as inversion conditions are best at that time of day.	Fogs and mists dispersed with ground equipment give satisfactory control when the weather is favorable but are not highly effective in strong winds, on still days or during the warmest part of the day. Airplane sprays are effective in light breezes and on still days, but may never reach the infested areas if strong winds are blowing or the weather is so hot that thermal air currents are rising.
Mosquito larvae	Streams, lakes, swamps, pools, ruts and water-containing receptacles around houses	Application from airplanes or ground equipment as emulsions, wettable powders, solutions or granules: a. DDT 0.05–0.4 lb/acre b. Methoxychlor 0.05–0.2 lb/acre c. Abate 0.05–0.1 lb/acre d. Chlorpyrifos 0.0125–0.05 lb/acre e. Lindane 0.1–0.15 lb/acre f. Fenthion 0.05–0.1 lb/acre g. Malathion 0.5 lb/acre h. Parathion 0.063–0.1 lb/acre i. Paris green 0.75 lb/acre	Larvicides are usually applied on a lb/acre basis and the concentration used varies with the type of dispenser. Where heavy vegetation cover is present, granules give the best penetration, but the other types of formulations are satisfactory for open terrain. Oil solutions are preferable in open terrain for species that are top feeders unless tender plants are present, while emulsions, wettable powders, and granules work better against species that are bottom feeders. *Mansonia* spp. can best be controlled by applying a herbicide such as the sodium salt of methyl chlorophenoxyacetic acid to their host plants.	Do not use insecticide on water intended for drinking by humans or animals. Parathion is extremely toxic and must be handled with care, but can be employed safely by experienced operators. Use all materials with care to avoid hazards to fish and wildlife.
Housefly adults	Enclosed spaces, as houses, barns, airplanes and the like	1. Space sprays or aerosols in oil solutions or emulsion concentrates: a. Ronnel 0.4% b. Naled 1% c. Dichlorvos 0.5% d. Malathion 2–4%	These insecticides should be released as a mist from a hand or power sprayer or an aerosol bomb after which the room should be closed for an hour. Spray into air for 4 sec/100 cu ft when using aerosol bombs. Thoroughly spray all parts of room with the hand or power sprayer. If a fast knockdown is desired, 0.1–0.25% pyrethrins + 1.2% of piperonyl butoxide or sulfoxide are often added.	Space sprays have no long-lasting effects and must be applied frequently. In using these insecticides, avoid contamination of animal food, water, milk or food-processing equipment.
		2. Residual sprays in oil solutions, emulsion concentrates or wettable powders: a. Diazinon 1% b. Naled 1% c. Methoxychlor 2.5–5% d. Fenthion 0.75–1.5% e. Ronnel 0.5–1% f. Ciodrin 1% g. Malathion 2.5%	Apply sprays to the interior and exterior of animal barns, dairy barns, hog houses, poultry houses and the like, as well as the screens, porches, doors and garbage cans around houses. Treat only those areas frequented by flies. Apply at 1–2 gal of spray/1000 sq ft.	Exclude animals while spraying barns. Some countries have placed restrictions on the use of insecticides around food-processing plants.

Table 72-1. THE CHEMICAL CONTROL OF ARTHROPODS OF MEDICAL IMPORTANCE *(Continued)*

Arthropod	*Place of Treatment*	*Chemical and Type of Formulation*	*Application Instructions*	*Precautions*
Housefly adults (cont.)		3. Baits containing insecticides and sweetening agents as sugar, malt or molasses: a. Trichlorfon 1–2% dry, 0.1% liquid b. Dichlorvos 1% dry, 0.1% liquid c. Diazinon 1–2% dry, 0.1% liquid d. Ronnel 1% dry, 2% liquid e. Naled 0.5% dry, 1.25% liquid f. Malathion 2% dry, 1.25% liquid	Baits are frequently used dry by coating granulated sugar or a mixture of 10% sugar and 90% corn meal with the insecticide. Liquid baits contain 10% sweetening agent and an insecticide in water. Apply 2–4 oz of dry bait/1000 sq ft or sprinkle the liquid bait lightly where the flies are feeding.	Baits do not have long residual action and must be applied frequently to maintain good control. Daily applications are needed until sufficient adults have been killed to reduce greatly the breeding potential. After several weeks the interval between treatments can be increased to once or twice each week.
Housefly larvae	Outdoors by spraying vegetation, manure and refuse	Sprays applied as emulsion concentrates or wettable powders: a. Dimethoate 1.25% b. Malathion 1–2% c. Dichlorvos 0.2% d. Ronnel 1% e. Diazinon 1%	Thoroughly cover decaying vegetation, manure and refuse using 10 gal/1000 sq ft. Pay particular attention to animal manure, privies and garbage.	Applications must be made once or twice each week to maintain good control.
Salt marsh sandflies, punkies, no-see-ums, biting midges (Family—CERATOPOGONIDAE [=HELEIDAE]) *Culicoides, Leptoconops* and *Styloconops* ssp.	1. Outdoors with space spray or fog for adults	Applications from airplanes, mist blowers or thermal aerosol machines as oil solutions, emulsion concentrates: a. Lindane 0.1–0.2 lb/acre b. Malathion 0.1–1.5 lb/acre c. DDT 0.2 lb/acre	Apply as directed for adult mosquitoes.	
	2. Salt marshes for larvae	Larvicides applied from airplanes as granules: a. Dieldrin 1 lb/acre	The treatments may be applied to the moist soil on salt marshes that are the principal source of larval breeding. One treatment may give control for as long as 1 year.	*Culicoides* may become resistant to these treatments very rapidly. Treatments must be used cautiously around water, as these heavy deposits of insecticide are very toxic to fish and fiddler crabs.
Eye gnats (Family CHLOROPIDAE)	Infested areas	DDT, lindane or malathion sprays	Temporary control of adults may be obtained by using DDT, lindane or malathion as sprays, mists or fogs as recommended for the control of adult mosquitoes.	Same as for mosquitoes.
Tsetse flies *Glossina* spp.	Outdoors by spraying vegetation or other resting places	1. Residual sprays applied as emulsion concentrates or wettable powders: a. DDT 5% b. Dieldrin 5%	Apply insecticides along river banks and to infested vegetation at rate of 18 gal of spray/mi with knapsack, compression or power sprayers. Make DDT applications at intervals of 2 wks until control is obtained. Dieldrin appears to be the better insecticide of the two, as one application usually produces control.	Same as for mosquitoes.

Table continued on the following page

Table 72–1. THE CHEMICAL CONTROL OF ARTHROPODS OF MEDICAL IMPORTANCE *(Continued)*

Arthropod	*Place of Treatment*	*Chemical and Type of Formulation*	*Application Instructions*	*Precautions*
Tsetse flies (cont.)		2. Aerosol or mist sprays applied as oil solutions or fogs from airplanes: a. DDT 0.2–0.4 lb/acre b. Lindane 0.03–0.1 lb/acre	Savannah woodlands can be treated successfully, even if they contain thickets, but it is preferable to do the spraying during leafless period of year. Droplets in 5 μm and 50 μm range needed, as large droplets impinge on trees and smaller droplets do not settle on insects.	Treatment is expensive and effective only for a limited period just after dawn and for a shorter period before dusk.
		3. Lindane aerosols applied from thermal aerosol generators	Apply to infested area as fog containing 1.5% of lindane.	These treatments should not be applied during the hottest part of the day while thermal currents are rising or in strong winds. They are much more effective between sunset and sunrise, when inversion conditions usually occur, and in light breezes.
Buffalo gnats, blackflies, (Family SIMULIIDAE)	Infested streams or rivers for larvae	1. Emulsifiable concentrates of DDT applied from a drip can	Treatments should be applied to moving water at 0.1 to 0.5 ppm of DDT for 30 min. Applications are made from a constant-flow injector at weekly or biweekly intervals. These treatments have given complete or almost complete control up to 160 mi downstream.	Excessive amounts of insecticide in the water may kill fish, so dosage recommendations should be followed closely.
		2. Emulsifiable concentrates, suspensions or oil solutions of DDT from airplanes	Treatments should be applied to moving streams at 0.1–0.2 lb of DDT/acre for a swath width of 100 ft, or at 0.13 ppm for 36 min.	
	Outdoor areas infested with adults	Oil solutions of DDT applied from airplanes or ground equipment	Fuel oil solutions containing 5–10% DDT can be applied to heavily infested areas at 0.4 lb/acre.	
Sandflies *(Phlebotomus* and *Lutzomyia* spp.)	Houses and outdoor harborages	DDT residual sprays	Apply DDT solution, emulsion or wettable powder spray to interior of houses and outdoor resting places such as stone walls at 100–300 mg of DDT/sq ft.	Make certain that residual deposits extend down to the floor, for some species sit on the lower parts of the wall.
Horseflies deerflies greenheads, breezeflies and mango flies (Family TABANIDAE)	Infested areas	1. DDT sprays 2. Lindane 0.5 lb/acre 3. Dieldrin 0.3 lb/acre 4. Malathion 6 oz/acre (ULV)	In limited areas some control of adult tabanids has been obtained with DDT applied as recommended for control of adult mosquitoes and lindane. Dieldrin has a larvicidal effect when applied to breeding areas.	
		INSECT REPELLENTS		
Repellents for flies, mosquitoes, gnats, mites, blackflies, sandflies, fleas, and ticks	Exposed surfaces of body and clothes	1. Diethyltoluamide (OFF, DEET)	1. Application on skin. Shake ½ teaspoonful into palm of hand, rub hands together and then apply in thin layer to face, neck, ears, hands and wrists. Do not get into eyes and mouth. 2. On clothes, spray or apply by hands. Effective for a number of days. Best all-around repellent.	Nontoxic. Very irritating to the eyes.
		2. Dimethyl phthalate.	Particularly effective against *Anopheles* and larval mites (chiggers). Use same as (1) above.	Same as above.
		3. Indalone	Same as (1) above. Best use against biting flies.	Same as above.
		4. 2-ethyl hexanediol-1, 3 (repellent 612)	Same as (1) above. Particularly effective against *Aedes*.	Same as above.

per square foot of cloth, or a total of 2½ ounces (5 tablespoonfuls) to a jacket (or shirt), trousers and socks of medium size. The underwear should not be treated. Benzyl benzoate is preferable for this purpose, as it is more resistant to leaching by water.

In the solution method, the repellent is dissolved in enough dry-cleaning fluid or other volatile solvent to wet the garment thoroughly without leaving any excess. About 3 pints are required for an outfit of heavy cotton cloth. After all parts of the garment have been saturated with the solution, the cleaning fluid is allowed to evaporate.

An emulsion can be made by mixing 2½ ounces (5 tablespoonfuls) of the repellent with 3 pints of water and ¼ ounce (1½ teaspoonfuls) of an emulsifier or 1 ounce (2 tablespoonfuls) of soap. All parts of the garments should be saturated with the emulsion, wrung lightly and dried thoroughly before wearing.

BARRIER METHOD. Considerable protection will be obtained by treating only the openings of the clothes—inside the neck band, fly and cuffs of shirts; inside the waist band, fly and cuffs of trousers; on the socks, both above the shoes and inside the shoe below the tongue. The material is applied by daubing, spraying or drawing the mouth of the bottle along the cloth to make a band ½ inch wide. Women's clothing may be protected in the same general way.

Flea Repellents. Diethyltoluamide is a superior flea repellent, particularly when used to impregnate socks and outer garments in the manner described for use against chiggers. Clothing impregnated with diethyltoluamide repels fleas for more than a week. Good temporary protection can be obtained by smearing or spraying the repellent on the socks and legs of trousers. Undecylenic (undecenoic) acid, *N*-propylacetanilide and benzyl benzoate are also good flea repellents; treatment with them remains effective through several days of ordinary wear.

Tick Repellents. None of the repellents mentioned above will provide complete protection against ticks, but several will afford a high degree of protection against one of the most annoying species, the lone star tick *(Amblyomma americanum)*. The socks and all the outer clothing should be treated by spraying or by the impregnation method described for use against chiggers. Repellents, in order of preference, are diethyltoluamide, Indalone, dimethyl carbate, dimethyl phthalate and benzyl benzoate. Treated clothing remains effective against ticks through several days of ordinary wear but begins to lose effectiveness after washing.

Precautions. The repellents discussed here have been found safe for use as recommended. Most are toxic if taken internally. Some people may be allergic to them and will show a rash or other minor skin reaction. Any repellent may cause smarting when applied to mucous membranes. Repellents should be kept out of the eyes, and therefore should not be applied too liberally on the forehead. Some repellents feel oily on the skin. Diethyltoluamide is the most acceptable cosmetically, and a 50 per cent solution in ethyl alcohol is preferred by many for this reason.

All the repellents mentioned here affect paints, varnishes and some plastics to varying degrees. They will damage a few types of synthetic cloth (for example, acetate rayon but not nylon), fingernail polish, and articles that are painted, varnished or made of certain plastics. Ethyl hexanediol has the least injurious effect, and diethyltoluamide is less injurious than the other materials.

REFERENCES

1. Anonymous. 1973. The use of viruses for the control of insect pests and disease vectors. Report of a Joint F.A.O./W.H.O. Meeting on Insect Viruses. Technical Report Series No. 531. World Health Organization, Geneva. 48 pp.
2. Smith, R. F. 1973. Considerations on the safety of certain biological agents for arthropod control. Bull. W.H.O. *48*:685–698.
3. Knipling, E. F. 1960. The eradication of the screwworm fly. Sci. Am. *203*:54–61.
4. Anonymous. 1973. Safe use of pesticides. 20th Report of the W.H.O. Expert Committee on Insecticides. Technical Report Series No. 513. World Health Organization, Geneva. 54 pp.
5. Billings, S. C. (ed.) 1974. Pesticide Handbook—Entoma. 25th ed. Entomological Society of America. College Park, Maryland. 312 pp.
6. Anonymous. 1973. Specifications for Pesticides Used

in Public Health. 4th ed. World Health Organization, Geneva. 333 pp.

7. Schaefer, C. M., and Wilder, W. H. 1972. Insect development inhibitors: a practical evaluation as mosquito control agents. J. Econ. Entomol. *65*:1066–1071.
8. Brown, A. W. A., and Pal, R. 1971. Insecticide Resistance in Arthropods. 2nd ed. Monograph Series No. 38. World Health Organization, Geneva. 491 pp.
9. Mallis, A. 1960. Handbook of Pest Control. 3rd ed. McNair-Dorland Co., New York. 1132 pp.
10. Anonymous. 1973. Communicable Disease Center report on public health pesticides. Pest Control *41*:17–50.
11. Anonymous. 1972. Vector control in international health. World Health Organization, Geneva. 144 pp.
12. Anonymous. 1971. Application and dispersal of pesticides. 18th Report of the W.H.O. Expert Committee on Insecticides. Technical Report Series No. 465. World Health Organization, Geneva. 66 pp.
13. James, M. T., and Harwood, R. F. 1969. Herm's Medical Entomology. 6th ed. MacMillan Co., New York. 484 pp.
14. Russell, P. F., Bradley, G. W., Hess, A. D., Mulrennan, J. A., and Stage, H. H. 1948. The Use of Aircraft in the Control of Mosquitoes. Am. Mosq. Cont. Assoc. Bul. No. 1. 46 pp.
15. Knipling, E. F. 1952. Ground Equipment and Insecticides for Mosquito Control. Am. Mosq. Cont. Assoc. Bul. No. 2. 116 pp.
16. Metcalf, C. L., and Flint, W. P. 1962. Destructive and Useful Insects. 4th ed. Revised by R. L. Metcalf. McGraw-Hill Book Co., Inc., New York. 1087 pp.
17. Smith, C. N., Gilbert, I. H., and Gouck, H. K. 1960. Use of Insect Repellents. 2nd ed. Agric. Res. Serv. U.S. Department of Agriculture, Circ. ARS–33–26. 7 pp.
18. Conn, H. F. (ed.). 1974. Current Therapy. W. B. Saunders Co., Philadelphia. 914 pp.

SECTION XII
Some Laboratory Diagnostic Methods

REVISED BY STANLEY H. ABADIE

CHAPTER 73
Methods and Procedures

I. General Procedures

INTRODUCTION

This section gives concise instructions for performing some of the laboratory tests used in the diagnosis of some important diseases. Examples have been chosen for their excellence in producing the desired results; some have been selected for their applicability to small laboratories with limited equipment. In fact, many of the tests may be performed in the field. For the details of elaborate laboratory procedures the reader is referred to standard texts on the subject.

1. PRESERVING AND PACKING PATHOLOGIC TISSUES FOR SHIPMENT

Formalin Fixation. Blocks of tissue of about 0.5 cm or less in thickness are dropped into 25 to 50 times their volume of 10 per cent formalin solution in distilled water (formaldehyde 37 per cent by weight is 100 per cent formalin). Fix for 1 or 2 days and transfer to 5 per cent formalin.

Zenker Fixation. Zenker's is one of the best fixatives for pathologic tissues.

Fixing Solutions

Solution A

Potassium dichromate	25 gm
Mercuric chloride	50 gm
Sodium sulfate (sometimes omitted)	10 gm
Distilled water	1000 ml

Solution B

Glacial acetic acid

Before use mix by volume—

Solution A	95 parts
Solution B	5 parts

This mixture deteriorates upon standing.

Procedure. Blocks of tissue of 0.5 cm thickness are left in fixative for 24 hours, then washed in running water for 24 hours. If piped water is not available the tissues may be washed in a brook in cheesecloth sacks; or, beakers containing tissues may be decanted frequently and refilled with water. After being washed, tissues are transferred to 50 per cent alcohol for 3 hours, then to 70 per cent for preservation and shipment. A pencilled note inside container should accompany tissue, indicating its nature and fixing agent and that it is preserved in 70 per cent alcohol but has not been treated with iodized alcohol.

Shipping. Fixed tissue blocks are wrapped in cheesecloth and either packed in cotton saturated with the preservative (usually 70 per cent ethyl alcohol) or placed directly in jars of the preservative that are completely filled with fluid and carefully stoppered.

2. PRESERVING AND PACKING PROTOZOA, HELMINTHS AND HELMINTH EGGS FROM FECES

Protozoan Cysts and Worm Eggs in Feces. Dilute feces with equal volume of warm (60°C, 140°F) 10 per cent formalin. It is important that the fecal material and formalin be well mixed. Caution should be taken not to boil the formalin. Allow to stand a few hours, decant and replace with 5 per cent formalin. Bottle, pack, and ship. Formalinized protozoan cysts stain well with iodine. Cysts of some protozoa and eggs remain well preserved for at least a year. Frequently cysts of *E. histolytica* and *I. butschlii* do not preserve satisfactorily.

Feces also may be preserved in PVA fixative and shipped (p. 825).

Fecal Smears. Coverglasses with fecal smears fixed in Schaudinn's fluid (p. 824) are packed for shipping in 70 per cent alcohol between lens paper in widemouth bottles completely filled with the alcohol. Include data giving source of material, method of fixation and whether it has been treated with iodine.

Smears may also be preserved in PVA fixative.

Helminths. Dead helminths of all types obtained at autopsy or roundworms from stools need only be washed in lukewarm physiologic salt solution and dropped into hot (80 °C, 176° F) 5 per cent formalin for preservation.

Live worms such as large tapeworms or ascarids may be allowed to die in cold water before fixation in hot 5 per cent formalin. If allowed to stand too long after death, degenerative changes (such as blistering or fraying of cuticle) will occur. Tapeworms may also be washed in physiologic salt solution, wrapped around a spool or a glass plate while still alive, and immersed in 3 per cent formalin. Small live nematodes and flukes will frequently become extremely distorted if dropped directly into fixatives; a preliminary fatiguing process consisting of prolonged shaking of the worms in physiologic salt solution is sometimes necessary. When relaxed they are dropped into 70 or 80 per cent alcohol made up with 3 to 5 per cent glycerin and heated to 60° C (140° F). The label should indicate the nature of the fixative so that the recipient of the shipment can mount the worms in glycerin merely by slow evaporation of the alcohol.

Pack for shipment as indicated for pathologic tissues. (See p. 805.)

3. PRESERVING AND PACKING ARTHROPODS FOR SHIPMENT

Insects and other arthropods of medical importance should be collected whenever possible for verification of their identification by specialists. Full data for each collection, such as date, locality, elevation, host, habitat and collector, should be included.

Aquatic Larvae, Especially Mosquito Larvae. 1. Kill in any manner to prevent distortion, such as immersion in hot water for 10 to 20 seconds, and then transfer to 70 per cent alcohol.

2. Pack carefully by placing larvae in a small vial or in short lengths of ordinary glass tubing. Fill tubes with alcohol and stopper with cotton, at both ends in the latter case, being careful to exclude *all* air bubbles. A number of such tubes may be packed in cotton in a larger alcohol-filled container that *should* contain an air bubble to allow for changes in pressure.

Adult Diptera, Especially Mosquitoes. 1. Collect several specimens of each sex and kill with chloroform or cyanide collecting tube. Adults that have been reared from immature stages should be kept alive for a day to allow the body to harden.

2. Adults are delicate and must be packed as soon as possible after killing by placing in pill boxes or the like between layers of cellucotton, lens paper, cleansing or soft toilet tissue. Pack to prevent movement. *Do not use absorbent cotton.* Include a few crystals of paradichlorobenzene.

3. The above applies to gnats, sandflies and other mosquitolike insects, although sandflies and blackflies may also be preserved in 70 per cent alcohol.

Other Arthropods. Large forms such as houseflies may be preserved in 70 per cent alcohol. Also use alcohol for all wingless forms, such as hard ticks, mites, fleas, spiders and maggots. Soft ticks may be shipped alive in well stoppered vials.

Shipping. Pack carefully in such a manner as to avoid breakage, and forward for identification.

4. MAKING THICK AND THIN BLOOD FILMS

1. Cleanse ear lobe or fingertip with gauze saturated with 70 per cent alcohol. In an emergency, rum or other strong spirits may be substituted. Dry with sterile gauze or allow to air dry.

2. Prick skin with a sterile Hagedorn needle, No. 11 Bard-Parker detachable blade or preferably a disposable blood lancet deeply enough to cause free flow of blood. Discard first drop.

3. Collect 3 or 4 small drops in small area near one end of clean glass slide. Stir them together with corner of another clean glass slide. Area covered by film should be the size of a dime; thickness such that newsprint can barely be read through it.

4. Make thin smear on remaining slide surface.

5. Place in slide box and allow to dry thoroughly in horizontal position. Thick

drop may require 2 hours or more to dry (especially in the tropics). Protect from dust, flies, cockroaches.

5. *USE OF ANTICOAGULANTS*

If large numbers of smears are desired from the same patient or if clotting is to be prevented, one of several anticoagulants may be used as follows:

Heller and Paul Anticoagulant Mixture

Potassium oxalate	0.8 gm
Ammonium oxalate	1.2 gm
Water	to 100 ml

1. Take 1 ml of above in test tube and evaporate water in oven, leaving crystalline residue.

2. Add 10 ml of blood to tube. This mixture has the advantage of preventing cell distortion.

Heparin. The exact quantity to be used is very small, not more than 2 mg per ml of blood. It may be dissolved in physiologic salt solution or alcohol, the liquid portion being subsequently evaporated as above. Tubes thus prepared are then ready for use.

Citrate. Two per cent sodium citrate in 0.85 per cent salt solution is an efficient anticoagulant. It is used in quantities up to 2 ml per 8 ml of blood (giving a 20 per cent solution of citrate). Blood thus rendered liquid may be used for parasite counts or other quantitative work only if the necessary mathematical adjustment due to its dilution is made. Other anticoagulants listed above do not alter the original blood volume significantly.

Sequester-Sol. This is a commercially available anticoagulant. The active ingredient is dipotassium ethylenediaminetetraacetate. It is used in a quantity of 1 drop to 5 ml of blood.

CAUTION: Large quantities of anticoagulant should not be used if blood is to be injected into experimental animals.

II. Methods of Examining Smears, Blood and Other Tissues[1]

1. *GRAM'S STAIN*

Materials

Ammonium oxalate—crystal violet solution:

Crystal violet (85% dye content, certified)	4 gm
Ethyl alcohol (95%)	20 ml

Dissolve the crystal violet in the alcohol.

Ammonium oxalate	0.8 gm
Water	80.0 ml

Dissolve the ammonium oxalate in the water. Dilute the crystal violet solution 1:10 with distilled water. Mix 1 part of the diluted crystal violet solution with 4 parts of ammonium oxalate solution.

Iodine solution:

Iodine	1 gm
Potassium iodide	2 gm

Dissolve in 5 ml of distilled water, then make up to 240 ml with water and add 60 ml of 5 per cent aqueous sodium bicarbonate. Prepare fresh solution if color loss is noted on standing.

Counterstain:

Safranin (2.5% solution in 95% alcohol)	10 ml
Water	100 ml

Procedure. 1. Stain 1 minute with the crystal violet solution.

2. Wash in water.

3. Apply iodine solution for 1 minute.

4. Wash in water.

5. Decolorize in 95 per cent alcohol for 30 seconds with gentle agitation, or until violet dye fails to appear in the alcohol. Wash in water. Acetone or equal parts acetone and alcohol may be employed as decolorizing agents, but care should be taken to wash with water as soon as the violet dye stops running, usually within a few seconds after applying the decolorizer.

6. Apply counterstain for 10 seconds.

7. Wash in water; dry without blotting.

2. GIEMSA'S STAIN FOR BLOOD PROTOZOA[2]

Stock Solution

Powdered stain	1.0 gm
Glycerin (C.P.)	66.0 ml
Methyl alcohol, absolute, acetone-free	66.0 ml

Grind powdered stain and glycerin together. When well mixed, dissolve stain in glycerin in a water bath at 55 to 60° C (131 to 140° F). When cool, add the methyl alcohol; allow to stand for 2 to 3 weeks, filter and store in small brown bottles. The addition of Triton X–100 to a concentration of 0.01 per cent enhances staining of parasites.

Preparation of Buffered Water. For this purpose two buffer solutions have been adopted: M/15 Na_2HPO_4 (disodium phosphate, anhydrous) and M/15 $NaH_2PO_4.H_2O$ (sodium acid phosphate).

These are made up as follows and may be kept indefinitely in separate Pyrex glass stoppered bottles.

Stock Buffer Solutions:

M/15 Na_2HPO_4 (disodium phosphate, anhydrous) 9.5 gm per liter

M/15 $NaH_2PO_4.H_2O$ (sodium acid phosphate) 9.2 gm per liter

From these stock solutions make the buffered water used in preparing stain and in rinsing stained specimens. Filter buffers before use. Buffered water is kept in well stoppered glass bottles and made up fresh each week. The pH of these solutions should be checked occasionally.

Buffered Water: (formula for 1 liter) In 900 ml Distilled Water:

pH	M/15 Na_2HPO_4	M/15 $NaH_2PO_4.H_2O$
6.8	49.6 ml	50.4 ml
7.0	61.1 ml	38.9 ml
7.2	72.0 ml	28.0 ml
7.4	80.3 ml	19.7 ml

Staining Procedure

Thin Smears

1. Fix thin smear by immersing in absolute methyl alcohol for a few minutes.

2. Then place smear in diluted stock Giemsa, 1 ml to 50 ml buffered water pH 7.0, for 45 minutes. *Older smears require a lower* pH.

3. Wash quickly in buffered distilled (or tap) water and stand on end to dry.

4. If smear appears too red use a more alkaline buffer; if too dark use a more acid buffer.

Thick Smears. Do not fix with methyl alcohol, but otherwise follow the procedure for staining thin smears. Wash gently for 2 minutes. Thick films are automatically laked while staining in an aqueous dilution of stain.

Thick and Thin Smears. These may be stained together on the same slide, *using caution not to fix the thick smear;* stain as outlined above.

3. WRIGHT'S STAIN FOR BLOOD[3]

Stock Solution

Stain (powdered)	0.3 gm
Glycerin (C.P.)	3.0 ml
Methyl alcohol, absolute, acetone free	97.0 ml

Grind powdered stain and glycerin together. When well mixed add the methyl alcohol and stir well. Place mixture in a tightly stoppered brown glass bottle for 2 to 3 weeks, then filter and the stain is ready for use. This stain improves considerably with age.

Staining Procedure

Thin Smears

1. Rule off area covered by the blood film with a wax pencil.

2. Cover dried film with stock stain for 1½ minutes (this fixes the blood film).

3. Add an equal amount of freshly distilled or buffered water (pH 6.8). Stain for 3 minutes.

4. Wash by flooding with distilled or buffered water. Stand on end to dry.

Thick Smears. In staining thick smears, it is first necessary to lake the red blood cells. This is done by simply immersing thick film in water until the hemoglobin stops running out and smear appears gray. Allow to dry, then stain as for thin films.

4. *FIELD'S RAPID METHOD FOR STAINING MALARIAL PARASITES IN THICK BLOOD FILMS*[4]

In this method thick blood films are stained in such a manner that the stained parasites and leukocytes are contrasted against a homogeneous background. After staining, differentiation of color is more clearly shown in lower edge of the film toward which the hemoglobin has drained. Reduced hemoglobin content of the blood increases the staining time necessary to as much as 10 seconds in cases of severe anemia.

Preparation of the Blood Films. Blood films should be about the size of a dime and not too thick. Films are ready to stain as soon as they are no longer obviously moist. Fixation is not necessary. Freshly prepared blood films stain better than when a day or two old.

Preparation of the Stains

Solution A	
Methylene blue	0.8 gm
Azur B (American stains)	0.5 gm
Disodium phosphate (anhydrous)	5.0 gm
Potassium phosphate, monobasic (anhydrous)	6.25 gm
Distilled water	500 ml

Solution B	
Eosin	1.0 gm
Disodium phosphate (anhydrous)	5.0 gm
Potassium phosphate, monobasic (anhydrous)	6.25 gm
Distilled water	500 ml

The phosphate salts are first dissolved; then the stain is added. Solution of the granular Azur B is aided by grinding in a mortar with a small quantity of the phosphate solution. Solutions of stain should be set aside for 24 hours, when, after filtration, they are ready for use. The same solutions may be used for many weeks without deterioration, but the eosin solution should be renewed when it becomes greenish from a slight carryover of methylene blue.

Staining Procedure. 1. Dip film for 1 second into solution A.

2. Remove from solution A and immediately rinse by waving *gently* in clean water for a few seconds until the stain ceases to flow from the film and the glass of the slide is free from stain.

3. Dip for 1 second into solution B.

4. Rinse by waving *gently* for 2 or 3 seconds in clean water.

5. Place vertically against a rack to drain and dry.

The concentration of the stain is adjusted for staining times of 1 second with an immediate wash of 5 seconds, but relative times may need slight adjustment to suit different batches of stain.

5. *RESTAINING OLD FILMS*[2]

Preparation of Blood Films for Restaining. Sometimes it becomes necessary to re-examine old blood films. Fading usually occurs in poorly stained films, or in those mounted in Canada balsam. Coverslips must be removed by soaking in xylene. Also remove all immersion oil. Smears mounted in diaphane probably cannot be restained.

Restaining Procedure. 1. Immerse cleaned smear in Giemsa for 2 to 6 hours, depending on the age of the film. Use 1 drop of Giemsa stock solution to distilled water that has been adjusted to a pH of 7.2.

2. Differentiate film in a 1 per cent solution of boric acid. This brings out any stippling.[2]

6. *HEMATOXYLIN STAINING OF THICK FILMS FOR MICROFILARIAE*

Hematoxylin stains the sheaths of microfilariae better than do Giemsa's or Wright's stains.

Preparation of Delafield's Hematoxylin

Hematoxylin crystals	4.0 gm
95% ethyl alcohol	25.0 ml

Dissolve the crystals in the alcohol and mix the solution with 400 ml of a saturated aqueous solution of ammonium alum.

Place in loosely capped container and keep in

a light airy location for 2 weeks. Then add mixture of

Methyl alcohol (acetone free)	100 ml
Glycerin	100 ml

Bottle and expose to direct sunlight for at least a month. Filter before use.

Staining Procedure. 1. Make a thick blood film as previously described or place centrifugalized sediment on glass slide. (See p. 806.)

2. When thoroughly dry, lake smear in tap water.

3. Allow to air dry.

4. Fix in equal parts of ether and 95 per cent alcohol for 10 minutes.

5. Allow to air dry.

6. Stain with Delafield's hematoxylin for 10 to 12 minutes.

7. Destain in water made slightly acid with HCl.

8. Wash in running water until blue color appears in film.

9. Air dry. Mount in any *neutral* mounting medium.

When microfilariae are observed in Giemsa-stained preparations they should be destained in acid alcohol, washed thoroughly and then stained according to the above directions.

7. MODIFIED GRAM'S STAIN FOR SPIROCHETES[1]

This stain was used originally for the spirochete of Vincent's infection but can be used also for relapsing fever organisms.

Procedure. 1. Fix smear (as swab smears from Vincent's infection or laked thick blood smears) by passing once or twice through flame.

2. Flood with gentian violet (1 per cent aqueous solution), add 5 drops of sodium bicarbonate (5 per cent solution, fresh or made previously with 1:20,000 merthiolate), allow to stand for 30 seconds.

3. Wash quickly in water.

4. Flood smear with iodine solution (iodine, 1 gm; potassium iodide, 2 gm; distilled water, 200 ml) for 1 minute.

5. Rinse slide in water, stand on end to air dry.

6. Examine with oil immersion lens. Spirochetes and fusiform bacilli stain dark purple.

8. FONTANA'S SILVER NITRATE METHOD FOR TREPONEMA AND LEPTOSPIRA[1]

Procedure. 1. Make film as thin as possible. Air dry.

2. Flood slide with fixative (formalin, 2 ml; glacial acetic acid, 1 ml; distilled water, 100 ml) for 1 or 2 minutes.

3. Wash 30 seconds in running water.

4. Flood slide with mordant solution (phenol, 1 gm; tannin, 1 gm; distilled water, 100 ml) and warm over flame for 30 seconds.

5. Wash 30 seconds in running water.

6. Flood slide with ammoniacal silver nitrate solution and steam gently for 30 seconds. (To prepare the silver nitrate solution dissolve 5 gm silver nitrate in 100 ml of distilled water. Remove 10 ml, and to the rest of the solution add, drop by drop, concentrated ammonia solution until the sepia precipitate that forms is dissolved. Then add enough more of the silver nitrate solution to produce a slight cloud, which persists after shaking.)

7. Wash 30 seconds in running water, blot dry and examine.

8. Spirochetes and leptospira appear as dark brown or black on a dark maroon field.

9. INDIA INK METHOD FOR SPIROCHETES AND CRYPTOCOCCUS

Procedure. 1. Mix a bacteriologic loop of fluid containing spirochetes or *Cryptococcus* with a small drop of India ink. Add a coverslip.

2. The cells of *Cryptococcus* and of spiro-

chetes will appear as clear figures against a dark background.

10. MACCHIAVELLO STAIN FOR RICKETTSIAE

Fixing and Staining Procedures. 1. Smear material to be stained on a clean glass slide.

2. Fix the smear by heat.

3. Flood with basic fuchsin 0.25 per cent for 5 minutes; drain.

4. Flood with citric acid 0.5 per cent and wash immediately with tap water.

5. Counterstain with methylene blue medicinal 1.0 per cent for 20 to 40 seconds. Rickettsiae appear bright red against a blue background. This stain is not useful in demonstrating rickettsiae of scrub typhus.

11. EXAMINATION OF FRESH BLOOD

Procedure. 1. Collect a small drop of blood from ear lobe or fingertip on slide.

2. Superimpose coverglass immediately; press gently to distribute blood evenly and thinly. Examine with the microscope.

3. Trypanosomes, microfilariae and spirochetes betray their presence by jostling the red cells. Malaria is recognized by pigment granules within the erythrocytes which, particularly in *Plasmodium vivax*, may be carried about by cytoplasmic streaming of the parasite.

12. EXAMINATION OF TISSUE ASPIRATES

Procedure. 1. Fluid aspirated from lymph nodes may also be examined in the fresh state for trypanosomes or microfilariae.

2. Aspirates from splenic punctures (kala-azar) or from the indurated margin of ulcers (dermal leishmaniasis) should be smeared and stained as blood smears. Examine for leishmanial bodies.

13. DARK FIELD ILLUMINATION FOR SPIROCHETES AND LEPTOSPIRAE[1]

General. Observation of living spirochetes in transmitted light is very difficult. Organisms should be brought into view by a special dark field condenser that gives concentrated oblique illumination, or by a "funnel stop" inside the oil immersion objective that reduces the amount of direct light. A special light source is needed as daylight is not sufficiently intense.

Adjustment of Apparatus. 1. Remove the ordinary condenser and insert the dark field condenser with its two lateral adjustment screws forward.

2. Adjust the source of light until a bright ring or spot appears on the upper surface of the condenser; the plane mirror is used.

3. With the low power objective, locate the top of the condenser and the ring etched on the surface of the condenser.

4. Manipulate the lateral adjustment screws until the ring is brought into the center of the field.

5. Remove the lower half of the oil immersion objective, insert the funnel stop with its small end toward the lens, and reassemble the objective.

Procedure. 1. Secure clean slides 1.45 to 1.55 mm thick and clean coverglasses.

2. Rim the coverglass with a small amount of petroleum jelly.

3. Place a small drop of the fluid to be examined on the center of the slide, apply the coverslip and press down to obtain a thin film, *avoiding bubbles.*

4. Lower the substage slightly and place a drop of immersion oil, free of bubbles, on the upper surface of the condenser.

5. Put the slide preparation on the mechanical stage and center the specimen.

6. Raise the substage until the oil is spread by contact with the slide.

7. Place a drop of immersion oil, free of bubbles, on the coverslip.

8. Lower the oil immersion objective and focus on the microorganisms, which should appear as bright objects against a black background. Adjust the light for bril-

liant illumination, reducing, if necessary, with the condenser diaphragm.

14. CENTRIFUGATION METHODS FOR TRYPANOSOMES

In Blood. 1. Mix 9 ml of blood and 1 ml of 6 per cent sodium citrate.

2. Centrifuge at 1500 rpm for 10 minutes.

3. Remove small amount of thin creamy layer between red cells and supernatant with a capillary pipette and examine; or

4. Transfer leukocytic cream and supernatant to another tube and spin at 1800 to 2000 rpm for 15 minutes.

5. Examine sediment directly under microscope; or

6. Make smears, lake, fix and stain with Giemsa.

In Cerebrospinal Fluid. 1. Spin 5 ml of spinal fluid at 1800 rpm for 15 minutes.

2. Examine sediment directly; or

3. Make smears, lake, fix and stain.

15. CENTRIFUGATION METHODS FOR NEMATODE LARVAE IN BLOOD AND SPINAL FLUID[5]

In Laked Blood. *Knott's Modified Survey Method.* 1. Collect exactly 1 ml of venous blood.

2. Mix with 10 ml of 2 per cent formalin in a 15 ml centrifuge tube. Blood lakes at once.

3. Centrifuge, or allow to sediment for 15 to 18 hours.

4. Decant supernatant fluid from sediment by quick tipping of tube so as to pour off surface bubbles.

5. Holding tube inverted, aspirate sediment with a capillary pipette.

6. Spread sediment into square area size of 22 mm coverglass; air dry.

7. Fix in equal parts of ether and 95 per cent alcohol for 10 minutes; air dry.

8. Stain with Delafield's hematoxylin for 40 to 60 minutes.

9. Rinse quickly in 0.05 per cent HCl.

10. Wash in running water until blue color appears in film; air dry.

11. Add immersion oil with or without coverglass and search for parasites under low power; confirm under oil.

In Citrated Blood. 1. Mix 5 ml of freshly drawn blood and 1 ml of 2.0 per cent sodium citrate made up in 0.85 per cent sodium chloride solution.

2. Centrifuge at 1000 rpm for 10 minutes.

3. Pass a fine pipette through the red cell sediment to remove material on bottom of tube.

4. Spread this sediment on a glass slide and examine for active microfilariae with low power of the microscope; also examine the buffy coat for microfilariae.

In Cerebrospinal Fluid. 1. Five to 15 ml of fluid is centrifuged at 1000 rpm for 5 or 10 minutes.

2. Examine sediment under low power of the microscope for living *Trichinella* larvae.

16. FILTER TECHNIQUE FOR DETECTION OF MICROFILARIAE IN BLOOD[6]

Materials

30 ml syringe
Swinney-25 filter holder, 25 mm
Millipore filter SCWPO 2500, 8 micron, 25 mm
Millipore filter pad, AP2002500, 25 mm
1:10,000 aqueous methylene blue

Procedure. 1. In a 30 ml syringe mix 2 to 3 ml of EDTA-treated venous blood with a lysing solution in a ratio of 10 ml of solution to each 1 ml of EDTA-treated blood.

2. Rotate or shake syringe until lysis occurs.

3. Attach filter holder to syringe and gently force solution through the filter.

4. A 5 ml syringe containing methylene

blue solution is then attached to filter holder and this solution forced through.

5. Remove filter, place on a glass slide and examine for stained microfilariae.

17. EXAMINING FOR SUPERFICIAL FUNGI[7]

Procedure. Hair should be removed from lesion by forceps; skin should be scraped from periphery of lesions or obtained from roof of vesicles with curved manicure scissors; nails should be scraped where friable or discolored, and detritus beneath nail collected. These materials should be cultured even though microscopic examination has failed to reveal the presence of fungi.

Microscopic Examination. 1. Clear collected material in 10 to 40 per cent potassium hydroxide by placing a small fragment of hair, skin or nail on slide in a drop of potassium hydroxide; add coverglass.

2. Heat gently over a low flame of Bunsen burner or alcohol lamp to hasten clearing process.

3. Examine under low or high dry power of a compound microscope; oil immersion is rarely needed.

Collected material should be cultured on Sabouraud's glucose agar slants and other appropriate media by placing two or three small fragments on each slant. (See p. 833 for further details.)

18. EXAMINING FOR SYSTEMIC FUNGI[7]

Sputum, pus and spinal fluid should be examined in the fresh state without the addition of a clearing agent to avoid artifact formation. A loop full of sputum or pus should be placed on a slide and gently pressed to a thin film under a coverglass. Spinal fluid itself may be examined directly or the centrifuged sediment may be examined. These materials should be mixed with a drop of India ink to demonstrate capsule formation if *Cryptococcus neoformans* is suspected (p. 810). Examine all preparations with reduced light from the microscopic condenser.

All material should be cultured on Sabouraud's glucose agar at room temperature and beef infusion blood agar at 37° C (98.6° F). (See p. 833 for additional media.) Hold all cultures for at least 3 weeks. If *Actinomyces israelii* is suspected, beef infusion glucose agar shake cultures or Brewer's thioglycollate medium should be inoculated to obtain a culture of this anaerobic fungus. (See p. 833 concerning cultures.)

19. LACTOPHENOL COTTON BLUE FOR STAINING FUNGI

Lactophenol cotton blue is prepared as follows:

Phenol crystals	20 gm
Lactic acid	20 ml
Glycerin	40 ml
Water	20 ml

Heat gently under a hot water tap to dissolve. Add 0.05 gm cotton blue (C_4 Poirrer).

Use as directed (p. 834) for staining fungi.

20. TRICHROME STAINING TECHNIQUE FOR PARASITES (FROM M. M. BROOKE)[1,8]

The trichrome technique is a rapid staining procedure that gives good results routinely.[9] The method is simple in that overstaining and differentiation are not necessary to bring out the morphologic details of the parasites nor is it necessary to mordant before staining. The stain solution is stable and may be used repeatedly, the lost volume being replaced by the addition of stock solution. Staining over 15 smears daily (in 50 ml of stain), however, tends to weaken the stain. Strength will return upon standing, if stain is allowed to evaporate in open air for 3 to 8 hours.

The staining of fresh and PVA-fixed material differs chiefly in the increased time required for the latter and the omission of the fixative step since the material in the PVA solution is already fixed. Both procedures are given below.

Stain Reactions (Trichrome). Thoroughly fixed and well stained *Entamoeba histolytica* cysts are blue-green tinged with purple; *Entamoeba coli* cysts, slightly more purplish. Background material usually stains green, resulting in a noticeable color contrast with the protozoa. Organisms in thick smears take the more neutral shades of red and green. In contrast with those stained with hematoxylin, such smears have a transparency that enables identification of imbedded protozoa. Protozoa and eggs are less subject to distortion, however, in thin smears. Eggs and larvae usually stain red and contrast strongly with green background. Thin-shelled eggs usually collapse when placed in mounting medium although some diagnostic features may be retained, especially if smear is examined immediately.

Large protozoa are readily picked up with a low power objective, using 10× oculars. Smaller forms (*Entamoeba hartmanni* and *Endolimax nana*) and those staining faintly are more visible with high dry and oil immersion lenses used with 7.5× eye pieces.

Nonstaining cysts and those staining predominantly red are most frequently associated with incomplete fixation. If unsatisfactorily stained organisms are obtained from specimens submitted in PVA-fixative, it usually indicates incomplete fixation associated with poor emulsification. Thorough emulsification of preferably *soft* stools will yield critically stained cysts and trophozoites. Degenerate forms stain pale green.

Mononuclear and polymorphonuclear leukocytes as well as *Blastocystis* present the same diagnostic problems as when stained with hematoxylin. The cytoplasm of pus and tissue cells, however, does stain more greenish.

Staining Procedure with Fresh Specimens

1. Schaudinn's fixative (Soln. 1)	5 min at 50°C (122°F), 1 hr at room temperature
2. 70% alcohol plus iodine (Soln. 2)	1 min.
3. 70% alcohol (1)	1 min
4. 70% alcohol (2)	1 min
5. Stain (Trichrome) (Soln. 5)	2–8 min
6. 90% alcohol, acidified (1 drop glacial acetic acid in 10 ml alcohol)	10–20 seconds or until stain barely runs from smear

Prolonged destaining in 90% alcohol (over 20 seconds) may differentiate organisms poorly, although larger trophozoites, particularly those of *E. coli* may require slightly longer periods of decolorization.

7. 95% or 100% alcohol	Rinsed twice
8. 100% alcohol or carbolxylene	1 min
9. Xylene	1 min or until refraction at smear-xylene interface ends

10. Mount with coverslip using Permount, Balsam, or other mounting media

Staining Procedure with PVA Films

1. 70% alcohol plus iodine (Soln. 2)	10 min
2. 70% alcohol (1)	3–5 min
3. 70% alcohol (2)	3–5 min
4. Stain (Trichrome) (Soln. 5)	6–8 min
5. 90% alcohol, acidified (1 drop glacial acetic acid in 10 ml alcohol)	10–20 seconds or until barely runs from smear
6. 95% alcohol	5 min
7. Carbolxylene	5–10 min
8. Xylene	10 min

9. Mount with cover slip using Permount, Balsam or other mounting media

See page 824 for technique for iron-hematoxylin staining of fecal smears.

21. GOMORI'S METHENAMINE–SILVER NITRATE STAIN FOR FUNGI AND PNEUMOCYSTIS

This is the recommended stain for the demonstration of *Histoplasma* and many other fungi and of *Pneumocystis.*

Tissue is fixed in 10 per cent formalin and may be sectioned in paraffin, celloidin or by frozen sections.

Reagents

5% Chromic acid:

Chromic acid	5.0 gm
Distilled water	100.0 ml

5% Silver nitrate solution:

Silver nitrate	5.0 gm
Distilled water	100.0 ml

3% Methenamine solution:

Hexamethylenetetramine, USP	3.0 gm
Distilled water	100.0 ml

5% Borax solution:

Borax (photographic grade)*	5.0 gm
Distilled water	100.0 ml

Stock methenamine–silver nitrate solutions:

Silver nitrate, 5% solution	5.0 ml
Methenamine, 3% solution	100.0 ml

A white precipitate forms but immediately dissolves on shaking. Clear solutions remain usable for months at refrigerator temperature.

Working methenamine–silver nitrate solution:

Borax, 5% solution	2.0 ml
Distilled water	25.0 ml
Mix and add:	
Methenamine–silver nitrate, stock solution	25.0 ml

1% Sodium bisulfite solution:

Sodium bisulfite	1.0 gm
Distilled water	100.0 ml

0.1% Gold chloride:

Gold chloride, 1% solution	10.0 ml
Distilled water	90.0 ml

This solution may be used repeatedly.

*Borax (Sodium Borate, anhy. reagent) obtained from Matheson Coleman & Bell Co., Norwood, Ohio.

2% Sodium thiosulfate (hypo) solution:

Sodium thiosulfate	2.0 gm
Distilled water	100.0 ml

Nuclear fast red solution:

Dissolve 0.1 gm of nuclear fast red in 5% solution of aluminum sulfate with heat. Cool, filter, add a grain of thymol.

Procedure

Run a Control Slide

1. Deparaffinize sections through 2 changes of xylene, and run through absolute and 95% alcohol to distilled water.
2. Oxidize in 5% chromic acid solution for 1 hour.
3. Wash in running tap water for a few seconds.
4. Rinse in 1% sodium bisulfite for 1 minute to remove any residual chromic acid.
5. Wash in tap water for 5 to 10 minutes.
6. Wash with 3 or 4 changes of distilled water.
7. Place in working methenamine-silver nitrate solution in oven at 60° C (140° F) for 70 minutes until section turns yellowish brown. Use paraffin-coated forceps to remove slide from this solution. Dip slide in distilled water and check with microscope for adequate silver impregnation. Fungi should be dark brown at this stage.
8. Rinse in 6 changes of distilled water.
9. Tone in 0.1% gold chloride solution for 3 minutes. Rinse in distilled water.
10. Remove unreduced silver with 2% sodium thiosulfate (hypo) solution for 2 to 5 minutes.
11. Wash thoroughly in tap water.
12. Counterstain with nuclear fast red solution for 7 minutes, wash.
13. Dehydrate with 2 changes of 95% alcohol, absolute alcohol, clear with 2 or 3 changes of xylene, and mount in Permount.

Results. *Histoplasma capsulatum* and many other fungi and *Pneumocystis carinii* will be sharply delineated in black. Acid-fast organisms and *Nocardia* also stain black. Mucin stains taupe to dark gray, while the inner parts of mycelia and hyphae are dark rose. The background stains pale green.

III. Methods For Obtaining And Examining Duodenal Fluid[10, 11]

1. STRONGYLOIDIASIS AND OTHER PARASITIC INFECTIONS

Procedure. 1. A standard Rehfuss tube with olive tip is used. Tube is passed *(through the mouth)* with the patient in a sitting position. It is passed until it reaches the stomach. This is indicated when the marking of *1 ring* on the tube is at the level of the patient's lips. Stomach contents are then aspirated (with a 30 ml syringe). Patient is then placed in a lying position on his right side. This position is very important. The patient is then instructed to swallow the tube farther down at a slow rate approximately 1 to 2 inches every 5 to 10 minutes—until the marking showing *3 rings* on the tube is at his lips. Usually during this period clear or cloudy gastric juice will flow and this may be discarded. After a period, which varies with each patient, a clear light yellow material will be seen. The patient then should be stimulated. Magnesium sulfate 33.3 per cent or olive oil may be used. Approximately 30 ml of 33.3 per cent magnesium sulfate is introduced into the duodenum through the tube and allowed to flow back into a test tube immediately. If the procedure has been properly carried out, dark bile will follow the returning magnesium sulfate. This procedure may be repeated as often as is necessary.

2. If difficulty is encountered in getting the tube into the duodenum, a few simple aids may be tried:

a. Use a pillow to elevate the patient's hips.

b. Turn the patient on his left side for 5 to 10 minutes; then return him to original position.

3. Two simple ways of determining the position of the tube are as follows:

a. The patient is given a small amount of water by mouth and a syringe is attached to the free end of the tube. If water can be aspirated, the tube is in the stomach and must be returned to stomach depth (that is, pulled out until the marking of *1 ring* is at the level of the patient's lips). The progressive swallowing process outlined above should then be repeated.

b. Attach a syringe to the free end of the tube and attempt to aspirate. If a vacuum is formed and you are unable to aspirate the fluid, it is safe to assume that the tube is in the duodenum or in the pylorus approaching the duodenum.

Identification of Intestinal Parasites. 1. Intestinal parasites may be found in A, B or C bile, but are detected most frequently in C bile (darkest bile). In most instances, the parasites are located in the mucoid content of the bile. They should be sought in the *mucus suspended in the bile* and in the sedimentated mucus. Some of the mucus usually settles to the bottom of the container after standing for a few minutes. Because of the viscosity of bile, centrifugation is of no significant aid in this procedure. The dark bile-stained drainage fluid may be placed in a conical sedimentation jar or in a pilsener glass. Transillumination of the fluid by placing a microscope lamp behind it aids in the visualization of the suspended mucus fragments, which should be examined microscopically. The floating and sedimentated mucus may be removed for examination by use of a large caliber pipette with a rubber bulb. The material is placed on a glass fecal slide and examined under low power. Several slides should be examined before calling the drainage fluid negative for strongyloidiasis.

2. The three parasites most frequently found are *Strongyloides stercoralis* rhabditiform larvae and/or embryonated eggs, *Giardia lamblia* trophozoites and hookworm eggs in various stages of cleavage.

Entero-Test.*[10, 11] With the fasting pa-

*Entero-Test is marketed by (Hedco) Health Development Corp., 2411 Pulgas Ave., Palo Alto, California.

tient seated, a swallow of water is offered to moisten the mouth and throat. The Entero-Test then is swallowed with water while holding the loop of the nylon thread. A piece of adhesive tape through the loop and attached to the face at one corner of the mouth will secure the line, which is left in place generally 3 to 4 hours. In over 95 per cent of reported cases the line has extended its full length in 4 hours. Some physicians prefer to leave the line in place 6 to 8 hours. The patient is instructed to drink a glass of water after the first and second hours. No other food or drink should be taken. When the capsule descends into the stomach the gelatin dissolves, leaving a miniature, weighted rubber bag that is carried by peristalsis into the duodenum. To remove the line the patient opens his mouth and raises his chin. The line then is withdrawn with a fairly rapid but gentle pull. During withdrawal the rubber bag separates from the line and later is passed unnoticed in the stool. The line is placed in a basin and the patient offered water to remove the taste of gastrointestinal contents. Normally the distal 60 to 90 cm of yarn is saturated with bile-stained mucus. This material may be scraped off into a small beaker by squeezing the line between two fingers of the gloved hand. Several drops of mucus are obtained. It may be useful, as well, to place some mucus from the esophageal and stomach segments of the line on slides and examine for exudative cells and fungi. To delineate the various segments clearly, place the still moist line on a flat surface and stroke over its length with the pH indicator stick. Compare the resulting colors with the chart provided. Usually the esophageal portion is neutral, the stomach acid, and the duodenal portion alkaline.

IV. Methods Of Examining Feces For Protozoa And Helminths[1]

1. DIRECT SMEARS—SALINE AND IODINE STAINED SMEARS[1]

Preparation of Iodine Stain (after D'Antoni). A suitable iodine stain may be prepared by mixing the following:

Potassium iodide	1.0 gm
Iodine crystals	Supersaturate
Distilled water	100 ml

Some prefer to add 1 ml of glacial acetic acid per 100 ml of water.

Procedure. 1. Place a drop of physiologic saline in the center of one half of the slide ($1\frac{1}{2} \times 3$ inch slide) and a drop of iodine stain on the other half.

2. Examine the stool for blood or mucus and carefully select material from those areas as well as from several others and spread it *evenly* throughout the saline over one coverglass width of the slide. Newsprint should be just legible through the smear after applying coverglass.

3. In the same manner additional fecal material is spread *evenly* in the drop of iodine stain.

4. A coverglass is then applied to each of the smears and the preparations are examined. This double smear preparation should always be employed when stools are examined microscopically.

5. The entire area of the double smear on the fecal slide should be examined *systematically* with low power. The high-dry magnification is employed to study objects suggestive of parasites. It is profitable even for experienced personnel to examine a part of each smear with the higher magnification. This will reduce the chances of overlooking small organisms. *Furthermore, a careful, methodical and diligent search is required, not merely a glance.* Frequently, amebae are not numerous in the stool.

6. The unstained (saline) side of a fecal smear is of greater value for detecting the presence of cysts or of trophozoites than the iodine-stained portion of the fecal smear. There is greater contrast between the refrac-

tile amebae and their background in the saline smear than in the iodine smear. In the latter, the amebae and the background both acquire a somewhat similar hue. Amebic trophozoites, if fresh and motile, are recognized principally in the saline portion of the smear. Cysts usually cannot be specifically identified in the unstained side, unless, as occasionally happens, chromatoid bars are present. Helminth larvae are more easily detected on the saline side because of their motility.

7. Iodine staining will kill trophozoites of protozoa and is not recommended for identifying worm eggs. However, it is invaluable in studying amebic and flagellate cysts, as nuclei and glycogen masses otherwise almost invisible are thereby stained.

2. "MIF" (MERTHIOLATE-IODINE-FORMALIN) STAIN AND FIXATIVE FOR INTESTINAL PROTOZOA AND HELMINTH EGGS (AFTER SAPERO AND LAWLESS)[12]

Both cysts and trophozoites are stained in a solution that also acts as an effective preservative.

For Staining the Cysts and Trophozoites of Fecal Specimens Brought to the Laboratory

Preparation

1. Place in a Kahn tube 1 ml of stain-fixative solution (sufficient for 25 fecal examinations) made up as follows: 0.125 ml formaldehyde solution (USP); 0.775 ml tincture of merthiolate (No. 99 Lilly 1:1000); and 0.10 ml, freshly prepared Lugol's solution 5 per cent (Merck Index). (Note: If Lugol's solution is over 1 week old, increase 0.10 ml to 0.125 ml; if over 2 weeks old, increase to 0.15 ml. Reduce merthiolate in same amount that Lugol's solution is increased. Do not use Lugol's over 3 weeks old.)

2. Place Kahn tube with 1 ml of stain, and a second Kahn tube containing distilled water in a rack. Put medicine dropper in each tube.

Procedure. Place a small drop of distilled water at one end of a glass slide; add equal size drop of stain solution. To this drop add feces and make a wet smear as described for the direct saline smear.

For Collection and Preservation of Specimens in Survey Studies, Hospital Wards, Homes, and for Mailing to a Laboratory. *Preparation.* Freshly prepare a 5 per cent Lugol's solution, and a stable stock "MF" solution containing 250 ml distilled water; 200 ml tincture merthiolate (No. 99 Lilly 1:1000); 25 ml solution formaldehyde, USP; 5 ml glycerin, to make 480 ml stock "MF" solution (store in brown bottle).

Procedure

1. Measure 2.35 ml "MF" stock solution into a standard Kahn tube and stopper with cork.

2. Measure 0.15 ml Lugol's solution (5 per cent) into a second Kahn tube and stopper with a rubber cork. The two tubes represent a collection unit.

3. Immediately upon collecting a stool, pour the "MF" solution into the Kahn tube containing the Lugol's solution. *The two solutions must not be combined until just prior to the addition of the fecal specimen.* Using an applicator stick, add and thoroughly stir into the solution a portion of feces about twice the volume of a medium-sized pea (about 0.25 gm). Do not overload with feces. Stopper the tube and record pertinent data on label.

4. To examine: With a medicine dropper, draw off a drop of fluid and feces from surface layer of sedimented feces. Observations indicate that most species of protozoa and helminth eggs tend to concentrate on the upper layer of the sedimented feces. Place drop on a glass slide. Mix the fecal particles in the drop thoroughly by means of an applicator stick, crushing any large particles. Cover and examine.

Preservation of Larger Samples of Feces for Teaching Purposes, or for Helminth Eggs or Protozoal Concentration Procedures. Use screw type cap vials to prevent evaporation. Feces, "MF" stock solution, and Lugol's solution, may be placed in vials in proportions as follows:

	AMOUNT OF FECES	"MF" SOLUTION	LUGOL'S SOLUTION
(small)	0.25 gm	2.35 ml	0.15 ml
(medium)	0.50 gm	4.70 ml	0.30 ml
(large)	1.00 gm	9.40 ml	0.60 ml

Lugol's solution should not be over 3 weeks old and should never be added to "MF" stock solution until just before the feces is to be added. Prior addition of iodine to "MF" stock solution will cause a dense precipitate to form upon standing.

Procedure

1. Remove a drop of intermixed fluid and feces from sedimented surface layer, make coverslip preparation and examine. Preparation may be ringed with sealing materials.

2. For flotation concentration of helminth eggs, replace supernatant fluid in vial specimen with saturated brine solution and proceed as usual for recovery of eggs.

Important Principles in Usage of Technique; Staining Characteristics. By placing feces in solution *within 5 minutes of passage,* the major disadvantage of loss of organisms and morphology deterioration which occur in most stools that are allowed to stand may be prevented. As an example, *D. fragilis* and flagellates, frequently largely lost in iron-hematoxylin–stained mounts, are recovered in undiminished density by immediate fixation in MIF solutions.

Staining

1. Staining reaction comprises an initial iodine phase, as seen in ordinary iodine preparations with the exception that both cysts and trophozoites are stained, and a subsequent eosin stage that gradually replaces the iodine. A reversal to the iodine phase, if desired, may be accomplished by addition of fresh Lugol's to specimen, i.e. by adding a drop of fresh MIF solution. In trophozoites from patients with amebic dysentery, red blood cells are even more readily defined than in fresh saline preparations.

2. Trophozoite forms stain immediately; cysts take stain more slowly. An increase in the strength of Lugol's, or use of a more freshly prepared Lugol's solution, will speed the staining time of cysts.

3. CONCENTRATION OF CYSTS AND EGGS BY ZINC SULFATE CENTRIFUGATION–FLOTATION (AFTER FAUST, ET AL.)[13]

This method is good for cysts of amebae and flagellates, and for some eggs. *Strongyloides* larvae likewise are usually brought to the surface. However, cysts are more distorted than with the formalin-ether sedimentation (MGL) technique. Caution must be taken to check the specific gravity of the zinc sulfate solution at frequent intervals. In areas with high humidity there is fluctuation in the specific gravity.

Procedure. 1. Thoroughly comminute a stool sample the size of a small pecan in 2 or 3 ml lukewarm tap water in a Wassermann tube and strain feces through one layer of wet gauze.

2. Add water to within 1/2 inch of the brim, stir thoroughly with applicator, centrifuge for 45 to 60 seconds at 2300 rpm.

3. Decant supernatant; fill with water and stir as before; centrifuge.

4. Repeat Step 3; may omit if supernatant is clear.

5. Decant water; replace with 1/4 tube of zinc sulfate solution (granular $ZnSO_4.7H_2O$ USP; dissolve 331 gm in 1 liter of water to give the solution a specific gravity of 1.180 – it should be checked with a hydrometer); stir thoroughly; fill to 1/4 inch of brim of tube and spin at 2500 rpm for 45 to 60 seconds. Allow centrifuge to stop smoothly. Wait 1 or 2 minutes.

6. Using a 3/16 inch bacteriologic loop, transfer the surface film onto a glass slide, and apply small coverglass.

7. Examine for cysts and eggs.

If the examination is intended for protozoan cysts, loop surface film into a drop of iodine solution.

4. CONCENTRATION OF CYSTS, EGGS AND LARVAE BY CENTRIFUGATION-SEDIMENTATION

Formalin-Ether Sedimentation – 406th MGL (Med. Gen. Lab.) Method (after Ritchie).[1, 14, 15] This is the method of choice for general use. It concentrates helminth larvae, eggs and protozoan cysts.

Preparation. Prepare a 10 per cent solution of formalin.

Procedure with Fresh Specimens

1. Partial comminution of entire stool, with an appropriate amount of water or saline, can be accomplished in the stool container. Add enough fluid to make it possible to recover 8 to 10 ml of strained emulsion which, when centrifuged, will yield 1/2 to 3/4 ml of fecal sediment.

2. Strain through two layers of moist gauze and collect in a 15 ml pointed centrifuge tube. A cone-shaped paper cup with the point cut off can be substituted for the glass funnel. (Straining may be omitted to simplify the procedure if desired.)

When time is of the essence, short cuts may be taken that generally result in a satisfactory specimen for examination. In such cases, substitute the following for Steps 1 and 2.

1a. Fill a 15 ml conical centrifuge tube half full of tap water or physiologic saline.

2a. Place approximately 2 ml of feces in the tube and mix, using a wooden applicator. Fill tube to within 1/2 inch of the top with additional water or saline and mix well again.

3. Centrifuge at 1500 rpm for 2 minutes or 1 minute at 2000 to 2500 rpm. Decant the supernatant fluid. Resulting sediment should be about 0.75 to 1.0 ml. Resuspend and repeat as in Step 2a if desired.

4. Add 10 per cent formalin to the sediment until the tube is one-half full; mix thoroughly with the aid of an applicator stick; *allow to stand for 5 minutes.*

5. Add about 3 ml of ether (until the tube is three-fourths full); stopper the tube (or use thumb or rubber finger cot) and *shake vigorously; remove the stopper or thumb carefully* to prevent spraying of material due to pressure within the tube. (If ether is not available, gasoline may be substituted.)

6. Centrifuge at 1500 rpm for about 2 minutes. Four layers should result: a small amount of sediment containing most of the parasites; a layer of formalin; a plug of fecal debris on top of the formalin; and a layer of ether at the top.

7. Free the plug of debris from the sides of the tube, by ringing with an applicator stick, and carefully decant the top three layers. Swabbing the sides of the tube with a cotton-tipped applicator stick gives a cleaner preparation for examination.

8. Mix the remaining sediment with the small amount of fluid that drains back from the sides of the tube. Drag sediment from tube on to a fecal slide by means of applicators. Prepare an iodine-stained mount of the sediment for microscopic examination.

The formalin-ether sedimentation technique is excellent for the detection and identification of protozoan cysts and helminth eggs and larvae of almost all intestinal parasites. The technique is also very useful for examining stools containing fatty substances that interfere with the performance of the zinc sulfate centrifugal flotation method. It is *not* satisfactory for trophozoites.

Formalin-Ether with Preserved Specimens (after Brooke).[8]

1. Formalinized specimens may also be prepared as described above using tap water. Straining may be omitted. Also omit Step 4.

2. Prepare iodine and unstained mounts in the usual manner for microscopic examination.

Acid–Sodium Sulfate–Triton NE*–Ether Concentration–AMS (Army Med. Sch.) Method (after Hunter et al.).[15,16] This method is recommended for the detection of helminth larvae and eggs. It is the method of choice for the detection of schistosome eggs.

Preparation

1. Prepare by adding approximately equal amounts of hydrochloric acid of a specific gravity of 1.089 (45 ml of concentrated HCl [37 per cent] and 55 ml of water) and sodium sulfate solution of a specific gravity of 1.080 (9.6 gm of anhydrous sodium sulfate to 100 ml of water), the final mixture having a specific gravity of 1.080.

2. In each solution, adjust to the proper specific gravity, if needed, before preparing the final mixture, which keeps 4 weeks or more.

---

*Triton NE (Triton = X 30) is a wetting agent that may be secured from Rohm & Haas Co., Philadelphia, Pennsylvania.

3. To insure the best possible results, it is advisable to dehydrate the sodium sulfate before using. Dry in desiccator or a hot air oven (2 hours at 130° C, 266° F) and cool in a desiccator.

Procedure

1. Partial comminution of the entire stool with an appropriate amount of water can be accomplished in the stool container. Add enough water so that it will be possible to recover 8 to 10 ml of strained emulsion, which, when centrifuged, will yield about 0.5 to 0.75 ml of fecal sediment.

2. Strain through two layers of gauze moistened with $HCl-Na_2SO_4$ mixture into a 15 ml pointed centrifuge tube. A cone-shaped paper cup with the point cut off can be substituted for a glass funnel.

3. Wash by brief centrifugation (1 minute at 2000 to 2500 rpm) with $HCl-Na_2SO_4$, decanting the supernatant each time and mixing the sediment with fresh $HCl-Na_2SO_4$; repeat twice or until the supernate is clear.

4. After decanting, add 5 ml of $HCl-Na_2SO_4$ plus 3 drops of Triton NE plus 3 ml of refrigerated ether. Shake for 30 seconds and centrifuge for 1 minute at 1500 rpm. Four layers should result: ether at top, plug of debris, acid–sodium sulfate solution and sediment.

5. Break ring at the interface with an applicator stick and decant.

6. Add tap water to the 0.1 mark, mix sediment, and pour as much as can be read onto a slide; cover with a 24 by 40 mm coverglass. An applicator may be used to draw the few drops of sediment to the lip of the tube, and is especially useful in controlling the amount of sediment that escapes onto the slide.

7. Examine under the low power of compound microscope. There should be a minimum of debris and the eggs should stand out clearly. Some mature eggs will exhibit viable miracidia.

5. *KATO THICK SMEAR TECHNIQUE*[18]

Non-moisture resistant cellophane paper with a 40 μm thickness is cut to a size of approximately 26 × 28 mm and used as a cover on the stool specimen to be examined. The cellophane strips should be soaked in solution A for at least 24 hours.

Solution A	
Distilled water	500 ml
Glycerin	500 ml
3% malachite green solution in water	5 ml

Since strong light is used during microscopic examination, the malachite green affords some protection to the eyes and the glycerin provides a clearer differentiation of the parasite eggs.

Sixty to 70 mg (roughly the size of a small bean) of stool are taken from various portions of the stool sample to be examined. This material is placed on a glass slide, covered with the wet, treated cellophane strip and pressed with the finger, a rubber stopper or other appropriate implement so that a stool film is formed between the cellophane and the slide. This is kept at room temperature for about 30 minutes for clearing. The parasite eggs are much easier to detect after this period. The prepared slide is then examined microscopically using 100× magnification. The intensity of light required is at least twice as much as is required for ordinary direct smears with a coverglass.

6. *ARTIFACTS*

It is always necessary to be alert to the possibility of confusing some yeast, plant, or tissue cells with diagnostic forms of helminths and protozoa, especially with amebae. Some of the more commonly encountered artifacts in stools are well illustrated in *The Color Atlas of Intestinal Parasites.*[15]

7. *QUANTITATION OF WORM INFECTIONS BY EGG COUNTS*[19]

Stoll's dilution method, the modified Stoll dilution method, Beaver's direct smear or McMaster technique may be used for the estimation of worm burden. They are mostly used for the evaluation of hookworm, *Ascaris* and *Trichuris* infections but may be applied to any worm infection in which eggs or larvae are more or less continuously added to the bowel stream. The main advantages in the Beaver direct smear method are that it is rapid and that it requires no correction for stool consistency. The chief disadvantage in the smear is that a calibrated, specially adapted photoelectric light meter is required. However, since smears made by experienced technicians are fairly uniform and nearly always contain between 1 and 2 mg of feces, worm infections can be determined roughly as heavy, moderate and light without the use of a light meter. Counts should not be made by either method on stools that are not made up of more or less normal fecal elements.

Stoll Dilution Method

Material

1. N/10 (0.4 per cent) sodium hydroxide solution.
2. Long-necked Erlenmeyer flask marked to indicate 56 ml and 60 ml levels.
3. Glass beads, slides and 22 × 30 mm coverglasses.
4. Pipette calibrated to deliver 0.075 ml.

Procedure

1. Fill flask to 56 ml mark with sodium hydroxide solution.
2. Add feces to bring contents up to 60 ml mark.
3. Add glass beads or BB shot to nearly fill flask and stopper it.
4. Allow to stand 12 to 24 hours with occasional shaking.
5. Shake to thoroughly mix and withdraw exactly 0.075 ml (or 0.15 ml).
6. Transfer to slide, cover and count eggs in entire preparation.
7. Eggs per preparation × 200 gives eggs per ml uncorrected.
8. Correct the count for stool consistency by multiplying uncorrected counts as follows: × 1, for hard-formed; × 1.5, for mushy-formed (can be cut with applicator but holds shape against stroke against container); × 2, for mushy (can be compressed by stroke against container); × 3, for mushy-diarrheic (takes shape of container but will not pour); × 4, diarrheic (can be poured).

Modified Stoll Dilution Method

Material

1. N/10 (0.4 per cent) sodium hydroxide solution.
2. 15 ml centrifuge tubes.
3. Pipette calibrated to deliver 0.1 ml.

Procedure

1. Fill centrifuge tube to 14 ml mark with sodium hydroxide solution.
2. Add feces to bring contents up to 15 ml mark.
3. Mix with wooden applicator stick.
4. If feces is hard, *allow to stand for several hours.*
5. Shake to thoroughly mix and quickly withdraw exactly 0.15 ml from middle of suspension.
6. Transfer to slide, cover and count eggs in entire preparation.
7. Eggs per preparation × 100 gives eggs per ml uncorrected. Corrections may be made as in Stoll Method.

Beaver Direct Smear Method.[15, 20] The ideal fecal smear for most purposes contains about 1 mg of feces in 1 drop of water or physiologic saline solution. Some workers prefer 2 mg smears.

Materials

1. Any type of photoelectric light meter having a galvanometer dial and cell window on the same face and calibrated.
2. An adapter (handmade from wood or similar material having a thickness of about 18 mm) to reduce the cell window to a circular opening 16 mm in diameter.
3. Gooseneck or other type of vertically adjustable lamp.

Calibration Procedure

1. Prepare 2N Na_2SO_4 and N/1 $BaCl_2$ solutions and mix each with ½ part pure glycerin.
2. Combine 1 part $BaCl_2$ mixture with 6 parts Na_2SO_4 mixture to give a white suspension of $BaSO_4$.
3. Place light meter apparatus directly under the lamp and adjust light to give an arbitrary whole number on the dial with a clean slide over the window.
4. Deliver 1 drop (0.05 ml) of the $BaSO_4$ suspension onto the slide above the window and spread just to cover the window.

5. The amount of reduction in the dial reading produced by the spread suspension (as compared with the clean slide) is that which will be produced by 1 mg of formed feces in one drop (0.05 ml) of water or normal saline solution.

6. Calibration of instrument for making 2 mg fecal smears is as above except 3 parts glycerinated Na_2SO_4 mixture to 1 part of the $BaCl_2$ mixture are used to give a $BaSO_4$ suspension twice as heavy.

Egg-count Procedure

1. Adjust light over meter to give arbitrary predetermined "zero point" with clean slide in place over window.

2. Place 1 drop of water or physiologic saline solution on slide and spread to just cover the window.

3. Add feces from applicator by stirring until dial is shifted to 1 mg point (or 2 mg as desired) determined by previous calibration.

4. Cover with 22 × 22 mm cover glass and count eggs in entire preparation.

5. Counts can be recorded as eggs/mg or eggs/gm (essentially the same as eggs/ml corrected to the formed stool basis). Infections giving counts of less than 5 hookworm or whipworm eggs, or less than 20 *Ascaris* eggs per mg feces, generally are regarded as light; counts above 25 for hookworm or whipworm and 50 for *Ascaris* indicate heavy infections. Interpretations must vary somewhat with circumstances such as age and condition of the patient, average bulk of the stool and duration of the infection.

McMASTER TECHNIQUE[17]

Material

McMaster egg-count slide
Spatula or disposable wood applicator
Hand sieve (aperture size ± 250 μm) type: commercial plastic tea sieve
Pasteur pipette (± 9 inc.) and rubber teats
Beakers, 100 ml
Cylinder measuring 100 ml
Densimeter
Saturated aqueous salt solution (density 1.200)

This is a very simple and accurate method, suitable for routine examination. It is, in principle, a flotation method using a special counting slide (McMaster cell).

Weigh out precisely 2 gm of fresh feces and place in suspension in 60 ml of saturated common salt solution. To remove the coarsest particles, the suspension can be poured through a sieve and the residue be well squeezed. However, the chance exists of eggs remaining in the residue.

Mix the suspension well by pouring it to and fro in two cups to get a completely homogenous division of eggs in the liquid. With a pipette, immediately fill the chambers of the egg-counting slide by slanting them to allow air bubbles to escape. After mixing well fill one chamber of the cell, after remixing fill the next chamber. After a few minutes eggs appear in the supernatant flotation liquid and attach to the coverglass. Under a low magnification of the microscope they can be easily counted. The older counting slides have two and the newer ones three chambers. Each chamber has a 10×10 mm square; the space between slides and coverglasses is 1.5 mm. Each chamber thus contains 0.15 ml liquid. Count at least two chambers and for best results four. The average number (X) of eggs recovered multiplied by 200 gives the number of eggs per gram of feces (EPG).*

The average number resulting from four counts is of value only when individual counts do not deviate more than 25 per cent of this average. Greater variations point to a poor homogenization of the mixture. In this case the figures are incorrect and the counting should be done again.

Cleaning Method

After use wash out immediately under spout of tap water.

Rinse in alcohol-ether.

Clean cell chamber with very fine brush (type: pipe cleaner brushes).

Rinse in alcohol-ether.

Rinse in ether.

Dry.

---

*$X \cdot \frac{60}{2} \cdot \frac{1}{0.15} = X \cdot 200$

8. *HEIDENHAIN'S IRON-HEMATOXYLIN STAINING OF FECAL SMEARS (MODIFIED FROM BROOKE)*[8]

This is the best method of staining protozoa in fresh feces. Properly prepared slides last many years. Both long and short methods are described. The standard long method gives excellent results if the procedure is carefully followed, especially with regard to destaining the organisms. If the fixative, mordant and stain are heated, considerable time can be saved. A special procedure is outlined for use in staining PVA fixed specimens (p. 825).

Staining Solutions

Schaudinn's Fluid

Saturated $HgCl_2$ solution in distilled water	64 ml
Absolute (or 95%) alcohol	32 ml
Acetic acid, glacial	4 ml

Iodine Alcohol

Prepare a stock solution by adding sufficient iodine crystals to 70% alcohol to produce a dark concentrated solution. For use, dilute some of stock solution with 70% alcohol until a port wine color is secured. Exact concentration is unimportant.

Mordanting Solution (Iron Alum)

Ferric ammonium sulfate	4 gm
Distilled water	100 ml

Hematoxylin Stain—Stock Solution

Hematoxylin powder	10 gm
Ethyl alcohol (95%)	100 ml

Dissolve powder in alcohol. Keep several weeks to ripen before use. Make staining solution by mixing 5 ml of stock solution with 100 ml of distilled water.

Procedure. 1. Make a thin fecal smear with a toothpick or applicator on a clean slide or coverglass. Dilute feces with physiologic saline if necessary. Immediately immerse slide in Schaudinn's fixative; the *smear must not be permitted to dry from this point until it is mounted.* However, if the staining schedule must be interrupted, before or after mordanting, the slides may be stored in 70 per cent alcohol for long periods. When interrupted between mordant and stain, store slides in 70 per cent alcohol, but repeat mordanting before completing staining.

2. Before a fecal smear dries, gently immerse in Schaudinn's fluid and proceed as follows:

	Rapid Method	*Long Method*
Schaudinn's	5 min at 50°C (122°F)	60 min at room temperature
50% alcohol	3 min at room temperature	
70% alcohol plus iodine (wine color)	5 min at room temperature	
50% alcohol	3 min at room temperature	
Tap water	3 min at room temperature	
4% mordant (iron alum)	10–20 min at 50°C (122°F)	12–24 hours unheated
2 changes in distilled or tap water	3 min (total)	
0.5% hematoxylin	5–10 min at 50°C (122°F)	12–24 hours unheated
1–2% mordant (iron alum) to destain	Usually 1–3 min	

Check carefully under microscope as this is the critical step; every 30 seconds rinse in water to slow down destaining process and observe under the low or high power of the microscope. The time varies with each smear even in same staining jar.

	Both Methods
Rinse in gently running tap water	5–30 min for permanent stain
70% alcohol containing a few drops of lithium carbonate	3 min unheated
95% alcohol	3–5 min unheated
Carbolxylene	3–5 min unheated
Xylene	3 min unheated

Mount with coverslip using Permount, Clarite, balsam or other *neutral* mounting media. Examine when dry.

Interpretation of Stain. 1. Well stained protozoa are grayish or bluish with black nuclei. In the ameba, chromatoid bars, red blood cells and bacteria stain black. Background appears blue-gray.

Trophozoites and cysts of protozoa are not usually distorted except in the cases of *Chilomastix and Trichomonas.* The latter especially tend to round up and so are atypical in appearance.

Organisms that do not stain well may have been poorly fixed. Fixing for 5 to 10 minutes in fixative warmed to 37° C (98.6° F) will largely overcome this, except for *E. coli,* which requires fixation for 30 minutes at 56° C (132.8° F). Fresh fixative, even though cold, yields sharper stained specimens but requires more time.

9. IRON GALLEIN AS A SUBSTITUTE FOR IRON HEMATOXYLIN[21]

Iron gallein as a substitute for iron hematoxylin may be used in staining various parasites.

Staining Solutions

Solution A

1 gm gallein in 20 ml glycol, followed by 80 ml of absolute alcohol

Solution B

4 gm iron alum
1.6 to 2 ml HCl
Distilled H_2O to make 100 ml (modified according to organism)

Staining Procedure

1. Bring paraffin sections to water.
2. Stain 5 to 20 min in iron gallein (depending on organism and fixation).
3. Counterstain with eosin or van Gieson's stain (time dependent on tissue).
4. Dehydrate quickly, proceed through xylol to mounting.

The best staining characteristics for *E. histolytica* trophozoites in tissue are obtained using a modification of solution B containing 1.6 ml of concentrated HCl for 5 to 10 min. *E. histolytica* trophozoites from feces are fixed in Schaudinn's solution and stained 20 min using 3.0 ml of concentrated HCl in solution B.

Balantidium coli trophozoites and *Onchocerca volvulus* adults in tissue are stained for 20 min using 2.5 ml of concentrated HCl in solution B.

10. POLYVINYL ALCOHOL-FIXATIVE METHOD FOR TROPHOZOITES OF INTESTINAL PROTOZOA (AFTER BROOKE AND GOLDMAN)[8]

This method is specifically designed to preserve trophozoites of amebae for long periods of time in a condition suitable for subsequent identification. It is fairly satisfactory for the detection of protozoan cysts.

Preparation. *PVA Fixative.* Add 5 gm of polyvinyl alcohol* to a mixture at room temperature of 1.5 ml glycerol, 5 ml glacial acetic acid, and 93.5 ml of Schaudinn's solution (2 parts of saturated aqueous mercuric chloride to 1 part of 95 per cent ethyl alcohol). Heat gently while stirring to about 75° C (167° F) or until the solution clears. Solution keeps for several months at least.

Saturated Aqueous Picric Acid Solution. Add 2 gm picric acid crystals to 100 ml of water; shake. Allow to stand for several days with intermittent shaking; add more crystals if all dissolve. Solution should be saturated in 3 to 4 days.

Procedure. *Fixation in Vial.* 1. Thoroughly mix 1 part of specimen in a vial containing 3 parts or more of PVA fixative.

2. Films for staining may be prepared immediately or months later by spreading a drop or two of the mixture on a microscope slide and allowing the smear to dry thoroughly (preferably overnight at 37° C, 98.6° F). Films should be of moderate thickness.

Fixation on Microscope Slides. 1. Mix thoroughly 1 drop of specimen with about 3 drops of PVA fixative on a microscope slide.

2. Spread the mixture over approximately one-third of the surface of the slide and allow to dry thoroughly.

Staining PVA Films (after Brooke). The Heidenhain staining technique should be modified as follows:

---

*PVA powder and solutions may be purchased in small quantities from Delkote, Inc., P.O. Box 1335, Wilmington, Delaware.

Place dry PVA film in 70% alcohol plus iodine	20 min
50% alcohol	10 min
Tap water	5 min
4% mordant (iron alum)	8–12 hrs
Tap water – 2 changes	3 min (total)
0.5% hematoxylin	8–12 hrs or overnight
Tap water – 2 changes	3 min (total)
Destain in saturated picric acid	15–20 min

(This step is critical. The slide should be removed at intervals, washed in water and examined under low and high powers of the microscope (not oil). The time required varies with the individual smear.)

Immerse in running tap water to stop destaining process	30 min
70% alcohol plus a few drops of lithium carbonate	10 min
95% alcohol	10 min
Carbolxylene	10 min

Mount with cover slip using Permount, Clarite, balsam or other *neutral* mounting media. Examine when dry.

Interpretation of stain essentially as described elsewhere for Heidenhain's (p. 825).

See page 813 for trichrome staining technique of fecal smears.

11. DIAGNOSIS OF PINWORM INFECTION[13]

Procedure. The most satisfactory means of diagnosing pinworm infection is by the recovery of eggs or female worms from the perianal region, as only 5 to 10 per cent of infected persons pass eggs in their stools.

Scotch Tape Method (after Graham). 1. Prepare a swab with a 4 inch strip of Scotch tape 3/4 to 1 inch in width and a standard 1 × 3 inch microscope slide. One-fourth inch of one end of the tape is folded upon itself to provide a nonadhesive area for handling. The remainder is applied to the slide with the gummed side down extending over the end and for about 1/2 inch on the undersurface of the slide. (See Fig. 48–14, p. 464.)

2. Employ the swab in the morning before bathing or bowel movement.

3. Hold the slide against a tongue depressor 1 inch below the end and lift the long portion of tape from the upper surface of the slide.

4. Loop the tape over the extended end of the depressor to expose the gummed surfaces. Hold the tape and slide against the depressor to provide tension and a firm support for the loop of Scotch tape.

5. Separate the buttocks and press the gummed surfaces against several areas of the perianal region.

6. Replace the tape on the slide (to which it has remained attached on the undersurface) and smooth the tape with cotton or gauze.

7. Examine the swab with the microscope for eggs (not adults) of *Enterobius vermicularis.*

8. A drop of toluene or xylol may be added to the slide before replacing the tape for clearing, if desired; however, the cells and detritus in uncleared preparations serve as guides for focusing on the correct optical plane.

12. FIXING AND STAINING TREMATODES

Many of the techniques recommended for one group of worms can be employed with equally satisfactory results for others. Three are outlined.

Fixing Solutions

1. Alcohol-Formol-Acetic (AFA) Fixative	
Formalin, commercial grade	10 ml
Alcohol, 95%	50 ml
Glacial acetic acid	5 ml
Distilled water	45 ml
2. Formalin	5–8%
3. Bouin's-Solution A. Saturated aqueous solution–picric acid	
Solution B	
Formalin	5 ml
Acetic acid	1 ml
Mix solutions A and B before use:	
Solution A	75 ml
Solution B	30 ml

Staining Solutions. Any of these will give consistently good results.

1. Semichon's Acetic Carmine

Acetic acid	50 ml
Distilled water	50 ml

Place in small flask; add excess carmine powder. Stopper flask with pierced stopper with thermometer, place in water bath, heat to 100°C (212°F) for 15 minutes. Cool, allow to settle, decant supernatant and filter.

2. Delafield's hematoxylin (p. 809)
3. Alum cochineal

Potassium alum	30 gm
Cochineal	30 gm
Distilled water	400 ml

Boil for 1 hour; cool and filter. Boil filter paper in 200 ml distilled water for 30 minutes; filter; add to first filtrate; boil 30 minutes. Filter and make up to 400 ml with distilled water.

Procedure. 1. Relax flukes by shaking vigorously in bottle half-filled with 1.0 per cent salt solution for 3 minutes.

2. Pour off liquid, replace with equal parts of 1 per cent salt solution and of fixative; shake vigorously for 3 minutes.

3. Drop the fixed trematodes into undiluted fixative for 3 to 12 hours.

4. Place in 70 per cent alcohol colored like port wine with iodine for 12 hours.

5. Place in 70 per cent alcohol for several hours to remove iodine.

6. Stain (diluted half and half with distilled water). The interval will vary with the stain used and the size of the specimen.

7. Decolorize in 70 per cent alcohol made slightly acid with a few drops of hydrochloric acid (about 0.5 to 1 per cent) until the internal structures are visible in transmitted light. Neutralize by repeated washings in 70 per cent alcohol.

8. Pass through 85 per cent, 95 per cent and 100 per cent alcohols and xylol allowing at least ½ hour in each.

9. Mount in balsam, clarite or other *neutral* mounting medium.

13. FIXING AND STAINING CESTODES

Fixing Solution

Alcohol–Formol–Acetic (p. 826)

Procedure. 1. Allow worms to lie in cold water until contractions have ceased, or wrap the worm about a spool (or glass plate) after washing in physiologic saline, or shake gently until relaxed.

2. Drop into fixative.

3. Cut out selected proglottids with sharp scalpel and place in water a few minutes before staining.

4. Proceed as described above for flukes, beginning with Step 6 (above), using Delafield's hematoxylin or Semichon's acetic carmine.

14. FIXING AND EXAMINING NEMATODES[22]

Roundworms may be killed and preserved by a variety of fixatives. In general, formalin, with few exceptions, is *not* recommended as a fixative due to its hardening properties.

Alcohol and Glycerin. Alcohol and glycerin are used to make a good fixative for all nematodes most effectively at 60 to 63°C (140 to 145.4° F); specimens may be stored in this solution indefinitely. The purpose of the glycerin is to protect the specimens from drying should the alcohol evaporate.

70% alcohol and 5% glycerin

95% ethyl alcohol	70 ml
Distilled water	25 ml
Glycerin	5 ml

In the examination of worms fixed in alcohol and glycerin it is necessary to *gradually* evaporate the alcohol and therefore bring the worms into a progressively higher concentration of glycerin; this process serves to clear the worms and render their internal structures readily visible.

Alcohol, Formalin, and Acetic Acid (AFA). A solution using alcohol, formalin, and acetic acid is an all-purpose fixative that is useful not only for nematodes but also for trematodes and cestodes. Best results are obtained when the fixative is used hot (60 to 63° C; 140 to 145.4° F). After fixation for 24 hours or longer, parasites can be transferred to an alcohol-and-glycerin mixture for prolonged storage.

Alcohol-formalin-acetic solution (AFA)

Formaldehyde	10 ml
95% ethyl alcohol	50 ml
Glacial acetic acid	5 ml
Distilled water	45 ml

Glacial Acetic Acid. Full-strength glacial acetic acid is extremely useful for the rapid killing of nematodes; they are killed almost instantly in an extended position. The acid has excellent clearing properties, so that the worms can be removed directly from the acid to a drop of water for study under the microscope; all organ systems are readily visible for identification. For prolonged storage, it is recommended that after killing the worms in acetic acid, they should be transferred to AFA for 24 hours and then to an alcohol-and-glycerin mixture.

Dilute Formalin. Although formalin is *not* recommended as a general fixative for nematodes, a dilute solution of 1 to 2 per cent formalin is recommended for adult *Ascaris.* Fixing adult *Ascaris* in higher concentrations of formalin may result in rupture of the worms due to changes in osmotic pressure. After fixation in the dilute formalin for a day or longer, the worms can be transferred to 10 per cent formalin for prolonged storage.

NOTE: It should be remembered that *Ascaris* eggs will continue to develop in 10 per cent formalin or lesser concentrations and will become infective and remain infective for several months or longer. Care should be exercised in handling such worms, especially if they are to be dissected.

V. Methods of Examining Urine

1. EXAMINING URINE FOR SCHISTOSOME EGGS

Procedure. 1. Collect urine sample in sedimentation glass for examination of eggs.

2. Allow to settle; pipette off bottom sediment to slide.

3. Examine microscopically for eggs of *S. haematobium.*

In infections with *Dioctophyma renale,* a kidney worm rarely infecting man, eggs may be found in urine sediment. Occasionally, microfilariae of *W. bancrofti* have been recovered from urine in cases of filariasis with chyluria. Microfilariae of *O. volvulus* may be observed in urine at times (p. 512).

2. EXAMINING URINE FOR SPIROCHETES

Spirochetes of relapsing fever, *Leptospira icterohemorrhagiae* or *L. canicola* sometimes may be found in urine.

Procedure. 1. Collect 30 to 50 ml of urine in a sterile vessel.

2. Centrifuge at 2000 rpm for 30 minutes.

3. Examine sediment under a dark field for spirochetes.

Refrigerate (but do not freeze) urine sample if urine must be transported great distances.

VI. Methods of Examining Sputum

1. EXAMINING SPUTUM FOR HELMINTH EGGS AND LARVAE

1. Mix sputum and 3 per cent sodium hydroxide solution in equal amounts.

2. Centrifuge at high speed.

3. Decant supernatant.

4. Examine sediment for eggs and larvae.

Instead of sodium hydroxide, Clorox (full strength) may be added in quantity sufficient to liquefy sputum.

2. ZIEHL-NEELSEN COLD STAIN FOR ACID-FAST BACILLI[1]

This stain is used to differentiate acid-fast and non-acid-fast organisms and depends upon a primary stain, decolorizer and counterstain.

Materials

Carbolfuchsin Cold Stain

Solution A	
Basic fuchsin (90% dye content)	0.3 gm
Ethyl alcohol (95%)	10.0 ml
Solution B	
Phenol	5.0 gm
Distilled water	95.0 ml
Mix solutions A and B	

1. Dissolve 3.5 gm basic fuchsin in 12.5 gm of pure phenol heated to 80°C (176°F) in boiling water bath.
2. Cool; add 25 ml of 95% alcohol and mix well.
3. Add 260 ml distilled water.
4. Slowly add 30 drops of 10% Tween 80 while stirring.
5. Filter and store; filter again before using.

Loeffler's Alkaline Methylene Blue

Solution A	
Methylene blue (90% dye content)	0.3 gm
Ethyl alcohol (95%)	30.0 ml
Solution B	
Dilute KOH (0.01% by weight)	100.0 ml
Mix solutions A and B; filter	

Procedure. 1. Stain dried smears 10 minutes with carbolfuchsin.

2. Rinse in tap water.

3. Decolorize in 95 per cent ethyl alcohol containing 3 per cent by volume of concentrated HCl, until only a suggestion of pink remains.

4. Wash in tap water.

5. Counterstain with Loeffler's alkaline methylene blue for about 1 minute.

6. Wash in tap water.

7. Dry and examine. Acid-fast organisms stain red, others blue.

VII. Culture Methods

1. MEMBRANE FILTER TECHNIQUE FOR DETECTION OF PATHOGENIC BACTERIA OR FUNGI[1]

Materials

Filter holder, Membrane filters, Absorbent pads — Obtainable from Millipore Filter Corporation, Watertown, Mass.
Filter flask
Vacuum source
Appropriate liquid medium, double strength
Petri dishes

Procedure. 1. The specimen (urine, spinal fluid, laked blood, or other) is filtered by means of suction through a previously sterilized membrane filter.

2. After the specimen has passed through the membrane filter, the filter is aseptically removed from the holder and placed in a sterile Petri dish on top of an absorbent pad that has been saturated with double strength liquid medium.

3. The plates are incubated in the usual manner. Colonies appear on the surface of the membrane filter analogous to their appearance on solid media. The advantages of this method are that a higher number of positive recoveries is obtained, growth appears faster and frequently in pure culture.

2. BOECK-DRBOHLAV'S LOCKE-EGG-SERUM MEDIUM[1]

This medium may be employed for the cultivation of *Entamoeba histolytica, Dientamoeba fragilis, Trichomonas hominis* and, to a limited extent, some other species of intestinal amebae and flagellates. Transfers are made every 48 hours. About 0.5 ml of the fluid medium at the bottom of the tube is used for each transplant.

Materials Required

1. *Eggs.*

2. *Sterile Ringer's Solution.* This is prepared according to the following formula:

Sodium chloride	(NaCl)	8.0 gm
Potassium chloride	(KCl)	0.2 gm
Calcium chloride	($CaCl_2$)	0.2 gm
Magnesium chloride	($MgCl_2$)	0.1 gm
Monosodium phosphate	(NaH_2PO_4)	0.1 gm
Sodium bicarbonate	($NaHCO_3$)	0.4 gm
Distilled water	(H_2O)	1000 ml

It is then autoclaved at 15 pounds pressure for 20 minutes and allowed to cool.

3. *Modified Sterile Ringer's Solution.* Prepared by adding 0.25 gm of Loeffler's Dehydrated Blood Serum* to 1000 ml of Ringer's solution, which should be made up in addition to the Ringer's solution of Step 2. Boil serum and Ringer's solution for 1 hour to facilitate solution of serum, filter, and autoclave for 20 minutes at 15 pounds pressure.

4. *Sterile Rice Flour.* The rice flour is sterilized by placing about 5 gm in a test tube and plugging it with cotton. It is distributed evenly and loosely over inner surface of tube by shaking, and then sterilized in horizontal position in dry heat at about 90° C (194° F) for 12 hours, using intermittent sterilization and allowing 4 hours for each period; flour remains white if not overheated.

Procedure. Wash four eggs thoroughly, rinse, and brush well with 70 per cent ethyl alcohol. Break into sterile Erlenmeyer flask containing glass beads and 50 ml of Ringer's solution. Emulsify completely by shaking. Place about 4 ml of this material in each test tube and sterilize as follows (using autoclave as inspissator): Place tubes in a preheated autoclave in such a position as to produce a slant of about 1.0 to 1.5 inches, close the door and vacuum exhaust valve, turn on the steam and open the outside exhaust valve. When steam appears from this valve, close it and allow the pressure to rise to 15 pounds; then shut off steam and allow pressure to decline to zero; remove media from autoclave. Repeat on three successive days, storing media at room temperature between sterilization.

To these sterile solid slants add enough modified Ringer's solution (about 5 or 6 ml) to cover egg slant completely. Incubate at 37.5° C (99.5° F) for 24 hours to determine sterility before adding the sterile rice flour. Flour is added by taking up 0.25 ml into a clean, sterile, dry, wide bore, 1 ml pipette and discharging it into the liquid medium by tapping the pipette against the inside wall of the tube. A flamed bacteriologic loop may also be used for this purpose. The tubes are again incubated at 37.5° C (99.5° F) for 24 hours to test for sterility.

*Instead of the Loeffler's Dehydrated Blood Serum, sterile human serum or sterile horse serum (inactivated and tricresol free) may be used, in which case the modified Ringer's solution should consist of 1 part serum to 8 parts of Ringer's solution. This solution is sterilized by passing through a Berkefeld filter and incubated at 37.5° C (99.5° F) to determine sterility before pouring onto egg slants.

3. CLEVELAND AND COLLIER'S MEDIUM FOR CULTIVATION OF AMEBAE

Materials

Bacto-Entamoeba medium
Horse serum
NaCl

Procedure. 1. Suspend 33 gm of the Bacto-Entamoeba medium in 1000 ml distilled H_2O and heat to boiling to dissolve completely.

2. Place in tubes and autoclave at 15 pounds pressure (120° C, 248° F) for 20 minutes.

3. Slant tubes. Test for sterility at 37.5° C (99.5° F). Overlay slants with sterile horse serum–saline solution (1:6 dilution). Add a 5 mm loop of sterile rice flour.

4. EGG YOLK MEDIUM FOR THE CULTIVATION OF AMEBAE (AFTER BALAMUTH)[1]

Materials

Dehydrated or fresh egg yolk
Liver extract (Lilly, No. 408)
Dibasic potassium phosphate (K_2HPO_4)

Potassium acid phosphate (KH_2PO_4)
Sodium chloride
Rice flour

Procedure. 1. Mix 36 gm of dehydrated egg yolk or the crumbled yolks of 4 hard boiled eggs with 36 ml of distilled water.

2. Add 125 ml of 0.8 per cent NaCl and mix with a rotary beater or Waring Blender.

3. Heat the mixture over boiling water for 20 minutes after the temperature has reached 80° C (176° F) and add distilled water to offset the loss by evaporation.

4. Filter. The mixture of the dehydrated yolks is difficult to separate through a Buchner funnel but may be passed through a double layer of muslin instead. If fresh eggs are used, the mixture may be filtered by suction through a Buchner funnel using ordinary filter paper.

5. Bring the filtrate to a volume of 125 ml by adding 0.8 per cent NaCl.

6. Autoclave at 15 pounds (120° C, 248° F) for 20 minutes.

7. Cool to below 10° C (50° F) and filter through a Buchner funnel.

8. Add to the filtrate an equal amount of M/15 potassium buffer adjusted to pH 7.5, prepared by diluting 1:15 a solution of M/1 dibasic potassium phosphate 4.3 parts and M/1 potassium acid phosphate 0.7 parts.

9. Add a 5 per cent crude liver extract (Lilly, No. 408) to give a final concentration of 0.5 per cent in order to insure rapid growth.

10. Autoclave and then refrigerate until dispensed in tubes containing 7 to 10 ml.

11. Prior to inoculation add a 5 mm loop of sterile rice flour.

5. NNN (NOVY, MACNEAL AND NICOLLE'S) MEDIUM FOR LEISHMANIA[1]

Materials

Bacto-Agar	14 gm
Sodium chloride	6 gm
Distilled water	900 ml
Sodium hydroxide solution	N/1
Rabbit (or guinea pig) defibrinated blood	10 ml

Procedure. To a flask containing 900 ml of distilled water add 14 gm of Bacto-Agar and 6 gm of sodium chloride. Bring to a boil and then neutralize with N/1 NaOH. Place 150 ml of the medium in 6 Erlenmeyer flasks and sterilize in autoclave for ½ hour at 12 pounds pressure. Store in refrigerator. Stock medium will keep for several months if stored at refrigerator temperatures.

Place one of the flasks containing 150 ml of stock medium in a boiling water bath; when agar has melted, cool medium to 50 to 55° C (122 to 131° F) and, using sterile technique, add 10 ml of defibrinated rabbit blood, mixing thoroughly. Pipette 5 ml of this medium into test tubes and slant tubes so as to produce a long slant. When slants have hardened, paraffin the cotton plugs and place in refrigerator for 12 hours, subsequently incubating tubes at 37.5° C (99.5° F) for 24 hours to test for sterility.

Antibiotics (penicillin 20 units per ml, streptomycin 40 units per ml) are usually introduced on inoculation of cultures to prevent bacterial overgrowth of the leishmanias.

6. DIPHASIC BLOOD-AGAR MEDIUM FOR TRYPANOSOMES AND LEISHMANIAS (NIH METHOD)

Materials

Bacto-Beef (Difco)	25.0 gm
Neopeptone (Difco)	10.0 gm
Bacto-Agar (Difco)	10.0 gm
Sodium chloride	2.5 gm
Distilled water	500 ml
Defibrinated rabbit blood	

Procedure. 1. Infuse Bacto-Beef and distilled water in water bath for 1 hour; heat mixture for 5 minutes at 80° C (176° F) to coagulate a portion of the protein.

2. Filter, using ordinary grade of filter paper.

3. Add Neopeptone, Bacto-Agar and sodium chloride.

4. Adjust the pH to 7.2–7.4 with NaOH.

5. Autoclave at 15 pounds, 120° C (248° F) for 20 minutes.

6. Cool until mixture may be held comfortably in the hand and add 10 per cent defibrinated rabbit blood. (For *Trypanosoma lewisi* add 30 per cent defibrinated rabbit blood.)

7. Dispense 5 ml per test tube, slant and cool.

8. Before inoculating, overlay the slants with 2 ml of sterile Locke's solution prepared by the following formula:

Sodium chloride	8.0 gm
Potassium chloride	0.2 gm
Calcium chloride	0.2 gm
Potassium phosphate (monobasic)	0.3 gm
Dextrose	2.5 gm
Distilled water	1000 ml

7. OFFUTT'S MEDIUM[23]

This medium is simple to prepare and all the materials are available in regular bacteriology laboratories. It can be made up in a relatively short time when needed. The addition of a sterile overlay makes it unnecessary to obtain a generous amount of water of condensation. All of the leishmanias, *T. cruzi, T. rangeli* and *T. lewisi* can be maintained on this medium on 14-day transfers. The use of antibiotics increases the effective diagnostic value of the medium by inhibiting bacterial growth.

While the blood-agar slants may be stored for several days before use, freshly prepared slants give better growth and are therefore recommended.

Materials

Bacto blood-agar base, dehydrated
Fresh rabbit blood, sterile and defibrinated
Sterile buffered normal saline or Locke's solution (pH 7.2 to 7.4)

Preparation. 1. Blood-agar base: The Bacto blood-agar base is prepared according to directions on the bottle and sterilized in flasks in 200 ml amounts. This medium can be stored in the refrigerator for several months if desired.

2. Medium for Use:

Melt one flask of the base and then cool it to 45 to 50° C (113 to 122° F).

Add aseptically 10 to 20 ml of the fresh, sterile, defibrinated blood.

Tube in 4 to 5 ml amounts in sterile test tubes.

Allow the medium to solidify in slants. (A fairly short slant with a deep butt is preferred.)

Add 0.5 to 1 ml of sterile Locke's solution or saline to each tube.

Test for sterility by incubating for 24 hours at 37° C (98.6° F).

Rubber stoppers or screw-caps are added after inoculation to prevent evaporation.

Procedure. Just before inoculating the medium, add 250 to 500 units of penicillin and streptomycin to the water of condensation.

8. CPLM (CYSTEINE-PEPTONE-LIVER-MALTOSE) MEDIUM FOR THE CULTIVATION OF TRICHOMONAS VAGINALIS (AFTER JOHNSON AND TRUSSELL)

Materials

Bacto-Peptone	32.0 gm
Bacto-Agar	1.6 gm
Cysteine HCl	2.4 gm
Maltose	1.6 gm
Liver infusion (Difco)	320 ml
Ringer's solution (NaCl 0.6%, $NaHCO_3$, KCl and $CaCl_2$ 0.01% each)	960 ml
Sodium hydroxide N/1	11–13 ml

Procedure. 1. Heat the mixture in a boiling water bath to melt the agar and filter through coarse filter paper.

2. Add 0.7 ml of 0.5 per cent aqueous methylene blue. Adjust the pH to 5.8 to 6.0 with N/1 HCl or N/1 NaOH.

3. Tube in 8 ml amounts and autoclave.

4. Cool; add 2 ml of sterile human serum.

5. Incubate for sterility for at least 4 days at 37.5° C (99.5° F) and store at room temperature until used.

9. MEDIUM FOR BALANTIDIUM COLI (AFTER REES AS MODIFIED BY LEVINE)

Materials

1. Make up a modified Ringer's solution as follows:

NaCl	6.50 gm
KCl	0.14 gm
$CaCl_2$	0.12 gm
$NaHCO_3$	0.20 gm
Na_2HPO_4	0.01 gm
Distilled water	1000 ml

2. Human, horse, rabbit or bovine serum.

3. Sterile rice flour (p. 830).

Procedure. 1. Make up modified Ringer's solution and sterilize in autoclave at 15 lb pressure for 10 minutes.

2. Add 25 ml of human, horse, rabbit or bovine serum aseptically to 500 ml of sterile Ringer's solution.

3. Tube in 8 ml quantities as aseptically as possible.

4. Add a 5 mm loop of sterile rice starch.

5. Incubate for 48 hours at 37° C (98.6° F) to test for sterility. Store sterile tubes in refrigerator.

6. Warm tubes to 37° C (98.6° F) in incubator before use.

7. Introduce inoculum to bottom of tube. Incubate at 37° C (98.6° F).

8. The protozoa grow in the bottom of the tube. Transfer every 72 hours.

10. HARADA AND MORI TEST TUBE CULTIVATION METHOD FOR NEMATODE LARVAE[24]

This method is useful for demonstration of larvae of *Ancylostoma duodenale, Necator americanus, Trichostrongylus orientalis* and *Strongyloides stercoralis.* Approximately 0.5 gm of feces is smeared on a narrow sheet of filter paper (3 cm × 16 cm). About 5 cm of space on one end and 1 cm (for handling) on the other end are left unsmeared. The filter paper is placed in a test tube 18 cm in height and 2 cm in diameter, with the unsmeared end (5 cm) toward the bottom. Two to 3 ml of water are introduced into the tube; then the opening is covered with a piece of polyethylene sheet that is held in place by a rubber band. The tube is kept in an incubator at 24 to 28° C (75.2 to 82.4° F) for about 10 days. Eggs of hookworm and certain other nematodes hatch on the filter paper and develop into infective larvae, which crawl out of the feces and migrate to the water. The tubes are examined under low power magnification for presence of larvae. If they are present, fluid is removed with a pipette and the larvae are identified under higher magnification. Incubation for 8 days at 30° C (86° F) provides the optimum condition for detection of *Strongyloides* larvae. Larvae usually are found much earlier than 8 days.

11. MEDIA FOR FUNGI

Materials

Sabouraud's glucose medium:

Glucose	20.0 gm
Neopeptone	10.0 gm
Agar	20.0 gm
Water	1000.0 ml

Keep in 10 ml quantities in stab tubes for poured plates as needed. Also, allow to harden into slants after autoclaving at 10 lb for 10 minutes. Chloromycetin (0.05 mg per ml) and cycloheximide (0.5 mg per ml) may be added to the medium before autoclaving. Cycloheximide should not be used if *Cryptococcus neoformans* is expected to be cultured from clinical materials.

Beef infusion agar (pH 7.4 to 7.6):

Beef infusion broth	1000.0 ml
Peptone	20.0 gm
Sodium chloride	5.0 gm
Agar	20.0 gm

Keep in 100 ml quantities in flasks. Melt and allow to cool to 45° C (113° F), add 5 ml of sterile blood, mix and pour into tubes for slants or sterile Petri dishes for plates. Test for sterility by incubating at 37.5° C (99.5° F) for 24 hours.

Add 10 units of penicillin and 30 units of streptomycin per ml of agar. Chloramphenicol (0.05 mg per ml) may be substituted for the streptomycin. This medium, with or without 6 per cent blood, is recommended for isolation of systemic fungi at 37° C (98.6° F).

Bacto-Mycobiotic Agar (Difco) is similar to Sabouraud's glucose medium and may be used exclusively for the isolation of dermatophytes. For systemic fungi, media without cycloheximide and chloramphenicol (Bacto-Brain Heart Agar) should be used in parallel with the Mycobiotic Agar.

Maintain cultures for mold-phase pathogens at room temperature for 3 weeks. For systemic pathogens, cultures should be incubated at both room temperature and 37° C (98.6° F) for a similar period of time. Transfers of growth from any bit of inoculum are made to fresh tubes for pure cultures. Cultures that cannot be readily identified should be maintained on Sabouraud's conservation medium to prevent degenerative loss of diagnostic morphologic characters.

Procedures. Yeastlike cultures are best examined by placing a bit of the culture on a slide in a drop of water and adding coverslip to the preparation. Filamentous cultures should be examined in a mounting medium. These cultures are examined by picking small fragments of the aerial growth from the agar surface by means of a straight inoculating wire bent slightly at the end. Place material on slide in a drop of lactophenol cotton blue (p. 813), tease or spread out gently with dissecting needles and add coverglass. Gentle heating of such a preparation will drive out air bubbles and allow greater penetration of the stain.

12. FLETCHER'S MEDIUM FOR LEPTOSPIRA

Materials

12%	Sterile rabbit serum in sterile distilled water	100.0 ml
2%	Nutrient agar	7.5 ml

Procedure. 1. Heat rabbit serum solution to 50° C (122° F).

2. Add melted nutrient agar.

3. Tube in 5 ml quantities and sterilize by heating at 56° C (132.8° F) for 1 hour on 2 successive days.

4. Incubate for sterility.

5. Inoculate with 0.03 ml of blood and incubate at 30° C (86° F).

6. Examine for leptospira on a dark field microscope on the 7th, 14th, 21st and 28th day. Then discard.

Bacto-Stuart Medium Base together with Bacto-Leptospira Enrichment may be substituted for the above.

13. TISSUE AND CELL CULTURE METHODS FOR THE ISOLATION, CULTIVATION AND IDENTIFICATION OF VIRUSES AND FOR THE ASSAY OF VIRAL ANTIBODIES[25]

Cell or tissue culture methods are usually faster and more convenient and accurate than animal inoculation methods for the cultivation and identification of viruses. Different technical methods are now used in different laboratories, and a standard procedure has not yet evolved. In addition, procedures will vary, depending upon the suspected viral agent.

Use of mammalian cell cultures for virus studies was begun with cultures in the form of outgrowths from explanted tissue fragments. This simplest method of culture may still be employed for pilot studies of new systems to determine what particular tissue or cells support virus replication. Commonly, the virus diagnostic laboratory uses trypsin-dispersed renal tissue (from a variety of animals), human amnion cells, or one or more of the established cell lines, such as HeLa. Infected cell cultures are microscopically examined for specific cytopathic effects of virus as evidenced by cellular destruction or formation of inclusion bodies. The type of cellular changes is sometimes suggestive of a particular group of viruses. For identification of the virus, the neutralization of the specific cytopathogenic effect by known antiserum is used. Infected cells may also be identified by use of specific antiviral antibody coupled with fluorescein.

Cell cultures can also be used to assay antibody. The same basic principle that underlies any virus neutralization test is employed, namely, that antibody will specifically neutralize the infectivity of virus. In this case, serial dilutions of serum are added to replicate cell cultures. A standard amount of virus is added to the tubes. After sufficient time has elapsed to permit destruction of cells in control tubes, the titer of antibody is determined by noting the highest dilution of the serum that prevents destruction of cells. Metabolic inhibition tests may also be employed to assay for antibody. For example, the pH color test utilizes the fact that, with continued cellular growth in the presence of an immune serum-virus mixture, acidic products of metabolism lower the pH of the medium. This effect is readily observed by incorporating a pH indicator such as phenol red in the medium. Conversely, cell death induced by virus leaves the medium and pH indicator unchanged.

VIII. Serologic And Immunologic Methods[1, 3]

1. METHODS OF COLLECTING MATERIAL FOR LABORATORY DIAGNOSIS OF NEUROTROPIC VIRUS DISEASES

Blood for Complement-Fixation and Neutralization Tests. 1. As soon as possible after the onset of illness, then again after approximately 3 and 6 weeks, collect 20 ml blood samples using sterile precautions.

2. Whole blood may be shipped, except in areas where sustained temperatures over 37.8° C (100° F) prevail. However, serum is preferable.

3. In the latter case separate serum from blood using aseptic technique.

4. Blood is shipped in 30 ml vacuum tubes if collected in them; blood or serum, in sterile Wassermann tubes with sterile rubber or cork stoppers sealed with adhesive.

CAUTION: The specimen should not be frozen unless serum is submitted.

Specimens for Isolation of the Virus. *Blood.* 1. Withdraw 12 ml of blood in dry, sterile syringe and distribute equally in 3 sterile Pyrex Wassermann tubes. Stopper tubes with sterile corks and seal with adhesive tape or fire seal if equipment is available.

2. Freeze contents by immersing tubes in a mixture of alcohol and dry ice. Rotate tubes while freezing; this distributes the contents over a greater surface area and prevents breakage from expansion of fluid. Wrap the tube or tubes in cotton and pack carefully in a vacuum bottle. Fill remainder of vacuum bottle with small pieces of dry ice. (Dry ice may be broken up by wrapping it in a piece of cloth and then crushing with a hammer.)

CAUTION: Do not touch dry ice with fingers. Use a forceps or spoon to fill bottle. Cut a small V-shaped slot longitudinally in vacuum bottle cork or place a large bore venipuncture needle through center of cork to allow escape of gaseous CO_2. A tiny hole should also be punched in the outer metal cap of bottle.

3. Stopper bottle and pack carefully.

Spinal Fluid. About 3 ml of spinal fluid should be placed in each of 3 sterile Pyrex Wassermann tubes. Stopper, freeze, and label as directed for blood.

Brain and Cord. 1. As soon as possible after death remove brain, with sterile precautions, before thorax and abdomen are opened.

2. Take several generous blocks from (I) temporal lobe including hippocampus, (II) motor cortex, (III) midbrain, (IV) thalamus, (V) pons and medulla, (VI) cerebellum, and (VII) cervical spinal cord.

3. Blocks of tissue for virus studies may be shipped frozen in dry ice or unfrozen in sterile 50 per cent buffered glycerin solution (see below). Freezing is preferable. Individual blocks of tissue are placed in separate, small, wide-mouth sterile bottles without added fluid, stoppered with sterile corks and sealed with adhesive tape. Freeze and pack in vacuum bottle as described for blood.

If shipment cannot reach the laboratory within 24 to 36 hours, the tissues should be shipped in buffered 50 per cent glycerin in a sterile stoppered container.

Preparation of Sterile Buffered Glycerin. 1. Citric acid 21 gm in 1000 ml double distilled water.

2. Anhydrous Na_2HPO_4 28.4 gm to 1000 ml double distilled water.

3. Take 9.15 ml of (1) and 90.85 ml of (2) to make 100 ml of buffered solution pH 7.4.

4. Mix equal parts of (3) and C. P. glycerin; fill specimen bottles half full, stopper with corks and sterilize at 15 lb steam pressure for 30 minutes.

2. METHODS OF COLLECTING MATERIAL FOR LABORATORY DIAGNOSIS OF RICKETTSIAL INFECTIONS

Excised tissue blocks (such as brain or testis) and blood specimens are frozen and packed as described above for suspected virus infections.

3. THE WEIL-FELIX REACTION

Theoretical Considerations. The Weil-Felix reaction is based on the agglutination of the O variant of certain strains of *Proteus X.* These strains appear in two growth phases designated as H (Ger. *Haut*) and O (Ger. *ohne Haut*). The H motile, flagellar form spreads rapidly over the surface of the medium; the O or nonmotile variant of the organism is used for the agglutination reaction, since it is this antigen that reacts "specifically" with sera from certain typhuslike rickettsial diseases. The H or motile variants will be agglutinated by many normal sera.

The three type strains of *Proteus X* in general use are X-2, X-19 and X-K.

The first two were isolated from the urine of patients ill with classic typhus: They originally appeared in the O phase. The origin of X-K is not entirely clear and was received by Dr. Kingsbury in Malaya from the National Type Cultures in London (the K denoting the so-called Kingsbury strain). An additional strain, X-L, isolated by Dr. Lima in an endemic center of "exanthematic typhus" at São Paulo, Brazil, is also frequently used. According to Felix this strain is of the X-19 type but also produces agglutinins for X-K, which is not true of the original X-19 strain.

X-19 is of the greatest diagnostic importance in louse-borne and flea-borne typhus.

X-K is the only strain agglutinated in the scrub typhus group.

In the Weil-Felix reaction for the spotted fever group, OX-2 as well as OX-19 should be used, as some sera agglutinate only the X-2 strain, and not frequently the agglutinin titer for OX-2 is as high as or higher than for OX-19.

Strains of *Proteus X* have also been recovered from the brain, bone marrow, spleen, liver, kidney, bile and heart blood. The organism is considered by Felix as the cultivable saprophytic stage of the specific infecting agent.

Cultivation of Proteus X Strains. The strains should be carried on fresh meat infusion agar adjusted to pH 6.8. All strains are in some degree unstable, i.e. there is a tendency to an O – OH (nonmotile to motile) reversion. This is most marked in the X-K strain and least in the X-2. Excess moisture hastens the reversion. Consequently, it is of greatest importance that all O variants be carried on a medium from which excess moisture has been removed by drying in the incubator for several days. To assure H variants, on the other hand, it is just as important that the medium have its full moisture content. Although media made from dehydrated preparations support a fairly heavy growth, cultures carried on such media may show a decreased agglutinability. It is essential that the antigens have been examined prior to routine use for reactivity with human antisera from individuals convalescent from spotted fever group and typhus group infections, as well as with normal human sera.

The Test. In the usual macroscopic tube test 0.5 ml of serial serum dilutions, 1:10, 1:20, and so on, are placed in a series of agglutination tubes and 0.5 ml of a 24-hour suspension of organisms killed by alcohol, phenol, formalin or by heat and standardized to MacFarland nephelometer reading No. 3 or to a "500" silica standard are added to each tube, thereby doubling the dilutions. The rack is shaken gently, placed at 37° C (98° F) for 2 hours and stored in the refrigerator for 48 hours. Twenty-four hours at refrigerator temperature gives only a slightly lower reading. Control sera should include normal human serum and known positive human convalescent serum containing the appropriate rickettsial antibodies.

The O agglutination results in a fine granular deposit often adhering to the walls of the tube. The H agglutination appears in large flocculi and is massed at the bottom of the tube.

Interpretation. Normal sera may show a low agglutinin titer for OX-K or OX-19, seldom for OX-2. If 2 or more successive serum samples are available, a sharp rise in titer is of definite significance. As a rule, serum taken during the first week will not show a titer higher than 1:80 or 1:160. This titer will then serve as a basis for later tests. When possible, second and third samples should be tested, the second taken on or about the tenth day, and the third at the end of the second or during the third week of the disease, or during early convalescence.

It must be remembered that, as in any serologic test, the Weil-Felix reaction is only an aid to diagnosis. It is only a part of the picture and should be interpreted as such. An occasional serum may show a relatively high titer in the absence of any apparent rickettsial infection.

Sera of infected guinea pigs do not give a Weil-Felix reaction.

4. METHODS OF COLLECTING MATERIAL FOR LABORATORY DIAGNOSIS OF SPIROCHETAL INFECTIONS

Blood. *Spirillum minus* of rat-bite fever does not live long after blood has been drawn, so animal inoculations have to be made almost immediately. The relapsing fever spirochetes and *Leptospira icterohemorrhagiae*, however, remain viable for a long time in sterile drawn blood, so that samples of whole blood for animal inoculation may be taken at the height of the febrile reaction and shipped in 30 ml vacuum collecting tubes or in sterile Wassermann tubes as described above for blood for complement fixation and neutralization tests in neurotropic viruses. Refrigeration, but not freezing, of the blood samples is recommended. When the samples reach the laboratory, grind clot in a mortar in physiologic salt solution under sterile conditions and inoculate into mice or other experimental animals.

Cerebrospinal Fluid. In cases of relapsing fever and *Leptospira icterohemorrhagiae* infection showing meningeal symptoms, the cerebrospinal fluid may contain spirochetes. Like blood, it is collected aseptically and shipped in sterile tubes to the laboratory where it is centrifuged for a half hour at 2000 rpm and the sediment examined in the dark field for spirochetes.

5. FORMOL-GEL TEST FOR KALA-AZAR (AFTER NAPIER)

This is a test for euglobulin, which is increased in kala-azar as well as in some other diseases.

The test in kala-azar is not ordinarily of diagnostic value until after the third to fifth month of the disease, and the reaction may remain positive for about 4 months after recovery.

Procedure. To 1 ml of clear serum of the patient add 1 or 2 drops full strength commercial formalin.

If serum becomes solidified and opaque like boiled egg white within 15 minutes, it is read as a strong positive. If a similar result is obtained within 24 hours, the reaction is still considered positive. If serum solidifies without becoming altogether opaque, the interpretation is doubtful. When serum remains clear it is read as a negative even though solidification occurs.

6. PRECIPITIN TEST TO DETERMINE SOURCE OF MOSQUITO BLOOD MEALS

1. Collect engorged female mosquitoes early in morning. Transport to laboratory in vials kept iced in vacuum jug.

2. Kill mosquito by chloroforming; place it on its back, head pointing away. With a small curved tissue forceps take hold

of mosquito near anterior end of abdomen and push lower abdomen against a small strip of filter paper of the harder sort (as Whatman No. 5), rupturing abdomen wall and stomach in such a manner that blood will be spread and absorbed by paper.

3. Write pertinent data as to date and place of collecting on remainder of the strip of filter paper.

4. Store strips in dry, cool, insect-proof place until tests can be made.

5. Cut off blood spot on filter paper into 2 to 3 ml of physiologic salt solution, and allow to soak for 1 hour at room temperature, shaking from time to time. If blood spot is unusually small, a smaller amount of saline solution should be used. It is not necessary to filter this solution but it should stand a while before the supernatant fluid is drawn off for precipitin test.

6. A few cubic millimeters of diluted, previously prepared antihuman serum is carefully pipetted into a small serum tube so as not to wet the sides above the serum level.

The dilution of the antihuman serum depends on its known titer. If the titer is from 3000 to 4000, a titer rarely attained in the rabbit, the serum should be diluted about 1:7. Sera of lower titer are diluted correspondingly.

7. The supernatant fluid from (5) is carefully layered onto the antihuman serum.

8. A cloudiness or opalescence at the interphase of the two fluids denotes a positive precipitin test, indicating that the mosquito had probably bitten man.

9. If the reaction does not occur immediately, inspect for 1 hour at intervals of 10 minutes.

10. Similar tests can be made with antihorse sera, antipig sera, and the like.

7. SERODIAGNOSIS OF PARASITIC DISEASES

Numerous immunodiagnostic tests for parasitic diseases are available for diagnostic purposes. A list of those which have been evaluated follows:

*1. Amebiasis	CF IH L
2. Chagas' Disease	CF IH IFA
3. African Trypanosomiasis	P
4. Leishmaniasis	ID CF IH P
5. Malaria	IFA
6. Toxoplasmosis	ID CF IH IFA
7. Ascariasis	BF IH
8. Filariasis	CF BF IH
9. Toxocariasis	CF BF IH
10. Trichinosis	ID CF BF IH L IFA P
11. Clonorchiasis	ID CF IH
12. Fascioliasis	CF IH
13. Paragonimiasis	ID CF
14. Schistosomiasis	ID CF IH IFA
15. Cysticercosis	CF IH
16. Echinococcosis	ID CF BF IH L IFA

For details of the tests, discussion of their sensitivity and specificity, and a listing of sources of antigen see Kagan and Norman.[1]

Commercial kits are available for some of these procedures. Their diagnostic application and usefulness vary and must be interpreted in conjunction with the individual clinical situation.

For details of the circumoval precipitin test for schistosomiasis see Reference 26 (p. 842).

8. REFERENCE DIAGNOSTIC SERVICES IN PARASITOLOGY TO STATE HEALTH DEPARTMENT LABORATORIES PERFORMED BY THE CENTER FOR DISEASE CONTROL OF THE PUBLIC HEALTH SERVICE (ATLANTA, GEORGIA 30333)†

1. Echinococcosis
2. Amebiasis
3. Toxoplasmosis

*ID, intradermal; CF, complement-fixation; BF, bentonite flocculation; IH, indirect hemagglutination; L, latex; IFA, indirect fluorescent antibody; P, precipitin.

†Specimens of serum must be sent to the local State Health Department Laboratory, which will transmit them to the CDC. The diagnostic specimens must not be sent to the CDC directly by the physician. The local health unit should be contacted regarding the procedure for collection of the specimens to be submitted.

4. Chagas' disease
5. Filariasis
6. Schistosomiasis
7. Cysticercosis
8. Trichinosis
9. Leishmaniasis
10. Visceral larva migrans
11. Strongyloidiasis
12. Paragonimiasis
13. Fascioliasis

IX. Miscellaneous

1. PARASITE COUNTS IN MALARIA (AFTER WILCOX)[2]

Procedure. There are both thick smear and thin smear methods of enumerating malaria parasites, but the former is recommended even for relatively inexperienced workers.

1. Make a thick smear at the same time the blood is drawn for a white count.
2. Fix and stain the thick film.
3. Count 100 white cells (or multiples of 100) on the thick film.
4. Count the malaria parasites seen in the same microscopic fields with the white cells.
5. Calculate the parasites per cubic millimeter of blood as below.

2. EXAMINATION OF FEMALE ANOPHELINE MOSQUITOES FOR MALARIAL PARASITES[27]

It is desirable under certain conditions to know whether mosquitoes contain oocysts on the stomach wall or whether the salivary glands contain sporozoites.

Procedure. 1. Kill female mosquitoes a few at a time with chloroform, carbon tetrachloride or tobacco smoke and identify species. It may be desirable to mount identical specimens for subsequent confirmation.

2. Do not dissect recently engorged mosquitoes. Remove legs and wings, dip quickly into 35 to 50 per cent alcohol and place at edge of drop of physiologic saline with head pointing away.

3. *Stomach Dissection.* Nick both sides of body wall of next to last abdominal segment so as partially to sever chitinous wall.

4. Transfix posterior thorax with needle, placing free needle on partially severed terminal abdominal segments, and exert gentle intermittent traction to draw out stomach, attached malpighian tubules and ovaries.

5. Carefully set aside thorax and head of mosquito in saline for subsequent examination.

6. Sever gut posterior to stomach, discarding attached malpighian tubules, intestine, ovaries and debris; transfer to a clean drop and carefully lower coverglass onto stomach.

7. Examine stomach wall for oocysts, which may be recognized as follows:

a. *Young oocysts* are clear, round, oval

$$\frac{x \text{ (No. of parasites per cu mm)}}{\text{White cell count per cu mm}} = \frac{\text{No. of parasites counted in the same fields with 100 white cells}}{\text{No. of white cells counted (100 in this case)}}$$

x = No. of parasites per cu mm of blood

Example:

$$\frac{x}{4000} = \frac{1200}{100}$$

$$100x = 4{,}800{,}000$$

$$x = 48{,}000$$

bodies, 6 to 12 μm in diameter, are more refractile than stomach cells, and contain minute pigment granules.

b. *Intermediate oocysts* are denser than stomach cells, 12 to 40 μm in diameter, and contain clumps of pigment.

c. *Mature oocysts* are 30 to 80 μm in diameter, show fine striations owing to enormous numbers of attenuated, spindle-shaped sporozoites, and are 12 to 44 μm in length. Pigment granules are not readily visible.

CAUTION: Protruding unpigmented stomach cells may be confused with immature oocysts of *Plasmodium.*

8. *Salivary Gland Dissection* (after Hunter, et al.).[27] Place head and thorax (or entire mosquito with wings and legs removed if it is being examined only for sporozoites) in a drop of physiologic saline tinted with methylene blue, with body pointing away.

9. Exert gentle pressure on anterior thorax so that neck bulges slightly, place second needle behind head and draw away from thorax.

10. Transfer head and attached tissue to a fresh drop of saline and search for blue-stained salivary glands under dissecting binocular or hand lens.

11. Tease out one or both trilobed glands and transfer carefully to a fresh drop on same side; gently lower coverglass.

12. Examine all 3 lobes of each gland carefully under a high dry lens for the characteristic sporozoites. If necessary confirm with oil immersion objective.

13. Crush glands by exerting pressure on cover with clean instrument; search again.

14. If glands are positive, remove coverglass and allow material on it and slide to dry. Fix both in methyl alcohol and stain with Giemsa's or Wright's stain. If desired, coverglass may be mounted smear side up on slide. Examine with high dry and oil immersion objective for sporozoites, which appear as slender blue-staining spindles with a central red chromatin dot.

3. EXAMINATION OF MOSQUITOES FOR FILARIAL WORMS

In areas where filariasis is endemic it is sometimes desirable to dissect mosquitoes to determine the per cent infected.

Procedure. 1. Proceed as in Steps 1 and 2 above.

2. Sever head and place in separate drop of saline. Carefully dissect thorax, teasing all tissues apart, add coverglass and examine for developing parasites.

3. Carefully dissect proboscis and head for presence of infective larvae, which are usually 0.1 mm or more in length.

4. MOUNTING ENTOMOLOGIC SPECIMENS FOR STUDY[28, 29]

Whole Mounts. Mosquito larvae, lice, fleas, mites, bedbugs and other small specimens not too heavily pigmented are usually cleared and mounted on glass slides for study by transmitted light. The following procedure, applicable specifically to mosquito larvae, may be modified, as necessary, for other forms:

Use of Potassium Hydroxide. Opaque or heavily chitinized specimens may require preliminary soaking in a 10 per cent solution of potassium hydroxide. Such treatment takes from a few minutes to several hours, depending on the condition of the specimens.

Mounting in Balsam. 1. Kill larvae by dropping into hot water (65.6 to 71.1° C or 150 to 160° F).

2. Dehydrate in alcohol as follows:

50% alcohol – 15 minutes
70% alcohol – 15 minutes
85% alcohol – 15 minutes
95% alcohol – 15 minutes
absolute alcohol – 10 minutes

(These time intervals are minimal – longer periods in each alcohol may result in better preparations.)

3. Clear in creosote, clove oil or xylene for approximately 10 minutes.

4. Mount in balsam under a coverglass.

This technique produces good permanent mounts.

If Euparal is used, the procedure is the same except that specimens do not require clearing but may be mounted directly from absolute alcohol.

Mounting in Berlese's Medium

FORMULA:

Gum arabic	8 gm
Water (distilled)	8 ml
Glycerin	5 ml
Chloral hydrate	70 gm
Glacial acetic acid	3 ml

Dissolve gum arabic in water and add other ingredients in order. Strain through muslin before use.

PROCEDURE. Specimens may be mounted in Berlese's medium directly from water, or if preserved in alcohol may be mounted after rinsing in water. The permanency of the mount may be increased by ringing the coverslip with a non-water-soluble material such as balsam or clear fingernail lacquer.

Mounting in Hoyer's Medium. This modification of Berlese's medium is now widely used by acarologists for mounting small, delicate mites after clearing in lactophenol.

FORMULAE

Lactophenol		*Hoyer's Medium*	
Lactic acid	50 pts	Distilled water	50 gm
Phenol crystals	25 pts	Gum arabic (crystals)	30 gm
Distilled water	25 pts	Chloral hydrate	200 gm
		Glycerin	20 gm

The Hoyer's medium is mixed and strained as noted for Berlese's medium above.

PROCEDURE. This is the same as for Berlese's medium after clearing for several hours in lactophenol and several rinses in water.

Maggots. Only the mouth hooks and posterior spiracles of most maggots are dissected off and mounted.

Ticks. Larval ticks may be punctured, cleared and slide mounted as above. Nymphs and adults are best preserved for study unmounted in 70 per cent alcohol as noted for large specimens below.

Pinned Specimens. Adult specimens of mosquitoes, flies, bees, wasps, ants, beetles, bugs and other groups may be mounted on insect pins in any of several ways. Such specimens require no special preservation and if kept in pest-proof boxes remain suitable for study for many years. The following techniques are recommended:

1. For larger insects (except COLEOPTERA), direct impalement through center of thorax is the most desirable procedure. Specimen is pushed up to within 1/4 inch of pinhead. This allows ample room below for small labels on which are written date and place of collection, collector's name and other pertinent data.

2. For beetles procedure is same, save that pin passes through base of right elytron (wing cover).

3. For smaller forms two techniques are employed:

   a. With small bugs, beetles and other species characterized by fairly rigid chitin and absence of body hair, use of small cardboard points is preferred. Thrust pin through broader end of point; add a small drop of shellac or similar material to fasten extremity of point to right side of insect's thorax.

   b. With more delicate forms possessing an abundance of hair on wings or body, very fine pins, termed "minuten nadeln," are recommended. Minuten, which are approximately 1/2 inch in length, are thrust up through one end of a small bit of cork, balsa wood or especially prepared cardboard which in turn is impaled on a standard pin in the usual manner. The point of the minuten is usually thrust up through the specimen from below, though some prefer insects be mounted in a lateral position.

Fluid Preservation of Large Specimens. Most ticks, spiders, scorpions, centipedes and larger larvae of all types do not lend themselves either to pinning or to mounting on slides. These are best preserved in vials containing 70 per cent alcohol or 4 per cent formaldehyde. For study they may be transferred to a watch glass and examined with a hand lens or binocular microscope.

REFERENCES

1. Lennette, E. H., Spaulding, E. H., and Truant, J. P. (eds.). 1974. Manual of Clinical Microbiology. 2nd ed. American Society for Microbiology, Washington, D.C. 970 pp.
2. Wilcox, A. 1960. Manual for the Microscopical Diagnosis of Malaria in Man. 3rd ed. P.H.S. Publication No. 796, Washington, D.C. 80 pp.
3. Bauer, J. D., Ackermann, P. G., and Toro, G. 1968. Bray's Clinical Laboratory Methods. The C. V. Mosby Co., St. Louis. 764 pp.
4. Russell, P. F., West, L. S., Manwell, R. D., and Macdonald, G. 1963. Practical Malariology. 2nd ed. Oxford University Press, New York. 750 pp.
5. Knott, J. 1935. The periodicity of the microfilaria of *Wuchereria bancrofti.* Preliminary report of some infection experiments. Trans. Roy. Soc. Trop. Med. Hyg. *29*:59–64.
6. Wylie, J. P. 1970. Detection of microfilariae by a filter technique. J. Am. Vet. Med. Assoc. *156*:1403–1405.
7. Rippon, J. W. 1974. Medical Mycology: The Pathogenic Fungi and the Pathogenic Actinomycetes. W. B. Saunders Co., Philadelphia. 587 pp.
8. Brooke, M. M. 1958. Amebiasis. Methods in Laboratory Diagnosis. U.S.P.H.S., Communicable Disease Center, Atlanta. 67 pp.
9. Wheatley, W. B. 1951. Rapid stain for intestinal amebae and flagellates. Am. J. Clin. Pathol. *21*:990–991.
10. Beal, C. B., Viens, P., Grant, R., and Hughes, J. 1970. Technique for sampling duodenal contents. Am. J. Trop. Med. Hyg. *19*:349–352.
11. Thomas, G. E., Goldsmid, J., and Wicks, A. 1974. Use of the enterotest duodenal capsule in the diagnosis of giardiasis. S. Afr. Med. J. *48*:2219–2220.
12. Sapero, J. J., and Lawless, D. K. 1953. The MIF stain preservation technique for the identification of intestinal protozoa. Am. J. Trop. Med. Hyg. *2*:613–619.
13. Faust, E. C., Russell, P. F., and Jung, R. C. 1970. Craig and Faust's Clinical Parasitology. 8th ed. Lea & Febiger, Philadelphia. 890 pp.
14. Ritchie, L. S. 1948. An ether sedimentation technique for routine stool examinations. Bull. U.S. Army Med. Dept. *8*:326.
15. Spencer, F. M., and Monroe, L. S. 1961. The Color Atlas of Intestinal Parasites. Charles C Thomas, Springfield, Illinois. 142 pp.
16. Hunter, G. W., III, Hodges, E. P., Jahnes, W. G., Diamond, L. S., and Ingalls, J. W., Jr. 1948. Studies on schistosomiasis. II. Summary of further studies on methods of recovering eggs of *S. japonicum* from stools. Bull. U.S. Army Med. Dept. *8*:128–131.
17. Parfitt, J. W. 1958. A technique for the enumeration of helminth eggs and protozoan cysts in feces from farm animals in Britain. Laboratory Practice. *7*:353–355.
18. Kato, K., and Mura, M. 1954. Comparative examinations. Jap. J. Parasitol. *3*:35. [Text in Japanese]
19. Stoll, N. R. 1961. Dilution egg counting for hookworm, *Ascaris. Trichuris,* etc. W.H.O. Mimeogr. Rept. 7 pp.
20. Beaver, P. C. 1950. The standardization of fecal smears for estimating egg production and worm burden. J. Parasit. *36*:451–456.
21. Deas, J., and Abadie, S. H. 1974. Iron gallein as a substitute for iron hematoxylin in parasitological staining. J. Parasit. *60*:1036.
22. Garcia, L. S., and Ash, L. R. 1975. Diagnostic Parasitology—Clinical Laboratory Manual. The C. V. Mosby Co., St. Louis. 110 pp.
23. Bodily, H. L., Updyke, E. L., and Mason, J. O. (eds.). 1970. *In* American Public Health Association. Coordinating Committee on Laboratory Methods. Diagnostic Procedures for Bacterial, Mycotic and Parasitic Infections; Technics for the Laboratory Diagnosis and Control of the Communicable Diseases. 5th ed. American Public Health Association, Inc., New York. 898 pp.
24. Hsieh, H. C. 1961. Employment of a test-tube filter-paper method for the diagnosis of *Ancylostoma duodenale, Necator americanus* and *Strongyloides stercoralis.* W.H.O. Mimeogr. Rept. 5 pp.
25. Lennette, E. H., and Schmidt, N. J. (eds.). 1969. Diagnostic Procedures for Viral and Rickettsial Infections. 4th ed. American Public Health Association, Inc., New York. 978 pp.
26. Newsome, J. 1964. Investigation of antischistosome opsonins in vivo. Trans. Roy. Soc. Trop. Med. Hyg. *58*:58–62.
27. Hunter, G. W., III, Weller, T. H., and Jahnes, W. G., Jr. 1946. An outline for teaching mosquito stomach and salivary gland dissection. Am. J. Trop. Med. *26*:221–228.
28. Middlekauff, W. W. 1944. A rapid method for making permanent mounts of mosquito larvae. Science. *99*:206.
29. Fairchild, G. B., and Hertig, M. 1948. An improved method for mounting small insects. Science. *108*:20–21.

Appendix

Distribution of Selected Communicable Diseases in the Tropical and Subtropical Areas of the World

ANNA C. GELMAN

This gazetteer includes the tropical and subtropical countries of the world classified according to contiguous geographic subdivisions which have similar disease patterns. The countries have been designated by their current names, footnotes indicating recent changes. References to disease occurrence and distribution are made in terms of current names.

Many of the diseases described in this book have been reported with varying degrees of frequency from the United States of America and do not normally pose a problem in recognition. They have been included in this gazetteer because it is possible for returning travelers, Peace Corps volunteers, business representatives, diplomats and missionaries, as well as foreign visitors or immigrants, to contract them elsewhere and to enter the United States before detectable signs and symptoms have appeared.

Other diseases have been included that may occur only infrequently or not at all in the United States. They may not be readily diagnosed unless a travel history has been elicited by a physician familiar with the geographic distribution of such diseases.

It is recognized that the reporting of communicable or other diseases is usually far from complete both here and abroad. Reported cases and special surveys offer, at best, a minimal estimate of the distribution of the various diseases. The data presented here are based primarily on the contents of the individual chapters of this book, on reports and publications of the World Health Organization and the Pan American Health Organization and on the most recent edition of the American Public Health Association publication *The Control of Communicable Diseases in Man.*

The new names of countries have been derived from publications of the United States Government Printing Office, and from information printed in the New York Times and the Official Associated Press Almanac 1973.

I. AMERICA

A. CENTRAL AMERICA, MEXICO, PANAMA

Belize, Canal Zone, Costa Rica, El Salvador, Guatemala, Honduras, Mexico, Nicaragua and Panama*

Helminth Diseases

Ancylostomiasis (hookworm) is widely reported from most of these countries. In 1963 Mexico reported 26,129 cases, the other countries a total of 6576. Helminth surveys conducted between 1950 and 1962 confirmed the presence of other intestinal

*Formerly British Honduras.

nematode infections, including **ascariasis, trichuriasis** and **strongyloidiasis** in the Canal Zone, Costa Rica, Honduras and Mexico.

Hydatid disease is endemic among the animals in Costa Rica, Guatemala and Nicaragua. In 1963 there were 6318 cases reported in swine in Guatemala and 278 in animals in Nicaragua. In 1972 there were 22 cases of human hydatidosis reported from Guatemala, 6 from Honduras and 1 from Panama (1971).

Helminth infections other than those named above that have been found in Central America are **visceral larva migrans** in Mexico, and infections with *Hymenolepis nana* in Costa Rica, Guatemala and Mexico. **Taeniasis,** endemic in Mexico, also occurs in Costa Rica, Guatemala and Honduras. **Trichinosis** occurs in Mexico and El Salvador, and **fascioliasis** in Mexico.

Dipylidiasis has been found in Guatemala, **schistosome cercarial dermatitis** in El Salvador and Mexico, and **sparganosis** in Belize. **Paragonimiasis** has been reported from the Canal Zone, Honduras, Costa Rica, El Salvador and Mexico.

Mosquito-borne filariasis, or **filariasis bancrofti,** occurs in a Caribbean coastal area of Costa Rica. **Filariasis ozzardi,** the midge-borne variety that is confined to the Western Hemisphere, has been found in Mexico (Yucatan) and Panama. **Onchocerciasis,** transmitted by the blackfly, is endemic in Guatemala; 6232 cases were reported in 1963. There is another focus in Mexico, from which 166 cases were reported in 1963. The 1958 to 1962 median in Mexico was 1855 cases. **Dipetalonemiasis,** midge-transmitted, has been reported from Panama.

Protozoan Diseases

Amebiasis, together with bacillary dysentery and other unspecified diarrheas, is endemic and widespread. In 1972 some 63,000 cases of amebiasis were reported from this region. Mexico alone provided some 48,000 of these, Honduras 7767 and El Salvador 4500. Other intestinal protozoan infections are also present.

Leishmaniasis (*Lutzomyia*-transmitted) is endemic in Mexico (Yucatan), Belize and Guatemala. It is present in the mucocutaneous form **chiclero ulcer** (*Leishmania mexicana*), and rarely in the visceral form. In 1963, 5 of the countries reported cases of unspecified leishmaniasis. Among these Costa Rica had 594 cases and Panama 111 cases. Guatemala, Honduras and Mexico also reported leishmaniasis in 1963.

Malaria is still a continuing problem. Although eradication programs are far advanced in Belize, Costa Rica, Panama and Canal Zone, and some urban areas have been declared free of risk of contracting malaria, collectively in 1974 these countries reported almost 100,000 cases of malaria. Among the countries responsible for many cases, El Salvador with some 67,000 cases. Mexico with some 175,000 cases and Nicaragua with some 5975 cases showed a noticeable increase over 1973.

Trypanosomiasis, the American variety, or **Chagas' disease** (transmitted by cone-nosed bugs) is widely distributed, although the reporting is of low frequency. In the 4-year period 1969 to 1972, there were 626 cases reported from El Salvador, 2 from Guatemala, 53 from Honduras and 67 from Panama. Seropositive cases with cardiopathy occur in Costa Rica.

Fungal Diseases

Tinea tonsurans and **tinea favosa** have been found in Mexico; **tinea imbricata** has been reported from Guatemala. Other mycotic diseases found in this region are **South American blastomycosis,** especially in Mexico; **coccidioidomycosis,** which occurs in Guatemala, Honduras and Mexico; and **histoplasmosis,** which has been found in the Canal Zone, Costa Rica, Belize, Guatemala and Honduras.

Bacterial Diseases

Anthrax has been reported from these countries. In 1972 El Salvador reported 35 cases, Guatemala 34, Mexico 20, and the Canal Zone 2 (1971).

Brucellosis is endemic among cattle in Costa Rica, El Salvador, Honduras, Nicaragua, Mexico and Panama. Sporadic human cases have been reported from most of these countries; however, in the first 5 months of 1973 Mexico reported 777 cases, 19 of which were in Juarez.

Bacillary dysentery or **shigellosis,** together with amebiasis and unspecified diarrheas, is endemic. In 1972 more than 15,000 cases were reported from this area.

Leptospirosis is present and is reported sporadically.

Leprosy is endemic in all of this area. In 1973 there were some 15,500 cases in the leprosy registers of these countries. Mexico alone accounted for more than 13,856. In 1972 there were some 792 newly identified cases reported from these countries.

Louse-borne relapsing fever has been reported. **Tick-borne relapsing fever** is present in Guatemala, Panama and Mexico.

The endemic treponematosis **pinta,** which is confined to areas of Latin America, is endemic in Mexico and affects large numbers of people. In 1962 there were 526 new cases reported. It has also been found in El Salvador, Guatemala, Honduras, Nicaragua and Panama.

Yaws has not been reported from most of Central America since 1955. In 1969, however, one case was reported from Panama and in 1970 one from Guatemala.

Typhoid fever is endemic. In 1974 the total reported from all the countries was approximately 4400.

Rickettsial Diseases

Epidemic typhus has been sporadically reported from this area. Between November 1971 and January 1972 there was an outbreak of **louse-borne typhus fever** involving 42 people in a small Indian village in northwest Guatemala. The last reported case for Mexico (8 cases) was in 1969. One case was reported by Costa Rica in 1974. **Murine** or **endemic typhus** is endemic in this area and has been reported from almost all these countries within the past decade.

Tick-borne spotted fevers have occurred in Panama and Mexico.

Viral Diseases

Arthropod-borne (arbo) virus infections are endemic in this region. Mosquito-borne encephalitides, including **western equine encephalitis, eastern equine encephalitis, Venezuelan equine encephalitis** and **St. Louis encephalitis,** are known to be present. In 1971 and 1972 there was an outbreak of arbovirus encephalitis in Mexico involving a total of 8695 reported cases (VEE was isolated); in these same years Belize reported 4, Costa Rica 22, Honduras 54 and Panama 7. *Phlebotomus*-transmitted **Changuinola fever** virus and mosquito borne **Ilheus virus** have also been found. **Sylvan yellow fever** periodically enters Panama from South America: in 1974, 4 cases were reported from the Province of Panama, district Chepo. Between 1951 and 1958 cases were reported from Central American countries.

Infectious hepatitis occurred in all of these countries in 1974. There were some 9000 cases reported in that year.

Rabies is endemic in this area. Cases are reported annually in both animals and humans. By August of 1974 there were 6 cases of **human rabies** reported in El Salvador and 4 in Guatemala, 2 in Honduras, 21 in Mexico and 2 in Nicaragua. **Animal rabies** had also been reported from these countries with a total of 2324 infections diagnosed in animals; laboratory-confirmed cases occurred in dogs, cats, cows and other domestic animals. In Panama there were also isolates from squirrels and a bat in 1963. Bats were found infected in the Canal Zone in 1963.

Trachoma is endemic in almost all of this region and is reported sporadically from many of the countries.

B. CARIBBEAN ISLANDS (WEST INDIES)

Barbados, Cuba, the Dominican Republic, Haiti, Jamaica, Trinidad and Tobago; British Antigua, the Bahamas, Bermuda, Dominica, Grenada, Montserrat, St. Lucia, St. Kitts, Nevis, Anguilla, St. Vincent, and many smaller islands; French Guadeloupe and Martinique; Netherlands Antilles; Puerto Rico and Virgin Islands

Helminth Diseases

Ancylostomiasis (hookworm) is widely reported from most of the West Indies. The presence of **ascariasis, trichuriasis, taeniasis, strongyloidiasis** and **hymenolepiasis nana** has been confirmed through recent surveys. In addition, **hymenolepiasis diminuta** has been found in Cuba, Grenada and Martinique; **sparganosis,** in Puerto Rico; **schistosome cercarial dermatitis,** in the West Indies; and **fascioliasis,** in Cuba. In 1962 cases of **filariasis** were reported from the Virgin Islands, Haiti, Trinidad and Tobago, Antigua, and St. Kitts: **filariasis bancrofti** is present throughout the West Indies, and **filariasis ozzardi** has occurred in Puerto Rico, St. Vincent and Dominica.

Dipetalonemiasis has been identified in Trinidad and Tobago.

Schistosomiasis is endemic in most of this area. In 1972, 68 cases were reported from Puerto Rico, 207 from the Dominican Republic, 432 from St. Lucia and 132 from Guadeloupe. Cases that occur in New York City are almost invariably traced to Puerto Rico or other of the West Indies.

Protozoan Diseases

Amebiasis is present in the Caribbean. It may be reported in conjunction with bacillary dysentery and other diarrheal diseases and not differentiated from them. However, in 1972 Cuba reported 2625 cases and Haiti 2410; proportionately fewer cases were reported from the other islands. Other intestinal protozoan infections are also present.

Malaria has virtually disappeared from the West Indies except for the island shared by Haiti and the Dominican Republic. In 1974 there were approximately 19,000 cases reported from Haiti and 248 from the Dominican Republic. These cases were being reported from rural areas.

Trypanosomiasis has been identified in Trinidad and Tobago.

Bacterial Diseases

Anthrax occurs among animals and humans in the West Indies. In 1972 there were 41 cases reported from Haiti and 11 from the U.S. Virgin Islands.

Brucellosis is present and occasionally reported from Cuba, Dominica, Puerto Rico, and the U.S. Virgin Islands.

Bacillary dysentery or **shigellosis** is endemic.

Between 1969 and 1972 **leptospirosis** was reported from Barbados, Puerto Rico, Haiti, Jamaica, Dominica, Trinidad and Tobago, St. Vincent and Guadeloupe.

Leprosy is present and reported from most of the West Indies. In 1972–1973 there were some 9268 cases in the active leprosy registers of the West Indies, and 662 new cases reported from 15 of them.

Endemic treponematoses occur in the West Indies. Cases of **pinta** have been reported from Cuba, Puerto Rico, Guadeloupe, the Virgin Islands, Haiti and the Dominican Republic.

Yaws is still occurring in the Caribbean. In 1972 cases were still being reported from the Dominican Republic, Haiti, Jamaica, Trinidad and Tobago, Dominica, Grenada, St. Lucia and St. Vincent.

Tetanus is reported from many of the Caribbean countries. The largest numbers of cases in 1972 were 384 from Haiti, 151 from Cuba, 11 from the Dominican Republic and 72 from Jamaica. A few cases were reported by each of the following as well: Barbados, Dominica, Grenada, Guadeloupe, Martinique, St. Lucia, St. Vincent and Puerto Rico.

Typhoid and **paratyphoid fevers** are endemic and are reported from most of the islands. In 1974, 1447 cases were reported from the following: Cuba, Haiti, the Dominican Republic, and to a lesser extent other islands.

Rickettsial Diseases

Murine typhus is present in the West Indies.

Viral Diseases

Between 1963 and 1972 there were some 700 cases of arthropod-borne **viral encephalitis** reported from Cuba, Dominica, Haiti, Jamaica, Trinidad and Tobago (EEE isolated in 1970), Bahamas, St. Lucia, St. Kitts, St. Vincent, and Puerto Rico. The viruses involved have been primarily mosquito-transmitted **eastern equine encephalitis** and **Venezuelan equine encephalitis. Caraparu, Guama, Catu, Oropouche, Mayaro** and **Ilheus fever,** caused by mosquito-transmitted viruses, have occurred in Trinidad.

Dengue fever occurs in epidemic and endemic forms in those areas still infested with *Aedes aegypti* mosquitoes, the vector. An outbreak that began in 1963–1964 is continuing and progressing. Puerto Rico has had three major outbreaks, one in 1963 affecting the northern part of the island, one in 1969 with the south primarily affected, and one in 1973 affecting primarily an area of the southwest. Other islands affected during this outbreak included Antigua, Barbados, Dominica, Dominican Republic, Grenada, Guadeloupe, Haiti, Jamaica, Martinique, Montserrat, Netherlands Antilles, St. Kitts, Nevis and Anguilla, St. Lucia, St. Vincent, and the British Virgin Islands.

Infectious hepatitis was reported from most of the West Indies in 1972. Cuba had the greatest number of cases, 14,294, and the Dominican Republic 850. Other figures reported were relatively low, some 200 cases in the other Caribbean islands.

There were a few cases of **human rabies** reported from Cuba, the Dominican Republic, Grenada and Haiti in 1971 and 1972.

Trachoma was reported in 1962 from the Dominican Republic and Haiti.

C. TROPICAL SOUTH AMERICA

Bolivia, Brazil, Colombia, Ecuador, French Guiana, Guyana, Peru, Surinam (Dutch Guiana) and Venezuela*

Helminth Diseases

Ancylostomiasis (hookworm) is endemic in most of South America. In 1962 Colombia reported more than 50,000 cases and Venezuela 232,000. The next year Peru reported 2721 cases. It has been estimated that in Surinam 20 to 30 per cent of the population are infected. There is evidence of its presence in Guyana, Brazil and French Guiana. Helminth surveys conducted between 1950 and 1962 have confirmed the presence of **ascariasis** and **trichuriasis** in Brazil, Colombia, French Guiana, Peru, Surinam and Venezuela; **hymenolepiasis nana** in Brazil and Peru; **strongyloidiasis** in Brazil, Colombia, French Guiana, Peru and Venezuela; **taeniasis** in Brazil, Colombia and Peru. **Fascioliasis** is present in Peru. **Paragonimiasis** is known in Brazil, Colombia, Ecuador, Peru and Venezuela. **Sparganosis** occurs in Colombia, Ecuador and Guyana. **Schistosome cercarial dermatitis** has been contracted in Colombia, Surinam and Venezuela, and **creeping eruption** has been found in all but Bolivia, Ecuador and Peru.

Filariasis bancrofti is endemic in Colombia (rare), Venezuela, portions of the Guianas and Brazil. **Filariasis ozzardi** is known to occur in the Guianas, Colombia and Venezuela.

Dipetalonemiasis occurs in Guyana, Surinam and Venezuela.

There are foci of **onchocerciasis** in Venezuela, Colombia and Surinam. In 1972 a new focus was found in Brazil near the Venezuelan border. This includes some of the northern Amazonas State and a large part of the Roraima Territory where the vector *Simulium* thrives. The first focus found in Colombia in 1970 was limited to locations along the Micay River, involving a relatively small area.

Hydatid disease is endemic in Ecuador, Bolivia, Brazil (Rio Grande do Sul) and Peru (Sierra). Colombia, French Guiana and Venezuela are apparently free. Studies of domestic animals show that infections are present in dogs, sheep, cattle, pigs and other animals. In Rio Grande do Sul, Brazil, 31.3 per cent of dogs and 22.1 to 38.6 per cent of sheep examined were found infected. In 1972, 134 human cases were reported in Peru.

Schistosomiasis is endemic in the northern and central regions of Venezuela, in large areas of Brazil and in the coastal region of Surinam. Reported cases do not reflect the extent of infection, which has been estimated at 6 million, principally in the rural areas. Reported cases between 1969 and 1972 consisted of 61 in Surinam and 1579 in Venezuela.

Protozoan Diseases

Amebiasis, together with other forms of dysentery, is widespread. In 1972 there were 12,609 cases of amebiasis reported from Venezuela, 782 from Bolivia and 909 from Peru. Other intestinal protozoan infections are also present.

Mucocutaneous and **visceral leishmaniasis** are endemic in all these countries. Approximately 1600 cases were reported in 1963 from Bolivia, Brazil, Colombia, Peru and Venezuela.

---

*Formerly British Guiana.

In 1972 it was conjectured that although there was still the risk of contracting **malaria** in rural regions, most of the urban areas were relatively safe. However, French Guiana and Surinam with some exceptions had areas of high risk in both rural and urban locations. Although an intensive eradication campaign is in progress, there were still some 71,000 new cases of malaria reported from these countries in 1974 (in contrast to 158,000 in 1972). All but Surinam and Brazil showed a decline from 1973.

American trypanosomiasis or **Chagas' disease** has been reported from all these countries except the Guianas. In 1972 there were 470 cases reported from Venezuela and 14 from Peru, and in 1971 Bolivia reported 114 new cases. It is, however, estimated that there are some 10 million people suffering from Chagas' disease in rural South America (several million of whom are in Brazil), and a million of these have Chagas' cardiopathies. Reporting is extremely poor and incomplete.

Fungal Diseases

The following are among the mycoses that are present in tropical South America: **coccidioidomycosis** occurs in Bolivia and Venezuela; **histoplasmosis** in Brazil; **South American blastomycosis** in all of South America, especially Brazil; and **tinea imbricata** in Brazil and Colombia.

Bacterial Diseases

Anthrax is reported annually from these countries. In 1970 Peru reported 60 cases, and in 1970 Colombia reported 7.

Bartonellosis is limited in its distribution to areas in Peru and Ecuador. In 1960, 237 cases were reported from Peru.

Brucellosis is reported from Colombia, Peru and Venezuela. Peru reported 1284 human cases in 1971. It is widespread among the cattle of Bolivia, Brazil, Peru, Colombia and Venezuela; among swine in Brazil, Ecuador and Venezuela; among goats in Peru; and among sheep in Brazil and Peru.

Bacillary dysentery or **shigellosis,** amebiasis, and other diarrheal diseases are very widespread.

Leprosy is endemic, and all these countries report new cases annually. In Brazil the total of registered cases in 1970 was 129,995; Colombia had 18,809 and Venezuela 14,595. In 1972 there was a total of 7738 new cases reported from these countries, 6411 of them from Brazil.

A few cases of **leptospirosis** were reported from Brazil and Venezuela. There is no accurate knowledge of the extent of leptospirosis in these countries except for the occasional reported case.

Plague is endemic in large areas of South America. In 1974, 14 human cases were reported from the Department of La Paz, Bolivia; 247 from the States of Bahia, Ceara and Pernambuco in Brazil; 8 from the Departments of Piura and Manbayeque in Peru. In other years cases were reported from the States of Alagoas, Rio de Janeiro, Minas Gerais, and Rio Grande do Norte in Brazil; from the Provinces of Chimborazo, Tungurahua, Manabi, Loja, Los Rios, El Oro, and Pichinch in Ecuador; from the Departments of Ancash, Trumbes, Cajamarca, and Amazonas in Peru; from the Departments of Santa Cruz and Chuquisaca in Bolivia; and from the States of Aragua and Miranda in Venezuela.

The endemic treponematoses, **pinta** and **yaws,** are present. **Pinta** occurs only in the Western Hemisphere and is endemic in tropical America, being especially prevalent in Peru and Venezuela. It also occurs in Brazil, Bolivia, Ecuador and the Guianas. It has been estimated that in Colombia there are more than half a million infected people. There are still endemic foci of **yaws** in parts of Bolivia, Brazil, Colombia, Venezuela, Ecuador, Guyana, Surinam and Peru. In 1972, 67 cases were reported from Colombia, 380 from Ecuador and 3 from Peru.

Louse-borne relapsing fever is sometimes reported from Bolivia, Brazil, Colombia and Peru. Four cases were reported in Colombia in 1960.

Tick-borne relapsing fever is present in Colombia, Ecuador and Venezuela.

Cases of **tetanus** are reported in sizeable numbers from these countries. In 1972 Brazil reported 2051 cases, Venezuela 761, Colombia 520, Peru 289, Bolivia 26, and French Guiana 2.

Typhoid fever is endemic. In 1974 some 15,000 cases were reported from these countries, chiefly from Brazil, Colombia, Ecuador and Peru.

Rickettsial Diseases

Epidemic or **louse-borne typhus fever** is reported from 4 of these countries. In 1973 there were 91 cases reported from Bolivia, Ecuador and Peru. The last reported cases for Colombia occurred in 1964.

Murine or **flea-borne typhus fever** was reported from Colombia, Ecuador, Peru and Venezuela in 1963.

Tick-borne spotted fever is present in Colombia and Brazil.

Viral Diseases

Arthropod-borne (arbo) virus infections transmitted through the bite of a mosquito are prevalent. In Brazil a whole series of fever-inducing arboviruses has been isolated. Among these are: **Mucambo fever** virus, **Apeu fever** virus, **Caraparu fever** virus, **Itaqui fever** virus, **Madrid fever** virus, **Marituba fever** virus, **Murutucu fever** virus, **Oriboca fever** virus, **Guama fever** virus, **Oropouche fever** virus, **Candiru fever** virus, **Mayaro fever** virus, and **Guaroa fever** virus. **Piry fever** virus transmitted by a soft tick is also present in Brazil. **Guaroa fever** virus has been isolated in Colombia as well as Brazil. **Dengue fever** occurs sporadically and in epidemic form and can break out wherever the vector is present. It has been reported from time to time from Colombia, Peru, Venezuela, Guyana and French Guiana. A serologic survey conducted in Colombia showed that between August 1971 and February 1972 there had been approximately 416,000 cases following the resurgence of *Aedes aegypti.*

Arthropod-borne encephalitis is also a problem. In Venezuela, in 1963, there was an epidemic of **Venezuelan equine encephalitis** involving 10,145 reported cases. In the same year cases were present among the animals in Guyana and Surinam. There is confirmed evidence that **western equine encephalitis** is present in Brazil and Guyana; **eastern equine encephalitis** in Brazil, Colombia and Guyana; **Venezuelan equine encephalitis** in Brazil, Colombia, Ecuador, Guyana, Venezuela and Peru (in 1973 Peru had 3693 reported cases and Venezuela 594; in 1972 Colombia reported 17 and Ecuador 4). **St. Louis encephalitis** occurs in Brazil, and **Ilheus fever** virus in Brazil, Colombia, Guyana, Surinam and Venezuela.

In 1974 there were 9 cases of **jungle yellow fever** reported from Brazil (and 40 in 1973), 11 from Bolivia and 7 from Colombia. In 1972 cases were reported from Venezuela and in 1973 from Bolivia and Peru. With the exception of eastern Brazil and some highland parts of Ecuador, Colombia, Peru and Bolivia, tropical South America is considered a yellow fever endemic area. Departments and States from which cases have been reported since 1974 include: Bolivia—Cochabamba, Santa Cruz and La Paz; Brazil—Acre, Amazonas, Maranhao, Mato Grosso and Minas Gerais; Colombia—Meta, Cundinamarca, Boyaca, Santander, Vaupes, Auraca; Peru—Huanuco and Puno; Venezuela—Apure, Barinas, Lara, Merida, Portugesa and Tachira; Surinam—District Marowijne.

Bolivian hemorrhagic fever caused by Machupo virus occurs in eastern Bolivia.

Infectious hepatitis is not too well reported. In the first 10 months of 1974, Bolivia reported 140 cases, French Guiana 15, Guyana 23, Peru 3462 and Venezuela 2334.

Rabies is endemic in animals in tropical South America. In 1972 there were 175 human rabies cases reported from all countries, excluding the Guianas: 17 of these cases occurred in Colombia, 18 in Ecuador, 5 in Peru, 4 in Venezuela and 105 in Brazil.

As of 1974 **smallpox** appears to have been eliminated from Brazil, its last stronghold in the Western Hemisphere.

Trachoma is endemic in the tropics. In 1962, 425 cases were reported from Surinam.

D. TEMPERATE SOUTH AMERICA

Argentina, Chile, Paraguay, Uruguay, Falkland Islands

Helminth Diseases

Ancylostomiasis (hookworm) is endemic. In 1963 there were 13,836 cases reported in Argentina and 14,760 in Paraguay. Helminth surveys conducted between 1950 and 1960 confirmed the presence of **ascariasis, trichuriasis, hymenolepiasis, taeniasis, strongyloidiasis** and **diphyllobothriasis** in Argentina and Chile. **Trichinosis** has been reported from Argentina, Chile and Uruguay. Other helminth infections found in these countries include: **schistosome cercarial dermatitis** in Argentina; **sparganosis** in Uruguay; **dipylidiasis** in Argentina and Chile. **Filariasis ozzardi** has been found in northern Argentina.

Hydatid disease is endemic in the domestic animals. In 1972 Argentina reported 233 human cases, Chile 827 and Uruguay 446. These 3 countries account for approximately 93 per cent of all human cases in the Americas.

Protozoan Diseases

Amebiasis, together with bacillary dysentery and unspecified diarrheas, occurs. Argentina, Uruguay and Chile reported cases in 1970. Other intestinal protozoan infections are also present.

Visceral and **mucocutaneous leishmaniasis** are endemic in Argentina and Paraguay. In 1963, 50 cases were reported from Argentina and 300 from Paraguay.

Chile, Uruguay and the Falkland Islands are currently free of **malaria.** However, Argentina still has some rural foci and Paraguay has some rural and urban areas of risk. In 1974 there were 145 new cases reported from Argentina and 92 from Paraguay.

American trypanosomiasis or **Chagas' disease** is endemic in these countries except for the Falkland Islands. Argentina reported 2860 cases in 1972. The other countries accounted for 9 additional cases.

Fungal Diseases

Mycotic infections that have been found include: **maduromycosis** present in Argentina; **coccidioidomycosis** in Argentina and Chile; **histoplasmosis** in Argentina.

Bacterial Diseases

Anthrax is reported annually from these countries. In 1972 Argentina reported 89 cases, Chile 74, Paraguay 20 and Uruguay 23.

Brucellosis is reported annually from these countries. In 1972, 1114 cases were reported by Argentina.

Bacillary dysentery together with amebiasis is endemic. In 1972 Argentina reported 88,615 cases of bacillary dysentery, Paraguay 245, and some were reported from Chile and Uruguay.

Leptospirosis has been found in Argentina and Chile.

Leprosy is endemic. A summary of the cases in the active registers of each country showed 9627 in Argentina, 4869 in Paraguay and 514 in Uruguay. The only cases in Chile are on Easter Island. In 1972 Argentina reported 596 new cases, Paraguay 321 and Uruguay 13.

Foci of **sylvatic plague** are present in the following localities in Argentina: Chanaritos, Telen, Las Toscas, Icano, Rio Seco and Quenquen. Between 1931 and 1955 the number of cases of **human plague** approximated 750. Since that time there has been only an occasional sporadic case so that Argentina is now considered practically free of human plague.

Tick-borne relapsing fever is present in northern Argentina and Chile.

There were 341 cases of **tetanus** reported from Argentina in 1972, 30 from Chile, 233 from Paraguay and 28 from Uruguay. In Paraguay, of 172 deaths, 80 per cent occurred in children aged less than one year.

Typhoid fever is endemic. In 1974 Argentina reported 1121 cases and Chile 4433.

Rickettsial Diseases

Louse-borne epidemic typhus fever has not been reported from Chile since 1966. **Flea-borne murine typhus** is present in Argentina and Chile.

Viral Diseases

Arthropod-borne (arbo) virus encephalitis has been reported from Argentina, Chile, Paraguay and Uruguay. Argentina averaged 500 cases of viral encephalitis annually between 1963 and 1972 (in 1972 isolations of WEE were made). **Western equine encephalitis, eastern equine encephalitis** and **St. Louis encephalitis** appear in Argentina. **Argentinian hemorrhagic fever** (Junin virus) occurs around Buenos Aires and other foci in Argentina. There were also 52 cases of viral encephalitis reported from Chile in 1972, 98 from Paraguay and 31 from Uruguay.

In 1974 there were 9 cases of **jungle yellow fever** reported from Amambay Province, Paraguay; in 1948 and 1966 there were outbreaks of jungle yellow fever in Argentina.

Infectious hepatitis is widespread. There were 15,500 cases reported from all these countries in 1974.

Human rabies is an important public health problem.

Trachoma has been reported from Argentina, Chile and Paraguay. In 1963 there were 369 cases reported in Argentina and 10 in Paraguay.

II. EUROPE

SOUTHERN EUROPE

Albania, Andorra, Bulgaria,* southern France, Gibraltar, Greece,* Italy, Malta and Gozo, Portugal mainland and the Azores and Madeira Islands, Rumania,* San Marino, Spain, Turkey-in-Europe,* Yugoslavia,* southern European U.S.S.R.†*

Helminth Diseases

Ancylostomiasis (hookworm) is endemic in southern Europe. Within the past decade it has been reported from Italy, Portugal and the Azores and Madeira islands and confirmed by survey in Spain, Rumania and Yugoslavia. **Ascariasis, trichuriasis** and **hymenolepiasis nana** have been found by survey to be present in Albania, Bulgaria, Spain, Greece, Italy, Portugal, Rumania, San Marino, Yugoslavia and southern France. **Taeniasis** has been found in Spain, Italy, Portugal, Rumania, San Marino, Yugoslavia and southern France.

Diphyllobothriasis occurs in Portugal and Rumania. It is also found in the Lake regions in Italy.

Fascioliasis was found in Spain, Italy and Rumania, and **strongyloidiasis** in Italy, Portugal, Rumania, San Marino and Yugoslavia.

Trichinosis is endemic in many parts of Europe where pork is consumed.

Schistosomiasis has been known to occur in isolated areas of Portugal. **Metagonimiasis** is present in man in Spain and in various Balkan States.

Trichostrongyliasis is a common parasitic infection in areas of Armenia (U.S.S.R.).

Hydatid disease occurs in southeastern Europe.

Filariasis bancrofti no longer occurs in Europe.

Protozoan Diseases

Amebiasis, together with bacillary dysentery and unspecified dysentery, is endemic and is reported from some of these countries. Other intestinal protozoan infections are also present.

Visceral leishmaniasis or **Mediterranean kala-azar** is present in the Mediterranean littoral, including southern Italy, France, Spain, Portugal, the Mediterranean islands, southern Russia (U.S.S.R.) and the Caucasian (U.S.S.R.) countries.

Cutaneous leishmaniasis occurs in the Mediterranean littoral, the Mediterranean islands, southern Italy, Spain, southern France and Greece.

A limited risk of contracting **malaria** still exists in Alexandria and Propouliou, Greece; otherwise the country is considered relatively free. Data from the U.S.S.R. are not readily available; however, the Ukrainian S.S.R. and Byelorussian S.S.R. are free of risk, although in some other areas some risk continues to exist.

---

*The Balkan States; parts of Rumania and Yugoslavia are included.

†Includes the Crimean Peninsula, southern Ukrainian S.S.R., Georgian S.S.R., Armenian S.S.R., Azerbaidzhanian S.S.R. and southern R.S.F.S.R.

Fungal Diseases

Mycotic diseases are present as in most areas of the tropical and subtropical world. **Tinea favosa** is not uncommon in the Balkans. Sporadic cases of **maduromycosis** have been reported from Italy and Greece.

Bacterial Diseases

Anthrax is being reported from some of these countries, including Greece, Italy, Bulgaria, Portugal, Rumania, Spain and Yugoslavia.

Brucellosis is endemic and has been reported from many of the countries. Notably, in 1971 Spain reported 6173 cases, Italy 3709, France 468 and Portugal 293.

Bacillary dysentery (shigellosis) is endemic together with amebiasis and unspecified dysentery. Cases have been reported from most of the countries.

In 1973, between August 27 and October 12 an epidemic of **cholera el Tor** occurred in Italy, in Naples and neighboring towns. During this time there were 127 confirmed cases reported from a total of 35 towns, and these occurred in the poorest and most crowded areas. This is part of the pandemic that started in 1961 in the Celebes. The assumption is that the infection spread from Tunisia to the Mediterranean coast. No more cases have been reported from Italy since then. In early May 1974, cholera appeared in Portugal. Cases were reported from the districts of Lisbon, Oporto, Setubal, Faro, Santarem, Beja, Braga, Aveiro and Colombia. By the end of November there had been 2241 reported cases. Eight cases were reported from Spain, 5 from France, and scattered imported cases elsewhere in Europe. Portugal was declared free from cholera on November 29, 1974.

Leptospirosis is present and has been reported from Greece, Italy, Portugal, Yugoslavia and France.

Leprosy is also present. In 1968 there were 3758 cases of leprosy on the leprosy register in Spain, 2164 in Greece, some 399 in France, 2676 in Portugal, 3958 in Turkey (European and Asiatic), 544 in Italy, and a few cases recorded for Albania, Rumania and Yugoslavia. It was also present in Malta and Gozo, and the Azores. In 1972 and 1973, 5 of these countries reported more than 200 new cases.

Louse-borne relapsing fever has not been reported in recent years but has occurred in areas where epidemic typhus was present.

Tick-borne relapsing fever is endemic in parts of southern Europe and has been reported from Spain, Portugal and the Caucasian countries of the U.S.S.R. It was reported from Spain in 1972 and 1973.

Endemic syphilis is present in the Balkans, especially Yugoslavia. W.H.O. Endemic Syphilis Control campaigns, conducted between 1949 and 1963, have included Yugoslavia.

Typhoid and **paratyphoid fevers** are endemic and were reported from almost all these countries. In 1972 Italy reported a total of 10,483 cases, of which 9083 were typhoid fever; Portugal reported 1130 cases, of which 1115 were typhoid fever; Greece reported 594 cases, of which 536 were typhoid fever; and Yugoslavia had 1398 cases, of which 826 were typhoid fever. The other countries also reported significant numbers of cases.

Rickettsial Diseases

Rickettsial disease reporting is very inadequate. In recent years there have been no cases of **epidemic typhus**; **Q fever** has been reported from Italy and Yugoslavia; **murine typhus** from Malta and Portugal; **boutonneuse fever** from Portugal and **Brill's disease** from Yugoslavia. In the first 6 months of 1974 Yugoslavia reported 22 cases of the latter condition.

Viral Diseases

Arthropod-borne (arbo) virus diseases occur in southern Europe. Mosquito-borne **Tahyna fever** is present in Yugoslavia, and **West Nile fever** in the Rhone River delta and other parts of the Mediterranean littoral.

Crimean hemorrhagic fever, tick-borne, is known in the Crimea, the lower Don and Volga River delta in the U.S.S.R.

Naples and **Sicilian phlebotomus fevers** are present in Italy.

Central European tick-borne encephalitis (diphasic meningoencephalitis) is found in central and eastern Europe from the Baltic to the Balkans.

Infectious hepatitis is endemic and widely reported. In 1972 Yugoslavia reported 25,438 cases, Italy reported 39,158, Portugal reported 658, with the others also reporting. In 1971 there were 14,895 cases reported from Bulgaria, 58,429 from Rumania and 9389 from Turkey.

Human rabies is sporadically reported. In 1963 a few cases were reported from Spain, Greece, Italy, Malta and Gozo, and Yugoslavia.

Trachoma has been endemic in these areas for a long time. In 1953 cases numbered in the thousands.

III. AFRICA

A. NORTHERN AFRICA

Algeria, Libya, Morocco, Tunisia, Spanish Sahara, Egypt, Canary Islands and Madeira

Helminth Diseases

Ancylostomiasis (hookworm), ascariasis, trichuriasis, hymenolepiasis nana, strongyloidiasis and **taeniasis** are present in this area.

Fascioliasis has been found in Egypt, and cases of **tropical eosinophilia, hydatid disease, heterophyiasis,** and **paragonimiasis** have also been identified.

Schistosomiasis is endemic and present across all of northern Africa from Egypt to Morocco. It is a major public health problem in the Nile Valley.

Filariasis bancrofti is endemic on the North African coast from Egypt to Morocco. In 1959 several cases were found in Libya and Egypt. A survey of 500,000 people conducted in 1955 revealed *Wuchereria bancrofti* infections to be endemic in the eastern part of the Delta region of Egypt, with low rates in the central and western parts of the Delta and Cairo. An occasional case has also been observed in Morocco. An occasional case of **dipetalonemiasis** is seen in Algeria and Tunisia.

Protozoan Diseases

Amebiasis together with bacillary and unspecified dysentery is reported in large numbers from all the countries. In most instances, there is no distinction made between them in reporting.

Both **visceral** and **cutaneous leishmaniasis** are present, although not to the same extent as in other parts of Africa.

Malaria is still endemic in North Africa; however, there are areas that have been declared free of risk. In Algeria there is no longer any risk in urban areas; in Egypt the risk is still present; in Libya the entire country has been declared free of risk except for two small foci in the southwest. Spanish Sahara has been declared free. Tunisia is also free of risk in urban areas except for the Gabes Governate.

Fungal Diseases

Mycotic diseases such as **maduromycosis, cladosporiosis, phycomycosis,** an African variety of **histoplasmosis** and, recently, **North American blastomycosis** have been identified in northern Africa.

Tinea favosa is known to occur in North Africa.

Bacterial Diseases

Brucellosis has been reported annually from all of northern Africa except Morocco.

Bacillary dysentery or **shigellosis,** together with amebiasis and unspecified dysenteries, is endemic and widespread in North Africa and reported annually from almost all the countries. In 1970 Morocco reported 40,715 cases of unspecified dysentery.

Cholera was reported from Morocco in 1971 (56 cases) and 1972 (7 cases). In 1972 Tunisia reported 4 cases and the following year, 60 cases, representing a small localized outbreak. In 1971 Algeria reported 109 cases; in 1972, 27 cases; in 1973, 39 cases and in 1974, 9 cases.

Cutaneous diphtheria is present in this entire area.

Leprosy is endemic. Recent surveys showed that Egypt had 28,611 cases on the leprosy register in 1968, with an attack rate of 2 per 1000. Tunisia had 153 cases on the register, and Morocco 3870 in 1966. New cases are still being reported.

Leptospirosis is often reported from Algeria.

In 1971 a case of **plague** was reported from Libya.

An occasional case of **relapsing fever** is reported, often not classified according to mode of transmission.

Among the endemic treponematoses, **endemic syphilis** or **bejel** has been found on the desert borders of northern Africa.

Typhoid and **paratyphoid fevers** are endemic in this area. In 1972 Morocco reported 1346 cases, Tunisia 904 and Morocco 9418.

Rickettsial Diseases

Louse-borne epidemic typhus is endemic in this area. In 1963, 263 cases of epidemic typhus were reported from Egypt; in 1962, 3 from Libya; and in 1961, 6 from Tunisia. In 1974 there were 7 cases reported from Algeria. **Boutonneuse fever** is endemic in most countries bordering the Mediterranean.

Viral Diseases

Arthropod-borne (arbo) virus infections are known in this area. The **Naples** and **Sicilian phlebotomus fever viruses, Quaranfil fever** tick-borne virus, and **Sindbis fever** mosquito-borne virus have been found in Egypt. The **West Nile fever** mosquito-borne virus occurs across the northern part of North Africa westward from Egypt.

Infectious hepatitis is present in northern Africa, but is not well reported. In 1972 Tunisia reported 952 cases.

Human rabies occurs sporadically. In 1962 there were 32 cases reported from Egypt.

Trachoma is extremely widespread in North Africa. According to some estimates, 40 to 50 per cent of the population of Tunisia is infected. In 1955 Algeria had more than one million cases, and Morocco approximately 250,000. Trachoma is also present in Libya and Egypt.

B. WESTERN AFRICA

Dahomey, Gambia, Ghana, Guinea, Guinea-Bissau, Ivory Coast, Liberia, Mali, Mauritania, Niger, Nigeria, Senegal, Sierra Leone, Togo, Upper Volta, Cape Verde Islands and islands of Sao Tome and Principe

Helminth Diseases

Ancylostomiasis (hookworm) is endemic in Gambia, Nigeria, Ghana, Ivory Coast, Liberia, Sierra Leone, Guinea-Bissau, Senegal, Cape Verde Islands and the islands of Sao Tome and Principe. Surveys conducted between 1950 and 1962 confirmed the presence of **ascariasis, trichuriasis, strongyloidiasis, hymenolepiasis nana** and **taeniasis** in most of these countries.

Dracunculiasis occurs in Dahomey, Gambia, Mauritania, Nigeria, Senegal, Togo and Upper Volta; **hydatid disease** is present in Liberia; **paragonimiasis, schistosomiasis** and **trichinosis** in Nigeria.

Filarial infections of all types are endemic here. **Filariasis bancrofti** and **loiasis** are present and widespread. **Onchocerciasis** is endemic throughout this area. In Togo in 1962 there were 1295 cases of onchocerciasis reported; in 1964 it was also reported from Mauritania, Nigeria, Senegal and Sierra Leone. Surveys verified its presence in large numbers in Dahomey, Ghana, Guinea, Ivory Coast, Liberia, Mali, Niger, Nigeria, Guinea-Bissau, Senegal, Sierra Leone and Upper Volta. **Dipetalonemiasis** is present in Nigeria, Ghana and Sierra Leone.

Protozoan Diseases

Amebiasis, together with bacillary dysentery and other unspecified dysenteries, is endemic in West Africa. In 1973 there were some 45,000 cases of amebic dysentery reported from many of these countries. Other intestinal protozoan infections are also present.

Cutaneous leishmaniasis has been found in Nigeria and on the West Coast of Africa as far south as Angola. **Visceral leishmaniasis,** known as **African kala-azar,** is also found in isolated areas across Africa to the West Coast south of the Sahara.

As of 1974 all these countries are still considered to be areas of high risk for **malaria.** In Senegal, the city of Dakar was felt to be free of risk between January and June.

African trypanosomiasis is endemic in all of these countries. In some, successful campaigns are being waged and the numbers of new infections are declining. In 1973, Mali reported 355 new cases, Togo more than 21, Senegal 10, Guinea-Bissau 38 and Guinea 55. In 1967, there were more than 2000 new cases in Nigeria, and 165 in Ghana.

Bacterial Diseases

Brucellosis has been reported from Mali, Mauritania, Niger, Senegal and Upper Volta. **Bacillary dysentery (shigellosis)** is also widespread in West Africa. In 1973 there were 15,000 cases of unspecified dysentery, and 8000 cases of bacillary dysentery in the reporting countries.

Since 1971 all these countries with the exception of Gambia, Guinea, Guinea-Bissau, Upper Volta, and the islands of Sao Tome and Principe have reported a number of cases of **cholera.** In 1974 alone they accounted for more than 2300 reported cases. In March 1975, Cape Verde Islands had 20 cases.

Leptospirosis has been reported from Ghana and Senegal.

Leprosy is endemic and very extensive throughout West Africa. The number of cases runs well over 300,000. Surveys conducted from 1966 to 1969 revealed that there were 120,510 cases on the leprosy register in Ivory Coast, 140,211 in Upper Volta, 100,803 in Mali, 302,611 in Nigeria, from 50,000 to 70,000 in Senegal and Guinea, 20,000 to 40,000 in Ghana and Dahomey, 5,000 to 20,000 in Gabon, Sierra Leone and Niger and between 600 and 1600 in Liberia, Mauritania and Cape Verde Islands. New cases reported in 1972 and 1973 were 462 in Dahomey, 538 in Guinea, 5213 in Mali, 2477 in Niger, 2507 in Senegal and 392 in Togo.

Tick-borne relapsing fever is endemic throughout tropical Africa. In 1962 and 1963 sporadic cases were reported from Dahomey and Nigeria. In May 1973, Mauritania reported 100 cases of relapsing fever, the vector not being mentioned. In 1974 Liberia reported the occurrence of more than 15 cases of **louse-borne relapsing fever.**

Typhoid fever and **paratyphoid fever** are also endemic and reported annually from most of the countries. **Yaws** programs have been in effect in Dahomey, Ghana, Guinea, Ivory Coast, Liberia, Mali, Nigeria, Senegal, Sierra Leone, Togo and Upper Volta. This area is one of the major endemic centers of yaws. Campaigns against **endemic syphilis** are being waged in Mali, Senegal and Upper Volta.

Rickettsial Diseases

Louse-borne epidemic typhus occurs sporadically in Liberia, Mauritania and the Gambia. Other rickettsial diseases have been reported from many of the countries.

Viral Diseases

Arthropod-borne (arbo) virus infections are present in West Africa. Mosquito-borne **Spondweni, Ilesha** and **dengue fevers** have been found in Nigeria. **Chikungunya fever** occurs in all of West Africa, **O'nyong-nyong fever** in Senegal and **Bunyamwera fever** in various areas of West Africa.

This region includes the **African yellow fever** endemic zone. The only countries not included in this zone are Mauritania, the northern part of Mali and Niger. Ghana, Nigeria and Sierra Leone were considered infected areas in 1972. At that time Ghana reported 4 cases (in 1973, 3 and in 1974, 1). Nigeria, which also continues to report cases periodically, reported 23 in 1974, but had 208 in 1969. In 1969 Mali reported 21 cases and Upper Volta 87. In 1970 Togo also reported some cases.

In 1973 cases of **infectious hepatitis** were reported from Guinea, Guinea-Bissau, Niger and Nigeria.

Lassa fever, a newly identified viral disease, has been found in Nigeria, Guinea, Sierra Leone, Liberia, Ivory Coast, Upper Volta and Mali. Case fatality was high in diagnosed cases. The disease is probably more prevalent than was heretofore supposed, since experience with serologic surveys seems to indicate that many mild, nonfatal, or subclinical cases have occurred without being recognized. It is very possible that the distribution coincides with that of a rodent, *Mastomys natalensis,* found to harbor the virus. Transmission is believed to be achieved either through contact with rodent urine, or by eating or handling infected rodents.

Rabies is endemic. Human rabies cases are reported annually from almost all the countries.

Smallpox is no longer being reported from this part of Africa.

Trachoma is endemic, and has been found in almost all the West African countries.

C. CENTRAL AFRICA

Burundi, Cameroon, Central African Republic, Chad, Congo (Brazzaville), Zaire, Rwanda, Cabinda, Gabon, Equatorial Guinea†*

Helminth Diseases

Ancylostomiasis (hookworm) is widespread throughout parts of Central Africa. Large numbers of cases have been reported from Cameroon, Congo (Brazzaville), Zaire, Burundi, Cabinda and Rwanda. In 1958 more than 476,000 cases were reported from Zaire. Helminth surveys conducted between 1950 and 1962 confirmed the presence of **ascariasis** and **trichuriasis** in Cameroon and Zaire. **Strongyloidiasis** was confirmed in Congo (Brazzaville) and **taeniasis** and **paragonimiasis** in Cameroon and Zaire.

Endemic centers of **dracunculiasis** are present in Cameroon and the Lake Chad region. **Tropical eosinophilia** is widespread.

Schistosomiasis (bilharziasis) is endemic in most of Central Africa. Surveys conducted in some areas of Zaire demonstrated infection rates far exceeding 50 per cent.

Various **filarial diseases** are present. Surveys conducted for evidence of filarial infections sometimes show conflicting findings. However, infections with one or all of the filaria *Wuchereria bancrofti, Loa loa, Dipetalonema perstans* and *D. streptocerca* are common in a wide geographic belt that includes all the Central African countries. **Onchocerciasis** also has a wide distribution in tropical Africa. The northern boundary is estimated at latitude 15° N and extends from Senegal to Ethiopia, the endemic area extending south of the equator to Angola in the west and Tanzania in the east. These geographic boundaries encompass the Central African countries. Detailed studies have been made in Chad, Cameroon and Zaire. **Dipetalonemiasis** has been identified in Cameroon, Equatorial Guinea, Zaire and Rwanda.

Protozoan Diseases

Amebiasis is endemic and extensive. In 1972 there were more than 55,000 cases of amebiasis reported from these countries. Other intestinal protozoan infections are also present. There are endemic foci of **cutaneous leishmaniasis** in Cameroon, Chad and Congo (Brazzaville). **Malaria** is also widespread and endemic. According to the most recent information, malaria is endemic in all these countries and none of the urban areas has been declared free of risk.

Trypanosomiasis has been reported from all these countries. Surveys and reporting of cases indicate a significant number of infections, although there has been a decline in the number of reported cases since 1947. Surveys conducted in 1967 and 1968 found that there were still active foci in Chad, Congo (Brazzaville), Central African Republic, Gabon, Burundi, Zaire, Rwanda and Cameroon. In 1973 Chad reported 15 new cases, Congo (Brazzaville) more than 42, Cameroon 19, Gabon more than 27 (82 cases were reported in 1972).

---

*Formerly Belgian Congo.

†Formerly Spanish Guinea; includes Rio Muni, Fernando Po, and others.

Fungal Diseases

Mycotic diseases are present in all of Africa. **Tinea imbricata** is common to this area.

Bacterial Diseases

In 1971, 22 cases of **anthrax** were reported by Rwanda.

Brucellosis is endemic here. Most of the countries report a few cases each year. **Bacillary dysentery (shigellosis),** together with amebiasis, is endemic and widespread. In 1972 there were more than 6000 cases of bacillary dysentery (and 55,000 cases of amebiasis) reported from these countries as well as a large number of cases of unspecified dysentery.

Some of these countries have been involved in the seventh **cholera** pandemic. In 1971 Chad reported 8236 cases and Cameroon 2411. In 1972 this had dropped to 5 cases for Chad and 362 for Cameroon. In 1973 Chad reported none, but in 1974, 338 cases occurred. Cameroon has had a steady decline in cases, 174 in 1973 and 82 in 1974.

Leptospirosis has been reported almost annually from Cameroon, Zaire and Equatorial Guinea. This area has an exceptionally large number of people suffering from **leprosy,** which is endemic in most of these countries. Reports are not available for all, but in 1968 a survey revealed the following: Cameroon had 55,559 cases on the leprosy register, a rate of 28.5 per 1000; Gabon had 11,253, a rate of 33.5 per 1000; Central African Republic had 31,380 on the register, Chad 35,617 and Congo (Brazzaville) 15,940; Zaire had 3000 inpatients and a rate of 116.3 per 1000. New cases for 1972 and 1973 totaled more than 5000.

In 1974 there were a few cases of **human plague** reported from Zaire. The disease is endemic in the animals of the area as is **tick-borne relapsing fever.** During the first 5 months of 1974 Rwanda reported 1268 cases of the latter, and Burundi, Zaire and Congo (Brazzaville) also reported a few cases.

Typhoid and **paratyphoid fevers** are reported from many areas, some 2700 cases having been listed in 1972.

This has been known as one of the large endemic centers of **yaws.** In 1957 several hundred thousand cases were reported from Cameroon, Zaire, Equatorial Guinea, Rwanda and Burundi. Between 1948 and 1965 some 19,780,000 people in Africa were treated for yaws. This included cases, contacts and latents during the W.H.O.–assisted yaws control campaigns. Surveys conducted in some parts of Africa reveal a gradual recrudescence of the disease, especially among children. Actual data were not available on yaws in the Central African countries.

Rickettsial Diseases

Louse-borne epidemic typhus is endemic in Burundi. In the first 7 months of 1974 there were 2825 cases of epidemic typhus reported from that country. Rwanda reported 2764 cases for the first 5 months of 1974, and Zaire and Chad each had a few cases. **Murine typhus, boutonneuse fever** and other members of the spotted fever group are occasionally reported.

Viral Diseases

Arthropod-borne (arbo) virus infections identified in this area include: **Nairobi tick-borne sheep disease;** mosquito-borne **chikungunya, West Nile** and **yellow fevers.** All of these countries are within the yellow fever endemic zone. In 1970 there were 10 cases reported from Zaire, and in 1971 one from Cameroon. A case of **Lassa fever** is reported to have originated in Central African Republic (Djema).

In spite of poor overall reporting of **infectious hepatitis,** there were more than 22,000 cases reported from Burundi, Chad, Gabon, Rwanda and Zaire in 1972.

Rabies is endemic in Cameroon, Central African Republic, Chad, Congo (Brazzaville) and Zaire, with human cases reported annually. **Smallpox** is no longer being reported from this area. Reporting of **trachoma** indicates that this disease is endemic in most of central Africa.

D. EASTERN AFRICA

Ethiopia, French Territory of Afars and the Issas, Kenya, Somalia, Sudan, Seychelles, Tanzania,† Uganda*

Helminth Diseases

Ancylostomiasis (hookworm) is endemic. In 1960 there were more than 80,000 cases reported from this area. Helminth surveys conducted in 1950 and 1962 confirmed the presence of **ascariasis, trichuriasis, strongyloidiasis** and **taeniasis** in almost all the countries. **Hymenolepiasis nana** infections were found in Sudan and Ethiopia. **Hydatid disease** is present in Ethiopia, Tanzania and Uganda. **Schistosomiasis** is endemic in most of eastern Africa.

Filariasis is widely distributed throughout most of these countries. Data from Ethiopia and Somalia are scant. However, surveys have established the presence of *Wuchereria bancrofti, Loa loa, Dipetalonema perstans* and probably *D. streptocerca* in the remaining countries. The distribution of each type of filaria depends on conditions suitable for vector survival. **Onchocerciasis** is endemic in Sudan, Kenya, Tanzania and Uganda. Rare cases occur in the French Territory of Afars and the Issas. *Wuchereria bancrofti* infections have been found in the Seychelles. **Dipetalonemiasis** has occurred in Tanzania and Uganda.

Protozoan Diseases

Amebiasis is reported, together with bacillary dysentery and other unspecified dysenteries. These exceed hundreds of thousands of cases annually. Other intestinal protozoan infections are also present. **Visceral leishmaniasis** or **kala-azar** is endemic in this area, especially in the Sudan. **Cutaneous leishmaniasis** or **Oriental sore** is endemic in Ethiopia and Sudan.

Malaria is endemic in these countries and, with few exceptions, rural and urban areas both pose a risk of contracting the disease. Free of risk are the Seychelles, the northern province of the Sudan, Kigesi in Uganda and a few of the urban areas in Uganda. There is very little risk in Mogadishu, Somalia.

African trypanosomiasis is endemic in Sudan, Kenya, Tanzania and Uganda. In 1973 Kenya reported more than 15 cases and Uganda 37, and in 1972 Tanzania 612. In 1965 the disease was also reported from the Sudan (27 cases), and in 1967, 11 cases were reported from Ethiopia. None has been reported from Somalia or the French Territory of Afars and the Issas. In Tanzania the cases came from the western *Glossina morsitans* belt.

Bacterial Diseases

Kenya reported 169 cases of **anthrax** in 1970, the Sudan 174, Uganda 98 and Tanzania 221. Cases have also been reported for 1971 and 1972 but the figures are not available.

Brucellosis is endemic in this area and has been reported from almost all the countries. **Bacillary dysentery** or **shigellosis** is widely reported. In 1970 the **cholera** pandemic moved into North and West Africa, entering through Ethiopia. In 1971 the French Territory of Afars and the Issas reported 439 cases, and in 1972, 8; Kenya reported 257 cases in 1971, 51 in 1972, none in 1973, but between December 27, 1974, and March 20, 1975, no fewer than 1260 cases occurred. Somalia had 88 cases in 1971, a few in 1972, and none since. Uganda reported 757 cases in 1971, and 3 cases early in 1975. In 1974 Tanzania reported 10 cases.

Leptospirosis is frequently reported from Kenya, Tanzania and Uganda.

Leprosy is endemic, and large numbers of cases are on record. Surveys conducted in 1966 and 1968 revealed that Tanzania had 101,159 cases of leprosy in the case register, Uganda 39,264, Kenya a rate of 20 per 1000, and Seychelles 87 cases. Prior records showed almost 11,000 cases in Ethiopia and more than 2000 in the Sudan, as well as

*Formerly French Somaliland.

†Formerly Tanganyika and Zanzibar.

some in Somalia. In 1972 the French Territory of Afars and the Issas reported 9 new cases, and in 1973 Kenya more than 80.

In 1972, 21 cases of **plague** were reported from Tanzania.

In 1964 there were almost 6000 cases of **louse-borne relapsing fever** in Ethiopia and 6 cases of **tick-borne relapsing fever** reported from Kenya. Sudan and Somalia have also reported tick-borne relapsing fever. **Yaws** was very widespread in all these countries, which participated in the W.H.O.-assisted yaws eradication program. Current data are not available but there is some evidence that there may be a recrudescence of the infection in children in some areas.

Typhoid and **paratyphoid fevers** are endemic and are annually reported from Ethiopia, the French Territory of Afars and the Issas, Kenya, Tanzania and Uganda.

Rickettsial Diseases

Louse-borne epidemic typhus has occurred in Ethiopia. In 1970 more than 2500 cases were reported. Uganda reported some cases in 1969. **Murine typhus** and other unspecified rickettsioses (which might be **tick-borne Kenya typhus** or **boutonneuse fever)** have been reported from Kenya and Ethiopia.

Viral Diseases

Arthropod-borne (arbo) virus infections have been found throughout this area. Mosquito-borne **Zika** and **Bwamba fevers** are present in Uganda. **Nairobi tick-borne sheep fever** occurs in Kenya. Mosquito-transmitted **chikungunya, o'nyong-nyong, Bunyamwera,** and **Rift Valley fevers** are found in all of East Africa. Mosquito-transmitted **West Nile fever** is present in the eastern part of Africa, from south to north.

Yellow fever occurs in some of these countries, which are within the yellow fever endemic zone. An estimated 100,000 cases with 30,000 deaths occurred in Ethiopia in the period 1960 to 1962.

Infectious hepatitis has been reported regularly from Ethiopia, Kenya, Seychelles, Somalia, the French Territory of Afars and the Issas, Tanzania and Uganda for at least 25 years.

A few cases of **human rabies** have been reported from Kenya, Sudan, Tanzania and Uganda. In all of Africa when the year 1975 commenced, this was the only region in which **smallpox** still occurred. In 1974 Ethiopia reported 4436 cases, and during January and February 1975 an additional 544. In 1974 Somalia reported 11 cases, and the French Territory of Afars and the Issas 13.

Trachoma is widespread and endemic.

E. SOUTHERN AFRICA

Angola, Botswana, Lesotho,† Malawi, Mozambique, Namibia (South West Africa), Rhodesia, Republic of South Africa, Swaziland, Zambia, Malagasy Republic, Comoro Archipelago, Mauritius, Reunion, St. Helena (including Ascension and Tristan da Cunha)*

Helminth Diseases

Ancylostomiasis (hookworm) is endemic in many of these countries. It has been reported from Zambia, Malawi, Mozambique, Rhodesia, Botswana, South Africa, Angola and Mauritius.

Filarial infections are present and widespread, and have appeared at some time or other in all but the Republic of South Africa, Namibia and Lesotho. **Filariasis bancrofti** is present in all these countries. **Onchocerciasis** has been found in Malawi, Malagasy Republic, Swaziland, Comoro Archipelago, Mauritius and Angola. **Dipetalonemiasis** occurs in Malawi and Rhodesia.

Helminth surveys conducted between 1950 and 1962 confirmed the presence of certain helminths in southern Africa. **Fascioliasis** has been found in Mozambique, and

---

*Formerly Bechuanaland.
†Formerly Basutoland.

ascariasis, trichuriasis, strongyloidiasis, hymenolepiasis nana and **taeniasis** in many of the mainland and island countries. **Dipylidiasis** was found in Zambia.

Schistosomiasis is endemic, especially in Angola, Malawi, Malagasy Republic, Mozambique, Rhodesia, Republic of South Africa, Mauritius and Reunion.

Protozoan Diseases

Amebiasis is endemic and reported in these countries. It is possible that some of the unspecified dysentery reported may include amebiasis. Other protozoan infections are also present. **Cutaneous leishmaniasis** or **Oriental sore** is reported as occurring in Angola. A few cases of **visceral leishmaniasis** are purported to have occurred in Mozambique.

Malaria is still quite prevalent. In 1974 all the countries except Lesotho, and the islands of St. Helena, Ascension and Tristan da Cunha, were still considered to be areas where malaria transmission could occur. However, the last indigenous cases of malaria in Mauritius occurred in 1965, and in 1973 this country was included in the W.H.O. register of countries where eradication has been achieved. Swaziland is considered to be free from risk in all but a few small areas near the border. In the Malagasy Republic, Ambositra, Antsirabe, Tananarive and some other urban areas are considered free of risk; and in Botswana, Ghanzi, Kgalagadi, Kweneng, Ngamiland, Ngwakeste, Ngwato and Tuli Block are considered to be without risk.

Trypanosomiasis is endemic in some of these countries. According to recent surveys it was still present in Malawi, Mozambique, Botswana, Rhodesia, Zambia and Angola. In 1972 and 1973, 10 cases were reported from Angola.

Bacterial Diseases

Angola, Rhodesia and the Republic of South Africa reported **anthrax** in 1972. Angola had 136 cases that year.

Brucellosis is reported frequently from Angola, Botswana, Lesotho, Mozambique, Malawi, Rhodesia, the Republic of South Africa and Zambia. **Bacillary dysentery** or **shigellosis** is endemic and widely reported, as are nonspecified dysenteries and amebiasis.

In 1974 there were 933 cases of **cholera** reported from Angola, 1228 from Malawi, 1018 from Mozambique, 753 from Rhodesia and 37 from the Republic of South Africa. In March 1975, the Comoro Archipelago reported 1000 cases.

Leprosy is widespread and reported from most of these countries. Surveys conducted in 1966, 1967 and 1968 found the following numbers of cases on the leprosy registers: Comoro Archipelago 326, a rate of 4.1 per 1000; Lesotho 348; Malagasy Republic 3351, a rate of 24.4 per 1000; Malawi 9368; Mozambique 62,669; Reunion 150; Zambia 18,363. Angola reported 929 new cases in 1972 and 1973, and Reunion 16. None has been reported from Namibia, St. Helena and Ascension. **Leptospirosis** has been reported from Botswana, Malagasy Republic, Mozambique, Malawi and Reunion.

Plague is endemic in this area. In 1972, 11 cases were reported from Lesotho, and in 1974, 39 from Malagasy Republic and 27 from Rhodesia. Cases have also been reported from Malawi, Namibia and the Republic of South Africa. **Tick-borne relapsing fever** is endemic in most of southern Africa and has been reported from almost all the mainland countries. Angola reported more than 9 cases during the first 6 months of 1974.

Endemic treponematoses including **endemic syphilis** and **yaws** have been present. Endemic syphilis is known in Botswana, and yaws is endemic in Angola, Botswana, the Comoro Archipelago, Malagasy Republic, Mozambique, Malawi and Zambia. In 1957 there were thousands of cases reported from these countries, but since that year the prevalence of these diseases has been reduced through the extensive eradication campaigns waged by W.H.O.

Typhoid and **paratyphoid fevers** are endemic here and regularly reported.

Rickettsial Diseases

Although **louse-borne epidemic typhus** has been reported from these countries in the past, since 1970 there have been no reported cases.

Murine typhus and **South African tick-borne typhus** (same as, or related to, **boutonneuse fever**) have been reported in recent years. Some illnesses designated only as rickettsioses have also been reported.

Viral Diseases

Arthropod-borne (arbo) virus fevers are present in southern Africa. Mosquito-borne viruses causing a variety of viral fevers including **Bunyamwera, chikungunya, Germiston, Spondweni, Sindbis** and **Wesselsbron** occur. In 1972 Angola reported 65 cases of yellow fever. **Rift Valley** mosquito-borne **fever** is also present. **West Nile fever** (mosquito-borne) occurs along the entire eastern half of the continent. **Quaranfil** tick-borne **fever** also occurs here.

Infectious hepatitis has been reported from most of the southern African countries in recent years. In 1972 Angola reported 984 cases, Mozambique 997, Reunion 1. **Human rabies** has been reported from all the countries except Namibia, Swaziland, Republic of South Africa, St. Helena and Ascension.

Smallpox is no longer being reported from this part of Africa. **Trachoma** is endemic in most of the mainland countries and has also been found in Mauritius.

IV. ASIA

A. SOUTHWEST ASIA

Bahrain, Cyprus, Iran, Iraq, Israel, Jordan, Kuwait, Lebanon, Oman, Qatar, Saudi Arabia, Syria, Turkey (Asiatic), United Arab Emirates,† Yemen (northern), Democratic Yemen (southern)‡*

Helminth Diseases

Surveys show that **ancylostomiasis (hookworm)** is endemic in southwest Asia. It was reported from Turkey and Iraq in 1961. **Dracunculiasis** is present in the Arabian peninsula, especially along the Red Sea coast. It also occurs in Iran and Iraq.

Filarial infections are present. **Filariasis bancrofti** has been found from coastal Arabia to India. A single focus remains in Alanya in Turkey. Filariasis was reported from Democratic Yemen in 1959 and established by survey as being endemic in Saudi Arabia. In Israel it was found among Indian immigrants. **Onchocerciasis** has been found in Yemen and Democratic Yemen.

Gnathostomiasis has been found in Israel. **Hydatid disease** is relatively common in this area. **Schistosomiasis** is endemic and widespread.

Helminth surveys conducted between 1950 and 1962 have confirmed the presence of **ascariasis, trichuriasis, hymenolepiasis** and **taeniasis** in Iraq, Iran, Israel, Jordan, Lebanon, Saudi Arabia, Syria, Turkey and Yemen. **Fascioliasis** has been found in Lebanon and Turkey, **clonorchiasis** and **diphyllobothriasis** in Turkey and Israel, and **strongyloidiasis** in Iraq, Israel, Jordan, Lebanon, Saudi Arabia and Turkey, and infrequently in Yemen.

Protozoan Diseases

Amebiasis is endemic in this area and reported from a number of countries. In most of the reports it has not been differentiated from bacillary dysentery. Other intestinal protozoan infections are also present.

Cutaneous leishmaniasis or **Oriental sore** occurs in the Arabian peninsula. It is present in Iran, Iraq, Israel and Syria. **Malaria** eradication campaigns are in progress, and some of these countries have been declared free of risk of acquiring malaria. These include all of Cyprus, Israel, Kuwait and Lebanon. Others are free in some areas and not in others. Among these are Saudi Arabia, where Jeddah, Mecca, Medina and Qatif are risk-free; Jordan, where the only risk remains in the Jordan valley and Karak lowlands; Turkey, where the only risk remains in Adiyaman, Edirne, Hakkari, Mardin, and Siirt Province; Yemen, where Hajja and Sada Provinces are risk-free; and Syria, in

---

*Formerly Muscat and Oman.
†Formerly Trucial Sheikhdoms.
‡Formerly Aden and Protectorate of South Arabia.

which country Damascus, Latakia, Deir-ez-zor and other urban areas are free but malaria risk is present elsewhere.

Bacterial Diseases

Anthrax has been reported annually from Iraq, Israel, Jordan, Lebanon, Syria and Turkey. Most cases are rare or sporadic, but in 1970 Iraq had 89 and Turkey 912.

Brucellosis has been reported from Iran, Iraq, Israel, Lebanon, Democratic Yemen and Turkey. **Bacillary dysentery (shigellosis),** together with amebiasis and unspecified dysentery, is endemic and widespread. In 1974, 91 cases of **cholera** were reported from Saudi Arabia; in 1972, cases had been reported from Saudi Arabia, Oman, Israel, Bahrain, Syria, Yemen and Democratic Yemen.

Leprosy is reported from most of these countries. Surveys conducted in 1965, 1968 and 1969 revealed that there were cases in the leprosy registers of most of these countries. Democratic Yemen had 206, Iran 5807, Cyprus 118, Jordan 20, Kuwait 128, Syria 185, Yemen 243 and Bahrain 11. In 1972 and 1973, 17 cases were reported from Bahrain, 9 from Democratic Yemen, 305 from Iran, 5 from Israel and 2 from Lebanon. **Leptospirosis** is present and is frequently reported from Cyprus and Israel. **Plague** is endemic in Iran and Iraq. There is an established focus of plague on the Yemeni-Saudi border in the district of Khawlan, Yemen. **Louse-borne relapsing fever** has not been reported recently except in Syria and Iran. **Tick-borne relapsing fever** is endemic in this region and is reported sporadically.

Endemic syphilis is present in all of Arabia. It occurs in Iraq, Syria and Turkey and is commonly known as **bejel. Typhoid** and **paratyphoid fevers** are endemic.

Rickettsial Diseases

The rickettsial diseases are endemic, but reporting is inadequate. **Epidemic typhus** has been reported from most of these countries in the past, but not recently. Cases of **murine typhus** and other rickettsial diseases, including **tick-borne typhus (boutonneuse fever)** in Cyprus and **scrub typhus** in Bahrain, have been reported from time to time.

Viral Diseases

Some of the arthropod-borne infections identified in southwest Asia are mosquito-borne **West Nile fever** in Israel, **Naples** and **Sicilian phlebotomus fever** in Iran and mosquito-borne **Sindbis fever** in Israel.

Infectious hepatitis is widely distributed and has been reported from many of these countries. Recent reporting has been almost limited to Bahrain, Iraq, Israel, Kuwait, Lebanon, Turkey and Democratic Yemen. In 1972 these countries reported some 12,500 cases of infectious hepatitis (undesignated). **Rabies** is endemic and has been reported from some of the countries in this area sporadically. **Smallpox** is no longer being reported from these countries. **Trachoma** is endemic, and past studies have revealed an exceptionally large number of cases of this disease. In 1953 there were approximately 500,000 cases reported from Iraq and 80,000 from Jordan. The other countries also had large numbers.

B. CENTRAL SOUTH ASIA

Afghanistan, Bangladesh, Bhutan, India,† Pakistan, Sri Lanka,‡ Tibet, Southeastern U.S.S.R.,§ Maldive Islands*

Helminth Diseases

Ancylostomiasis (hookworm) is endemic in this area. Cases were reported from India and Sri Lanka in 1960, and helminth surveys conducted between 1950 and 1962 confirmed its presence in Pakistan and Nepal. **Dracunculiasis** is found in Afghanistan, Pakistan, the western half of India and portions of southeastern U.S.S.R.

---

*Formerly East Pakistan.

†Including Kashmir and Sikkim, both incorporated into India in 1975.

‡Formerly Ceylon.

§Turken S.S.R., Tadzik S.S.R., Kirghiz S.S.R., Uzbek S.S.R. and Kazakh S.S.R.

Filariasis bancrofti and **malayi** occur in this area; filariasis malayi has been reported from India, filariasis bancrofti from Nepal, India, Sri Lanka and the Maldive Islands.

The presence of **ascariasis, trichuriasis, strongyloidiasis** and **taeniasis** has been confirmed by surveys in Pakistan, India and Tibet. **Echinostomiasis, gastrodisciasis, paragonimiasis, hymenolepiasis diminuta** and **gnathostomiasis** have been found in India; **hymenolepiasis nana** and **fasciolopsiasis** in India and Pakistan; and **opisthorchiasis** in India and Sri Lanka. A small focus of **schistosomiasis** in India may still exist.

Protozoan Diseases

Amebiasis, together with bacillary dysentery, is very widespread. In 1958 India reported more than 1 million deaths from dysentery, without differentiation into types. Some individual States reported cases of amebiasis, in 1957 Madras having 40,831 cases and in 1954 West Bengal reporting approximately 250,000 cases. Other intestinal protozoan infections are also present.

Cutaneous leishmaniasis or **Oriental sore** and **visceral leishmaniasis** or **kala-azar** are present in parts of India, Pakistan, and southeastern U.S.S.R. **Malaria** transmission can take place in most of central south Asia. Great efforts have been made to lessen the risk in India and in neighboring countries. However, in spite of the fact that there are many States in which progress has been made, India is still considered to be an area of high risk. Sri Lanka has a few areas free of risk (Galle, Kalutara partially, Colombo), as have Nepal and the Maldive Islands.

Fungal Diseases

A variety of mycotic diseases has been identified in central South Asia. Included are **tinea favosa** (overall), **tinea imbricata** recognized in southern India and Sri Lanka, and **maduromycosis** and **rhinosporidiosis** in India and Sri Lanka.

Bacterial Diseases

Brucellosis has been reported from Sri Lanka and India. Classic **cholera** is endemic in India and Bangladesh, with many cases reported annually. In 1966 cholera el Tor was reported from Afghanistan and southeastern U.S.S.R., having first spread to 15 Asian countries from the Celebes islands of Indonesia where it first appeared in 1961. In 1974 it was reported from Sri Lanka, 4180 cases; India, 20,948 cases; Nepal, 8 cases; Bangladesh, 5498. Although the other countries in this region reported cases in previous years, they did not do so in 1974.

Bacillary dysentery or **shigellosis** is endemic and widespread and reported from all the major countries in this area. In 1957 there were more than 340,000 cases of bacillary dysentery reported from Madras in India. In 1959 in Rajasthan, India, there were 95,927 cases of bacillary dysentery among the 340,000 cases of unspecified dysentery reported.

Leprosy is endemic and extensive. It has been estimated that India and China together hold one-half of the world total of 5 to 10 million sufferers from leprosy. Surveys conducted in 1970 showed 857,284 cases on the leprosy registers of these countries. Afghanistan had approximately 500, Bhutan 450, Sri Lanka 4673, Nepal (in 1966) 2640, Pakistan 13,000, Bangladesh 3119. In 1973 Pakistan reported 364 new cases.

Leptospirosis occurs in Sri Lanka. **Sylvatic plague** is present in central Asia. In 1964 there were 109 cases of **human plague** reported from some of the Indian states.

Tick-borne relapsing fever is endemic in parts of central south Asia including Afghanistan, India, Pakistan and southeastern U.S.S.R. Foci of **louse-borne relapsing fever** may yet be present in these same countries.

The endemic treponematoses, **endemic syphilis** and **yaws,** are present. There is a focus of **bejel** or **endemic syphilis** in India. Yaws is endemic in Sri Lanka and India where campaigns against it have been waged by W.H.O. In 1957 there were 700 cases reported from Sri Lanka.

Typhoid and **paratyphoid fevers** are endemic. Sri Lanka reported more than 2500 cases in 1972.

Rickettsial Diseases

There is a focus of **endemic** or **louse-borne typhus** in Afghanistan. In 1963 there were 39 cases reported. Other rickettsioses are commonly reported from Sri Lanka. **Boutonneuse fever** is present in India. **Scrub typhus** or **tsutsugamushi disease** is present in India and its adjacent islands in the Indian Ocean and Bay of Bengal, in Pakistan and in Sri Lanka.

Viral Diseases

Arthropod-borne (arbo) virus infections ranging from mild febrile illness to hemorrhagic fever and encephalitis are present. **Naples** and **Sicilian phlebotomus fever** has been found in Pakistan; mosquito-borne **Sindbis, chikungunya, West Nile** and **dengue 1** and **4 fevers** are present in India; **Kyasanur Forest disease,** a tick-borne hemorrhagic fever, is present in parts of India; **Central Asian** tick-borne **hemorrhagic fever** in Kazakh and Uzbek S.S.R., and mosquito-borne **Japanese B encephalitis** in India.

Human rabies cases have been annually reported from most of these countries. The concerted effort to eradicate **smallpox** is having its effect, and the disease has gradually been confined to a few circumscribed areas. Except for the focus in Ethiopia, in 1974 it was reported only from India, where 187,815 cases occurred in 346 villages, 336 of which were located in the 3 States Bihar, U.P., and Assam; from Bangladesh, where 16,485 cases occurred; from Nepal, 1550 cases; and from Pakistan, 7859 cases. During the first 10 weeks of 1975, cases have been reported only from Bangladesh (3708), India (1222) and Nepal (80). The relatively high mortality rates occurring particularly in Bangladesh may be attributed in part to the adverse effects of malnutrition. **Trachoma** is present as in most of Asia.

C. SOUTHEAST ASIA

Burma, Brunei, Khmer Republic, Indonesia,† Laos, Malaysia,‡ Singapore, Portuguese Timor, Thailand, North and South Vietnam, Philippine Islands*

Helminth Diseases

Ancylostomiasis (hookworm) and other soil-transmitted helminth infections such as **ascariasis, trichuriasis** and **strongyloidiasis** are endemic. West Malaysia (at that time Malaya) reported more than 16,000 cases of ancylostomiasis in 1958.

Schistosomiasis japonica is endemic in Thailand, Indonesia (Celebes) and some of the Philippine Islands. **Creeping eruption** caused by *Ancylostoma braziliense* has been reported from Burma, Indonesia (Java), West Malaysia, Thailand and the Philippines. **Gnathostomiasis** is known from Java, West Malaysia and Thailand, where it is endemic.

Clonorchiasis occurs in Vietnam. **Dracunculiasis** has been found in limited areas of Indonesia.

Echinostomiasis is present in the Philippines and Indonesia (Java and Celebes). **Eosinophilic meningitis** has been identified in West Malaysia, and **tropical eosinophilia** in West Malaysia and the Philippines.

Fasciolopsiasis is widely distributed, especially in Thailand, Vietnam, West Malaysia, Sumatra and Borneo. **Heterophyiasis** and **hydatid disease** have been found in the Philippines and **opisthorchiasis** in Thailand. **Paragonimiasis** is present in Thailand, Vietnam, Malaysia, Indonesia, the Philippines and most of Southeast Asia.

Sparganosis has been reported from Vietnam and Indonesia and **taeniasis** from Vietnam and Singapore. **Hymenolepiasis nana** occurs in Singapore; **hymenolepiasis diminuta** and **dipylidiasis** infrequently in the Philippines. **Filariasis bancrofti** and **malayi** are widespread in all of Southeast Asia.

---

*Formerly Cambodia.

†Including Irian Jaya (formerly Netherlands New Guinea).

‡Comprising West Malaysia (the former Malaya) and East Malaysia (Sabah and Sarawak in Borneo).

Protozoan Diseases

Amebiasis, together with bacillary dysentery and unspecified dysentery, is endemic and widespread and reported from almost all the countries. Reporting is sporadic, but in 1972 Khmer Republic noted 1842 cases of amebiasis and West Malaysia 592. Unspecified dysentery, which includes bacillary as well as amebic, was reported from Sarawak (1378 cases) and the Philippines (20,513 cases). In other years reports were made by the other countries in this region.

Malaria still remains a great problem in this region although some areas are now considered free of risk. The only country declared entirely free is Brunei. In Burma malaria can be contracted in most of the country except for the Rangoon Division, and most urban areas are considered relatively free. The Khmer Republic is a risk area with the exception of Kirivong Town, and the provinces of Kandal, Preyveng, Scay-Rieng, Takeo (excluding Kirivong Division), and the Phnom-Penh Municipality. Indonesia is also an area of risk with the exception of Dajakarta-Raya, Surabaja and Regencies. Laos has only one area free of risk, Vientiane. In Malaysia, the towns of Kota Kinabalu and Sandakan in Sabah are free of risk, the urban areas of Sarawak are considered free, there is no risk in the capital, Kuala Lumpur, and Georgetown (Penang State) and the Malacca Municipality are free of malaria. Portuguese Timor poses a definite risk. In Thailand there are now some 14 provinces and parts of 33 other provinces that are considered free of malaria. North Vietnam and South Vietnam are areas of risk. In Singapore malaria can be contracted except in the City District in the south of the island. The Philippines are areas of risk, except in the principal cities where the risk is negligible and on the islands of Leyte, Cebu and the northern part of Luzon.

Fungal Diseases

Mycotic infections are widespread. **Histoplasmosis** has been identified in Java and the Philippines, **phycomycosis** in Indonesia, and **tinea imbricata** in Malaysia.

Bacterial Diseases

Brucellosis is periodically reported from West Malaysia and Sabah. **Bacillary dysentery** or **shigellosis** is endemic and extensively reported from almost all the countries, but not so extensively as amebiasis.

Cholera, both classic and el Tor, is present in Southeast Asia. In 1961 cholera el Tor appeared in the Celebes (Sulawesi) in Indonesia. From there it has spread to many countries. In 1974 there were 1923 cases reported from Burma, 133 from the Khmer Republic, 139 from South Vietnam, 1490 from Thailand, 36,237 from Indonesia, 265 from Malaysia, 8 from Singapore and 730 from the Philippines. These countries have been reporting cholera regularly.

Leptospirosis has been regularly reported from some of these countries, especially Malaysia (West and East) and Singapore. In 1972 it was reported from Brunei.

Leprosy is very widespread and the registered cases alone number in the hundreds of thousands. Surveys conducted in 1968 found 199,065 cases on the Burma register, 26,759 in the Philippines, 6802 in Khmer Republic, 2018 in Laos, 52,250 in Indonesia, 5460 in Malaysia and 97,379 in Thailand. In 1972 the Philippines reported 617 new cases, and in 1973, 28 new cases were reported from Khmer Republic, 3 from Laos and 86 from Singapore. **Plague** is endemic in some of the countries. In 1974, 217 cases were reported from Burma, some from Khmer Republic and 830 from South Vietnam.

Typhoid fever is endemic and reported from almost all of Southeast Asia. In 1972 there were 1500 cases reported from these countries, together with 5500 cases of undifferentiated typhoid/paratyphoid fever. These countries are within the **yaws** endemic zone. Control projects have been conducted in Malaysia, Laos, Indonesia including Irian Jaya, Thailand and Khmer Republic. In 1957 there were 49,000 cases recorded in the Philippines and 104,000 in Thailand. It is expected that the incidence of yaws has been greatly reduced by now.

Rickettsial Diseases

Scrub typhus or **tsutsugamushi disease** is endemic in all of Southeast Asia, especially Burma, South Vietnam, Malaysia, Thailand, Celebes in Indonesia and the Philippines. In 1971 scrub typhus was reported from Malaysia, some 40 cases being notified during the first half of that year in West Malaysia and additional cases occurring in Sarawak and Sabah. There were also some cases of the disease reported from the Philippines in 1972.

Viral Diseases

Arthropod-borne virus infections present in Southeast Asia include mosquito-borne **Japanese B encephalitis** in Burma, Thailand, Malaysia, Portuguese Timor and Indonesia; mosquito-borne **West Nile fever** in Malaysia and Borneo; **dengue fever,** including dengue hemorrhagic fever, in Thailand, Malaysia, Vietnam and the Philippines; **Sindbis fever** and **chikungunya fever** in Thailand and Malaysia. **Viral encephalitis** was reported from the Khmer Republic in 1972 (74 cases), Laos (11 cases) and the Philippines (263 cases).

Infectious hepatitis type unspecified has been reported from many of these countries, among those reporting being Brunei, Khmer Republic, Indonesia, Malaysia, South Vietnam, Singapore and the Philippines. **Rabies** is endemic and **human rabies** has been periodically reported from Khmer Republic, South Vietnam, Thailand, Malaysia and the Philippines. In 1963 the latter reported 218 cases. **Smallpox** is no longer being reported from these countries.

D. EAST ASIA

Peoples Republic of China, Republic of China (Taiwan†), Republic of Korea (south), Democratic Peoples Republic of Korea (north), Mongolian Peoples Republic, Hong Kong, Portuguese Macao, Japan,‡ Siberian U.S.S.R.*

Helminth Diseases

Ancylostomiasis (hookworm) has been reported from Hong Kong, Portuguese Macao and Japan, and surveys have placed it in China (Peoples Republic and Taiwan), Korea (north and south) and Japan (Ryukyu Islands). **Ascariasis, trichuriasis** and **strongyloidiasis** are present as well. **Trichostrongyliasis** is a common helminth infection in Japan, Korea and China (Peoples Republic and Taiwan).

Filariasis is widely distributed in southern China and Taiwan, Korea (south), Hong Kong, southern Japan and the Ryukyu Islands. Both **filariasis bancrofti** and **malayi** are present. **Schistosomiasis japonica** is present in parts of China (Peoples Republic and Taiwan) and Japan, and **schistosome cercarial dermatitis** in Japan. **Fasciolopsiasis** is present in southern China (Peoples Republic), the Republic of Korea and Japan.

Clonorchiasis is endemic and widely distributed in southeastern China (Peoples Republic) and in Taiwan, in north and south Korea, and in Japan. **Paragonimiasis** is found throughout East Asia, including Manchuria.

Creeping eruption is present in Taiwan and Hong Kong; **gnathostomiasis** is found in China and Japan; **eosinophilic meningitis** occurs in Taiwan and **tropical eosinophilia** in China. **Heterophyiasis** occurs in China (Peoples Republic and Taiwan), in south Korea and in Japan. **Metagonimiasis** is endemic in China, and present in Japan and parts of the Siberian U.S.S.R. **Echinostomiasis** has been found in Canton, China, and in Japan.

Opisthorchiasis is said to be present in Japan. **Taeniasis saginata** and **solium** are present, depending on the availability of pork or beef. **Diphyllobothriasis** occurs in Japan, Manchuria and parts of Siberia. **Sparganosis** is present in China (Peoples Republic and Taiwan), south Korea and Japan. **Hymenolepiasis nana** has been identified in the Republic of Korea and Japan, and **hymenolepiasis diminuta** in China and Japan. **Dipylidiasis** has occurred in China.

Protozoan Diseases

Amebiasis, together with bacillary dysentery and unspecified dysentery, is widespread and has been reported from Hong Kong, Portuguese Macao, Japan, Korea and

---

*The mainland.

†Also known as Formosa.

‡Includes the Ryukyu Islands (with Okinawa).

the Ryukyu Islands in recent years. Other intestinal protozoan infections are also present. **Visceral leishmaniasis** or **kala-azar** is present in southern China and in Manchuria.

Malaria is still being reported from this region although some of the countries are already free of the disease. In 1972, Japan, Macao, Mongolia and the Ryukyu Islands were assumed to be free. The position is uncertain regarding the Peoples Republic of China and the Siberian U.S.S.R. In Hong Kong, Hong Kong Island, Kowloon and West Kowloon are free of risk. There is little information available concerning the Democratic Peoples Republic of Korea but it is generally considered to be in the malaria risk category. There is a risk in the Republic of Korea, but no longer in the urban areas such as Seoul and the provinces of Cheju-Do, Cholla-Namdo, Cholla-Pukto, Chungchong-Namdo, Chungchong-Pukto, Kangwon-Do and Kyongsang-Namdo.

Fungal Diseases

A variety of mycotic diseases is present in East Asia. Among them are **tinea favosa** and **imbricata** found in China, and **cladosporiosis** and **histoplasmosis** found in Japan.

Bacterial Diseases

Japan reported 3 cases of **anthrax** in 1972.

Cholera is present in this area. Cases of cholera el Tor occurred in the Republic of Korea, Hong Kong, Portuguese Macao and Japan in 1963. In 1964 Hong Kong, the Republic of Korea and Macao were involved. Although some of these countries (the Republic of Korea, Hong Kong, Macao and Japan) had been involved in the 1961 pandemic, there have been no reported cases since 1970. **Brucellosis** has been reported from Japan and Macao.

Bacillary dysentery is very widespread. **Leprosy** is endemic in many of the countries of East Asia. A survey of leprosy registers conducted in 1968 revealed that the Republic of Korea had 37,571 cases on record, Japan 10,307 and the Republic of China (Taiwan) 4361. In 1962 there were 3924 cases on the Hong Kong register. In 1973, 100 new cases were reported from Hong Kong, and in 1972 one from Macao and 90 from Japan.

Plague is endemic in China, Mongolian Peoples Republic and Manchuria (U.S.S.R.). **Tick-borne relapsing fever** is present in western China. **Tularemia** has been found only in Japan, which is one of its endemic centers. **Typhoid** and **paratyphoid fevers** are endemic and have been reported annually from the Republic of China (Taiwan), the Republic of Korea, Hong Kong, Portuguese Macao, Japan and the Ryukyu Islands.

Rickettsial Diseases

Scrub typhus (tsutsugamushi disease) is endemic in all of East Asia. In 1964 there was an outbreak of **louse-borne epidemic typhus** in the Republic of Korea, but none has been reported recently.

Viral Diseases

Among the arthropod-borne virus infections that have been identified in East Asia are mosquito-borne **dengue fever** in Japan, **Omsk** tick-borne **hemorrhagic fever** in western Siberia (U.S.S.R.), **Far Eastern** or **Korean** mite(?)-transmitted **hemorrhagic fever** in Korea and China, **Russian spring-summer** tick-borne **encephalitis** in eastern Siberia and China, and **Japanese B encephalitis** from Japan, Korea and many eastern areas of Asia.

Infectious hepatitis is present and has been reported from Hong Kong (883 cases in 1970), Japan (479 cases in 1970), Republic of China (20 cases in 1972), Macao (409 cases in 1971), and the Ryukyu Islands. **Human rabies** was reported from Taiwan in 1958 and the Republic of Korea in 1963.

In 1953 Japan had reported 123,008 cases of **trachoma** and the Ryukyu Islands 2043. It is known to be endemic in Korea, China, Japan and some of the Ryukyu Islands.

V. OCEANIA

Australia, Cook Islands, Fiji, French Polynesia, Gilbert and Ellice Islands, Guam, Hawaii, Marshall Islands, Nauru, New Caledonia, New Hebrides, New Zealand, Papua New Guinea, Pitcairn Island, Samoa (American), Samoa (Western), Solomon Islands, Tahiti, Tonga, Wallis and Futuna, and many other islands*

Helminth Diseases

Ancylostomiasis (hookworm) has been reported from Australia, Solomon Islands, Fiji and New Zealand. Surveys have also placed it in Papua New Guinea, Cook Islands, French Polynesia, Western Samoa and the Marshall Islands. Helminth surveys conducted between 1950 and 1962 found **ascariasis, trichuriasis** and **hymenolepiasis nana** present in Australia, the latter condition also occurring in the Cook Islands and French Polynesia, and **ascariasis, trichuriasis** and **strongyloidiasis** endemic in the Cook Islands, French Polynesia, New Guinea and Western Samoa. Trematode diseases have been found in the Cook Islands.

Paragonimiasis is present in New Guinea. **Diphyllobothriasis** occurs in New Guinea and Papua. **Schistosome cercarial dermatitis** has been found in New Zealand. **Tropical eosinophilia** occurs in the Samoas. **Eosinophilic meningitis** or **rodent lungworm infection** occurs in Australia, Fiji, Guam, New Caledonia, the Marshall Islands, the Caroline Islands, Hawaii, the Marianas, Ponape, Tahiti, and Truk.

Filariasis bancrofti has been reported from French Polynesia, Fiji, and New Caledonia. In 1956 Fiji reported 2 cases of **onchocerciasis.** Cases of **filariasis** have also been found occasionally in New Guinea and New Zealand.

Protozoan Diseases

Amebiasis, together with bacillary dysentery, has been reported annually from almost all of Oceania. Other intestinal protozoan infections are also present. An outbreak of **balantidiasis** occurred in the Truk district of Micronesia Trust Territory in 1971, involving 110 people.

As of 1975, the only countries in Oceania in which there remained a risk of contracting **malaria** were Papua New Guinea, the Solomon Islands and New Hebrides.

Fungal Diseases

Tinea imbricata is present in the South Pacific islands. Other mycotic infections are also present but not reported.

Bacterial Diseases

Anthrax is reported periodically from Australia, Papua New Guinea and French Polynesia.

Brucellosis has been reported annually from Australia, Fiji, French Polynesia, New Zealand and occasionally from Guam.

Bacillary dysentery is endemic and has been reported almost annually from all of Oceania.

In July 1974, 6 cases of **cholera** were reported from Guam. This was a common source outbreak limited to a group of people who had eaten fish caught in Agana Bay.

Leprosy is endemic and occurs throughout Oceania, including the larger countries of Australia, Papua New Guinea, Fiji and New Zealand, and the smaller ones such as Nauru and Wallis and Futuna. A survey conducted in 1968 showed more than 8400 people on the leprosy registers of this area. This excluded Hawaii, where in 1969 a survey showed 555 people on the leprosy register. In 1972 and 1973 an additional 288 new cases were reported from 8 of the countries composing Oceania, exclusive of Hawaii. **Leptospirosis** has been reported from Australia, French Polynesia, New Zealand, New Caledonia, Wallis and Futuna, Guam, Tonga and other Pacific islands.

Typhoid and **paratyphoid fevers** are endemic and have been reported annually from almost all the areas that report to the W.H.O. **Yaws** was endemic in the islands.

---

*Also known as French Oceania.

Tonga, Western Samoa, Cook Islands, Fiji, the Gilbert and Ellice Islands, New Hebrides and the Solomon Islands were included in the W.H.O. yaws control campaigns conducted from 1949 to 1963.

Rickettsial Diseases

Endemic or **murine typhus** has been reported annually from Australia and Hawaii. **Q fever** has been reported from Australia. Sporadic cases of **murine typhus** have been reported from New Caledonia and other rickettsial diseases from New Hebrides.

Scrub typhus is endemic in the southwest Pacific islands, the northeast coast of Australia and adjacent islands as far east as Espiritu Santo. It has also been reported from Papua New Guinea. A mild rickettsial disease resembling rickettsialpox has been reported from Queensland, Australia, and is called **Queensland tick typhus.**

Viral Diseases

Arthropod-borne (arbo) virus infections have been found in Oceania. Mosquito-borne **Japanese B encephalitis** is present in the western Pacific islands from Japan to Guam; **Murray Valley encephalitis,** in Australia and New Guinea. In 1973, 12 cases of **viral encephalitis** were reported from Fiji, 2 from New Hebrides and a few from other Pacific islands.

Dengue fever is present in Oceania, especially in New Guinea, and previously in northern Australia and Hawaii. An outbreak of dengue-1 fever occurred in the Marshall Islands during March, April and May 1974. **Kunjin fever** and **Sindbis fever** are found in Australia.

Infectious hepatitis has been reported annually from parts of Oceania. The highest number of reported cases, 6118, was from Australia in 1972. In 1973 New Zealand reported 3363 cases. Fiji, French Polynesia, New Caledonia, New Hebrides and various Pacific islands accounted for some 1459 cases in 1973. Other countries reporting were Nauru, Guam, Tonga, Solomon Islands, Gilbert and Ellice Islands, Niue, and Papua New Guinea. In 1963 **human rabies** was reported from most of Oceania. This region currently is free of **smallpox**, but **trachoma** is endemic.

PRINCIPAL SOURCES OF DATA

Hunter, Swartzwelder, and Clyde. 1976. Tropical Medicine. 5th ed.

Pan American Sanitary Bureau: Health Conditions in the Americas. 1969–1972.

Pan American Sanitary Bureau: Weekly Epidemiological Report, Vols. 44–47, 1972–1975.

U.S. Department of Health, Education, and Welfare: Center for Disease Control. Morbidity and Mortality Weekly Reports.

U.S. Department of Health, Education, and Welfare. Health Information for International Travel 1974. Supplement to Morbidity and Mortality Report, Vol. 23 (September 1974).

World Health Organization: Epidemiological and Vital Statistics Report. 1955–1974.

World Health Organization: W.H.O. Chronicle, and W.H.O. Technical Report Series. Various numbers, 1964–1974.

Index

Note: Page references in *italics* indicate illustrations; page references to tables include the designation (t).